Cardiac Arrhythmias 2003

Springer
Milan
Berlin
Heidelberg
New York
Hong Kong
London
Paris
Tokyo

Cardiac Arrhythmias 2003

Edited by

Antonio Raviele

Proceedings of the
8th International Workshop
on Cardiac Arrhythmias

(Venice, 5-8 October 2003)

Springer

Antonio Raviele, MD
Divisione di Cardiologia
Ospedale Umberto I
Via Circonvallazione 50
I-30174 Venezia Mestre

Springer-Verlag Italia
a member of BertelsmannSpringer Science+Business Media GmbH

ISBN 88-470-0231-1

Library of Congress Cataloging-in-Publication Data: Applied for

Cover design: Simona Colombo, Milan
Typesetting: Graphostudio, Milan

SPIN: 10955390

Preface

The field of cardiac arrhythmias has been evolving so fast during the last years that scientific meetings are frequently necessary to present technological advances, to communicate results of relevant and innovative researches, to assess the impact of recently developed diagnostic and therapeutical tools, to discuss controversial aspects, and to reach a consensus on the most appropriate evaluation and management of specific problems. This is the main reason why in 1988 we started to organize a biannual International Workshop on Cardiac Arrhythmias. Since then many editions of the workshop have taken place and over the years the fame and popularity of the event have increased continuously.

This book contains the Proceedings of the Eighth Edition of the Workshop held in Venice at the Fondazione Giorgio Cini from the 5th to the 8th of October 2003. During the meeting all the principal aspects of the different arrhythmias, from epidemiology to physiopathology, electrogenetic mechanisms, diagnosis, prognosis, treatment, pshycological implications and economic costs have been discussed among the numerous experts and participants.

The book is divided in thirteen sections, each dedicated to a different topic: atrial fibrillation: clinical aspects and cardioversion; medical treatment of atrial fibrillation: rhythm control and rate control; atrial fibrillation: electrical therapy, transcatheter and surgical ablation; atrial fibrillation: prevention of thromboembolic complications; supraventricular tachyarrhythmias: diagnosis and treatment; ventricular arrhythmias and sudden death; implantable cardioverter defibrillator: practical aspects, indications and cost-effectiveness; out-of-hospitals cardiac arrest and public access defibrillation; syncope: current evaluation and management; sick sinus syndrome: clinical aspects and pacing issues; hemodynamics and cardiac pacing; cardiac resynchronization therapy: mechanisms, technical and clinical aspects; pacemaker/ICD complications: detection and management.

In my opinion, the book represents a comprehensive and modern overview of all pertinent aspects of cardiac arrhythmias and should be of interest not only to electrophysiologists and experts of the sector but also to general cardiologists, internists and medical students. I hope it will contribute to a better diffusion of current knowledge on cardiac arrhythmias and motivate researches in this field.

Many recognized authors have contributed to this volume. I am deeply indebted to all of them. Without their dedicated efforts and talents this book would not have been completed. I also wish to express my appreciation to Springer-Verlag and its staff, in particular Donatella Rizza, Executive Editor, for the great professionalism and meticulous attention to all the details of the editorial process. I am especially grateful to Rita Reggiani, Project Manager of Adria Congrex, for the exceptional skill and enthusiasm in preparing the workshop. Moreover, I would like to thank my colleagues at Umberto I Hospital, Drs. De Piccoli, Di Pede, Bonso, Gasparini, Giada, Themistoclakis, Zuin, Rigo for their support in the organization of the meeting and their scientific collaboration over the years.

Also the personal involvement and help of Gloria Leandro, Susanna Orbolato, Stefania Damiani and other members of the secretarial and nurse staff at my institution is sincerely appreciated. A special word of gratitude to my mentor, professor Piccolo, whose example and advices continue to represent an inestimable guidance and stimulus. Finally, my sincere thanks to my wife Carmen and my children, Francesca and Michele. Their continuous encouragement, assistance and patience helped me during the long hours of preparing the meeting and editing the book.

Antonio Raviele

Table of Contents

ATRIAL FIBRILLATION: CLINICAL ASPECTS AND CARDIOVERSION

Sympathetic and Vagal Fibrillation: Do They Exist?
F. Lombardi, F. Tundo, F. Colombo, S. Belletti, D. Tarricone 3

"Lone" Atrial Fibrillation in Athletes: A Consequence Of Long-Term Intensive Sport Practice
F. Naccarella, F. Furlanello , A. Bertoldi, S. Sdringola Maranga, G. Lepera, R. Cappato 11

Predicting Atrial Fibrillation in Patients with Hypertension: Can We Do It?
R.G. Tieleman, H.J.G.M. Crijns 23

What is the impact of Atrial Fibrillation on the Clinical Course of Hypertrophic Cardiomyopathy?
F. Cecchi, I. Olivotto 29

Atrial Fibrillation in Heart Failure: Prognostic Significance and Management
G.V. Naccarelli, B.J. Hynes, D. Wolbrette, M. Khan, L. Bhatta, S. Samii, J. Luck 37

Atrial Fibrillation After Cardiac Surgery: What's All the Fuss About?
D.G. Wyse 43

"Pill in the Pocket": How Effective and Safe Is this Strategy for Treatment of Recurrences of Atrial Fibrillation?
A. Capucci, G.Q. Villani, G. Rusticali, M.F. Piepoli 51

Cardioversion of Recent Onset Atrial Fibrillation: Which Drug to Prefer in the Individual Patient?
P.E. Vardas, E.M. Kanoupakis 57

Pretreatment with Antiarrhythmic Drugs: Is It Useful to Avoid Immediate and Early Postcardioversion Recurrences?
G. L. Botto, M. Luzi, A. Sagone 65

Is Echocardiography Useful to Predict Successful Cardioversion of Atrial Fibrillation and Long-Term Maintenance of Sinus Rhythm?
B. De Piccoli 71

Does the Policy of Repeated Early Cardioversion for Recurrences of Atrial Fibrillation Work?
E. Bertaglia 79

MEDICAL TREATMENT OF ATRIAL FIBRILLATION: RHYTHM CONTROL AND RATE CONTROL

Which Is the Ideal Drug for Chronic Prophylaxis of Atrial Fibrillation?
G. Boriani, M. Biffi, I. Diemberger, C. Martignani, C. Camanini, C. Valzania, G.Domenichini, I. Corazza, A. Branzi 85

ACE Inhibitors and Angiotensin Receptor Blockers: a New Effective Non-Conventional Approach to Prevent Atrial Fibrillation
A.H. Madrid, C. Escobar, J.M.G. Rebollo, I. Marín, E. Bernal, L. Limón, S. Nannini, J. Peng, C. Moro 93

Rate Control of Atrial Fibrillation: By How Much Should the Ventricular Rate be Lowered?
P. Alboni, L. Gianfranchi, G. Fucà, F. Pacchioni, G. Corbucci 99

Ablate and Pace: Is This Still a Valid Option?
M. Brignole 107

Transvascular Parasympathetic Stimulation for Ventricular Rate Control During Atrial Fibrillation: A Bionic Approach
P. Schauerte, M. Schmidt, T. Schimpf, J. Plisiene, M. Zarse, K. Mischke ... 117

Management of Atrial Fibrillation: Is it Already Time to Update the Recent ACC/AHA/ESC Guidelines?
D. G. Wyse 127

ATRIAL FIBRILLATION: ELECTRICAL THERAPY, TRANSCATHETER AND SURGICAL ABLATION

Atrial Fibrillation Suppression: What Role Does It Have?
A. Schuchert 137

Dual-chamber ICDs: How Effective and Safe Are They in the Treatment of Atrial Tachyarrhythmias?
J. Kautzner, P. Peichl 141

Ablation of Atrial Fibrillation: Are We Still "Learning While Burning"?
J.A. Salerno-Uriarte, R. De Ponti, M. Tritto, M.E. Lanzotti, R. Marazzi, G. Spadacini, P. Moretti 149

Ablation of Atrial Fibrillation: Is a Cure at Hand?
B. K. Lee, M. M. Scheinman 159

Atrial Fibrillation: Anatomical Guidance Is Superior to Electrophysiological Guidance for Ablation
C. Pappone, V. Santinelli 167

Atrial Fibrillation: Catheter Laser Balloon Ablation
A. Bonso, S. Themistoclakis, A. Rossillo, A. Raviele 173

Isolation of Pulmonary Veins Using Cryothermal Technologies
A. C. Skanes, A. D. Krahn, R. Yee, G. J. Klein 177

Ablation of Atrial Fibrillation by Radiofrequency: Circular Energy Delivery
T. Lewalter, H. Bielik, J. Schrickel, A. Bitzen, J.O. Schwab, A. Yang, B. Lüderitz 189

Catheter Ablation of Atrial Fibrillation: What Are the Risks and Complications and How Do We Avoid Them?
S. Themistoclakis, A. Bonso, A. Rossillo, A. Raviele 195

Risk Stratification and Prevention of Thromboembolism: What Is the Role of Intracardiac Echocardiography?
A. Rossillo, N.F. Marrouche, E.B. Saad, O. Wasni, M. Bhargava, D. Bash, S. Beheiry, M. Wexman, B. Strunk, E. Pisanò, R. Fanelli, A. Bonso, S. Themistoclakis, D. Erciyes, W.I. Saliba, R.A. Schweikert, J. Brachmann, A. Raviele, A. Natale 205

Radiofrequency and Microwave Ablation of Atrial Fibrillation During Open Heart Surgery: What Are the Long-Term Results?
A. Venturini, V. Cutaia, A. Asta, D. Mangino, R. Moretti, E. Polesel, A. Terrini, C. Zussa 215

Minimally Invasive Surgical Approach to Radiofrequency Ablation of Atrial Fibrillation: Is the Game Worth the Candle?
C. Piorkowski, G. Hindricks, H. Kottkamp 221

ATRIAL FIBRILLATION: PREVENTION OF THROMBOEMBOLIC COMPLICATIONS

What Is the Best Practical Scheme for Initiating Oral Anticoagulant Treatment in Outpatients with Atrial Fibrillation?
R. Cazzin, P. Serra, C. Fusilli 231

How Intense Should Anticoagulation Be at the Time of Cardioversion to Reduce the Risk of Thromboembolism?
N. Baldi, V.A. Russo, V. Morrone, L. Di Gregorio, L. Liconso, G. Polimeni .. 235

Warfarin Underuse for Nonvalvular Atrial Fibrillation: How to Adjust Our Aims?
G. Di Pasquale, E. Cerè, A. Lombardi, B. Sassone, S. Biancoli, R. Vandelli .. 241

SUPRAVENTRICULAR TACHYARRHYTHMIAS: DIAGNOSIS AND TREATMENT

Palpitations of Unknown Origin: How Frequent Are Supraventricular Arrhythmias?
F. Giada, A. Raviele 251

Acute Termination of Atrial Flutter: Class III Drugs or Transesophageal Pacing?
A. Bonso, S. Themistoclakis, A. Rossillo, A. Raviele 257

Atrial Flutter Induced by Class IC Drugs/Amiodarone: What Are the Long-term Results of Cavo-tricuspidal Isthmus Ablation?
P. Delise, N. Sitta, L. Corò, L. Sciarra, E. Marras 263

Non-Isthmus-Dependent Atrial Flutter: How to Locate and Ablate the Re-entry Circuit
I. Mangat, M. M. Scheinman 271

Complex Supraventricular Tachycardia Ablation: What Is the Role of Alternative Technology?
M. Tritto, R. De Ponti, G. Spadacini, M. Lanzotti, P. Moretti, B. Molinari, R. Marazzi, J. A. Salerno-Uriarte 285

Late Atrial Tachyarrhythmias After Repair of Congenital Heart Disease What is the Mechanism and How Can They Be Localized and Ablated?
R. Mantovan 293

Late Atrial Arrhythmias as a Complication After Valvular Heart Surgery: Is There A Place for Prevention?
D. Mangino, A. Asta, A. Venturini, E. Polesel, R. Moretti, A. Terrini, C. Zussa .. 301

VENTRICULAR ARRHYTHMIAS AND SUDDEN DEATH

Coffee Enhances Sympathetic Activity and Induces Cardiac Arrhythmias: True or False?
G. Zuin, E. Piccolo, F. Di Pede, M. Celestre, A. Raviele 309

Is the Cause of Arrhythmogenic Right Ventricular Cardiomyopathy Congenital or Acquired?
C. Basso, A. Rampazzo, B. Bauce, F. Calabrese, G. Danieli, A. Nava, M. Valente, G. Thiene 313

Is ICD Implantation Useful in Patients with Arrhythmogenic Right-ventricular Cardiomyopathy?
D. Corrado, L. Leoni, G. Buja, G. Thiene, on behalf of the Investigators of the Defibrillator in Arrhythmogenic Right Ventricular Cardiomyopathy/Dysplasia in North Italy (DARVIN) Study 323

What is the Prevalence, Incidence and Prognostic Value of Brugada-type Electrocardiogram in the General Population?
H. Sakurada, H. Okazaki, T. Tejima 331

Brugada Syndrome or Brugada Mimicry?
R.N.W. Hauer 335

Ventricular Tachycardia or Conduction Disease: What Is the Mechanism of Death in Brugada Syndrome?
G. Buja, L. Leoni, D. Corrado, C. Basso, B. Bauce, A. Nava, S. Iliceto, G. Thiene 339

Idiopathic Ventricular Tachycardia: Is Radiofrequency Ablation the First Line Therapy?
D. J. Callans 347

Ventricular Tachycardia from the Aortic Cusps: Localization and Ablation
F. E. Marchlinski, D. Lin, S. Dixit, J. Jacobson, W. Sauer, M. McKernan, J. F. Ren 357

Extreme Left Vetricular Hypertrophy: An Indicator of Increased Risk of Sudden Death in Hypertrophic Cardiomyopathy
P. Bernabò, C. Autore, P. Spirito 371

Does a Maximum Left Ventricular Thickness Greater than 30 mm Identify Patients with Hypertrophic Cardiomyopathy at Risk of Sudden Death?
I. Olivotto, F. Cecchi 375

Drug-Induced Torsade de Pointes. Role of Genetic Factors
N. El-Sherif, G. Turitto 379

Identifying Patients at High Risk for Sudden Cardiac Death: Is Low Ejection Fraction Alone Enough, or Do We Need Additional Testing?
S.M. Narayan,M.E. Cain 387

What Is The Prognostic Value of Non-Sustained Ventricular Tachycardia in Patients Without Severely Depressed Ejection Fraction After Myocardial Infarction?
G. Turitto, N. El-Sherif 397

Mechanical/Surgical Revascularization in Patients with Ventricular Fibrillation and Coronary Artery Disease: Is It Enough, or Do We Also Need an Implantable Cardioverter Defibrillator?
M. Lunati, M. Paolucci, G. Magenta, G. Cattafi, R. Vecchi, M. Schirru, T. Di Camillo 405

Surgical Revascularization in Patients with "Ischemia-related" Ventricular Fibrillation: Is It Sufficient to Prevent Sudden Death?
R.N.W. Hauer 413

New-onset Ventricular Tachyarrhythmias After Cardiac Surgery: Significance and Treatment
G. Crescenzi, S. Benussi, G. Landoni, O. Alfieri 415

Electrophysiologically Guided Antiarrhythmic Surgery for Treatment of Frequently Recurrent Ventricular Tachycardia: What Role Does It Have Today?
R. De Ponti, J. A. Salerno-Uriarte 419

Heart Transplantation in Frequently Recurrent Drug-Refractory Tachyarrhythmias: is it Worthwhile?
D. G. Benditt, V. Tholakahalli, S. Sakaguchi, C. Ermis, M.-T. Olivari, F. Lü 427

Ablation of Unstable Ventricular Tachycardia
F.E. Marchlinski, D. Lin, H. Nayak, A.M. Russo, H. Hsia, S. Dixit, E. Gerstenfeld, D. Callans, W. Pulliam, S. Siddique, S. Del Castillo, E. Zado 433

Ablation of Ventricular Tachycardia: Can the Current Results be Improved Using Intracardiac Echocardiography?
D. J. Callans, J.-F. Ren 451

IMPLANTABLE CARDIOVERTER DEFIBRILLATOR: PRACTICAL ASPECTS, INDICATIONS AND COST-EFFECTIVENESS

Left Ventricular Dysfunction and Electrophysiologic Study in the Primary and Secondary ICD Trials
D. S. Cannom 463

New Evidence from the Secondary Endpoints of the MADIT II Study
S. L. Higgins 469

The Real Economic Impact of the MADIT-II Study on the European Medical Community
G. Boriani, M. Biffi, C. Martignani, C. Camanini, C. Valzania, I. Diemberger, C. Greco, A. Branzi 475

Post-infarction Patients with Left Ventricular Ejection Fraction of 30%–40%, Non-sustained Ventricular Tachycardia, and without Inducible Tachyarrhythmias: Is ICD Therapy Necessary?
H. U. Klein, S. Reek, C. Geller, A.Auricchio 481

Secondary Prevention of Sudden Death in Post-Infarction Patients: When is ICD Implantation Really Cost-Effective?
S. R. Raj, R. S. Sheldon 489

Primary Prevention of Sudden Death in Post-Infarction Patients: When ICD Implantation is Really Cost-effective
S.C. Hammill 497

Cost-Effectiveness of ICD Implantation in Clinical Settings Different From Ischemic Heart Disease: What Do We Know?
G. Boriani, M. Biffi, C. Martignani, C. Greco, C. Camanini, C. Valzania, I. Diemberger, F. Cecaro, A. Branzi 505

Expanding ICD Indications: Can We Afford It?
M. Santini, M. Russo, R. Ricci, C. Pignalberi, B. Magris, L. Santini 511

Waveform Flexibility: The Present and Future Solution for Clinically Effective Defibrillation
M. W. Kroll 519

Lessons from the Lower Energy Safety Study (LESS): Is One Ventricular Fibrillation Induction Adequate for ICD Implant?
S. L. Higgins 527

Inappropriate Defibrillator Therapies: Do Dual-chamber Devices Really Provide a Remedy?
T. Kurita, K. Satomi, A. Taguchi, W. Shimizu, K. Suyama, N. Aihara, S. Kamakura, K. Niwaya, J. Kobayashi 535

Should Antiarrhythmic Drugs Be Administered After First Appropriate ICD Shock, and If So, Which Ones?
G. Abali, K. Aytemir, A. Oto 541

Quality of Life in Patients with ICD: Is It Improved or Worsened?
B. Lüderitz 547

OUT-OF-HOSPITALS CARDIAC ARREST AND PUBLIC ACCESS DEFIBRILLATION

Public Use of AEDs in Europe: Where Are We Now and Where Are We Going?
D. Chamberlain, L. Bossaert, S. Davies, M. Colquhoun 555

Use of AED by Lay People in Patients with Out-of-Hospital Cardiac Arrest: How Does It Impact Survival?
A. Capucci, D. Aschieri 563

In-Hospital Cardiac Arrest: Are We Well Enough Equipped and Prepared to Face It?
M. Santomauro, L. Ottaviano, A. Borrelli, C. Riganti, L. Quagliata, A. Costanzo, C. Liguori, D. Da Prato, M. Chiariello 569

Mild Therapeutic Hypothermia for Treatment of Cardiac Arrest: Current Results and Future Perspectives
W. Behringer, M. Holzer, F. Sterz 579

SYNCOPE: CURRENT EVALUATION AND MANAGEMENT

Distinguishing Syncope From Seizures: How Useful is the Clinical History?
R. S. Sheldon 589

Diagnosis of Neurally Mediated Syncope: Might Use of the Implantable Loop Recorder Replace the Tilt-table Test? A Positive View
A. Moya 595

Unexplained Syncope: Can We Predict the Outcome of Prolonged Monitoring with the Implantable Loop Recorder?
A. D. Krahn, G. J. Klein, R. Yee, A. C. Skanes 599

Patients with Structural Heart Disease, Syncope of Unknown Origin and Suspected Ventricular Tachycardia: ICD Implantation or "Wait and See" Strategy?
C. Menozzi, N. Bottoni, M. Brignole 607

Vasovagal Syncope, Orthostatic Hypotension and Postural Orthostatic Tachycardia Syndrome: Is There a Connection?
A.Gonzalez-Hermosillo, M.F. Marquez, A. Kostine, K. Jauregui-Renaud, M. Cardenas 615

Water Drinking to Prevent Orthostatic Hypotension and Neurally Mediated Syncope: Mechanisms and Benefits
C.J. Mathias, T.M. Young 625

Physical Counterpressure Maneuvers to Prevent and Abort Vasovagal Syncope: A Novel Effective Treatment?
N. van Dijk, C.T.P. Krediet, I.G.J.M. de Bruin, J.J. van Lieshout, W. Wieling 633

Isometric Arm Contraction at the Onset of Prodromal Symptoms: a New First-line Treatment for Vasovagal Syncope?
M. Brignole, F. Croci, C. Menozzi, A. Solano, P. Donateo, D. Oddone, E. Puggioni, G. Lolli 641

To Pace or not to Pace for Neurally Mediated Syncope: Do We Know the Answer? A Positive View
F. Giada, A. Raviele 651

To Pace or Not to Pace for Neurally Mediated Syncope: Do We Know the Answer? A Negative View
O. Oseroff 655

Patient-Activated Implantable Drug Pump for Treatment of Vasovagal Syncope: Is It Time for Clinical Use?
A. Raviele, F. Giada 659

SICK SINUS SYNDROME: CLINICAL ASPECTS AND PACING ISSUES

Genetics of Sinus Node Disease
E. Schulze-Bahr, D. Etzrodt, H. Wedekind, G. Breithardt, D. Isbrandt 667

Sleep Apnea: New Insights
M.G. Bongiorni, G. Giannola, E. Gronchi, E. Soldati, G. Arena, E. Hoffmann, M. Mariani 679

Remodeling of Sinus Node Function Produced by Supraventricular Tachyarrhythmias: What Are the Clinical Implications?
P.E. Vardas, H.E. Mavrakis 685

Drug-Induced Bradycardia: When Is a Pacemaker Warranted?
I.E. Ovsyshcher, N. Gulko 691

Permanent Pacing Treatment: Conventional DDDR, Antitachycardia Pacing or Atrial Defibrillator?
M. Santini, R. Ricci, C. Pignalberi, M. Russo, B. Magris, L. Santini 697

HEMODYNAMICS AND CARDIAC PACING

Hemodynamic Assessment with Implantable Pacemakers: How Feasible and Reliable Is It?
R. Chirife 705

Hemodynamic Sensors: Their Impact in Clinical Practice
E. Occhetta, A. Magnani, M. Bortnik, G. Francalacci, F. Di Gregorio, C. Vassanelli 713

Haemodynamic Pacing: When Is It Selectively Indicated?
J. Clémenty, S. Reuter, P. Bordachar, S. Garrigue, P. Jaïs, M. Haïssaguerre .. 719

Can Hemodynamic Sensors Ensure Physiological Rate Control?
G. Gasparini, A. Curnis, M. Gulizia, E. Occhetta, A. Corrado, G. Mascioli, L. Bontempi, G.M. Francese, A. Magnani, M. Bortnik, F. Di Gregorio, A. Barbetta, F. Monese, A. Raviele 725

Transvalvular Impedance: Does It Allow Automatic Capture Detection?
M.G. Bongiorni, E. Soldati, G. Arena, F. Di Gregorio, A. Barbetta, F. Monese, M. Mariani 733

What Are the Keys to Hemodynamic Improvement in Heart Failure Patients?
R. Ricci, G. Ansalone, C. Pignalberi, M. Russo, B. Magris, L. Santini, M. Santini 741

Atrioventricular Delay in Heart Failure Patients: How to Manage It
H. O. Luttikhuis 745

Cardiac Resynchronisation and Haemodynamic Monitoring: the Living-CHF Study
J. Clémenty, for the BEST-CARE Study Group 753

Heart Failure Therapy Driven by Implantable Sensors: What May We Expect?
G. Plicchi, E. Marcelli 759

CARDIAC RESYNCHRONIZATION THERAPY: MECHANISMS, TECHNICAL AND CLINICAL ASPECTS

Reverse Structural and Contractile Remodeling without Reverse Electrical Remodeling by Biventricular and Right Ventricular Apex Pacing in Dogs with Chronic AV Block
M. Peschar, M. A. Vos, F. W. Prinzen 767

How Are Perfusion and Adrenergic Innervation of the Left Ventricle Affected in Paced Patients?
E.N. Simantirakis, P.E. Vardas 777

Cardiac Resynchronization Therapy: The Low Voltage Road or the High Voltage Road?
G. Boriani, M. Biffi, C. Martignani, C. Camanini, C. Valzania, I. Diemberger, D. Saporito, P. Bartolini, A. Branzi 785

Cardiac Resynchronization Therapy: What Are the Benefits of Digital Pacemakers?
G. Fröhlig, P. Wohlgemuth, N.M. van Hemel, A. Vincent 793

Cardiac Resynchronization Therapy: What Device Data Do We Need for Optimal Patient Treatment?
S. Sermasi, G. Corbucci, M. Marconi, M. Mezzetti, G. Piovaccari 799

How to Identify Patients Most Likely to Respond to Cardiac Resynchronization Therapy
M. M. Gulizia, G. M. Francese 805

Upgrading from Right Ventricular Apical Pacing to Biventricular Pacing
M. H. Schoenfeld 815

Cardiac Resynchronisation Therapy in Patients with Atrial Fibrillation: Are Results as Good as in Patients with Sinus Rhythm?
C. Linde 823

Patients with Heart Failure and Right Bundle Branch Block or Nonspecific Intraventricular Conduction Disturbances
Can They Benefit from Cardiac Resynchronization Therapy?
S. Garrigue, P. Bordachar, S. Reuter, M. Hocini, P. Jaïs, M. Haïssaguerre, J. Clémenty 829

Which Left Ventricular Stimulation Site Is Best for Cardiac Resynchronisation Therapy?
F. Nacci, F. Fino, E. Spennati, V.F. Napoli, S. Favale 837

Permanent His Bundle Pacing: A Good Unconventional Mode of Right Ventricular Pacing?
E. Occhetta, M. Bortnik, G. Francalacci, A. Magnani, C. Piccinino, C. Vassanelli 843

Cardiac Resynchronization Therapy: Is Atrial Resynchronization Important with Biventricular Pacing?
F. Di Pede, G. Gasparini, M. Celestre, G. Zuin, B. De Piccoli, A. Raviele ... 851

Impact of Cardiac Resynchronization Therapy on Mortality: What Do We Expect from Ongoing Trials?
M. Lunati, M. Paolucci, G. Magenta, G. Cattafi, R. Vecchi, M. Schirru, T. Di Camillo 857

COMPANION Study: Rationale
D. S. Cannom 861

Pharmacological Therapy in COMPANION Study: Compliance and Dosage
A. Boccanelli, G. Cacciatore 865

The Lesson from the COMPANION Study: How Large Is the Patient Population That May Benefit?
E.G. Gronda, M. Mangiavacchi, D. Pini, L. Genovese, L. Tomaello, B. Andreuzzi, A. Municinò 877

PACEMAKER/ICD COMPLICATIONS: DETECTION AND MANAGEMENT

How to Detect and Manage Pacemaker/ICD Failure and Infections
M.G. Bongiorni, G. Arena, E. Soldati, G. Giannola, E. Gronchi, G. Sgarito, M. Mariani 885

Pacemaker/ICD Lead Extraction Using the Excimer Laser Sheath: What Are the Advantages and What Are the Risks?
G. Gasparini, A. Rossillo, F. Giada, A. Corrado, A. Raviele 897

How to Detect and Treat superior Vena Cava Obstruction Caused by Multiple Pacing/ICD Leads?
G. Chiarandà, A. Busà, G. Muscio, A. Lazzaro, L. Cavarra, T. Regolo 903

Lead-Related Thrombi in Patients with Pacemaker/ICD: What Is the Prevalence, Clinical Significance, and Recommended Management?
R.M. Polimeni, G. Meduri, A. Amato, D. Baccellieri 909

Effects of Electromagnetic Interference on Implanted Cardiac Devices
M. L. Blitzer, M. H. Schoenfeld 911

Subject Index 919

List of Contributors

ABALI G., 541
AIHARA N., 535
ALBONI P., 99
ALFIERI O., 415
AMATO A., 909
ANDREUZZI B., 877
ANSALONE G., 741
ARENA G., 679, 733, 885
ASCHIERI D., 563
ASTA A., 215, 301
AURICCHIO A., 481
AUTORE C., 371
AYTEMIR K., 541
BACCELLIERI D., 909
BALDI N., 235
BARBETTA A., 725, 733
BARTOLINI P., 785
BASH D., 205
BASSO C., 313, 339
BAUCE B., 313, 339
BEHEIRY S., 205
BEHRINGER W., 579
BELLETTI S., 3
BENDITT D.G., 427
BENUSSI S., 415
BERNABÒ P., 371
BERNAL E., 93
BERTAGLIA E., 79
BERTOLDI A., 11
BHARGAVA M., 205
BHATTA L., 37
BIANCOLI S., 241
BIELIK H., 189
BIFFI M., 85, 475, 505, 785
BITZEN A., 189
BLITZER M. L., 911
BOCCANELLI A., 865
BONGIORNI M.G., 679, 733, 885
BONSO A., 173, 195, 205, 257
BONTEMPI L., 725
BORDACHAR P., 719, 829
BORIANI G., 85, 475, 505, 785
BORRELLI A., 569
BORTNIK M., 713, 725, 843
BOSSAERT L., 555
BOTTO G. L., 65
BOTTONI N., 607
BRACHMANN J., 205
BRANZI A., 85, 475, 505, 785
BREITHARDT G., 667
BRIGNOLE M., 107, 607, 641
BUJA G., 323, 339
BUSÀ A., 903
CACCIATORE G., 865
CAIN M.E., 387
CALABRESE F., 313
CALLANS D.J., 347, 451
CALLANS D, 433
CAMANINI C., 85, 475, 505, 785
CANNOM D. S., 463, 861
CAPPATO R., 11
CAPUCCI A., 51, 563
CARDENAS M., 615
CATTAFI G., 405, 857
CAVARRA L., 903
CAZZIN R., 231
CECARO F., 505
CECCHI F., 29, 375
CELESTRE M., 309, 851
CERÈ E., 241

Chamberlain D., 555
Chiarandà G., 903
Chiariello M., 569
Chirife R.,705
Clémenty J., 719, 753, 829
Colombo F., 3
Colquhoun M., 555
Corazza I., 85
Corbucci G.,99, 799
Corò L., 263
Corrado A., 725, 897
Corrado D., 323, 339
Costanzo A., 569
Crescenzi G., 415
Crijns H.J.G.M., 23
Croci F., 641
Curnis A., 725
Cutaia V., 215
Da Prato D., 569
Danieli G., 313
Davies S., 555
de Bruin I.G.J.M., 633
De Piccoli B., 71, 851
De Ponti R., 149, 285, 419
Del Castillo S., 433
Delise P., 263
Di Camillo T., 405, 857
Di Gregorio F., 713, 725, 733
Di Gregorio L., 235
Di Pasquale G., 241
Di Pede F., 309, 851
Diemberger I., 85, 475, 505, 785
Dixit S., 357, 433
Domenichini G., 85
Donateo P., 641
El-Sherif N., 379, 397
Erciyes D., 205
Ermis C., 427
Escobar C., 93
Etzrodt D., 667
Fanelli R., 205
Favale S., 837
Fino F., 837
Francalacci G., 713, 843
Francese G.M., 725, 805
Fröhlig G., 793
Fucà G., 99
Furlanello F., 11
Fusilli C., 231
Garrigue S., 719, 829
Gasparini G., 725, 851, 897
Geller C., 481
Genovese L., 877
Gerstenfeld E., 433
Giada F., 251, 651, 659, 897
Gianfranchi L., 99
Giannola G., 679, 885
Gonzalez-Hermosillo A., 615
Greco C., 475, 505
Gronchi E., 679, 885
Gronda E.G., 877
Gulizia M., 725, 805
Gulko N., 691
Haïssaguerre M., 719, 829
Hammill S.C., 497
Hauer R.N.W., 335, 413
Higgins S. L., 469, 527
Hindricks G., 221
Hocini M., 829
Hoffmann E., 679
Holzer M., 579
Hsia H., 433
Hynes B.J., 37
Iliceto S., 339
Isbrandt D., 667
Jacobson J., 357
Jaïs P., 719, 829
Jauregui-Renaud K., 615
Kamakura S., 535
Kanoupakis E.M., 57
Kautzner J., 141
Khan M., 37
Klein G.J., 177, 599
Klein H.U., 481
Kobayashi J., 535
Kostine A., 615
Kottkamp H., 221
Krahn A.D., 177, 599
Krediet C.T.P., 633
Kroll M.W., 519

Kurita T., 535
Landoni G., 415
Lanzotti M., 285
Lanzotti M.E., 149
Lazzaro A., 903
Lee B. K., 159
Leoni L., 323, 339
Lepera G., 11
Lewalter T., 189
Liconso L., 235
Liguori C., 569
Limón L., 93
Lin D., 357, 433
Linde C., 823
Lolli G., 641
Lombardi A., 241
Lombardi F., 3
Lü F., 427
Luck J., 37
Lüderitz B., 189, 547
Lunati M., 405, 857
Luttikhuis H.O., 745
Luzi M., 65
Madrid A.H., 93
Magenta G., 405, 857
Magnani A., 713, 725, 843
Magris B., 511, 697, 741
Mangat I., 271
Mangiavacchi M., 877
Mangino D., 215, 301
Mantovan R., 293
Marazzi R., 149, 285
Marcelli E., 753
Marchlinski F.E., 357, 433
Marconi M., 799
Mariani M., 679, 733, 885
Marín I., 93
Marquez M.F., 615
Marras E., 263
Marrouche N.F., 205
Martignani C., 85, 475, 505, 785
Mascioli G., 725
Mathias C.J., 625
Mavrakis H.E., 685
McKernan M., 357
Meduri G., 909
Menozzi C., 607, 641
Mezzetti M., 799
Mischke K., 117
Molinari B., 285
Monese F., 725, 733
Moretti P., 149, 285
Moretti R., 215, 301
Moro C., 93
Morrone V., 235
Moya A., 595
Municinò A., 877
Muscio G., 903
Naccarella F., 11
Naccarelli G.V., 37
Nacci F., 837
Nannini S., 93
Napoli V.F., 837
Narayan S.M., 387
Natale A., 205
Nava A., 313, 339
Nayak H., 433
Niwaya K., 535
Occhetta E., 713, 725, 843
Oddone D., 641
Okazaki H., 331
Olivari M.-T., 427
Olivotto I., 29, 375
Oseroff O., 655
Oto A., 541
Ottaviano L., 569
Ovsyshcher I.E., 691
Pacchioni F., 99
Paolucci M., 405, 857
Pappone C., 167
Peichl P., 141
Peng J., 93
Peschar M., 767
Piccinino C., 843
Piccolo E., 309
Piepoli M.F., 51
Pignalberi C., 511, 697, 741
Pini D., 877
Piorkowski C., 221
Piovaccari G., 799

Pisanò E., 205
Plicchi G., 753
Plisiene J., 117
Polesel E., 215, 301
Polimeni G., 235
Polimeni R.M., 909
Prinzen F.W., 767
Puggioni E., 641
Pulliam W., 433
Quagliata L., 569
Raj S. R., 489
Rampazzo A., 313
Raviele A., 173, 195, 205, 251, 257, 309, 651, 659, 725, 851, 897
Rebollo J.M.G., 93
Reek S., 481
Regolo T., 903
Ren J.-F., 357, 451
Reuter S., 719, 829
Ricci R., 511, 697, 741
Riganti C., 569
Rossillo A., 173, 195, 205, 257, 897
Russo A.M., 433
Russo M., 511, 697, 741
Russo V.A., 235
Rusticali G., 51
Saad E.B., 205
Sagone A., 65
Sakaguchi S., 427
Sakurada H., 331
Salerno-Uriarte J.A., 149, 285, 419
Saliba W.I., 205
Samii S., 37
Santinelli V., 167
Santini L., 511, 697, 741
Santini M., 511, 697, 741
Santomauro M., 569
Saporito D., 785
Sassone B., 241
Satomi K., 535
Sauer W., 357
Schauerte P., 117
Scheinman M.M., 159, 271
Schimpf T., 117
Schirru M., 405, 857
Schmidt M., 117
Schoenfeld M. H., 815, 911
Schrickel J., 189
Schuchert A., 137
Schulze-Bahr E., 667
Schwab J.O., 189
Schweikert R.A., 205
Sciarra L., 263
Sdringola Maranga S., 11
Sermasi S., 799
Serra P., 231
Sgarito G., 885
Sheldon R.S., 489, 589
Shimizu W., 535
Siddique S., 433
Simantirakis E.N., 777
Sitta N., 263
Skanes A.C., 177, 599
Solano A., 641
Soldati E., 679, 733, 885
Spadacini G., 149, 285
Spennati E., 837
Spirito P., 371
Sterz F., 579
Strunk B., 205
Suyama K., 535
Taguchi A., 535
Tarricone D., 3
Tejima T., 331
Terrini A., 215, 301
Themistoclakis S., 173, 195, 205, 257
Thiene G., 313, 323, 339
Tholakahalli V., 427
Tieleman R.G., 23
Tomaello L., 877
Tritto M., 149, 285
Tundo F., 3
Turitto G., 379, 397
Valente M., 313
Valzania C., 85, 475, 505, 785
van Dijk N., 633
van Hemel N.M., 793
van Lieshout J.J., 633
Vandelli R., 241
Vardas P.E., 57, 685, 777

VASSANELLI C., 713, 843
VECCHI R., 405, 857
VENTURINI A., 215, 301
VILLANI G.Q., 51
VINCENT A., 793
VOS M.A., 767
WASNI O., 205
WEDEKIND H., 667
WEXMAN M., 205
WIELING W., 633
WOHLGEMUTH, P. 793
WOLBRETTE D., 37
WYSE D.G., 43, 127
YANG A., 189
YEE R., 177, 599
YOUNG T.M., 625
ZADO E., 433
ZARSE M., 117
ZUIN G., 309, 851
ZUSSA C., 215, 301

ATRIAL FIBRILLATION:
CLINICAL ASPECTS AND CARDIOVERSION

Sympathetic and Vagal Fibrillation: Do They Exist?

F. Lombardi, F. Tundo, F. Colombo, S. Belletti, D. Tarricone

Background

Atrial fibrillation is a major clinical problem, not only because it involves a growing number of patients with different arrhythmia-related symptoms, but also because of its social and economic impact. Patients with atrial fibrillation are characterised by such symptoms as palpitations and dyspnoea, are limited in their exercise capability and are at high risk of thromboembolic events [1]. Current figures indicate that almost 4% of all hospital admissions are due to symptoms related to atrial fibrillation and its complications.

From a clinical point of view, atrial fibrillation can be classified as paroxysmal when episodes are of short duration and self terminating, persistent when pharmacological or electrical interventions are required to terminate the arrhythmia and, finally, permanent when pharmacological and nonpharmacological interventions become useless to terminate this arrhythmia or to maintain sinus rhythm and efforts are directed at controlling ventricular response (Fig. 1). It is commonly supposed that the time elapsing from the onset of the paroxysmal type to the emergence of the permanent form of this arrhythmia is extremely variable and influenced by several factors, such as the presence or absence of structural heart disease, the presence of atrial dilatation and the duration of the fibrillatory state, which is one of the major determinants of the extent of electrical, mechanical and anatomical remodelling [1–3].

It can be assumed that some resistance to atrial fibrillation is present in the normal heart and disappears with the occurrence of the cardiac structural abnormalities that characterise patients with chronic atrial fibrillation. In patients with paroxysmal atrial fibrillation trigger factors have a critical role. Recent evidence suggests that rapid focal activity at the junction between the pulmonary veins and the atrium, at the level of the Marshall ligament or at the junction between the superior vena cava and the right atrium plays a critical

Cardiologia, Dipartimento di Medicina, Chirurgia e Odontoiatria, Ospedale San Paolo, University of Milan, Italy

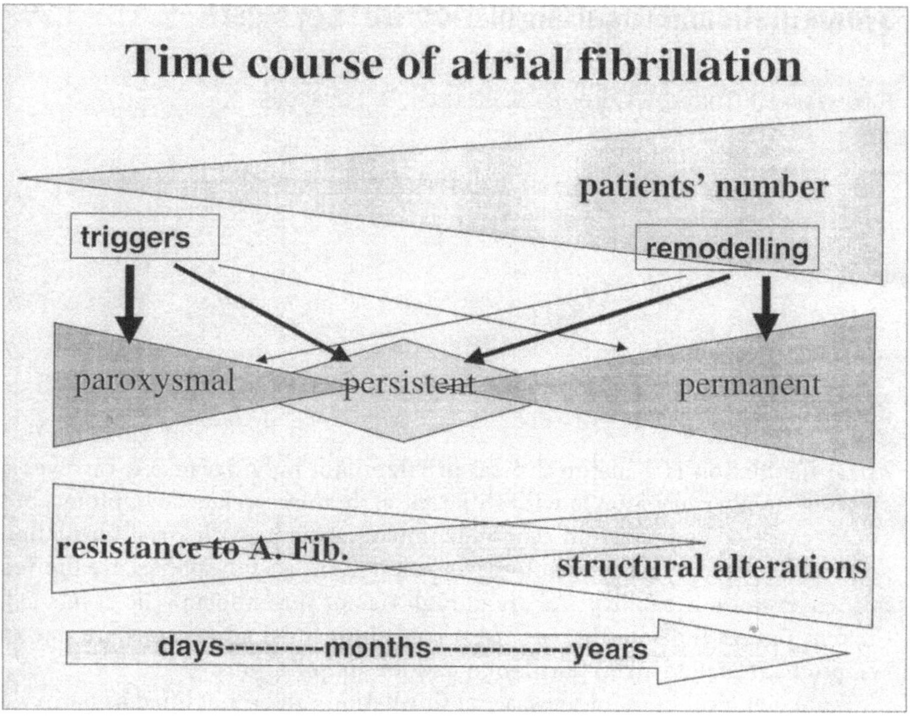

Fig. 1. Schematic illustrating the time-course of atrial fibrillation from its initial paroxysmal manifestations to the permanent phase characterised by critical structural alterations of the atria

part in the initiation of atrial fibrillation [4]. However, for fibrillatory activity to be maintained in the atria, involvement of a critical mass is necessary. In patients with no structural heart disease, most episodes of atrial fibrillation are self-terminating because the relative atrial mass is insufficient to maintain the fibrillatory waves in the absence of those electrophysiological and anatomical alterations that can affect the core size of re-entry by changing atrial conduction velocity and refractoriness. In these patients it is possible that repetitive bouts of focal activity are necessary to reinitiate and perhaps to perpetuate atrial fibrillation.

A factor that is often not adequately considered is the role of the autonomic nervous system and, in particular, the pro-arrhythmic effects of sympathetic or vagal activation. In experimental models of atrial fibrillation it has been possible to observe that both sympathetic and vagal activations are capable of reducing atrial refractoriness and therefore of favouring the onset of re-entrant mechanisms. This effect on atrial refractoriness was observed both during an increase in atrial cycle length secondary to vagal activation and during a shortening of atrial cycle length secondary to sympathetic activation.

Changes in action potential duration and refractoriness could produce pro-arrhythmic effects not only in the induction but also in the perpetuation of atrial fibrillation. In addition, the possibility that the continuous and nonphysiological variations in cardiac cycle duration during atrial fibrillation episodes might affect autonomic control mechanisms and atrial and ventricular remodelling, thus favouring the maintenance of arrhythmia, cannot be excluded.

An abnormal autonomic modulation has been consistently reported before the onset of atrial fibrillation when heart rate variability has been studied in the minutes preceding the onset of arrhythmia. A loss of the fractal-like characteristic of the variability signal before paroxysmal atrial fibrillation episodes was also described.

Less information is available on the effects of the continuous nonphysiological variations in cardiac cycle that are typical of the fibrillatory state on autonomic control mechanisms. This aspect, which is substantially unknown, involves several points of interest. The ventricular response to atrial fibrillation is considered to reflect the filtering properties of the atrioventricular node. Additional factors, such as characteristics of fibrillatory waves, abnormalities of intra-atrial conduction, extent of left-ventricular diastolic dysfunction, presence of mitral regurgitation and beat-to-beat variations in stroke volume, are likely to be involved.

The aim of the present study is to evaluate the predictive value of distinct patterns of variation in cardiac cycles during atrial fibrillation in relation to the maintenance of sinus rhythm after electrical cardioversion.

In the last few years, several studies have been conducted with the aim of verifying the existence of a link between atrial fibrillation episodes and the autonomous nervous system. In most instances, particularly in subjects with paroxysmal atrial fibrillation, a pro-arrhythmic role of sympathetic or vagal activation was recognised. The inference, however, was mainly based on analysis of the environmental context in which atrial fibrillation was initiated. Accordingly, exercise-induced atrial fibrillation was considered to depend upon sympathetic activation, whereas arrhythmic episodes occurring during rest or in the night were classified as of vagal origin [5].

Heart Rate Variability Before Atrial Fibrillation Episodes

A simple method that allows evaluation of the autonomous nervous system and its relationship with atrial fibrillation is the analysis of heart rate variability (HRV) on Holter recordings during sinus rhythm preceding the onset of the arrhythmia. Herweg et al. [6] used spectral techniques to analyse heart rate variability on Holter recordings of 29 patients during sinus rhythm just before the onset of episodes of paroxysmal atrial fibrillation. Patients were divided into two groups: 17 patients had night-time episodes and 12 patients, day-time episodes. Samples taken 5, 10 and 20 min before AF onset were compared. An increase in the high-frequency (HF) component of HRV, reflecting an enhanced parasympathetic activity, was evident in the minutes preceding most episodes of atrial fibrillation. However, day–night differences were observed: the increase in HF component was more consistently seen before nocturnal episodes, and mostly in younger patients with structurally normal hearts ("lone fibrillators").

Dimmer et al. [7] analysed changes in sympathovagal balance in the hour preceding atrial fibrillation during 35 episodes of paroxysmal atrial fibrillation recorded in 26 patients who underwent coronary artery bypass surgery. In this study, HRV was evaluated with both time- and frequency-domain methodologies. It was shown that the LF/HF ratio was significantly lower in the first 30 min, with a subsequent progressive increase in the last few minutes immediately preceding the onset of atrial fibrillation, as a result of a reduction in the power of the HF component. These findings led the authors to conclude that a shift in the autonomic balance with a loss of vagal tone and a moderate increase in sympathetic tone was characteristic of the time immediately before atrial fibrillation onset.

Similar findings were also reported by Wen et al., who studied 12 patients with paroxysmal atrial flutter [8]: analysis of the HRV in the frequency domain demonstrated an increase in the normalised value of the low-frequency (LF) component and in the LF/HF ratio and a decrease in the normalised value of the HF component. These changes started 6 min before the onset of episodes of paroxysmal atrial flutter, thus suggesting a shift in sympathovagal balance toward a sympathetic predominance.

Other authors [9] evaluated the LF/HF ratio 30, 20, 10 and 2 min before the onset of 17 episodes of atrial fibrillation. There were no significant differences in the HF values before the onset of PAF, but the LF/HF ratio increased progressively from about 30 min to just before the onset. Therefore, sympathetic nervous activity increased progressively before the onset of atrial fibrillation, but parasympathetic nervous activity showed no significant changes.

In a recent study published by Bettoni and Zimmermann [10], a more consistent number of patients was analysed. A total of 147 episodes of sustained paroxysmal atrial fibrillation (> 30 min) were recorded and submitted to time-domain and frequency-domain HRV analyses. In the frequency-domain analysis, a significant increase in HF components and a progressive decrease in LF components were observed before the initiation of the arrhythmia. The LF/HF ratio showed a linear increase until 10 min before paroxysmal atrial fibrillation, followed by a sharp decrease immediately before the arrhythmia onset, suggesting a primary increase in adrenergic tone followed by a late parasympathetic activation buffering the adrenergic predominance. No difference was observed in these HRV changes according to whether structural heart disease was present or absent. The study results allowed the authors to conclude that the occurrence of paroxysmal atrial fibrillation depends heavily on variations in autonomic tone, with a primary increase in adrenergic tone followed by an abrupt shift towards vagal predominance.

Regarding the trigger mechanisms initiating paroxysmal atrial fibrillation,

Vikman et al. [11] studied 22 patients without structural heart disease, to test the hypothesis that reduced complexity in R-R interval dynamics may precede the spontaneous onset of the arrhythmia. Traditional HRV measures and approximate entropy were analysed before 62 episodes of paroxysmal atrial fibrillation. An increase in the predictability of R-R interval dynamics was consistently observed in the minutes preceding the onset of the arrhythmic episodes. Thus, altered dynamic behaviour of cardiac interbeat intervals was considered an important trigger of atrial fibrillation in subjects without structural heart disease.

All the above studies seem therefore to support the hypothesis that the autonomous nervous system has an important role in the genesis and the maintenance of the atrial fibrillation and that this effect is more detectable in subjects with no evidence of organic heart disease.

Autonomic Control Before and After Episodes of Paroxysmal Atrial Fibrillation

The effect of restored sinus rhythm on autonomic control mechanisms in patients with paroxysmal atrial fibrillation is largely unknown [12]. We therefore analysed Holter recordings containing episodes of paroxysmal atrial fibrillation lasting more than 30 s, examining the role of the autonomous nervous system in mechanisms of initiation and maintenance of atrial fibrillation and also the role of the restoration of sinus rhythm. The main purpose of the study was to evaluate the changes in the indexes of sympathetic activation before and after paroxysmal atrial fibrillation episodes. In addition, we evaluated the pattern of onset of the arrhythmia and the possible relations between R-R interval preceding the arrhythmia and the coupling interval and between these and the mean ventricular response of atrial fibrillation. The presence of a pseudo-regularisation of the ventricular response in the last part of the arrhythmic episodes before spontaneous recovery of sinus rhythm was also evaluated.

We analysed 110 arrhythmic episodes each lasting at least 30 s. The mean age of the population was 67±10 years (range 47–87 years). The pharmacological therapy included digoxin in 4 patients, class I anti-arrhythmic drugs in 17 patients, β-blockers in 8 patients, class III anti-arrhythmic drugs in 13 patients, and calcium antagonists in 7 patients; 29 patients were receiving no therapy. The clinical characteristics of individual patients were: systemic hypertension in 35%, coronary artery disease in 19%; sick sinus syndrome in 8%; valvular disease in 8%; and lone AF in 30%.

Two-channel 24-h electrocardiographic recordings were analysed using a commercially available digital scanner (Synetec, V 1.20, Ela Medical, Paris, France). The ECG was digitally sampled at 128 samples per second, and data were then transferred from the scanner to an IBM PC-compatible computer for HRV analysis. Data relating to 75 patients and 110 episodes of PAF were used to estimate the spectral power of short-term variability (250–350 cycles) during the control period, about 5 min of sinus rhythm immediately preceding the onset of atrial fibrillation and after its spontaneous termination. Details on the performance of spectral computations and a discussion of the physiological interpretation of spectral components have already been published elsewhere [13–15]. Arrhythmic episodes were divided into day-time (0601–2100 hours) and night-time (2101–0600 hours) episodes on the basis of the moment of onset. Patients were also divided into two groups on the basis of the prevalence of a LF or a HF component, the cut-off value used for the LF/HF ratio being ≥ 2, which is known to reflect a shift in the sympathovagal balance toward a sympathetic activation [16–18].

The mean duration of atrial fibrillation episodes was 154 ± 20 min (range 0.5–1020 min). Sixty-five episodes (59%) occurred during the day; 45 episodes (41%) started during the night.

On the basis of the presence or absence of a 'short-long-short' sequence before atrial fibrillation was initiated, the arrhythmic episodes were classified in type 1 (T1, n=37) and type 2 (T2, n=73). The analysis of the HRV in relation to the type of onset revealed a greater increase in the LF component in T1 than in T2 onset (61.8 ± 4.1 vs 53 ± 3.2). Furthermore, the duration of AF episodes with T1 onset was significantly shorter than that of episodes with T2 onset (68 ± 16 versus 197 ± 27 min, $P < 0.001$). Conversely, no significant difference between the day- and night-time episodes was discovered in the duration (165 ± 16 versus 146 ± 24 min) or between the mean values for RR, variance, LF, HF and LF/HF ratio.

When patients were classified according to a cut-off value of > 2 for the LF/HF ratio, signs of sympathetic predominance were observed in 73 cases, whereas a parasympathetic predominance was detectable in the remaining 37 events. Moreover, when we analysed HRV in the minutes immediately following the spontaneous recovery of sinus rhythm, patients with an initial LF/HF ratio ≥ 2 presented a significant increase in the HF components and a reduction of the LF components and of the LF/HF ratio, whereas patients with an initial LF/HF ratio < 2 showed an increase in LF component and in LF/HF ratio toward values consistent with a more physiological sympathovagal balance.

Finally, when the standard deviation and the coefficient of variation of RR interval in the early, middle and final parts of the arrhythmic episode were compared no differences were observed, indicating the absence of any pseudo-regularisation of ventricular response before spontaneous termination of paroxysmal atrial fibrillation episodes.

Conclusions

Our results are in good agreement with those of previous studies, suggesting that alterations in autonomic control mechanisms are frequently detectable in the minutes preceding the onset of paroxysmal atrial fibrillation. In most instances, signs of sympathetic activation and of reduced vagal modulation are well in evidence, whereas in about one-third of the episodes parasympathetic control mechanisms appear to prevail. Immediately after spontaneous recovery of sinus rhythm, signs of sympathetic activation are no longer evident but are replaced by an HRV pattern consistent with a more physiological modulation of sinus node. Also, in patients with signs of vagal activation before atrial fibrillation episodes a more physiological sympathovagal balance is present at the end of the arrhythmic episodes. It remains to be assessed whether the observed changes in autonomic control mechanisms might contribute to the termination of the arrhythmic events or simply reflect the haemodynamic consequences of the arrhythmia. Nevertheless, the minutes preceding and following atrial fibrillation episodes appear to be characterised by fluctuations in sympathovagal balance with variable shifting toward distinct pattern of autonomic imbalance.

Acknowledgements. This work was supported in part by the 2002 national grant from MIUR.

References

1. Zipes DP (1997) Atrial fibrillation. A tachycardia-induced cardiomyopathy. Circulation 95:562–564
2. Ausma J, Wijffels MCEF, Thonè F et al (1997) Structural changes of atrial myocardium due to sustained atrial fibrillation in the goat. Circulation 96:3157–3163
3. Levy S, Campbell RW, Camm AJ et al, on behalf of the Working Group on Arrhythmias of the European Society of Cardiology (1998) Atrial fibrillation: current knowledge and recommendations for management. Eur Heart J 19:1294–1320
4. Honjo H, Boyett MR, Niwa R et al (2003) Pacing-induced spontaneous activity in myocardial sleeves of pulmonary veins after treatment with ryanodine. Circulation 107:1937–1943
5. Coumel P (1994) Autonomic arrhythmogenic factors in paroxysmal atrial fibrillation. In: Olsson SB, Alessie MA, Campbell RW (eds) Atrial fibrillation: mechanism and therapeutic strategies. Futura, Armonk pp 171–184
6. Herweg B, Dalal P, Nagy B, Schweitzer P (1998) Power spectral analysis of heart period variability of preceding sinus rhythm before initiation of paroxysmal atrial fibrillation. Am J Cardiol 82:869–874
7. Dimmer C, Tavernier R, Gjorgov N et al (1998) Variations of autonomic tone preceding onset of atrial fibrillation after coronary artery bypass grafting. Am J Cardiol 82:22–25
8. Wen Z-C, Chen S-A, Tai-T, Huang JL, Chang MS (1998) Role of autonomic tone in facilitating spontaneous onset of typical atrial flutter. J Am Coll Cardiol 31:602–607
9. Tomoda Y, Uemura S, Fujimoto S et al (1998) Assessment of autonomic nervous activity before the onset of paroxysmal atrial fibrillation. Am J Cardiol 31:11–17
10. Bettoni M, Zimmermann M (2002) Autonomic tone variations before the onset of paroxysmal atrial fibrillation. Circulation 105:2753–2759
11. Vikman S, Makikallio TH, Yli-Mayry S et al (1999) A decrease in complexity of R-R interval dynamics precedes the spontaneous onset of atrial fibrillation. Pacing Clin

Electrophysiol 22 [pt II]:A48
12. Lombardi F, Tundo F (2002) Autonomic nervous system and atrial fibrillation. G Ital Aritmol Cardiostimol 5:23–27
13. Pagani M, Lombardi F, Guzzetti S et al (1986) Power spectral analysis of heart rate and arterial pressure variabilities as a marker of sympathovagal interaction in man and conscious dog. Circ Res 59:178–197
14. Malliani A, Pagani M, Lombardi F, Cerutti S (1991) Cardiovascular neural regulation explored in the frequency domain. Circulation 84:482–492
15. Task Force of the European Society of Cardiology and the North American Society of Pacing and Electrophysiology (1996) Heart rate variability. Standards of measurement, physiological interpretation, and clinical use. Circulation 93:10431065
16. Lombardi F (2000) Chaos theory, heart rate variability, arrhythmic mortality. Circulation 101:8–10
17. Lombardi F, Colombo A, Basilico B et al (2001) Heart rate variability and early recurrence of atrial fibrillation after electrical cardioversion. J Am Coll Cardiol 37:157–162
18. Lombardi F (2002) Clinical implications of present physiological understanding of HRV components. Card Electrophysiol Rev 6:245–249

"Lone" Atrial Fibrillation in Athletes: A Consequence Of Long-Term Intensive Sport Practice

F. Naccarella[1], F. Furlanello[2,3], A. Bertoldi[4], S. Sdringola Maranga[5], G. Lepera[1], R. Cappato[6]

Introduction

Atrial fibrillation (AF) in both the paroxysmal and persistent atrial forms has been documented both in normal hearts without signs of demonstrable cardiac disease [1-67] and, since 1990, also in some professional and competitive athletes, by Furlanello et al. [4–17, 68–73], Maron and Mitchell [11], Fenici et al. [41] Zeppilli [42], and Naccarella and Brachetti [20, 67]. A useful classification from the diagnostic and therapeutic points of view is the following:

1. Lone vagal AF associated with severe sinus bradycardia and cardiac pauses [19, 20, 29, 30, 33–38]
2. Lone sympathetic AF induced only by strenuous physical activity or exercise test or psychological stress. [24, 36–38]
3. A mixture of 1 and 2 [19, 20, 24]
4. AF associated with supraventricular tachycardia (RSVT) [20–27]
5. AF associated with Wolff–Parkinson–W ite (WPW) syndrome or cardiac pre-excitation syndromes [21–27, 32]
6. "Familial "lone AF [29–31, 43–49]

The most important and recently discovered mechanism involved in lone AF induction in normal hearts is documented spontaneously occurring electrical activity in the pulmonary veins [1–3, 53–57]. So-called "ectopic" AF originates from ectopic activity arising from pulmonary veins, due to the persistence and propagation of sleeves of normal atrial myocardial tissue into the orifices of the four pulmonary veins. The tissue has been documented to be present for 10–15 mm mainly inside the superior right and left pulmonary veins [1–3, 53–57]. Other sites or multiple sites of origin have also been docu-

[1] Cardiology Department, Azienda USL Citta' di Bologna, Cardiology DH DS, Bologna., Italy; [2] Cardiology and Arrhythmology Department, Policlinico San Donato, Milan, Italy; [3] Cardiology Department, Villa Bianca Hospital, Trento, Italy; [4] Cardiology Department, Santa Chiara Hospital, Trento, Italy; [5] Cardiology Department, Hermann Memorial Hospital, Houston, Texas, USA; [6] Cardiology-Centro Aritmologia Clinica ed Elettrofisiologia, Policlinico San Donato, Milan, Italy

mented [60–63]. Other mechanisms, such as differences in vagal tonus or vagal hypertonia as a consequence of excessive and prolonged training, have been documented as a cause of lone AF in professional overtrained athletes, as in subjects without demonstrated heart disease (NDHD) [4–14, 20, 67].

Criteria for the Evaluation of Athletic Eligibility

Careful evaluation of professional athletes to identify lone AF and to exclude other associated structural heart disease or electrical disorders such as WPW syndrome or other cardiac pre-excitation syndromes has been advised by international and Italian guidelines, and has been carried out in recent years [10–14, 20, 37–40, 41, 42, 68–73]. A methodology for the clinical evaluation of these subjects and identification of parameters of clinical relevance and risk stratification has been proposed in the US, and the Italian guidelines for the evaluation of eligibility for competitive sport have been defined and recently updated [20, 39, 40, 68–73]. The evaluation, as proposed by Furlanello et al. [10–14, 68–73] and by our group in Bologna [20, 29–31, 51, 52, 67] many years ago, should include all the noninvasive procedures aimed at identifying the mechanisms and electrophysiological characteristics of arrhythmias, the triggering or etiologic factors, and the hemodynamic sequelae or related symptoms [20, 39, 40]. These are:

1. Noninvasive or invasive electrical diagnostic tests
2. Imaging techniques (echocardiography, MRI, others)
3. Laboratory tests, including screening for acute or chronic myocarditis, hormonal disorders, electrolyte imbalances, and use of illicit substances [4–14, 20, 39, 40, 67]

Long-lasting or serial 24-h, 12-lead Holter monitoring is very useful only for frequently occurring AF/atrial flutter (AFL) to document the mechanisms of initiation and interruption of AF/AFL. Concomitant evaluation of the site(s) of origin of ectopic atrial beats could be of interest to elucidate the mechanisms and identify the most appropriate modalities of treatment and the site of mapping and ablation [1–3, 35, 57–62].

Personal Experience

The largest experience in this field has been collected by Furlanello et al. [4–14, 64, 66, 68–73].This experience can be summarized into two parts. The first part, in the preablation era (1974–1998) [8], and the second part, in the ablation era (1998–2003) [4–14, 64, 66, and unpublished data), have been reported in different papers and are summarized in Tables 1–5.

Results

Furlanello's large database on arrhythmias in competitive athletes, which to date includes almost 2503 athletes, 285 of them elite athletes, is reported in Table 1. Almost 29.5% showed supraventricular arrhythmias. The majority of these were RSVT or WPW syndrome (10%).

Table 1. Young competitive athletes with arrhythmias (1974–2003): Furlanello' s data. [4–14, 64, 66, and unpublished data]

	No. of athletes	Male	Female	Average age (years)	Follow-up (months)
Total athletes	2503	2160	343	21.7±7	3–180
Elite athletes	285	248	37	24.2±8	3–170

Among elite athletes with arrhythmias, 29.5 % had supraventricular arrhythmias, 57% ventricular arrhythmias, 8.2% bradyarrhythmias, and 5.3% unidentified arrhythmias

AF or AFL or both have been documented in a "significant minority" of athletes. Some elite athletes with disabling AF/AFL have been successfully treated for recurrences with radiofrequency catheter ablation (RFCA); one became eligible for competitive athletic activity and the others for noncompetitive sporting activity, even at "the beginning of the ablation era" [17, 18] (Table 2).

Table 2. Patient population of athletes in the ablation era (1998-2003): Furlanello's data [4–14, 64, 66, and unpublished data]

No. of athletes	Elite athletes	Mean age (years)	Male	Female	SV arrhythmias	AF/AFL
343	80%	22±7	310	33	96/343 (28%)	17/343 (4.9%)

SV, supraventricular

To turn to Furlanello's most recent athlete patient population, in the modern and more accurate "ablation era," 343 consecutive arrhythmic athletes have been evaluated, more than 80% of them elite athletes and the majority of whom were male. Supraventricular arrhythmias were documented in 28% of the subjects (Tables 2 and 3).

Seventeen of 343 (4.9%) cases of AF or AF associated with AFL have been identified. The clinical characteristics are reported in Table 3, from which it can be seen that 7 (41%) of the 17 (5/7 were elite athletes) were successfully treated with RFCA of AFL and AF substrates, with encouraging results in terms of resumption of competitive practice by the athletes, with no sequelae at all. In the case of sporadically occurring spontaneous episodes of AF/AFL, detraining and temporary discontinuation of athletic activity was the preferred and most useful clinical decision [4–14, 64, 66, 68–73, and unpublished data].

Table 3. Athletes with AF/AFL treatment and follow up in the ablation era: Furlanello's data (unpublished data)

Observations	Treatment	Follow-up
17 athletes (9/17 (53%) elite type) all male with: - 8 AF alone (47%) - 6 in association with AFL (35%) - 3 with AFL alone (18%)	Mean age at first observation of AF/AFL = 30.2 years	
2 (12%) elite athletes with underlying arrhythmogenic heart disease (1 AFL)	Alive on hybrid treatment (one ICD, one RFCA for VT plus AA drugs)	
4 (23%) AF/AFL (sporadic episodes)	Detraining	No recurrences, eligible for athletic activity
7 (41%) (5/7 are elite athletes) with AF alone or with AFL	4 RFCA for both AFL and AF 2 RFCA of AFL	4 no recurrences, eligible for athletic activity 2 on AA drugs, noncompetitive sport activity
3 AF alone (no organic heart disease)	Recurrences no detraining	No eligibility
1 chronic AF (elite rugby player)	Warfarin treatment	Noncompetitive sport activity, 10 years' follow-up

ICD, implantable cardioverter-defibrillator; *VT*, ventricular tachycardia; *AA*, antiarrhythmic

In our own experience [20, 67, and unpublished data] of professional and nonprofessional athletes, lone AF is rarely (<1%) documented as the sole arrhythmia. Conversely, in arrhythmia patients, AF/NDHD was found in 175/1856 subjects (Table 4). AF associated with mild organic disease, rheumatic heart disease, acute or chronic myocarditis, WPW syndrome, or RVDC or Brugada syndrome was excluded.

Table 4. AF in semiprofessional and professional athletes and young subjects with non-demonstrated heart disease (AF/NDHD). Naccarella's data [20, 67, and unpublished data], 1990-2003

		AF	AF/NDHD
Athletes observed	456	6/456 (<1%)	5/6 (83%)
Arrhythmia patients	2789	1856 (67%)[a]	175/1856 (9%)[b]

[a] Both paroxysmal and chronic AF/AFL, to be entered in the Euro Heart Survey on atrial fibrillation; [b] AF/NDHD atrial fibrillation /nondemonstrable heart disease or minal heart disease

Table 5. AF in athletes [20, 67, and unpublished data]

	Age	Sport	Characteristics of AF/AFL symptoms	Neurovegetative state	Treatment	Follow-up
1 AB	18	Soccer	Sporadic but familial	Vagal hypertonus	Detraining	No recurr.
2 SA	32	Running walk	Monthly episodes, disabling	Sympathetic drive effort inducible	Ablation (serial) ectopic AF	AA drugs recurr.
3 PR	28	Road racing	2 episodes	Effort-inducible	AA drugs	Spont. int
4 CM	29	Water polo	Frequent syncopal TR, enlarged RA, previous acute myocarditis	Vagal hypertonus,	Detraining	Ablation? Not eligible
5 LA	43	Cross country skiing	SSS	Vagal hypertonus	PP	Not eligible
6 FG	39	Tennis	PAF >2 episodes	Effort and rest episodes	Hyperthyroidism therapy	Eligible

Recurr., recurrences; *familial*, familial, early in life, occurrence in different members; *spont. int.*, episodes of short duration with spontaneous interruption in 20–30 min, after sport or effort termination, nondisabling episodes; *TR*, tricuspid regurgitation; *RA*, right atrium; *ectopic AF*, ectopic origin originating from left atrium; *not eligible*, not eligible for sport activity; *SSS*, sick sinus syndrome, associated atrial disease; *PP*, permanent pacing; *PAF*, paroxysmal AF

Only 9% of our cases of AF were without any demonstrated heart disease; one showed important tricuspid regurgitation and a dilated right atrium, and one was suffering from thyroid hyperfunction. (Similar data on the incidence of lone AF have been reported for arrhythmia patients by Capucci, Santini, and others, with percentages ranging from 5% to 34% [20, 27, 41, 42, 57].) Patients with moderate atrial dilatation and mild dilated cardiomyopathy or hypertensive cardiomyopathy were excluded. Furthermore, some of the 175 lone AF subjects developed over time signs of myocardial ischemia or a positive treadmill test, or developed moderate to severe blood hypertension and/or a hypertensive cardiomyopathy [20, 67, and unpublished data] (Table 4).

A detailed analysis of six observations of ours is reported in Table 5. The subjects can be divided in those with sporadic (spontaneous regression of PAF and no recurrences over time) and those with frequently occurring or highly symptomatic episodes. In our series we also observed two patients with syncope [29–31] not only related to AF but associated with a vagal hypertonus producing a sudden drop in blood pressure due to massive vasodilation (case 4) and SSS (case 5), as reported in the literature in young and sometimes middle-aged apparently healthy subjects [20, 27, 29, 31, 41, 42]. These subjects should be appropriately treated with an ablation procedure [4–14, 53–61] and allowed, after a period of follow-up without recurrences, to perform sport activity again, or be treated with a hybrid therapy and withdrawal from competitive sport, temporarily or, sometimes, for ever. We have also observed some familial, cases and we agree with Brugada [20, 43, 49, 67] and other authors [43–49] that in some cases lone AF can be a genetically determined disease with hereditary aspects.

Discussion and Comments

From Furlanello's experience it is evident that episodes of AF alone or in association with AFL can be documented even in competitive high-level athletes [4–14, 20, 67, 68–73, and unpublished data]. Seventeen out of 343 were documented in the most recently collected arrhythmic athletic population excluding WPW syndrome (Tables 2 and 3). In Furlanello's population it can be observed that all are male subjects as in the previous reports [6, 9]. The mean age of subjects with AF/AFL is higher (31 vs 22 years) than that of the whole athlete population (Tables 2 and 3).

The arrhythmia seems to be related to the duration over time and the intensity of sport practice and intensity of training. Sometimes, though rarely, AF/AFL can be the first sign of an underlying heart disease. The arrhythmia mechanisms and the possible underlying cardiac disease should be always adequately investigated with all the appropriate noninvasive diagnostic procedures to rule out an underlying myocardial or systemic disease [68–73]. Recently it has been realized that some illicit drugs may induced AF in athletes, e.g., stimulants, including cocaine, cannabinoids, alcohol, β_2-agonists, and anabolic steroids [73]. A laboratory workup is always necessary.

Accurate mapping of initiating mechanisms is appropriate for ablation purposes [1-3, 18, 53–61].

In some of these athletes with sporadically occurring episodes of AF, athletic activity should be temporarily discontinued and resumed after an adequate period of detraining (the duration of which should be individually assessed in each case). Usually these subjects can return to competitive sport activity without any other pharmacological or nonpharmacological treatment [6–9 and unpublished data].

The majority of these subjects, those with recurrences of AF/AFL not compatible with athletic eligibility, should be adequately treated with RFCA [particularly electrical disconnection of multiple pulmonary veins (PVs)]. Today, this can be considered a curative approach in many instances and in numerous athletes. Only one subject has been left in chronic AF, because of the patient's wish not to have cardiac ablation performed.

"The pill in the pocket approach" to paroxysmal AF can be used only in selected cases with sporadic episodes.

Acknowledgements.Particular thanks to Donatella Orlando, FDP, in Bologna for preparing the manuscript. Thanks also to Sdringola Maranga, MD, and to Elena Cuomo, PhD, for selecting the references at the Library and the Permanent Education Center of the Maggiore Hospital, Azienda USL Citta' di Bologna, Bologna.

References

1. Haïssaguerre M, Jais P, Shah DC et al (1998) Spontaneous initiation of atrial fibrillation by ectopic beats originating in the pulmonary veins. N Engl J Med 339:659–666
2. Hwang C, Wu T-J, Doshi RN, Peter CT, Chen P-S (2000) Vein of Marshall cannulation for the analysis of electrical activity in patients with focal atrial fibrillation. Circulation 101:1503–1505
3. Hindricks G, Kottkamp H (2001) Simultaneous noncontact mapping of left atrium in patients with paroxysmal atrial fibrillation. Circulation 104:297–303
4. McGovern BA, Liberthson R (1996) Arrhythmias induced by exercise in athletes and others. S Afr Med J 86(Suppl 2):C78–C82
5. Zehender M, Meinertz T, Keul J et al (1990) ECG variants and cardiac arrhythmias in athletes: clinical relevance and prognostic importance. Am Heart J 119:1378–1394
6. Biffi A, Piovano G, Verdile L et al (1997) Prognostic evaluation on supraventricular arrhythmias in athletes. In: Pelliccia A, Caselli G, Bellotti P (eds) Advances in sport cardiology. Springer, Berlin New York Milan, pp 40–44
7. Delise P, Bonso A, Cor L et al (1992) Electrophysiologic substrates of idiopathic atrial fibrillation in the general population and in athletes. New Trends Arrhyth 8:719–724
8. Coelho A, Palieo E, Ashley W et al (1990) Tachyarrhythmias in young athletes. J Ambul Monit 3/4:269–281
9. Bertoldi A, Furlanello F, Fernando F et al (1993) Cardioarrhythmologic evaluation of symptoms and arrhythmic manifestations in 110 top level consecutive professional athletes. New Trends Arrhythm 9:199–209

10. Furlanello F, Bettini R, Bertoldi A et al (1991) Competitive sports and cardiac arrhythmias. In: Luderitz B, Saksena S (eds) International electrophysiology. Futura, Mount Kisco, NY, pp 41–47
11. Maron BJ, Mitchell J (1994) 26th Bethesda Conference. Recommendations for determining eligibility for competition in athletes with cardiovascular abnormalities. J Am Cardiol 24:848–899
12. Murgatroyd FD, O'Farrel D, Ward DE et al (1993) Who gets paroxymal atrial fibrillation? Clinical features in 222 patients from the Craft multi-centre registry. (Abstract) In: Olson SB, Allessie MA, Campbell RWF (eds) Atrial fibrillation mechanisms and novel therapeutic strategies. Abstracts book. Lund p 7
13. Epstein AE, Mile WM, Bendin DG et al (1996) Personal and public safety issues related to arrhythmias that may affect consciousness: implications for regulation and physician recommendations. Circulation 94:1147–1166
14. Coumel PR (1994) Autonomic arrhythmogenic factors in paroxysmal atrial fibrillation. In: Ollson SB, Allessie MA, Campbell RWF (eds) Atrial fibrillation mechanisms and therapeutic strategies. Futura, Armonk, NY, pp 171–185
15. Furlanello F, Bertoldi A, Bettini R et al (1992) Life-threatening tachyarrhythmias in athletes. Pacing Clin Electrophysiol 15:1403–1411
16. Furlanello F, Bertoldi A, Dallago M et al (1998) Atrial fibrillation in athletes. J Cardiovasc Electrophysiol 9:563–568
17. Bertoldi A, Furlanello F, Fernando F et al (2002) Risk stratification in elite athletes with arrhythmias. G Ital Aritmol Cardiostim 5:218–219
18. Cappato R, Negroni S, Furlanello F et al (2002) Efficacy of a probabilistic approach, step-wise RF catheter ablation approach for the curative treatment of atrial fibrillation. G Ital Aritmol Cardiostim 5:281–228
19. Wijffels MC, Kirchhof CJ, Dorland R, Alessie MA (1995) Atrial fibrillation begets atrial fibrillation. A study in awake chronically instrumented goats. Circulation 92:1954–1968
20. Bracchetti D, Naccarella F (2002) Cuore e sport. Linee guida per l'idoneità all'attività sportiva agonistica. Centro Scientifico
21. Brembilla-Perrot B, Marçon F, Bosser G et al (2001) Paroxysmal tachycardia in children and teenagers with normal sinus rhythm and without heart disease. Pacing Clin Electrophysiol 24:41–45
22. Benson DW, Dunningan A, Benditt DG et al (1983) Transesophageal study of infant with supraventricular tachycardia. Electrophysiologic characteristics. Am J Cardiol 52:1002–1006
23. Brembilla-Perrot B, Spatz F, Khaaldi E et al (1990) Value of esophageal pacing in the evaluation of supraventricular tachycardia. Am J Cardiol 65:322–330
24. Brembilla-Perrot B, Terrier De La Chaise A, Pichenè M et al (1989) Isoprenaline as an aid to the induction of catecholamine-dependent supraventricular tachycardia. Br Heart J 61:322–330
25. Slama R, Coumel Ph, Mottè G et al (1975) Tachycardies paroxystiques liées à un syndrome de Wolff Parkinson White inapparent. Nouv Press Med 45:169–172
26. Garson A, Gillette PC (1981) Electrophysiologic studies of supraventricular tachycardia in children. Prediction of specific mechanism by noninvasive features. Am Heart J 102:383–388
27. Biffi A, Ammirati F, Caselli G et al (1993) Usefulness of transesophageal pacing during exercise for evaluation of palpitations in top-level athletes. Am J Cardiol 72:922–926
28. Pongiglione G, Saul P, Dunningan A et al (1988) Role of transesophageal pacing in

evaluation of palpitations in children and adolescents. Am J Cardiol 66:566–570
29. Driscoll DJ, Jacobsen SJ, Porter CNJ et al (1997) Syncope in children and adolescents. Am J Cardiol 29:1039–1045
30. Beder SD, Cohen MH, Riewenschneider TA (1985) Occult arrhythmias as the etiology of unexplained syncope in children with structurally normal hearts. Am Heart J 109:309-313
31. Leitch JW, Klein GT, Yee R et al (1992) Syncope associated with supraventricular tachycardia. An expression of tachycardia rate or vasomotor response. Circulation 85:1064–1071
32. Bayès de Luna A, Furlanello F, Maron BJ, Zipes DP (2000) Arrhythmias and sudden death in athletes. Dev Card Med 1–126
33. Lin P-H, Huang J-L, Ting C-T, Chen S-A (2001) Respiration and initiation of atrial fibrillation. J Cardiovasc Electrophysiol 12:979
34. Chou H-H, Lin K-H, Luqman N, Kuo C-T (2003) Prolonged ventricular asystole, sinus arrest, and paroxysmal atrial flutter-fibrillation: an uncommon presentation of vasovagal syncope. Pacing Clin Electrophysiol 26:914–917
35. Miyamoto K-J, Tsuchihasashi K, Uno K et al (2001) Studies on the prevalence of complicated atrial arrhythmias, flutter and fibrillation in patients with reciprocating supraventricular tachycardia before and after successful catheter ablation. Pacing Clin Electrophysiol 24:969–978
36. Taneja T, Windhagen Mahnert B, Passman R, Goldberger J, Kadish A (2001) Effects of sex and age on electrocardiographic and cardiac electrophysiological properties in adults. Pacing Clin Electrophysiol 24:16–21
37. Report of the American College of Cardiology (2002) Management of patients with atrial fibrillation. In ACC/AHA/ESC Pocket Guidelines, pp 1–75
38. Report of the American College of Cardiology (2001) ACC/AHA/ESC Guidelines for the management of patients with atrial fibrillation: executive summary. ACC/AHA/ESC Guidelines Executive Summary 38:4. 1–19
39. Comitato organizzativo cardiologico per l'idoneità allo sport (ANCE-ANMCO-FMSI-SIC-SIC SPORT) (1995) Protocolli cardiologici per il giudizio di idoneità allo sport agonistico. Casa Editrice Internazionale, pp 1–75
40. Comitato organizzativo cardiologico per l'idoneità allo sport (ANCE-ANMCO-FMSI-SIC-SIC SPORT) (2003) Protocolli cardiologici per il giudizio di idoneità allo sport agonistico. Casa Editrice Internazionale, pp 430–437
41. Fenici RR, Brisinda D, Fenici P, Zinzi D, Delise P (2201) La sindrome da preeccitazione cardiaca e l'ablazione transcatetere delle aritmie. In: Cardiologia dello sport. Casa Editrice Scientifica Internazionale
42. Zeppilli P (2003) Cardiologia dello sport. Casa Editrice Scientifica Internazionale, pp 1–590
43. Brugada R, Roberts E (2000) Familial atrial fibrillation. In: Molecular genetics of cardiac electrophysiology, vol 7. Kluwer Academic, Dordrecht, pp 90–98
44. Feinberg WM, Blackshear JL, Laupacis A, Kronmal R, Hart RG (1995) Prevalence, age distribution, and gender of patients with atrial fibrillation. Arch Intern Med 155:469–473
45. Wolff L (1943) Familial auricular fibrillation. N Engl J Med 229:396–397
46. Poret P, Mabo P, Deplace C et al (1996) Isolated atrial fibrillation genetically determined? A propos of a familial history. Arch Mal Coeur Vaiss 89:1197–1203
47. Beyer F, Luhmer PT, Bertram H, Kallfeltz HC (1993) Familial idiopathic atrial fibrillation with bradyarrhythmia. Z Kardiol 82:674–677
48. Brugada R, Bachinski LL, Hill R, Roberts R (1998) Familial atrial fibrillation is a gene-

tically heterogeneous disease. J Am Coll Cardiol 31:349 A
49. Berul CI, Towbin JA (2000) Molecular genetics of cardiac electrophysiology. Kluwer Academic, Dordrecht, pp 1–201
50. Mark estes III NA, Salem DN, Wang PJ (1999) Sudden cardiac death in the athlete. Futura, Armonk, NY, pp 1–350
51. Palmieri M, Bracchetti D (2002) Il paziente con fibrillazione atriale. In: Atti del Convegno di Aggiornamento in Cardiologia dello Sport, pp 69–78
52. Palmieri M, Bracchetti D (2002) Atti del Convegno di Aggiornamento in Cardiologia dello Sport, pp 1–203
53. Karch MR, Ndrepepa G, Schneider MAE et al (2003) Single chamber atrial fibrillation involving only the left atrium: implications for maintenance and radiofrequency ablation therapy. Pacing Clin Electrophysiol 26:883–981
54. Schweikert RA, Lugones AP, Kanagaratnam L et al (2001) A simple method of mapping atrial premature depolarization triggering atrial fibrillation. Pacing Clin Electrophysiol 24:22–27
55. Wang T-D, Chen W-J, Su S-S, Su T-C, Chen M-F, Liau C-S, Lee Y-T (2001) Increased levels of tissue plasminogen activator antigen and factor VIII activity in nonvalvular atrial fibrillation: relation to predictors of thromboembolism. J Cardiovasc Electrophysiol 12:877–884
56. Schuessler RB (2001) Does size matter? J Cardiovasc Electrophysiol 12:875–876
57. Santini M (2002) Non pharmacological treatment of atrial fibrillation. Arianna Editrice, pp 1–325
58. Lau C-P, Tse H-F (2001) Early reinitiation of atrial fibrillation after electrical defibrillation: a new electrophysiological phenomenon. Pacing Clin Electrophysiol 24:1581–1582
59. Maounis T, Kyrozi E, Katsaros K et al (2000) The prognostic significance of atrial arrhythmias recorded early after cardioversion for atrial fibrillation. Pacing Clin Electrophysiol 24:1076–1081
60. Wu T-J, Doshi RN, Huang H-L et al (2002) Simultaneous biatrial computerized mapping during permanent atrial fibrillation in patients with organic heart disease. J Cardiovasc Electrophysiol 13:571–577
61. Erdogan A, Carlsson J, Neumann T et al (2001) Quality-of-life in patients with paroxysmal atrial fibrillation after catheter ablation: results of long-term follow-up. Pacing Clin Electrophysiol 26:678–684
62. Leclercq J-F, De Sisti A, Fiorello P et al (2000) Is dual better than single site atrial pacing in the prevention of atrial fibrillation? Pacing Clin Electrophysiol 23:2101–2107
63. De Ambroggi L (2002) Atrial fibrillation in 2000 electrocardiology. Proceedings of the XXVII International Congress in Electrocardiology, Milan, 27 June–1 July 2002
64. Furlanello F, Cappato R., De Ambroggi L (2003) Evaluation of the arrhythmic athlete. Proceedings of a one-day workshop, Milan, 3 March 2003
65. (2003) Atrial fibrillation and arrhythmic syndromes. In: Atti del Convegno "Esperienze a confronto" II giornata livornese di Medicina dello Sport. 30–31 May 2003, pp 1–75
66. Furlanello F (2003) Atrial fibrillation. In: Proceedings of the Italian Congress of the SIC SPORT. Montecatini, 16–17 June 2003, pp 1–96
67. Naccarella F (2003) Dati preliminari del registro prospettico italiano RETE MIDAS–Medtronic, Milan, 3 March 2003 "Fibrillazione atriale ed aritmie negli atleti di calcio e basket"
68. Furlanello F, Fernando F, Galassi A, Bertoldi A (2001) Ventricular arrhythmias in

apparently healthy athletes. In: Malik M (ed) Risk of arrhythmia and sudden death. BMJ Books, London, pp 316–324

69. Furlanello F, Bertoldi A, Galassi A et al (1999) Management of severe cardiac arrhythmic events in elite athletes. Pacing Clin Electrophysiol 22:A 165
70. Furlanello F, Bertoldi A, Dallago M et al (1998) Atrial fibrillation in elite athletes. J Cardiovasc Electrophysiol 98(Suppl):563–568
71. Furlanello F, Bertoldi A, Fernando F, Biffi A (2000) Competitive athletes with arrhythmias. Classification, evaluation and treatment. In: Bayes de Luna A, Furlanello F, Maron BJ, Zipes DP (eds) Arrhythmias and sudden death in athletes. Kluwer Academic, Dordrecht, pp 89–105
72. Furlanello F, Bertoldi A, Dallago M et al (1994) Atrial fibrillation in top-level athletes. In: Olsson SB, Allessie MA, Campbell RWF (eds) Atrial fibrillation: mechanisms therapeutic strategies. Futura, Armonk, NY, pp 203–204
73. Furlanello F, Bentivegna S, Cappato R, De Ambroggi L (2003) Arrhythmogenic effects of illicit drugs in athletes. Submitted for publication in IHJ 2003

Predicting Atrial Fibrillation in Patients with Hypertension: Can We Do It?

R.G. Tieleman, H.J.G.M. Crijns

Introduction

Hypertension is a silent disorder, which is usually asymptomatic. However, long-standing hypertension increases the risk of developing cardiovascular complications, such as stroke, renal failure, peripheral atherosclerosis, coronary artery disease, and heart failure [1]. Systolic blood pressure is a stronger predictor of cardiovascular complications than diastolic pressure [2], and systolic hypertension in isolation has an especially high complication rate [3]. The reduction of morbidity and mortality by prevention of these potentially serious cardiovascular complications is the primary aim of treatment for hypertension [1]. One complication that is not often mentioned in hypertension research is atrial fibrillation (AF). The development of AF in a hypertensive patient may have serious impacts on symptoms and prognosis, since it has been demonstrated that AF independently increases morbidity and mortality rates [4-6], and worsens the quality of life. On the other hand, in many AF patients, hypertension is the main cause of the arrhythmia.

Since the treatment of AF has its limitations, prevention of AF in a population at risk is preferred. For this purpose, the hypertensive patient at increased risk for the development of AF should be identified. In this way, preventive measures such as regular ECG monitoring and the initiation of antithrombotic therapy or rate-control medication could be advised in a selected group of patients, as indicated. Furthermore, in a group with a known increased risk for AF primary prevention studies on the development of AF could be performed.

Epidemiology of Hypertension and AF

Hypertension is a common disorder in the western world, approximately 25%

Department of Cardiology, University Hospital Maastricht, The Netherlands of the US population being affected [7]. AF is another common disorder, although on a different scale. Its prevalence increases with age, from approximately 0.5% at 50-59 years to 5% at the age 70-79 years, and almost 9% at 80-89 years [5, 8]. In several large-scale population-based studies, the development of AF was related to multiple risk factors, such as age, hypertension, valvular and ischaemic heart disease, left-ventricular hypertrophy, heart failure, left atrial enlargement, obesity or thyrotoxicosis [4-6, 9, 10]. Because hypertension is so common in the general population, it is the most important risk factor, accounting for more AF cases than any other risk factor [5]. In the recently published AFFIRM and RACE studies, 50% of the AF patients had hypertension as (one of the) underlying disease(s) [11, 12]. In the Manitoba follow-up study [4], a long-term follow-up study of healthy male air crew recruits, 7.5% of the 3,983 patients developed AF during 154,131 patient-years of observation. The relative risk of AF in the hypertensive men 1.42 fold that in the normotensive men. In a recent report by Verdecchia et al. [13], who followed 2,482 initially untreated hypertensive patients for up to 16 years, the incidence of a first episode of AF was 0.5% per year. During a mean follow-up of 5.4 years, AF became chronic in one-third of these subjects.

Why Is it Important to Predict the Occurrence of AF?

As mentioned above, AF is associated with increased morbidity and mortality [4-6]. Among the complications are tachycardia-induced congestive heart failure, and thromboembolic complications such as ischaemic stroke. Heart failure can be prevented and treated by rate-control medication such as β blockers and verapamil. Aspirin and warfarin are advised in the prevention of stroke in the case of AF [14]. However, it is estimated that up to 50% of patients with AF are asymptomatic [15]. In fact, tachycardiomyopathy and stroke may be the first symptoms of AF and, especially in the case of the latter, anticoagulative therapy may come too late. Mortality studies describe a 1.5- to 2-fold increase in the rate of death in AF patients, independently of concomitant diseases [4-6].

Furthermore, once AF has developed it is often very difficult to treat. Repeated cardioversions and administration of antiarrhythmic drugs can not prevent that a large subset of patients will eventually cease to maintain sinus rhythm [16]. In fact, this so-called rhythm control was not able to improve morbidity and mortality over that achieved with rate control in the recently published RACE and AFFIRM trials [11, 12]. Part of the problem in these trials stemmed from the fact that with current treatment modalities only 40-60% of the patients maintain sinus rhythm during follow-up. Furthermore, the combination of hypertension and rhythm control in AF appeared to be a dangerous duo, with an increased incidence of the combined end-point of morbidity and mortality in the RACE study [11]. *Prevention* of AF may therefore be preferable to optimising its *treatment*.

Mechanisms by Which Hypertension Can Cause AF

The exact mechanism by which hypertension causes AF is not known. The general opinion is that hypertension gives rise to left ventricular hypertrophy and (diastolic) left ventricular dysfunction. In parallel with the situation of experimentally induced heart failure in a dog model of rapid ventricular pacing [17], this may increase the susceptibility to AF due to left atrial dilatation and subsequent fibrosis of the left atrial tissue. Fibrosis may lead to decreased conduction velocity and an increased path length of activation. Together with the increase in atrial size, this creates favourable conditions for a re-entry arrhythmia such as AF. Whether hypertension also increases triggers for AF, for example by increasing the number of PACs, is not known.

Predictors of AF

Even though the precise pathological mechanism by which hypertension causes AF is not known, several risk factors have been identified from epidemiological and observational studies.

Demographic Variables

Age is the most important predictor of AF in the general population [5, 8]. Verdecchia et al. [13] demonstrated in a hypertensive population that the 61 subjects who developed AF were older than the 2,421 patients who did not (51±12 versus 59±10 years, respectively; $p<0.01$) and had higher systolic blood pressure (144±15 mmHg versus 137±15 mmHg, respectively; $p< 0.01$). Although some population-based studies claim an increased incidence of AF in males, this recent report did not reveal any sex difference in either group (53.2% versus 52.5%, respectively; not significant). The prevalence of diabetes mellitus (7.1% versus 9.8%) and that of cigarette smoking (22.8% vs 23.0%) were also similar.

Echocardiographic Variables

Population-based studies such as the Framingham and the Manitoba follow-up studies have demonstrated that left-ventricular hypertrophy is an independent predictor of AF [4, 7]. In an echocardiographic study of 8,056 cardiological patients (with and without hypertension), we found that during a median follow-up of 3 years, 514 patients developed AF [18]. As in the general population, an increase in left ventricular wall thickness increased the likelihood of incident AF. Starting at 1% in the absence of left-ventricular hypertrophy (8 mm), the incidence of AF increased by 0.5% for every 1-mm increment in LV wall thickness (Fig. 1). However, on multivariate analysis, the only independent predictors of AF found were age, left-ventricular ejection fraction and left atrial size.

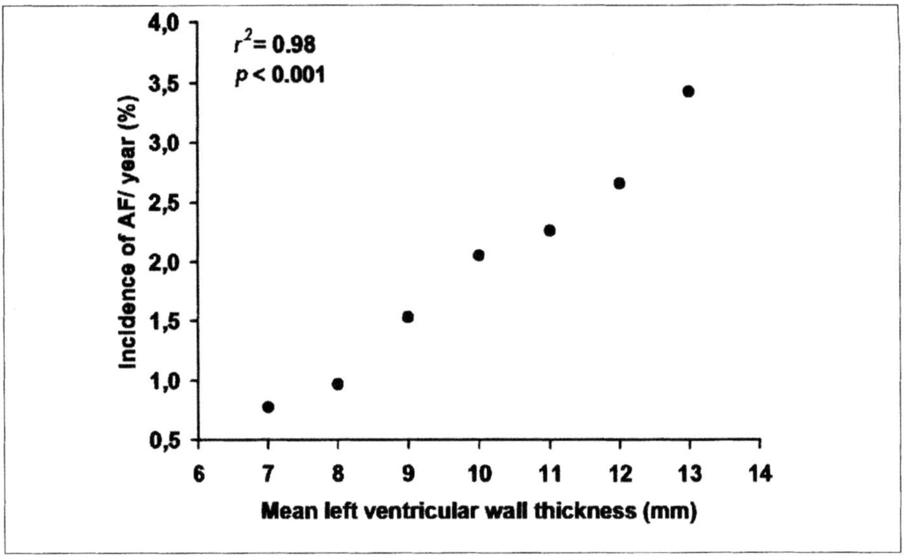

Fig. 1. Correlation between left ventricular wall thickness and incidence of atrial fibrillation (AF) during a median follow-up of 3 years in cardiological patients undergoing echocardiography [18]

In the hypertensive population studied by Verdecchia et al. [13], independent predictors of new acute AF were age and LV mass. Independent predictors of recurrent or chronic AF were age, LA diameter, and left ventricular hypertrophy. When adjusted for age, left ventricular hypertrophy combined with left-atrial dilatation was associated with the highest incidence of AF.

Electrocardiographic Variables

In parallel with the echocardiographic findings, electrocardiographic (ECG) signs of left-ventricular hypertrophy increase the risk of AF [5]. As mentioned above, one of the mechanisms by which hypertension-induced left-ventricular hypertrophy can cause AF may be the development of atrial dilatation and atrial fibrosis. In accordance with this theory, a prolonged P-wave duration has been shown to predict AF in several patient populations [19, 20]. Atrial late potentials as detected by the high-resolution signal-averaged electrogram of the P-wave may also help in predicting AF in hypertension [21-24]. Furthermore, several reports have been published on the predictive value of P-wave dispersion as a predictive marker of AF [19, 20, 24-27].

In the study by Verdecchia et al. [13], ECG signs of left-atrial dilatation were also associated with a 2-fold increased risk of AF after adjustment for age (RR 2.17, 95% CI 1.18 - 4.01). However, after control for LV mass, the association was lost.

Conclusions

At present, it is clear that hypertensive heart disease is one of the most important risk factors for AF. However, the exact mechanism of the development of AF in these patients is not clear. Population and hospital-acquired database studies have revealed an important role for age, degree of LV hypertrophy, LV function, and left atrial size. Despite these risk factors, more studies are needed to identify charateristics with a high positive predictive value, so that preventive strategies against the development of AF can be evaluated.

Reference

1. Chobanian AV, Bakris GL, Black HR et al (2003) The seventh report of the Joint National Committee on Prevention, Detection, Evaluation, and treatment of High Blood Pressure: the JNC 7 Report. JAMA 289:2560-2571
2. Kannel WB (2000) Elevated systolic blood pressure as a cardiovascular risk factor. Am J Cardiol 85:251-255
3. Staessen JA, Gasowski J, Wang JG et al (2000) Risks of untreated and treated isolated systolic hypertension in the elderly: meta-analysis of outcome trials. Lancet 355:865-872
4. Krahn AD, Manfreda J, Tate RB, Mathewson FA, Cuddy TE (1995) The natural history of atrial fibrillation: incidence, risk factors, and prognosis in the Manitoba Follow-Up Study. Am J Med 98:476-484
5. Kannel WB, Wolf PA, Benjamin EJ, Levy D (1998) Prevalence, incidence, prognosis, and predisposing conditions for atrial fibrillation: population-based estimates. Am J Cardiol 82:2N-9N
6. Benjamin EJ, Wolf PA, D'Agostino RB, Silbershatz H, Kannel WB, Levy D (1998) Impact of atrial fibrillation on the risk of death: the Framingham Heart Study. Circulation 98:946-952
7. Burt VL, Whelton P, Roccella EJ et al (1995) Prevalence of hypertension in the US adult population. Results from the Third National Health and Nutrition Examination Survey, 1988-1991. Hypertension 25:305-313
8. Furberg CD, Psaty BM, Manolio TA, Gardin JM, Smith VE, Rautaharju PM (1994) Prevalence of atrial fibrillation in elderly subjects (the Cardiovascular Health Study). Am J Cardiol 74:236-241
9. Kannel WB, Abbott RD, Savage DD, McNamara PM (1982) Epidemiologic features of chronic atrial fibrillation: the Framingham study. N Engl J Med 306:1018-1022
10. Psaty BM, Manolio TA, Kuller LH et al (1997) Incidence of and risk factors for atrial fibrillation in older adults. Circulation 96:2455-2461
11. Van Gelder IC, Hagens VE, Bosker HA et al (2002) A comparison of rate control and rhythm control in patients with recurrent persistent atrial fibrillation. N Engl J Med 347:1834-1840
12. Wyse DG, Waldo AL, DiMarco JP et al (2002) A comparison of rate control and rhythm control in patients with atrial fibrillation. N Engl J Med 347:1825-1833
13. Verdecchia P, Reboldi G, Gattobigio R et al (2003) Atrial fibrillation in hypertension: predictors and outcome. Hypertension 41:218-23
14. Fuster V, Ryden LE, Asinger RW et al (2001) ACC/AHA/ESC guidelines for the management of patients with atrial fibrillation: executive summary. A report of the

American College of Cardiology/ American Heart Association Task Force on Practice Guidelines and the European Society of Cardiology Committee for Practice Guidelines and Policy Conferences (Committee to Develop Guidelines for the Management of Patients With Atrial Fibrillation): developed in collaboration with the North American Society of Pacing and Electrophysiology. J Am Coll Cardiol 38:1231-1266

15. Page RL, Tilsch TW, Connolly SJ et al (2003) Asymptomatic or "silent" atrial fibrillation: frequency in untreated patients and patients receiving azimilide. Circulation 107:1141-1145
16. Van Gelder IC, Crijns HJ, Tieleman RG et al (1996) Chronic atrial fibrillation. Success of serial cardioversion therapy and safety of oral anticoagulation. Arch Intern Med 156:2585-2592
17. Li D, Fareh S, Leung TK, Nattel S (1999) Promotion of atrial fibrillation by heart failure in dogs: atrial remodeling of a different sort. Circulation 100:87-95
18. Neven K, Tieleman RG, Cheriex EC, Crijns HJGM (2002) The degree of left ventricular hypertrophy predicts the incidence of atrial fibrillation (abstract). Eur Heart J 23:138
19. Dilaveris PE, Gialafos EJ, Sideris SK et al (1998) Simple electrocardiographic markers for the prediction of paroxysmal idiopathic atrial fibrillation. Am Heart J 135:733-738
20. Dilaveris PE, Gialafos EJ, Andrikopoulos GK et al (2000) Clinical and electrocardiographic predictors of recurrent atrial fibrillation. Pacing Clin Electrophysiol 23:352-358
21. Fukunami M, Yamada T, Ohmori M et al (1991) Detection of patients at risk of paroxysmal atrial fibrillation during sinus rhythm by P-wave triggered signal-averaged electrogram. Circulation 83:162-169
22. Klein M, Evans SJ, Blumberg S, Cataldo L, Bodenheimer MM (1995) Use of P-wave-triggered, P-wave signal-averaged electrocardiogram to predict atrial fibrillation after coronary artery bypass surgery. Am Heart J 129:895-901
23. Cecchi F, Montereggi A, Olivotto I et al (1997) Risk for atrial fibrillation in patients with hypertrophic cardiomyopathy assessed by signal averaged P-wave duration. Heart 78:44-49
24. Dilaveris PE, Gialafos EJ, Chrissos D et al (1999) Detection of hypertensive patients at risk for paroxysmal atrial fibrillation during sinus rhythm by computer-assisted P wave analysis. J Hypertens 17:1463-1470
25. Dilaveris P, Batchvarov V, Gialafos J, Malik M (1999) Comparison of different methods for manual P wave duration measurement in 12-lead electrocardiograms. Pacing Clin Electrophysiol 22:1532-1538
26. Ciaroni S, Cuenoud L, Bloch A (2000) Clinical study to investigate the predictive parameters for the onset of atrial fibrillation in patients with essential hypertension. Am Heart J 139:814-819
27. Ozer N, Aytemir K, Atalar E et al (2000) P wave dispersion in hypertensive patients with paroxysmal atrial fibrillation. Pacing Clin Electrophysiol 23:1859-1862

What Is the Impact of Atrial Fibrillation on the Clinical Course of Hypertrophic Cardiomyopathy?

F. Cecchi, I. Olivotto

Introduction

Atrial fibrillation (AF) is the most common sustained arrhythmia in patients with hypertrophic cardiomyopathy (HCM), with a reported prevalence ranging from 10% to 28% [1-13]. In a recent study involving 480 patients with HCM followed up at two institutions for over 9 years, AF was documented in 22% of patients, with an incidence of 2% new cases per year [4]. Comparison with the general population shows that the likelihood of developing AF is 4-6 times in HCM patients at any given age. AF became progressively more common with age in HCM patients, and particularly after the age of 60 years; the mean age at onset of the arrhythmia was 54 years for paroxysmal AF and 57 years for chronic AF [4]. However, over one-third of patients with AF developed their arrhythmia before the age of 50 years, and these patients were at greater risk of clinical deterioration and HCM-related death than were patients with AF onset later in life [4]. Finally, postoperative AF occurred following surgical septal myectomy in approximately 30% of patients in one series [13].

AF often occurs in patients who are already symptomatic, but may occasionally be the initial presenting symptom leading to the diagnosis of HCM [4]. At the clinical onset, AF is often in its paroxysmal form, which may later become chronic; however, patients presenting with established, chronic AF as the first manifestation of the arrhythmia are not uncommon (Fig. 1).

AF and Functional Limitation

The clinical consequences associated with acute onset of AF in HCM are variable, ranging from a total lack of symptoms to syncope or pulmonary edema. In most cases, patients with acute AF show sudden and severe clinical deterio-

Regional Referral Center for Myocardial Diseases, Azienda Ospedaliera Careggi, Florence, Italy

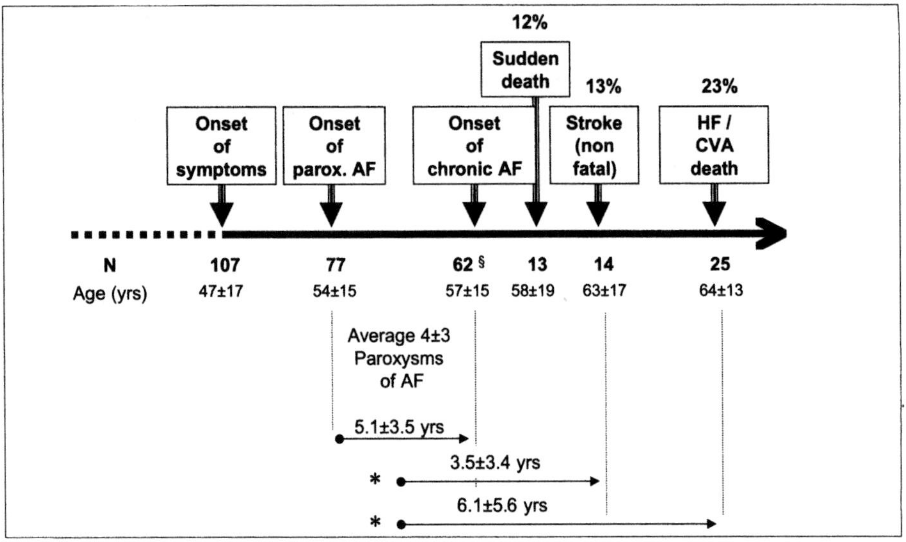

Fig. 1. Sequence of events in 107 patients with hypertrophic cardiomyopathy (HCM) and atrial fibrillation (AF). The diagram is designed to illustrate the average time-course of atrial fibrillation in relation to outcome. * calculated from date of first documented AF, paroxysmal or chronic; § 32 with previous documented paroxysmal AF and 45 without. Data from [4]

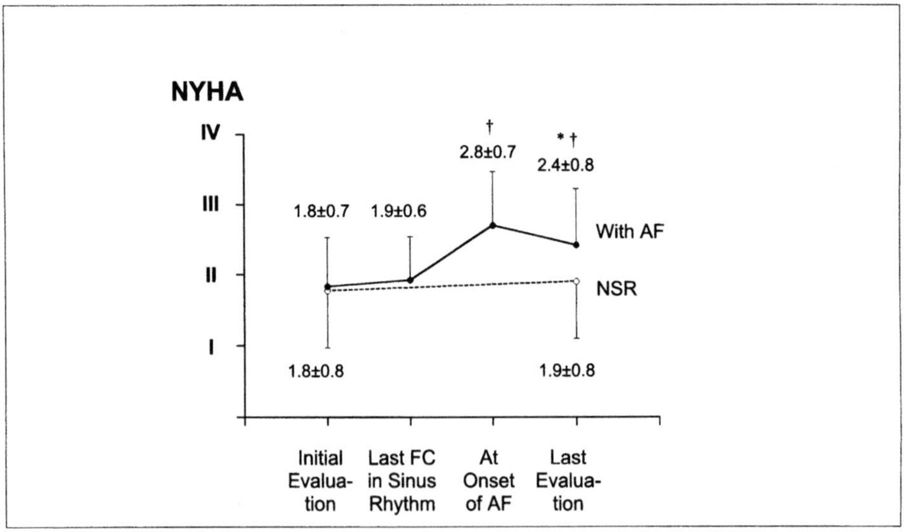

Fig. 2. Impact of AF on symptoms and functional status. When compared with the matched group of patients in sinus rhythm (NSR; n=133), AF patients (n=107) were found to have developed significantly greater functional limitation during follow-up, both in the first hours after initial onset of the arrhythmia and in the long term. FC, NYHA functional class; *p<0.001 vs patients in sinus rhythm; † p<0.001 vs patients with AF at diagnosis. Data from [4]

ration, owing to the combined effects of the loss of atrial systole, increased ventricular rate, and left-ventricular diastolic impairment [4,10-11] (Fig. 2).

In the long term, patients with AF experience significant symptomatic impairment and functional limitation compared with patients in sinus rhythm, despite receiving standard treatment for ventricular rate control. Indeed, the likelihood that patients with AF would be in NYHA class III-IV by the end of a 9-year follow-up period were almost 3 times that for patients who remained in sinus rhythm [4].

Impact on Outcome

Among the limited number of existing studies, most reveal an adverse outcome associated with AF in HCM populations [3-6]. Only in one study was no difference in survival found between patients with and without AF, in spite of generally more severe clinical impairment and higher risk of thromboembolic complications in the AF group [12]. Nevertheless, the low survival rates of the HCM patients in sinus rhythm who were used as controls may have concealed an adverse effect of AF in this study [12].

In our experience, AF is a key determinant of unfavorable outcome, being associated with an almost 4-fold increase in cardiovascular mortality independent of other important clinical variables, such as age and NYHA functional class [4]. Annual HCM-related mortality was 3% among AF patients, versus 1% among matched patients in sinus rhythm; the prognosis was even more unfavorable among those AF patients who had experienced the onset of the arrhythmia at a younger age (≤50 years). The impact of AF on outcome appears to be more pronounced in HCM patients than in the general population or in patients with other heart diseases [14].

Overall risk of HCM-related mortality was not significantly related to the qualitative (paroxysmal versus chronic) or quantitative (number of paroxysmal episodes) manifestations of AF [4]. Nevertheless, patients developing chronic AF, as opposed to exclusively paroxysmal AF, were found to have a higher combined probability of HCM-related death, functional impairment, and stroke [4].

It is noteworthy that, while associated with a marked increase in heart failure- and stroke-related death, AF did not appear to represent a consistent trigger of sudden and unexpected death in HCM patient populations [4, 15]. On the other hand, a circumstantial association between AF and sudden death is suggested by the observation that about 20% of those HCM patients who had survived a documented cardiac arrest showed supraventricular arrhythmias (including AF) at the onset of symptoms preceding the collapse [16]. Indeed, AF with rapid ventricular conduction is capable of degenerating into ventricular fibrillation, as the result of a combination of electrophysiological instability and ischemia [17, 18].

HCM patients with left ventricular outflow obstruction appear to be highly dependent on active atrial contribution for LV filling, and are therefore particularly susceptible to the adverse consequences of AF. The combination of basal left ventricular outflow obstruction and AF more than doubles the risk of cardiovascular mortality compared with that of patients with non obstruction [3, 4].

AF and Risk of Embolic Stroke

Stroke and other cardioembolic events are well-recognized causes of disability and death in HCM patients, and are robustly associated with AF [4-6, 15, 19-21]. Among HCM patients with AF, the risk of stroke is 8-fold that of patients in sinus rhythm [4, 21], with no significant difference between patients with chronic or paroxysmal AF. Moreover, among patients with paroxysmal AF, the risk appears to be independent of the number of AF episodes [4]. Thus, patients with only a single AF paroxysm may be at risk for embolic complications just as much as patients who have experienced multiple episodes or have long-standing AF. Fortunately, stroke was rarely the first clinical manifestation of AF in HCM [21].

The primary determinant of cardioembolic events related to AF is undoubtedly the slow and sluggish flow within the LA, which predisposes to clot formation. Moreover, particularly in the elderly, AF may predispose patients to ischemic stroke by causing localized impairment of cerebral blood flow secondary to reduced cardiac output [22]. In addition, AF is associated with a hypercoagulable state similar to that observed in patients with heart failure, which is probably mediated by an increase in catecholamine levels. Such a hypercoagulable state has been documented in HCM patients by an increase in factors VIII:C and VIIIR:Ag and in platelet aggregation rate [23, 24]. As a consequence, both paroxysmal and chronic AF represent clear indications to oral anticoagulation in HCM patients [1, 2, 4]. Specifically, the threshold for initiation of anticoagulant treatment in HCM should be low and independent of the number of documented AF episodes [4]. Nevertheless, such clinical decisions often need to be tailored in the individual patient, with due consideration for his or her risk of hemorrhagic complications, lifestyle modification, and expected compliance [25].

Maintenance of Sinus Rhythm vs Rate Control

Current treatment strategies for AF in HCM patients are largely based on standard guidelines developed for patients with other cardiac conditions [25]. In HCM patients with recent onset of AF, early reversal to sinus rhythm is desirable for its beneficial hemodynamic effects. Therefore, an aggressive approach to AF with pharmacological or electrical cardioversion in association with prophylactic antiarrhythmic treatment (and anticoagulation) may prevent or delay AF-related complications. In a retrospective study, low-dose amiodarone treatment has been found to have several advantages over conventional antiarrhythmic treatment (including digoxin, verapamil, β blockers and class I agents), including a lower number of cardioversion attempts and embolic complications and longer intervals of sinus rhythm maintenance before AF recurrence [12]. Low-dose amiodarone treatment has been shown to be safe for long-term administration in HCM patients with ventricular arrhythmias [26, 27]. The efficacy and safety of other class III agents including sotalol and dofetilide is still unknown in HCM patients. In addition, the use of implantable devices, such as multisite pacemakers or dual-chamber defibrillators for the management of AF has had some promising results, but has not been systematically tested in HCM [28].

When maintenance of sinus rhythm is not feasible, and in this subpopulation conservative strategies directed at ventricular rate control represent a necessary alternative [25]. Recent evidence suggests that optimal control of ventricular rate may be equivalent to sinus rhythm maintenance in terms of outcome [29]. However, whether these results also apply in the case of HCM patients in still not known, and any default extrapolation should therefore be avoided.

In patients who have gone into chronic AF, adequate rate control can be obtained with β-adrenergic blocking agents, verapamil or diltiazem, or amiodarone, each of which can be used alone or in combination. Digitalis, which is contraindicated in patients with outflow obstruction, can be used in patients without obstruction, particularly in the presence of systolic dysfunction and in the end-stage phase [2, 25]. However, in our experience, digitalis is often incapable of maintaining adequate rate control during exercise in HCM patients. Finally, in patients with persistently elevated ventricular rates associated with functional limitation, atrioventricular node ablation with implantation of a rate-responsive pacemaker is an effective alternative for rate control [25].

Acknowledgements. This work was supported by grants from the Italian Ministry for Scientific and Technologic Research (grant COFIN 2002).

References

1. Maron BJ (1997) Hypertrophic cardiomyopathy. Lancet 350:127-133
2. Spirito P, Seidman CE, McKenna WJ, Maron BJ (1997) The management of hypertrophic cardiomyopathy. N Engl J Med 336:775-785
3. Maron MS, Olivotto I, Betocchi S et al (2003) Effect of left ventricular outflow tract obstruction on clinical outcome in hypertrophic cardiomyopathy. N Engl J Med 348:295-303
4. Olivotto I, Cecchi F, Casey SA et al (2001) Impact of atrial fibrillation on the clinical course of hypertrophic cardiomyopathy. Circulation 104:2517-2524
5. Cecchi F, Olivotto I, Montereggi A et al (1995) Hypertrophic cardiomyopathy in Tuscany: clinical course and outcome in an unselected population. J Am Coll Cardiol 26:1529-1536
6. Maron BJ, Casey SA, Poliac L et al (1999) Clinical course of hypertrophic cardiomyopathy in a Regional United States Cohort. JAMA 281:650-655

7. Cecchi F, Montereggi A, Olivotto I et al (1997) Risk for atrial fibrillation in patients with hypertrophic cardiomyopathy assessed by signal-averaged P-wave. Heart 78:44-49
8. McKenna WJ (1983) Arrhythmia and prognosis in hypertrophic cardiomyopathy. Eur Heart J 4[Suppl F]:225-234
9. Savage DD, Seides SF, Maron BJ et al (1979) Prevalence of arrhythmias during 24-hour electrocardiographic monitoring and exercise testing in patients with obstructive and nonobstructive hypertrophic cardiomyopathy. Circulation 59:866-875
10. McKenna WJ, England D, Doi YL et al (1981) Arrhythmia in hypertrophic cardiomyopathy. I. Influence on prognosis. Br Heart J 46:168-172
11. Glancy DL, O'Brien KP, Gold HK, Epstein SE (1970) Atrial fibrillation in patients with idiopathic hypertrophic subaortic stenosis. Br Heart J 32:652-659
12. Robinson KC, Frenneaux MP, Stockins B et al (1990) Atrial fibrillation in hypertrophic cardiomyopathy: a longitudinal study. J Am Coll Cardiol 15:1279-1285
13. Ommen SR, Thomson HL, Nishimura RA et al (2002) Clinical predictors and consequences of atrial fibrillation after surgical myectomy for obstructive hypertrophic cardiomyopathy. Am J Cardiol 89:242-244
14. Benjamin EJ, Wolf PA, D'Agostino RB et al (1998) Impact of atrial fibrillation on the risk of death. The Framingham Heart Study. Circulation 98:946-952
15. Maron BJ, Olivotto I, Spirito P et al (2000) Epidemiology of hypertrophic cardiomyopathy-related death: revisited in a large non-referral based patient population. Circulation 102;858-864
16. Cecchi F, Maron BJ, Epstein SE (1989) Long-term outcome of patients with hypertrophic cardiomyopahy successfully resuscitated after cardiac arrest. J Am Coll Cardiol 13:1283-1288
17. Stafford WJ, Trohman RG, Bilsker M et al (1986) Cardiac arrest in an adolescent with atrial fibrillation and hypertrophic cardiomyopathy. J Am Coll Cardiol 7:701-704
18. Lopez Gil M, Arribas F, Cosio FG (2000) Ventricular fibrillation induced by rapid atrial rates in patients with hypertrophic cardiomyopathy. Europace 2:327-332
19. Furlan AJ, Craciun AR, Raju NR, Hart N (1984) Cerebrovascular complications associated with idiopathic hypertrophic subaortic stenosis. Stroke 15:282-284
20. Di Pasquale G, Andreoli A, Lusa AM et al (1990) Cerebral embolic risk in hypertrophic cardiomyopathy. In: Baroldi G, Camerini F, Goodwin J (eds) Advances in Cardiomyopathies. Springer, Milan, pp. 91-96
21. Maron BJ, Olivotto I, Bellone P et al (2002) Clinical profile of stroke in 900 patients with hypertrophic cardiomyopathy. J Am Coll Cardiol 39:301-307
22. Lavy S, Stern S, Melamed E et al (1980) Effect of chronic atrial fibrillation on regional cerebral blood flow. Stroke 1:35-38
23. Longo G, Cecchi F, Grossi A et al (1984) Coagulation and platelet function in hypertrophic cardiomyopathy. Thromb Haemost 51:299
24. Yarom M, Lewis BS, Lijovetsky G et al (1982) Platelet studies in patients with hypertrophic cardiomyopathy. Cardiovasc Res 16:324-330
25. Fuster V, Ryden LE, Asinger RW et al (2003) ACC/AHA/ESC Guidelines for the Management of Patients With Atrial Fibrillation: Executive Summary: a report of the American College of Cardiology/American Heart Association Task Force on Practice Guidelines and the European Society of Cardiology Committee for Practice Guidelines and Policy Conferences. Circulation 104:2118-2150
26. McKenna WJ, Oakley CM, Krikler DM, Goodwin JF (1985) Improved survival with amiodarone in patients with hypertrophic cardiomyopathy and ventricular tachycardia. Br Heart J 53:412-416

27. Cecchi F, Olivotto I, Montereggi A et al (1998) Prognostic value of nonsustained ventricular tachycardia and efficacy of amiodarone treatment in an unselected patient population with hypertrophic cardiomyopathy. Heart 79:331-336
28. Friedman PA, Dijkman B, Warman EN et al (2001) Atrial therapies reduce atrial arrhythmia burden in defibrillator patients. Circulation 104:1023-1028
29. Wyse DG, Waldo AL, DiMarco JP et al (2002) Atrial fibrillation follow-up investigation of rhythm management (AFFIRM) investigators. A comparison of rate control and rhythm control in patients with atrial fibrillation. N Engl J Med 347:1825-1833

Atrial Fibrillation in Heart Failure: Prognostic Significance and Management

G.V. Naccarelli, B.J. Hynes, D. Wolbrette, M. Khan, L. Bhatta, S. Samii, J. Luck

Atrial Fibrillation in CHF: Prognostic Significance

Patients with congestive heart failure (CHF) have a poor prognosis and are at increased risk of dying suddenly or from progressive pump dysfunction. Atrial and ventricular arrhythmias commonly occur in patients with CHF and are a significant source of symptoms, morbidity, and mortality. Atrial fibrillation occurs in up to 9% of patients over the age of 80 and in 15%–30% of patients with CHF [1]. The prevalence of atrial fibrillation increases with progression of NYHA heart failure class from less than 10% in NYHA class I to almost 50% in NYHA class IV CHF [2].

Although patients with atrial fibrillation and CHF have up to a three-fold increase in cardiovascular mortality compared to patients with sinus rhythm [3, 4], it is uncertain whether the presence of atrial fibrillation serves as an independent predictor of a worse prognosis in CHF patients. Several retrospective studies have addressed the prognostic significance of atrial fibrillation in CHF patients and the results of these studies have been conflicting [5–10]. Whether atrial fibrillation is the cause or simply a coexisting marker of hemodynamic deterioration or both is not well delineated. However, it has been demonstrated that there is a significant improvement in left ventricular systolic function after catheter ablation of the atrioventricular junction in patients with chronic, rapid atrial fibrillation who have a tachycardia-induced cardiomyopathy [11]. If the clinical and hemodynamic changes of atrial fibrillation seen in heart failure patients are so dramatic, it is puzzling that atrial fibrillation has not been reported as an independent predictor of a worse prognosis in patients with CHF. The AFFIRM trial demonstrated that maintenance of sinus rhythm did not improve survival compared to rate control and anticoagulation and suggests that rate control can serve as a primary therapy in high-risk atrial fibrillation patients, or as a secondary therapy if rhythm con-

Division of Cardiology and the Penn State Cardiovascular Center, Penn State University College of Medicine, Hershey, Pennsylvania, USA

trol is ineffective [12]. However, AFFIRM included only a small number of patients with left ventricular dysfunction and heart failure. In order to discern better whether maintenance of sinus rhythm in CHF patients portends a better prognosis, another prospective international multicenter trial, the AF-CHF trial, is enrolling patients to evaluate the effect of atrial fibrillation therapy on cardiovascular mortality in patients with heart failure [13]. The trial is designed to include 1450 patients with a left ventricular ejection fraction (LVEF) below 35% and a history of atrial fibrillation, who will be randomized to rhythm control or rate control strategies.

Role of Antiarrhythmic Drugs in Maintaining Sinus Rhythm in CHF

For maintenance of sinus rhythm, amiodarone has been shown to have a 66% efficacy rate of maintaining sinus rhythm at 1 year compared to 50% efficacy rates for class IA, IC, and other class III drugs [14, 15]. Based on safety data from survival trials in patients with structural heart disease, the ACC/AHA/ESC guidelines for the management of patients with atrial fibrillation recommend amiodarone or dofetilide when prevention of atrial fibrillation in heart failure is the goal [16]. In post-myocardial-infarction patients, sotalol, amiodarone, and dofetilide are the drugs of choice. In patients with structural heart disease and left ventricular dysfunction, class I drugs should be avoided because of the excess mortality secondary to these drugs noted in the CAST and SPAF trials.

Results from the GESICA and CHF-STAT trials suggest that amiodarone improves survival in patients with nonischemic heart failure, and has at least a neutral effect on those with ischemic heart failure. Data from the Congestive Heart Failure–Survival Trial Antiarrhythmic Therapy (CHF-STAT) [17] database demonstrated that amiodarone converted atrial fibrillation to sinus rhythm in 31%, whereas only 8% converted to sinus rhythm in the placebo group ($p=0.002$). Amiodarone also statistically reduced the ventricular response at 2 weeks (20% reduction, $p=0.001$) better than the control group. The development of atrial fibrillation was lower during amiodarone therapy (4.1% versus 8.4% in the placebo group). In addition, a lower mortality rate ($p=0.04$) was seen in patients receiving amiodarone who converted to sinus rhythm, than in amiodarone-treated patients who remained in atrial fibrillation.

In the DIAMOND-CHF trial, among 391 patients who had atrial fibrillation at baseline, conversion to sinus rhythm was more frequent with dofetilide (12% at 1 month and 44% at 12 months) than with placebo (1% at 1 month and 13% at 12 months; $p<0.001$) [18]. In DIAMOND-AF, 148 (59%) of 249 dofetilide-treated patients converted to sinus rhythm, versus 86 (34%) of 257 placebo patients [19]. Maintenance of sinus rhythm with dofetilide over 1 year was 79%, compared to only 42% maintenance of sinus rhythm in placebo-treated patients ($p<0.001$). Even though dofetilide had no effect on all-cause mortality, conversion to sinus rhythm was associated with a significant reduction in mortality (risk ratio *RR* 0.44; $p<0.0001$). Treatment with dofetilide was also associated with a significantly lower risk ratio versus placebo for either all-cause (*RR* 0.70; $p\leq0.005$) or heart failure rehospitalization (*RR* 0.69; $p\leq0.02$).

In some patients with atrial fibrillation, restoration or maintenance of sinus rhythm fails and rate control of the ventricle along with oral anticoagulation is mandated. However, rate control may be difficult in patients with heart failure who cannot tolerate the negative inotropy of high doses of β-blockers or calcium channel blockers.

Role of Nonarrhythmic Pharmacologic Therapy

With the persistence of atrial fibrillation or progression of CHF, left atrial volume increases over time [20]. Such dilatation can alter stretch-activated channels and provoke stretch-induced arrhythmias [21, 22]. Dilatation can augment synthesis of angiotensin II, which is known to induce myocyte hypertrophy, increase L-type calcium current, and decrease I_{to}, resting membrane potential, and action potential amplitude and duration, resulting in increased afterdepolarizations [23]. Blockade of angiotensin II has protective effects by preventing shortening of the atrial effective refractory period during rapid atrial pacing [24]. In addition, atrial fibrillation is associated with a down-regulation of atrial angiotensin II type I and an up-regulation of type II proteins [25]. These basic facts have had added support from clinical trials suggesting that angiotensin-converting enzyme inhibitors (trandolapril in the TRACE study) [26] and angiotensin receptor blockers (irbesartan) [27] have a role in preventing atrial fibrillation. Whether the benefit of the above agents was secondary to an angiotensin-related mechanism or decreasing stretch-induced atrial fibrillation is not known.

Management of Atrial Fibrillation in CHF

Most patients deserve at least one attempt to convert and maintain sinus rhythm. Spontaneous conversion is likely with rate control measures in patients with recent-onset atrial fibrillation. Further treatment should be based on the likelihood of recurrences and the absence or presence of structural heart disease. In coronary artery disease, sotalol, dofetilide, and amiodarone, and in nonischemic cardiomyopathy, dofetilide and amiodarone are drugs of choice for the maintenance of sinus rhythm. All patients with left ventricular systolic dysfunction should also be treated with β-blockers and angiotensin-converting enzyme inhibitors. In patients with CHF, digoxin, diuretics, and spironolactone should be used when appropriate. In addition, patients with class III/IV CHF and intraventricular conduction disturbances should be considered for cardiac resynchronization therapy. Finally, proper rate control and antiembolic treatment are required in all patients.

References

1. Hynes BJ, Luck JC, Wolbrette DL et al (2003) Atrial fibrillation in patients with heart failure. Curr Opin Cardiol 18:32–38
2. Maisel WH, Stevenson LW (2003) Atrial fibrillation in heart failure: epidemiology, pathophysiology, and rationale for therapy. Am J Cardiol 91:2D–8D
3. Benjamin EJ, Wolf PA, D'Agostino RB et al (1998) Impact of atrial fibrillation on the risk of death: the Framingham Heart Study. Circulation 98: 946–952
4. Krahn AD, Manfreda J, Tate RB, Mathewson FA, Cuddy TE (1995) The natural history of atrial fibrillation: incidence, risk factors, and prognosis in the Manitoba follow-up study. Am J Med 98:476–484
5. Middlekauff HR, Stevenson WG, Stevenson LW (1991) Prognostic significance of atrial fibrillation in advanced heart failure: a study of 390 patients. Circulation 84:40–48
6. Carson PE, Johnson GR, Dunkman WB et al, for the V–HeFT VA Cooperative Studies Group (1993) The influence of atrial fibrillation on prognosis in mild to moderate heart failure. Circulation 87:VI102–V110.
7. Dries DL, Exner DV, Gersh BJ et al (1998) Atrial fibrillation is associated with an increased risk for mortality and heart failure progression in patients with asymptomatic left ventricular systolic dysfunction: a retrospective analysis of the SOLVD trials. J Am Coll Cardiol 32:695–703.
8. Stevenson WG, Stevenson LW, Middlekauff HR et al (1996) Improving survival for patients with atrial fibrillation and advanced heart failure. J Am Coll Cardiol 28:1458
9. Mahoney P, Kimmel S, DeNofrio D, Wahl P, Loh E (1999) Prognostic significance of atrial fibrillation in patients at a tertiary medical center referred for heart transplantation because of severe heart failure. Am J Cardiol 83:1544–1547
10. Mathew J, Hunsberger S, Fleg J et al, for the Digitalis Investigative Group (2000) Incidence, predictive factors, and prognostic significance of supraventricular tachyarrhythmias in congestive heart failure. Chest 118:914–922
11. Brignole M, Menozzi C, Giafranchi L et al (1998) Assessment of atrioventricular junction ablation and VVIR pacemaker versus pharmacologic treatment in patients with heart failure and chronic atrial fibrillation. Circulation 98:953–960
12. The Atrial Fibrillation Follow-Up Investigations of Rhythm Management (AFFIRM) Investigators (2002) A comparison of rate control and rhythm control in patients with atrial fibrillation. N Engl J Med 347:1825–1833
13. Roy D, for the AF–CHF Trial Investigators (2002) The Atrial Fibrillation and Congestive Heart Failure Trial (abstract). Europace 3:A–11
14. Roy D, Talajic M, Dorian P et al, for the Canadian Trial of Atrial Fibrillation Investigators (2000) Amiodarone to prevent recurrence of atrial fibrillation. N Engl J Med 342: 913–920
15. Naccarelli GV, Wolbrette DL, Khan M et al (2003) Old and new antiarrhythmic drugs for converting and maintaining sinus rhythm in atrial fibrillation: comparative efficacy and results of trials. Am J Cardiol 91:15D–26D
16. Fuster V, Rydén LE, Asinger RW, Cannom DS et al (2001) ACC/AHA/ESC guidelines for the management of patients with atrial fibrillation: executive summary: a report

of the American College of Cardiology/American Heart Association Task Force on Practice Guidelines and the European Society of Cardiology Committee for Practice Guidelines and Policy Conferences. (Committee to Develop Guidelines for the Management of Patients With Atrial Fibrillation). J Am Coll Cardiol 38:1231–1265
17. Deedwania PC, Singh BN, Ellenbogen K et al, for the Department of Veterans Affairs CHF-STAT Investigators (1998) Spontaneous conversion and maintenance of sinus rhythm by amiodarone in patients with heart failure and atrial fibrillation. Observation for the veterans affairs congestive heart failure survival trial of antiarrhythmic therapy (CHF-STAT). Circulation 98:2574–2579
18. Torp-Pederson C, Moller M, Bloch-Thomsen PE et al (1999) Dofetilide in patients with congestive heart failure and left ventricular dysfunction. Danish Investigations of Arrhythmia and Mortality on Dofetilide Study Group. N Engl J Med 341:857–865
19. Pederson OD, Bagger H, Keller N et al, for the Danish Investigations of Arrhythmia and Mortality ON Dofetilide Study Group (2001) Efficacy of dofetilide in the treatment of atrial fibrillation-flutter in patients with reduced left ventricular function: a Danish Investigations of Arrhythmia and Mortality ON Dofetilide (DIAMOND) substudy. Circulation 104:292–296
20. San Fillippo AJ, Abascol VM, Sheehan M et al (1990) Atrial enlargement as a consequence of atrial fibrillation: a prospective echocardiographic study. Circulation 82:792–797
21. Solti F, Vecsey T, Kékesi V, Juhász-Nagy A (1989) The effect of atrial dilatation on the genesis of atrial arrhythmias. Cardiovasc Res 23:882–886
22. Tomaselli GF, Marbán E (1999) Electrophysiological remodeling in hypertrophy and heart failure. Cardiovasc Res 42:270–283
23. Allessie MA, Boyden PA, Camm AJ et al (2001) Pathophysiology and prevention of atrial fibrillation. Circulation 103:769–777
24. Nakashima H, Kumagai K, Urata H et al (2000) Angiotensin II antagonist prevents electrical remodeling in atrial fibrillation. Circulation 101:2612–2617
25. Goette A, Arndt M, Rocken C et al (2000) Regulation of angiotensin II receptor subtypes during atrial fibrillation in humans. Circulation 101:2678–2681
26. Pederson OD, Bagger H, Kober L, Torp-Pedersen C (1999) Trandolapril reduces the incidence of atrial fibrillation after acute myocardial infarction in patients with left ventricular dysfunction. Circulation 100:376–380
27. Madrid AH, Bueno MG, Rebollo JMG et al (2002) Use of irbesartan to maintain sinus rhythm in patients with long-lasting persistent atrial fibrillation. A prospective and randomized study. Circulation 106:331–336

Atrial Fibrillation After Cardiac Surgery: What's All the Fuss About?

D.G. Wyse

Introduction

The topic of atrial fibrillation after recent cardiac surgery has been one of intense interest for at least the past decade. Entire books have been written on this subject [1]. The reasons behind such intense interest are not entirely clear. However, the major driving factor seems to be the demonstrated relationship between post-operative atrial fibrillation and length of stay in hospital after surgery. Particularly in North America, there is a tremendous financial incentive to shorten the length of stay in hospital after cardiac surgery. The "current wisdom" is that if atrial fibrillation can be prevented, the average length of stay in hospital after cardiac surgery will be shortened. In the opinion of this author, the "current wisdom" is extremely naïve, unlikely to be correct and a more pragmatic approach would be preferable in the quest to shorten length of stay after cardiac surgery. The reasons for this opinion will be outlined below.

Factors Associated With Post-operative AF

The peak incidence of atrial fibrillation after cardiac surgery is on the second post-operative day, with the vast majority of cases beginning between day 1 and day 4 after surgery. There are a large number of factors statistically related to the likelihood of developing post-operative atrial fibrillation [2] and some of these are presented in Table 1. However, it is not exactly clear why some patients get atrial fibrillation after their surgery. Although many of the same factors that are associated with atrial fibrillation in other settings are also associated with atrial fibrillation after cardiac surgery, it is generally felt by experts that additional factors come into play in this particular circumstance. In the classification of atrial fibrillation in the recent ACC/AHA/ESC treatment

Division of Cardiology, Department of Cardiac Sciences, University of Calgary/Calgary Health Region, Alberta, Canada

Table 1. Some factors associated with development of atrial fibrillation post-operatively

Factors	
Prior atrial fibrillation	Pre-operative chronic obstructive pulmonary disease
Male gender	Cardiomegaly on chest x-ray
Prolonged P-wave on electrocardiogram	Decreased LVEF
Pre-operative treatment with beta-blocker	Elevated LVEDP
Pre-operative congestive heart failure	Intra-operative factors*
Pre-operative hypertension	Post-operative factors*
Older age	And so on

*Many of these
LVEDP, left ventricular end-diastolic pressure; *LVEF*, left ventricular ejection fraction

guidelines post-operative atrial fibrillation is separated from other situations in which this common tachyarrhythmia occurs [3]. One potentially important and relatively unique factor in the etiology of atrial fibrillation after cardiac surgery is post-operative inflammation, particularly when it involves the pericardium. Indeed, there is clear evidence that C-reactive protein, a well-recognized marker for inflammation, rises after heart surgery, peaking on the second post-operative day [4], coincident with the peak incidence of post-operative atrial fibrillation. There is a strong correlation between increased C-reactive protein with the occurrence of post-operative atrial fibrillation with an r^2-value of over 0.4 ($r = 0.64$, $p = 0.0037$) [4], indicating that over 40% of post-operative atrial fibrillation is explained by this one factor. Although the cause of atrial fibrillation is multi-factorial in this setting, such a prominent role for inflammation is relatively unique, although it is important in other clinical settings of inflammation of the heart and pericardium.

A number of associations have been made between post-operative atrial fibrillation and clinical morbidity. Patients that have post-operative atrial fibrillation are more likely to have a stroke, congestive heart failure, myocardial infarction, ventricular tachyarrhythmia, receive a pacemaker and die [1]. Finally, the average length of stay in the hospital is 3 to 4 days longer for patients that have post-operative atrial fibrillation [1]. The problem that has arisen has to do with the assimilation of this information and Figure 1 illustrates three possible scenarios. Panel A is the simplest conceptual formulation. In it, a factor ("X") causes atrial fibrillation, which in turn leads to morbidity and increased length of stay. In this simple scheme, eliminating the atrial fib-

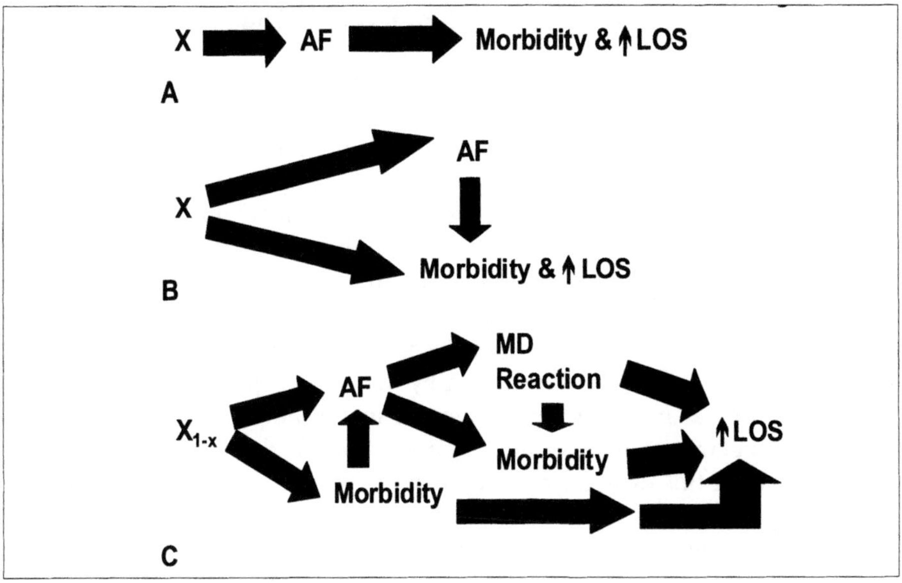

Fig. 1. Three different schema depicting potential relationships between post-operative atrial fibrillation (*AF*) and length of stay (*LOS*) in hospital are shown. "X" indicates causative factors for atrial fibrillation. The complexity of the relationships increases in panels A through C

rillation would have a major impact on morbidity and length of stay. Panel B is slightly more complex. In this scheme, "X" causes both atrial fibrillation and directly contributes to morbidity and increased length of stay. Of course, atrial fibrillation itself then contributes to the morbidity and increased length of stay. In the latter scheme, eliminating atrial fibrillation still has an important, albeit somewhat lessened, effect on morbidity and length of stay. Finally, panel C adds several more levels of complexity, including the possibility that there are many causes of atrial fibrillation and morbidity; that morbidity can itself then cause atrial fibrillation; and finally that how a physician reacts to the development of morbidity and atrial fibrillation can contribute to the increase length of stay in hospital. It is quite likely that the last situation is much closer to the truth than either of the other two. Finally, it must be emphasized that a statistical association is simply two factors somehow related to one another and does not establish cause and effect. It is particularly important to recognize that even in a multivariate model that no adjustment can be made for factors that have not been measured. In fact, a recently unpublished report from the University of Toronto found that atrial fibrillation was one of 18 factors that seem to independently predict an increased length of stay in hospital after cardiac surgery. Undoubtedly the more things we measure, the more associations we will find and the less likely we will have a better understanding of how to explain this complex set of interrelationships.

Review of Therapies Tested in Randomized Clinical Trials

With this background it is instructive to review the therapies that have been tested and their impact on length of stay in hospital after cardiac surgery. Fortunately, these have been reviewed recently and extensively in a meta-analysis [5]. The therapy that has been most intensively investigated has been the use of beta-blockers. The use of these agents is partly related to the observation that discontinuation of beta-blocker therapy at the time of cardiac surgery (once a common practice) was noted to be associated with and increased the likelihood of post-operative atrial fibrillation (Table 1). The sum of the evidence is that beta-blocker therapy (excluding sotalol) reduces the risk of post-operative atrial fibrillation by over 60% [5]. It might be reasoned that the additional antiarrhythmic action of sotalol would increase the efficacy of this particular beta-blocker but the meta-analysis data suggest the magnitude of effect of this drug is approximately the same as that of the other beta-blockers [5]. There has been a lot of interest in the use of amiodarone for the prophylaxis of post-operative atrial fibrillation but this potent antiarrhythmic drug appears to be no more effective than beta-blockers [5]. The other therapy that has been evaluated in randomized clinical trials is atrial pacing, either left, right or bi-atrial pacing. These pacing therapies have shown relative risk reductions from about 30 to 60% [5]. A wide variety of other therapies, including magnesium, anti-inflammatory agents and anti-oxidants have been incompletely evaluated. Needless to say, this multi-factorial problem is unlikely to respond to any single therapy and several of the therapies tested so far have shown remarkable efficacy.

Effect of Therapies on Length of Stay

It is even more interesting to examine the effect of therapies with demonstrated efficacy for preventing post-operative atrial fibrillation on the average length of stay in hospital after cardiac surgery. Such an analysis shows that therapies that reduce the risk of post-operative atrial fibrillation by more than 60% (beta-blockers, sotalol, amiodarone) reduce the average length of stay by less than one day and in some cases the difference is not statistically significant (beta-blockers, sotalol) [5]. Indeed, the therapy associated with the greatest reduction in length of stay (bi-atrial pacing) is the one that has been studied the least. These findings suggest that there are other important factors that come into play in the determination of length of stay after cardiac surgery. Furthermore, it is unlikely that prevention of atrial fibrillation in itself will lead to a reduction in length of stay. In the opinion of this writer, concomitant illness and physician reaction to atrial fibrillation are the major reasons for the increased length of stay after cardiac surgery in those who develop post-operative atrial fibrillation.

Synthesis of the Current State of Knowledge

A review of the information about atrial fibrillation after cardiac surgery suggests a number of conclusions. The first is that post-operative atrial fibrillation has a multi-factorial etiology and, therefore, no one therapy is likely to be completely effective. Furthermore, observational studies suggest that in the vast majority of patients this is a self-limited problem that disappears within 2 weeks [6]. Atrial fibrillation after cardiac surgery is associated with a number of problems but it is entirely unclear what is the "cause" and what is the "effect". Another therapeutic approach seems more appropriate at this time, particularly with recent evidence showing that attempts to restore and maintain sinus rhythm in other settings have no impact on morbid events [7-9].

A Pragmatic Approach

A simpler approach is outlined in Figure 2 and is based on that taken in a previous observational study [6]. That rather small study showed that most (90%) of the patients treated with simple rate control were in sinus rhythm within two weeks after discharge [6]. The main limitations of this small observational study are that the patients were all hemodynamically stable and the only treatment for thromboembolism prophylaxis was aspirin. There was only one stroke but the number of patients studied was small [6]. The scheme in Figure 2 simply divides patients with atrial fibrillation after cardiac surgery into those who are hemodynamically stable and those who are not. For the hemodynamically unstable patient, immediate cardioversion followed by amiodarone treatment for 6 to 8 weeks is recommended. When stroke risk factors are present, subcutaneous low molecular weight heparin and warfarin are administered as soon as it is deemed safe to do so. The patient is discharged as soon as they are medically fit. The low molecular weight heparin is discontinued as soon as the INR (International Normalized Ratio) is therapeutic. The warfarin must be continued for 4 weeks after stopping the amiodarone and the patient must be assessed for recurrence of atrial fibrillation at that point and again 3 to 6 months after stopping the amiodarone. When atrial fibrillation returns, long-term treatment is determined according to the guidelines for recurrent atrial fibrillation [3].

A simpler treatment is undertaken in those that are hemodynamically stable (Figure 2). That is, if the patient is not on a beta-blocker and without a contraindication for beta-blockers, one is started. This treatment is augmented (or substituted for) with intravenous digoxin and/or a calcium channel-blocker to achieve a resting heart rate less than 100 beats per minute. Again, low molecular weight heparin and warfarin are used when there are stroke risk factors and the patient is discharged when heart rate control is achieved. In this case, the patient is assessed again in 2 weeks and if the atrial fibrillation has resolved, the warfarin is discontinued 4 weeks after documentation of the

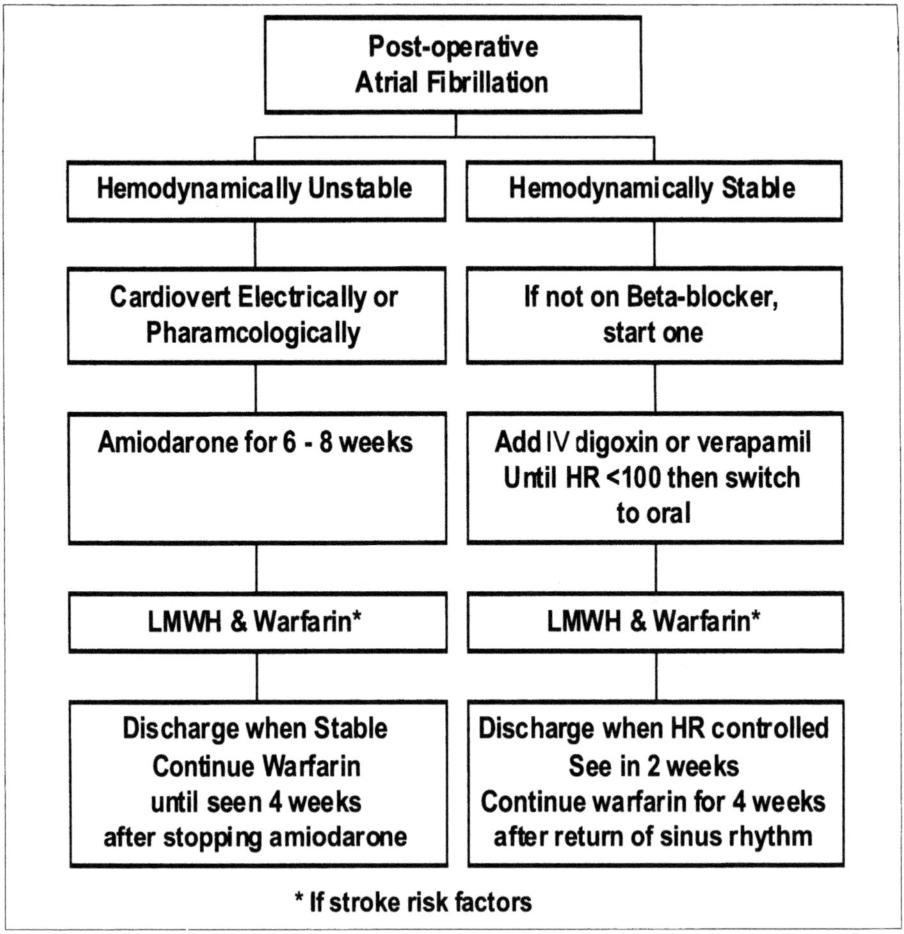

Fig. 2. A simple scheme to expeditiously deal with atrial fibrillation after cardiac surgery is depicted. *HR*, heart rate; *LMWH*, low molecular weight heparin; *IV*, intravenous

return of sinus rhythm. Long-term treatment of persistent atrial fibrillation is according to the guidelines and whether this is the first episode of atrial fibrillation or a recurrence [3].

References

1. Atrial Fibrillation After Cardiac Surgery, (2000), Ed. J. Steinberg, Kluwer Academic Publishers, Norwell, MA, USA, 02061
2. Aranki SF, Shaw DP, Adams DH et al (1996) Predictors of atrial fibrillation after coronary artery surgery. Current trends and impact on hospital resources. Circulation 94:390-397
3. Fuster V, Ryden LE, Asinger RW et al (2001) ACC/AHA/ESC guidelines for the mana-

gement of patients with atrial fibrillation: executive summary: a report of the American College of Cardiology/American Heart Association Task Force on Practice Guidelines and the European Society of Cardiology Committee for Practice Guidelines and Policy Conferences (Committee to Develop Guidelines for the Management of Patients with Atrial Fibrillation). Circulation 104:2118-2150
4. Bruins P, te Velthuis H, Yazdanbakhsh AP et al (1997) Activation of the complement system during and after cardiopulmonary bypass surgery: postsurgery activation involves C-reactive protein and is associated with post-operative arrhythmia. Circulation 96:3542-3548
5. Crystal E, Connolly SJ, Sleik K, Ginger TJ, Yusuf S (2002) Interventions on prevention of post-operative atrial fibrillation in patients undergoing heart surgery: a meta-analysis. Circulation 106:75-80
6. Myers MG, Alnemri K (1998) Rate control therapy for atrial fibrillation following coronary artery bypass surgery. Can J Cardiol 14:1363-1366
7. Hohnloser SH, Kuck KH, Lilienthal J (2000) Rhythm or rate control in atrial fibrillation – Pharmacological Intervention in Atrial Fibrillation (PIAF): a randomized trial. Lancet 356:1789-1794
8. The AFFIRM Investigators (2002) A comparison of rate control and rhythm control in patients with a trial fibrillation. New Engl J Med 347:1825-1833
9. van Gelder IC, Hagens VE, Bosker HA et al (2002) A comparison of rate control and rhythm control in patients with recurrent persistent atrial fibrillation. New Engl J Med 347:1834-1840

"Pill in the Pocket": How Effective and Safe Is this Strategy for Treatment of Recurrences of Atrial Fibrillation?

A. Capucci, G.Q. Villani, G. Rusticali, M.F. Piepoli

Introduction

Atrial fibrillation (AF) is a very common type of arrhythmia, which is considered to be the most frequent arrhythmia leading to hospital admission [1]. Several substrates underlie this arrhythmia, and different mechanisms are involved in its onset: it is a clinical challenge because there are several diagnostic and therapeutic options, making it a money- and time-consuming entity.

In the era of rationalization of healthcare costs, a strategy of outpatient management of patients with recurrent AF should be considered. This option requires a careful selection of low-risk patients who can be trained in recognition of the symptoms of AF and in administration of the therapy following confirmation that this therapy is safe. No pharmacological strategies have proved effective in reducing the frequency of readmissions to hospital.

In most cases AF is considered a benign clinical entity, so that in the choice of a "home-care" strategy safety is the first issue that clinicians and practitioners should consider.

The clinical experience recorded so far with different pharmacological strategies is reviewed below.

Oral Antiarrhythmic Therapy in AF

At present several pharmacological options are available for outpatient treatment of AF paroxysms.

Quinidine

This agent has long been considered the treatment of choice in AF, with success rates ranging from 30% to 90% in different series (mean 70%) and a mean

Cardiology Department, "Guglielmo da Saliceto" General Hospital, Piacenza, Italy time to recovery of sinus rhythm of 6 h [2, 3]. Because of its capability to facilitate conduction through the A-V node, quinidine needs to be given in association with agents that slow A-V conduction (typically digoxin). Use of this class IA agent is limited by the relatively high incidence of side effects: gastrointestinal disturbances may occur in up to 40% of cases, while a pro-arrhythmic effect has been demonstrated in about 4% of patients, with major arrhythmias occurring up to 48 h after the recovery of sinus rhythm [4]. These side effects limit the use of quinidine in a protected, hospital setting.

Flecainide

Several studies have demonstrated the efficacy of this class IC agent to restore sinus rhythm when administered intravenously, with success rates ranging from 60% to 90% [5–9] (Table 1).

The favorable pharmacological profile of the drug, with a good oral absorption, suggests that flecainide may be considered for oral outpatient therapy.

In a population of 37 consecutive patients with paroxysmal AF our group has shown the higher efficacy of a single oral loading dose of 200 mg of flecainide in restoring sinus rhythm (95%) than of placebo (21%); none of our patients experienced adverse effects [10]. We have demonstrated that flecainide (300 mg) is more effective than amiodarone (1,800 mg/day) in restor-

Table 1. Efficacy of flecainide

Reference	Type of study	No. of patients	Dose	Efficacy (%-time)	Adverse events
[5]	Double blind, controlled	102	2 mg/kg	57-1 h, 67-6 h	Hypotension (11); TdP (1)
[6]	Comparative	90	2 mg/kg	96	Hypotension (2); A-V block (4)
[7]	Comparative, controlled, cross-over	80	1.5 mg/kg in 15 min	92	Hypotension (2); A-V block (1)
[8]	Comparative, prospective	30	2 mg/kg in 10 min	80	Hypotension (2); A-V block (2)
[9]	Comparative, double blind, controlled	98	2 mg/kg	59-2 h	Hypotension (8); A-V block (1)

TdP, Torsade de pointe

ing sinus rhythm in a population of 60 patients with paroxysmal AF, with success rates of 91% for flecainide, 37% for amiodarone, and 48% for placebo. No side effects were reported in any of these three study groups [11].

In a comparative, controlled study on 243 patients with AF, Botto et al. [12] demonstrated that a single, 300-mg oral dose of flecainide restored sinus rhythm in 59% of cases within 4 h after drug administration. In the same study transient atrial flutter with A-V conduction ≥2:1 before restoration of sinus rhythm was observed in 9% of patients.

When considering oral flecainide for the treatment of paroxysms of AF the possibility of synchronized, rapid arrhythmias, such as 1:1 atrial flutter, must be underlined; a period of monitoring until sinus rhythm is achieved should be the rule. In addition, sympathetic activation may reduce the antiarrhythmic effect of the drug [13–15].

Propafenone

This class IC antiarrhythmic has been shown to be effective in the treatment of AF when administered intravenously (2 mg/kg), with success rates ranging from 43% to 81% (mean 60%) [16, 17]. Recent studies have evaluated the possibility of oral administration of a loading dose of propafenone in the treatment of acute episodes of AF. We compared oral propafenone (600 mg, followed by 300 mg after 8 h if necessary) with quinidine (1,350 mg in 24 h) associated with digoxin (1,125 mg in 24 h) for the restoration of sinus rhythm checked 12 h after therapy. The mean time to restoration of sinus rhythm was 267 ± 238 min for propafenone and 648 ± 631 min for the combination of quinidine+digoxin; 1 patient in the propafenone group experienced a syncope, which was attributed to ortostatic hypotension secondary to the occurrence of 1:1 atrial flutter [18]

The efficacy of oral propafenone (300 mg) or flecainide (300 mg) was compared with that of placebo in the treatment of recent AF [19]. The study population was made up of 181 patients: after 3 h, sinus rhythm was restored in 51% of patients treated with propafenone and in 59% of those treated with flecainide; 6 h after drug administration sinus rhythm was present in 72% of the propafenone group and 78% of the flecainide group. The mean time to restoration of sinus rhythm was 158 ± 109 min for flecainide and 165 ± 119 min for propafenone. Atrial flutter with 1:1 A-V conduction was observed in 2 flecainide-treated patients, and atrial flutter with 2:1 A-V conduction in 6 patients altogether (2 treated with flecainide, 4 in the propafenone group) [16].

Safety of the oral loading dose of propafenone (600 + 300 mg 8 h apart) was evaluated and compared with the safety of the loading doses of the associations digitalis+quinidine and propafenone+quinidine in 246 patients in the "Safety Antiarrhythmic Therapy Evaluation – SATE" study [19]. The results of this study showed that propafenone restored sinus rhythm within a mean of 4 ± 4 h; quinidine+digitalis, in 5.4 ± 4.5 h; and propafenone+digitalis, in 5 ± 8.6 h. All patients rested in bed for the entire observation period, and all possible sympathetic stimuli were avoided. Pro-arrhythmic effects of the study drugs and associations are summarized in Table 2.

In low-risk patients, i.e., those without myocardial or coronary disease, who had experienced recent AF, oral propafenone associated with absolute bedrest seems to be a safe and effective way of restoring sinus rhythm.

Table 2. Pro-arrhythmic effects of the study drugs and drug combination in the SATE study [19]

	Quinidine-digoxin	Propafenone-digoxin	Propafenone	Placebo
NSVT	1	4	0	0
2:1 AFl	9	13	12	3
1:1 AFl	0	0	0	0
BBB	2	2	3	0
SAB	2	0	2	0

NSVT, nonsustained ventricular tachycardia; *AFl*, atrial flutter; *BBB*, bundle branch block; *SAB*, sinus atrial block

Soltalol

The efficacy and safety of oral sotalol (160-mg loading dose and 320 mg daily as maintenance) were evaluated in patients with AF of recent onset and compared with those of quinidine [20]. Sotalol was effective in restoring sinus rhythm in 20% of patients after 1 week of treatment, and quinidine, in 60% of cases treated. No major side effects were observed in the sotalol group, while 4 episodes of ventricular tachycardia, 2 of which degenerated into ventricular fibrillation, occurred after the restoration of sinus rhythm with quinidine, confirming an unsatisfactory safety profile of the latter drug.

Clinical Experience of Outpatient Treatment of AF

Few data are available on clinical experience of outpatient treatment of patients with supraventricular arrhythmias instituted with the aim of minimizing the need for emergency hospital admission during recurrences of tachycardia.

Alboni et al. [21] tested the efficacy of two drug treatments, flecainide and the combination of diltiazem and propranolol, vs placebo, each administered as a single oral dose for termination of the arrhythmic episodes, as first-line treatments in patients with infrequent and well-tolerated episodes of paroxysmal supraventricular tachycardia. First they evaluated the efficacy of different treatments during electrophysiological studies, administering the drugs in a random order after the induction of arrhythmia. Conversion to sinus rhythm occurred within 2 h in 52%, 61%, and 94% of patients receiving placebo, flecainide, and diltiazem/propanolol (D/P), respectively ($P<0.001$). Four patients (1 receiving placebo, 1 D/P, and 2 flecainide) had hypotension and 4 (3 treated with D/P, and 1 with flecainide) a sinus rate of <50 beats/min following interruption of the arrhythmia. Patients were discharged home with a single oral dose of the drug treatment (flecainide or D/P) found at the time of acute testing to be most effective. Twenty-six patients were discharged with D/P, and 5 with flecainide. During 17 ± 12 months of follow-up, the treatment was successful in 81% of D/P patients and in 80% of flecainide patients, as all the arrhythmic episodes were interrupted within 2 h without admission to hospital. In the remaining patients, a failure occurred during one or more episodes because of drug ineffectiveness or drug unavailability. One patient had syncope after D/P ingestion. During follow-up, the percentage of patients calling for emergency assistance was significantly lower than in the year before enrolment (9% vs 100%, $P< 0.0001$).

Villani et al. [22] also evaluated the reproducibility of the oral loading dose of propafenone in restoring sinus rhythm in patients with frequent episodes of persistent AF. In a population of 62 patients treated in hospital, a reproducible efficacy (93%) of antiarrhythmic treatment was observed, without significant adverse events. We have concluded that this therapeutic approach may be suggested for selected patients with demonstrated reproducibility of this antiarrhythmic therapy who were able to recognize the AF recurrences correctly and to manage the therapy themselves (i.e., dietary intake, bedrest).

Conclusions

On the basis of the available results, the pill-in-the-pocket" strategy appears to be of questionable practicability in daily clinical routine, because of the lack of safety data in large cohorts of patients. Furthermore, the selection criteria for patients to receive outpatient drug treatment are not clearly established: the major open issues that should be addressed as priorities are the clinical reproducibility and the electrophysiological evaluation. A trial supported by the Associazione Italiana Cardiostimolazione is currently ongoing, and its results will contribute the clarification of the real impact of this therapeutic strategy in AF therapy.

References

1. Furberg CD, Bruco MP, Manclio TA et al, for the CHS Collaborative Research Group (1994) Prevalence of atrial fibrillation in elderly subjects (the Cardiovascular Health Study). Am J Cardiol 74:236–241
2. Borgeat A, Goy JJ, Maendly R et al (1986) Flecainide versus quinidine for conversion

of AF to sinus rhythm. Am J Cardiol 58:496–501

3. Negrini M, Gibelli G, De Ponti C (1990) Confronto fra amiodarone e chinidina nella conversione a ritmo sinusale della fibrillazione atriale di recente insorgenza. G Ital Cardiol 20:207–213
4. Roden DM, Woosley RL, Primm RK (1986) Incidence and clinical features of the quinidine-associated long QT syndrome: implications for patient care. Am Heart J 111:1088–1093
5. Donovan KD, Dobb GJ, Cooms LJ et al (1992) Efficacy of flecainide for the reversion of acute onset AF. Am J Cardiol 70:50A–55A
6. Kingma JH, Suttorp MJ (1992) Acute pharmacologic conversion of AF and flutter: the role of flecainide, propafenone and verapamil. Am J Cardiol 70:56A–61A
7. Madrid AH, Moro C, Marin-Huerta E (1993) Comparison of flecainide and procamide in cardioversion of AF. Eur Heart J 14:1127–1131
8. Barranco F, Sanchez M, Rodriguez J et al (1994) Efficacy of flecainide in patients with supraventricular arrhythmias and respiratory insufficency. Int Care Med 20:42–44
9. Donovan HD, Power BM, Hockings BE et al (1995) Intravenous flecainide versus amiodarone for recent onset AF. Am J Cardiol 75:693–697
10. Villani GQ, Rosi A, Piepoli M et al (1990) Efficacia del trattamento orale con flecainide nella fibrillazione atriale parossistica: correlazione con le concentrazioni plasmatiche. G Ital Cardiol 20:564–568
11. Capucci A, Lenzi T, Boriani G et al (1992) Effectiveness of loading oral flecainide for converting recent onset AF to sinus rhythm in patients without organic heart disease or with only systemic hypertension. Am J Cardiol 70:69–72
12. Botto GL, Bonini W, Broffoni G et al (1994) Regular ventricular rhythms before conversion of recent onset AF to sinus rhythm. Pacing Clin Electrophysiol 17:2114–2117
13. Sihm J, Hansen FA, Rasmussen J et al (1990) Flecainide acetate in atrial flutter and fibrillation. The arrhythmogenic effects. Eur Heart J 11:145–148
14. Ahsan A, Aldridge R, Bowes R (1993) 1:1 Atrioventricular conduction in atrial flutter with digoxin and flecainide. Int J Cardiol 39:88-90
15. Helmy I, Scheinman NM, Herre JM et al (1990) Electrophysiologic effects of isoproterenol in patients with reentrant atrioventricular tachycardia treated with flecainide. J Am Coll Cardiol 16:1649–1655
16. Suttorp MJ, Kingma HJ, Jessurun ER et al (1990) The value of class 1C antiarrhythmic drugs for acute conversion of paroxysmal AF or flutter to sinus rhythm. J Am Coll Cardiol 16:1722–1730
17. Capucci A, Boriani G, Rubino I et al (1994) A controlled study on oral propafenone versus digoxin plus quinidine in converting recent onset AF to sinus rhythm. Int J Cardiol 43:305–313
18. Capucci A, Boriani G, Botto GL et al (1994) Conversion of recent-onset AF by a single oral loading dose of propafenone and flecainide. Am J Cardiol 74:503–505
19. Capucci A, Villani GQ, on behalf of SATE Investigators (1995) Propafenone oral loading dose plus digitalis in converting AF to sinus rhythm: a placebo-controlled multicenter study (abstract). Eur Heart J 92:I-775
20. Hohnloser SH, van de Loo A, Baedeker F (1995) Efficacy and proarrhythmic hazards of pharmacologic cardioversion of AF: prospective comparison of sotalol versus quinidine. J Am Coll Cardiol 995:852–858
21. Alboni P, Tomasi C, Menozzi C et al (2001) Efficacy and safety of out-of-hospital self-administered single oral drug treatment in the management of infrequent well-tolerated paroxysmal supraventricular tachycadia. J Am Coll Cardiol 37:548–553
22. Villani GQ, Marrazzo N, Rosi A et al (2001) Loading oral propafenone in paroxysmal AF: reproducibility and speed of effect (abstract). Eur Heart J 22 [Suppl]:327

Cardioversion of Recent Onset Atrial Fibrillation: Which Drug to Prefer in the Individual Patient?

P.E. Vardas, E.M. Kanoupakis

The management of atrial fibrillation (AF) still represents one of the therapeutic challenges of modern cardiology. This arrhythmia is extremely common, particularly in elderly persons and in patients with organic heart disease, and carries the risk of embolic complications, especially cerebrovascular accidents [1, 2].

Notwithstanding the controversy relating to the publication of recent studies which compare the strategies of rate control versus rhythm control [3, 4], there is a concept supporting the prompt restoration and maintenance of sinus rhythm whenever possible. Experimental studies [5, 6] suggest that remodeling of the atria during AF can lead to persistent electrical and structural changes that may develop within a relatively short period. This finding suggests that cardioversion should be performed as early as possible after the onset of the arrhythmia. Prompt treatment may result in a higher success rate in restoring sinus rhythm and may prevent recurrences of AF. Several potential benefits of this strategy include relief of symptoms, prevention of tachycardia-induced dysfunction, improved exercise capacity and quality of life, and a possible reduction in embolic risk and improved survival.

The main steps for the acute treatment of AF include rate control, termination of AF, and maintenance of sinus rhythm and anti-embolic therapy. Digitalization is often used to control the ventricular response. Although safe, it often takes hours and is less useful when there is an acute need to slow the ventricular response quickly. Intravenous β-blocking agents or calcium antagonists are faster and more effective than digitalis for controlling the ventricular rate [7, 8]. Combination therapy is often required [9].

Most reversions after the administration of atrioventricular (AV) nodal-blocking agents result from spontaneous conversion. Spontaneous and placebo conversion rates are as high as 50%–70% over the first 24 h after presentation with symptoms [10, 11]. Patients with recent-onset AF of less than 24–48 h duration have the highest spontaneous reversion rates. Thus, rate control with

Department of Cardiology, Heraklion University Hospital, Heraklion, Crete, Greece spontaneous conversion to sinus rhythm may represent the most cost-effective approach to patients who present with recent-onset AF [12].

Patients who do not revert spontaneously within a short period are good candidates for cardioversion. Cardioversion may be achieved by either pharmacologic or electrical means. The success rate of electrical cardioversion varies between 70% and 90% [13]. Immediate electrical cardioversion is indicated in patients with AF and a rapid ventricular response who have evidence of acute myocardial ischemia or symptomatic hypotension, angina, or heart failure that do not respond promptly to pharmacologic measures [13]. Otherwise, pharmacologic cardioversion may be attempted, thus avoiding the inconvenience of general anesthesia. For this purpose, class I and class III antiarrhythmic drugs have been studied.

Quinidine, an alkaloid derived from cinchona bark, was first used in Europe in 1918 to terminate recent-onset AF. Today, quinidine is less often used for this indication because its safety has been questioned after reported cases of sudden death. However, other class IA antiarrhythmic drugs have been tested. The results of a study in our department suggest that intravenous procainamide (1 g over 30 min, followed by an infusion of 2 mg/min over 1 h) is an effective and safe means for the rapid termination of AF of recent onset and that its success rate is inversely related to the size of the left atrium. However, the drug is ineffective in the conversion of AF lasting more than 48 h [14].

More recently, class Ic drugs, oral flecainide or propafenone, have been used in recent-onset AF to restore sinus rhythm [15]. Success rates as high as 91% were recently reported with a single oral dose of 300 mg flecainide [16]. This was significantly higher than the success rates with the placebo (48%) during an observation period of 8 h. In other reports the success rates with flecainide ranged between 67% and 95%. Studies with oral propafenone (600 mg as a single dose) showed success rates as high as 81% at 12 h, which was significantly better than the placebo (33%) or the combination of oral quinidine and intravenous digoxin (50%) [17, 18].

In a comparison of intravenous propafenone (2 mg/kg) and intravenous flecainide over a 10-min period in patients with AF of less than 6 months' duration, Suttorp et al. [19] reported better results (90%) with flecainide than with propafenone (55%). Pharmacologic conversion with sodium channel blockers carries the risk of converting AF to atrial flutter and ventricular proarrhythmia because the slowing of atrial rate may allow 1:1 propagation through the AV node. This phenomenon may be facilitated by the anticholinergic action of certain sodium channel blockers such as quinidine and disopyramide.

Among the class III agents, amiodarone was the first to be used. Its reported efficacy in converting AF is heterogeneous, and it has multiple extracardiac side effects. Its relatively good tolerance in the setting of heart failure and ischemic heart disease contributes to the popularity of this drug.

Intravenous amiodarone 5 mg/kg over a 10- to 30-min period followed by the infusion of 500 mg over a 24-h period has been reported to be associated with a high success rate [20]. This treatment is generally used for patients with AF and acute myocardial infarction or with left ventricular dysfunction in whom class Ic drugs are contraindicated.

In a prospective, randomized, controlled study, we aimed to assess the effectiveness and safety of amiodarone as a first-choice drug in the treatment of patients with recent onset AF [21]. The results of our own study were more encouraging than any previously reported [22–27]. According to our findings, patients with AF lasting less than 24 h had a high probability of conversion (>95%) with amiodarone, regardless of left atrium size.

Our good results are probably due to the fact that in this study amiodarone was used as the first-choice drug. The high serum levels of amiodarone and desethylamiodarone–higher than the levels reported by other studies–which we achieved after the first 24 h of treatment are also likely to have been a significant factor. In contrast, the duration of treatment does not appear to play a significant role in the cardioversion of recent-onset AF, since all our patients in this category who converted did so within the first 24 h.

However, in a placebo-controlled study in our department intravenous propafenone (2 mg/kg over 15 min followed by 10 mg/kg over the next 24 h) and intravenous amiodarone (300 mg intravenously over 1 h, followed by 20 mg/kg over the next 24 h, plus 1800 mg/day orally, in three divided doses) were compared in the management of AF of recent onset [28]. Conversion to normal sinus rhythm occurred in 36 of 46 patients (78.2%) receiving propafenone, in 40 of 48 patients (83.3%) receiving amiodarone, and in 27 of the 49 (55.10%) controls ($p<0.02$ drug vs placebo, NS between drugs). The mean time to conversion was 2±3 h for propafenone, 7±5 h for amiodarone, and 13±9 h for placebo ($p< 0.05$). Patients who converted had smaller atria than those who did not (diameter: 42.7±5 vs 47.2±7 mm, $p<0.001$ for all). Both drugs were equally effective and safe for the rapid conversion of recent-onset AF to sinus rhythm. However, propafenone offered the advantage of more rapid conversion than amiodarone.

The main findings of a very recent meta-analysis [29] confirm our results, demonstrating that amiodarone facilitates conversion of recent-onset AF to sinus rhythm (with a 44% superiority in efficacy compared with placebo), but with a delay of 8–24 h until the onset of antiarrhythmic activity. This efficacy is comparable to that of class Ic agents at 24 h after drug administration, although class Ic drugs showed a more rapid onset of action, with some effect already apparent at 1–2 h after administration.

Even if cardioversion may be delayed compared with class Ic drugs, amiodarone has the advantage of promptly slowing a rapid ventricular rate [30]. This may be due to predominant β-adrenergic and calcium channel blockade observed early after intravenous amiodarone injection, the class III effect being least identifiable at this stage [31].

No serious side effects were reported with amiodarone. Class Ic drugs have the potential of inducing atrial flutter with 1:1 AV conduction, but this occurred only exceptionally (in three patients on flecainide). Thus, both amiodarone and class Ic drugs seem to be safe in the population studied. However, there is evidence that class I drugs may increase mortality in a subset of patients who may benefit most from cardioversion, i.e., those with severe underlying myocardial dysfunction or ischemic heart disease [32]. Amiodarone should also be used with caution in these patients, as profound hypotension may be induced by intravenous or high-dose oral loading [33]. The incidence of extracardiac side effects due to short-term administration of amiodarone is not well defined. However, most of the toxicity of the drug seems to be dose-dependent and related to chronic treatment [34].

The issue of dosage and route of administration is difficult to assess, as protocols varied widely between studies. It seems, furthermore, that intravenous and oral amiodarone do not have the same electrophysiologic effects, possibly owing to cumulative effects and/or active metabolites [35]. With the appearance of AF in patients under chronic treatment with oral amiodarone the clinician is faced with the choice of the appropriate method of cardioversion. Since intravenous amiodarone exhibits different electrophysiologic properties than when the drug is taken orally over a long period, we performed a study, first, to assess the efficacy and safety of intravenous amiodarone administered to patients with recent-onset AF who were receiving long-term amiodarone therapy and, second, to investigate the electrophysiologic effects of such a combined therapy [36].

Within the 24 h of infusion 87% of patients receiving intravenous amiodarone and 59% receiving placebo ($p<0.05$) had converted to normal sinus rhythm. The median time to arrhythmia termination after the initiation of infusion was 11 h for amiodarone and 22 h for the placebo. No serious side effects of the intravenous administration were observed. This high conversion rate could be explained by the additional electrophysiologic effects of intravenous loading with amiodarone that we observed in patients under chronic oral treatment with that drug. Prolongation of refractoriness was seen in all patients who underwent electrophysiologic study after intravenous loading, without any effect on repolarization, AV conduction, or sinus node function.

An alternative to amiodarone and class Ic drugs is ibutilide, a novel antiarrhythmic agent that prolongs action potential duration by enhancing sodium exchange during phase 2 of the action potential. It has efficacy in terminating recent-onset AF and atrial flutter, making this a potentially useful drug in the emergency room setting [37]. However, there was an 8.3% incidence of polymorphic ventricular tachycardia, which sometimes required electrical cardioversion.

Dofetilide is another new class III antiarrhythmic agent that is effective in cardioverting AF [38]. It prolongs action potential duration almost twice as much in the atria as in the ventricles. In a randomized trial comparing intravenous dofetilide with amiodarone and placebo in patients with AF of up to 2 months' duration, dofetilide achieved a higher cardioversion rate than amiodarone and placebo (35%, 4%, and 4% of patients respectively). However, the follow-up period in that study was only 3 h, which may have been insufficient to show efficacy of amiodarone. Furthermore, 8% of the patients receiving dofetilide had torsades de pointes. These new class III agents are most useful for cardioverting atrial flutter, with efficacy rates of over 50% [38, 39].

Conclusions

Before considering antiarrhythmic drug treatment one should bear in mind that up to 60% of patients with recent-onset AF spontaneously cardiovert to sinus rhythm within 24 h. Pharmacologic cardioversion is considered in symptomatic patients who are hemodynamically stable. In unstable patients pharmacologic cardioversion should be avoided because of drug side effects. Electrical cardioversion may be useful, but in any case, rate-controlling drugs should be administered. For this purpose amiodarone is useful since it may serve two goals: rate control and cardioversion. Basically, all antiarrhythmic drugs can convert short-lasting AF to sinus rhythm. However, efficacy differs, and the most successful agents are flecainide and propafenone. Therefore, class Ic antiarrhythmic drugs are the first choice for pharmacologic cardioversion of AF.

In clinical practice, amiodarone is a reasonable alternative to class Ic drugs and may be the drug of choice in the setting of ventricular dysfunction and ischemic heart disease. In these patients amiodarone can be useful, although the time to conversion is relatively long. Most of the data are on intravenous amiodarone, and more studies using oral administration need to be carried out. Ibutilide is moderately effective but associated with a significant risk of torsades de pointes. These class III agents tend to be much more effective in atrial flutter.

References

1. Kannel WB, Abbot RD, Savage DD et al (1982) Epidemiologic features of chronic atrial fibrillation: the Framingham study. N Engl J Med 306:1018–1022
2. Wolf PA, Abbott RD, Kannel WB (1991) Atrial fibrillation as an independent risk factor for stroke. The Framingham Study. Stroke 22:983–988
3. Wyse DG, Waldo AL, DiMarco JP et al, Atrial Fibrillation Follow-up Investigation of Rhythm Management (AFFIRM) Investigators (2002) A comparison of rate control and rhythm control in patients with atrial fibrillation. N Engl J Med 347:1825–1833
4. Van Gelder IC, Hagens VE, Bosker HA et al, Rate Control versus Electrical Cardioversion for Persistent Atrial Fibrillation Study Group (2002) A comparison of rate control and rhythm control in patients with recurrent persistent atrial fibrillation. N Engl J Med 347:1834–1840
5. Allessie M, Rensma PPL, Lammers WJEP et al (1989) The role of refractoriness, conduction velocity and wavelength in initiation of atrial fibrillation in normal dogs. In: Attuel P, Coumel P, Janse MJ (eds) The atrium in health and disease. Futura, Mount Kisco, NY, p 27–41

6. Wijfells MC, Kirchhof CJHJ, Dorland R et al (1995) Atrial fibrillation begets atrial fibrillation. A study in awake chronically instrumented goats. Circulation 92:1954–1968
7. Farshi R, Kistner D, Sarma JSM, Longmate JA, Singh BN (1999) Ventricular rate control in chronic atrial fibrillation during daily activity and programmed exercise: a crossover open-label study of five drug regimens. J Am Coll Cardiol 33: 304–310
8. Klein HO, Kaplinsky E (1986) Digitalis and verapamil in atrial fibrillation and flutter: is verapamil now the preferred agent? Drugs 31:85–197
9. David D, Segni ED, Klein H (1979) Inefficacy of digitalis in the control of heart rate in patients with chronic atrial fibrillation: beneficial effect of an added beta-adrenergic blocking agent. Am J Cardiol 4:1378–1382
10. Dell'Orfano JT, Patel H, Wolbrette DL, Luck JC, Naccarelli GV (1999) Acute treatment of atrial fibrillation: spontaneous conversion rates and cost of care. Am J Cardiol 83:788–790
11. Danias PG, Caulfield TA, Weigner MJ, Silverman DI, Manning WJ (1998) Likelihood of spontaneous conversion of atrial fibrillation to sinus rhythm. J Am Coll Cardiol 313:588–592
12. Naccarelli GV, Dell'Orfano JT, Wolbrette DL, Patel H, Luck JC (2000) Acute cost-effective management of atrial fibrillation: role of rate control, spontaneous conversion, cardioversion, and antiembolic therapy. Am J Cardiol 85:36D–45D
13. Fuster V, Rydén LE, Asinger RW et al (2001) ACC/AHA/ESC guidelines for the management of patients with atrial fibrillation: executive summary: a report of the American College of Cardiology/American Heart Association Task Force on Practice Guidelines and the European Society of Cardiology Committee for Practice Guidelines and Policy Conferences (Committee to Develop Guidelines for the Management of Patients With Atrial Fibrillation). J Am Coll Cardiol 38:1231–1265
14. Kochiadakis GE, Igoumenidis NE, Solomou MC et al (1998) Conversion of atrial fibrillation to sinus rhythm using acute intravenous procainamide infusion. Cardiovasc Drugs Ther 12:75–81
15. Capucci A, Tiziano L, Boriani G et al (1992) Effectiveness of loading oral flecainide for converting recent-onset atrial fibrillation to sinus rhythm in patients without organic heart disease or with only systemic hypertension. Am J Cardiol 70:69–72
16. Crijns HJGM, van Vijk M, van Gilst WH et al (1988) Acute conversion of atrial fibrillation to sinus rhythm: clinical efficacy of flecainide acetate. Comparison of two regimens. Eur Heart J 9:634–639
17. Capucci A, Boriani G, Rubino I et al (1994) A controlled study on oral propafenone versus digoxin plus quinidine in converting recent onset atrial fibrillation to sinus rhythm. Int J Cardiol 43:305–311
18. Boriani G, Biffi M, Capucci A et al (1997) Oral propafenone to convert recent-onset atrial fibrillation in patients with and without underlying heart disease. A randomized controlled trial. Ann Intern Med 126:621–624
19. Suttorp MJ, Kingma HJ, Jessurun ER et al (1990) The value of class 1C antiarrhythmic drugs for acute conversion of paroxysmal atrial fibrillation or flutter to sinus rhythm. J Am Coll Cardiol 16:1722–1727
20. Galve E, Rius T, Ballester R et al (1996) Intravenous amiodarone in the treatment of recent-onset atrial fibrillation. Results of a randomized, controlled trial. J Am Coll Cardiol 27:1079–1082
21. Vardas PE, Kochiadakis GE, Igoumenidis NE et al (2000) Amiodarone as a first-choice drug for restoring sinus rhythm in patients with atrial fibrillation: a randomized, controlled study. Chest 117:1538–1545

22. Pritchett ELC (1992) Management of atrial fibrillation. N Engl J Med 326:1264–1271
23. Management of patients with atrial fibrillation (1996) A statement for healthcare professionals from the subcommittee on electrocardiography and electrophysiology, American Heart Association. Circulation 93:1262–1277
24. Nattel S (1995) Newer developments in the management of atrial fibrillation. Am Heart J 130:1094–1106
25. Falk RH (1994) Current management of atrial fibrillation. Curr Opin Cardiol 9:30–39
26. Hou ZY, Chang MS, Chen CY et al (1995) Acute treatment of recent-onset atrial fibrillation and flutter with a tailored dosing regimen of intravenous amiodarone. Eur Heart J 16:521–528
27. Levy S (1994) Amiodarone as a first-line drug in the treatment of atrial fibrillation: The Protagonist Viewpoint. Cardiovasc Drugs Ther 8:769–771
28. Kochiadakis GE, Igoumenidis NE, Simantirakis EN et al (1998) Intravenous propafenone versus intravenous amiodarone in the management of atrial fibrillation of recent onset: a placebo-controlled study. Pacing Clin Electrophysiol 21:2475–2479
29. Chevalier P, Durand-Dubief A, Burri H et al (2003) Amiodarone versus placebo and classic drugs for cardioversion of recent-onset atrial fibrillation: a meta-analysis. J Am Coll Cardiol 41:255–262
30. Blanc JJ, Voinov C, Marek M (1999) Comparison of oral loading dose of propafenone and amiodarone for converting recent-onset atrial fibrillation. PARSIFAL Study Group. Am J Cardiol 84:1029–1032
31. Kowey PR, Marinchak RA, Rials SJ, Filart RA (1997) Intravenous amiodarone. J Am Coll Cardiol 29:1190–1198
32. Schwartz A, Shen E, Morady F et al (1983) Hemodynamic effects of intravenous amiodarone in patients with depressed left ventricular function and recurrent ventricular tachycardia. Am Heart J 106:848–856
33. Gottlieb SS, Riggio DW, Lauria S et al (1994) High dose oral amiodarone loading exerts important hemodynamic actions in patients with congestive heart failure. J Am Coll Cardiol 23:560–564
34. Jafari-Fesharaki M, Scheinman MM (1998) Adverse effects of amiodarone. Pacing Clin Electrophysiol 21:108–120
35. Wellens J, Brugada P, Abdollah H, Dassen WR (1984) A comparison of the electrophysiologic effects of intravenous and oral amiodarone in the same patient. Circulation 69:120–124
36. Kanoupakis EM, Kochiadakis GE, Manios EG et al (2003) Pharmacological cardioversion of recent onset atrial fibrillation with intravenous amiodarone in patients receiving long-term amiodarone therapy: is it reasonable? J Interv Card Electrophysiol 8:19–26
37. Stambler BS, Wood MA, Ellenbogen KA et al (1996) Efficacy and safety of repeated intravenous doses of ibutilide for rapid conversion of atrial flutter or fibrillation. Ibutilide Repeat Dose Study Investigators. Circulation 94:1613–1621
38. Falk RH, Pollak A, Singh SN, Friedrich T (1997) Intravenous dofetilide, a class III antiarrhythmic agent, for the termination of sustained atrial fibrillation or flutter. Intravenous Dofetilide Investigators. J Am Coll Cardiol 29:385–390
39. Bianconi L, Castro A, Dinelli M et al (2000) Comparison of intravenously administered dofetilide versus amiodarone in the acute termination of atrial fibrillation and flutter: a multicentre, randomized, double-blind, placebo-controlled study. Eur Heart J 21(15):1265-1273

Pretreatment with Antiarrhythmic Drugs: Is It Useful to Avoid Immediate and Early Postcardioversion Recurrences?

G. L. Botto, M. Luzi, A. Sagone

Introduction

In patients with atrial fibrillation (AF), restoration of sinus rhythm (SR) may eliminate symptoms and prevent left ventricular dysfunction [1]. Electrical cardioversion is the most effective way to convert persistent AF to SR, since its efficacy is very close to 100% success in the biphasic shock era [2]. Unfortunately, because of the high recurrence rate, particularly in the first few hours after cardioversion, only 30% of patients maintain SR for 6 months or more without antiarrhythmic drug prophylaxis [3]. These findings provide the rationale for pretreatment and long-term prophylaxis with antiarrhythmic agents, although there are some concerns about the risk-benefit ratio of these drugs.

Antiarrhythmic Drugs to Facilitate Electrical Cardioversion

The majority of patients will be successfully cardioverted with DC shock alone. The procedure itself may restore SR in up to 95% of patients with persistent AF, using external biphasic shock [2]. While standard practice dictates that DC shock alone should be attempted before antiarrhythmic agents are added, empirical pretreatment with drugs is becoming more common. Studies looking at administration of antiarrhythmic agents before electrical cardioversion are typically small, and rarely placebo-controlled.

Recently, Oral et al. [4] examined ibutilide in facilitating transthoracic cardioversion. Ibutilide successfully cardioverted 100% of the patients who underwent pharmacological pretreatment, compared to 72% of those who did not receive the agent. Those in whom SR was not achieved with electrical cardioversion alone were later successfully cardioverted when ibutilide was added

Department of Cardiology, Sant' Anna Hospital, Como, Italy

before the electrical procedure. Two patients (3%) who received ibutilide suffered from polymorphic ventricular tachycardia (neither resulting in increased mortality).

The use of class IC drugs or amiodarone as pretreatment for electrical cardioversion will be discussed later in the present paper.

Time Course of Recurrences of Atrial Fibrillation

The most relevant clinical problem after successful cardioversion is the risk of recurrences, which is particularly high in the first minutes to hours following electrical cardioversion using either internal [5] or external [6] methods. The phenomenon has only recently been described, with the various forms acquiring their different own acronyms: recurrence may occur in a very early phase (minutes) after electrical shock: IRAF (*i*mmediate *r*ecurrence of *a*trial *f*ibrillation); in a subacute phase (first 24–48 h to 7–14 days): ERAF (*e*arly *r*ecurrence of *a*trial *f*ibrillation); or weeks to months following the successful procedure: LRAF (*l*ate *r*ecurrence of *a*trial *f*ibrillation) [1].

Immediate and Early Recurrences of Atrial Fibrillation

The phenomena of IRAF and ERAF are difficult to characterize: data from the literature on the outcome of electrical cardioversion do not usually distinguish shock failure from IRAF or IRAF from ERAF. However, two important concepts are implicated and may strongly interact to produce these phenomena. First, a growing number of patients have AF initiated, and possibly maintained, by an ectopic focus of repetitive atrial activity [7]. Secondly, AF itself causes changes in cellular electrophysiology that have the effect of further increasing the tendency to fibrillation [8], and there is a reversal of this electrophysiological remodeling after a certain period of SR [9]. The first of these two concepts relates to the triggers for initiation of the AF and the second to the substrate predisposing to and maintaining the arrhythmia.

The most important atrial parameter related to AF-induced electrical remodeling is the refractory period. During control, early premature beats do not induce any arrhythmia. After a few hours of AF, the atrial refractory period is shortened and a premature stimulus is followed by a short run of rapid atrial responses. Twenty-four hours of AF further shorten the atrial refractory period, and now early premature beats trigger paroxysms of AF [8]. Some studies have tested the efficacy of drug treatment before cardioversion in preventing AF relapse. Antiarrhythmic agents may act in two ways: reducing atrial refractoriness maladaptation, or preventing premature supraventricular beats.

Pretreatment with Class IV Drugs

Intracellular calcium overload is the most important mechanism sustaining electrophysiological remodeling. Animal experiments have shown that calcium channel blockade significantly prevents the shortening of atrial refractoriness when given before short episodes of artificially induced AF [10]. If in humans too, electrical remodeling is related to intracellular calcium overload, the frequency of relapse might be lowered by drugs that lower the intracellular calcium concentration.

Tieleman et al. [11], using transtelephonic monitoring, studied 61 patients who underwent successful cardioversion for persistent AF. Being on intracellular-calcium-lowering medication preceding the cardioversion was the only significant variable related to maintenance of SR.

De Simone et al. [12] were the first to demonstrate, in a randomized fashion, the beneficial effect of oral pretreatment with verapamil, combined with an antiarrhythmic drug, in reducing the incidence of ERAF after external or internal electrical cardioversion. They found a higher incidence of AF recurrences in patients who received propafenone alone before electrical cardioversion than in patients in whom propafenone was combined with verapamil, suggesting that intracellular-calcium-lowering drugs reduce electrical remodeling, which may in turn lead to a more rapid recovery after cardioversion.

More recently, the final result of the VERAF study [13] clearly demonstrated that verapamil alone, in patients who were not taking antiarrhythmic agents at the moment of cardioversion and in the whole follow-up, is highly effective in reducing IRAF and ERAF after successful cardioversion, whereas the drug is ineffective in preventing arrhythmia recurrences occurring in the long run.

Pretreatment with Class IA and Class III Drugs

There is a clear evidence that any tendency to atrial ectopic activity is exaggerated in the early period following cardioversion.

Bianconi et al. [6] tested the efficacy of propafenone in a placebo-controlled study involving 100 patients, comparing two different strategies: pretreatment with oral propafenone, or propafenone only after cardioversion. Pharmacological conversion before DC shock was obtained in 6% of the subjects. Propafenone did not exert any significant effect on the success rate of the procedure. Arrhythmia recurrence was significantly reduced within 10 min after cardioversion (0% vs 17% in the placebo group) and also within 24 h and 48 h. After cardioversion, the incidence of supraventricular ectopic beats was higher in the placebo patients.

Oral amiodarone is the most effective in long-term maintenance of SR compared to propafenone or sotalol [14]. However, its use around electrical cardioversion of AF may be difficult because amiodarone loading requires at least 4–6 weeks to reach therapeutic plasma levels, and during the first weeks of treatment patients may be at risk of recurrences.

Capucci et al. [15] randomized 92 patients with persistent AF and organic heart disease to receive pretreatment with oral amiodarone at a dosage of 400 mg/day for 1 month before and 200 mg/day for 2 months after cardioversion or oral diltiazem 180 mg/day for 1 month before and 2 months after cardioversion. In the amiodarone group, 25% of patients reversed to SR before the procedure, and amiodarone pretreatment increased cardioversion efficacy. ERAF was similar in the different groups, while at 2 months the recurrence rate was lower in the amiodarone-treated patients (32% vs 52%–56%). It is possible to suppose the beneficial effect of amiodarone to be acting either via the prolongation of the atrial refractoriness and/or via the reduction in intracellular calcium concentration. Both these mechanisms may have affected the atrial remodeling phenomenon.

Pretreatment with Nonantiarrhythmic Drugs

The development of a therapy directed against remodeling could mark an important change in the management of patients who are going to receive electrical cardioversion to reverse AF to SR.

A recent study performed on animals [16] demonstrated for the first time that angiotensin II contributes to atrial electrical remodeling. In this study, the shortening of the atrial refractory period during rapid pacing was prevented by treatment with candesartan or captopril but increased by angiotensin II. The results of the first prospective and randomized study performed in humans [17] showed that adding the angiotensin II receptor blocker irbesartan to amiodarone is more effective in the maintenance of sinus rhythm after cardioversion of persistent atrial fibrillation than is amiodarone alone, suggesting that angiotensin II receptor antagonists could play a role in preventing atrial remodeling. Irbesartan reduced the immediate recurrence of atrial fibrillation (no patient had recurrence during a time window of 1 h after cardioversion) and the subacute recurrences during the first weeks. This class of drug could prevent or modify atrial remodeling by modifying electrical parameters, but also by decreasing atrial stretch or preventing atrial fibrosis (a possible second factor involved in the genesis of structural atrial remodeling).

Conclusions

Antiarrhythmic pharmacotherapy may effectively supplement electrical cardioversion of AF in two ways. After DC cardioversion alone has failed, antiarrhythmic agents may be given before the procedure to facilitate cardioversion. Ibutilide and amiodarone have proven most effective in this regard.

If AF recurs, antiarrhythmics may be given, after a second cardioversion attempt, to improve maintenance of SR. The mechanism underlying early recurrence of AF is unclear for the majority of patients, but is probably multifactorial. Contributing factors may include electrophysiological remodeling, which strongly interacts with triggering factors such as atrial ectopic beats, both probably modulated by the autonomic nervous system.

The administration of class IC and class III antiarrhythmic drugs has a favorable effect in reducing early recurrences, mainly by reducing the incidence of atrial ectopic beats, which is counterbalanced by the possibility of postcardioversion bradyarrhythmias. An alternative approach could be pretreatment with verapamil or angiotensin II blockers, given alone or together with antiarrhythmic drugs, to reduce the maladaptation of electrophysiological parameters induced by AF itself.

However, future randomized, prospective studies are needed to establish the real role of verapamil and angiotensin II antagonists in preventing AF recurrences, particularly regarding their possible favorable effect when given together with antiarrhythmic drugs.

Amiodarone is the most effective agent in maintenance of SR in the long run, but the benefit gained may not outweigh the threat of the associated side effects.

References

1. ACC/AHA/ESC guidelines for the management of patients with atrial fibrillation (2001) J Am Coll Cardiol 38:1266i–ixx
2. Mittal S, Ayati S, Stein KM et al (2000) Transthoracic cardioversion of atrial fibrillation. Comparison of rectilinear biphasic versus damped sine wave monophasic shocks. Circulation 101:1282–1287
3. Van Gelder IC, Crijins HJGM, Lie KI (1992) Characteristics of patients with chronic atrial fibrillation and prediction of successful DC electrical cardioversion. In: Kingma JH, Van Hemel NM, Lie KL (eds) Atrial fibrillation: a treatable disease? Kluwer Academic, Amsterdam, pp 67–86
4. Oral H, Souza JJ, Michaud GF et al (1999) Facilitating transthoracic cardioversion of atrial fibrillation with ibutilide pretreatment. N Engl J Med 340:1849-54
5. Timmermans C, Rodriguez LM, Smeets JLRM et al (1998) Immediate reinitiation of atrial fibrillation following internal defibrillation. J Cardiovasc Electrophysiol 9:122–128
6. Bianconi L, Mennuni M, Lukic V et al (1996) Effects of oral propafenone administration before electrical cardioversion of chronic atrial fibrillation: a placebo-controlled study. J Am Coll Cardiol 28:700–706
7. Jais P, Haissaguerre M, Shah DC et al (1997) A focal source of atrial fibrillation treated by discrete radiofrequency ablation. Circulation 95:572–576
8. Wijffels MCEF, Kirchhof CJHJ, Dorland R et al (1995) Atrial fibrillation begets atrial fibrillation: a study in awake chronically instrumented goats. Circulation

92:1954–1968
9. Yu WC, Lee SH, Tai CT et al (1999) Reversal of atrial electrical remodeling following cardioversion of long standing atrial fibrillation in man. Cardiovasc Res 42:470–476
10. Tieleman RG, De Langen CDJ, Van Gelder IC et al (1997) Verapamil reduces tachycardia-induced electrical remodeling of the atria. Circulation 95:1945–1953
11. Tieleman RG, Van Gelder IC, Crijins HJGM et al (1998) Early recurrence of atrial fibrillation after electrical cardioversion: a result of fibrillation-induced electrical remodeling of the atria? J Am Coll Cardiol 31:167–173
12. De Simone A, Stabile G, Vitale DF et al (1999) Pre-treatment with verapamil in patients with persistent or chronic atrial fibrillation who underwent electrical cardioversion. J Am Coll Cardiol 34:810–814
13. Botto GL, Belotti G, Cirò A et al, on behalf of the VERAF study group (2002) Verapamil in prevention of early recurrence of atrial fibrillation: final results of the VERAF study. Eur Heart J 23:660
14. Roy D, Talajic M, Dorian P et al, for the Canadian Trial of Atrial Fibrillation Investigators (2000) Amiodarone to prevent recurrence of atrial fibrillation. Canadian Trial of Atrial Fibrillation Investigators. N Engl J Med 342:913–920
15. Capucci A, Villani GQ, Aschieri D et al (2000) Oral amiodarone increases the efficacy of DC cardioversion in restoration of sinus rhythm in patients with chronic atrial fibrillation. Eur Heart J 21:66–73
16. Nakashima H, Kumagai K, Urata H et al (2000) Angiotensin II antagonist prevents electrical remodeling in atrial fibrillation. Circulation 101:2612–2617
17. Madrid AH, Bueno MG, Rebollo JMG et al (2002) Use of ibesartan to maintain sinus rhythm in patients with long-lasting persistent atrial fibrillation. A prospective randomized study. Circulation 106:331–336

Is Echocardiography Useful to Predict Successful Cardioversion of Atrial Fibrillation and Long-Term Maintenance of Sinus Rhythm?

B. De Piccoli

Introduction

Atrial fibrillation (AF) is the most frequently sustained arrhythmia; it occurs in 2%–4% of people aged over 60 years and in almost 9% of octogenarians [1]. People affected by AF exhibit a higher risk of heart failure and, above all, of embolic events [2]. It is not definitively established whether sinus rhythm restoration and maintenance warrant a better prognosis than chronic persistence of the arrhythmia combined with optimal control of the heart rate and anticoagulation therapy to prevent thromboembolism [3], but nevertheless in common clinical practice cardioversion is proposed in order to improve cardiac function and survival [4].

Rate of Success of Cardioversion

Formerly such clinical parameters as the age of the patient, the underlying cardiac disease and, above all, the duration of AF were adopted as predictors of the success of a cardioversion [5]. The importance of the duration of the arrhythmia has been also recently emphasized by Corrado et al. [6], who demonstrated more frequent successful cardioversion in people whose arrhythmia lasted less than 4 weeks than in those with AF lasting for more than 4 weeks or of an unknown duration. Furthermore, Pàlinkàs et al. [7] demonstrated a higher success rate in patients with AF lasting less than 2 weeks.

After the introduction of transthoracic echocardiography (TTE) into clinical practice, such parameters as left atrial size or left ventricle size and function could be investigated and related to cardioversion, and were shown to correlate poorly with success of sinus rhythm (SR) restoration [8]. More recently,

Department of Cardiology, Umberto I Hospital, Mestre–Venice, Italy

transesophageal echocardiography (TEE) has enabled the anatomical and functional aspects of the left atrial appendage (LAA) to be investigated [9]. By this means, LAA Doppler flow patterns were found to be predictive of embolic events [10, 11] as well as of successful cardioversion [12]. Although some authors [13] have disagreed with these conclusions, at present the outflow velocity of the LAA is considered a predictive indicator of successful restoration of SR by cardioversion. Pàlinkàs et al. [7] have recently suggested that we can expect a high rate of SR restoration in patients with a peak outflow velocity of LAA during AF that is greater than 31 cm/s (p=0.0013).

Prediction of SR Maintenance After Cardioversion: Analysis Before Cardioversion

The clinical and echocardiographic parameters previously described were also used to predict maintenance of SR after successful cardioversion. Dittrich et al. [14] observed that the persistence of SR at 1 month after cardioversion was related to a short duration of AF (<3 months vs >12 months, $p<0.05$). Weigner et al. [15] observed a higher rate of persistence of SR at 1 year in patients with a duration of AF of less than 3 months in comparison to patients with a longer duration of the arrhythmia (68.8% vs 51.3%).

In 1976 Henry et al. [16] observed a longer persistence of SR in subjects with left atrial dimensions of less than 45 mm; conversely, Dittrich et al. [14] reported that left atrial area and long axis dimension, calculated by two-dimensional echocardiography, were significantly larger in subjects remaining in SR than in those who reverted to AF at 1 month after cardioversion (28±7 vs 24±5 cm^2 and 65±9 vs 59±8 mm respectively, in both cases $p<0.05$). In both papers there was a large overlap between the compared groups of patients.

Doppler flow patterns of the LAA calculated by TEE have proven to be stronger predictors of SR maintenance than TTE indices. Verhorst et al. [17] in 1997 used TEE to study 62 patients with AF before their first successful cardioversion. One year later, 58% of the analyzed subjects continued to be in SR; their outward LAA Doppler flow velocity before cardioversion was 36±15 cm/s, whereas the velocity in patients who reverted to AF was 19±8 cm/s ($p<0.0005$). In the study by Verhorst et al. the predictive value of the LAA outflow velocity for the maintenance of SR at 1 year was stronger than the clinical variables and the size of the atrium.

In a recent work on this subject from our institution [18] we analyzed both the outward and the inward Doppler flow of the LAA during AF, considering the fibrillatory flow waves with both the maximal (highest) and the minimal (lowest) velocity. One month after cardioversion, 55% of patients maintained SR; the sum of the outward and inward velocity of both the maximal and minimal pulse Doppler fibrillatory waves of these patients was significantly higher (88.10±24.98 vs 59.25±11.73 cm/s and 28.7±3.07 vs 23±4.99 cm/s, respectively) than that observed in patients who reverted to AF.

Omran et al. [19] in 1998 observed that a peak emptying velocity of the LAA that was below 36 cm/s had a sensitivity of 82% and a specificity of 83% for predicting recurrence of AF.

More recently, Antonielli et al. [20] documented that the negative and positive predictive values of a mean LAA emptying velocity greater than 40 cm/s for assessing preservation of SR 1 year after cardioversion were 66% and 73% respectively.

Thus, echocardiographic evaluation, above all by TEE, performed before cardioversion exhibits a good predictive value for SR maintenance in the short and middle term.

Prediction of SR Maintenance After Cardioversion: Analysis After Cardioversion

Echocardiographic analyses performed soon after cardioversion are scarce [21, 22] and have not focused on predicting AF recurrence. In the above-cited study from our institution [18] we considered the echo parameters recorded soon before as well as 5–10 min after the electrical shock delivery; the latter indices were analyzed in order to test whether both the mechanical contraction of LA and the contraction and relaxation of LAA recorded during the heaviest stunning [23] of these structures could be predictive of SR maintenance 1 month after cardioversion, when about 57% of AF recurrences take place [24]. For this purpose we calculated by TTE the A-wave peak velocity (A-peak vel.) and the A wave velocity-time integral (A-VTI) of the Doppler mitral flow. By TEE we calculated the fractional area change of the LAA (LAA FAC), the spontaneous echocontrast score (SEC score), and the following LAA Doppler flow parameters: the sum of peak velocities and durations of the outward and inward ($A+A_1$) end-diastolic flow and the sum of peak velocities and durations of the outward and inward ($E+E_1$) early diastolic flow, the former with regard to the contraction, the latter to the conduit phase of the appendage mechanics. We also calculated the following Doppler flow parameters of the pulmonary veins: peak velocity and VTI of both systolic (S) and diastolic (D) components, and the ratios between S and D and S VTI and D VTI.

Table 1 reports the postcardioversion results of the analyzed parameters in patients who maintained SR at 1 month after cardioversion and in those who reverted to AF. A-wave peak velocity and VTI of the mitral flow, recorded by TTE, were significantly higher in the first than in the second group. Similarly, the TEE Doppler flow parameters of the LAA, with regard to both the contraction and the conduit phase, were higher in the first than in the second group.

The differences between TEE parameters were more significant than the differences between TTE parameters; furthermore, the differences between the two groups of patients were more significant after than before cardioversion (Table 2).

Table 1. Comparison of the values of the echocardiographic parameters recorded after DC shock in the two groups of patients

	Sinus rhythm (10 patients)	Atrial fibrillation (8 patients)	*p*
TTE:			
LV EF (%)	50.17±6.34	45.06±6.4	0.180
Mitral flow:			
A peak velocity (cm/s)	30.10±5.24	20.50±6.32	0.003*
A VTI (cm)	2.83±0.91	1.89±0.32	0.014*
TEE:			
LAA FAC (%)	14±5.87	16.88±7.97	0.270
SEC score (+)	2±0.82	2.38±0.52	0.257
LAA flow:			
A+A1 peak velocity (cm/s)	58.2±17.02	31.25±9.27	0.001*
A+A1 duration (ms)	162.70±27.01	133.75±5.31	0.002*
E+E1 peak velocity (cm/s)	25.00±4.5	19.33±4.08	0.024*
E+E1 duration (ms)	101.90±35.15	53.33±16.33	0.006*
PVF:			
S peak velocity (cm/s)	35.3±19	22.1±12	0.310
S VTI (cm)	5.51±3	5.95±3.56	0.792
D peak velocity (cm/s)	40.18±16.46	36±16.02	0.376
D VTI (cm)	11.2±3.1	9.3±3.6	0.118
S peak velocity/ D peak velocity	0.87±0.13	0.61±0.4	0.478
S VTI/ D VTI	0.53±0.32	0.65±0.48	0.410

A, End-diastolic mitral flow; A+A1, sum of the end-diastolic contraction and relaxation of LAA; E+E1, sum of the early diastolic forward and reverse flow of LAA; EF, ejection fraction; FAC, fractional area change; LV, left ventricle; PVF, pulmonary venous flow; D, diastolic flow; S, systolic flow; SEC, spontaneous echo contrast; VTI, velocity-time integral; +, SEC score. *Differences are significant where $p<0.05$. Modified from De Piccoli et al. [18]

Figure 1 shows the scatterplot of the indices most closely related to SR maintenance: an A-wave peak velocity of the mitral flow greater than 28 cm/s, an $A+A_1$ peak velocity greater than 43 cm/s, duration of LAA greater than 140 ms, and an $E+E_1$ duration greater than 85 ms were closely related to persistence of SR at 1 month after cardioversion. Other parameters such as LV ejection fraction, LAA FAC, SEC score, and the pattern of the pulmonary venous flow did not exhibit significant differences between the patients who maintained SR and those who reverted to AF.

Table 2. Comparison of the values of the echocardiographic parameters recorded before DC shock in subjects who maintained SR and in those who reverted to AF 30 days after cardioversion

	Sinus rhythm (10 patients)	Atrial fibrillation (8 patients)	*p*
TTE:			
LV EF (%)	48.13 ± 7	49.2 ± 3.7	0.680
LA area (cm2)	20.8 ± 4.5	28.13 ± 5.11	0.009*
TEE:			
LAA FAC (%)	22.87 ± 8.36	24.8 ± 15.6	0.714
SEC score (+)	0.9 ± 0.7	1.2 ± 0.7	0.125
LAA flow			
Peak velocity (cm/s), + and –, of max. wave	88.10 ± 24.98	59.25 ± 11.73	0.010*
Duration (ms), + and –, of max. wave	168.7 ± 41.3	160 ± 61.9	0.860
Peak velocity (cm/s), + and –, of min. wave	28.7 ± 3.06	23 ± 4.99	0.010*
Duration (ms), + and –, of min. wave	97.6 ± 27.73	82.5 ± 24.66	0.392
PVF:			
S peak velocity (cm/s)	40.6 ± 22	24.6 ± 22.81	0.120
S VTI (cm)	7 ± 2.62	4.8 ± 1.64	0.155
D peak velocity (cm/s)	48.87 ± 16.46	43 ± 13.02	0.540
D VTI (cm)	10.5 ± 4	8.2 ± 4.38	0.408
S peak velocity/D peak velocity	0.8 ± 0.4	0.58 ± 0.4	0.286
S VTI/ D VTI	0.73 ± 0.32	0.6 ± 0.38	0.802

EF, ejection fraction; LA, left atrium; LAA, left atrial appendage; LV, left ventricle; MAX, Maximal; MIN, minimal fibrillatory waves; PVF, pulmonary venous flow; D, diastolic flow; S, systolic flow; SEC, spontaneous echo contrast; VTI, velocity-time integral; (+), SEC score; + and –, sum of the forward and reverse flow. *Differences are significant where p<0.05. Modified from De Piccoli et al. [18]

Hypothetical Influence on Anticoagulation

The parameters we found to be predictive of AF recurrence are similar to those involved in the risk stratification of embolic events [25] related to cardioversion. Thus, if we are able to identify these indices during AF and, above all, soon after SR restoration, when the mechanical function of the LA and LAA are heavily compromised by stunning, we could adopt a shorter period of anticoagulation. Current recommendations regarding anticoagulation therapy

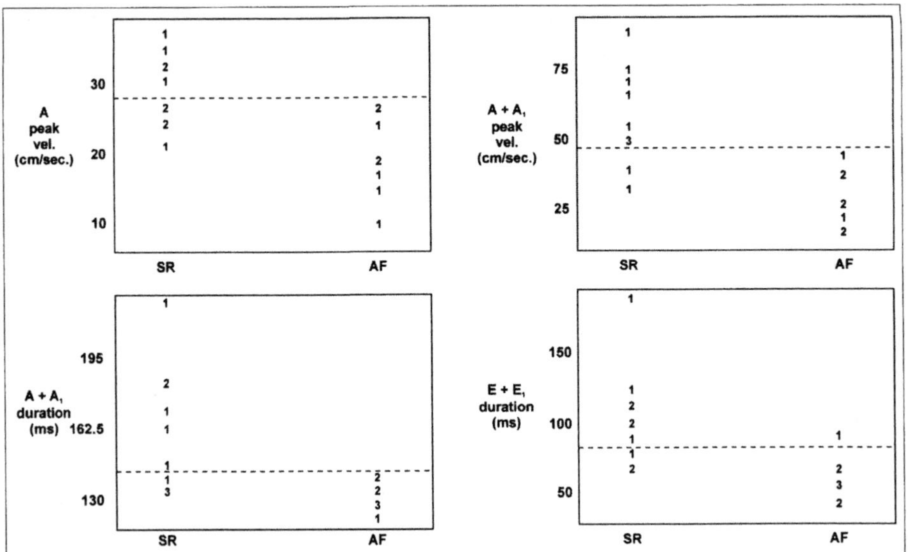

A = end-diastolic mitral flow. A+A1 = sum of the end-diastolic contraction and relaxation flow of the left atrial appendage.
E+E1 = sum of the early diastolic forward flow and reverse flow of the left atrial appendage.
Numbers contained in the rectangles represent the numbers of subjects corresponding to the value of the parameter considered.
The dotted line separates the subjects who maintained SR.

Fig. 1. Scatterplot of the data of the four postcardioversion parameters most closely correlated to persistence of SR 30 days after DC shock. Modified from De Piccoli et al. [18]

involve a long period of oral treatment [26]; this carries the risk of possible hemorrhagic complications and is often difficult to manage. Previous authors who performed TEE studies in patients undergoing cardioversion, proposed a brief period of anticoagulation treatment before the procedure. If we could also use postcardioversion indices of the recovery and long persistence of the optimal kinetics of the LA and LAA, we could propose a shorter period of anticoagulation after cardioversion as well.

Conclusions

Analysis of the above-mentioned studies allows us conclude that echocardiography constitutes an useful tool to predict the rate of success of cardioversion and the maintenance of SR after the procedure. Doppler indices of LAA emptying and filling are more predictive than the anatomical and functional aspects of LA. The parameters of LA and LAA function recorded soon after electrical shock delivery appear to be more related to SR maintenance than to precardioversion indices. These conclusions could have profitable implications for anticoagulation therapy after SR restoration.

References

1. Kannel WB, Wolf PA (1992) Epidemiology of atrial fibrillation. In: Falk RH, Podrid P (eds) Atrial fibrillation: mechanisms and management. Raven, New York, pp 81–92
2. Benjamin EJ, Wolf PA, D'Agostino RB et al (1998) Impact of atrial fibrillation on the risk of death. The Framingham heart study. Circulation 98:946–952
3. Wyse DG, Anderson JL, Antman EM et al (1997) Atrial fibrillation follow-up investigation of rhythm management: The AFFIRM study design. Am J Cardiol 79:1198–1202
4. Pritchett ELC (1992) Management of atrial fibrillation. N Engl J Med 326:1264–1271
5. Hall JI, Wood DR (1968) Factors affecting cardioversion of atrial arrhythmias with special reference to quinidine. Br Heart J 30:84–90
6. Corrado G, Beretta S, Tadeo G et al (2000) Early cardioversion of atrial fibrillation and atrial flutter guided by transoesophageal echocardiography: a single centre 8.5-year experience. Europace 2:119–126
7. Pàlinkàs A, Antonielli E, Picano E et al (2001) Clinical value of left atrial appendage flow velocity for predicting cardioversion success in patients with non-valvular atrial fibrillation. Eur Heart J 22:2201–2208
8. Silverman DI, Manning WJ (1998) Role of echocardiography in patients undergoing elective cardioversion of atrial fibrillation. Circulation 98:479–486
9. Steward JB, Khandheria BK, Oh JK et al (1988) Transesophageal echocardiography: technique, anatomic correlations, implementation and clinical applications. Mayo Clin Proc 63:649–680
10. Pozzoli M, Febo O, Torbicki A et al (1991) Left atrial appendage dysfunction: a cause of thrombosis? Evidence by transesophageal echocardiography Doppler studies. J Am Soc Echocardiogr 4:435–441
11. Mügge A, Kuhn H, Nikuta P et al (1994) Assessment of left atrial appendage function by biplane transesophageal echocardiography in patients with nonrheumatic atrial fibrillation: identification of a subgroup of patients at increased thromboembolic risk. J Am Coll Cardiol 23:599–607
12. Mitusch R, Garbe M, Schmücker G et al (1995) Relation of left atrial appendage function to the duration and reversibility of nonvalvular atrial fibrillation. Am J Cardiol 75:944–947
13. Perez Y, Duval AM, Carville C et al (1997) Is left atrial appendage flow a predictor for outcome of cardioversion of nonvalvular atrial fibrillation? A transthoracic and transesophageal echocardiographic study. Am Heart J 134:745–751
14. Dittrich HC, Erickson JS, SchneidermanT et al (1989) Echocardiographic and clinical predictors for outcome of elective cardioversion of atrial fibrillation. Am J Cardiol 63:193–197
15. Weigner MJ, Thomas LR, Patel U et al (2001) Early cardioversion of atrial fibrillation facilitated by transesophageal echocardiography: short-term safety and impact on maintenance of sinus rhythm at 1 year. Am J Med 110:694–702
16. Henry W, Morganroth J, Pearlman A et al (1976) Relation between echocardiographically determined left atrial size and atrial fibrillation. Circulation 53:273–279
17. Verhorst PMJ, Kamp O, Welling RC et al (1997) Transesophageal echocardiographic predictors for maintenance of sinus rhythm after electrical cardioversion of atrial fibrillation. Am J Cardiol 79:1355–1359

18. De Piccoli B, Rigo F, Ragazzo M et al (2001) Transthoracic and transesophageal echocardiographic indices predictive of sinus rhythm maintenance after cardioversion of atrial fibrillation: an echocardiographic study during direct current shock. Echocardiography 18:545–552
19. Omran H, Jung W, Schimpf R et al (1998) Echocardiographic parameters for predicting maintenance of sinus rhythm after internal atrial defibrillation. Am J Cardiol 81:1446–1449
20. Antonielli E, Pizzuti A, Palinkas A et al (2002) Clinical value of left atrial appendage flow for prediction of long-term sinus rhythm maintenance in patients with nonvalvular atrial fibrillation. J Am Coll Cardiol 39:1443–1449
21. Grimm RA, Stewart WJ, Maloney JD et al (1993) Impact of electrical cardioversion of atrial fibrillation on left atrial appendage function and spontaneous echo contrast: characterization by simultaneous transesophageal echocardiography. J Am Coll Cardiol 22:1359–1366
22. Fatkin D, Kuchar DL, Thornburn CW, Feneley MP (1993) Transesophageal echocardiography before and during direct current cardioversion of atrial fibrillation: evidence for "atrial stunning" as a mechanism of thromboembolic complications. J Am Coll Cardiol 23:307–316
23. Piccolo E, De Piccoli B (1998) Stunning atriale post-fibrillazione atriale. Cardiologia 43:577–579
24. Tieleman RG, Van Gelder IC, Crijns HJG et al (1998) Early recurrence of atrial fibrillation after electrical cardioversion: a result of fibrillation-induced electrical remodelling of the atria? J Am Coll Cardiol 31:167–173
25. Garcia-Fernandez MA, Torrecilla EG, San Roman D et al (1992) Left atrial appendage Doppler flow patterns: implications on thrombus formation. Am Heart J 124:955–961
26. Laupacis A, Albers G, Dunn M et al (1992) Antithrombotic therapy in atrial fibrillation. Chest 102(Suppl):426S–433S

Does the Policy of Repeated Early Cardioversion for Recurrences of Atrial Fibrillation Work?

E. Bertaglia

Introduction

Atrial fibrillation (AF) is a very common arrhythmia, which increases in prevalence in patients more than 60 years old. Over time, it tends to become persistent or permanent, even if no underlying structural heart disease is present. The success rate of electrical cardioversion and the maintenance of sinus rhythm are highly dependent on the duration of the previous AF episode. After electrical cardioversion only 20%–40% of patients maintain sinus rhythm for the first year [1]. The highest incidence of recurrences is seen during the first month after cardioversion, particularly within the first 5 days, when AF recurs in up to 40% of patients [2].

The mechanism of early relapses seems to be different from that of late recurrences. A possible explanation for early relapses is remodeling of the atria: AF itself causes progressive electrophysiological and structural changes to the atria and modification of the autonomic innervation, which initiate or perpetuate AF [3]. Serial electrical cardioversion is often used to maintain sinus rhythm in patients with persistent AF. However, its usefulness is still debated [4, 5]. We have recently demonstrated the efficacy of a policy of serial electrical cardioversion after early AF recurrences [6].

Mechanisms of Early Relapses of Atrial Fibrillation

Recently, many studies have demonstrated the high rate of AF recurrence within the first few days after conversion to sinus rhythm. Restoration of sinus rhythm after AF is accompanied by the persistence of a high vulnerability to AF, which can easily recur [3]. To date, many reports have demonstrated in animal models and humans that this high vulnerability is related to atrial electro-

Dipartimento di Cardiologia, Ospedale Civile, Mirano, Italy

physiological changes occurring during AF. Atrial electrical remodeling includes shortening of the atrial effective refractory period, reversal of the physiological rate adaptation of the refractory period, spatial dispersion of atrial refractoriness, and reduction of conduction velocity. These changes have been reported to commence within a few minutes of the onset of AF and to be progressive. The time course of reversibility of the electrophysiological modifications that characterize atrial electrical remodeling has been seen to depend closely on the duration of AF. It is well established that after short periods (minutes or hours) of AF, atrial electrical remodeling resolves within a few minutes. By contrast, it has not yet been established how long the remodeling phenomenon lasts after long-standing AF (weeks or months).

Many mechanisms have been proposed to explain atrial electrical remodeling. The roles of ischemia, shifts in vagal or sympathetic tone, mechanical stretching of the atrial wall, increase in plasma natriuretic factor, and increase in outward potassium current have not been confirmed. By contrast, cytosolic calcium overload has been suggested as an important mediator of this phenomenon [7].

The duration of AF may have implications for the underlying cellular mechanisms involved in the cytosolic calcium overload. Changes in ionic pump activity or phosphorylation of ion channels occur within seconds or minutes after a change in heart rate. Only if the heart rate remains altered for days do processes other than metabolic adaptation come into play. Down-regulation of the L-type calcium channel and of Ca^{2+}-ATPase has been reported after 3 months of AF. Thus, in a later phase of AF, the decrease in the L-type calcium channel and in calcium uptake by Ca^{2+}-ATPase further contributes to the cytosolic calcium overload and to the shortening of the action potential duration. After several weeks of AF, structural changes may contribute to the maintenance of AF. The increase in mitochondrial size and disruption of the sarcoplasmic reticulum may further increase cytosolic calcium overload [7].

Clinical Studies on Serial Electrical Cardioversion Strategy

A policy of serial electrical cardioversion is often used to maintain sinus rhythm in patients with persistent AF. However, few studies have evaluated its usefulness. Moreover, in previous studies, either the follow-up duration was short or cardioversion was combined with serial antiarrhythmic drug treatments. Van Gelder et al. followed up for 3.7±1.6 years 236 patients after a first episode of AF lasting more than 24 h [4]. After 12 months, about 15% of patients who did not undergo repeated electrical cardioversion were in sinus rhythm, as against 40% of patients who had undergone more than one cardioversion. No further advantage in terms of maintenance of sinus rhythm was observed after the fourth electrical cardioversion.

More recently, two studies have evaluated the efficacy of serial electrical cardioversion in patients with persistent AF and early AF relapses. Fynn et al.

evaluated 45 patients with persistent AF and without antiarrhythmic treatment [8]. Up to three internal electrical cardioversions were performed as soon as possible after AF relapse, and patients were followed up for 1 month. Despite evidence of reversal of atrial electrical remodeling, only 17% of the patients who underwent repeated internal electrical cardioversion maintained sinus rhythm for 1 month.

Our group evaluated 90 patients who underwent a successful external electrical cardioversion for persistent AF. The patients, all on antiarrhythmic treatment, were randomly assigned in a 1:1 fashion to up to two repetitions of electrical cardioversion in the event of relapse of AF detected within 1 month of the previous cardioversion, or to nontreatment of AF relapses. After cardioversion AF recurred in 40% of patients during the first 30 days of follow-up: in 1% within 6 h, and in 28% within 7 days. At 12-month follow-up, 55% of patients randomized to receive repeat electrical cardioversion were in sinus rhythm, as against only 30% of patients randomized to nontreatment of AF recurrences ($p<0.03$) (Fig. 1)

By contrast, only 17% of patients treated by Fynn et al. with serial internal electrical cardioversion were in sinus rhythm at the 1-month examination [8]. The absence of antiarrhythmic treatment and the longer mean duration of AF in patients enrolled by Fynn et al. might explain this discrepancy.

At the same time, our results showed that repetition of more than one electrical cardioversion after early AF recurrence has limited clinical value. Sinus rhythm was maintained in 43% of patients who had only one repeat cardioversion, while only one of the seven patients (14%) who underwent a second repeat cardioversion was in sinus rhythm after 1 week.

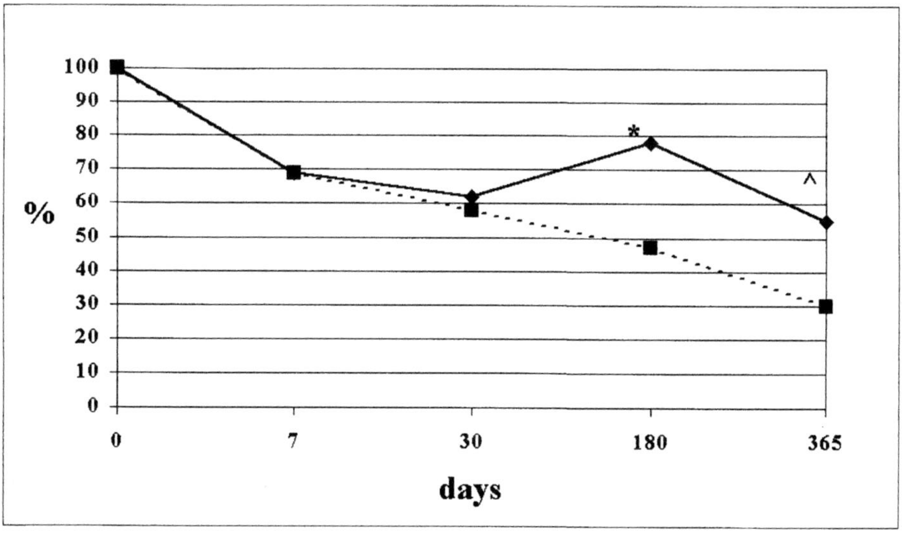

Fig. 1. AF-free survival curves of patients randomized to undergo repeat electrical cardioversions (u) or to nontreatment of AF recurrences (n) during the study period. * $p<0.005$; ^ $p<0.03$. (Reproduced from [6], with permission)

As discussed above, in patients with persistent AF, recovery from atrial electrical remodeling ranged from 12 to 72 h. Thus, the useful effect of our policy in maintaining sinus rhythm does not seem to be related to prevention of atrial electrical remodeling, as cardioversion was repeated too late after AF recurrence. Indeed, in patients with long-lasting AF, prevention of atrial electrical remodeling by means of prompt repetition of cardioversion did not produce any reduction in AF recurrences [8]. The question remains as to what kind of atrial remodeling prevention (ultrastructural, structural?) may be obtained by our successful serial electrical cardioversion policy [7].

Clinical Implications

Recently, two studies have evaluated the efficacy of serial electrical cardioversion in patients with persistent AF and early AF relapses. The findings from these studies disagreed. Perhaps a policy of repetition of electrical cardioversion after early recurrence of AF should be combined with the best antiarrhythmic treatment (preferably amiodarone) to increase persistence of sinus rhythm. Repetition of more than one cardioversion after early AF relapse has no clinical benefit.

References

1. Prystowsky EN, Benson DW, Fuster V et al (1996) Management of patients with atrial fibrillation. Circulation 93:1262–1277
2. Tieleman RG, Van Gelder I, Crijns HJ et al (1998) Early recurrences of atrial fibrillation after electrical cardioversion: a result of fibrillation-induced electrical remodeling of the atria? J Am Coll Cardiol 31:167–173
3. Wijffels MC, Kirchof CJ, Dorland R, Allessie MA (1995) Atrial fibrillation begets atrial fibrillation. Circulation 92:1954–1968
4. Van Gelder I, Crijns HJ, Tieleman RG et al (1996) Chronic atrial fibrillation. Success of serial cardioversion therapy and safety of oral anticoagulation. Arch Intern Med 156:2585–2592
5. Van Gelder I, Crijns HJ (1997) Cardioversion of atrial fibrillation and subsequent maintenance of sinus rhythm. Pacing Clin Electrophysiol 20(Pt II):2675–2683
6. Bertaglia E, D'Este D, Zerbo F, Zoppo, F, Delise P, Pascotto P (2002) Success of serial electrical cardioversion of persistent atrial fibrillation in maintaining sinus rhythm. Eur Heart J 23:1522–1528
7. Allessie MA (1998) Atrial electrophysiologic remodeling: another vicious circle? J Cardiovasc Electrophysiol 9:1378–1393
8. Fynn SP, Todd DM, Hobbs WJ, Armstrong KL, Fitzpatrick AP, Garratt CJ (2002) Clinical evaluation of a policy of early repeated internal cardioversion for recurrence of atrial fibrillation. J Cardiovasc Electrophysiol 13:135–141

MEDICAL TREATMENT OF ATRIAL FIBRILLATION: RHYTHM CONTROL AND RATE CONTROL

Which Is the Ideal Drug for Chronic Prophylaxis of Atrial Fibrillation?

G. Boriani, M. Biffi, I. Diemberger, C. Martignani, C. Camanini, C. Valzania, G. Domenichini, I. Corazza, A. Branzi

Prevention of Atrial Fibrillation Recurrences

A series of antiarrhythmic agents have been demonstrated to be highly effective in terminating recent-onset atrial fibrillation, class IC agents being the most effective [1, 2]. In contrast with the high efficacy shown in treating recent-onset atrial fibrillation, results obtained in preventing recurrences of atrial fibrillation are scanty [3–6]. Table 1 summarizes reported data from the literature. As shown, the percentage of patients who maintain sinus rhythm without arrhythmia recurrence under placebo treatment is around 30% after 3-6 months and around 20%–25% after 12 months. Antiarrhythmic agents may increase the percentage of patients who maintain sinus rhythm, but the overall efficacy is limited and, except for amiodarone, no more than 50% of the treated patients are free from arrhythmia recurrences after 6–12 months. For amiodarone, efficacy rates of 75%–78.5% at 6 months and of 50%–73% at 12 months have been reported.

Flecainide

The efficacy of flecainide in increasing time to the first atrial fibrillation recurrence and reducing atrial fibrillation burden is supported by two placebo-controlled studies [7, 8]. Moreover, other randomized studies [9, 10] evidenced comparable efficacy to that of quinidine, coupled with fewer side effects. Flecainide was shown to be effective in postponing the first recurrence of atrial fibrillation (in comparison with untreated patients) without the occurrence of severe ventricular proarrhythmia or sudden death, as reported by Van Gelder et al. [11]. Side effects were predominantly related to negative dromotropism and occurred in five patients (9%). Moreover, in the same study flecainide (200 mg daily) was superior to long-acting quinidine (1100 mg daily) in preventing recurrent atrial fibrillation after cardioversion.

Institute of Cardiology, University of Bologna, Italy

Table 1. Drugs used for preventing atrial fibrillation recurrences and sinus rhythm maintenance following cardioversion of atrial fibrillation

Drug	Sinus rhythm maintenance			
	At 1 month (%)	At 3 months (%)	At 6 months (%)	At 12 months (%)
Quinidine	65	44–75	27–58	23–51
Disopyramide	–	72	44–50	54
Procainamide	–	39	–	25
Propafenone	54	44	40	–
Flecainide	–	44	–	34–42
Amiodarone	–	–	75–78.5	50–73
Sotalol	–	49–50	46–50	37–46
Dofetilide	–	58–74	51–71	40–66
Placebo	58	15–56	19–35	0–45

Amiodarone

The efficacy of amiodarone for maintenance of sinus rhythm after atrial fibrillation conversion has been supported by many studies, but its relatively high incidence of side effects [12] justifies the common use of this agent as a second-line or last-resort option, with the important exception of heart failure. The efficacy of amiodarone in maintaining sinus rhythm was compared to the efficacy of propafenone and sotalol in the CTAF study [13]. This study enrolled a population in which 46% of patients had had a first episode of paroxysmal atrial fibrillation and 54% a persistent form of atrial fibrillation (in which at least half of the previous episodes required pharmacological or electrical intervention to resolve). Amiodarone prevented further attacks beyond the first month in a significantly higher proportion of the study population than did propafenone and sotalol (69% vs 39%, $p<0.001$). However, a higher incidence of side effects occurred in patients treated with amiodarone (18% vs 11%). The efficacy of amiodarone in paroxysmal atrial fibrillation refractory to one or more type I agents has been evaluated in uncontrolled observational studies [14–16]. Considering its side effect profile, amiodarone should only be used cautiously as a first-line agent in paroxysmal atrial fibrillation. As already mentioned, heart failure is an exception since amiodarone is superior to the other agents in terms of relative risks and benefits.

Few randomized studies have been performed to assess the efficacy of amiodarone for maintenance of sinus rhythm after cardioversion in patients with persistent atrial fibrillation. In a study of a cohort of postcardioversion patients [17], the group treated with amiodarone showed a significantly lower incidence of atrial fibrillation relapses in comparison with the patients who were given quinidine, and this was coupled with fewer side effects (although amiodarone side effects tend to occur later in the follow-up).

In a single-crossover study performed by Kerin et al. [18] amiodarone proved again to be superior to quinidine in achieving conversion of atrial fibrillation and long-term maintenance of sinus rhythm. Amiodarone was also better tolerated [18 of 27 amiodarone-treated patients (67%) were in sinus rhythm at 9 months vs 2 of 17 patients (12%) taking quinidine]. There are a large number of uncontrolled studies on amiodarone [14, 15, 19–23]. In a study involving 110 patients [14] with refractory atrial fibrillation or atrial flutter previously unsuccessfully treated with a median of two type I agents, amiodarone treatment was associated with recurrence during a 5-year follow-up in 9% of patients with persistent atrial fibrillation and in 40% of those with paroxysmal atrial fibrillation. Overall, a series of uncontrolled studies showed that amiodarone is an effective last-resort agent.

Dofetilide

Dofetilide is a rather new antiarrhythmic agent which is approved for use in the USA but not in Europe. Its efficacy in preventing atrial fibrillation and atrial flutter has been supported by two large-scale, double-blind, randomized studies [24, 25]. The reported conversion rates in the combined population of the SAFIRE-D (Symptomatic Atrial Fibrillation Investigative Research on Dofetilide) [24] and EMERALD [25] studies achieved by the administration of 125, 250, and 500 μg twice a day were respectively 6%, 10%, and 30% within 72 h (87% conversions obtained within 30 h). In these two studies the maintenance of sinus rhythm also appeared to be dose-dependent: in SAFIRE-D 40%, 52%, and 66% of patients in the three dosage groups respectively were in sinus rhythm at 6 months, compared with 21% of those in the placebo group [24]. In the EMERALD trial, 51%, 57%, and 71% of patients were free from atrial fibrillation relapses of regimens of 125, 250, and 500 μg daily, respectively, compared with approximately 25% in the placebo group and 60% of those receiving sotalol [25].

To reduce the risks of proarrhythmia, dofetilide treatment should be initiated in the hospital with dose titration based on renal function and cautious monitoring of the QT interval. In the above-mentioned studies the incidence of torsades de pointes was 0.8%, with a prevalent clustering in the first 3 days.

Proarrhythmic Effects

Today there is major concern over the risk of potentially fatal ventricular proarrhythmic effects caused by antiarrhythmic agents employed for a relatively benign arrhythmia such as atrial fibrillation [26, 27]. Indeed, an important issue that has emerged in last 15 years is the awareness of the risks related to drugs used for maintaining sinus rhythm.

The proarrhythmic risks of quinidine were assessed by a meta-analysis of six randomized trials on quinidine after atrial fibrillation cardioversion [28].

Although more effective in preventing recurrences than placebo, quinidine was associated with a three-fold increase in mortality risk (2.9% versus 0.8%). Caution has been suggested in interpreting these data in view of the limitations of meta-analysis, the possibility that concomitant treatment with digoxin or diuretics may have conditioned quinidine-related risks, the finding that the precise mode of death was not available for a significant proportion of deaths, and the fact that sudden death occurred only in 3 out of 12 patients who died on quinidine. The most typical quinidine-related proarrhythmic effect is torsades de pointes, the occurrence of which is associated with marked QT interval prolongation and is favored by hypokalemia, but is not related to quinidine dose [26]. The occurrence of torsades de pointes is favored by bradycardia or by a relatively slow heart rate, and for this reason during treatment with class IA agents (quinidine, disopyramide, procainamide) it occurs more often after termination of atrial fibrillation, when sinus rhythm is restored. In view of these findings, the use of quinidine has been restricted in recent years, and in patients who need to be treated with this drug, careful monitoring of QT interval changes in the first days of treatment is required. Initiation of treatment during an in-hospital stay is recommended in patients at higher risk of proarrhythmia [27, 29].

Sotalol, a β-blocker with class III antiarrhythmic activity, may also cause torsades de pointes, but the risk is dose-dependent, being around 1% for dosages between 160 and 240 mg daily and 4%–5% for dosages higher than 480 mg daily [26].

Class IC antiarrhythmic drugs (flecainide, propafenone) have a marked effect on conduction velocity, and like class IA agents may organize and slow the rate of atrial fibrillation, converting it into atrial flutter. In some cases the atrial rate is slow enough to allow 1:1 atrioventricular conduction, thus with rapid ventricular response, wide QRS complexes simulating ventricular tachycardia, and risk of hemodynamic impairment [26]. This proarrhythmic effect is favored by adrenergic stimulation and has been reported in 3%–5% of patients treated with flecainide or propafenone [26].

The risk of ventricular proarrhythmia, such as sustained ventricular tachycardia or ventricular fibrillation, during treatment with antiarrhythmics for supraventricular arrhythmias seems to be generally low, but patients with significant left ventricular dysfunction are potentially at higher risk.

For amiodarone, a low risk of ventricular proarrhythmic effects has been reported, even in patients with structural heart disease [30]. Amiodarone has little or no negative inotropic effect and is usually tolerated in patients with congestive heart failure. The mortality rate associated with amiodarone treatment is around 0.4%, comparable to that of control patients.

Other proarrhythmic effects, such as aggravation of sinus node disease in the brady–tachy syndrome or occurrence of high-degree atrioventricular block in patients with previous conduction disease, may occur with virtually any antiarrhythmic drug and are of great importance in elderly subjects.

In clinical practice, awareness of the problem of proarrhythmic effects is essential in order to prevent them, to identify them promptly, and to solve them. Some categories of patients who are at higher risk of proarrhythmia and can be identified are: (1) patients with previous myocardial infarction; (2) patients with overt or previous congestive heart failure; (3) patients with significant left ventricular dysfunction; (4) patients with previous conduction disease or sinus node dysfunction; (5) patients with electrolyte impairment; (6) patients with concomitant renal or hepatic insufficiency; and (7) patients of advanced age. For these patients, the effective need for antiarrhythmic treatment must be evaluated and the most appropriate drug selected [26, 29], accompanied by close monitoring of the patient in the first 2–3 days of treatment. In some cases it has been recommended that treatment should be started during hospitalization [27, 29]. In-hospital initiation is mandatory for dofetilide, in view of the potential risk of excessive QT prolongation at the beginning of treatment.

Noncardiac Adverse Effects

Noncardiac adverse effects cause intolerance, thus restricting patient compliance. However, these effects are usually reversible after drug withdrawal. For amiodarone, noncardiac toxicity has limited the widespread use of the drug. Some of its side effects, including hypo- or hyperthyroidism, are not dose-related. The most serious adverse effect of amiodarone is pulmonary toxicity, which occurs more frequently in older patients and when daily dose is higher than 300 mg daily. Unfortunately, the lowest effective dose of amiodarone which can be considered at very low risk of toxicity has still to be defined.

Choice of Antiarrhythmic Drugs in Different Clinical Conditions

The choice of an antiarrhythmic drug in clinical practice is based on proper evaluation of the patient's clinical condition and of the underlying heart disease, with special regard to the presence or absence of left ventricular dysfunction or heart failure. The choice of the most appropriate antiarrhythmic agent is based on a series of considerations that include (1) evaluation of the type of underlying heart disease and of the degree of hemodynamic impairment; (2) knowledge of the pharmacokinetic and pharmacodynamic properties of a specific antiarrhythmic agent, with particular regard to its hemodynamic effects; (3) knowledge of the proarrhythmic risk and of the other adverse effects that a specific agent may provoke in a specific clinical subset; and (4) assessment of the risk-benefit ratio of a specific antiarrhythmic agent. Therefore, a wide range of factors condition our choices and an agent such as flecainide, which is a first-choice treatment in patients without structural heart disease, has no specific indication to be used in a patient with ischemic heart disease with a previous myocardial infarction and left ventricular dysfunction.

In accordance with general considerations, a series of suggestions may help in the choice of the most appropriate antiarrhythmic agent for preventing atrial fibrillation recurrences, as shown in Table 2. This approach appears of landmark importance in clinical practice. Although alternative, nonpharmacological approaches for atrial fibrillation treatment have been proposed, antiarrhythmic agents will continue to be used given the incidence of this arrhythmia and its wide spectrum of clinical expression.

Table 2. Suggestions for the choice of antiarrhythmic agents (AA) for prevention of atrial fibrillation recurrences

	No structural heart disease or minimal heart disease	Hypertension/ left ventricular hypertrophy	Ischemic heart disease/previous myocardial infarction	Dilated cardiomyopathy/ heart failure
Patient's risk of proarrhythmia	Low	High	Moderate	High
First choice drug	Flecainide/ propafenone	Flecainide/ propafenone	Sotalol	Amiodarone
Second choice drug	Sotalol/ dofetilide	Amiodarone	Amiodarone/ dofetilide	Dofetilide
Gray zone	Amiodarone/ quinidine	Sotalol/ dofetilide	Propafenone	The other AA agents

References

1. Boriani G, Biffi M, Capucci A et al (1997) Oral propafenone to convert recent-onset atrial fibrillation in patients with and without underlying heart disease. A randomized, controlled trial. Ann Intern Med 126:621–625
2. Boriani G, Biffi M, Capucci A et al (1998) Conversion of recent-onset atrial fibrillation to sinus rhythm: effects of different drug protocols. Pacing Clin Electrophysiol 21:2470–2474
3. Boriani G, Biffi M, Branzi A et al (1998) Pharmacological treatment of atrial fibrillation: a review on prevention of recurrences and control of ventricular response. Arch Gerontol Geriatr 27:127–139
4. Jung F, DiMarco JP (1998) Treatment strategies for atrial fibrillation. Am J Med 104:272–286
5. Van Gelder IC, Crijns HJ (1998) Cardioversion of atrial fibrillation and subsequent maintenance of sinus rhythm. Pacing Clin Electrophysiol 20:2675–2683

6. Allessie MA (1998) Atrial electrophysiologic remodeling: another vicious circle? J Cardiovasc Electrophysiol 9:1378–1393
7. Anderson JL, Gilbert EM, Alpert BL et al (1989) Prevention of symptomatic recurrences of paroxysmal atrial fibrillation in patients initially tolerating antiarrhythmic therapy. A multicenter, double-blind, crossover study of flecainide and placebo with transtelephonic monitoring. Flecainide Supraventricular Tachycardia Study Group. Circulation 80:1557–1570
8. Pietersen AH, Hellemann H (1991) Usefulness of flecainide for prevention of paroxysmal atrial fibrillation and flutter. Danish-Norwegian Flecainide Multicenter Study Group. Am J Cardiol 67:713–717
9. Naccarelli G, Dorian P, Hohnloser SH et al (1996) Prospective comparison of flecainide versus quinidine for the treatment of paroxysmal atrial fibrillation/flutter. Am J Cardiol 77:53A–59A
10. van Wijk LM, den Heijer P, Crijns HJ et al (1989) Flecainide versus quinidine in the prevention of paroxysms of atrial fibrillation. J Cardiovasc Pharmacol 13:32–36
11. Van Gelder IC, Crijns HJ, Van Gilst WH et al (1989) Efficacy and safety of flecainide acetate in the maintenance of sinus rhythm after electrical cardioversion of chronic atrial fibrillation or atrial flutter. Am J Cardiol 64:1317–1321
12. Vorperian VR, Havighurst TC, Miller S et al (1997) Adverse effects of low dose amiodarone: a meta-analysis. J Am Coll Cardiol 30:791–798
13. Roy D, Talajic M, Dorian P et al (2000) Amiodarone to prevent recurrence of atrial fibrillation. Canadian Trial of Atrial Fibrillation Investigators. N Engl J Med 342:913–920
14. Chun SH, Sager PT, Stevenson WG et al (1995) Long-term efficacy of amiodarone for the maintenance of normal sinus rhythm in patients with refractory atrial fibrillation or flutter. Am J Cardiol 76:47–50
15. Horowitz LN, Spielman SR, Greenspan AM et al (1985) Use of amiodarone in the treatment of persistent and paroxysmal atrial fibrillation resistant to quinidine therapy. J Am Coll Cardiol 6:1402–1407
16. Tuzcu EM, Gilbo J, Masterson M et al (1989) The usefulness of amiodarone in management of refractory supraventricular tachyarrhythmias. Cleve Clin J Med 56:238–242
17. Vitolo E, Tronci M, Larovere M et al (1981) Amiodarone versus quinidine in the prophylaxis of atrial fibrillation. Acta Cardiol 36:431–434
18. Kerin NZ, Faitel K, Naini M (1996) The efficacy of intravenous amiodarone for the conversion of chronic atrial fibrillation: amiodarone vs quinidine for conversion of atrial fibrillation. Arch Intern Med 156:49–53
19. Opolski G, Stanislawska J, Gorecki A et al (1997) Amiodarone in restoration and maintenance of sinus rhythm in patients with chronic atrial fibrillation after unsuccessful direct-current cardioversion. Clin Cardiol 20:337–340
20. Gosselink AT, Crijns HJ, Van Gelder IC et al (1992) Low-dose amiodarone for maintenance of sinus rhythm after cardioversion of atrial fibrillation or flutter. JAMA 267:3289–3293
21. Gold RL, Haffajee CI, Charos G et al (1986) Amiodarone for refractory atrial fibrillation. Am J Cardiol 57:124–127
22. Blevins RD, Kerin NZ, Benaderet D et al (1987) Amiodarone in the management of refractory atrial fibrillation. Arch Intern Med 147:1401–1404
23. Brodsky MA, Allen BJ, Walker CJ 3rd et al (1987) Amiodarone for maintenance of sinus rhythm after conversion of atrial fibrillation in the setting of a dilated left atrium. Am J Cardiol 60:572–575

24. Singh S, Zoble RG, Yellen L et al (2000) Efficacy and safety of oral dofetilide in converting to and maintaining sinus rhythm in patients with chronic atrial fibrillation or atrial flutter: the symptomatic atrial fibrillation investigative research on dofetilide (SAFIRE–D) study. Circulation 102:2385–2390
25. Greenbaum RA, Campbell TJ, Channer KS et al (1998) Conversion of atrial fibrillation and maintenance of sinus rhythm by dofetilide: the EMERALD (European and Australian Multicenter Evaluative Research on Atrial Fibrillation Dofetilide) Study. Circulation 98:1663–I
26. Falk RH (1998) Proarrhythmia in patients treated for atrial fibrillation or flutter. Ann Intern Med 117:141-150
27. Waldo AL, Prystowsky EN (1998) Drug treatment of atrial fibrillation in the managed care era. Am J Cardiol 81:23C–29C
28. Coplen SE, Antman EM, Berlin JA et al (1990) Efficacy and safety of quinidine therapy for maintenance of sinus rhythm after cardioversion. A meta-analysis of randomized control trials. Circulation 82:1106–1116
29. Fuster V, Ryden LE, Asinger RW et al (2001) ACC/AHA/ESC guidelines for the management of patients with atrial fibrillation: executive summary. A report of the American College of Cardiology/ American Heart Association Task Force on Practice Guidelines and the European Society of Cardiology Committee for Practice Guidelines and Policy Conferences (committee to develop guidelines for the management of patients with atrial fibrillation): developed in collaboration with the North American Society of Pacing and Electrophysiology. J Am Coll Cardiol 38:1231–1266
30. Middlekauff HR, Wiener I, Saxon LA et al (1992) Low-dose amiodarone for atrial fibrillation: time for a prospective study? Ann Intern Med 116:1017–1020

ACE Inhibitors and Angiotensin Receptor Blockers: a New Effective Non-Conventional Approach to Prevent Atrial Fibrillation

A.H. Madrid, C. Escobar, J.M.G. Rebollo, I. Marín, E. Bernal, L. Limón, S. Nannini, J. Peng, C. Moro

The Problem of Atrial Fibrillation

Atrial fibrillation is the most frequent arrhythmia found in clinical practice. Atrial fibrillation doubles mortality and increases the risk of stroke. The early appearance of electrical remodeling is followed by structural remodeling of the atrial tissue. In the past decade, arrhythmologists have been encouraged to investigate the etiology and pathophysiology of this type of frequent arrhythmia. These investigations have resulted in new concepts on the initiation and perpetuation of this arrhythmia. New techniques are being developed for its treatment. However, the majority of patients are candidates for the traditional treatment: antiarrhythmic drugs and/or electrical cardioversion. Direct current cardioversion of persistent atrial fibrillation is the most effective treatment for the restoration of sinus rhythm, but it may be hampered by a high percentage of recurrences. Many of the recurrences are probably the clinical consequence of electrical remodelling [1, 2], due to the changes in refractory period of atrial muscle and/or due to abnormal activity occurring inside the pulmonary veins. This could explain the drug-resistance of long-standing atrial fibrillation.

Studies With Non-Antiarrhythmic Drugs

Some studies with non antiarrhythmic drugs have demonstrated a positive effect to prevent episodes of atrial fibrillation, both in humans and in animals. Pedersen et al. [3] investigated the effect of Trandolapril on the incidence of atrial fibrillation in patients with reduced left ventricular function. Trandolapril reduced the risk of developing atrial fibrillation by 55 %. Angiotensin converting enzyme (ACE) inhibitors could be effective based on

Arrhythmia Unit, Ramón y Cajal Hospital, Department of Medicine, Alcalá University, Madrid, Spain their favorable effects on cardiovascular fibrosis and apoptosis [4]. The study carried out by Nakashima et al. [5] demonstrated for the first time that angiotensin II contributes to atrial electrical remodeling. In their study, the shortening of the atrial refractory period during rapid pacing was prevented by treatment with Candesartan or Captopril, but increased by angiotensin II. Other recent studies have demonstrated the ability of Losartan to regress fibrosis in hypertensives with biopsy-proven myocardial fibrosis, independently of its antihypertensive efficacy. This suggest that blockade of the angiotensin II type AT_1 receptor is associated with inhibition of collagen type I synthesis and regression of myocardial fibrosis [6] (Fig. 1). Thus, data from studies with ACE inhibitors provide evidence that the renin-angiotensin-aldosterone system plays a role as a mediator of atrial remodeling in atrial fibrillation. These are the reasons why we performed the study: "Use of Irbesartan to maintain sinus rhythm in patients with long-lasting persistent atrial fibrillation. A prospective and randomised study [7]". This study has evaluated the effect of treatment with the AT_1 receptor blocker, Irbesartan, to maintain sinus rhythm after conversion from persistent atrial fibrillation. On the other hand, several trials have previously evaluated the safety of low-dose Amiodarone, and have shown that it can be used safely with appropriate monitoring [8, 9].

In our study, patients must have had an episode of persistent atrial fibrillation (> 7 days). These patients were then randomised and scheduled for electrical cardioversion. Two groups were compared: group I, treated with amiodarone and group II, treated with amiodarone plus Irbesartan. The primary end point was the length of time to a first recurrence of atrial fibrillation. A total of 186 patients were enrolled in the study. 154 were analysed by intention to treat analysis. Seventy-five patients were randomly allocated to group I and 79 patients to group II. After two months of follow-up, in the intention to treat

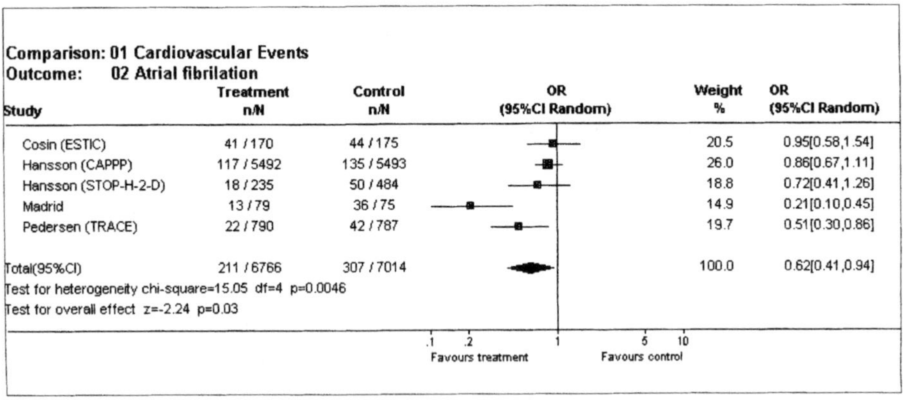

Fig. 1. Comparison of ACE inhibitors/angiotensin receptor blockers versus other treatment on the incidence of new or recurrent atrial fibrillation, excluding the STOP-H-2 trial and including the published sub-study of this trial, with the elderly and diabetic patients (STOP-H-2-D). The result is statistically significant (p=0.03)

analysis, the group treated with Irbesartan had a lower number of patients with recurrent atrial fibrillation (Kaplan - Meier analysis, 84.79 % vs 63.16 %, p=0.008). The Kaplan-Meier analysis of time to first recurrence during the follow-up period (median time 254 days, range 60-710 days) also showed that patients treated with Irbesartan had a greater probability of remaining free of atrial fibrillation (79.52 % vs 55.91 %, p=0.007).

The results of this prospective and randomized study showed that an angiotensin II receptor blocker, Irbesartan (a long-acting AT_1 receptor antagonist, with a high affinity for the AT_1 receptor), added to Amiodarone was more effective in the maintenance of sinus rhythm in patients with persistent atrial fibrillation cardioverted to sinus rhythm. Most of the benefit of Irbesartan occurred during the first 2 months after conversion. After that, the two curves seem to be parallel. This is similar to some recent studies and points to the importance of the remodeling just after cardioversion [10]. Moreover, after categorizing the failures of electrical cardioversion and recurrences, we demonstrated that Irbesartan reduced the immediate recurrence of atrial fibrillation and the so-called subacute recurrences during the first weeks [11].

There are multiple possible mechanisms by which Irbesartan (or ACE inhibitors) may have antiarrhythmic efficacy. These include decrease of wall stress, modulation of refractoriness, interference with ion currents, modification of sympathetic tone and stabilization of electrolyte concentrations. Further evidence of a positive interaction between antagonists of type I receptors of angiotensin II and potassium channel blockers comes from some recent studies, including Irbesartan, where transmembrane action potentials and currents have been evaluated [12, 13]. The results have demonstrated that at therapeutic concentrations Losartan modified the cardiac delayed rectifier hKv 1.5, HERG and Ks currents. These effects suggest possible antiarrhythmic (and/or proarrhythmic) properties.

The modern clinical approach in the fight against atrial fibrillation involves an early intervention to restore sinus rhythm, therefore preventing atrial remodeling. This approach is now being questioned by the publication of two important studies; one American [14] and the other European [15]. Their results pointed out that there was no advantage in survival of rhythm control versus rate control in an elderly population (around the age of 60 in both studies). The study AFFIRM tried to show which of the two approaches to the treatment of atrial fibrillation could be better: cardioversion with antiarrhythmic drugs to maintain sinus rhythm, or the use of rate-controlling drugs. They conducted a randomized, multicenter comparison of these two treatment strategies in patients with atrial fibrillation and a high risk of stroke or death. Younger patients without risk factors for stroke were not included in these studies. Furthermore, the proportion of patients using betablockers in the rhythm-control group was significantly smaller than that in the rate-control group. This difference is important, because betablockers improve the prognosis in many patients with the same clinical characteristics as the patients included in the AFFIRM trial. In both groups, but mostly in the rhythm-control group, the majority of strokes occurred after Warfarin had been stopped or when the international normalized ratio was subtherapeutic. Furthermore, non antiarrhythmic drugs to prevent recurrences, like Irbesartan, were not used or controlled. The advantage of remaining in sinus rhythm was probably offset by the adverse effects of multiple antiarrhythmic drugs used in these studies (quinidina, felcainide, moricizine, disopiramide, amiodarone, popafenone, or combinations). More than a decade ago, Coplen et al. [16], published the results of a meta-analysis with Quinidine. The evidence was clear that Quinidine was effective in preventing recurrences, but with an increase in mortality (typical odds ratio 2.98, $p < 0.05$).

The treatment against atrial fibrillation has recently begun with new cardioprotective agents capable of preventing remodeling [7] or modifying ionic channels [13]. We should not forget that catheter ablation has demonstrated a solution for many arrhythmias. Some cases of atrial fibrillation could be prevented and cured by ablation of the supraventricular tachycardia substrates and the pulmonary veins' foci while achieving isolation from the left atrial myocardium.

The data from the AFFIRM and RACE trials confirm that rate-control is an acceptable approach, depending upon the specific clinical circumstances. We have to remind that most patients with atrial fibrillation should be chronically anticoagulated. In patients who are highly symptomatic, rate-control may be insufficient to control symptoms. In this setting, rhythm-control should be attempted more aggressively.

We have conducted a meta-analysis of all randomized controlled clinical trials that compared angiotensin receptor blockers and/or ACE inhibitors with either placebo or conventional therapy in patients with either hypertension, heart failure, ischemic heart disease or diabetes mellitus. The pooled outcome was the development of atrial fibrillation. Five trials involving a total of 19,675 patients were included (8736 randomized to active therapy and 10939 to control). Overall, there was no significant statistical difference in the pooled development of atrial fibrillation between the treatment and control group (odds ratio: 0.70; 95 % confidence interval: 0.47 to 1.05; test for overall effect $z = -1{,}71$ $p = 0.09$). However, after the inclusion of the higher risk patients of a trial reported separately (STOP-H-2), involving a total of 13,780 patients (6,766 randomized to active therapy and 7,446 to control), there was a significant statistical difference in the pooled development of atrial fibrillation (odds ratio: 0.62; 95 % confidence interval: 0.41 to 0.94; test for overall effect $z = -2.24$ $p = 0.03$).

Conclusions

There is no doubt that new randomized and controlled studies, most probably with the combination of two drugs like antiarrhythmics and non antiarrhythmic drugs, are needed to reach a definitive answer for the treatment of atrial fibrillation. The pretreatment of patients with atrial fibrillation who undergo electrical cardioversion is very important and will be the subject for continuous improvement.

References

1. Allessie MA (1998) Atrial electrophysiological remodeling: another vicious circle? J Cardiovasc Electrophysiol 9:1378-1393
2. Wijffels MCEF, Kirchhof CJHJ, Dorland R, Allessie MA, Begets AF (1995) A study in awake chronically instrumented goats. Circulation 92:1954-1968
3. Pedersen OD, Bagger H, Køber L, Torp-Pedersen C (1999) Trandolapril reduces the incidence of atrial fibrillation after acute myocardial infarction in patients with left ventricular dysfunction. Circulation 100:376-380
4. Fortuño MA, Ravassa S, Etayo JC, Diez J (1998) Overexpression of Bax protein and enhanced apoptosis in the left ventricle of spontaneously hypertensive rats. Effects of AT_1 blockade with losartan. Hypertension 32:280-286
5. Nakashima H, Kumagai K, Urata H et al (2000) Angiotensin II Antagonist Prevents Electrical Remodeling in Atrial Fibrillation. Circulation 101:2612-2617
6. López B, Querejeta R, Varo N et al (2001) Usefulness of serum carboxy-terminal propeptide of procollagen type I in assessment of the cardioreparative ability of antihypertensive treatment in hypertensive patients. Circulation 104: 286-291
7. Madrid AH, Bueno MG, Rebollo JM et al (2002) Use of irbesartan to maintain sinus rhythm in patients with long-lasting persistent atrial fibrillation. a prospective and randomized study. Circulation 106:331-336
8 Roy D, Talajic M, Dorian P et al (2000) Amiodarone to prevent recurrence of atrial fibrillation. Canadian Trial of Atrial Fibrillation Investigators. N Engl J Med 342(13):913-920
9. Kochiadakis GE, Igoumenidis NE, Marketou ME et al (1998) Low-dose amiodarone versus sotalol for suppression of recurrent symptomatic atrial fibrillation. Am J Cardiol 81:995-998
10. Kühlkamp V, Schirdewan A, Stangl K et al (2000) Use of metoprolol CR/XL to maintain sinus rhythm after conversion from persistent atrial fibrillation. J Am Coll Cardiol 36:139-146
11. Crijns HJGM, Van Noord T, Van Gelder IC (2001) Recurrence of atrial fibrillation and the need for new definitions. Eur Heart J 22:1769-1771
12. Caballero R, Delpón E, Valenzuela C et al (2002) Losartan and its metabolite E3174 modify cardiac delayed rectifier K+ currents. Circulation 101:1199-1205
13. Moreno I, Caballero R, Gonzalez T et al (2003) Effects of irbersartan on cloned potassium channels involved in human cardiac repolarization. J Pharmacol Exp Ther :304
14. Wyse DG, Waldo AL, DiMarco JP et al (2002) A comparison of rate control and rhythm control in patients with atrial fibrillation. N Engl J Med 347(23):1825-1833
15. Van Gelder IC, Hagens VE, Bosker HA et al (2002) A comparison of rate control and rhythm control in patients with recurrent persistent atrial fibrillation. N Engl J Med 347(23):1834-1840
16. Coplen SE, Antman EM, Berlin JA, Hewitt P, Chalmers TC (1990) Efficacy and safety of quinidine therapy for maintenance of sinus rhythm after cardioversion. A meta-analysis of randomized control trials. Circulation 82(4):1106-1116

Rate Control of Atrial Fibrillation: By How Much Should the Ventricular Rate be Lowered?

P. Alboni[1], L. Gianfranchi[1], G. Fucà[1], F. Pacchioni[1], G. Corbucci[2]

Heart rate (HR) should be neither too high, since it can be responsible for tachycardia-induced cardiomyopathy [1, 2], nor too low, since it can facilitate the appearance of heart failure, at least in old people with heart disease [3, 4]. Moreover, mounting evidence shows that an elevated resting sinus rate is a predictor of cardiovascular morbidity and mortality. In fact, in multivariate analysis, a high sinus rate emerged as an independent predictor of mortality in the general population [5], in elderly subjects [6], and in selected groups of patients with hypertension [7] or myocardial infarction [8]. At present the prognostic value of resting HR in patients with chronic atrial fibrillation (AF) is unknown; however, it should be expected to be the same.

To date, no clear demonstration of the "optimal HR" for any particular activity has been made. Some contributions have been offered by studies carried out in pacemaker patients, where the relationship between pacing rate and cardiac output (CO) has been investigated [9, 10]. Results suggest that a three-phase relationship exists between CO and pacing rate at rest and during constant exercise. When starting at a low rate, increasing the pacing rate leads to an increase in CO (phase I), then little change in CO (phase II), after which further increases in the pacing rate lead to a decrease in CO (phase III). In patients with impaired left ventricular function phase II may be absent or reduced. To find the optimal HR, consideration has to be given to the fact that the higher the HR, the greater the energy consumption. Increasing HR not only decreases the efficiency of the heart, but reduces diastolic time. As coronary impedance is lower during diastole than systole, its average value will increase if the diastolic time is decreased, especially in the endocardial tissue. Coronary blood flow occurs mainly during diastole; therefore maximizing the diastolic interval is important. From this it follows that the optimum HR is the lowest one at which maximum CO is achieved (i.e., the onset of phase II). However, in the clinical setting, definition of this exact point appears unrealistic. Moreover, the bound-

[1]Division of Cardiology and Arrhythmologic Center, Cento (Fe), Italy, and [2]Vitatron

aries of phase II have been defined and the optimal rate lies within this rate band [10]. The mean of the optimal rate bands has also been calculated at each workload [10]. This has been shown to vary both individually and with the workload, increasing with greater loads in a nonlinear fashion. Of more clinical concern is the lack of correlation between optimal HR and age or predicted peak HR. The variability of this mean rate means that the "optimal HR" for one individual will be suboptimal in another. Therefore, the data obtained by this technique appear to be of very little utility in the clinical setting.

Heart Rate in Patients with Atrial Fibrillation

In some studies HR and exercise capacity have been investigated in the same patients during both AF and sinus rhythm, and this allows each patient to serve as his or her own control. Atwood et al. [11] investigated 11 patients (mean age 59 years); mean HR was significantly higher during AF at rest (105 ± 13 versus 66 ± 9 beats/min), during submaximal workload (156 ± 26 versus 109 ± 18 beats/min, p <0.001), and during maximal exercise (192 ± 24 versus 144 ± 21 beats/min, p <0.001). Similar results were reported by Ostermaier et al. [12]. Ueshima et al. [13] compared maximal HR in 79 male patients with AF (mean age 64 years) who were classified into five groups: lone AF, hypertension, ischemic heart disease, cardiomyopathy or history of heart failure, and valvular heart disease. The mean maximal HR was about 20 beats/min higher than that estimated for age. Maximal HRs were particularly high in patients with lone AF and in those with hypertension (190 ± 7 and 187 ± 8 beats/min, respectively). The mean maximal HR observed among subjects with lone AF was higher than that in patients with heart failure (164 ± 5 and 162 ± 8 beats/min, respectively; p <0.05). In these studies resting, submaximal, and maximal HRs showed marked variations from patient to patient.

Exercise capacity has been investigated by some authors in the same patients during both sinus rhythm and AF. Atwood et al. [11], in a small group of patients, observed at maximal exertion a slightly reduced exercise capacity during AF. In fact maximal minute ventilation, carbon dioxide production, oxygen pulse, and respiratory exchange ratio were significantly lower when patients were in AF (minute ventilation 73 ± 17 versus 81 ± 16 l/min, p <0.05; carbon dioxide production 1.9 ± 0.6 versus 2.3 ± 0.7 l/min, p <0.01; respiratory exchange ratio 1.0 ± 0.1 versus 1.1 ± 0.6, p <0.01). In the 63 patients reported by Ostermaier et al. [12] the exercise capacity of the whole group during sinus rhythm was 426 ± 180 s and decreased to 402 ± 168 during AF. A similar trend was observed in the patients with lone AF and in those with structural heart disease. Exercise capacity declined in both young (≤ 64 years) and older patients (–22 s versus –27 s, p = NS). Patients with left ventricular dysfunction who developed AF had a 72-s decline in exercise capacity compared with 12-s decline in patients with normal left ventricular function. The difference did not reach statistical significance; however, the group with left ventricular dysfunction (7 patients) may have been too small. These results show that the development of chronic AF results in only a mild decrease in cardiovascular performance as reflected by exercise duration. This effect seems to occur to a similar extent in all groups of patients and is unrelated to the underlying heart condition. However, there are not enough data to draw conclusions about the patients with left ventricular dysfunction or heart failure. Other authors [13, 14] evaluated the response of patients with chronic AF to exercise and observed a lower exercise capacity in the patients with structural heart disease than in those with lone AF, and concluded that exercise impairment in patients with AF is due to underlying heart disease and not to the arrhythmia itself. In the absence of a control group (patients in sinus rhythm) this conclusion is only apparently contrasting. However, it must be underlined that among the various groups of patients there is marked individual variability with regard to the increase in resting and exercise HR and the decrease in exercise tolerance after the appearance of AF. Moreover, it has been reported that some patients with AF show a marked increase of HR during the early part of the exercise test and others only during the late part [15].

The above data show that in patients with AF, a high HR should be lowered in order to reduce the risk of tachycardia-induced cardiomyopathy and other cardiovascular events (prognostic task) and to improve, at least in some patients, exercise capacity (hemodynamic task). Therefore, we should control HR. But what is meant by "control" of HR? When applied to the HR in AF, the term "controlled" is generally used loosely to mean "not excessive". In the ACC/AHA/ESC guidelines [16], the HR is generally considered controlled when it ranges between 60 and 80 beats/min at rest and between 90 and 115 beats/min during moderate exercise, as proposed by Resnekov and McDonald [17] and Atwood et al. [18]. Rawles [19] investigated the slope of CO/HR in patients with AF and found it to be positive in all patients with a resting HR below 80 beats/min and negative in 40% of those with a HR greater than 90 beats/min. In Rawles' opinion, in AF the HR can be regarded as "controlled" when the CO/HR is positive and "uncontrolled" when the slope is negative, that is, when a rise in HR would lead to decreased CO. So defined, HR at rest was controlled in every patient when the HR was less than 90 beats/min, in 73% of patients when it was 90–140 beats/min, and uncontrolled in every case when it was greater than 140 beats/min. The mean predicted value of HR for maximum CO was 122 beats/min, with wide individual variation ranging from 60 to 200 beats/min.

A range this wide precludes any definition of a general rule. During AF the effects of a controlled HR on hemodynamics are difficult to predict because of the complex relationship between diastolic ventricular filling time, HR, and the loss of atrial systole, and these effects seem to be different from patient to patient at rest and above all during exercise. In this regard, no accepted criteria for "optimal HR during exercise" exist in patients with chronic AF. Corbelli et al. [15] defined a maximal HR as good if it was greater than 85% and less than 115% of the maximal predicted HR. These limits defined two standard deviations from the mean of a normal population in sinus rhythm. However, no specific experimental or clinical data are available to support this definition.

In a recent study, Zhang et al. [20] determined in 14 dogs, after induction of AF, the hemodynamic changes at each level of HR slowing, using a method for computerized vagally controlled HR slowing. Four target average HR levels, corresponding to 75%, 100%, 125%, and 150% of the sinus cycle length, were achieved by computer feedback algorithm. Slowing the HR to the sinus rate or slightly faster (average RR interval in the range of 75%–100% of the sinus cycle length) appeared to yield best overall results. In fact, rapid irregular electrical activation of the ventricles during AF resulted in many aborted beats, that is, electrical activation without subsequent stroke volume. In such beats, left ventricular contraction resulted in an insufficient left ventricular pressure, less than the diastolic arterial blood pressure level. As a result, the aortic valve did not open and no blood was ejected from the left ventricle. With producing HR slowing, these aborted beats were dramatically reduced and all the hemodynamic variables improved. These results suggest that during AF the HR should be rather slow, similar to the HR observed during normal sinus rhythm. These data appear very interesting; however, they were obtained in dogs and cannot be directly translated into the clinical setting.

Some authors [21, 22] have tried to define optimal HR during AF by an analysis of ventricular efficiency by means of ventriculoarterial coupling. In accordance with this method, left ventricular properties are quantified using the slope and volume axis intercept of the linear end-systolic pressure–volume relationship. At present, these data appear only speculative.

Heart Rate Reduction by Cardiovascular Drugs

Some cardiovascular drugs such as digoxin, β-blockers, and calcium antagonists (verapamil and diltiazem) are widely used for HR slowing in patients with chronic AF. Digoxin slows resting HR by 13%–24%, but generally fails to control HR during exercise [23–25]. The drug does not significantly change exercise capacity [25].

β-Blockers have been shown to be effective in reducing resting HR and HR during exercise. Reductions in maximal HR have been demonstrated in the order of 25–40 beats/min, ranging from 22% to 33% [26–32]. Control of the exercise is generally thought to make the heart more efficient by increasing ventricular filling time and therefore end-diastolic volume, leading to an increase in stroke volume. On the other hand, HR control by β-blockade has resulted in reduction of oxygen uptake (VO_2), CO, and exercise time by 15%–20% in some studies [27, 29, 32], although β-blockade has had minimal effects in others [30, 31]. These data suggest a compensatory mechanism of high HRs during maximal exercise in patients with chronic AF. However, the effects of β-blockade on maximal HR, VO_2, and exercise capacity varied considerably from patient to patient.

Verapamil and diltiazem slow resting and exercise HR, and the effect of these two drugs is of similar magnitude [33]. The reduction of maximal HR after calcium antagonist administration appears lower than after β-blockade, ranging from 12% to 20% [33–36]. In some studies maximal VO_2 and exercise tolerance slightly improved after oral administration of verapamil or diltiazem [33, 37]; in other studies neither diltiazem nor verapamil was reported to change exercise tolerance [34, 36]. As after β-blockade, there was marked variability from patient to patient in maximum HR response and exercise capacity.

Conclusions

Definitions of optimal HR in chronic AF have been made on the basis of electrocardiographic and hemodynamic data (exercise capacity), and results of experimental and clinical studies suggest that resting HR should be similar to that observed during normal sinus rhythm, at least in most patients. However, even if controlled at rest, HR markedly varies from subject to subject during moderate or maximal exercise. Moreover, another important point to be considered is *the clinical presentation* and *the symptoms,* in particular *palpitation.*

At present it is not clear whether target HR differs in the presence or absence of heart disease. However, because of different types of hemodynamic involvement, in some diseases, such as aortic or mitral insufficiency, a rather high HR is preferable and in others, such as mitral stenosis or coronary heart disease, a rather low HR is recommended. A very important point is the target HR in patients with heart failure and AF. The optimal HR has never been clearly defined; however, several data suggest that the HR should be rather slow, at least in most patients [38].

Improvement of symptoms remains a mandatory task in order to improve quality of life; Holter recording or effort test can be useful in some patients in order to adequately treat palpitation or dyspnea during moderate exercise. As previously mentioned, some cardiovascular drugs are available with different effects on exercise HR.

In conclusion, an optimal HR does not exist in patients with AF; HR should be controlled individually on the basis of electrocardiographic and hemodynamic findings and, above all, the presence of symptoms.

References

1. Keane JF, Plauth WH, Nadas AS (1974) Chronic ectopic tachycardia of infancy and childhood. Am Heart J 84:748–757
2. Peters KG, Kienzle MG (1988) Severe cardiomyopathy due to chronic rapidly conducted atrial fibrillation: complete recovery after restoration of sinus rhythm. Am J Med 85:242–244
3. Alboni P, Menozzi C, Brignole M et al (1997) Effects of permanent pacemaker and

oral theophylline in sick sinus syndrome. The THEOPACE study: a randomized controlled trial. Circulation 96:260–266
4. Alboni P, Brignole M, Menozzi C, Scarfò S (1999) Is sinus bradycardia a factor facilitating overt heart failure? Eur Heart J 20:252–255
5. Kannel WB, Kannel C, Paffenbarger RS, Cupples LA (1987) Heart rate and cardiovascular mortality: the Framingham study. Am Heart J 113:1489–1494
6. Aronow WS, Ahn C, Mercando AD et al (1996) Association of average heart rate on 24-hour ambulatory electrocardiograms with incidence of new coronary events at 48-month follow-up in 1311 patients (mean age 81 years) with heart disease and sinus rhythm. Am J Cardiol 78:1175–1176
7. Gillman MW, Kannel WB, Belanger A, D'Agostino RB (1993) Influence of heart rate on mortality among persons with hypertension: the Framingham study. Am Hear J 125:1148–1154
8. Zuanetti G, Hernandez-Bernal F, Rossi A et al (1999) Relevance of heart rate as a prognostic factor in myocardial infarction: the GISSI experience. Eur Heart J 1:52H–57H
9. Geddes LA, Wessale JL (1991) Cardiac output, stroke volume and pacing rate: a review of the literature and a proposed technique for selection of the optimum pacing rate for an exercise responsive pacemaker. J Cardiovasc Electrophysiol 2:408–415
10. Payne G, Spinelli J, Garrat CJ, Skehan JD (1997) The optimal pacing rate: an umpredictable parameter. Pacing Clin Electrophysiol 20:866–873
11. Atwood JE, Myers J, Sullivan M et al (1989) The effect of cardioversion on maximal exercise capacity in patients with chronic atrial fibrillation. Am Heart J 118:913–918
12. Ostermaier RH, Lampert S, Dalla Vecchia L, Ravid S (1997) The effect of atrial fibrillation and the ventricular rate control on exercise capacity. Clin Cardiol 20:23–27
13. Ueshima K, Myers J, Ribisl PM et al (1993) Hemodynamic determinants of exercise capacity in chronic atrial fibrillation. Am Heart J 125:1301–1305
14. Atwood JE, Myers J, Sullivan M et al (1988) Maximal exercise testing and gas exchange in patients with chronic atrial fibrillation. J Am Coll Cardiol 11:508–513
15. Corbelli R, Masterson R, Wilkoff BL (1990) Chronotropic response to exercise in patients with atrial fibrillation. Pacing Clin Electrophysiol 13:179–187
16. ACC/AHA/ESC guidelines for the management of patients with atrial fibrillation (2001) Eur Heart J 22:1852–1923
17. Resnekov L, McDonald L (1971) Electroconversion of lone atrial fibrillation and flutter including hemodynamic studies at rest and on exercise. Br Heart J 33:339–350
18. Atwood JE, Myers J, Sandhu S et al (1989) Optimal sampling interval to estimate heart rate at rest and during exercise in atrial fibrillation. Am J Cardiol 63:45–48
19. Rawles JM (1990) What is meant by a "controlled" ventricular rate in atrial fibrillation? Br Heart J 63:157–161
20. Zhang Y, Mowrey KA, Zhuang S et al (2002) Optimal ventricular rate slowing during atrial fibrillation by feedback AV nodal-selective vagal stimulation. Am J Physiol Heart Circ Physiol 282:H1102–H1110
21. Sunagawa K, Maughan WL, Sagawa K (1985) Optimal arterial resistance for the maximal stroke work studied in isolated canine left ventricle. Circ Res 56:586–595
22. Nobuoka S, Hatano S, Nagashima J et al (2002) Determination of the target ventricular rate in patients with atrial fibrillation by evaluation of ventriculoarterial coupling. Tex Heart Inst 29:100–104
23. Lang R, Klein HO, Weiss E et al (1983) Superiority of oral verapamil therapy to digoxin in treatment of chronic atrial fibrillation. Chest 83:491–499
24. Beasley R, Smith DA, McHaggie DJ (1985) Exercise heart rate at different serum

digoxin concentration in patients with atrial fibrillation. Br Med J 290:9–11

25. Zarowitz BJ, Gheorghiede M (1992) Optimal heart rate control for patients with chronic atrial fibrillation: are pharmacological choices truly changing? Am Heart J 123:1401–1403
26. Yahalom J, Klein H, Kaplinsky E (1977) Beta-adrenergic blockade as adjunctive oral therapy in patients with chronic atrial fibrillation. Chest 71:582–592
27. Di Bianco R, Morganroth J, Freitag JA et al (1984) Effects of nadolol on the spontaneous and exercise-provoked heart rate of patients with chronic atrial fibrillation receiving stable dosages of digoxin. Am Heart J 108:1121–1127
28. Molajo AO, Coupe MO, Bennet DH (1984) Effect of Corwin (ICI 118587) on resting and exercise heart rate and exercise tolerance in digitalised patients with chronic atrial fibrillation. Br Heart J 52:392–395
29. Atwood JE, Sullivan M, Forbes S et al (1987) Effects of beta-adrenergic blockade on exercise performance in patients with chronic atrial fibrillation. J Am Coll Cardiol 10:314–320
30. Zoble RG, Brewington J, Olukotun AY et al (1987) Comparative effects of nadolol-digoxin combination therpay and digoxin monotherapy for chronic atrial fibrillation. Am J Cardiol 60:39D–45D
31. Wong CK, Lau CP, Leung WH et al (1990) Usefulness of labetalol in chronic atrial fibrillation. Am J Cardiol 66:1212–1215
32. Atwood JE, Myers J, Quaglietti S et al (1999) Effect of betaxolol on the hemodynamic, gas exchange, and cardiac output to exercise in chronic atrial fibrillation. Chest 115:1175–1180
33. Lundstrom T, Ryden L (1990) Ventricular rate control and exercise performance in chronic atrial fibrillation: effects of diltiazem and verapamil. J Am Coll Cardiol 16:86–90
34. Channer KS, Papouchado M, James MA, Pitcher DW, Rees JR (1987) Towards improved control of atrial fibrillation. Eur Hear J 8:141–147
35. Steinberg JS, Katz RJ, Bren GB, Buff LA, Varghese PJ (1987) Efficacy of oral diltiazem to control ventricular response in chronic atrial fibrillation at rest and during exercise. J Am Coll Cardiol 9:405–411
36. Lewis RV, Irvine N, McDevitt DG (1988) Relationships between heart rate, exercise tolerance and cardiac output in atrial fibrillation: the effects of treatment with digoxin, verapamil and diltiazem. Eur Heart J 9:777–781
37. Lang R, Klein HO, Di Segni E et al (1983) Verapamil improves exercise capacity in chronic atrial fibrillation: double-blind crossover study. Am Heart J 105:820–825
38. Kjekshus J, Gullestad L (1999) Heart rate as therapeutic target in heart failure. Eur Heart J (Suppl 1):H64–H69

Ablate and Pace: Is This Still a Valid Option?

M. Brignole

A Pragmatic Approach

Atrioventricular (AV) junction ablation (producing AV block) followed by implantation of a pacemaker is a well-established, generally accepted, treatment for patients affected by atrial fibrillation (AF) that is not controlled by antiarrhythmic drugs. Nevertheless, ablation and pacing is a palliative treatment. Indeed, in contrast to other ablative procedures, i.e., those used for the treatment of AV-nodal re-entrant tachycardia and accessory by-pass tracts, in which the ablation can be considered curative, AV junction ablation cannot eliminate the electrophysiological substrate of the disease and only works indirectly by controlling the irregular and fast ventricular rate. In other words, an old disease (uncontrolled AF) is replaced by another disease (iatrogenic AV block and pacemaker dependence). Moreover, the procedure is necessarily associated with a pacemaker implant, and there is a small but definite risk of of short- and long-term complications from the ablative therapy and pacemaker implantation. For these reasons, many cardiologists and electrophysiologists have concerns about wide use of this new treatment and some refute the wisdom of its introduction into clinical practice. It must be remembered that the typical candidate for ablation and pacing is an elderly patient who has frequent (even daily) episodes of symptomatic paroxysmal AF; is very distressed by the arrhythmia, which greatly limits the quality of life; and has been treated unsuccessfully for many years with multiple drug therapies. Apart from AF, frequently no structural heart disease is found, suggesting that rapid and irregular rhythms are the most likely contributory factors in the symptomatology. What should we do for these patients when drugs fail?

Department of Cardiology, Arrhythmologic Centre, Ospedali del Tigullio, Lavagna, Italy

Ablation and Pacing Therapy Compared with the Other Nonpharmacological Therapies

Theoretically, other nonpharmacological therapies that aim to preserve or restore sinus rhythm should be preferred; these may include atrial pacing (single or multi-site), endocardial ablation of AF foci, and atrial defibrillation. Nevertheless, their role has yet to be fully defined, and without further clinical evaluation they must still be considered investigational [1]. Moreover, five recent randomized controlled studies - the PIAF, AFFIRM, RACE, PAF 2, and STAFF pilot [2-6] - have definitely shown that: (1) rhythm control therapy, compared with rate control, cannot reduce mortality and major morbidity (stroke, thromboembolisms, etc.) rates, which on the contrary were higher with rhythm control, albeit not significantly, probably because of the side effects of the therapy necessary for the maintenance of the sinus rhythm; and (2) rate control therapy can lead to an improvement of quality of life and of physical performance similar to that achieved with rhythm control. Thus, rate control therapy is a good alternative to rhythm control therapy when this latter is difficult to achieve. It is anticoagulant therapy, and not antiarrhythmic therapy that makes it possible to prevent stroke and other thromboembolisms. The patient with AF has a similar risk of stroke to the patient in either sinus rhythm or AF. The logical inference of these studies is that the scope of any antiarrhythmic therapy of AF must be addressed exclusively to reduction of symptoms and improvement of the quality of life. What is the best therapy? The therapy that allows achievement of the best clinical results with the lowest risk of complications and the lowest costs. Advantages and disadvantages of each nonpharmacological therapy should be evaluated in order to offer each individual patient the best available treatment.

Ease of Performance

AV junction ablation can be obtained by way of a right-sided or a left-sided approach. The greater body of experience available with right-sided approaches and the higher prevalence of complications following left-sided catheterization have made the right-sided approach the approach of choice. When this fails, left-sided ablation is performed during the same session (sequential approach) or in another surgical session. Left-side ablation may be easier and it requires fewer applications of radiofrequency, but it requires arterial catheterization [7-9]. In expert hands, the efficacy of complete AV block produced with a sequential approach is usually >95% [7-13]; regression of AV block late after ablation (which requires a second procedure on a different day) occurs in about 0-7% of cases [7, 11, 12, 14-16]. Periprocedural complication rates (including malignant ventricular arrhythmias) are generally less than

2%, and the frequency of procedure-related death is estimated at 0.1% [17, 18]. Most patients who die in the periablation observation period are reported to have severely depressed left-ventricular function with very low ejection fractions in association with chronic (permanent) AF [1].

Established Clinical Efficacy

Paroxysmal AF

Uniform data from some small, uncontrolled studies [19-22] and from two randomized controlled trials [14, 23] definitely show that in patients affected by severely symptomatic recurrent (paroxysmal and persistent) AF which is not controlled by pharmacological therapy, ablation and pacing is highly effective and superior to drug therapy in controlling their symptoms and improving their quality of life. After ablation, palpitations, the most specific symptom of paroxysmal AF, were virtually abolished in more than 80% of patients; the mean improvement in the score of specific symptoms of AF (e.g. effort dyspnea, exercise intolerance, easy fatigue) varied from 30% to 80% according to the indexed parameter. Although arrhythmia was paroxysmal, patients were also expected to report a great improvement in general, physical, emotional, and social indexes of their health-related quality of life and not only in arrhythmia-specific parameters, and the quality of life scores approached those of asymptomatic subjects.

Chronic AF

A few uncontrolled studies [10, 20, 21, 24, 25] have suggested a beneficial effect of AV junction ablation during long-term follow-up in patients with chronic AF, in terms of improved quality of life and cardiac function. In two randomized controlled trials [26, 27], ablation and pacemaker treatment were evaluated against medical treatment during a long follow-up period. The ablative treatment was superior to drug therapy in controlling specific symptoms, although its efficacy was lower than that observed in the intrapatient comparison, as some improvement was also observed in the medically treated control patients. Improvement was greater for the specific symptoms of the disease (palpitations, effort dyspnea, exercise intolerance, easy fatigue, and chest discomfort) than for the indexes of health-related quality of life, which failed to confirm any statistically significant benefit. However, the studies were unable to show a benefit of the treatment on cardiac performance or on progression of the disease when evaluated by echocardiography and exercise test.

Finally, improvements in cardiac function and clinical status have been shown when AV junction ablation is associated with cardiac resynchronization pacing in patients with heart failure and AF [28-31].

Who Are the Ideal Candidates for Ablation and Pacing?

Pharmacological therapy remains the initial therapy of choice in patients with AF.

Paroxysmal AF [32]

Ablation and pacing can be proposed for patients with paroxysmal AF that is not controlled by antiarrhythmic drugs. Antiarrhythmic therapy is considered ineffective not only when AF recurs despite the best antiarrhythmic therapy, but also when the recurrences are so frequent or cause such severe symptoms that the patients' quality of life is greatly impaired.

Alternatively, patients may be exposed to a risk of life-threatening complications, such as syncope, cardiac arrest or acute heart failure.

Ablation and pacing is also generally accepted for patients with the bradycardia-tachycardia syndrome who are already being treated with a pacemaker.

Finally, ablation and pacing may be indicated as an alternative to drug therapy when there is a risk of severe side effects or when side effects are not tolerated.

Persistent AF

The indications for ablation and pacing are less clear in persistent AF, because efforts must be made to restore and maintain sinus rhythm. Ablation and pacing is contraindicated when there is evidence of an electrophysiologic substrate amenable to a curative procedure (e.g., focal AF, AF associated with AV accessory pathway, atrial flutter, AV nodal re-entrant tachycardia).

Chronic AF

Symptomatic uncontrolled ventricular rate

In conjunction with cardiac resynchronization therapy, ablation and pacing is indicated in patients with heart failure with left-ventricular desynchronized contraction (generally due to the presence of left bundle block), in whom the rate control obtained by means of the AV junction ablation is essential before left-ventricular pacing can be implemented.

Investigation continues into whether it is indicated, in conjunction with cardiac resynchronization therapy, in patients with heart failure and narrow QRS complex.

How Many Potential Candidates Are There for Ablation and Pacing?

Atrial fibrillation is by far the most frequent type of arrhythmia. It has been calculated that it affects 1.6-2% of the general population. It is particularly frequent in the elderly, in males and in patients with heart disease; the prevalence of AF approaches 10% in men and women who have cardiovascular disease and are over 65 years of age [33, 34]. Thus, we can estimate that, in Europe, at least 8.2 million out of a total population of 513 million inhabitants are affected by AF. About 40% of these have paroxysmal/persistent AF, and in 12% their AF is considered intractable despite multiple-drug therapy [35]. Therefore, we can calculate that in Europe about 396,000 patients (216,000 over 65 years) are affected by paroxysmal AF that is not controlled by drug therapy. Permanent forms are even more frequent, but how many of those concerned could benefit from ablation and pacing is still unknown. Given this high prevalence, its treatment has socioeconomic and organizational implications that go beyond the remit of the electrophysiologist.

In practice, the number of patients actually undegoing catheter ablation therapy seem to be very low in comparison. For example, in 2001, only 0.5% of patients affected by AF (476 cases) underwent ablation and pacing in Italy [36].

Mode of Pacing

In patients with paroxysmal AF, AV junction ablation creates an iatrogenic condition only rarely found in other patients, namely the presence of total AV block and paroxysmal atrial tachyarrhythmias. The aim of permanent cardiac pacing should therefore be, to restore AV synchrony during episodes of sinus rhythm and provide an adequate increase in ventricular rate in response to physical activity during episodes of AF. These criteria are met by a DDDR mode-switching device. The VVIR mode, which is adequate during episodes of AF, is not adequate during periods of sinus rhythm, as it does not maintain AV synchrony and may cause pacemaker syndrome. Ablation and DDDR mode-switching pacing produces more symptomatic benefit than VVIR pacing [23].

VVIR is the preferred mode in patients who have permanent AF, and probably also in those patients with persistent AF who are at high risk of developing permanent AF following AV junction ablation, i.e., those aged over 75 years or those who have previously undergone DC cardioversion [37, 38].

Cardiac resynchronization pacing therapy should be considered in patients with heart failure or severe systolic dysfunction

Failure of Ablation and Pacing Treatment

In contrast to the excellent results observed in most cases, ablation and pacing treatment is clinically unsuccessful in a minority of patients. In the case of paroxysmal AF, this occurred in 14% of the patients in the Italian study [14] and in 7% of Kamalvand's cases [39]. There are several possible explanations for this contrasting behavior. Careful analysis of a patient's follow-up records has sometimes suggested that AF recurrences were only partially responsible for the subjective perception of palpitations. It is quite possible that their symptoms after ablation were also related to DDDR pacing per se or to its inappropriate programming or to the adverse hemodynamic effect of electrostimulation from the apex of the right ventricle. Moreover, Weber et al. [40] found that a psychiatric illness accounts for the etiology of palpitations in nearly one-third of all cases. It is possible that a depressive status (which is frequently associated) may decrease the threshold of subjective perception of nonphysiological rhythms.

Among patients with congestive heart failure, hemodynamic deterioration soon after ablation was observed in 7% of Vanderheiden's cases [41] and in 9% of Twindale's cases [42]. The presence of significant mitral regurgitation before ablation and a very low value of the ejection fraction were identified as predictors of this adverse event [35]. Although this finding was not confirmed in two randomized studies [26, 27], it is commonly accepted that pacing from the apex of the right ventricle is not optimal, since it provides a nonphysiological asynchronous contraction that results in a decrease in cardiac performance [43, 44]. This suggests that the beneficial hemodynamic effect of regularization of heart rhythm is counteracted by adverse haemodynamic effect of nonphysiological pacing. In patients with severe congestive heart failure, both left-ventricular pacing alone and biventricular pacing improved symptoms and cardiac performance in patients with chronic AF who underwent AV junction ablation [28-31]. A recent study [45] assessed the effects of upgrading to biventricular pacing in 20 patients with congestive heart failure who had had a prior AV junction ablation and right-ventricular pacing for chronic atrial fibrillation performed a mean of 26 months before. A mean of 17 months after the upgrading procedure, the NYHA functional class improved by 29% (from 3.4 to 2.4), the number of hospitalizations per year decreased by 81% (from 1.9/year to 0.4/year), and the scores on the Minnesota Living with Heart Failure Questionnaire decreased by 33% (from 78 to 52). The left-ventricular ejection fraction increased by 44% (from 21% to 31%).

How can candidates be selected for cardiac resynchronization therapy? Who will benefit the most? There are no definite criteria to date, and the simplest univentricular right pacing should be the preferred mode of pacing. On the other hand, we know from the literature that predictors of poor outcome after AV junction ablation are ejection fraction <30%, congestive heart failure, moderate to severe mitral regurgitation, and lack of acute improvement immediately after ablation [42], and that upgrading to biventricular pacing is effective in patients with congestive heart failure with low ejection fraction who have had a prior AV junction ablation and right-ventricular pacing [45]. When the above risk factors are present resynchronization therapy can be offered immediately at the time of AV junction ablation.

Long-term Follow-up

Data on the long-term effects of this treatment on morbidity and survival are now available from several studies.

There is a high rate of progression to permanent AF following ablation and pacing of initially paroxysmal or persistent forms (roughly 20% per year) [37, 38]. Nevertheless, the PAF2 study [5] has shown that progression to permanent AF is not associated with a worse outcome or with worsening of the clinical symptoms; thus, the complete control of ventricular rhythm provided by ablation and pacing seems to be the most important objective and the importance of preserving atrial contraction is probably not so great.

There is no evidence to date to suggest that ablation and pacing increases thromboembolic risk in patients with AF, and a large long-term retrospective study has shown a fairly low rate of thromboembolic events after ablation (roughly 1% per year) [46]. These data have been confirmed in a recent large meta-analysis [47]. Anticoagulant therapy should, therefore, be prescribed according to current guidelines.

Finally, the results of randomized controlled studies [14, 23, 26, 27], of two case-control studies [15, 48], and of a large meta-analysis [47] do not document an increased risk of death, especially sudden death, either early or late after ablation. In particular, in the absence of underlying heart disease, survival among patients with AF after AV junction ablation was similar to the expected survival in the general population [48] and long-term survival was similar for patients with AF regardless of whether they underwent ablation or drug therapy [15, 48]. Thus, in conclusion, the late outcome after ablation and pacing therapy is more likely to be attributable to the natural course of the underlying disease than to an adverse effect of the ablation and pacemaker treatment.

Conclusions

In conclusion, ablation and pacing therapy is the best rate control therapy available for paroxysmal and permanent AF. It is easy to perform, has a low complication rate, is highly effective in controlling specific symptoms, improves the quality of life, does not affect cardiac performance, has a low embolic risk, and does not increase morbidity or mortality during the long-term follow-up. In addition, ablation and pacing therapy is well accepted by the patients, involves a relatively low cost, and has been performed worldwide over the last 20 years. Its efficacy and safety can be considered established. Nevertheless, as it is a palliative (not curative) treatment and creates an iatrogenic AV block, its use must be reserved for a very small minority of AF patients who are severely symptomatic and whose AF is refractory to drug therapy.

References

1. Prystowsky E, Benson DW, Fuster V et al (1996) Management of patients with atrial fibrillation. A statement for healthcare professionals from the Subcommittee on Electrocardiography and Electrophysiology, American Heart Association. Circulation 93:1262-1277
2. Hohnloser S, Kuck KH (2000) Rhythm or rate control in atrial fibrillation. Pharmacological intervention in atrial fibrillation. Lancet 356:1789-1794
3. Wyse DG, Waldo AL, DiMarco JP (2002) A comparison of rate control and rhythm control in patients with atrial fibrillation. N Engl J Med 347:1825-1833
4. van Gelder IC, Hagens VE, Bosker HA (2002) A comparison of rate control and rhythm control in patients with recurrent persistent atrial fibrillation. N Engl J Med 347:1834-1840
5. Brignole M, Menozzi C, Gasparini M et al (2002) An evaluation of the strategy of maintenance of sinus rhythm by antiarrhythmic drug therapy after ablation and pacing therapy in patients with paroxysmal atrial fibrillation. Eur Heart J 23:892-900
6. Carlsson J et al (2001) Mortality and stroke in rate vs rhythm control in AF: the STAF Pilot Study. J Am Coll Cardiol 38:A595
7. Trohman R, Simmons T, Moore S et al (1992) Catheter ablation of the atrioventricular junction using radiofrequency energy and a bilateral cardiac approach. Am J Cardiol 70:1438-1443
8. Souza O, Gursoy S, Simonis F et al (1992) Right-sided versus left-sided radiofrequency ablation of the His bundle. Pacing Clin Electrophisiol 15: 1454-1459
9. Kalbfleisch S, Williamson B, Man C et al (1993) A randomized comparison of the right- and left-sided approaches to ablation of the atrioventricular junction. Am J Cardiol 72:1406-1410
10. Brignole M, Gianfranchi L, Menozzi C et al (1994) Influence of atrioventricular junction radiofrequency ablation in patients with chronic atrial fibrillation and flutter on quality of life and cardiac performance. Am J Cardiol 74: 242-24611
11. Geelen P, Brugada J, Andries E et al (1997) Ventricular fibrillation and sudden death after radiofrequency catheter ablation of the atrioventricular junction. Pacing Clin Electrophisiol 20:343-348
12. Darpo B, Walfridsson H, Aunes M et al (1997) Incidence of sudden death after radiofrequency ablation of the atrioventricular junction for atrial fibrillation. Am J Cardiol 80:1174-1177
13. Marshall H, Griffíth M (1999) Ablation of the atrioventricular junction: technique, acute and long-term results in 115 consecutive patients. Europace 1: 26-29
14. Brignole M, Gianfranchi L, Menozzi C et al (1997) An assessment of atrioventricular junction ablation and DDDR mode-switching pacemaker versus pharmacological treatment in patients with severely symptomatic paroxysmal atrial fibrillation. A randomized controlled study. Circulation 96:2617-262
15. Olgin J, Scheinman M (1993) Comparison of high energy direct current and radiofrequency catheter ablation of the atrioventricular junction. J Am Coll Cardiol 21:557-564
16. Morady F, Calkins H, Langberg J et al (1993) A prospective randomized comparison of direct current and radiofrequency ablation of the atrioventricular junction. J Am Coll Cardiol 21:102-109
17. Hindricks G and MERFS investigators (1993) The Multicentre European Radiofrequency Survey (MERFS): complications of radiofrequency catheter ablation of arrhythmias. Eur Heart J 14:1644-1653

18. Scheinman M (1994) Patterns of catheter ablation practice in the United States: results of the 1992 NASPE survey. Pacing Clin Electrophisiol 17:873-875
19. Kay GN, Bubien RS, Epstein AE et al (1988) Effect of catheter ablation of the atrioventricular junction on quality of life and exercise tolerance in paroxysmal atrial fibrillation. Am J Cardiol 62:741-744
20. Jensen SM, Bergfeldt L, Rosenquist M (1995) Long-term follow-up of patients treated by radiofrequency ablation of the atrioventricular junction. Pacing Clin Electrophisiol 18:1609-1614
21. Fitzpatrick AD, Kourouyan HD, Siu A et al (1996) Quality of life and outcomes after radiofrequency His-bundle catheter ablation and permanent pacemaker implantation: impact of treatment in paroxysmal and established atrial fibrillation. Am Heart J, 131:499-507
22. Bubien RS, Knotts-Dolson SM, Plumb VJ et al (1996) Effect of radiofrequency catheter ablation on health-related quality of life and activities of daily living in patients with recurrent arrhythmias. Circulation, 94:1585-1591
23. Marshall H, Harris Z, Griffith M et al (1999) Prospective randomized study of ablation and pacing versus medical therapy for paroxysmal atrial fibrillation. Effects of pacing mode and mode-switch algorithm. Circulation 99:1587-1592
24. Rosenquist M, Lee M, Mouliner L et al (1990) Long-term follow-up of patients after transcatheter direct current ablation of the atrioventricular junction. J Am Coll Cardiol 16:1467-1474
25. Natale A, Zimerman L, Tomassoni G et al (1996) Impact on ventricular function and quality of life of transcatheter ablation of the atrioventricular junction in chronic atrial fibrillation with a normal ventricular response. Am J Cardiol 78:1431-1433
26. Brignole M, Menozzi C, Gianfranchi L et al (1998) Assessment of atrioventricular junction ablation and VVIR pacemaker versus pharmacological treatment in patients with heart failure and chronic atrial fibrillation. A randomized controlled study. Circulation 98:953-960
27. Weersoorija R, Davis M, Powell A et al (2003) The Australian intervention randomized control of rate in atrial fibrillation trial (AIRCRAFT). J Am Coll Cardiol (in press)
28. Etienne Y, Mansourati J, Gilard M et al (1999) Evaluation of left ventricular based pacing in patients with congestive heart failure and atrial fibrillation. Am J Cardiol 83:1138-1140
29. Leclerq C, Victor F, Alonso C et al (2000) Comparative effects of permanent biventricular pacing for refractory heart failure in patients with stable sinus rhythm or chronic atrial fibrillation. Am J Cardiol 85:1154-1156
30. Lupi G, Brignole M, Oddone D et al (2000) Effects of left ventricular pacing on cardiac performance and quality of life in patients with drug-refractory heart failure. Am J Cardiol 86:33-36
31. Leclercq C, Walker S, Linde C et al (2002) Comparative effects of permanent biventricular and right-univentricular pacing in heart failure patients with chronic atrial fibrillation. Eur Heart J 23: 1780-1787
32. Brignole M, Gammage M, Jordaens L et al (1999) Sutton R. Report of a study group on ablate and pace therapy for paroxysmal atrial fibrillation. Europace 1:8-13
33. Furberg C, Psaty B, Manolio T (1994) Prevalence of atrial fibrillation in elderly subjects (the cardiovascular Heart Study). Am J Cardiol 74:236-241
34. Kannel W, Abbott R, Savage D (1983) Coronary heart disease and atrial fibrillation: The Framingham Study. Am Heart J 106:389-396
35. Crjins HJ, van Gelder IC, van Gilst WH et al (1991) Serial antiarrhythmic drug treatment to maintain sinus rhythm after electrical cardioversion for chronic atrial fibril-

lation or atrial flutter. Am J Cardiol 68:335-341
36. Inama G (2002) Attività dei laboratori di elettrofisiologia italiani nel 2001. G Ital Aritm Cardiostim 5:231-237
37. Gribbin GM, Bourke JP, McComb J (1998) Predictors of atrial rhythm after atrioventricular node ablation for the treatment of paroxysmal atrial arrhythmias. Heart 79:548-553
38. Gianfranchi L, Brignole M, Menozzi C et al (1998) Progression of permanent atrial fibrillation after atrioventricular junction ablation and dual-chamber pacemaker implantation in patients with paroxysmal atrial tachyarrhythmias. Am J Cardiol 81:351-354
39. Kamalvand K, Tan K, Kotsakis A (1997) Is mode switching beneficial? A randomised study in patients with paroxysmal atrial tachyarrhythmias. J Am Coll Cardiol 30:496-504
40. Weber BE, Kapoor WN (1996) Evaluation and outcome of patients with palpitations. Am J Med, 100:138-148
41. Vanderheiden M, Goethals M, Anguera I et al (1997) Hemodynamic deterioration following radiofrequency ablation of the atrioventricular conduction system. Pacing Clin Electrophisiol 20:2422-2438
42. Twidale N, Manda V, Nave K et al (1998) Predictors of outcome after radiofrequency catheter ablation of the atrioventricular node for atrial fibrillation and congestive heart failure. Am Heart J 136:647-657
43. Zile M, Blaustein A, Shimizu G et al (1987) Right ventricular pacing reduces the rate of left ventricular relaxation and filling. J Am Coll Cardiol 10:702-709
44. Ausubel K, Furman S (1985) The pacemaker syndrome. Ann Intern Med 103:420-429
45. Leon A, Greenberg J, Kanaru N et al (2002) Cardiac resynchronization in patients with congestive heart failure and chronic atrial fibrillation. J Am Coll Cardiol 39:1258-1263
46. Gasparini M, Mantica M, Brignole M et al (1999) Thromboembolism after atrioventricular node ablation and pacing: long term follow-up. Heart 82:494-498
47. Wood M, Brown-Mahoney C, Kay GN et al (2000) Clinical outcomes after ablation and pacing therapy for atrial fibrillation. Circulation 101:1138-1144.
48. Ozcan C, Jahangir A, Friedman PA et al (2001) Long-term survival after ablation of the atrioventricular node and implantation of a permanent pacemaker in patients with atrial fibrillation. N Engl J Med 344:1043-1051

Transvascular Parasympathetic Stimulation for Ventricular Rate Control During Atrial Fibrillation: A Bionic Approach

P. Schauerte[1], M. Schmidt[2], T. Schimpf[1], J. Plisiene[1], M. Zarse[1], K. Mischke[1]

Of all arrhythmias atrial fibrillation (AF) is the most frequent, with a prevalence of 5–9% among the older population [1]. AF accounts for most rhythm-related hospital treatments [2]. Recently, equal outcomes have been reported for treatment strategies aiming at the restoration and maintenance of sinus rhythm (rhythm control) or at persistence of AF with ventricular rate control [3, 4], provided that the patients are sufficiently anticoagulated. Ventricular rate control, however, is a significant problem as the chaotic bombardment of the atrioventricular (AV) node by the fibrillating wavelets causes almost unpredictable sequences of ventricular activation, leading to both tachycardic and bradycardic episodes. Particularly during physical exertion, the adaptation of the heart rate to an increasing physical demand is impaired and often results in excess tachycardia. This adds to the reduced exercise capacity which is already impaired by the loss of the atrial contribution to ventricular filling. Therefore, pharmacological therapy with negative dromotropic drugs is necessary in the vast majority of AF patients in whom rate control is pursued. Unfortunately, this is often a trade-off, because the patients may experience symptomatic bradycardia despite effective suppression of tachycardic episodes, leading to pacemaker implantation in a substantial proportion of patients. Even more importantly, apart from cardiac glycosides, most of the drugs that exert negative dromotropic effects also have significant ventricular negative inotropic and vasodilating properties at dosages which effectively decrease the rapid ventricular rate during AF. This limits their benefit in patients with congestive heart failure or arterial hypotension. Cardiac glycosides, in turn, have limited rate-slowing effects during rapid ventricular rates caused by physical activity [5].

How does nature control conduction? In addition to the intrinsic decremental conduction properties of the AV node and its inputs, the autonomic nervous system plays a key role in the dynamic control of AV conduction.

[1]Department of Cardiology, and [2]Department of Cardiovascular and Thoracic Surgery, University of Technology, Aachen, Germany

Sympathetic and parasympathetic neurons form a dense network throughout the AV node and its borders which allows instantaneous and automatic adaptation of AV conduction to changing physiological or pathophysiological states [6, 7]. The present chapter will demonstrate how the distinct anatomy of the parasympathetic innervation of the AV node in humans offers the opportunity to stimulate these nerves electrically with intracardiac electrode catheters, thereby rendering a novel therapeutic means of controlling ventricular rate during AF without negative inotropic or vasodilating side effects.

Methods

The study was performed at the University of Technology in Aachen, Germany. Neural stimulation was attempted during electrophysiological studies in 26 patients. The baseline rhythm was sinus rhythm in 20 patients and AF in 6 patients. Tetrapolar electrode catheters (Torq, Medtronic Inc., Minneapolis, Minn., USA) were placed in the high right atrium and the right ventricular apex for pacing and sensing, respectively. In addition, an octapolar electrode catheter (Cordis Corp., Calif., USA) was positioned at the His bundle.

Most parasympathetic nerves which innervate the AV node accumulate epicardially between the ostium of the coronary sinus (CS), the entrance of the inferior vena cava into the right atrium, and the low right atrium (Fig. 1). This inferior vena cava–inferior atrial ganglionated plexus contains axons that preferentially innervate the AV node, but also contains some fibers that innervate adjacent atrial myocardial tissue [8–13]. Transvascular or transmyocardial electrical nerve stimulation occurs at relatively high stimulation frequencies of 10–50 Hz. Such high-frequency stimulation of the inferior vena cava–inferior atrial ganglionated plexus during sinus rhythm inevitably excites atrial myocardial tissue, thereby inducing and maintaining AF. Therefore, during sinus rhythm or atrial tachycardias, high-frequency electrical stimuli (200 Hz) have to be delivered within the atrial refractory period. To explore such a stimulation algorithm, the atria were paced from the proximal CS and the high-frequency nerve stimulation trains (train duration: 50 ms) were coupled to the pacing stimulus at a delay of 20 ms.

After the introduction of a deflectable decapolar electrode catheter (Cordis Corp.) through the femoral vein, the tip of the catheter was advanced into the CS so that the most proximal pair of electrodes was situated in the CS ostium (Fig. 1). Subsequently, parasympathetic nerve stimulation (PS) was performed over each of the five bipole pairs of the decapolar electrode catheter starting with the most proximal electrode pair. In order to quantify a negative dromotropic effect during PS, the antegrade Wenckebach period was determined during PS at different stimulation voltages (10 to 30 V in 5-V steps). In five patients, PS at 30 V was repeated after muscarinergic blockade with 1 mg atropine i.v..

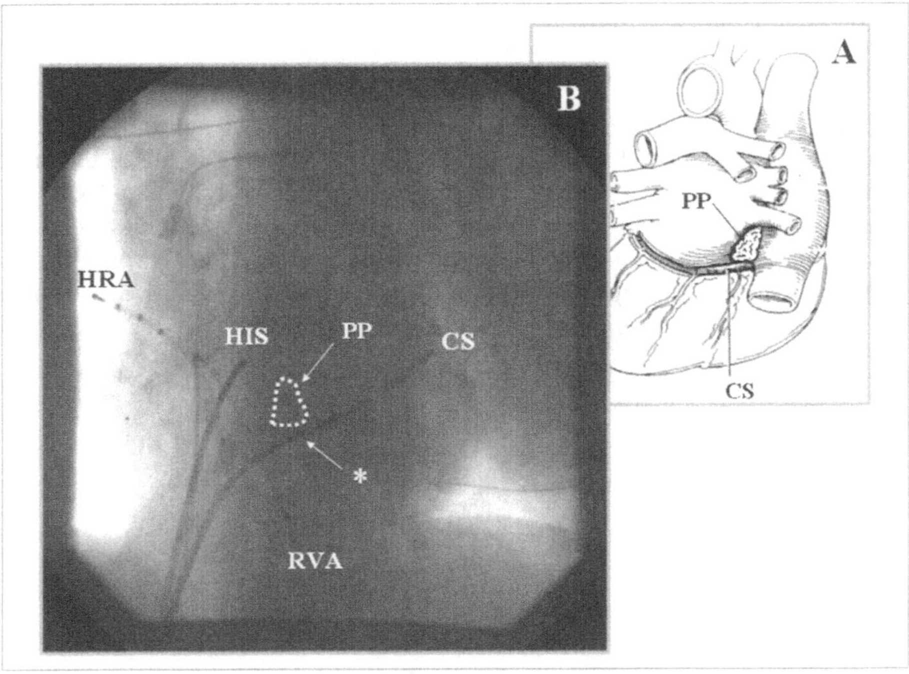

Fig. 1. A Schematic dorsal view of the heart. The parasympathetic plexus (PP) which innervates the atrioventricular node is localized epicardially at the cranial aspect of the ostium of the coronary sinus (CS). B 30° left anterior oblique view of a decapolar electrode catheter in the CS. Transvascular parasympathetic stimulation (PS) from the proximal electrode pair (*) resulted in high-degree atrioventricular (AV) block as long as PS was ongoing. HRA, catheter in the high right atrium; RVA, catheter in the right ventricular apex; HIS, His bundle catheter

During AF nerve stimulation can be delivered in short packages of 200-Hz stimuli as described above. Alternatively, stimulation can be performed at more optimal stimulation frequencies of 20 Hz because the induction of AF is no longer an issue in these patients. Therefore, in six patients with chronic persistent AF, PS in the CS at a frequency of 20 Hz was delivered to slow the ventricular rate during AF.

Statistical Analysis

All data are expressed as mean ±1 standard deviation. Repeated measure ANOVA was used to test whether the nerve stimulus strength affected the antegrade Wenckebach cycle length. For individual comparison of the antegrade Wenckebach cycle length with the baseline values a paired Student's *t*-test was applied. Probability values of 0.05 or less were considered significant.

Results

Parasympathetic Nerve Stimulation During Sinus Rhythm

As soon as the CS was engaged with a multielectrode catheter, the inferior interatrial ganglionated plexus could be easily stimulated in all 26 patients. Importantly, PS in the CS did not induce ventricular arrhythmias. Electrical stimulation with 200 Hz in the atrial myocardial refractory period avoided the induction of AF while effectively exciting parasympathetic nerves which innervate the AV node. During sinus rhythm PS prolonged AV conduction, as shown in Fig. 2. The negative dromotropic effect could almost be "titrated," as shown

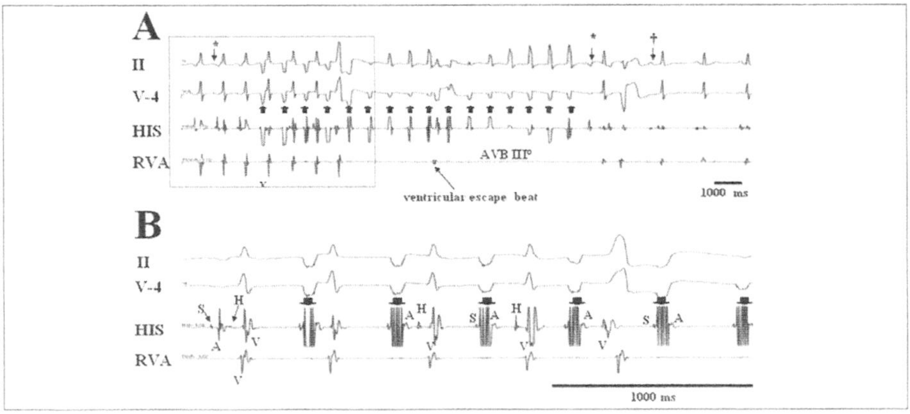

Fig. 2A, B. Third-degree AV block during PS in the proximal CS. A Surface ECG leads II and V-4 are shown. HIS represents a His bundle electrogram whereas RVA shows an electrogram from the right ventricular apex. The atria were paced from the same electrode pair within the ostium of the CS over which nerve stimuli were delivered (note the negative P-waves in surface ECG lead II: *). The arrows indicate short nerve stimulation trains (50 ms train duration) of high-frequency stimuli (200 Hz) which were coupled to the pacing stimuli with a delay of 20 ms to ensure nerve stimulation within the local atrial myocardial refractory period. Due to the high voltage (20 V) of the high-frequency stimulation trains, huge electrical artifacts are also visible in the surface ECG (arrows). After the fifth PS train AV block III with a ventricular escape beat occurred. Immediately after PS was terminated (after last arrow) 1:1 AV conduction resumed. The last negative P-wave after cessation of PS (*) is still a paced beat from the CS which is conducted with a prolonged P–R interval. Following this beat atrial pacing was discontinued and sinus rhythm resumed, as can be seen from the now upright P-waves in lead II (†). B Magnification of the onset of PS as marked by the box in A. The first beat is a stimulated beat from the proximal CS (A, atrial signal; H, His bundle deflection; V, ventricular signal). Starting with the second paced beat, a high-frequency (200-Hz) stimulation train (arrow) lasting 50 ms is coupled to the pacing stimulus (S) with a delay of 20 ms, which allows the delivery of the high-frequency stimuli within the local atrial refractory period. In the His bundle recording, an increasing prolongation of the A–H interval can be seen with increasing numbers of nerve stimulation trains until supra-His AV block III occurs after the fifth nerve stimulation train. (Reproduced from [14], with permission)

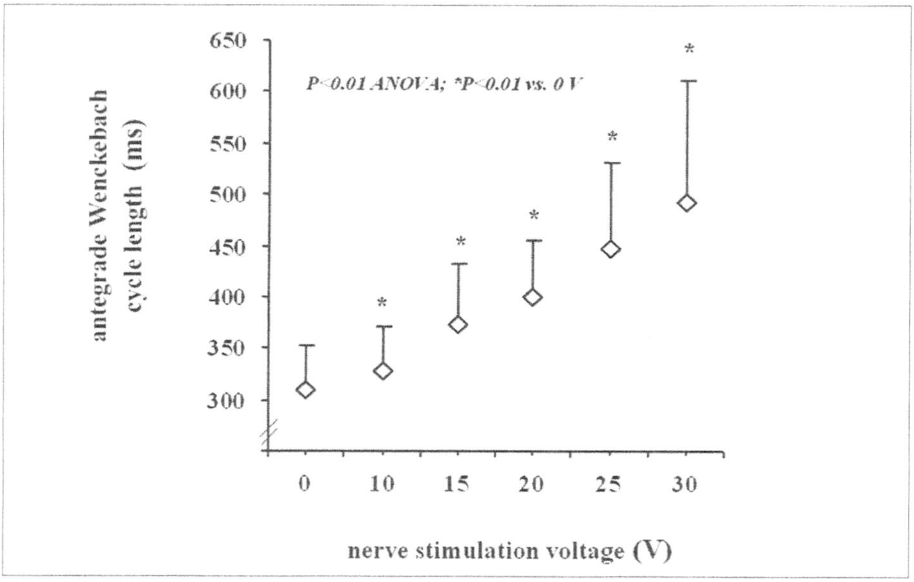

Fig. 3. Influence of the nerve stimulation voltage on the antegrade Wenckebach cycle length during PS in the CS: as the stimulation voltage increases, an increase in the antegrade Wenckebach cycle length is seen ($p<0.01$, ANOVA). *: $p<0.01$ compared to baseline. (Reproduced from [14], with permission)

by a graded increase in the antegrade Wenckebach cycle length during increasing nerve stimulation voltages (Fig. 3). Atropine abolished the negative dromotropic effect.

Parasympathetic Nerve Stimulation During Atrial Fibrillation

In six patients with chronic persistent AF, PS in the CS led to a significant ventricular rate slowing, as illustrated in Fig. 4a. The rate slowing completely vanished after muscarinergic blockade with atropine (Fig. 4B). The negative dromotropic effect could almost be titrated by choosing an appropriate stimulation voltage as shown in Fig. 5.

PS per se did not decrease aortic pressure, as shown in Fig. 6. When PS at a stimulus intensity that resulted in slowing of the ventricular rate during AF was performed during ventricular pacing at a constant cycle length (higher than the ventricular rate during AF), no decrease in aortic pressure was observed.

PS in the CS also evoked chest discomfort, which was, however, less than previously observed during stimulation in the superior vena cava [14]. The degree of pain perception correlated to the magnitude of the nerve stimulation voltage. The discomfort was reported to be located behind the sternum. Of interest, in some patients slight negative dromotropic effects could be obtained

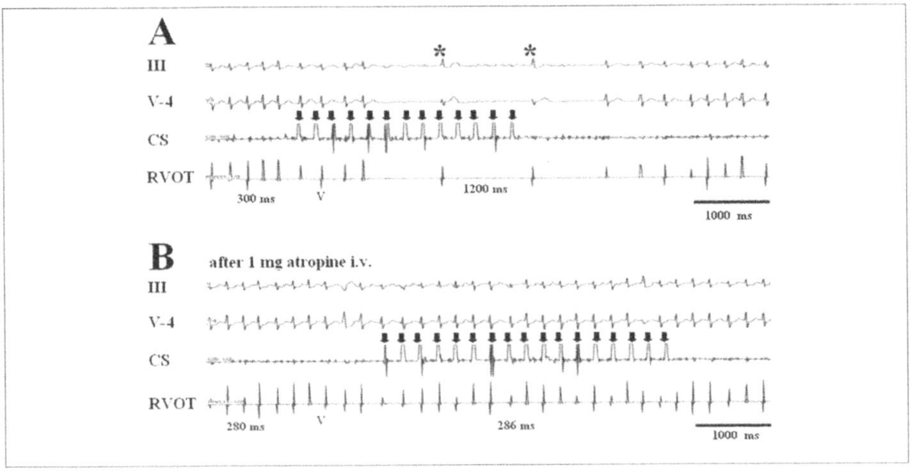

Fig. 4A, B. PS during AF. Surface ECG leads II and V-4 are shown. CS, coronary sinus electrogram; RVOT, right ventricular outflow tract electrogram. A Without PS the shortest R–R interval during AF was 300 ms. The black arrows indicate the PS trains that were delivered via the CS catheter (CS-7-8, not shown because of the stimulation artifacts). PS consisted of brief trains (50 ms duration) of high-frequency stimuli (200 Hz) (arrows). Shortly after the onset of PS, AV block III with two ventricular escape beats (*) occurred. After cessation of PS, rapid AV conduction resumed. B After 1 mg of atropine the PS effect completely dissipated. (Reproduced from [14], with permission)

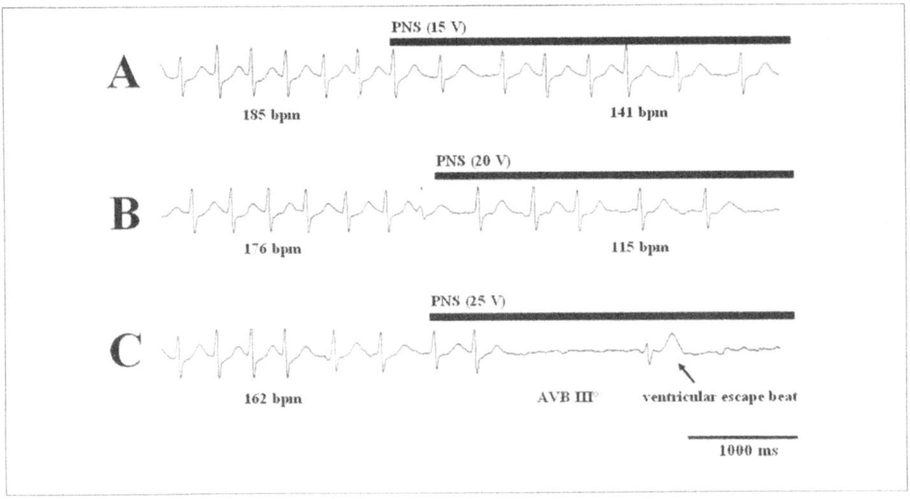

Fig. 5A–C. PS (PNS) in the proximal CS in a patient with AF. The horizontal bars indicate the duration of PS. Continuous PS at 20 Hz was applied. Mean heart rates with and without PS are given. From A to B the stimulation strength was increased from 15 to 25 V, resulting in a graded decrease of the ventricular rate during AF until AV block III occurred at 25 V (C)

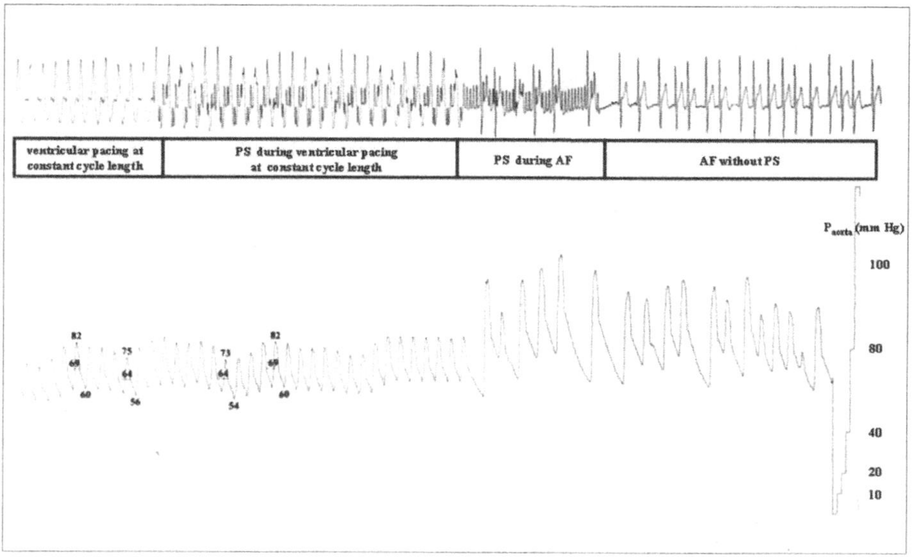

Fig. 6. Hemodynamic effects of PS in a patient with AF. To document the effect of PS on arterial blood pressure, the ventricle was first paced at a constant cycle length. After initiation of PS no overall decrease of blood pressure was observed. After discontinuation of ventricular pacing, AF led to a slower irregular ventricular rate. Once PS during AF was terminated, rapid AV conduction during AF resumed

without sensations of discomfort. In most instances, the pain quality was described as a deep visceral pain. Notably, pain during attempted PS did not occur at ineffective CS sites at which negative dromotropic effects could not be achieved during PS.

Discussion

In selected patients, transvascular PS may open a nonpharmacological approach to selectively enhance cardiac parasympathetic tone. In this way ventricular rate during AF can be controlled as intended. The immediate onset or cessation of the negative dromotropic effect once PS is initiated or terminated makes this technique especially attractive for ventricular rate control during AF as it may offer the opportunity to control AV conduction on a beat-to-beat basis. In addition, the characteristics of the dose-response curves allow precise adjustment of the ventricular rate during AF.

Importantly, no negative inotropic side effects are obtained in humans, which renders the technique especially attractive for rate control in CHF patients, as most of the commonly available drugs for rate control decrease left ventricular contraction force or lower arterial blood pressure. However, there are several other concerns which arise. Rate control by PS via a hypothetical chronic device requires the implantation of a combined neurostimulator–pacemaker with capabilities of neurostimulation and ventricular sensing. This raises the question whether simple AV nodal ablation and implantation of a VVIR pacemaker might be equally effective for ventricular rate control during AF but easier to accomplish. This issue has recently been addressed by Mazgalev's group in dogs [15]. The investigators observed that PS appeared to be hemodynamically more favorable than AV nodal ablation and ventricular pacing as it allowed intraventricular conduction via the specialized conduction system, thereby giving a normal ventricular contraction pattern.

Another concern is long-term efficacy of neural stimulation. Although we observed in animals a preserved negative dromotropic effect over 24 h of continuous PS (Fig. 7) [16], it remains to be elucidated whether transvascular or transmyocardial nerve stimulation effects can be maintained over several weeks or months. Of note, preliminary animal data indicate that a negative dromotropic effect can be evoked over 6 months with epicardial stimulation electrodes which had been implanted surgically after thoracotomy [17].

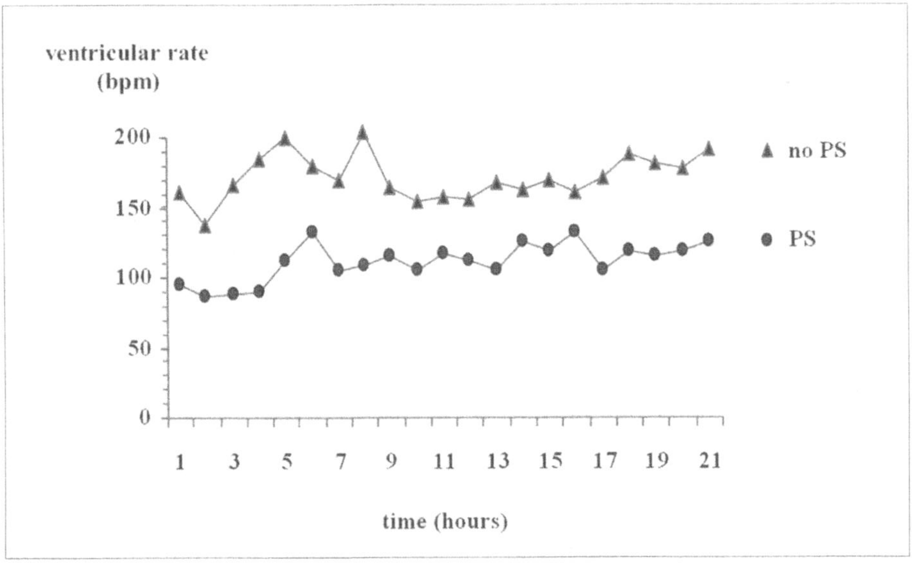

Fig. 7. Continuous cardiac PS at 20 Hz and 25 V in the coronary sinus over 20.5 h in a dog. Every 30 min PS was stopped for 30 s to measure the ventricular rate without PS. The ventricular rate (R–R interval) during AF is plotted versus time. Circles represent the ventricular rate with PS and triangles the rate without PS. The effect of ventricular rate slowing during AF slightly diminished in the first 3 h of PS but then remained fairly constant. After 20.5 h there was still a considerable decrease of the ventricular rate during PS as compared to no PS. The latter was determined during a 30-s period of no PS. (Reproduced from [16], with permission)

By far the most relevant concern, however, relates to the observation of sensations of discomfort which arise in most cases whenever efferent parasympathetic nerves which innervate the AV node are stimulated in *conscious* nonsedated humans. The intensity of these sensations correlate well to the magnitude of the negative dromotropic effect. Attempts are currently being undertaken to adjust the stimulation intensity below the pain threshold to enable a clinically sufficient rate drop with little sensation. Clinical experiments to date, however, indicate that the corridor for efferent stimulation while avoiding afferent excitation is very narrow if present at all. While assuming that afferent nerve projections might be less present close to the AV node or the His bundle, we have also stimulated these areas in awake nonsedated patients with electrode catheters. Although limited in numbers, it turns out that PS in these areas cannot avoid simultaneous afferent and efferent nerve stimulation. The negative dromotropic effect during high-frequency stimulation in the midseptal (supposed AV-nodal) region or at the atrial insertion to the His bundle yielded considerably lower negative dromotropic effects and in parallel less pain sensation. Thus, stimulation at anatomically distinct areas close to the compact AV node or to the His bundle cannot avoid *afferent* nerve stimulation in man. This leaves the mechanistic question of why afferent nerves arising from pain receptors travel through the AV-nodal region and whether they arise from the AV node or just pass through the area.

The dilemma of concomitant afferent nerve excitation during efferent PS has not yet been resolved and remains the major hurdle to be overcome before PS can become a valuable tool for ventricular rate control during AF.

References

1. Kannel WB, Wolf P (1992) Epidemiology of atrial fibrillation. In: Falk RH, Podrid PJ (eds) Atrial fibrillation: mechanism and management. Raven, New York
2. Feinberg WM, Blackshear JL, Laupacis A, Kronmal R, Hart RG (1995) Prevalence, age distribution, and gender of patients with atrial fibrillation. Arch Intern Med 155:469–473
3. Van Gelder IC, Hagens VE, Bosker HA et al (2002) A comparison of rate control and rhythm control in patients with recurrent persistent atrial fibrillation. N Engl J Med 347:1834–1840
4. Wyse DG, Waldo AL, DiMarco JP et al (2002) A comparison of rate control and rhythm control in patients with atrial fibrillation. N Engl J Med 347:1825–1833
5. David E, Segni ED, Klein HO, Kaplinsky E (1979) Inefficacy of digitalis in the control of heart rate in patients with chronic atrial fibrillation: beneficial effect of an added beta adrenergic blocking agent. Am J Cardiol 44:1378–1382
6. Randall WC, Ardell JL, Calderwood D, Milosavljevic M, Goyal SC (1986) Parasympathetic ganglia innervating the canine atrioventricular nodal region. J Auton Nerv Syst 16:311–323
7. Dahlstrom A, Mya-Tu M, Fuxe K, Zetterstrom BE (1965) Observations on adrenergic innervation of dog heart. Am J Physiol 209:689–692

8. Pauza DH, Skripka V, Pauziene N et al (2000) Morphology, distribution, and variability of the epicardiac neural ganglionated subplexuses in the human heart. Anat Rec 259:353–382
9. Lazzara R, Scherlag BJ, Robinson MJ, Samet P (1973) Selective in situ parasympathetic control of the canine sinuatrial and atrioventricular node. Circ Res 32:393–401
10. Wallick DW, Martin PJ (1990) Separate parasympathetic control of heart rate and atrioventricular conduction of dogs. Am J Physiol 259:H536–542
11. Yuan BX, Ardell JL, Hopkins DA Losier AM, Armour JA (1994) Gross and microscopic anatomy of the canine intrinsic cardiac nervous system. Anat Rec 239:75–87
12. Schauerte P, Scherlag BJ, Scherlag MA, Jackman WM, Lazzara R (2000) Transvenous parasympathetic nerve stimulation in the inferior vena cava and atrioventricular conduction. J Cardiovasc Electrophysiol 11:64–69
13. Schauerte P, Scherlag BJ, Pitha J et al (2000) Transvascular radiofrequency current catheter ablation of parasympathetic cardiac nerves abolishes vagally mediated atrial fibrillation. Circulation 28:2774–2780
14. Schauerte P, Mischke K, Plisiene J et al (2001) Catheter stimulation of cardiac parasympathetic nerves in humans. A novel approach to the cardiac autonomic nervous system. Circulation 104:2430–2435
15. Zhuang S, Zhang Y, Mowrey KA et al (2002) Ventricular rate control by selective vagal stimulation is superior to rhythm regularization by atrioventricular nodal ablation and pacing during atrial fibrillation. Circulation 106:1853–1858
16. Schauerte P, Scherlag BJ, Scherlag MA et al (1999) Ventricular rate control during atrial fibrillation by cardiac parasympathetic nerve stimulation. A transvenous approach. J Am Coll Cardiol 34:2043–2050
17. Bharati S, Zhang Y, Mazgalev TN (2003) Localized hypertrophy of nerves as a result of long-term selective AVN vagal stimulation. Pacing Clin Electrophysiol 26(4-II):1030 (abstract)

Management of Atrial Fibrillation: Is it Already Time to Update the Recent ACC/AHA/ESC Guidelines?

D. G. Wyse

Introduction

The current ACC/AHA/ESC were formulated in 1999-2000 and the executive summary was published in 2001 [1]. The full text of the guidelines is available on the websites of the American College of Cardiology, American Heart Association, European Society of Cardiology and the North American Society of Pacing and Electrophysiology. It is the policy of these organizations to review the guidelines annually and make a decision to revise them or withdraw them from distribution. Almost three additional years of relevant research are now available since the original guidelines were developed. In that time some important new information has become available and it is anticipated that an effort to revise the guidelines will be mounted soon. In the discussion below, some of the areas in need of revision will be discussed. Several areas not specifically discussed could also be updated.

One purpose of the guidelines that is under-appreciated is to highlight areas of deficiency in the knowledge base that is the foundation of the guidelines. In the ensuing 3 years since the guidelines were formulated, new areas of deficiency in the knowledge base have also appeared and some of these areas will also be highlighted.

Classification

Classification of atrial fibrillation has been a contentious issue, and an important milestone in the guidelines and elsewhere [2] has been to reach an international consensus on a clinical classification for atrial fibrillation that is simple, easy to remember and useful at the bedside. The current classification scheme is time-based and divides an episode of atrial fibrillation into its two

Division of Cardiology, Department of Cardiac Sciences, University of Calgary/Calgary Health Region, Alberta, Canada

basic forms: paroxysmal (stops by itself) and persistent (lasts longer than 7 days or is terminated by cardioversion). Two additional categories are identified because they have important implications for management. They are new onset and permanent atrial fibrillation. It is important to note that atrial fibrillation with a reversible cause, such as recent heart surgery or pericarditis, are excluded in this scheme. There are several points about the scheme that need emphasis (Table 1). The first is that it is a scheme that is better suited for classification of a single episode of atrial fibrillation than for classification of a patient. Another is that "new onset" is not necessarily the first episode of atrial fibrillation, but rather is the first episode documented electrocardiographically. Often, previous episodes have occurred but were asymptomatic or, symptomatic but not distinguished from other causes of the symptoms of atrial fibrillation. The persistent atrial fibrillation category may include some episodes that really are paroxysmal atrial fibrillation that were cardioverted within 7 days and that may have stopped by themselves if the intervention had not been undertaken. Finally, permanent atrial fibrillation does not mean that sinus rhythm cannot be restored. Rather, it means a determination has been made to make no attempt or no further attempts to restore and maintain sinus rhythm.

An important new area of deficiency in our knowledge base has emerged from the need to classify patients with recurrent atrial fibrillation rather than classifying episodes of atrial fibrillation. It seems quite clear that in at least one of the techniques currently used for electrical isolation of the pulmonary veins for the treatment of recurrent atrial fibrillation, the long-term results are quite different for those patients with the paroxysmal form of atrial fibrillation in comparison to those with the persistent form of atrial fibrillation [3]. This emerging issue raises the question of whether or not the current scheme can be used to classify patients rather than episodes (Table 1). It is relatively easy to see how the current scheme can be transformed to a classification of patients in the case of new onset and permanent atrial fibrillation. However, even in these cases, some new onset atrial fibrillation patients will progress to have recurrent atrial fibrillation and, less commonly, some permanent atrial fibrillation patients may return to recurrent episodes of paroxysmal or persistent atrial fibrillation. More importantly, we do not have a consensus about how to categorize a patient with recurrent episodes of atrial fibrillation as paroxysmal or persistent. It is relatively simple when all episodes of atrial fibrillation are paroxysmal, or all episodes of atrial fibrillation are persistent. However, how does one classify a patient who has some episodes of each type of atrial fibrillation? Additional factors to be considered include whether or not a threshold number of episodes need to occur before a patient can be classified as paroxysmal, or persistent and over what period of time are episodes used in the classification. There are little or no objective data to help with these decisions and it seems clear that any definitions will be arbitrary and may have to include an "indeterminate" category and a "mixed" category. This area of the guidelines needs to be clarified more because it is a gap in knowledge rather than because there has been new knowledge.

Table 1. Considerations in making changes in the classification scheme for atrial fibrillation in the current guidelines: classification of episodes vs. patients

Issue	Comment
Current Scheme	
Best suited to classification of an episode of AF	Not dissimilar to angina
New onset is not the same as first episode	Earlier episodes may be asymptomatic or undocumented by ECG
Persistent may include some paroxysmal	Cardioverted before self-termination occurs
Permanent does not mean sinus rhythm cannot be restored	A judgment has been made to make no attempt or no further attempt
Potential Areas for Change	
Do patients always have episodes that are always paroxysmal or persistent?	Probably a small proportion are but will probably need a "mixed" category
Is a patient category likely to change over time?	Likely and therefore a recent time window (e.g., one year) should be used for categorization
Should there be a period of time during which episodes are catalogued?	A short but recent period of time results in better characterization
Should a minimum number of documented episodes be required?	A larger number results in better characterization but more frequent use of "indeterminate"

AF, atrial fibrillation; *ECG*, electrocardiography

Rate Vs. Rhythm

The issue of whether or not to treat atrial fibrillation with the rate control strategy or the rhythm control strategy is one about which there has been a considerable amount of new data [4-7]. The current guidelines suggest that the initial selection of this strategy be based on the presence or absence of disabling symptoms – disabling symptoms favoring selection of the rhythm control strategy [1]. In this respect, the guidelines were probably prescient, in that the consistency of the data from the recently completed trials indicates that there is no clear advantage of the rhythm control strategy with respect to morbid events such as death, stroke and embolic events [4, 6-7].

Whether or not there is an advantage for the rhythm control strategy with respect to quality of life and relief of symptoms is less clear. Although no difference in quality of life between the two strategies was demonstrated, in one of the trials the rhythm control strategy resulted in a greater distance walked on a six-minute walk test [4]. Furthermore, it has been noted that the degree of symptoms among the patients enrolled in these trials may have been low. In the three larger trials [4, 6-7], patients with predominately persistent and symptomatic atrial fibrillation were enrolled but it seems likely that a high proportion of patients with disabling symptoms were not enrolled. On the other hand, the fourth study enrolled only highly symptomatic patients with paroxysmal atrial fibrillation who all had a DDDR pacemaker and atrioventricular junction ablation [5]. In that study, there was no further improvement in quality of life over this rate control therapy when drugs were used to try and maintain sinus rhythm, although it must be admitted that drugs were not very successful in maintaining sinus rhythm in these patients [5].

Further studies are necessary in other groups of patients under-represented in these trials to clarify some of these issues and such a study is in progress for patients with congestive heart failure [8]. Subgroup analysis of the largest trial [6] does suggest that in some patients the rate control strategy may be particularly advantageous. In the meantime, it is possible to suggest alteration of the current scheme for a large number of patients with recurrent atrial fibrillation and one potential alteration is illustrated in Figure 1.

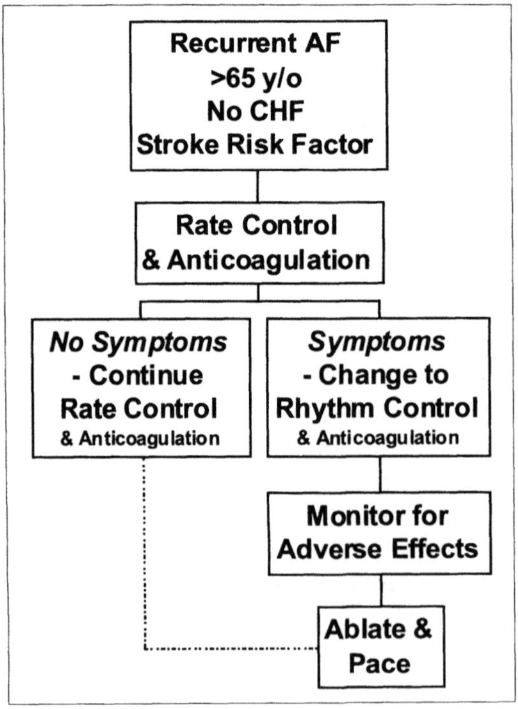

Fig. 1. A potential alteration of the current guidelines based on the results of the rate vs. rhythm trials

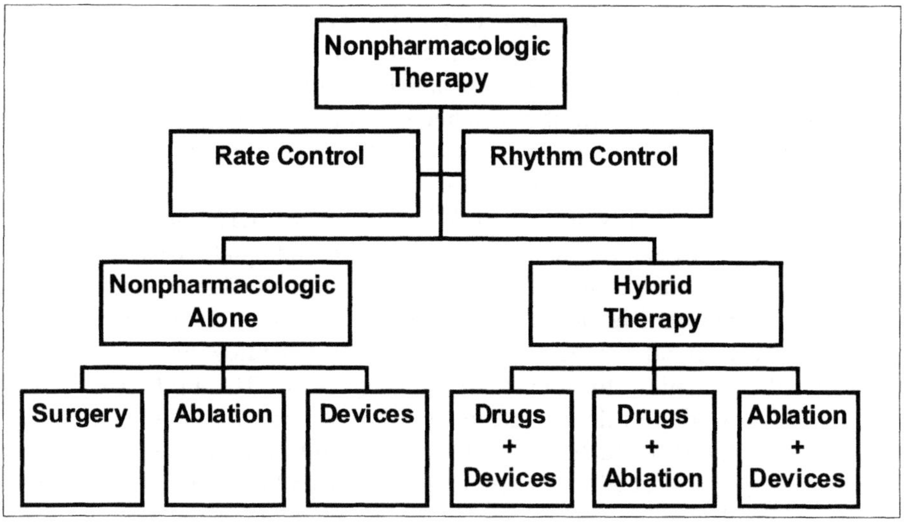

Fig. 2. One possible scheme for organization of the available data and discussion on nonpharmacologic and hybrid therapies used for treatment of atrial fibrillation

Nonpharmacologic Therapy

Although extensive consideration was given to nonpharmacologic therapies, particularly radiofrequency ablative therapy, in the preparation of the guidelines, very little of this discussion was provided in the published executive summary. Furthermore, much less attention was given to device therapies and hybrid therapies. The ACC/AHA Subcommittee on Data Standards for Atrial Fibrillation has defined a hybrid therapy as a combination of drug therapy with one or more nonpharmacologic therapy, or the combination of one or more nonpharmacologic therapies (unpublished). Although these approaches remain to be more thoroughly tested in randomized controlled trials, much progress has been made in these areas in the past 3 years. Even though the incremental new information may be relatively small, this area would benefit from a more organized approach and development of a framework. One possible framework is presented in Figure 2.

Antithrombotic Therapy

Another area wherein there are substantial new data is the area of antithrombotic therapy. The first development has been the evidence from the randomized trials of rate versus rhythm control showing that maintenance of sinus rhythm, at least with currently available therapies, does not remove the risk of stroke in patients with risk factors [4, 5-7]. The majority of strokes in these studies occurred in patients who discontinued their warfarin or whose International Normalized Ratio (INR) was subtherapeutic, regardless of which strategy was used for rhythm management [6]. Thus, it is important to emphasize in the guidelines that warfarin therapy should not be discontinued in those patients with recurrent atrial fibrillation and stroke risk factors, even when is seems that sinus rhythm has been restored and maintained according to patient symptoms. It is probably unlikely that even periodic 24-hour ambulatory electrocardiographic monitoring is adequate to guarantee that atrial fibrillation has been totally abolished. Whether or not permanent monitoring with an implanted electronic device will provide adequate assurance of the permanence of sinus rhythm remains to be established. One of the frequently encountered ambiguities for many physicians in the current guidelines for antithrombotic therapy is the distinction between the guidelines for cardioversion and the guidelines for long-term anticoagulation. The guidelines for cardioversion note that anticoagulation can be discontinued 3 weeks after cardioversion without adequate emphasis on the need to continue anticoagulation indefinitely in patients with risk factors for stroke and likelihood of recurrence of atrial fibrillation. At the present time, pharmacologic therapy for maintenance of sinus rhythm is not an adequate assurance in these patients.

Another point that is emerging has to do with the utility of the current schemes for selection of patients at high risk for stroke. There are presently 4 published schemes for determination of risk for stroke in patients with atrial fibrillation [9-12]. The problem is that these were all developed from a particular data set and they have never been evaluated in another data set. Recent unpublished data that tested the four schemes on a data set of patients taking aspirin alone suggests that the number of patients at truly high risk (≥4 strokes per 100 patient years) is much lower than previously thought. If this data withstands peer review it will be important because it may mean that warfarin may not be needed in a substantial number of patients who have a competing high risk for bleeding. The Atrial Fibrillation Treatment Guidelines Subcommittee needs to evaluate these data.

Finally, there is also emerging data that there are suitable alternatives to warfarin, such as ximelagatran. These new findings also need to be incorporated into the guidelines.

Conclusions

The published data that led to the formulation of the current guidelines for the treatment of atrial fibrillation was current up to and including the year 2000. Management of atrial fibrillation is an extremely active area of investigation. There have now been 3 additional years of data accumulation. Given this data accumulation and further data appearing during the period during which the Subcommittee would meet, it is probably time to re-convene the Subcommittee. Furthermore, one of the purposes of the guidelines is to identify areas of knowledge in which there is a void. Since the guidelines were developed, there are probably new areas that need to be identified. In this discussion four areas that need specific attention in any revision of the guidelines are highlighted: classification of patients with atrial fibrillation, application of the rate control versus rhythm control strategies, nonpharmacologic and hybrid therapies and antithrombotic therapy.

References

1. Fuster V, Ryden LE, Asinger RW et al (2001) ACC/AHA/ESC guidelines for the management of patients with atrial fibrillation: executive summary: a report of the American College of Cardiology/American Heart Association Task Force on Practice Guidelines and the European Society of Cardiology Committee for Practice Guidelines and Policy Conferences (Committee to Develop Guidelines for the Management of Patients with Atrial Fibrillation). Circulation 104:2118-2150
2. Levy S, Camm AJ, Saksena S et al (2003) International consensus on nomenclature and classification of atrial fibrillation. A collaborative project of the Working Group on Arrhythmias and Working Group on Cardiac Pacing of the European Society of Cardiology and the North American Society of Pacing and Electrophysiology. Europace 5:119-122
3. Oral H, Knight BP, Tada H et al (2002) Pulmonary vein isolation for paroxysmal and persistent atrial fibrillation. Circulation. 105:1077-1081
4. Hohnloser SH, Kuck KH, Lilienthal J (2000) Rhythm or rate control in atrial fibrillation - Pharmacological Intervention in Atrial Fibrillation (PIAF). Lancet 356:1789-1794
5. Brignole M, Menozzi C, Gasparini M et al (2002) An evaluation of the strategy of maintenance of sinus rhythm by antiarrhythmic drug therapy after ablation and pacing therapy in patients with paroxysmal atrial fibrillation. Eur Heart J 23:892-900
6. The AFFIRM Investigators (2002) A comparison of rate control and rhythm control in patients with atrial fibrillation. New Engl J Med 347:1825-1833
7. van Gelder IC, Hagens VE, Bosker HA (2002) A comparison of rate control and rhythm control in patients with recurrent persistent atrial fibrillation. New Engl J Med 347:1834-1840
8. The AF-CHF Investigators (2002) Rationale and design of a study assessing treatment strategies of atrial fibrillation in patients with heart failure: the Atrial Fibrillation and Congestive Heart Failure (AF-CHF) trial. J Am Heart 144:597-607
9. Atrial Fibrillation Investigators (1994) Risk factors for stroke and efficacy of antithrombotic therapy in atrial fibrillation. Arch Intern Med 154:1449-1457
10. Stroke Prevention Atrial Fibrillation III Writing Committee (1998) Patients with nonvalvular atrial fibrillation at low risk of stroke during treatment with aspirin: Stroke Prevention in Atrial Fibrillation III Study. JAMA 279:1273-1277
11. Albers GW, Dalen JE, Laupacis A et al (2001) Antithrombotic therapy in atrial fibrillation. Chest 119(Suppl 1):194-206
12. Gage BF, Waterman AD, Shannon W et al (2001) Validation of clinical classification schemes for predicting stroke: results from the National Registry of Atrial Fibrillation. JAMA 285:2864-2870

ATRIAL FIBRILLATION: ELECTRICAL THERAPY, TRANSCATHETER AND SURGICAL ABLATION

Atrial Fibrillation Suppression: What Role Does It Have?

A. Schuchert

Present-day pacemaker therapy is not only used to prevent bradycardia or asystole in cases of advanced AV block or sick sinus syndrome. More recent proposed indications for permanent cardiac pacing are the prevention of paroxysmal atrial fibrillation and cardiac resynchronization therapy in patients with heart failure.

As to preventing paroxysmal atrial fibrillation, AAI and dual-chamber pacing effectively prevented atrial fibrillation compared to VVI pacing [1–3]. Another observation was that more frequent atrial pacing is associated with a decrease in atrial fibrillation in patients with paroxysmal atrial tachyarrhythmias and standard pacing indications [4–6]. Because the patients in these studies had received conventional dual-chamber pacemakers, the lower atrial pacing rate was increased above the mean sinus rate. This approach has a potential limitation in patients with a normal sinus rate. Since the lower atrial rate in these patients has to be programmed to 75–90 bpm, many patients do not tolerate the high atrial rates during long-term follow-up. More recent dual-chamber pacemakers offer two solutions. One approach is continuously to compare the lower atrial pacing rate with the present sinus rate, and the pacemaker delivers an atrial pacing rate slightly above the present sinus rate. The other solution is to deliver a higher atrial rate after the pacemaker has detected specific triggers such as atrial premature contractions or the spontaneous termination of atrial fibrillation.

An algorithm implementing the first approach is the AF Suppression™ algorithm provided by St. Jude Medical devices. The algorithm is designed continuously to monitor the intrinsic atrial activity and stimulate the atrium slightly above the patient's intrinsic rhythm in an attempt to "control" the atrium. The algorithm increases the atrial rate as soon as two intrinsic beats are detected within any of 16 consecutive cardiac cycles. The lower rate overdrive controls the degree of overdrive stimulation in the lower end of the pacing rate range

Medical Clinic III, Hamburg-Eppendorf University Hospital, Hamburg, Germany

(45–59 bpm); it is set at 10 bpm. The Upper Rate Overdrive is effective in the upper end of the pacing rate range (150–180 bpm); it is set at 5 bpm. The maximum overdrive pacing rate is limited by the maximum sensor rate regardless of the sensor activation. The AF Suppression™ rate is always equal to or higher than the sensor-indicated rate. The number of Overdrive Pacing Cycles defines for how many cycles overdrive stimulation will be applied before the rate is decreased to search for the underlying rate. The settings are 15, 20, 25, 30, 35, and 40 cycles, with a nominal setting of 15 cycles. After delivering the programmed number of overdrive pacing cycles at a rate slightly above the intrinsic rhythm, the algorithm increases the cycle length in order to search for intrinsic rhythm. The Dynamic Rate Recovery determines the rate decrease from overdrive pace rate to base rate. It has a value of 8 ms for rates above 100 bpm and of 12 ms for rates from 45 to 100 bpm.

The AF Suppression™ algorithm was prospectively studied in the multicenter Adopt A study [7]. The Adopt A study included patients with a sick sinus syndrome who had a class I pacing indication and a documented history of atrial arrhythmia. After implantation of the DDDR pacemaker the patients were randomized to the Dynamic Atrial Overdrive (DAO) algorithm either *on* (n=130) or *off* (n=158). During 6 months' follow-up the patients recorded the frequency of symptomatic episodes of atrial arrhythmia verified with an event recorder. The algorithm increased the percentage of atrial pacing from 68% to 93%. The atrial fibrillation burden was 1.86% in the therapy group compared to 2.49% in the control group, which is a 25% reduction. There was a greater reduction (36%) if the patients with atrial fibrillation for more than 30 days after implantation were excluded.

The ADOPT-ALL study is a randomized, crossover-controlled, prospective, single-blinded study in 250 patients with a history of paroxysmal atrial fibrillation [8]. The primary objective is to determine whether the group utilizing the DAO algorithm will spend less time in automatic mode switch (AMS) as detected from the AMS diagnostic counter than those without DAO. Frequency of AMS episodes higher than 275 bpm are used to calculate atrial fibrillation burden. In a preliminary analysis 145 patients were enrolled, and 33 had completed 6 months' follow-up. AMS burden was 98 min/day during DAO *off* and reduced during DAO *on* by 23% to 76 min/day. Atrial fibrillation burden was 66 min/day in the control group and 39 min during DAO *on*, which is a 40% reduction. These preliminary data indicate the efficacy of the algorithm in reducing AMS burden and atrial fibrillation burden.

The OASES (Overdrive Atrial SEptum Stimulation) trial was presented at the 24th Annual North American Society of Pacing and Electrophysiology (NASPE) Scientific Sessions. The prospective multicenter trial included patients with paroxysmal atrial fibrillation and a class I or II pacemaker indication. The AF Suppression™ algorithm significantly reduced atrial fibrillation, and even better results were obtained when the atrial lead was placed in the low atrial septum. Atrial fibrillation burden was lowered by nearly 50%, from a mean of 76.0 min in the AF Suppression *off* group to a mean of 38.9 min in the AF Suppression *on* group (p=0.033). In the group of patients with atrial leads placed in the low atrial septum versus the atrial appendage, the reduction was even greater (p<0.037) from a mean of 78.1 min in the AF Suppression *off* group to a mean of 22.0 min in the AF Suppression *on* group, a 72% reduction in atrial fibrillation burden (p=0.027). In addition, the quality of life results increased significantly (p<0.001) when AF Suppression was *on* compared to *off* as calculated by Aquarel and SF 36.

The other solution, to pace intermittently after the detection of specific triggers, has not yet been studied alone. At present, the triggered algorithms have been evaluated in combination with a continuously pacing algorithm. In the studies presented so far, e.g., the ATTEST and ASPECT studies, all pacing functions programmed *on* were compared to all pacing functions *off* [9, 10]. The activation of all pacing functions had no significant beneficial effects on the atrial fibrillation burden [9, 10]. The lack of any beneficial effect indicated that simple activation of all pacing functions available in such pacemakers seems not to be effective, probably because these algorithms could have both pro- and antiarrhythmic effects at various times.

In December 2002, the AFFIRM and RACE study were published. Both studies evaluated the outcome of medical rhythm control versus rate control in patients with paroxysmal and persistent atrial fibrillation [11, 12]. The main outcome was that patients with atrial fibrillation do not have improved survival from medical rhythm control. For this reason, the revised aim of rhythm control is to reduce and avoid symptoms related to atrial fibrillation.

Another finding of the two studies was that the rhythm and the rate control groups had the same frequency of stroke. A possible explanation could be that silent or asymptomatic episodes of atrial fibrillation did occur and were not harmful in patients who had not received anticoagulation treatment. As a clinical consequence, anticoagulation treatment should be prescribed in all patients with atrial fibrillation and a medium or high risk for stroke.

Preventive pacing for atrial fibrillation requires reliable monitoring of the atrial rhythm in order to assess the efficacy of the AF Suppression™ algorithm. The extended diagnostic counters of the present-day dual-chamber pacemakers store the atrial rate histogram and duration in the automatic mode switch. These counters could be misleading if atrial oversensing, e.g., R-wave far-field sensing or P-wave undersensing, occurred. Newer pacemakers are able to verify the onset of an atrial tachyarrhythmia by stored intracardiac electrograms. An additional advantage of these diagnostic pacemaker counters is their detection of asymptomatic episodes of atrial fibrillation, which can help to tailor anticoagulation in selected patients.

For clinical impact, in several prospective, randomized studies the AF Suppression™ algorithm significantly and effectively reduced the frequency of paroxysmal atrial fibrillation in patients with standard pacing indications. The algorithm is easy to activate and simple to program on hospital discharge or during a follow-up visit. The AF Suppression™ algorithm should be programmed *ON* in patients with a history of atrial tachyarrhythmia and could be considered for patients at high risk of a new onset of atrial fibrillation. These are patients with sick sinus syndrome and, probably, heart failure patients undergoing cardiac resynchronization therapy.

References

1. Andersen HR, Nielsen JC, Thomsen PEB et al (1997) Long-term follow-up of patients from a randomised trial of atrial versus ventricular pacing for sick sinus syndrome. Lancet 350:1210–1216
2. Connolly SJ, CR Kerr, M Gent et al (2000) Effects of physiologic pacing versus ventricular pacing on the risk of stroke and death due to cardiovascular causes. N Engl J Med 342:1385–1391
3. Lamas GA, Lee KL, Sweeney MO et al (2002) Mode selection trial in sinus-node dysfunction ventricular pacing or dual-chamber pacing for sinus-node dysfunction. N Engl J Med 346:1854–1862
4. Attuel P, Pellerin D, Muciga J, Coumel PH (1988) DDD pacing: an effective treatment modality for recurrent atrial arrhythmias. Pacing Clin Electrophysiol 11:1647–1654
5. Garrigue S, Barold SS, Cazeau S et al (1998) Prevention of atrial arrhythmias during DDD pacing by atrial overdrive. Pacing Clin Electrophysiol 21:1751–1759
6. Saksena S, Prakash A, Ziegler P et al, for the DAPPAF Investigators (2002) Improved suppression of recurrent atrial fibrillation with dual-site right atrial pacing and antiarrhythmic drug therapy. J Am Coll Cardiol 40:1140–1150
7. Carlson MD, Gold MR, Ip J et al, for the ADOPT Investigators (2001) Dynamic atrial overdrive pacing decreases symptomatic atrial arrhythmia burden in patients with sinus node dysfunction. Circulation 104:II-1–II-1088
8. Beinhauer A, Vock P, Nobis H et al (2001) AF suppression by atrial dynamic overdrive pacing in the ADOPT-ALL trial. P2965. Eur Heart J 22 Abstr Suppl 554
9. Lee MA, Weachter R, Pollak S et al for the ATTEST Investigators (2003) The effect of atrial pacing therapies on atrial tachyarrhythmias burden and frequency. J Am Coll Cardiol 41:1926-1932
10. Padeletti L, Purerfellner H, Adler S et al (2002) Atrial septal lead placement and atrial pacing algorithms for prevention of paroxysmal atrial fibrillation: ASPECT study results. NASPE Abstract no 659
11. Wyse DG, Waldo AL, DiMarco JP et al, The Atrial Fibrillation Follow-up Investigation of Rhythm Management (AFFIRM<de>) Investigators (2002) A comparison of rate control and rhythm control in patients with atrial fibrillation. N Engl J Med 347:1825–1833
12. Van Gelder IC, Hagens VE, Bosker HA et al, the Rate Control versus Electrical Cardioversion for Persistent Atrial Fibrillation Study Group (2002) Comparison of rate control and rhythm control in patients with recurrent persistent atrial fibrillation. N Engl J Med 347:1834–1840

Dual-chamber ICDs: How Effective and Safe Are They in the Treatment of Atrial Tachyarrhythmias?

J. Kautzner, P. Peichl

Introduction

The rapid development of internal cardioverter defibrillator (ICD) technology in the late 1990s resulted in the construction of sophisticated dual-chamber devices. Initially, the rationale behind their introduction was the possibility of sequential pacing for bradyarrhythmia whenever required, thus avoiding the need for parallel pacemaker implantation. At the same time, the use of an atrial lead was viewed as an opportunity to improve discrimination between supraventricular and ventricular arrhythmias. The experience obtained with atrial defibrillators and in studies on pacing prevention of atrial fibrillation was subsequently also exploited in novel ICD devices. Now, as they have such a powerful tool available, some clinicians suggest the use of dual-chamber devices in all ICD candidates who are in sinus rhythm [1]. Indeed, most ICDs currently implanted in the USA are dual-chamber devices [2]. On the other hand, there is mounting evidence that such an approach is not devoid of risk. Therefore, the purpose of this review is to discuss the pros and cons of dual-chamber ICDs.

Therapy for Atrial Tachyarrhythmia

Apart from when indicated by bradyarrhythmia, dual-chamber ICDs are most frequently used when it is thought they will decrease the incidence of supraventricular tachyarrhythmias, with the intention of treating these effectively. In this context, it has been reported that 20–25% of patients receiving an ICD for the treatment of ventricular tachyarrhythmias have a history of paroxysmal atrial fibrillation [3, 4]. In addition, even ICD patients with no such history appear to present with their first episode of paroxysmal atrial fibrillation

Department of Cardiology, Institute for Clinical and Experimental Medicine, Prague, Czech Republic

after the implant at an annual rate of approximately 2.6% [4]. Atrial fibrillation may not only trigger inappropriate therapy, but also induce ventricular arrhythmia, worsen heart failure, or be associated with thromboembolism. Therefore, novel dual-chamber ICDs offer a significant advance in arrhythmia management in ICD recipients. Schoels et al. [5] summarized extensive clinical experience obtained in a multicenter trial on the safety and efficacy of a dual-chamber ICD (Medtronic 7250 Jewel AF). They analyzed data from 293 patients over a follow-up period of 7.9±4.7 years and observed no failures in detecting and treating ventricular arrhythmias; at the same time, they found 95% positive predictive accuracy for the detection of atrial episodes. The efficacy of atrial antitachycardia pacing and high-frequency (50 Hz) pacing was 55% and 17%, respectively. High-frequency burst pacing terminated 16.8% of episodes classified as atrial fibrillation, while atrial defibrillation was successful in 76% of cases. More extensive experience with the same device was published by Adler et al. [6], who demonstrated an overall pacing efficacy of 48% for termination of atrial tachyarrhythmia episodes. Pacing successfully terminated 59% of atrial tachycardia episodes, but only 30% of atrial fibrillation episodes. Surprisingly, 63% of the treated episodes were classified as atrial tachycardias and not as atrial fibrillation, even though the vast majority of patients concerned had a history of atrial fibrillation. More recently, data from the Italian registry of patients with a Medtronic 7250 Jewel AF device have also provided support for these figures [7]. Out of 414 treated episodes, 159 (38.4%) were classified by the device as atrial fibrillation, while 225 (61.6%) were described as atrial tachycardia. Clinicians classified these episodes as atrial fibrillation in 46.4%, atrial tachycardia in 47.1% and sinus rhythm in 6.5%. Accordingly, the success rate of pacing therapy (burst and ramp pacing, 50-Hz burst) in the treatment of atrial tachycardias reached 71%. Furthermore, a 50-Hz burst was able to terminate even atrial fibrillation in 36.2% of cases. The overall efficacy of atrial antitachycardia pacing therapy was 54%. Atrial shock proved effective in 62.5% for termination of atrial fibrillation, and no ventricular tachyarrhythmias were observed. Results of a substudy on the ability of the dual-chamber ICD to reduce the burden of spontaneous atrial tachyarrhythmias were reported by Friedman et al. [8]. ICD patients were randomized to 3-month periods with atrial therapies "on" and "off" and subsequently crossed over. Atrial therapies resulted in a reduction of the atrial tachyarrhythmia burden from a mean of 58.5 h to 7.8 h per month. The median difference in burden was highly significant (p=0.007), and there was a trend towards a reduction in the frequency of episodes of atrial arrhythmia (p=0.07). To summarize the above experience, it seems that atrial therapies provided by dual-chamber ICDs are both safe and reasonably effective in the treatment of supraventricular tachyarrhythmias.

Atrial Fibrillation Prevention Algorithms

Pacing algorithms to prevent atrial fibrillation are based predominantly on suppression of the atrial premature beats that play an important part in its initiation. At present, different variants are under clinical evaluation, and several preliminary reports have shown a reduced frequency of arrhythmia [1, 9]. While this is encouraging, similar studies are limited by frequent patient exclusion, there are problems with the implementation of these algorithms in the presence of far-field ventricular sensing in the atrial lead, and it is uncertain whether the burden reduction is related to pacing prevention or to antitachycardia pacing itself. Thus, in the absence of a well-controlled randomized trial, the efficacy of prevention algorithms remains uncertain.

Dual-chamber Efficacy in Discrimination

The advent of dual-chamber ICDs has offered the potential advantage that these devices could substantially reduce or even avoid inappropriate therapies through better discrimination of arrhythmias. Clinical studies in patients with single-chamber ICDs have demonstrated that inappropriate therapy is delivered in 20-30% cases [10, 11]. Such inappropriate therapy may be associated with pain and/or psychological stress [12], and can even lead to death [13]. The most frequent cause is supraventricular tachyarrhythmia erroneously identified by the device as ventricular tachycardia or ventricular fibrillation. The actual benefits of new dual-chamber ICDs have been investigated in relatively few studies. Most of these have concentrated on safety at implantation, involved only small numbers of patients, and been restricted to devices obtained from one manufacturer only. More recent studies show increased specificity of detection algorithms and a significant reduction in the frequency of inappropriate therapies due to supraventricular tachyarrhythmias [14, 15]. However, Kühlkamp et al. [16] demonstrated that new dual-chamber detection algorithms did not reduce the frequency of inappropriate therapies compared with the single-chamber ICD supplied by the same manufacturer. In the study of Deisenhofer et al. [17], the overall incidence of inappropriate therapies was 10.1% in 16 of 92 patients, and in 13 of them the error was due to inaccurate detection of supraventricular tachyarrhythmia. Randomized comparison with single-chamber ICD failed to demonstrate any major advantage of a dual-chamber detection algorithm over enhanced criteria in single-chamber ICD.

Risks Associated with Dual-chamber ICDs

While the effectiveness of ICDs has predominantly been established with single-chamber backup pacing, a number of currently implanted ICDs incorporate dual-chamber pacing. In this context, we should ask whether one can simply extrapolate the data on efficacy of these devices to mortality benefit and whether there are any additional risks related to the use of dual-chamber devices in a typical ICD population.

Consideration of these concerns is prudent in the light of data about the potentially deleterious effect of right-ventricular pacing in patients with bradyarrhythmias, especially when associated with left-ventricular dysfunction (Fig. 1). Andresen et al. [18] evaluated the differences between AAI and VVI

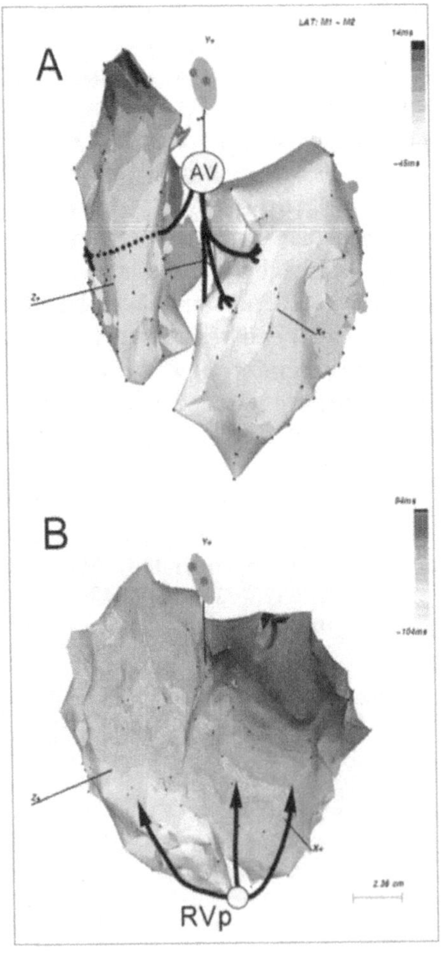

Fig. 1. Electroanatomical activation maps of both ventricles in left anterior oblique view and caudal tilt in: **A** subject with normal ventricular conduction and **B** a patient with right ventricular pacing (maps are coded in grey scale with the lightest tinge being the earliest, while the darkest shade corresponds to very late activation). Note almost simultaneous early activation of both the left ventricular septum and the right ventricular anterior wall in a normal patient (drawing suggests location of the AV node and branching of the conduction system). The activation wavefront subsequently spreads towards the left lateral wall, and finally, towards the apex. On the contrary, right ventricular apical pacing reverses completely activation sequence of the left ventricle, with early activation of the apex spreading towards the base (*arrows*), leading to variable degree of electromechanical dyssynchrony

pacing among patients with sick sinus syndrome. AAI pacing was associated with slightly better survival and a lower occurrence of severe heart failure. Similarly, in the Pacemaker Selection in the Elderly Study [19] VVI was compared with DDD pacing, revealing no difference in overall outcome as reflected in the incidence of cardiovascular events or deaths. The only difference favoring DDD pacing was found in terms of better quality of life. Recent data from the MOST (Mode Selection Trial in Sinus Node Dysfunction) trial suggested that an increased number of hospitalizations for heart failure was associated with the prevalence of more than 40% right-ventricular pacing, and not with the pacing mode per se [20].

The only ICD trial that included dual-chamber ICDs, MADIT II [21], reported that the incidence of new or worsened heart failure was higher in the ICD group than in the conventional therapy group (19.9% vs 14.9%; $p = 0.09$). These data suggest that unnecessary right-ventricular stimulation in patients with left-ventricular dysfunction may promote progression of heart failure. On the other hand, patients with heart failure and a need for ICD therapy are known to suffer more frequently with atrial tachyarrhythmias, low cardiac output and/or symptomatic bradycardia in the presence of drugs with negative chronotropic potential. In such a population, dual-chamber ICDs could offer potential benefits. The DAVID trial was designed to find whether this is so [22]. A total of 506 patients in whom there was a primary or secondary indication for ICD therapy and who had evidence of ventricular dysfunction underwent implantation of dual-chamber ICD and were randomized to either ventricular back-up pacing only (VVI, 40 bpm lower rate) or dual-chamber rate-responsive pacing (DDDR, 70 bpm lower rate). The trial was terminated early because the incidence of new or worsened congestive heart failure was greater in the DDDR group. At the 18-month follow-up, DDDR patients had an approximately 60% higher relative probability of death or hospitalization for new or worsened heart failure than did VVI patients (p=0.03). None of the patients had a primary indication for bradycardia pacing, and the mode of pacing thus resulted in a different percentage of ventricular paced beats. In the VVI group, pacing accounted for approximately 1% of all beats, whereas in the DDDR group nearly 60% of all beats were paced. This suggests that ventricular dyssynchrony resulting from right-ventricular apical pacing was responsible for most of the detrimental effect of DDDR pacing. This seems to outbalance all other potential benefits of dual-chamber devices.

Regardless of its potentially detrimental use in patients with heart failure, there is limited information on the long-term safety of dual-chamber ICDs. In this respect, somewhat disturbing data were published by Takahashi et al. [23], who compared the frequency of complications in single-chamber and in dual-chamber ICDs in 178 patients. Twelve (16%) of the 74 patients with dual-chamber ICDs presented with a total of 16 major complications, compared with 6 (6%) of the 104 patients with single-chamber ICDs (p=0.01).

Could Biventricular ICDs Solve the Problem?

So far, there are no data on the prophylactic use of biventricular pacing in patients with symptoms classed as lower than NYHA functional class III. Based on preliminary results of the COMPANION (Comparison of Medical Therapy, Pacing, and Defibrillation in Heart Failure) Trial showing a highly significant (43%) reduction in mortality in patients with heart failure and NYHA class III or IV, we can expect an expansion of the indication for sophisticated dual-chamber ICDs with biventricular pacing [24].

Conclusions

When all the above aspects are considered together, it seems prudent to restrict the use of dual-chamber devices predominantly to ICD patients who have conventional pacemaker bradyarrhythmic indication. The proportion of such patients is estimated at up to 30% [25]. At present, there is no clearly documented data supporting the use of dual-chamber devices in subjects with primary indication for ICD implantation. Those with frequent atrial tachyarrhythmias at the time of ICD implantation may be among the few exceptions. Patients who need an ICD and present with more advanced heart failure (NYHA class III/IV) appear rather to be candidates for dual-chamber ICD with biventricular pacing.

References

1. Santini M, Ricci R (2001) Atrial fibrillation coexisting with ventricular tachycardia: a challenge for dual chamber defibrillators. Heart 86:253-254
2. Product market mix of dual-chamber and single-chamber ICDs. Available at http://imshealth.com.
3. Schmitt C, Montero M, Melichercik J (1998) Significance of supraventricular tachyarrhythmias in patients with implanted pacing cardioverter defibrillators 17:295-302
4. Best PJ, Hayes DL, Stanton MS (1999) The potential usage of dual chamber pacing in patients with implantable cardioverter defibrillators. Pacing Clin Electrophysiol 22:79-85
5. Schoels W, Swerdlow CD, Jung W et al (2001) Worldwide clinical experience with a new dual-chamber implantable cardioverter-defibrillator system. J Cardiovasc Electrophysiol 12:521-528
6. Adler SW, Wolpert C, Warman EN et al (2001) Efficacy of pacing therapies for treating atrial tachyarrhythmias in patients with ventricular arrhythmias receiving a dual-chamber implantable cardioverter-defibrillator. Circulation 104:887-892
7. Ricci R, Pignalberi C, Disertori M et al (2002) Efficacy of a dual chamber defibrillator with atrial antitachycardia functions in treating spontaneous atrial tachyarrhytmias in patients with life-threatening ventricular tachyarrhytmias. Eur Heart J 23:1471-1479

8. Friedman PA, Dijkman B, Warman EN et al (2001) Atrial therapies reduce atrial arrhythmia burden in defibrillator patients. Circulation 104:1023-1028
9. Prakash A (2002) Pacing for the prevention of atrial fibrillation. Curr Opin Cardiol 17:73-81
10. Pinski SL, Fahy GJ (1995) The proarrhythmic potential of implantable cardioverter-defibrillators. Circulation 92:1651-1664
11. Weber M, Block M, Brunn J et al (1996) Inadequate therapies with implantable cardioverter-defibrillators – incidence, etiology, predictive factors and prevention strategies. Z Kardiol 85:809-819
12. Lüderitz B, Jung W, Deister A et al (1993) Patient acceptance of implantable cardioverter-defibrillator in ventricular tachyarrhythmias. Pacing Clin Electrophysiol 16:1815-1821
13. Birgetsdotter-Green U, Rosenqvist M, Lindemans FW et al (1992) Holter documented sudden death in a patient with an implanted defibrillator. Pacing Clin Electrophysiol 15:1008-1014
14. Lavergne T, Daubert JC, Chauvin M et al (1997) Preliminary clinical experience with the first dual chamber pacemaker defibrillator. Pacing Clin Electrophysiol 20:182-188
15. Trappe HJ, Achtelik M, Pfitzner P et al (1999) Single-chamber versus dual-chamber implantable cardioverter-defibrillators: indications and clinical results. Am J Cardiol 83(5B):8D-16D
16. Kühlkamp V, Dornberger V, Mewis C et al (1999) Clinical experience with the new detection algorithms for atrial fibrillation of a defibrillator with dual chamber sensing and pacing. J Cardiovasc Electrophysiol 10:905-915
17. Deisenhofer I, Kolb C, Ndrepepa G et al (1999) Do current dual chamber cardioverter defibrillators have advantages over conventional single chamber cardioverter defibrillators in reducing inappropriate therapies: a randomized, prospective study. J Cardiovasc Electrophysiol 12:134-142b
18. Andresen HR, Nielsen JC, Thomsen PE et al (1997) Long-term follow-up of patients from a randomized trial of atrial versus ventricular pacing for sick-sinus syndrome. Lancet 350:1210-1216
19. Lamas GA, Orav EJ, Stambler BS et al (1998) Quality of life and clinical outcomes in elderly patients treated with ventricular pacing as compared with dual chamber pacing. Pacemaker Selection in the Elderly Investigators. N Engl J Med 338:1097-1104
20. Sweeney M, Hellkamp A, Greenspon A et al (2002) Baseline QRS duration ≥ 120 milliseconds and cumulative percent time ventricular paced predicts increased risk of heart failure, stroke, and death in DDDR/paced patients with sick sinus syndrome in MOST (abstract). Pacing Clin Electrophysiol 25:690
21. Moss AJ, Zareba W, Hall WJ et al (2002) Prophylactic implantation of a defibrillator in patients with myocardial infarction and reduced ejection fraction. N Engl J Med 346:877-883
22. The DAVID Trial Investigators (2002) Dual-chamber pacing or ventricular backup pacing in patients with an implantable defibrillator: The Dual Chamber and VVI Implantable Defibrillator (DAVID) Trial. JAMA 288:3115-3123
23. Takahashi T, Bhandari A, Watanuki M et al (2002) High incidence of device-related and lead-related complications in the dual-chamber implantable cardioverter defibrillator compared with the single-chamber version. Circ J 66:748-750
24. Bristow MR, Saxon LA, Boehmer J et al Cardiac resynchronization therapy (CRT) reduces hospitalizations, and CRT+an implantable defibrillator (CRT-D) reduces mortality in chronic heart failure: preliminary results of the COMPANION Trial. www.uchsc.edu/cvi

25. Proclemer A, Della Bella P, Facchin D et al (2001) Indications for dual-chamber cardioverter defibrillators at implant and at 1 year follow-up: a retrospective analysis in the single-chamber defibrillator era. Europace 3:132-135

Ablation of Atrial Fibrillation: Are We Still "Learning While Burning"?

J.A. Salerno-Uriarte[1], R. De Ponti[1], M. Tritto[2], M.E. Lanzotti[1], R. Marazzi[1], G. Spadacini[2], P. Moretti[2]

During the 1990s, the concept of "learning while burning" was introduced and developed by Callans et al. in a series of articles [1–3]. In these papers, the authors expressed the idea that catheter ablation (burning), far from marking the end of pathophysiological investigation, may be viewed as a tool to provide unique and new information (learning) about arrhythmia substrates. Earlier, since with the introduction of catheter ablation electrophysiology had focused more and more on procedural efficacy and case volume, Smith and Cain [4] showed the possible detrimental development from electrophysiology to "electrotechnology," with loss of research, investigation, and learning–teaching, which has always surrounded the field of cardiac electrophysiology. Recently, the "learning while burning" concept has been revisited and applied [5] to the pathophysiology of atrial fibrillation, where, although the experience of pulmonary vein ablation contributes to the increase of our knowledge day by day, much still remains to be understood of the ultimate mechanism of the arrhythmia. On the other hand, it has been pointed out that trying to elucidate the mechanism of human atrial fibrillation appears as frustrating as being the translator at the Tower of Babel [6], meaning that the pathophysiology of this arrhythmia may present multiple aspects in different clinical and electrophysiological settings, difficult to investigate in humans. In the present paper, we attempt to revisit some aspects of the experience in catheter ablation of atrial fibrillation, trying to point out what we have learnt and what we still have to learn to improve our knowledge and, hopefully, results. For reasons of brevity, only catheter ablation for electrical isolation of the pulmonary veins with an electrophysiological end-point [7] is considered.

[1]University of Insubria–Varese, Department of Cardiovascular Sciences, Ospedale di Circolo e Fondazione Macchi, Varese, and [2]Department of Cardiology "Mater Domini", Castellanza, Italy

Learning Before Burning

Circular mapping tools placed at the venoatrial junction are widely used to identify pulmonary vein potentials, whose disappearance or dissociation represents the end-point of the ablation procedure as proposed by Haïssaguerre [7]. Valuable preablation electrophysiological studies [8, 9] using these mapping catheters evidence great heterogeneity in conduction properties and refractoriness, which suggests the presence of abnormal and unique electrophysiological characteristics of pulmonary vein myocardial fibers. In fact, in patients with atrial fibrillation as compared to control patients, the effective refractory period of the myocardial sleeves in the pulmonary veins is shorter than the value in the left atrium; similarly, the effective refractory period in the pulmonary veins is significantly shorter in patients with atrial fibrillation than in control patients [8]. Furthermore, programmed electrical stimulation in the pulmonary veins results in decremental conduction with possible change in the circumferential activation sequence of the pulmonary vein [8, 9]. In our experience, a 64-pole basket catheter (Constellation, Boston Scientific) is used for high-density mapping in the pulmonary veins first, before ablation, to evaluate their pattern of electrical activation and then, during ostial ablation, to monitor the atrium-to-vein conduction. By using a computerized mapping system (QMS2, Boston Scientific), analysis of the local activation time in each of the 57 bipolar recordings from the basket catheter is performed and polar isochronal maps are generated. From these high-density mapping data we learnt that the electrical activation of the pulmonary veins during sinus or a left-paced rhythm may be complex, reflecting the mesh-like arrangement of fibers, which has been described on histology in humans [10]. In fact, our analysis shows that the pattern of pulmonary vein activation during sinus or a left-paced rhythm can be of two different types (Fig. 1): in the first type, the vein activation is predominantly longitudinal (i.e., from the atrium-to-vein conduction breakthrough the impulse follows predominantly a direction parallel to the long axis of the vein), whereas in the second type it is predominantly transverse (i.e., the activation direction is predominantly perpendicular to the long axis of the vein). Limited areas of transverse conduction can also be observed in veins with a predominantly longitudinal pattern and vice versa. Interestingly, although these preliminary data refer only to 37 pulmonary veins in 19 patients, the activation pattern is likely to be patient-specific, since, when multiple veins are mapped in the same patient, the activation pattern is the same in all of them in the vast majority of the patients. Furthermore, as also shown in Fig. 1, this method allows simultaneous identification on a single beat of the multiple atrium-to-vein conduction breakthroughs, which may be particularly useful in case of early atrial fibrillation recurrence after DC shock cardioversion. No less than two and no more than three breakthroughs have been identified per vein, each breakthrough showing a discrete and definite extension at the venoatrial junction.

Firing activity originating from the pulmonary veins can be reproducibly

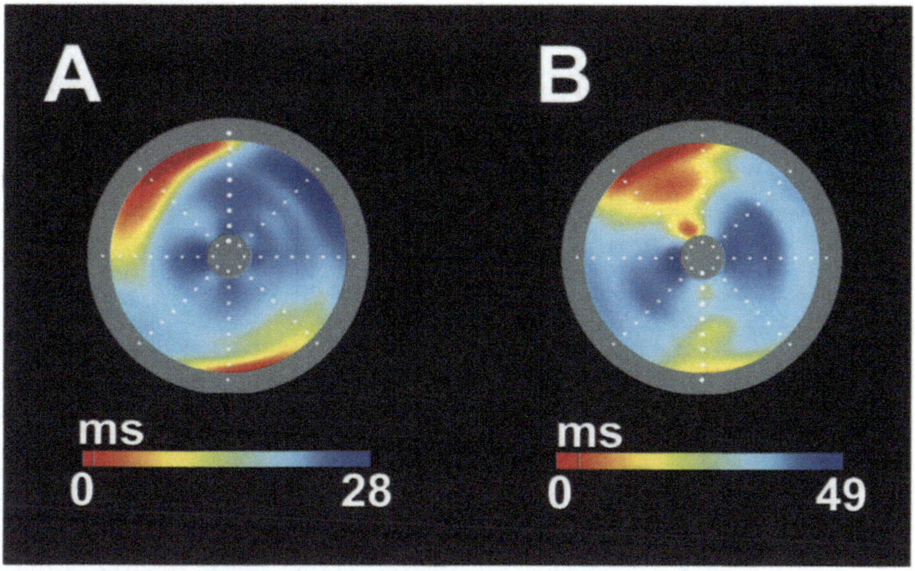

Fig. 1. Isochronal polar high-density map of a right superior (panel A) and of a left superior (panel B) pulmonary vein during sinus rhythm in two different patients. In each map, as well as in Fig. 3, the *inner circle* identifies the distal electrodes of the basket catheter, whereas the *outer circle* corresponds to the vein orifice, where the proximal electrodes are placed. The colors *red* and *purple* identify earliest and latest activation, respectively, considering the time of the earliest activated pulmonary vein potential as time 0. The range of values (in milliseconds) are indicated on the scale. In panel A, the two *red* areas at 9–12 o'clock and at 5–6 o'clock of the pulmonary vein orifice indicate the two breakthroughs of atrium-to-vein conduction. The pattern of vein activation is predominantly transverse, since the activation proceeds from the breakthroughs in a direction perpendicular to the long vein axis. Two breakthroughs are also identified in the case shown in panel B: the predominant breakthrough is located at 10–12 o'clock, whereas the second and less obvious breakthrough may be identified at 6 o'clock. In this case, the vein activation is predominantly longitudinal, since the activation proceeds from the breakthrough straight towards the distal part of the vein

observed in the same vein and in the same patient only in a limited number of cases. Nevertheless, these observations may contribute to clarify the mechanism and the pattern of atrial fibrillation at its onset in this subset of patients. Recently, it has been reported that, when ectopic activity from pulmonary veins is reproducibly observed in a form of bigeminy [11], ectopies conducted to the atrium have a significantly longer coupling interval than do those that remain concealed in the vein, suggesting that a critical value of refractoriness at the venoatrial junction may be responsible for this phenomenon. Figure 2 reports an example of this phenomenon, recorded in our laboratory in a left inferior pulmonary vein. As highlighted by the dotted lines, the activation

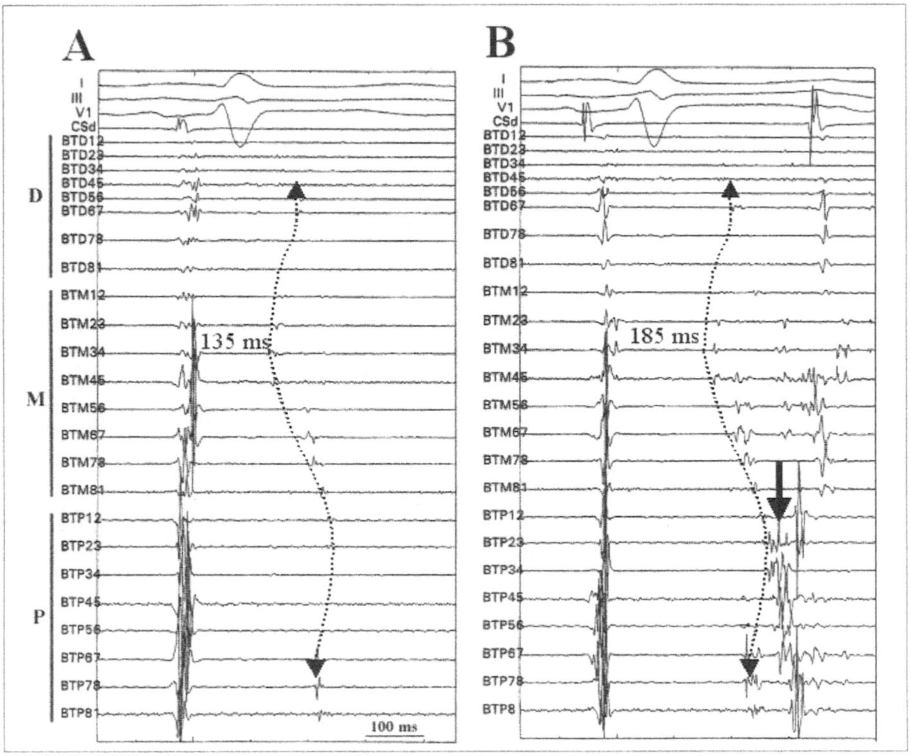

Fig. 2. Example of concealed (panel **A**) and manifest (panel **B**) ectopic beat originating from a left inferior pulmonary vein. From *top* to *bottom*, leads I, III, V1, bipolar recording of the coronary sinus electrogram (CSd), and eight bipolar recordings from a distal (D), medium (M), and proximal (P) cross-section of the basket catheter are shown. In panel A, ectopy is confined in the vein with no propagation to the atrial myocardium. The activation sequence of the ectopic beat is evidenced by the dotted arrow and the coupling interval to the previous sinus beat is 135 ms. Panel B shows another ectopy occurring in the same vein and patient. Here, the activation sequence is very similar to the one shown in panel A, but the coupling interval is longer (185 ms) and now the ectopic beat is conducted to the atrium, with the earliest atrial activation indicated by the *vertical arrow*

sequence of the concealed ectopy is identical to the one of the conducted ectopy, although the coupling interval is reproducibly shorter in the first case. In our experience, the basket catheter in combination with the QMS2 mapping system has been also used for high-density mapping of the ectopic activity arising from pulmonary veins and triggering atrial fibrillation (Fig. 3). A preliminary analysis of the isochronal maps obtained shows that in the majority of the cases the sites of earliest activation of the ectopic activity are multiple and the spatial distribution, as well as the activation times, suggests a multifo-

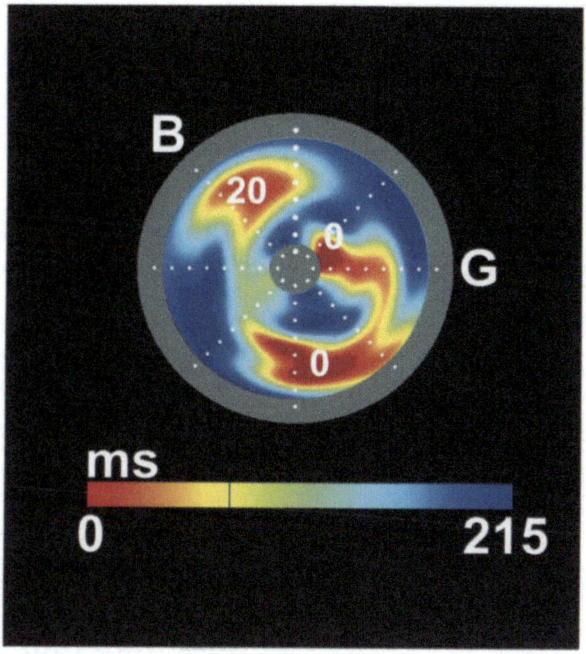

Fig. 3. Isochronal polar high-density map of the same right superior pulmonary vein as shown in A in Fig. 1, during ectopic activity originating from this vein. Upon onset of atrial fibrillation, three areas of earliest, almost synchronous activation are observed in different regions of the vein, with a clear multifocal activation pattern. Interestingly, at 4–5 o'clock a very proximal, ostial focus is observed. *B* and *G* refer to the names of the splines of the basket catheter, the electrograms from which are shown in Fig. 4

cal origin of the ectopy. Furthermore, the pattern of ectopic activation in a given pulmonary vein and in a given patient is very reproducible, being almost identical in all the recorded ectopies. Interestingly, in about half of the cases, at least one ectopic focus is located in the proximal part of the vein (Fig. 3), and this underlines the need for a very proximal line of isolation in these cases. A final peculiar observation in high-density mapping is that, upon initiation of atrial fibrillation, in the multiple foci of earliest activation a fragmented fibrillatory activity is already present (Fig. 4) and "drives" the onset of the arrhythmia; the earliest ectopic activation shows a minimum and almost fixed value of coupling interval to the preceding sinus beat. Longer F–F cycles are observed in late-activated areas of the vein, with a pattern in favor of a passive role of these sites upon onset of atrial fibrillation. These as well as other authors' data (see below) may shed some light on the arrhythmogenesis of atrial fibrillation, suggesting that, possibly, a combination of triggered activity and local reentry may take place in multiple, although very limited, areas of the vein and be the "primum movens" of the arrhythmia, with a combination of active "driving" areas and passive "driven" zones.

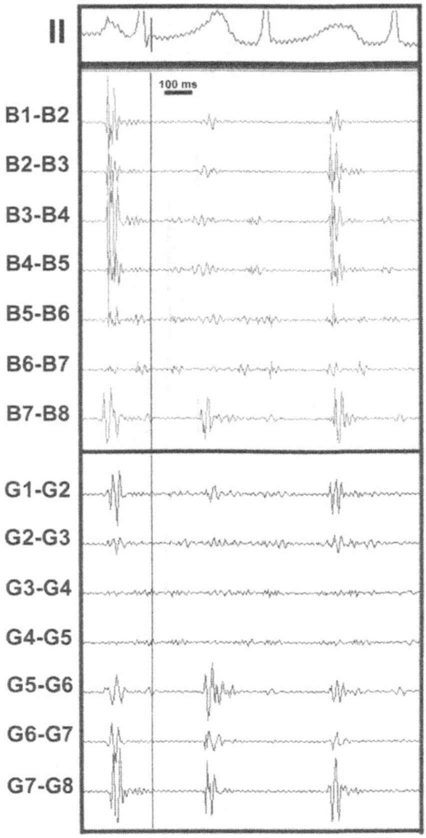

Fig. 4. High-density mapping of the onset of atrial fibrillation in the right superior pulmonary vein shown in Figs. 1 (panel A) and 3. From *top* to *bottom*, lead II is shown together with bipolar electrograms obtained from seven contiguous bipoles (from distal to proximal) in splines B and G, whose position is indicated in the previous figure. The *uninterrupted vertical line* is arbitrarily traced at the end of the QRS complex of the last sinus beat; the *short vertical lines* indicate the beginning of activation in each tracing. In the areas of earliest activation (B5–B6, B6–B7; G2–G3, G3–G4, G4–G5), indicated as *red* areas in Fig. 3, an early, fragmented fibrillatory activity is recorded at the onset of atrial fibrillation. Conversely, in later activated areas (B1–B2, B2–B3; G6–G7, G7–G8), shown in *blue* in Fig. 3, discrete atrial deflections and longer F–F cycles are observed

Learning While Burning

Although electrical isolation of the pulmonary vein is usually performed in sinus rhythm or coronary sinus pacing after identification of the atrium-to-vein conduction breakthroughs, it has been recently reported that pulmonary vein isolation is also feasible during sustained atrial fibrillation, when DC shock cardioversion is unable to restore stable sinus rhythm [12, 13]. Interestingly, this approach taught us that a disorganized activation pattern during atrial fibrillation is less frequently observed in the inferior pulmonary veins than in the superior pulmonary veins, which are considered to be more active in triggering atrial fibrillation. Furthermore, progressive elimination by radiofrequency energy delivery of the conduction fascicles from the left atrium to pulmonary veins results in a transition from a disorganized to a more and more organized activation pattern before pulmonary vein isolation, which eventually allows restoration of stable sinus rhythm [13]. As pointed out by the authors, this observation correlates well with what was originally described by Garrey in 1914: when an isthmus of conduction is narrowed during fibrillation, fibrillatory activity disappears and a more organized pattern is observed. This intriguing concept that complex interactions occur at the venoatrial junction to produce atrial fibrillation is corroborated by the observation that ostial disconnection of the pulmonary vein is associated with suppression of the ectopic bigeminy activity, reproducibly recorded inside the vein before ablation [11].

The recent observation of occurrence of confined atrial fibrillation in isolated common left pulmonary veins, although rare, may contribute to shed further light on the underlying mechanism of atrial fibrillation [14]. In these cases, the dissociated intrinsic pulmonary vein rhythm after ostial isolation was enhanced by orciprenaline infusion, up until a repetitive local response with a fixed coupling interval to the dissociated rhythm appeared and eventually produced a nonsustained fibrillation solely affecting the isolated common left pulmonary veins, with no alteration of the stable sinus rhythm observed in the atria. As already mentioned before, this observation too is in favor of the combination of two arrhythmogenic mechanisms, namely triggered activity and reentry, as the underlying mechanism of focal atrial fibrillation, which is very sensitive to autonomic tone variation induced by orciprenalin infusion [14, 15].

While ablating the breakthroughs of atrium-to-vein conduction, we learnt that in some cases it is difficult to block these fascicles surrounding the pulmonary veins. Usually, the more proximal the line of ablation is, the more difficult the conduction interruption appears. This problem may be also related to the use of low-power radiofrequency energy in this area, to prevent pulmonary vein stenosis (see below). In our experience, in some cases the lesion created at the sites of atrium-to-vein conduction may be unstable and prone to resumption of conduction. In fact, the acute intravenous administration of adenosine in 62 pulmonary veins in a series of consecutive patients after achievement of acute electrical isolation showed transient or persistent resumption of atrium-to-vein conduction in 35% of the veins, with an activation pattern similar to baseline. Further radiofrequency ablation at the conduction breakthroughs permanently eliminated atrium-to-vein conduction in all cases. These data, although on the one hand they provide evidence that adenosine injection can be a useful test to identify those cases prone to conduction recurrence, on the other highlight that low-power radiofrequency energy may produce an unstable and partial lesion of the myocardial sleeves, which surround the pulmonary veins. Therefore, research on alternative systems for energy delivery (cooled-tip radiofrequency energy ablation) or on alternative energy sources should continue.

Learning After Burning

Early in the experience of pulmonary vein ablation, we learnt that radiofrequency energy delivery at the orifice or inside a vein may produce significant lumen reduction. This phenomenon is related to the heat-induced contraction of the pulmonary veins, is associated with collagen denaturation [16], and correlates with the amount of energy delivered [17] and the lesion extension [18]. Distal ablation inside the pulmonary vein, as performed at the beginning of the experience of atrial fibrillation ablation, was associated with a 5.6-fold higher risk of stenosis than ostial ablation [19]. Several methods, such as transesophageal Doppler echocardiography, spiral computed tomography, and three-dimensional contrast-enhanced magnetic resonance imaging [17–22], are used to evaluate the presence of postprocedure stenoses and their evolution during follow-up. From these data we learnt that, although on the one hand mild stenosis may remain unchanged or regress, significant stenosis (>50% of the lumen) may progress to a high-grade stenosis in the first months of follow-up [17, 18]; at a 2-year follow-up, significant pulmonary vein stenosis/occlusion is observed in up to 28% of the cases in a limited patient series [19]. Although significant pulmonary vein stenosis may remain asymptomatic, one should not underestimate the importance of this complication, which is at risk of developing into high-degree stenosis or even complete pulmonary vein occlusion – a condition which is highly symptomatic, frequently misdiagnosed [23], and not permanently treated by stenting [20]. As we evaluate methods to avoid pulmonary vein stenosis, such as intracardiac echo monitoring during the ablation procedure [24] and the use of other energy sources, at present a safe approach for pulmonary vein isolation should include the delivery of a limited amount of radiofrequency energy only at the atrial aspect of the vein orifice and the effort to identify, when possible, and isolate only the culprit pulmonary veins.

Another peculiar observation during follow-up is that, unlike other supraventricular arrhythmias, early postprocedure recurrences do not preclude delayed cure of the arrhythmia after the first months of follow-up [25]. It could be speculated that in these cases, the irritative effect of the acute lesion may be responsible for early recurrence, whereas healing of the ostial lesion leads to magnification of the effect of ablation.

Finally, another interesting finding in the follow-up of patients who are partially responsive after the first pulmonary vein ablation procedure is a significant reduction of the postprocedure atrial fibrillation burden, with shortening of the duration of atrial fibrillation recurrences as compared to the preablation period. This observation, in conjunction with the one of "non-random" termination of atrial fibrillation during ostial ablation [12] and of rapid focal pulmonary vein activation during atrial fibrillation [26], suggests that pulmonary veins are involved not only in the initiation, but also in the perpetuation of the arrhythmia.

Concluding Remarks

Over the last few years, the amount of data gathered in the experience of catheter ablation for atrial fibrillation has helped both to refine the ablation technique and to formulate some plausible hypotheses on the underlying arrhythmogenic mechanism of atrial fibrillation in humans. However, to date, we are still "learning while burning," and there are still "more questions than answers" [27]. In general, there are too many options for treating atrial fibrillation, all with suboptimal results, and it is axiomatic that an inverse relationship exists between knowledge of the pathophysiology of an arrhythmia and the number of proposed therapies to cure it [6]. Thus, from this point on, the best way to proceed could be "learning *before* burning," and to plan good basic and clinical prospective research that aims to clarify the still unexplained issues of atrial fibrillation in humans.

References

1. Callans DJ, Schwartzman D, Gottlieb CD, Marclinski FE (1994) Insights into the electrophysiology of ventricular tachycardia gained by the catheter ablation experience: "learning while burning." J Cardiovasc Electrophysiol 5:877–894
2. Callans DJ, Schwartzman D, Gottlieb CD, Marclinski FE (1995) Insights into the electrophysiology of atrial arrhythmias gained by the catheter ablation experience: "learning while burning, Part II." J Cardiovasc Electrophysiol 6:229–243
3. Callans DJ, Schwartzman D, Gottlieb CD, Marclinski FE (1996) Insights into the electrophysiology of accessory pathway-mediated arrhythmias provided by the cather ablation experience: "learning while burning, Part III." J Cardiovasc Electrophysiol 7:877–904
4. Smith JM, Cain ME (1993) Radiofrequency catheter ablation for supraventricular tachycardias. J Cardiovasc Electrophysiol 4:390–392
5. Shivkumar K (2002) Mechanism of arrhythmias: are we still "learning while burning"? J Cardiovasc Electrophysiol 13:393–394
6. Prystowsky EN (2001) When technology exceeds knowledge, is success a reasonable expectation? J Cardiovasc Electrophysiol 12:1284–1285
7. Haïssaguerre M, Jaïs P, Shah DC et al (2000) Electrophysiological end point for catheter ablation of atrial fibrillation initiated from multiple pulmonary vein foci. Circulation 101:1409–1417
8. Jaïs P, Hocini M, Macle L et al (2002) Distinctive electrophysiological properties of pulmonary veins in patients with atrial fibrillation. Circulation 106:2479–2485
9. Tada H, Oral H, Ozadyn M et al (2002) Response of pulmonary vein potentials to premature stimulation. J Cardiovasc Electrophysiol 13:33–37
10. Ho SY, Cabrera JA, Tran VH et al (2001) Architecture of the pulmonary veins: relevance to radiofrequency ablation. Heart 86:265–270
11. Reithmann C, Dorwarth U, Gerth A et al (2002) Pulmonary vein bigeminy: electrophysiological characteristics and results of catheter ablation. J Interv Card Electrophysiol 7:233–241
12. Oral H, Knight BP, Ozadyn M et al (2002) Segmental ostial ablation to isolate the pulmonary veins during atrial fibrillation: feasibility and mechanistic insights. Circulation 106:1256–1262
13. Macle L, Jaïs P, Scavée C et al (2003) Electrophysiologically guided pulmonary vein isolation during sustained atrial fibrillation. J Cardiovasc Electrophysiol 14:255–260
14. Willems S, Weiss C, Risius T et al (2003) Dissociated activity and pulmonary vein fibrillation following functional disconnection: impact for the arrhythmogenesis of

focal atrial fibrillation. Pacing Clin Electrophysiol 26:1363–1370
15. Chen SA, Tai CT, Yeh HI, Chen YJ, Lin CI (2003) Controversies in the mechanism and ablation of pulmonary vein atrial fibrillation. Pacing Clin Electrophysiol 26:1301–1307
16. Kok LC, Everett TH 4th, Akar JG, Haines DE (2003) Effect of heating on pulmonary veins: how to avoid pulmonary vein stenosis. J Cardiovasc Electrophysiol 14:250–254
17. Purerfellner H, Cihal R, Aichinger J, Martinek M, Nesser HJ (2003) Pulmonary vein stenosis by ostial irrigated-tip ablation: incidence, time course, and prediction. J Cardiovasc Electrophysiol 14:158–164
18. Dill T, Neumann T, Ekinci O et al (2003) Pulmonary vein diameter reduction after radiofrequency catheter ablation for paroxysmal atrial fibrillation evaluated by contrast-enhanced three-dimensional magnetic resonance imaging. Circulation 107:845–850
19. Arentz T, Jander N, von Rosenthal J et al (2003) Incidence of pulmonary vein stenosis 2 years after radiofrequency catheter ablation of refractory atrial fibrillation. Eur Heart J 24:963–969
20. Ernst S, Ouyang F, Goya M et al (2003) Total pulmonary vein occlusion as a consequence of catheter ablation for atrial fibrillation mimicking primary lung disease. J Cardiovasc Electrophysiol 14:366–370
21. Saad EB, Cole CR, Marrouche NF et al (2002) Use of intracardiac echocardiography for prediction of chronic pulmonary vein stenosis after ablation of atrial fibrillation. J Cardiovasc Electrophysiol 13:986–989
22. Scharf C, Sneider M, Case I et al (2003) Anatomy of the pulmonary veins in patients with atrial fibrillation and effects of segmental ostial ablation analyzed by computed tomography J Cardiovasc Electrophysiol 14:150–155
23. Saad EB, Marrouche NF, Saad CP et al (2003) Pulmonary vein stenosis after catheter ablation of atrial fibrillation: emergence of a new clinical syndrome. Ann Intern Med 138:634–638
24. Marrouche NF, Martin DO, Wazni O et al (2003) Phased-array intracardiac echocardiography monitoring during pulmonary vein isolation in patients with atrial fibrillation. Impact on outcome and complications. Circulation 107:2710–2716
25. O'Donnell D, Furniss SS, Dunuwille A, Bourke JP (2003) Delayed cure despite early recurrence after pulmonary vein isolation for atrial fibrillation. Am J Cardiol 91:83–85
26. Kumagai K, Yasuda T, Tojo H et al (2000) Role of rapid focal activation in the maintenance of atrial fibrillation originating from the pulmonary veins. Pacing Clin Electrophysiol 23:1823–1827
27. Hindricks G, Kottkamp H (2002) Potential benefits, risks, and complications of catheter ablation of atrial fibrillation: more questions than answers. J Cardiovasc Electrophysiol 13:768–769

Ablation of Atrial Fibrillation: Is a Cure at Hand?

B. K. LEE, M. M. SCHEINMAN

Introduction

The treatment of atrial fibrillation (AF) is one of the most vexing and frustrating problems in cardiology. It is the most common sustained cardiac arrhythmia and its prevalence is increasing [1, 2]. Even with treatment, AF is associated with considerable morbidity and mortality and is the most common cause of embolic stroke [3]. Recently, we have gained new insights into the mechanisms of AF that have made a significant impact on our approach to treatment. We now recognize that rapidly firing foci in the pulmonary veins play a critical role in the initiation and maintenance of AF [4]. Radiofrequency ablation (RFA) to electrically isolate these foci has become an increasingly popular new approach for the treatment of AF. In this chapter, we review the evolution of AF ablation, the methodology of pulmonary vein isolation for AF and the results of this new approach.

Background

In 1959, Moe et al. proposed the hypothesis that AF is sustained by the presence of multiple reentrant wavelets propagating simultaneously in the atria [5]. Subsequently, Allessie et al. substantiated the multiple wavelet hypothesis in animal and human studies [6]. Based on this understanding of AF, Cox et al. developed a surgical approach to AF called the maze procedure. The maze procedure involved creating long linear barriers to conduction in the atria which compartmentalize the atria and prevent maintenance of reentry. The long term success rate of the maze procedure is high at approximately 90% [7]. However, despite multiple modifications of the maze procedure, the morbidity and mortality of the procedure remains significant. This has prevented widespread

Cardiac Electrophysiology Service, Division of Cardiology, University of California, San Francisco, California, USA application of the procedure. Notably, electrically isolating the pulmonary veins from the rest of the left atrium has been retained in each update of the maze procedure.

Percutaneous catheter-based approaches to AF originally tried to mimic the maze procedure by using RFA to create linear lines of block in the atria. However, it has become evident that using catheters to create linear lesions in order to develop complete barriers to conduction is extremely difficult [8]. Most published series have indicated long procedure times and significant complication rates. Therefore, excitement for this percutaneous catheter-based approach has waned.

In 1998, Hassaguerre et al. made a seminal discovery that renewed interest in pecutaneous catheter-based approaches to AF. They found that rapidly firing foci in the pulmonary veins are the predominant trigger of AF. By ablating these foci, they were able to cure AF in a subset of patients [4]. It appears that these rapidly firing foci which trigger AF are found in short sleeves of atrial tissue that extend into the pulmonary veins. It is hypothesized that these atrial sleeves are arrhythmogenic because of their embryonic origin. They come from tissue that gives rise to the conduction system and thus may be subject to automaticity [9, 10].

Based on Hassaguerre et al.'s discovery, there was a major paradigm shift in the approach to AF. Instead of just trying to alter the substrate which allows maintenance of AF, we now sought to eliminate the triggers which initiate AF. Many centers started to do AF ablation by mapping and ablating the ectopic focus responsible for initiating AF. This often involved doing RFA inside one or more pulmonary veins. Rarely the ectopic focus would be localized to other regions such as the superior vena cava, ligament of Marshall, coronary sinus or other atrial structures and be targeted for ablation [11-15]. However, there were several limitations to the focal approach to pulmonary vein ablation. First, induction of atrial ectopy is required by this approach for mapping. Unfortunately, in up to 30% of patients no sufficient ectopy can be induced for mapping [16]. Many cardioversions are frequently necessary. Furthermore, this approach did not have a clear endpoint since it is uncertain if elimination of all sources of ectopy, or if elimination of only sources of ectopy that trigger AF during mapping is necessary. Finally, in many of the reported series, many patients needed multiple procedures and the recurrence rate following focal ablation was generally high (up to 60%) [17].

Given the limitations of focal ablation, almost all centers have modified their approach and now try to achieve electrical isolation of the pulmonary veins. In this approach, RFA is generally applied at the ostium rather than inside of the pulmonary veins. The goal is to ablate the atrial sleeves at their site of entry into the pulmonary vein and electrically disconnect the distal portion of the sleeve from the left atrium. This electrically isolates the rapidly firing foci in the pulmonary vein and the prevents these triggers from conducting into the atria and initiating AF. In the following sections, we detail the general approach to electrical isolation of the pulmonary veins.

Patient Selection

Pulmonary vein isolation is a complex and invasive procedure, and therefore, it is typically reserved for patients who are drug refractory and symptomatic. At our center, except in special circumstances, we require that patients fail at least two antiarrhythmic medications and are symptomatic before we entertain pulmonary vein isolation. Most centers favor patients with paroxysmal AF since reported series have generally shown better results with patients with paroxysmal rather than chronic AF. However, Morrouche at al. found in their series that the results were similar irrespective of duration of AF if all pulmonary veins could be isolated [18].

Patient Preparation

Since there can be extensive variation in pulmonary vein anatomy, imaging of the pulmonary veins is often performed beforehand to guide the procedure. An MRI or CT scan may reveal the presence of more than the usual four pulmonary veins or common orifices of the upper and lower pulmonary veins [16]. Furthermore, imaging can serve as a baseline for comparison when screening for pulmonary vein stenosis following ablation. Oral anticoagulants are stopped a few days prior to the procedure. A transeophageal echocardiogram is performed just before the procedure to exclude a thrombus in the left atrial appendage which would make the procedure too risky.

Pulmonary Vein Isolation Procedure

The procedure is performed in the cardiac electrophysiology laboratory and typically takes between three to five hours. At our center, we prefer having an anesthesiologist present for conscious sedation. Catheters are placed in the coronary sinus, right atrium, and the His position. Two transseptal punctures are performed to allow access to the left atrium for a pulmonary vein mapping catheter and an ablation catheter. Heparin is started after both transseptal punctures have been done. Activated clothing time (ACT) is checked every 20 minutes and is typically maintained above 280 while catheters are on the left side of the heart.

A loop mapping catheter is then introduced into one of the pulmonary veins just beyond the ostium (Fig. 1). This catheter allows circumferential mapping of the pulmonary vein. Although most centers are using loop mapping catheters, at our center, we have started using a basket catheter for mapping (Fig. 2). The basket catheter allows for 3-dimensional mapping which is helpful in identifying the ostium. Electrical mapping of the pulmonary vein is typically done in sinus rhythm, but may also be done in AF if sinus rhythm is not maintained after cardioversion. The electrograms from the loop mapping

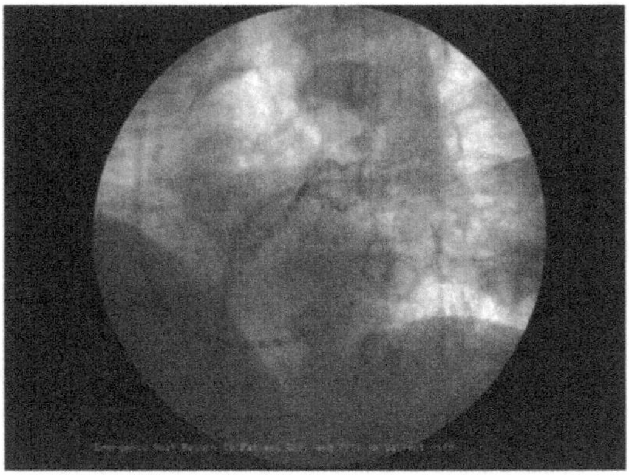

Fig. 1. Loop mapping catheter in the left upper pulmonary vein

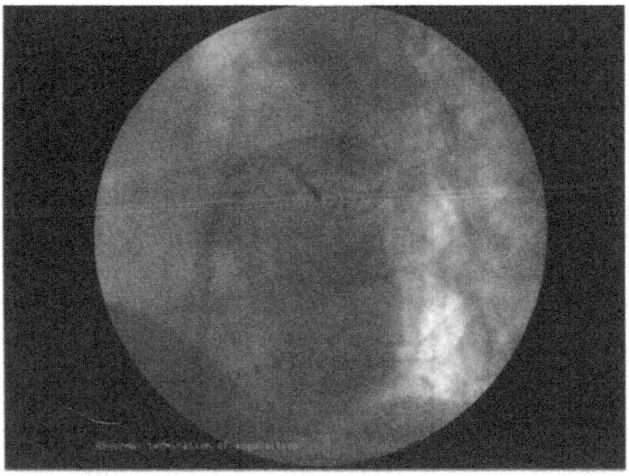

Fig. 2. A basket mapping catheter in the left lower pulmonary vein

catheter show sharp local potentials at the sites where the atrial sleeves extend into the pulmonary vein. Occasionally, pacing from the right atrium, coronary sinus, or the left atrial appendage allows better delineation of the sharp local potentials. The targeted site for ablation is at the ostium just proximal to the electrode with the earliest local potential (Fig. 3). Presumably, this is one site where the conduction enters and exits the pulmonary vein.

RFA energy is delivered using powers up to approximately 30 W. Successful ablation of an atrial sleeve is indicated by a change in the activation sequence of the local potentials, or complete elimination of all the local potentials. If the

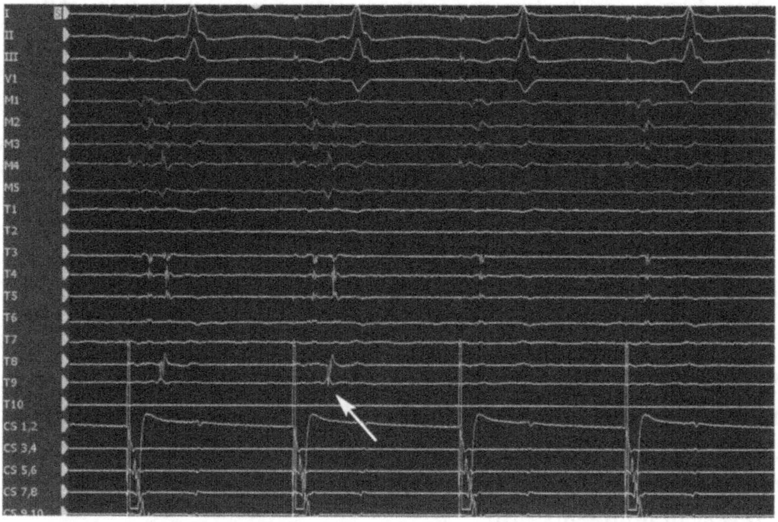

Fig. 3. CS pacing to delineate sharp local potentials. The earliest potential is at T9 (*arrow*). Ablation at T9 eliminates all local potentials in the latter half of the tracings. The remaining sharp potentials are probably from the left atrial appendage

activation sequence has changed, presumably, the targeted site has been ablated and now conduction into the pulmonary vein occurs via a different atrial sleeve. Conduction originating from a different sleeve forms another pattern of activation and therefore, a different site of earliest activation to target. This new site of earliest activation is then targeted. This process is repeated until all local potentials are eliminated suggesting that the pulmonary vein has been entirely electrically isolated. In our experience, the pulmonary vein can be isolated with ablation along less than 50% of the circumference of the pulmonary vein ostium. Elimination of all local potentials is a readily identifiable endpoint for the isolation of a particular pulmonary vein. Most centers attempt to isolate all four of the pulmonary veins. Successful isolation of all the pulmonary veins has been associated with lower rates of recurrence [19].

After isolation of all the pulmonary veins, isoproterenol may be infused and pacing *maneuvers* may be performed to elicit other foci of ectopic beats that may trigger AF. These sites may also be mapped and targeted for RFA. Some centers also routinely electrically isolate the superior vena cava at the end of the procedure using an approach similar to that used for isolation of the pulmonary veins.

After completion of the case, the patient is monitored overnight on a telemetry unit. Oral anticoagulants are typically restarted. The patient usually can be discharged the following day.

It should be noted that in the immediate post-procedure period (up to 12 weeks), early recurrence of AF does not necessary indicate failure of the procedure. This may be a period of increased atrial irritablility which resolves as the RFA lesions mature. Because of this early recurrence, we typically continue antiarrhythmic medicines for at least 3 months following the procedure. Many of these patients with early recurrence become free of AF at long-term follow-up.

Results

Reported success rates for pulmonary vein isolation range from 22 to 86% [20, 21]. At least part of the variation in success rates results from differences in patient selection and variation in the number of pulmonary veins targeted for isolation. At centers which attempt to isolate all the pulmonary veins, the success rate is generally around 70 to 80% in terms of eliminating AF episodes in the first year of follow-up [16].

Since pulmonary vein isolation is a relatively new approach to AF ablation, long-term results are unavailable. It should be noted that if the success seen at one-year follow-up were not durable, the utility and applicability of pulmonary vein isolation for AF would need to be reassessed.

Risks

In general, the risk of major complication is very low. The risk of thromboembolic events and tamponade is less than 0.5% [19]. However, pulmonary stenosis is a potential complication of pulmonary vein isolation, which may be underappreciated. The reported rates of pulmonary vein stenosis has ranged from 0 to 42% [19]. Imaging by CT scanning or MRI at 3 months is useful for assessing the presence of pulmonary vein stenosis. Most centers now limit RFA to powers less than 30 W, which seems to have reduced rates of pulmonary vein stenosis to less than 2% [19].

Conclusions

The discovery that rapidly firing foci in the pulmonary veins is the predominant trigger for AF has taken us to a new era in RFA for the treatment of AF. The focus of percutaneous catheter-based approaches has shifted from modifying the atrial substrate that maintains AF to eliminating the focal triggers. Pulmonary vein isolation has become a well-established procedure, which is being performed at many centers throughout the world. At centers where isolation of all the pulmonary veins is the goal, the results at early follow-up have been generally very favorable.

So have we found a cure for AF? The answer depends on how cure is defined. If cure is defined as one year free of AF, then yes, we do have a cure for AF in selected patients. If cure is defined as durable freedom from AF beyond one year without long-term complications, then it is too early to tell. Nevertheless, with many centers now performing pulmonary vein isolation, the answer to this question will be forthcoming. We should know if pulmonary vein isolation is a safe and durable cure for AF in the coming years.

References

1. Wolf PA et al (1996) Secular trends in the prevalence of atrial fibrillation: The Framingham Study. Am Heart J 131(4):790-795
2. Feinberg WM et al (1995) Prevalence, age distribution, and gender of patients with atrial fibrillation. Analysis and implications. Arch Intern Med 155(5): 469-473
3. Chugh SS et al (2001) Epidemiology and natural history of atrial fibrillation: clinical implications. J Am Coll Cardiol 37(2):371-378
4. Haissaguerre M et al (1998) Spontaneous initiation of atrial fibrillation by ectopic beats originating in the pulmonary veins. N Engl J Med 339(10): 659-666
5. Moe, G.K (1968) A conceptual model of atrial fibrillation. J Electrocardiol 1(2):145-146
6. Allessie MA, Bonke FI, F.J. Schopman FJ (1997) Circus movement in rabbit atrial muscle as a mechanism of tachycardia. III. The "leading circle" concept: a new model of circus movement in cardiac tissue without the involvement of an anatomical obstacle. Circ Res 41(1):9-18
7. Cox JL et al (1996) An 8 1/2-year clinical experience with surgery for atrial fibrillation. Ann Surg 224(3):267-273; discussion 273-275
8. Olgin JE et al (1997) Electrophysiological effects of long, linear atrial lesions placed under intracardiac ultrasound guidance. Circulation 96(8):2715-2721
9. Blom NA et al (1999) Development of the cardiac conduction tissue in human embryos using HNK-1 antigen expression: possible relevance for understanding of abnormal atrial automaticity. Circulation 99(6):800-806
10. DeRuiter MC et al (1995) In normal development pulmonary veins are connected to the sinus venosus segment in the left atrium. Anat Rec 243(1):84-92
11. Chen SA et al (2000) Radiofrequency catheter ablation of atrial fibrillation initiated by pulmonary vein ectopic beats. J Cardiovasc Electrophysiol 11(2):218-227
12. Tsai CF et al (2000) Initiation of atrial fibrillation by ectopic beats originating from the superior vena cava: electrophysiological characteristics and results of radiofrequency ablation. Circulation 102(1):67-74
13. Natale A et al (2000) Catheter ablation approach on the right side only for paroxysmal atrial fibrillation therapy: long-term results. Pacing Clin Electrophysiol 23(2):224-233
14. Natale A et al (2000) Ablation of right and left atrial premature beats following cardioversion in patients with chronic atrial fibrillation refractory to antiarrhythmic drugs. Am J Cardiol 85(11):1372-1375
15. Hwang C, Karagueuzian HS, Chen PS (1999) Idiopathic paroxysmal atrial fibrillation induced by a focal discharge mechanism in the left superior pulmonary vein: possible roles of the ligament of Marshall. J Cardiovasc Electrophysiol 10(5)636-648

16. Saad EB, Marrouche NF, Natale A (2002) Ablation of focal atrial fibrillation. Card Electrophysiol Rev 6(4):389-396
17. Tsai CF, Tai CT, Chen SA (2003) Pulmonary vein ablation: role in preventing atrial fibrillation. Curr Opin Cardiol 18(1):39-46
18. Marrouche NF et al (2002) Circular mapping and ablation of the pulmonary vein for treatment of atrial fibrillation: impact of different catheter technologies. J Am Coll Cardiol 40(3):464-474
19. Jais P et al (2002) Ablation therapy for atrial fibrillation (AF): past, present and future. Cardiovasc Res 54(2):337-346
20. Oral H et al (2002) Pulmonary vein isolation for paroxysmal and persistent atrial fibrillation. Circulation 105(9):1077-1081
21. Chen SA et al (1999) Initiation of atrial fibrillation by ectopic beats originating from the pulmonary veins: electrophysiological characteristics, pharmacological responses, and effects of radiofrequency ablation. Circulation 100(18):1879-1886

Atrial Fibrillation: Anatomical Guidance Is Superior to Electrophysiological Guidance for Ablation

C. Pappone, V. Santinelli

Electrophysiologically guided ablation was the initial strategy applied in patients with focal atrial fibrillation (AF), but electroanatomical mapping systems have had an increasingly important role in successful elimination of both paroxysmal and chronic AF [1–3]. Currently, targets for ablation of AF are increasingly being selected on the basis of anatomical considerations [4–14]. Therefore, ablation strategies that are based more on anatomical considerations than on mapping are needed to improve the efficacy of catheter ablation of AF. It has become accepted that detailed anatomical knowledge of the number, size, and shape of the pulmonary veins (PVs), especially the atriopulmonary junction and the tributaries and branching pattern of the PVs, is of critical importance in PV ablation for AF. Recent experimental studies have demonstrated a correlation between anatomy and electrical activation; in particular, segmental muscle disconnection, a differential muscle narrowing at PV–LA junctions, and complex fiber orientations within the PV provide robust anatomical bases for conduction disturbances at the PV–LA junction and complex intra-PV conduction patterns. Consequently, new technologies, including the CARTO system using detailed anatomical images, have become available for catheter guidance and mapping, and their practicability has been validated by our group [2, 3]. Therefore, the importance of anatomically based catheter ablation procedures is now well recognized. Catheter ablation of isthmus-dependent atrial flutter, which is based strictly on anatomical criteria, is regarded as the first-line therapy in atrial flutter. Similarly, the results of catheter ablation for AF have become better and better as procedures have been based increasingly on anatomical considerations. Therefore, future mapping technology that provides more specific anatomical information on critical areas will ultimately result in catheter ablation becoming first-line therapy for both paroxysmal and chronic AF.

Department of Cardiology, Cardiac Electrophysiology, San Raffaele University Hospital, Milan, Italy

Electrophysiologically Guided Ablation Strategy

Over the past few years, the electrophysiologically guided ablation strategy has been focused on the development of several catheter ablation techniques and ablation systems to achieve higher success rates than have been obtained with the anatomically guided strategy. This technique was first applied by Haisseguerre et al. after they demonstrated the focal origin of AF within the pulmonary veins (PVs). In his initial mapping studies, Haissaguerre showed that a rapidly firing focus within or close to the PVs was the mechanism of arrhythmia in most patients with paroxysmal AF [1]. However, this initial focal approach immediately showed important limitations, even in experienced laboratories. A first obstacle was the difficulty in mapping the focus if the patient is in AF or has no consistent firing. A second obstacle was the frequent existence of multiple foci, leading to high recurrence rates, and the appearance of new foci following the procedure. In addition, it was uncertain whether the appropriate end-point of the focal approach should be the elimination of atrial premature beats, the inability to induce AF, or both. Finally, stenosis of the PVs was a frequent complication of the focal ablation [15]. On the other hand, severe PV stenosis after isolation of PVs may be minimally symptomatic, emerging as a new and alarming syndrome characterized by respiratory symptoms that frequently mimic more common disease, often leading to erroneous diagnostic and therapeutic procedures [16]. From the initial experience of the Bordeaux group, very different strategies of mapping and targeting ectopic foci within PVs for successful ablation prevented widespread acceptance of focal ablation. In particular, some investigators sequentially mapped each of the four PVs targeting ectopic firings from PVs, while others only targeted ectopic foci that actually precipitated AF. Other investigators placed catheters simultaneously in each of the four PVs to identify arrhythmogenic foci. The efficacy of electrophysiologically guided ablation in the general population with chronic AF is limited, while among patients in whom PVs are the dominant triggers reinitiating chronic AF the elimination of PV potentials by ostial RF applications results in stable sinus rhythm in 60% [17]. Recently, the original approach has been modified and catheter ablation is performed at the PV ostium guided by circumferential mapping data obtained using a steerable circular multipolar catheter (LASSO catheter) designed to fit just inside the PV ostium [18, 19]. Advantages of this approach include an easily defined end-point for catheter ablation, a marked reduction in the risk of PV stenosis because of the ostial location of the RF applications, and the intuitive value of having an electrode catheter to mark the orifice of the PV. After evaluation of the perimetric distribution and the activation sequence of PV potentials, ostial ablation was performed in segments showing the earliest activation, with the end-point of PV disconnection. The extent of perimetric ablation was therefore less than the actual muscle coverage, thereby minimizing the risk of PV stenosis. Although in 73% of the 70 study patients complete elimination of AF was achieved without antiarrhythmic therapy, 44% of patients had AF recurrences after only a 4-month follow-up [18]. As a result, multiple ablation sessions were required because of unmasked foci from the ostial edge or atrial tissue. The main limitation of this approach is the improper alignment of the mapping catheter, with the well-known irregular geometry of PVs making interpretation of the electrograms recorded challenging. In addition, catheter "drift" may give the operator a mistaken idea of the ostial position. Finally, this technique may not be applicable to RF ablation outside the ostia of the PV, which may require complete circumferential lesions to induce distal disconnection.

Anatomically Guided Ablation Strategy

At the same time as Haisseguerre's focal ablation strategy emerged, we became the first to propose a highly effective anatomically based ablation strategy for curing both paroxysmal and chronic AF to the electrophysiological community [2, 3]. We first used a nonfluoroscopic electrogeometric mapping system able to reconstruct the anatomy of venous–atrial junction to demonstrate the safety and efficacy of this strategy by the creation around and outside the PV ostia of a long line encircling all PVs [2]. This anatomical system makes it possible to tailor the number and size of lesions to the complex morphology of the PV–LA junction to disconnect PVs by eliminating PVs ostial potentials and electrical activity inside the lesion during pacing outside the ablation lines. In addition, as with surgery, we can reduce the "electrically active" atrial tissue by involving substantial parts of the posterior LA wall with profound atrial electroanatomical remodeling, as expressed by voltage abatement (<0.1 mV) inside and around the encircled areas. Most importantly, the efficacy of this anatomical system strategy was similar regardless of whether patients had paroxysmal or chronic AF. The fact that our technique was able to eliminate AF regardless of its duration or the presence of structural heart disease indicates that substrate ablation other than trigger ablation is important for restoration of a stable sinus rhythm in the general population with chronic AF. Elimination of both triggers and arrhythmogenic substrate may lead to stable sinus rhythm, which can reverse the atrial remodeling induced by chronic AF, thus preventing AF recurrences. This hypothesis is consistent with the good results obtained with RF applications around the ostia of the PVs during mitral valve surgery, as documented by the restoration of sinus rhythm in approximately 80% of chronic AF patients with dilated atria [17]. These observations suggest that atrial size may not itself be a major determinant in suppressing AF. In our experience, among patients with both paroxysmal and permanent AF, the only predictive criterion for a successful ablation was the amount of post-RF low-voltage encircled area [3]. Therefore, it is likely that our purely anatomical approach, when effective, results in profound atrial electroanatomical remodeling involving the LA posterior wall to the point that the substrate for AF is no longer present. Our experience was innovative because a 3D electroanatomical nonfluoroscopic mapping system (CARTO) was used for the first time. Unlike electrophysiologically based ablation, the CARTO system reduces the time required for the procedure by eliminating the need for mapping spontaneous or induced arrhythmias and would be effective in preventing recurrent AF attributable to multiple PV foci, even if new foci may emerge at some future time. An additional advantage of the CARTO system is that lesions can be tailored to the varying PV–LA junction features, unlike novel circumferential ablation catheters with a prefixed size and design, which are difficult to accommodate in ostia with larger diameters, eccentric shape, or a complex proximal PV branching pattern, as recently reported [14]. We demonstrated in a large cohort of patients (251, of whom 179 had paroxysmal AF and 72, chronic AF) that a purely anatomical ablation strategy is highly effective and safe. Major complications (cardiac tamponade) occurred in only 0.8% of patients, without embolic events or PV stenosis, and, after a 1-year follow-up, freedom from AF recurrence was 80% overall, 86% for paroxysmal AF, and 68% for permanent AF, with a minority of these patients taking medication [3]. As far as the repeatability of our approach is concerned, we are fully aware that this is a considerable problem. A potential limitation of an anatomically guided approach is the possibility of creating nontransmural lesions, which increases the risk of proarrhythmic re-entrant circuits in some patients. We believe that for future optimum ablation strategies, some problems remain to be solved. It is necessary to find a more detailed imaging system to visualize the PV–LA junction as precisely as possible so as to obtain quantitative data allowing stratification of the procedural and clinical success. In addition, it is important to perfect current catheter technology to improve coaxial movement of the tip, not only to perform effective lesions in a complex area, i.e., the PV–LA junction, but also to reduce the time needed for the procedures. Finally, it is advisable to test other forms of energy, such as saline-irrigated or cooled radiofrequency (RF) energy, microwave energy, or cryoablation to reduce the risk of charring, thromboembolism, and pulmonary hypertension.

References

1. Haissaguerre M, Jais P, Shah DC et al (1998) Spontaneous initiation of atrial fibrillation by ectopic beats originating in the pulmonary veins. N Engl J Med 339:659–666
2. Pappone C, Rosanio S, Oreto G et al (2000) Circumferential radiofrequency ablation of pulmonary vein ostia: a new anatomic approach for curing atrial fibrillation. Circulation 102:2619–2628
3. Pappone C, Oreto G, Rosanio S et al (2001) Atrial electroanatomic remodeling after circumferential radiofrequency pulmonary vein ablation: efficacy of an anatomic approach in a large cohort of patients with atrial fibrillation. Circulation 104:2539–2544
4. Kato R, Lickfett L, Meininger G et al (2003) Pulmonary vein anatomy in patients undergoing catheter ablation of atrial fibrillation: lessons learned by use of magnetic resonance imaging. Circulation 107:2004–2010

5. Ho SY (2003) Pulmonary vein ablation in atrial fibrillation: does anatomy matter? J Cardiovasc Electrophysiol 14:156–157
6. Honjo H, Boyett MR, Niwa R et al (2003) Pacing-induced spontaneous activity in myocardial sleeves of pulmonary veins after treatment with ryanodine. Circulation 107:1937–1943
7. Weerasooriya R, Macle L, Jais P, Hocini M, Haissaguerre M (2003) Pulmonary vein ablation using the LocaLisa nonfluoroscopic mapping system. J Cardiovasc Electrophysiol 14:112
8. Wittkampf FH, Vonken EJ, Derksen R et al (2003) Pulmonary vein ostium geometry: analysis by magnetic resonance angiography. Circulation 107:21–23
9. Solomon SB, Dickfeld T, Calkins H (2003) Real-time cardiac catheter navigation on three-dimensional CT images. J Interv Card Electrophysiol 8:27–36
10. Mangrum JM, Mounsey JP, Kok LC, DiMarco JP, Haines DE (2002) Intracardiac echocardiography-guided, anatomically based radiofrequency ablation of focal atrial fibrillation originating from pulmonary veins. J Am Coll Cardiol 39:1964–1972
11. Ho SY, Cabrera JA, Tran VH et al (2001) Architecture of the pulmonary veins: relevance to radiofrequency ablation. Heart 86:265–270
12. Moubarak JB, Rozwadowski JV, Strzalka CT et al (2000) Pulmonary veins-left atrial junction: anatomic and histological study. Pacing Clin Electrophysiol 23:1836–1838
13. Hocini M, Ho SY, Kawara T et al (2002) Electrical conduction in canine pulmonary veins: electrophysiological and anatomic correlation. Circulation 105:2442–2448
14. Scharf C, Sneider M, Case I et al (2003) Anatomy of the pulmonary veins in patients with atrial fibrillation and effects of segmental ostial ablation analyzed by computed tomography. J Cardiovasc Electrophysiol 14:150–155
15. Arentz T, Jander N, von Rosenthal J et al (2003) Incidence of pulmonary vein stenosis 2 years after radiofrequency catheter ablation of refractory atrial fibrillation. Eur Heart J 24:963–969
16. Saad EB, Marrouche NF, Saad CP et al (2003) Pulmonary vein stenosis after catheter ablation of atrial fibrillation: emergence of a new clinical syndrome. Ann Intern Med 15:138:634–638
17. Haissaguerre M, Jais P, Shah DC et al (2000) Catheter ablation of chronic atrial fibrillation targeting the reinitiating triggers. J Cardiovasc Electrophysiol 11:2–10
18. Haissaguerre M, Shah DC, Jais P et al (2000) Electrophysiological breakthroughs from the left atrium to the pulmonary veins. Circulation 102:2463–2465
19. Oral H, Knight BP, Ozaydin M et al (2002) Segmental ostial ablation to isolate the pulmonary veins during atrial fibrillation: feasibility and mechanistic insights. Circulation 106:1256–1262

Atrial Fibrillation: Catheter Laser Balloon Ablation

A. Bonso, S. Themistoclakis, A. Rossillo, A. Raviele

Recently many studies have reported that the left atrium has a central role in the initiation and maintenance of atrial fibrillation (AF); the most arrhythmogenic areas of the left atrium are in the pulmonary veins, atriovenous junctions, and contiguous atrial regions [1–3]. Electrical isolation of the pulmonary veins seems to be the most effective ablation technique for patients with AF [4, 5].

Various kinds of techniques have been employed to obtain electrical disconnection of the pulmonary veins. Electrical segmental, circumferential, and anatomical disconnection have been proposed [1–5]. Radiofrequency catheter ablation has been extensively applied. Various types of catheters for radiofrequency ablation have been utilised with tip electrodes of 4 mm, 4 mm cooled, and 8 mm [5]. Results have been verified after the procedure with demonstration of both entry block and exit block in the pulmonary veins using multipolar mapping catheters. Entry block has been defined as the absence of pulmonary vein potentials during sinus rhythm and pacing from the distal coronary sinus. When evaluating the left pulmonary veins, pacing from the distal coronary sinus and from the proximal left auricula entry often has been performed to separate the far-field potential of the left atrium from the local pulmonary vein potential.

The overall success rate of these techniques (with or without antiarrhythmic drugs) ranges from 60% to 92% for patients with paroxysmal or persistent, drug-refractory, symptomatic AF and from 60% to 89% for patients with permanent AF. Recurrences demonstrate recovery of conduction from left atrium to pulmonary vein [1–7]. In patients in whom pulmonary vein isolation is not sufficient to eliminate AF, adjunctive therapy with (previously ineffective) antiarrhythmic drugs can increase the success rate by 5%–20%, whatever ablation technique is used. This behaviour is probably because the antiarrhythmic drugs are more effective on areas of arrhythmogenic substrate that have been

Division of Cardiology, Cardiovascular Department, Umberto I Hospital, Mestre–Venice, Italy

partially electrically disconnected. In our experience, with 37 patients with symptomatic paroxysmal, persistent, and permanent AF who underwent intracardiac echocardiography-guided pulmonary vein isolation, after a follow-up of 4.5±2 months 65% had no AF recurrences without antiarrhythmic drugs and 21% remained in sinus rhythm while taking previously ineffective antiarrhythmic drugs.

Although the high success rate is very encouraging for widespread use of this approach, some limitations of radiofrequency ablation have nevertheless been noted: (1) So far, the efficacy of the pulmonary disconnection has depended on the manual skill and expertise of the operator. (2) To produce a continuous line of conduction block, radiofrequency energy requires contact between the electrode and endocardium throughout. (3) Lesions are limited in depth and can cause endocardial disruption and thrombus formation. Therefore, some serious potential complications can be related to the procedure. The most significant complications are pulmonary vein stenosis, thromboembolic events, pericardium effusion or tamponade, and phrenic nerve paralysis. The incidence of pulmonary vein stenosis has been reported to range from 3% to 42 % depending on the ablative technique used and the method of assessment [8]. Thromboembolic events occur in up to 2.8% of the patients [9]. However, with technological progress the main complications related to this procedure are becoming progressively less.

Among the major difficulties in providing energy ablation are how to define a vein ostium accurately in a three-dimensional view and the wide anatomical variability of the structures. Pulmonary angiography, transoesophageal echocardiography, three-dimensional non-fluoroscopic mapping (Carto system) and, more recently, magnetic resonance imaging [10], three-dimensional computed tomography [11], and phased-array intracardiac echocardiography [7] have been used to reconstruct the real structure of the posterior left atrial wall and the pulmonary veins. In addition, two-dimensional echocardiography was also used to monitor power during radiofrequency ablation [7]. These techniques help to achieve correct positioning of ablating catheters to the atriovenous junction of the pulmonary veins and to better control the onset of complications.

Because of the limitations of conventional radiofrequency ablation in creating large or linear lesions, alternative energy sources have been used as possible methods of catheter ablation.

Modified radiofrequency energy, cryoablation [12], and microwave, ultrasound [6], and laser technologies [13] may be able to create longer, deeper, and more controlled lesions. In order to create a continuous circumferential lesion around venous ostia, first a catheter balloon was made which was inflated at the ostium of the pulmonary vein, and a contrast venogram was performed to demonstrate complete occlusion of the vein with the balloon [6]. Circumferential ultrasound ablation isolation of the pulmonary veins was performed in 33 patients by means of the Atrionix circumferential ultrasound vein ablation system. Acute procedural success was obtained with the ultrasound balloon system in 73% of patients and longer-term cure (22-month follow-up) in 36%. The ostial anatomy of the veins, very different in each patient, may have affected the delivery of ultrasound energy to achieve circumferential lesions. Reconfiguration of the system to overcome the shortcomings identified in the initial experience could increase its performance [14].

Laser energy has been proposed as an alternative to radiofrequency energy for ablation of ventricular tachycardia [15, 16] or to disconnect the pulmonary veins, as some experiments with animals demonstrated [17]. Lesions demonstrated coagulation necrosis with smooth, well-demarcated borders, and most lesions are transmural or near-transmural in thickness. No animal suffered cardiac perforation, hypotension, haemopericardium, damage to cardiac valves, or cavitation effect from any of the ablations [15]. Diode laser produces *controlled low energy ablation* and can be delivered through a range of optical fibre configurations including *loop balloons* to produce thin continuous lesions [17]. The use of optical fibres for laser delivery also provides an option for reflectance spectroscopy as a feedback mechanism on both contact and lesion progression in real time [17]. The use of a balloon catheter positioned under two-dimensional endocardial echocardiographic control at the left atrial junction of the pulmonary veins should overcome the limitations of previous experience [6, 14]. Employing a balloon, laser energy can probably circumferentially electrically disconnect pulmonary veins in a high percentage of patients with a low number of complications.

The possibility of performing linear defined circumferential lesions around the orifice of pulmonary veins through a laser balloon is currently under investigation in our centre and many others.

References

1. Haïssaguerre M, Jais P, Shah DC et al (1998) Spontaneous initiation of atrial fibrillation by ectopic beats originating in the pulmonary veins. N Engl J Med 339:659–666
2. Chen SA, Hsieh MH, Tai CT et al (1999) Initiation of atrial fibrillation by ectopic beats originating from the pulmonary veins: electrophysiological characteristics, pharmacological responses and effects of radiofrequency ablation. Circulation 100:1879–1886
3. Haïssaguerre M, Shah DC, Jais P (2000) Electrophysiological breakthroughts from the left atrium to the pulmonary veins. Circulation 102: 2463–2465
4. Pappone C, Oreto G, Rosanio S et al (2001) Atrial electroanatomic remodeling after circumferential radiofrequency pulmonary vein ablation: efficacy of an anatomic approach in a larg cohort of patients with atrial fibrillation. Circulation. 104:2539–2544
5. Marrouche NF, Dresing T, Cole C et al (2002) Circular mapping and ablation of the pulmonary vein for treatment of atrial fibrillation: impact of different catheter technologies. J Am Coll Cardiol 40:464–474
6. Natale A, Pisano E, Shewchik J et al (2000) First human experience with pulmonary vein isolation using a through-the-balloon circumferential ultrasound ablation system for recurrent atrial fibrillation. Circulation 102:1879–1882

7. Marrouche NF, Martin DO, Wazni O et al (2003) Phased array intracardiac echocardiography monitoring during pulmonary vein isolation in patients with atrial fibrillation: impact on outcome and complications. Circulation 107:2710–2716
8. Saad EB, Marrouche NF, Saad CP et al (2003) Pulmonary vein stenosis after catheter ablation of atrial fibrillation: emergence of a new clinical syndrome. Ann Intern Med 138:634–638
9. Zhou L, Keane D, Reed G et al (1999) Thromboembolic complications of cardiac radiofrequency catheter ablation: a review of the reported incidence, pathogenesis and current research directions. J Cardiovasc Electrophysiol 10:611–620
10. Tsao HM, Yu WC, Cheng HC et al (2001) Pulmonary vein dilation in patients with atrial fibrillation: detection by magnetic resonance imaging. J Cardiovasc Electrophysiol 12:809–813
11. Tada H, Oral H, Knight BP, Moradt F (2002) Three-dimensional computed tomography of the pulmonary veins. J Cardiovasc Electrophysiol 13:521
12. Gaita F, Gallotti R, Calò L et al (2000) Limited posterior atrial cryoablation in patients with chronic atrial fibrillation undergoing valvular heart surgery. J Am Coll Cardiol 36:159–166
13. Keane D, Ruskin J (1999) Linear atrial ablation with a diode laser and fiberoptic catheter, Circulation 100:e59–e60
14. Saliba W, Wilber D, Packer D et al (2002). Circumferential ultrasound ablation for pulmonary vein isolation: analysis of acute and chronic failures. J Cardiovasc Electrophysiol 13:957–961
15. Keane D (2002) New catheter ablation techniques for the treatment of cardiac arrhythmias. Card Electrophysiol Rev 6:341–348
16. Wagshall A, Abela GS, Maheshwari A et al (2002) A novel catheter design for laser photocoagulation of the myocardium to ablate ventricular tachycardia. J Interv Card Electrophysiol 7:13–22
17. D'Avila A, Splinter R, Svenson RH et al (2002) New perspectives on catheter-based ablation of ventricular tachycardia complicating Chagas' disease: experimental evidence of the efficacy of near infrared lasers for catheter ablation of Chagas' VT. J Interv Card Electrophysiol 7:23–38

Isolation of Pulmonary Veins Using Cryothermal Technologies

A. C. Skanes, A. D. Krahn, R. Yee, G. J. Klein

Introduction

Elimination of pulmonary venous triggers can eliminate paroxysmal atrial fibrillation in 70-80% of selected patients [1-3]. This is achieved in most centers by isolation of 3 to 4 pulmonary veins at the pulmonary venous atrial junction. A major obstacle to the widespread dissemination of this procedure is the risk of significant pulmonary venous stenosis [4, 5]. Rates of severe symptomatic stenosis in high volume centers vary, but remain in the range of 1-8% [4-7]. Symptomatic stenosis can be very problematic [8]. Milder asymptomatic stenosis may be more prevalent and of unknown significance. Acute as well as chronic occlusions have also been described [8, 9]. The incidence of stenosis in general practice may be underestimated. As such, a new technology that can effectively and permanently isolate the pulmonary veins without producing stenosis would be highly desirable.

A number of new technologies show promise of a more effective, more rapid and safer method of performing pulmonary venous (PV) isolation [10]. Many of the new technologies, including ultrasound, laser and microwave induce ablation via thermal injury. Cryoablation is unique in that the mechanism of cellular injury is different from thermal injury and may have some characteristics that make it safer [11]. This chapter will review the mechanism of cryothermal cellular injury especially as it contrasts to radiofrequency ablation. The progress made towards cryoablative PV isolation and future directions will then be reviewed.

Mechanism of PV Stenosis

Little is known as to the mechanism of formation of this unique iatrogenic complication of atrial fibrillation ablation. In the only animal study of

Arrhythmia Service, University of Western Ontario, London, Ontario, Canada radiofrequency-induced pulmonary vein stenosis, aggressive ablation produced significant stenosis in 22 out of 33 ablated veins [12]. This is much higher than that seen clinically. This study used more aggressive ablation than used clinically and no anticoagulation or anti-platelet therapy was used. Histopathologic examination demonstrated both progressive endovascular contraction, organizing thrombus and intimal proliferation in 80% of veins at 10-14 weeks.

Radiofrequency lesions are known to cause endothelial disruption, with subendothelial collagen exposure and platelet activation [12-15]. Endothelial disruption and subsequent platelet activation results in neo-intimal proliferation in coronary arteries. If one uses this as a model of the effects of endothelial disruption, it may have parallels with PV stenosis. It seems plausible that radiofrequency-induced endothelial disruption contributes to stenosis.

Endovascular contraction has also been demonstrated in patients. Acute reduction of PV diameter has been demonstrated during radiofrequency ablation. Haines et al. used intracardiac echo to document the response [7]. Four out of 64 patients (6.3 %) developed greater than 50 % reduction in PV area immediately following ablation, as measured by planimetry on the echo image. This corresponds to an acute 30 % reduction in diameter due to a combination of edema and thermally-mediated contracture. This study is by no means unique in demonstrating acute reduction in PV diameters, but the real-time echocardiographic monitoring makes it highly illustrative. Thermal injury, induced by radiofrequency, has recently been shown to produce calcium-mediated *irreversible* contracture in papillary muscle preparations [16]. Such contracture appears to be temperature sensitive, with greater contracture recorded at progressively higher temperatures. Importantly, this appears to be the result of lesions produced with power and temperatures used clinically. While edema is expected to resolve over time, thermally-mediated contracture may not. Hence, the course of acute changes after ablation may be highly variable and may be the initial events that are recognized later as stenosis. The rate of PV stenosis has also been reported to be temperature-sensitive; the widely applied limit of 50-5°C during ablation being djacent to the limit for causing PV stenosis [17].

Thermal injury produces denaturation of extracellular proteins, especially collagen [18-19]. Importantly, thermally-induced collagen shrinkage has been well documented in animal and human studies [20-22]. In fact, orthopedic studies have taken advantage of radiofrequency energy to cause thermally-induced collagen shrinkage as a possible repair for patients with anterior cruciate ligament laxity [20]. The method, power and target temperature in these studies overlap with those used clinically. There is no question that similar changes in the extracellular matrix are produced during radiofrequency ablation. However, as most clinical ablation lesions produced outside of the pulmonary veins are focal and small, these effects are without obvious consequence. When near circumferential lesions are produced within the tubular confines of the pulmonary veins, collagen shrinkage may result in endovascular contracture.

The contribution of each of the phenomena to chronic symptomatic stenosis remains speculative. Nonetheless, it is reasonable that new technologies that limit these phenomena may result in less pulmonary vein stenosis. Cryothermal ablation holds much promise in this regard due to its unique mechanism of cellular injury.

Mechanism of Cryoablation

The mechanisms of cellular death associated with tissue freezing are well studied because of the utility in cryosurgery, both in the cardiovascular realm and others [11]. There are immediate cellular effects as well as late effects that determine the lesion produced.

Direct Cell Injury

Extracellular Ice (Solution effect injury)
As cells are cooled at a relatively slow rate, extracellular ice begins to form. This results in a hyperosmotic extracellular environment, that in turn draws water from the cells [11]. This phenomenon occurs at a moderate temperature of −20 °C when applied sufficiently slowly to allow intracellular to extracellular water shifts to occur. Hypertonic stress causes cellular shrinkage and damage to membrane and cellular constituents. Upon re-warming, reversal of these effects results in cellular swelling sufficient to disrupt cellular membranes. If sufficient in duration, cooling to this level of freezing will result in cellular death. If these effects are small by cooling to mild temperatures (0° to -10 °C), fully reversible effects can be produced. This has been well documented in the surgical literature and has been termed “ice mapping”. Clinically, the ability to test the functionality of a potential ablation target prior to permanent destruction has obvious appeal. This will be developed further below.

Intracellular Ice
If tissue temperature is dropped further to −40 °C or beyond, especially if cooled at rapid rates, intracellular water will freeze forming intracellular ice. This is considered lethal to cells, as it causes major and irreversible disruption of intracellular organelles and cellular membranes. In the early re-warming phase, coalescence of ice crystals into larger ice crystals causes further disruption of intracellular organelles and cellular membranes.

Vascular Injury

Within the zone of frozen tissue, cryothermy is known to have profound effects on the microvasculature. As tissue is cooled, vasoconstriction occurs and as the tissue freezes, circulation ceases altogether within the frozen tissue. Upon re-warming there is a hyperemic vasodilation, with increased vascular permeability and localized edema. Damage to the endothelium within the frozen tissue results in microthrombi and microcirculatory arrest within the lesion within 30-45 minutes. By 4 hours after thawing, small blood vessels are occluded. This loss of blood supply results in ischemic necrosis and a dense uniform lesion. It is generally accepted that this is a major mechanism of cryolesion formation during tissue freezing, although it is impossible to distinguish this mechanism of cell death from that of intracellular ice formation.

Important Characteristics of Cryolesions

The mechanism of cellular injury compared to radiofrequency (RF) ablation produces clinically important differences. The degree of endothelial disruption with cryothermy is known to be less than in standard RF lesions. This was recently evaluated by Dubuc et al. who compared standard temperature-guided RF lesions with catheter-based cryolesions in a canine preparation [13]. Despite pre-treatment with ASA and standard heparin protocols, the cryolesions were associated with substantially less endothelial disruption and overlying thrombus formation. This is a well-accepted characteristic of cryolesions produced in an open manner at surgery and now confirmed for cryolesions produced with catheters [23-25]. Cryoablation also results in dense homogenous fibrosis with a well-demarcated border zone. The lesions are non-arrhythmogenic and preserve the underlying extracellular collagen matrix and tensile strength [26]. Hence, the degree of endovascular contracture may in fact be reduced in comparison to RF.

Safety in the Pulmonary Veins

As with all new technologies, cryoablation has been delivered in the pulmonary veins both as a focal approach, initially by our group and then others, for successful isolation [27, 28]. Also under investigation by our group is the use of a circular cryoablation catheter for PV isolation [29].

Animal Studies

Cryolesions have been produced within the coronary sinus using surgical cryoprobes with little short-term thrombus or long-term stenosis [30]. We have produced coronary sinus lesions using catheter-based cryothermy in a swine model without the production of significant thrombus, venous stenosis or damage to the adjacent artery [31, 32]. Aggressive focal cryoablation at the pulmonary venous in goats did not induce stenosis over a three-month follow-up (D. Keane et al., Massachusetts General Hospital, personal communication). Likewise, circumferential cryoablation of the pulmonary veins of dogs did not induce any PV contracture in 9 dogs acutely, or stenosis in 4 dogs in chronic follow-up [33].

Preliminary Human Studies

Our laboratory has performed pulmonary vein isolation using both focal and circular cryoablation catheters. In all, 33 pulmonary veins, guided by ice mapping, were isolated in 16 patients using one or both techniques. PV diameters using spiral CT scans performed three months following cryoablation demonstrated no reduction in PV diameter (14 ± 3 mm versus 14 ± 2 mm, p=0.2). As a control, non-ablated pulmonary venous diameters were 14 ± 4 mm pre-ablation and 15 ± 3 mm post-ablation [29-34]. An international registry has accumulated significant experience with cryoablation in the pulmonary veins and we await the evaluation of the effects on the pulmonary veins when applied to larger numbers of patients.

Specific Cryoablation Strategies and Tools

Focal Ablation (Figs. 1, 2)

As with radiofrequency, focal cryoablation has been delivered at the PV atrial junction to isolate the pulmonary veins. Initial animal work using the 7Fr Cryocath Freezor™ catheter (Cryocath Technologies, Montreal, Canada) suggested that isolation could be achieved with fewer lesions than that required with RF. We evaluated this in our laboratory in 5 patients. While Lasso-guided PV isolation was indeed feasible, the number of lesions was not reduced as compared to RF. In fact, as the cryolesions were each 4 minutes in duration, the isolation of a single vein required up to four times as long. Similar results have been reported by Tondo et al. where 44 out of 52 (84%) of PVs were acutely isolated using a mean of 10-18 lesions per vein [27]. Like our experience, the procedure times of 4.2 hours were long. At short follow-up of 3 + 1 month, 61% of patients were free of atrial fibrillation. A similar approach has been reported by Tse et al. using a 10Fr catheter produced by CryoCor (San Diego, Ca.) [35]. Despite a larger catheter tip, the results were qualitatively similar in 22 patients. A total of 55 veins (2.8 per patient) were isolated. At short follow-up, 80% were arrhythmia free and 45% without anti-arrhythmic drugs. Long procedure times (6 ± 0.2 hours) were also recorded, despite the larger catheter tip. Importantly, the accumulated evidence has documented no PV stenosis across all experiences. All in all, the early cryoablation experience has demonstrated safety of ablation at or within the initial part of the PVs, as well as feasibility, but with long procedure times and modest success rates.

Circumferential (Fig. 3)

As experience demonstrated that cryoablation within the pulmonary veins was safe, a circular linear ablation catheter was produced (Arctic Circler, Cryocath Technologies) to sit within the first few millimeters of the vein to produce circumferential ablation. This catheter is currently undergoing evaluation in our

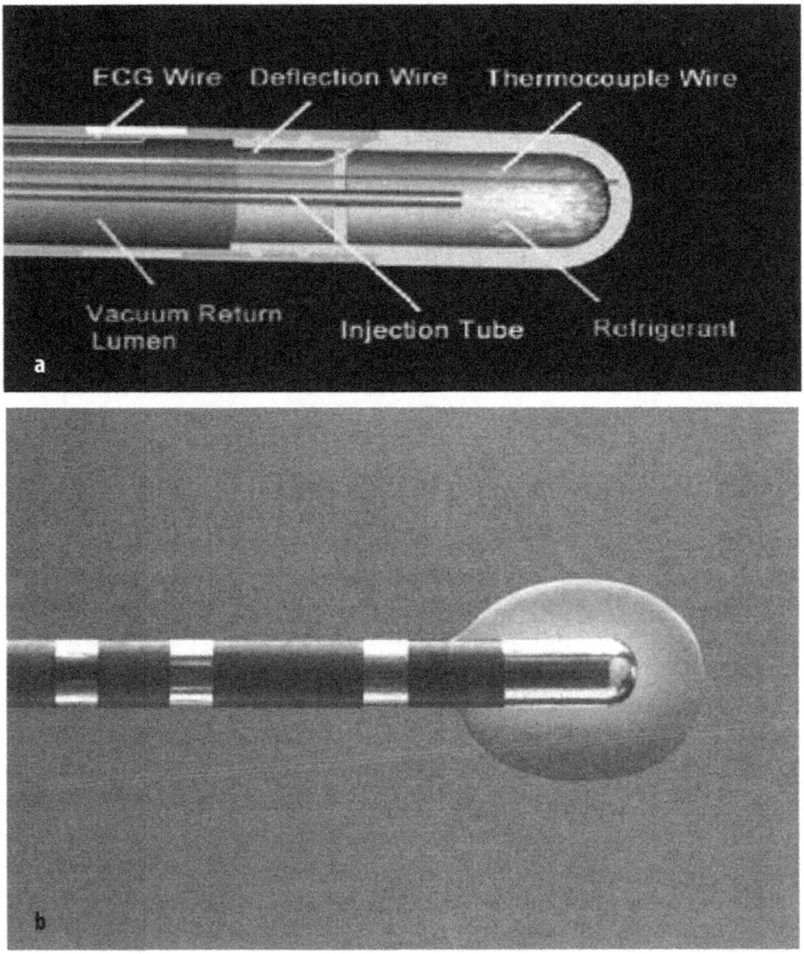

Fig. 1. Focal 7Fr cryoablation catheter. Panel A shows a schematic representation of a cryoablation catheter. Liquid refrigerant (nitrous oxide) is delivered under pressure into the hollow tip via a small injection tube. As a phase change takes place from liquid to gas, cooling occurs. The gaseous refrigerant is removed through a co-axial vacuum tube. Thermocouple and deflection wires are as a standard RF catheter. Panel B shows ice formation on the tip of a 7Fr cryoablation catheter (Freezor™) that has been placed in a saline bath. Reproduced with permission from Cryocath Technologies Inc., Montreal Canada

and other laboratories. The current iteration is a 7Fr catheter with maximal cooling temperatures to −80 °C. Within the cooling segment, a nitinol strut causes the circler to self-expand upon cooling to fully engage vein diameters of 18 to 30 mm. Complete clinical evaluation should be reported in the coming months. Experience in our hands with the initial prototype demonstrated modest efficacy, (7 out of 9 had elimination of atrial fibrillation on previously

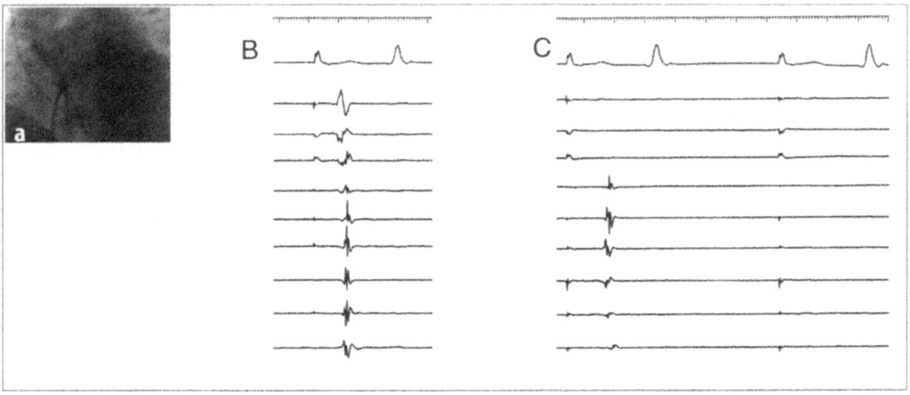

Fig. 2. Pulmonary vein isolation with a focal cryoablation catheter. Panel A demonstrates a fluoroscopic image of Lasso™-guided focal cryoablation in the right upper pulmonary vein. Panel B shows pulmonary venous electrograms as recorded by a Lasso™ catheter at baseline during distal coronary sinus pacing. Panel C shows isolation of the pulmonary vein during cryoablation with sudden elimination of pulmonary vein electrograms on two consecutive beats

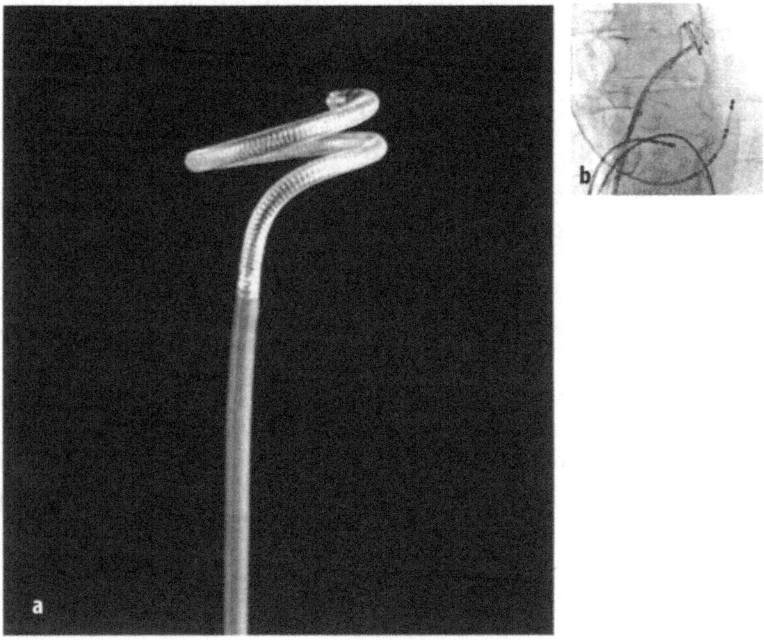

Fig. 3. 7Fr circular pulmonary vein cryoablation catheter (Arctic Circler™, Cryocath Technologies Inc., Montreal Canada). Panel A shows the catheter, while panel B shows deployment in the left upper pulmonary vein with a Lasso™ catheter placed distally in the vein for simultaneous monitoring of cryothermal delivery

ineffective drugs) with successful isolation of 19 of 22 veins (2.4 per patient). No acute venous contracture was seen on venography and no stenosis was seen as evaluated by spiral CT at 3 months [29, 34]. An international registry will continue to compile data of efficacy and safety on the use of this technology. Results of this registry will be available relatively soon. Despite the modest efficacy results as compared to that published for RF, enthusiasm for cryoablation continues based on the safety profile, especially with the continued publication of cases of PV stenosis and occlusion [8, 36].

Cryothermal Balloon

The highly variable anatomy of the pulmonary veins provides a significant challenge for any balloon-based technology. This has been highlighted by the initial use of the over-the-wire ultrasound balloon experience (Atrionix) [10, 37]. By design, this technology works best when the shaft of the catheter sits coaxial to the pulmonary vein. This may be a significant challenge to any operator, even when assisted by intracardiac ultrasound. On the other hand, a cryothermal balloon overcomes this, as the entire balloon can freeze and adhere to the adjacent tissue. As such, the perimeter of the balloon in closest apposition to the vein becomes the source of ablation irrespective of orientation in the vein. Preliminary work in a canine preparation by Avitall et al. has demonstrated feasibility and safety [38]. The lesions are transmural, circumferential and without overlying thrombus. Moreover, as the heat source of the pulmonary venous flow is occluded by the balloon, transmural lesions within the thick atrium adjacent to the vein can be achieved, unlike with previous non-occlusive technologies. Further safety and engineering challenges are required prior to the successful deployment of such a balloon in humans. There is obvious concern of rupture of the balloon with egress of nitrous oxide into the circulation. Nitrous oxide is a highly soluble gas in plasma. Nonetheless, a large bolus of gas at body temperature would act as a gas embolism until complete dissolution occurred. There are further issues as to producing balloons of sufficient variability in size to accommodate the highly variable anatomy. The above discussion not withstanding, a cryothermal balloon prototype is expected in the next 6-12 months.

Linear Lesions

The major focus of ablation of atrial fibrillation is the pulmonary veins. Some centers have begun to add linear ablation lesions to successful isolation of all veins. As patients with more challenging substrates are tackled, long linear lesions will almost certainly be required. The unique characteristics of cryothermal lesions, with less endothelial disruption and platelet activation, make this technology ideal for linear ablation, especially in the presence of sluggish atrial flow. As more versatile and more powerful catheters are produced, it is expected that linear ablation catheters will be used to produce long continuous transmural ablation lesions with greater safety than RF.

Conclusions

Extensive surgical experience has taught us much about the unique features of cryothermal ablation. Our center recognized the safety profile of this technology as being ideal for ablation near the AV node, within the coronary sinus or adjacent to coronary arteries, as well as within the pulmonary veins. Mounting evidence continues to confirm the absence of pulmonary venous stenosis with this technology. At the present time, the efficacy of cryothermal pulmonary vein isolation is limited. As the technology continues to improve, with newer designs and more powerful systems, the efficacy will approach that of RF, but with a safety profile that will make it a more applicable technology to the widespread application of pulmonary vein isolation.

References

1. Haissaguerre M, Jais P, Shah DC et al (1998) Spontaneous initiation of atrial fibrillation by ectopic beats originating in the pulmonary veins. N Engl J Med 339:659-666
2. Oral H, Knight BP, Tada H et al (2002) Pulmonary vein isolation for paroxysmal and persistent atrial fibrillation. Circulation 105:1077-1081
3. Marrouche NF, Dresing T, Cole C et al (2002) Circular mapping and ablation of thepulmonary vein for treatment of atrial fibrillation. Impact of different catheter technologies. J Am Coll Cardiol 40:464-474
4. Chen SA, Hsieh MH, Tai CT et al (1999) Initiation of atrial fibrillation by ectopic beats originating from the pulmonary veins: electrophysiological characteristics, pharmacological responses, and effects of radiofrequency ablation. Circulation 100:1879-1886
5. Chen SA, Yu WC, Tai CT (2000) Editorial comment: can we avoid pulmonary vein stenosis following ablation of atrial fibrillation? J Interv Card Electrophysiol 4:633-634
6. Haissaguerre M, Jais P, Shah DC et al (2000) Electrophysiological end point for catheter ablation of atrial fibrillation initiated from multiple pulmonary venous foci. Circulation 101:1409-1417
7. Mangrum JM, Mounsey JP, Kok LC et al (2002) Intracardiac echocardiography-guided, anatomically based radiofrequency ablation of focal atrial fibrillation originating from pulmonary veins. J Am Coll Cardiol 39:1964-1972
8. Ernst S, Ouyang F, Goya M et al (2003) Total pulmonary vein occlusion as a consequence of catheter ablation for atrial fibrillation mimicking primary lung disease. J Cardiovasc Electrophysiol 14:366-370
9. Packer DL, Peterson LA, Monahan KH et al (2002) Relationship between the degree of pulmonary vein narrowing and symptoms in pulmonary vein stenosis: Where is the symptom threshold? PACE 25:560 (Abstract)
10. Natale A, Pisano E, Shewchik J et al (2000) First human experience with pulmonary vein isolation using a through- the-balloon circumferential ultrasound ablation system for recurrent atrial fibrillation. Circulation 102:1879-1882
11. Gage AA, Baust J (1998) Mechanisms of tissue injury in cryosurgery. Cryobiology 37:171-186
12. Taylor GW, Kay GN, Zheng X et al (2000) Pathological effects of extensive radiofrequency energy applications in the pulmonary veins in dogs. Circulation 101:1736-1742

13. Khairy P, Chauvet P, Lehmann J et al (2003) Lower incidence of thrombus formation with cryoenergy versus radiofrequency catheter ablation. Circulation in press
14. Yamane T, Jais P, Shah DC et al (2000) Efficacy and safety of an irrigated-tip catheter for the ablation of accessory pathways resistant to conventional radiofrequency ablation. Circulation 102:2565-2568
15. Chauvet P, Santoianni D, Tanguay J et al (2001) Cryoablation produces less endothelial thrombus than RF ablation. Circulation (Abstract)
16. Everett TH, Nath S, Lynch C et al (2001) Role of calcium in acute hyperthermic myocardial injury. J Cardiovasc Electrophysiol 12:563-569
17. Haissaguerre M, Jais P, Shah DC et al (2000) Electrophysiological end point for catheter ablation of atrial fibrillation initiated from multiple pulmonary venous foci. Circulation 101:1409-1417
18. Chen SS, Wright NT, Humphrey JD (1997) Heat-induced changes in the mechanics of a collagenous tissue: isothermal free shrinkage. J Biomech Eng 119:372-378
19. Arnoczky SP, Aksan A (2002) Thermal modification of connective tissues: basic science considerations and clinical implications. J Am Acad Orthop Surg 8:305-313
20. Carter TR, Bailie DS, Edinger S (2002) Radiofrequency electrothermal shrinkage of the anterior cruciate ligament. Am J Sports Med 30:221-226
21. Deak G, Romhanyi G (1967) The thermal shrinkage process of collagen fibres as revealed by polarization optical analysis of topooptical staining reactions. Acta Morphol Acad Sci Hung 15:195-208
22. Gorisch W, Boergen KP (1982) Heat-induced contraction of blood vessels. Lasers Surg Med 2:1-13
23. Klein GJ, Guiraudon GM, Perkins DG et al (1984) Surgical correction of the Wolff-Parkinson-White syndrome in the closed heart using cryosurgery: a simplified approach. J Am Coll Cardiol 3:405-409
24. Klein GJ, Guiraudon GM, Perkins DG et al (1985) Controlled cryothermal injury to the AV node: feasibility for AV nodal modification. Pacing Clin Electrophysiol 8:630-638
25. Szabo TS, Jones DL, Guiraudon GM et al (1987) Cryosurgical modification of the atrioventricular node: a closed heart approach in the dog. J Am Coll Cardiol 10:389-398
26. Klein GJ, Harrison L, Ideker RF et al (1979) Reaction of the myocardium to cryosurgery: electrophysiology and arrhythmogenic potential. Circulation 59:364-372
27. Tondo C, Fassini G, De Martino G et al (2002) Catheter isolation of the pulmonary veins by cryothermal ablation: Preliminary results. PACE 25:612(Abstract)
28. Wong T, Markides V, Chow AWC et al (2002) Percutaneous cryoablation pulmonary vein isolation to treat atrial fibrillation. PACE 25:552(Abstract)
29. Skanes AC, Klein GJ, Yee R, Krahn AD (2002) Initial experience with a novel circular cryoablation catheter for pulmonary vein isolation. Circulation (Abstract)
30. Bredikis J, Bredikis A (1985) Cryosurgical ablation of left parietal wall accessory atrioventricular connections through the coronary sinus without the use of extracorporeal circulation. J Thorac Cardiovasc Surg 90:199-205
31. Skanes AC, Jones D, Teefy P et al (2002) Cryoablation of accessory pathways via the distal coronary sinus: Safety and feasibility in a swine model. PACE 25:660 (Abstract)
32. Yagi T, Nakagawa H, Khammar GS et al (2001) Safety and efficacy of cryo-ablation in the canine coronary sinus. Circulation (Abstract)
33. Arruda M, Azegami K, Wang Z et al (2002) Circumferential cryoablation of pulmonary veins using a novel spiral catheter. PACE 25:592 (Abstract)
34. Skanes AC, Klein GJ, Yee R, Krahn AD (2002) Cryoablation does not cause pulmonary vein stenosis. Can J Cardiol (Abstract)

35. Tse H-F, Rodriguez L-M, Geller C et al (2002) Long-term safety and efficacy of transvenous cryoablation for pulmonary vein isolation for atrial fibrillation. PACE 25:551(Abstract)
36. Leite L, Asirvathaam S, Hammill SC et al (2002) Clinical and electrophysiologic predictors of pulmonary vein stenosis following radiofrequency catheter ablation for atrial fibrillation. PACE 25:559 (Abstract)
37. Saliba W, Wilber D, Packer D et al (2002) Circumferential ultrasound ablation for pulmonary vein isolation: analysis of acute and chronic failures. J Cardiovasc Electrophysiol 13:957-961
38. Avitall B, Urboniene D, Rozmus G et al (2003) New cryotechnology for electrical isolation of the pulmonary veins. J Cardiovasc Electrophysiol 14:281-286

Ablation of Atrial Fibrillation by Radiofrequency: Circular Energy Delivery

T. Lewalter, H. Bielik, J. Schrickel, A. Bitzen, J.O. Schwab, A. Yang, B. Lüderitz

Introduction

Pulmonary vein (PV) ablation has entered the therapeutic armamentarium as a curative intervention in a subset of patients with focal atrial fibrillation (AF) [1]. Clinical application of this therapy is mainly limited by the potential risks of pericardial tamponade, thromboembolic events, and PV stenosis. The development of PV stenosis has been documented after these procedures, especially when radiofrequency (RF) delivery is performed within the vein and when circumferential burns with multiple applications are neccessary [2, 3]. There is evidence that when energy applications are limited to the PV ostium or left atrium to the PV transition area, and when patients do not require a full-circumference PV burn, PV stenosis is observed less frequently than with distal-intravenous RF delivery [4]. Therefore, identification of a circumscribed left atrial to PV breakthrough during sinus rhythm or atrial pacing may offer the chance of delivering more 'focal' RF, rather than a full-circumference RF application. In addition, RF energy delivery should be limited to the PV ostium, which means methods of verifying the position of the ablation catheter are needed.

We report about a new, deflectable guiding sheath and microcatheter system that make it possible check the catheter position by repetitive contrast medium injection given via the guiding sheath in order to find a "true" ostial position, and also on the use of coronary sinus (CS) extrastimulus pacing, which has recently been described as a helpful maneuver for breakthrough identification [5, 6].

The Naviport Guiding Sheath for Repetitive Contrast Injection

The Naviport catheter, an 8-F deflectable soft-tip guiding sheath, needs to be

Department of Medicine-Cardiology, University of Bonn, Germany

advanced to the left atrium through an additional guiding catheter, which is used for transseptal puncture. After the Naviport has then been advanced to the left atrium and the transseptal sheath withdrawn to the inferior vena cava, pre-ablation PV angiography can be performed via the Naviport. The left-sided and the right upper PVs are usually easy to approach even with fixed-curve catheters; however, the right lower PV is often difficult to reach owing to its position relative to the interatrial septum. In a consecutive series of seven patients who underwent a left-sided ablation procedure with the Naviport guiding sheath for recurrent focal AF at the University of Bonn, there was no problem performing angiography of the right lower PV in each patient and advancing additional catheter material into the same vein when desired (Fig. 1). For intubation of the right lower PV, the deflectability of the catheter tip was its most important feature (Fig. 2). In the seven consecutive patients the Naviport guding sheath was combined with a 4-F fixed-wire catheter with eight 6-mm coiled platinum electrodes in a looped configuration (Revelation Helix, Cardima Inc.) for both PV mapping and ablation [7]. In all patients all four PVs underwent pre-ablation angiography. In three patients the right lower PV was either smaller than 15 mm or did not exhibit PV potentials, so that ablation was not performed in this vessel, whereas all remaining 25 PVs

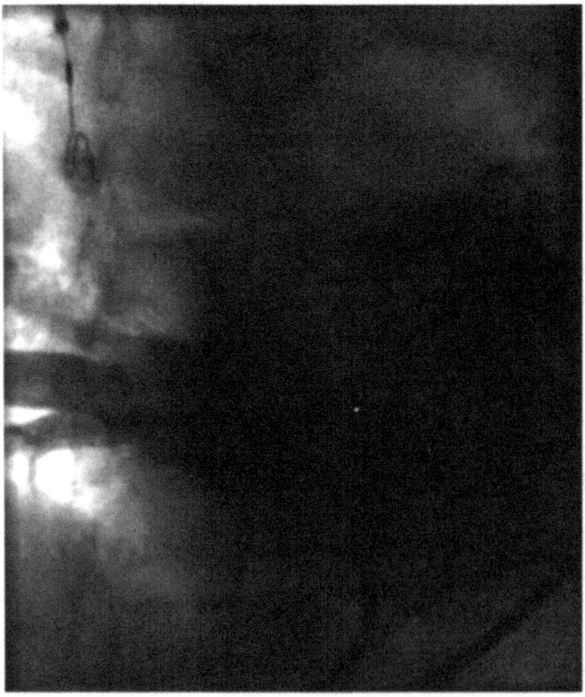

Fig. 1. Angiography of the right lower pulmonary vein (PV). X-ray in RAO 30° view depicts angiography of the right lower PV using the Naviport guiding sheath

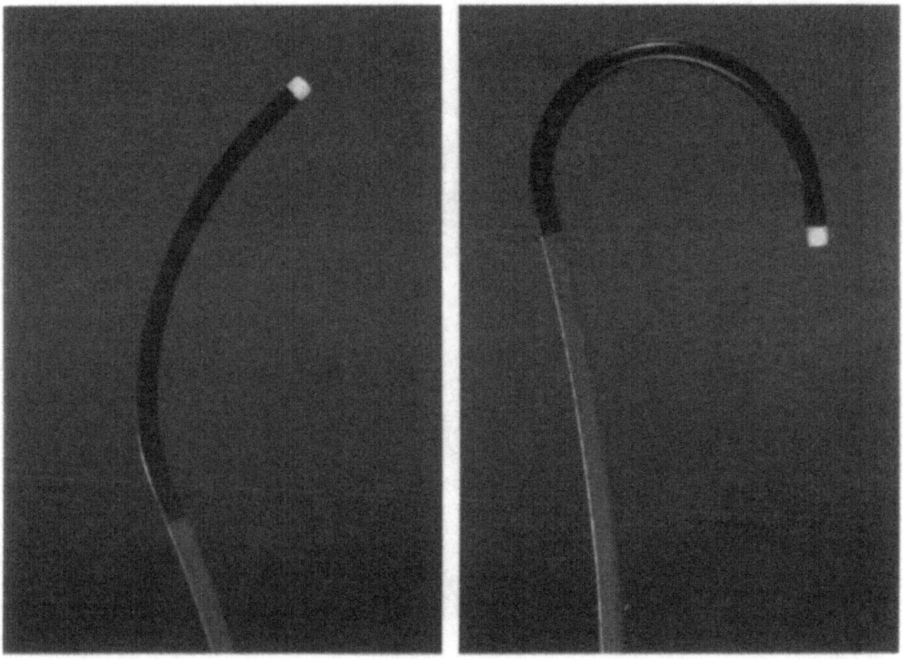

Fig. 2. Deflectable soft-tip Naviport guiding sheath

were mapped and ablated. We compared the first 'best guess' catheter position of the Helix catheter, as guided by the pre-ablation angiography, with the need for catheter replacement following a contrast medium injection via the guiding sheath with the catheter in its 'best guess' PV position. It is possible to inject contrast medium injection via the guiding sheath after the mapping and ablation catheter has been advanced through this sheath, because the inner lumen of the Naviport is 6 F, whereas the outer diameter of the Helix Revelation catheter s only 4 F, leaving enough space for contrast flow (Fig. 3).

In 22 out of 25 PVs in seven patients, angiography with the ablation catheter in place led to catheter replacement: in 12 PVs a too-distal catheter position more than 5 mm from the assumed PV ostium was the reason for catheter replacement. In 3 PVs, early vessel branching with the catheter crossing a branching area made it necessary to change position. In the case of 3 PVs, at least parts of the Helix catheter were located outside the PV and in 4, the angiography revealed inadequate wall contact.

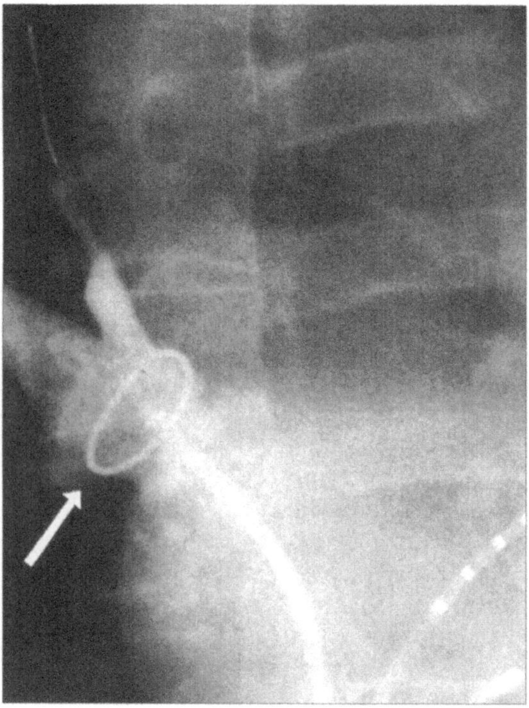

Fig. 3 Catheter position in the right upper PV. X-ray in RAO 30° view depicts the octapolar Revelation Helix catheter positioned in the ostium of the right upper PV (*white arrow*) during injection of contrast medium via the guiding sheath. Standard diagnostic catheters are placed in the right atrium at the bundle of His and the coronary sinus for atrial pacing maneuvers

Coronary Sinus Extrastimulus Pacing for Identification of Left Atrial to PV Breakthrough

Looped mapping catheters in ostial positions often exhibit a greater amount of fusion between the left atrial and the PV signal than catheters in a more distal position inside the PV. Fixed-rate coronary sinus (CS) pacing is a known and helpful maneuver that can be used to separate the left atrial from the PV signal [8]. However, even with fixed-rate CS pacing, left atrial-to-PV breakthrough identification can still be difficult. For such cases, CS extrastimulus pacing was recently described as a pacing technique that can lead to an additional 'reduction' of the left atrial-to-PV breakthrough area [5, 6]: 25 PVs (10 right, 15 left) were mapped using the 4-F fixed-wire Revelation Helix catheter with a distal loop of eight 6-mm electrodes. For mapping and ablation the electrode loop was positioned in the PV ostium perpendicular to the longitudinal PV axis. The electrical breakthrough (EBT) area was identified as those electrodes indicating the earliest PV signals during CS pacing. The reduction of two or more EBT electrodes was defined as a significant benefit in EBT identification: in 22 of the 25 PVs, mapped PV potentials were observed. When fixed-rate pacing was performed, the EBT area was identified in a mean of 4.2±1 electrodes, whereas using extrastimulus pacing, EBT area could be significantly reduced to 2.3±0.8 electrodes. In 13 of the 22 PVs mapped (59%), extrastimulus pacing was beneficial in the identification of the EBT as the primary target for RF delivery. The authors conclude that CS extrastimulus pacing induces intra-PV decremental conduction properties, allowing the identification of a more localized and smaller EBT area as the primary target for RF delivery and may therefore help to limit intrapulmonary RF delivery.

Conclusions

Identification of ostial PV potentials is crucial to allow the delivery of limited and localized, rather than full-circumference RF ablation in focal AF. Fixed-rate pacing from the distal CS or the left atrium has been demonstrated to be effective and helpful in unmasking PV potential in about two-thirds of all patients undergoing left-sided PV ablation [8]. In addition, identification of the most limited left atrial-to-PV breakthrough area is desired, as the 'minimal necessary' tissue target for RF delivery [4].

We report on a new deflectable guiding sheath and microcatheter system, which makes it possible to verify the catheter position by repetitive contrast medium injection given via the guiding sheath to find a true ostial position. However, in these locations identification of the left atrial-to-PV breakthrough area is frequently more difficult than in a distal PV location. For such cases CS extrastimulus pacing has been recently described as a helpful maneuver for the identification of breakthrough [5, 6].

References

1. Haissaguerre M, Jais P, Shah D, Takahashi A, Hocini M, Quiniou G, Garrigue S et al (1998) Spontaneous initiation of atrial fibrillation by ectopic beats originating in the pulmonary veins. N Engl J Med 339:659-666
2. Yu WC, Hsu TL, Tai CT, Tsai CF, Hsieh MH, Lin WS, Lin YK et al (2001) Acquired pulmonary vein stenosis after radiofrequency catheter ablation of paroxysmal atrial fibrillation. J Cardiovasc Electrophysiol 12:887-892
3. Gerstenfeld EP, Guerra P, Sparks PB, Hattori K, Lesh MD (2001) Clinical outcome after radiofrequency catheter ablation of focal atrial fibrillation triggers. J Cardiovasc Electrophysiol 12:900-908
4. Haissaguerre M, Shah D, Jais P, Hocini M, Yamane T, Deisenhofer I, Chauvin M et al (2000) Electrophysiological breakthroughs from the left atrium to the pulmonary veins. Circulation 102:2463-2465
5. Lewalter T, Burkhardt D, Chun S, Schimpf R, Bielik H, Schrickel J, Shlevkov N, Yang A, Lüderitz B (2002) Decremental intravenous pulse propagation during extrastimulus pacing: relevance for catheter ablation of focal atrial fibrillation. Europace 4:411-415
6. Burkhardt D, Schimpf R, Bielik H, Schrickel J, Shlevkov N, Yang A, Schwab JO, Lüderitz B, Lewalter T (2002) Decremental pulmonary vein conduction: relevance for

ablation in focal atrial fibrillation. Pacing Clin Electrophysiol 25/4:abs 727

7. Lewalter T, Burkhardt D, Bielik H, Schrickel J, Yang A, Shlevkov N, Schimpf R, Schwab JO, Lüderitz B (2002) Circumferential pulmonary vein mapping and ablation in focal atrial fibrillation: single catheter technique. J Interv Card Electrophysiol 7:165-170
8. Hocini M, Shah DC, Jais P, Haissaguerre M, Peng JT, Yamane T, Deisenhofer I et al (2000) Concealed left pulmonary vein potentials unmasked by left atrial stimulation. Pacing Clin Electrophysiol 23:1832-1835

Catheter Ablation of Atrial Fibrillation: What Are the Risks and Complications and How Do We Avoid Them?

S. THEMISTOCLAKIS, A. BONSO, A. ROSSILLO, A. RAVIELE

Atrial fibrillation (AF) is the most common cardiac arrhythmia, with a prevalence of between 2% and 4% in the general population over 60 years old and an increasing incidence with age [1]. Its presence causes a rise in morbidity and mortality rates due to the increase of embolic risk and loss of atrial function with a consequent decrease in cardiac performance. Very often AF is associated with disabling symptoms–such as palpitations, exercise intolerance, and fatigue–that can influence the quality of life significantly. In patients affected by persistent or permanent AF with rapid ventricular response, the persistent high rate may produce a tachycardiomyopathy that can be reversible when sinus rhythm is restored or the ventricular rate is controlled. This arrhythmia is also a significant social financial burden. In the USA, AF causes more hospital admissions than any other arrhythmia, accounting for a nearly 1 million hospital days per year [2].

The clinical importance and the high cost of AF create a need for effective treatment. Various management strategies are currently employed, including rate control, cardioversion, maintenance of sinus rhythm, and stroke prevention. Pharmacological treatment strategies directed at the prevention of the recurrence of AF are frequently ineffective or should be withdrawn because of adverse effects including ventricular proarrhythmia.

Catheter ablation of AF has been recently described as an effective curative treatment overall in patients with paroxysmal and persistent AF and is becoming more widely available. This therapy was first applied by making linear lesions in the right and/or left atrium. However, the treatment of AF with linear lesion ablation, in particular in the right atrium, has been demonstrated have a poor efficacy [3]. In fact, only 6%–25% of patients with idiopathic or paroxysmal AF treated with linear right atrial ablation remained free of symptomatic AF in the absence of antiarrhythmic drugs after a follow-up of 6–21 months [4–7]. Studies of linear left atrial ablation had discordant results. Two

Division of Cardiology Umberto I Hospital, Mestre–Venice, Italy

studies reported 40%–58% success rates without antiarrhythmic drugs [4, 6] but these results were not reproduced in a third study, where none of patients had a successful outcome after treatment [7]. Moreover, linear ablation of AF shows complications, with a magnitude of related risk that is not yet clear in view of the small number of studies available [3]. The most common complication reported with linear ablation in the left and/or right atrium has been pericardial effusion, which occurred in less than 11% of patients. In about 8% of patients treated with linear ablation in the right atrium sinus node dysfunction occurred. Two serious complications restricted to left atrial ablation are cerebral infarction (up to 8%) and pulmonary vein stenosis, the incidence of which is unclear. Symptomatic pulmonary vein stenosis was reported by Robbins et al. [8] in 2 of 18 patients (11%) treated with linear right and left atrial ablation but was not observed in any of the published series of patients who underwent linear ablation of AF.

A few years ago, Haïssaguerre et al. [9] demonstrated that atrial ectopic beats within the pulmonary veins were responsible for the initiation of AF in most patients. In the past 5 years, various techniques have been proposed to effectively abolish the pulmonary vein firing responsible for initiating and maintaining AF. The first approach was to target the site of origin of firing within the pulmonary vein directly [9, 10]. However, the early experience with focal ablation within the pulmonary vein indicated that the recurrence rate was high and the success rate modest, associated with serious complications such as a high percentage of pulmonary vein stenosis [3, 9, 10]. This complication was observed in up to 42% of patients [10], and with severe pulmonary vein stenosis reported in up to 14% [19], the long-term sequelae of even mild or moderate stenosis is unknown [3].

Recently, different approaches have been developed to electrically confine the triggers in the pulmonary veins (pulmonary vein isolation). The overall success rate (with or without antiarrhythmic drugs) of this procedure is increasing progressively and at present ranges from 51% to 92% for patients with paroxysmal or persistent AF and from 51% to 89% for patients with permanent AF [9–16]. However, although the high success rate is very encouraging for widespread adoption of this approach, complications such as cardiac tamponade (up to 2%), cerebrovascular accident (up to 5%), pulmonary vein stenosis (ranging from 0% to 36 %, depending on the ablative technique used and the method of assessment), coronary embolism (up to 5%), hemopneumothorax (up to 3%), and pericardial effusion (up to 3%) can still be observed [9–21].

The most serious complications are pulmonary vein stenosis or thromboembolic events. Animal data have shown that acute pulmonary vein stenosis are the result of denaturation of collagen, which occurs at 65 °C [22]. In contrast, chronic luminal narrowing of the pulmonary vein from extensive radiofrequency ablation was a result of an inflammatory response with progressive intimal proliferation, collagen replacement of necrotic myocardium, endovascular contraction, and proliferation of elastic lamina over the study period of 14 weeks [23].

The clinical presentation of this complication is various; frequently the pulmonary vein stenosis is asymptomatic, especially when a mild or moderate degree of stenosis is present or a single vein is involved [21]. The symptoms, when present, appear to be largely respiratory in origin, mimicking more common lung diseases (such as asthma, pneumonia, lung cancer, and pulmonary embolism) and can be under-recognized.

Saad et al. [21] reported that 18 (5%) of 335 patients treated with pulmonary vein isolation developed severe pulmonary vein stenosis, defined as a luminal narrowing by more than 70%. Forty-eight percent of these patients were asymptomatic. Among the symptomatic patients, shortness of breath was the most frequent symptom (44%), followed by persistent cough (39%), hemoptysis (28%), and pleuritic pain (22%). These symptoms may be explained by the slowly increased intravascular pressure in the pulmonary circulatory system. Vascular resistances in the affected lung segment may be elevated by the reduction or absence of flow through the stenotic pulmonary vein.

Other authors also described drug-refractory pneumonia in patients with pulmonary vein occlusion after ablation [24]. Ernst et al. [24] explain these symptoms by a lesser degree of ventilation associated with a less perfused lung segment. These poorly perfused and ventilated segments offer ideal conditions for bronchopulmonary infections.

It seems that symptom severity was not related only to the degree of stenosis but also to the number of stenotic pulmonary veins. Radiographic findings were abnormal in 50% of patients with severe stenosis and mainly represented by lung consolidation and left pleural effusion (78% and 56% of patients respectively) [21]. In the same report symptoms improved spontaneously over time in 50% of patients and were related to improvement in the radiographic abnormalities detected, although other hemodynamic compensatory mechanisms (such as development of collaterals) may also play a role.

CT scan and MRI of the pulmonary veins can reveal the correct diagnosis and lead to appropriate therapy. However, in the previously cited study [21] pulmonary vein angiography (the diagnostic gold standard) confirmed total venous occlusion in only one of seven patients who had such findings on CT scan. This might have important implications for planning pulmonary vein interventions, considering that in the presence of total occlusion the dilatation procedure is more challenging, if it can be performed at all. Therefore, the sensitivity and specificity of these noninvasive techniques need to be studied further.

Currently, we cannot offer a validated treatment to patients who have developed severe pulmonary vein stenosis. Pulmonary vein balloon angioplasty with stenting is the most widely used interventional strategy [21, 22] and is recommended in affected patients because lesions can progress to total occlusion, precluding dilatation and potentially resulting in hemodynamic compromise. However, the follow-up after pulmonary vein dilatation showed a high incidence of severe restenosis (ranging from 33% to 100% [21, 22]). Thus, pulmonary vein stenosis is one of the most serious complications after a pulmonary vein ablation procedure, with limited treatment options, and rigorous efforts have been made in the attempt to prevent them.

Pulmonary vein stenoses were minimized by delivering the radiofrequency energy at the pulmonary vein–left atrium junction. Haïssaguerre et al. [11] reported that the incidence of stenosis (defined as a diameter reduction >50% detected by angiography early after ablation) was 5.5% after a mean follow-up of 8 months. The prevalence of pulmonary vein stenosis was the highest for the left inferior pulmonary vein (7% of left inferior pulmonary veins versus 1.5% of all other pulmonary veins, $p<0.05$) and when the maximum delivered radiofrequency power reached 45 W. With limitation of power to below 30 W at the ostium, the authors did not observed pulmonary vein stenosis in a short-term follow-up.

The same authors reported, in another study, the absence of pulmonary vein stenosis in 70 patients treated with pulmonary vein ostial segmental ablation guided by a circumferential mapping catheter (mean follow-up 4±5 months) [12].

The incidence of pulmonary vein stenosis in a long-term follow-up was evaluated by Arentz et al. [13]. Two years after radiofrequency ablation, 9 of 47 patients (19%) followed with transesophageal echocardiography and/or magnetic resonance imaging experienced pulmonary vein stenosis of greater than 50%. A complete pulmonary vein occlusion was observed in 4 (8.5%). However, the ablation was performed within the vein in about 50% of patients. Dividing patients treated with ostial ablation from those ablated within the vein, the incidences of pulmonary vein stenosis were 8% and 45%, respectively. It was interesting to note that in this study the temperature and power setting were almost the same as those suggested by Haïssaguerre et al. [11, 12] to reduce the risk of pulmonary vein stenosis (55 °C and 30–35 W, respectively).

Purerfellner et al. [14] performed the pulmonary vein isolation with circumferential mapping and an angiography-guided approach using an irrigated-tip catheter for the ablation in the attempt to reduce charring and thrombus formation. However, a luminal narrowing by greater than 20% was observed in 7 (18%) of 37 patients and severe pulmonary vein stenosis in 2 of them (5%). In this series the irrigated-tip catheter did not reduce the risk of pulmonary vein stenosis and the risk of stroke (2.7%) compared with other studies focused on ostial pulmonary vein isolation. It is important to note that affected pulmonary veins exhibiting luminal narrowing by less than 50% within 3 months showed no further progression as assessed by serial CT scan at 1-year follow-up [14].

Marrouche et al. [19] evaluated the impact of different catheter technologies (4-mm tip, 8-mm tip, and cooled-tip ablation catheters) on the safety and efficacy of ostial pulmonary vein isolation. Despite the smaller number of patients treated with the 8-mm tip catheter, this technology appeared to be superior to the other two in terms of AF recurrences, fluoroscopy, and procedure time. Although no complications were detected in the group operated on using the 8-mm tip catheter, this group was too small and no significant differences were observed compared with the patients treated with the other two catheters.

Despite the efforts made to better define the pulmonary vein ostia and to perform the ablation outside the vein, this target may be difficult to reach with a simple fluoroscopic landmark because of the complex three-dimensional relationship of the pulmonary veins and the left atrium, and may require integration of data from a variety of different techniques.

Pappone et al. [15] proposed an anatomic approach for circumferential pulmonary vein ablation. For this purpose, they used a nonfluoroscopic navigation system (Carto) to perform a real-time 3D left atrium map. The pulmonary vein ostia were defined by fluoroscopic visualization of the mapping catheter tip entering the cardiac silhouette with spontaneous decrease in impedance and appearance of atrial potential. However, as the same authors described, the definition of the true pulmonary vein ostia may also be difficult with Carto, and they do not rule out that a separate pulmonary vein branch could be missed in some patients [15]. Nevertheless, performing circumferential lines with contiguous focal radiofrequency lesions at a distance of greater than 5 mm from the identified pulmonary vein ostia, they obtained a success rate of 80% after a follow-up of 10 months without pulmonary vein stenosis (at transesophageal echocardiography) or thromboembolic episodes. However, these data were not confirmed in other studies. Kanagaratnam et al. [16], performing the ablation at the ostium of the pulmonary vein (defined using the Carto system and angiography), documented with CT scan pulmonary vein stenoses in 36% of patients (severe and moderate pulmonary vein stenoses were seen in 10% and 19% of patients, respectively). In our experience on 16 patients treated with circumferential pulmonary vein isolation, as previously described [15], no pulmonary vein stenosis were observed. However, complete success, defined as the absence of AF recurrences, was observed in only 28% of patients after a follow-up of 7 mouths.

Recently, Marrouche et al. [20] evaluated the effectiveness of intracardiac echocardiography (ICE) to improve the long-term success rate and minimize the complications. Pulmonary vein isolation was performed using circular mapping alone (group 1), circular mapping and ICE (group 2), or circular mapping and ICE with titration of radiofrequency energy directed by visualization of microbubbles with ICE (group 3). The ICE was also used to define the ostium, to ensure a correct circular mapping position and appropriate energy delivery at this site. In patient group 3 ablation was performed with energy delivery titration by monitoring microbubble formation. Two types of bubble pattern were described in this report: scattered microbubbles (type 1), reflecting early tissue overheating, and a brisk shower of dense microbubbles (type 2), reflecting an impending impedance rise. In this group of patients power was titrated upward (5-W increments), watching for formation of type 1 bubbles. When this bubble pattern was seen, energy was titrated down by 5-W decrements until microbubble generation subsided. Energy delivery was immediately terminated when type 2 bubbles were seen. In this study ICE-guided pulmonary vein isolation with energy titration was more effective than ICE-guided pulmonary vein isolation with a fixed power setting or angiography-guided circular mapping alone (success rates were 90%, 83%, and 80% respectively after a mean follow-up of 14 months). Moreover, the pulmonary vein isolation under ICE-guide and microbubble energy monitoring decreased the risk of complications compared to the other groups. Severe pulmonary vein stenosis were not observed in this group of patients, but were documented in 3.5% and 1.8% of groups 1 and 2 respectively. Moderate (50%–70%) pulmonary vein stenosis were also reduced in group 3 compared with groups 1 and 2 (2.5%, 5%, and 4.5% respectively). No cerebrovascular events were detected in group 3, compared with 3.5% and 3% of embolic events observed in the groups 1 and 2 respectively. These authors also observed that the pulmonary vein ostium defined angiographically was found to correlate with the ICE-defined pulmonary vein ostium only in 15% of pulmonary veins. In the other 85% of cases ICE showed that placement of circular mapping based on angiography was inaccurate and distal to the true pulmonary vein–left atrium ostium (5±3 mm within the vein).

ICE is also useful to evaluate catheter tip–tissue contact, helping to avoid delivering energy with poor contact between the ablation catheter tip and the endocardial surface, which may result in increased power output, inefficient lesion formation, and increased risk of coagulum formation [20]. Showers of dense microbubbles preceded rises in impedance by 3–5 s, and it has been demonstrated that an increase in impedance is associated with increased risk of coagulum formation and endothelial and subendothelial layer injury. Therefore, by monitoring the power titration with ICE, preventing type 2 bubbles, it is possible to avoid improper lesion formation, and this could explain the lower occurrence of severe pulmonary vein stenosis observed with this approach. Marrouche et al. [20] demonstrated a poor correlation between microbubble formation and delivered energy parameters (power and temperature); type 1 and type 2 bubbles were observed for different power and temperature settings without significant differences in the range of 20–50 W or 20–50 °C. On the basis of these data, the low energy setting (<30 W) does not exclude the possibility of improper lesion formation and the risk of pulmonary vein stenosis or cerebrovascular accident. In our electrophysiology lab, 41 patients with symptomatic paroxysmal (19 patients), persistent (17 patients), and permanent AF (5 patients) underwent pulmonary vein and superior vena cava isolation under ICE and circular mapping guide with energy monitoring as previously described. All four pulmonary veins were isolated in every patient. Complete isolation of the superior vena cava was obtained in 37 patients (90%). After a mean follow-up of 6±2,6 months the success rate was 90% (37 patients), with a complete success (defined as the absence of AF recurrences in the follow-up without antiarrhythmic drugs) in 27 patients (66%) and a partial success (defined as the absence of AF recurrences in the follow-up with previously ineffective antiarrhythmic drugs) in 10 (24%). The radiofrequency energy delivered during the ablation ranged from 30 to 100 W. The procedure was complicated in one case with a cerebrovascular embolic event that occurred in one of the first patients treated with this approach. No severe pulmonary vein stenosis were observed during the procedure or in the follow-up.

Recently Kok et al. [25] reported the occurrence of stroke after AF ablation in 3 of 56 (5%) patients. In this report all 3 patients who developed stroke were more than 60 years old and 2 of them had a prior history of transient ischemic attacks. This percentage is high compared with previous reports in which the incidence of cerebrovascular events, including transient ischemic attacks, was up to 2.7% [3, 10, 11, 13–20]. Therefore, the authors hypothesized that the risk of stroke from radiofrequency ablation of AF might be higher in older patients, especially in those with a history of transient ischemic attacks. A similar observation was made in our series, where a cerebrovascular event was detected in a 74- year-old patient with a previous history of transient ischemic attacks, maintaining activated clotting time (ACT) around 250 s and using two large 8.5F sheaths in the left atrium. However, in our opinion there are other possible reasons for the high percentage of stroke reported by Kok et al. [25], as follows:

1. The intravenous heparin administration started after successful double trans-septal catheterization with the first sheath, which remained in the left atrium without anticoagulation. Moreover, the ACT was not always maintained above 300 ms in the affected patients (the lowest ACT recorded ranged between 219 and 274 s).
2. The use of two large 8.5F sheaths instead of 8F in the left atrium for an extended period of time might promote clot formation despite anticoagulation.

Kok et al. [25] performed the ablation under ICE with radial cross-sectional imaging and limited penetration (single frequency of 9 MHz). Therefore, structures distal to the echo catheter (such as the pulmonary vein ostia or catheter–tissue interface) were difficult to detect, and this may explain why bubble formation was not seen in this study. Marrouche et al. [20], using a phased-array ICE with frequency adjustable from 5.5 to 10 MHz, were able to see the more distal structures and the bubble formation at good resolution; no thromboembolic complications were observed in the group of their patients in whom power titration was guided by microbubble formation. By contrast, embolic events were detected when pulmonary vein isolation was performed using circular mapping alone or circular mapping and intracardiac echography without microbubble monitoring (3.5% and 3% of patients, respectively). Continuous ICE monitoring can be also able to visualize char or thrombus formation allowing to take adequate countermeasures.

In conclusion, at present the integration of data from a variety of different technologies (ICE, angiography, fluoroscopy, and circular mapping catheter) seems to be the most effective strategy to avoid serious complications such as pulmonary vein stenosis or cerebrovascular events detected during radiofrequency ablation of AF. The target of the ablation must be the pulmonary vein–left atrium junction, and more distal energy delivery must be carefully avoided. The indication for this procedure should be cautious in patients suspected to be at increased risk of severe complication (i.e., older patients with a previous history of cerebrovascular events). Aggressive anticoagulation with heparin should be maintained during the procedure.

Alternative sources of energy (ultrasound [17, 18], cryoablation, laser energy) and new catheters (through-the-balloon circumferential ablation technology) have been developed in the attempt to reduce the risk of complications without a decrease in efficacy. However, further studies are need to demonstrate that these technologies are able to fulfill these goals.

References

1. Kannel W, Wolff P, Benjamin E, Levy D (1998) Prevalence, incidence, prognosis, and predisposing conditions for atrial fibrillation: population-based estimates. Am J Cardiol 82:2N–9N
2. Murgatroyd FD, Camm AJ (1993) Atrail arrhythmias. Lancet 341:1317–22
3. Scheinman MM, Morady F (2001) Nonpharmacological approaches to atrial fibrillation. Circulation 103:2120–2125
4. Haissaguerre M, Jais P, Shah DC et al (1996) Right and left atrial radiofrequency catheter ablation therapy of paroxysmal atrial fibrillation. J Cardiovasc Electrophysiol 7:1132–1144
5. Gaita F, Riccardi R, Calo L et al (1998) Atrial mapping and radiofrequency catheter ablation in patients with idiopathic atrial fibrillation. Circulation 97:2136–2145
6. Pappone C, Oreto G, Lamberti F (1999) Catheter ablation of paroxysmal atrial fibrillation using a 3D mapping system. Circulation 100:1203–1208
7. Ernst S, Schlutter M, Ouyang F et al (1999) Modification of the substrate for maintenance of idiopathic human atrial fibrillation: efficacy of radiofrequency ablation using nonfluoroscopic catheter guidance. Circulation 100:2085–2092
8. Robbins IM, Colvin EV, Doyle TP et al (1998) Pulmonary vein stenosis after catheter ablation of atrial fibrillation. Circulation 98:1769–1775
9. Haissaguerre M, Jais P, Shah DC et al (1998) Spontaneous initiation of atrial fibrillation by ectopic beats originating in the pulmonary veins. N Engl J Med 339:659–666
10. Chen SA, Hsieh MH, Tai CT et al (1999) Initiation of atrial fibrillation by ectopic beats originating from the pulmonary veins: electrophysiological characteristics, pharmacological responses and effects of radiofrequency ablation. Circulation 100:1879–1886
11. Haïssaguerre M, Jais P, Shah DC et al (2000) Electrophysiological end point for catheter ablation of atrial fibrillation initiated from multiple pulmonary vein foci. Circulation 101:1409–1417
12. Haïssaguerre M, Shah DC, Jais P (2000) Electrophysiological breakthroughs from the left atrium to the pulmonary veins. Circulation 102:2463–2465
13. Arentz T, Jander N, von Rosenthal J et al (2003) Incidence of pulmonary vein stenosis 2 years after radiofrequency catheter ablation of refractory atrial fibrillation. Eur Heart J 24:963–969
14. Purerfellner H, Cihal R, Aichinger J et al (2003) Pulmonary vein stenosis by ostial irrigated-tip ablation: incidence, time course and prediction. J Cardiovasc Electrophysiol 14:158–164

15. Pappone C, Oreto G, Rosanio S et al (2001) Atrial electroanatomic remodeling after circumferential radiofrequency pulmonary vein ablation: efficacy of an anatomic approach in a large cohort of patients with atrial fibrillation. Circulation 104:2539–2544
16. Kanagaratnam L, Tomassoni G, Schweikert R et al (2001) Empirical pulmonary vein isolation in patients with chronic atrial fibrillation using a three-dimensional non-fluoroscopic mappig system: long-term follow-up. Pacing Clin Electrophysiol 24:1774–1779
17. Natale A, Pisano E, Shewchik J et al (2000) First human experience with pulmonary vein isolation using a through-the-balloon circumferential ultrasound ablation system for recurrent atrial fibrillation. Circulation 102:1879–1882
18. Saliba W, Wilber D, Packer D et al (2002) Circumferencial ultrasound ablation for pulmonary vein isolation: analysis of acute and chronic failures. J Cardiovasc Electrophysiol 13:957–961
19. Marrouche NF, Dresing T, Cole C et al (2002) Circular mapping and ablation of the pulmonary vein for treatment of atrial fibrillation: impact of different catheter technologies. J Am Coll Cardiol 40:464–474
20. Marrouche NF, Martin DO, Wazni O et al (2003) Phased array intracardiac echocardiography monitoring during pulmonary vein isolation in patients with atrial fibrillation: impact on outcome and complications. Circulation 107:2710–2716
21. Saad EB, Marrouche NF, Saad CP et al (2003) Pulmonary vein stenosis after catheter ablation of atrial fibrillation: emergence of a new clinical syndrome. Ann Intern Med 138:634–638
22. Kok LC, Everett TH, Akar JG et al (2003) Effect of heating on pulmonary veins: how to avoid pulmonary vein stenosis. J Cardiovasc Electrophysiol 14:250–254
23. Taylor GW, Kay GN, Zheng X et al (2000) Pathological effects of extensive radiofrequency energy applications in the pulmonary veins in dogs. Circulation 101:1736–1742
24. Ernst S, Ouyang F, Goya M et al (2003) Total pulmonary vein occlusion as consequence of catheter ablation for atrial fibrillation mimicking primary lung disease. J Cardiovasc Electrophysiol 14:366–370
25. Kok LC, Mangrum JM, Haines DE et al (2002) Cerebrovascular complication associated with pulmonary vein ablation. J Cardiovasc Electrophysiol 13:764–767

Risk Stratification and Prevention of Thromboembolism: What Is the Role of Intracardiac Echocardiography?

A. Rossillo[1], N.F. Marrouche[2], E.B. Saad[2], O. Wasni[2], M. Bhargava[2], D. Bash[2], S. Beheiry[3], M. Wexman[3], B. Strunk[3], E. Pisanò[4], R. Fanelli[4], A. Bonso[1], S. Themistoclakis[1], D. Erciyes[2], W.I. Saliba[2], R.A. Schweikert[2], J. Brachmann[5], A. Raviele[1], A. Natale[2]

Introduction

Pulmonary vein isolation is becoming the treatment of choice for symptomatic atrial fibrillation (AF) that is refractory to drugs [1–3]. However, thromboembolic complications are an important limitation of this approach [4], occurring in up to 2.8% of the patients. Alternative energy sources such as cryoablation and ultrasound have the potential to improve the safety of the procedure by preventing disruption of the endothelial surface during energy delivery [5, 6].

On the other hand, most procedures are still performed with radiofrequency (RF) energy. When this source is used thromboembolic complications occur despite the limitation of temperature and impedance.

In this study, we observed the charring and thrombus formation rate with different anticoagulation protocols and the possible role of intracardiac echo in reducing the frequency and severity of these complications.

Methods

Patients

From January 1998 to December 2002, 783 patients (mean age 54 years, 83.6% males) underwent catheter-based pulmonary vein (PV) isolation for treatment of drug-refractory, symptomatic AF. Demographic characteristics are presented in Table 1. Antiarrhythmic drugs and oral anticoagulants were discontinued five half-lives and 5 days before the ablation, respectively. In all but 3 patients amiodarone was withdrawn 4–5 months before the procedure. Informed consent was obtained from all patients before the procedure, and collection and analysis of the data were approved by the institutional review board committee.

[1]Department of Cardiology, Umberto I Hospital, Mestre, Venice, Italy; [2]Center for Atrial Fibrillation, Cleveland Clinic Foundation, Cleveland, Ohio, USA; [3]Department of Cardiology, Marin Heart Center, San Francisco, Calif., USA; [4]Department of Cardiology, Casa Sollievo della Sofferenza, S.Giovanni Rotondo, Italy; [5]Department of Cardiology, Klinikum Coburg, Coburg, Germany

Table 1. Demographic characteristics

Characteristic	All patients (N=783)
Age: years (mean ± SD)	54.0±11.0
Male sex: n (%)	655 (83.6)
AF duration: years (mean ± SD)	6±4.5
Left atrial size: (cm; mean ± SD)	4.4±2.4
Left-ventricular ejection fraction (%; mean ± SD)	53±8
Structural heart disease: n (%)	327 (45.8)
Antiarrhythmic drugs: n (range)	3 (1–7)
Paroxysmal AF: n (%)	429 (54.7)
Persistent AF: n (%)	98 (12.5)
Permanent AF: n (%)	256 (32.8)

Description of the Procedure

Patients came to the electrophysiology laboratory in the fasting state. Immediately before the procedure transesophageal echocardiography was performed in all study patients to exclude the presence of left atrial thrombus. An 8- or 14-pole catheter was placed in the coronary sinus from the right internal jugular vein. The proximal electrodes were positioned between the superior vena cava and the high crista terminalis, while the distal electrodes were in the coronary sinus. A transesophageal recording lead was used to record activation of the left atrial posterior wall. Mapping of left atrium and the PVs was performed after the left atrium had been reached via the transseptal approach.

Isolation of the PVs was performed utilizing previously described strategies [3, 6, 7]:

1. Ultrasound balloon system (Atrionix, Inc). Energy was adjusted to maintain a target interface temperature of at least 60°C.
2. Electroanatomical mapping (Biosense-Webster, Diamond Bar, Calif.) with radiofrequency lesions delivered around the circumference of the veins by means of a 4mm-tip catheter in a temperature-controlled mode.
3. Distal isolation guided by circular mapping. Isolation was attempted by targeting recorded PV potentials with a 4-mm tip in a temperature-controlled mode.
4. Ostial isolation guided by PV angiography. Isolation was performed in a temperature-controlled mode.
5. Ostial isolation guided by intracardiac echocardiography (ICE). Ablation was performed with a 4-mm-tip or cooled-tip catheter in a temperature-controlled mode.
6 Ostial isolation guided by ICE associated with power titration directed by formation of microbubbles with cooled- or 8-mm-tip catheter. The delivery

of RF energy was controlled by progressively increasing power (watts) until scattered microbubbles were observed by ICE.

When type-I bubbles were seen, energy was immediately titrated downward by 5-W decrements until the microbubbles subsided. Energy delivery was also discontinued if microbubble generation did not settle. This was considered an early manifestation of tissue overheating. Energy delivery was immediately interrupted if brisk generation of microbubbles was observed in the left atrial cavity, although an effort was made to avoid this phenomenon.

Anticoagulation Protocols

Anticoagulation therapy with heparin i.v. infusion was restarted after the first transseptal puncture with a 5,000-IU i.v. bolus plus continuous infusion at 1000 IU/h. A second bolus of 3,000 IU was administered after the second puncture.

In groups 1–4, the infusion of heparin was maintained during the ablation procedure to achieve an activation coagulation time of 250–300 seconds.

In groups 5 and 6 the activated clotting time (ACT) was maintained about 350–400 s for all the procedure. In the 180 patients in group 5 ACT was maintained about 300–350 sec. and an infusion of eptifibatide was given at 135 μg/kg as an i.v. bolus, followed by infusion at 0.5 μg/kg per min, adjusted to achieve greater than 85–90% suppression of platelet aggregation (Ultegra, Accumetrics).

Ineffective Radiofrequency Energy Delivery Monitoring

RF energy monitoring was considered ineffective when the generation of microbubbles was not prevented or could not be controlled owing to poor visualization of the area of interest or to operator error.

Follow-up

At the end of the procedure a single dose of aspirin was administered and the anticoagulation therapy was restarted. An arrhythmia transmitter was given to all patients before hospital discharge for detection of AF recurrences.

Clinical visits with ECG and Holter monitoring were made at 3, 6 and 12 months after the procedure. A spiral computed tomography was also performed at 3 months and whenever any patient experienced symptoms compatible with PV stenosis having developed.

Statistical Analysis

Continuous variables are expressed as mean ± SD. Continuous variables were compared by means of the paired t-test. Categorical variables were compared by Fisher's exact test. Results with $P<0.05$ were considered statistically significant.

Results

In all patients all the four pulmonary veins were isolated. In group 1 a mean ± SD of 16.9 ± 12.3 ultrasound energy applications were delivered per patient, and there was a mean of 6.7 ± 4.7 applications per vein.

In groups 2–4 a clot was detected on the ablation catheter at the end of the procedure in 68 patients (42.5%). In 13 patients (2.2%) an echo-dense mobile structure on the mapping catheter (lasso) was detected by ICE during the ablation procedure. The mapping catheter was immediately removed from the left atrium. Scarring was seen in 8 patients (2.5%) in group 5 and in 5 (1.8%) in group 6.

In the patients in group 6 scarring was observed only when adequate energy titration was not achieved by monitoring microbubbles, whether because of operator error or because the imaging quality in the area targeted by ablation was inadequate.

In all patients the presence of an echo-dense mobile structure on the circular mapping catheter appeared to be correlated with scarring on the catheter.

In this study we were able to detect thrombus or fibrin formation on the catheter deployed in the left atrium in 4 patients. In 3 patients a heparin infusion was not correctly administered, and ACT ranged between 250 and 280 sec, and in 1 patient the heparin infusion line was inadvertently closed.

Complications

The overall incidence of cerebrovascular accidents was 1.4% (11/783).

Anticoagulation protocols including platelet inhibitors did not prevent cerebrovascular accidents, as shown in Fig. 1. However, higher degrees of

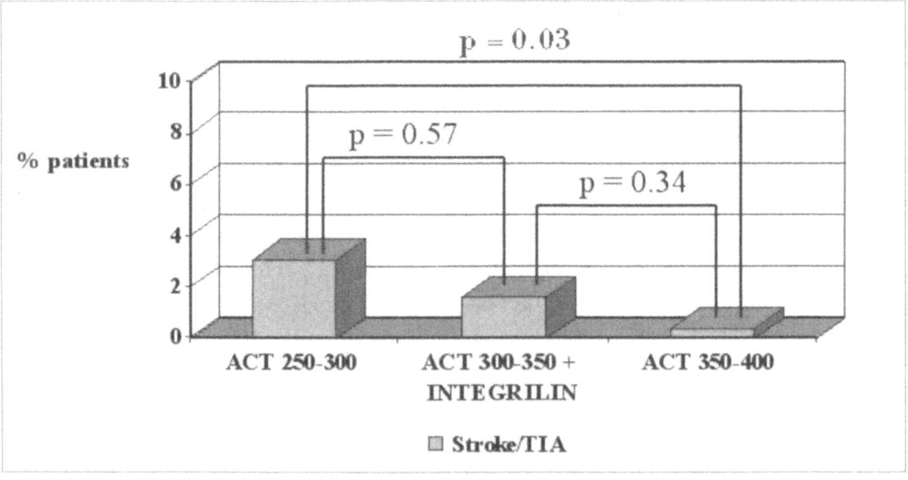

Fig. 1. Distribution of embolic events by anticoagulation protocol

heparinization with ACT between 350 and 400 s were associated with a slight reduction in the frequency of periprocedural embolic events.

One patient in group 1 experienced a periprocedural cerebellar embolic stroke. No evidence of clot or PV thrombosis was seen after the procedure on either the transesophageal echocardiogram or the MRI scan.

Ten patients (2%) experienced embolic events, including stroke and transient ischemic attacks (TIA), with temperature-guided energy delivery, while no cerebrovascular events were detected with ICE-guided power-titrated energy delivery, as reported in Fig. 2. The details of our results are shown in Table 2.

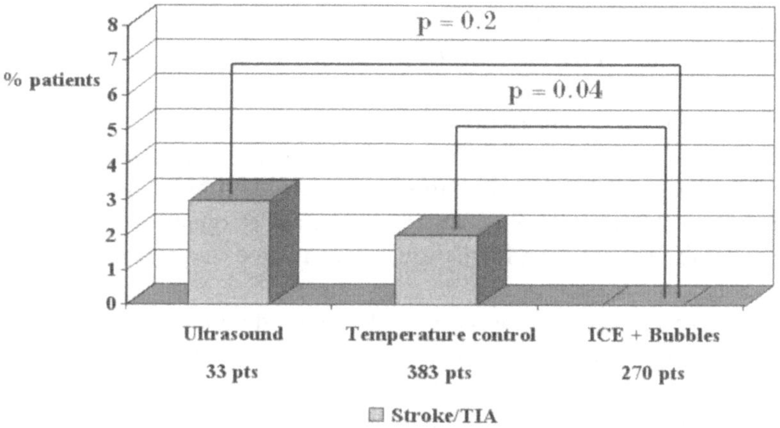

Fig. 2. Distribution of embolic events by energy delivery strategy (pts patients)

Table 2. Main results

	No. of patients	ACT 250–300	ACT 300–350 + integrilin	ACT 350–400	No. with scarring	No. with CVA
CUVA	33	33				1
CARTO	71	71			31	3
Distal PVI	25	25			12	0
Proximal PVI	64	64			25	2
ICE	320		180		5	3
				140	3	2
ICE + bubbles	270			270	5	0

CUVA, ultrasound ballon catheter; *PVI*, pulmonary vein isolation; *CVA*, celebrovascular accident; *ICE*, ultracardiac echocardiography

Discussion

The use of excessive power during RF catheter ablation may result in thromboembolic and other complications, which are especially important in the case of left-side procedures. Thus, a reliable method of achieving more accurate energy delivery is needed.

Thromboembolic Complications

Several cases involving neurological [8–11], pulmonary [12, 13], coronary [14], and peripheral artery [12] thromboembolic complications after RF ablation have been reported. Scientific evidence to support strategies for prevention of thromboembolic complications in patients undergoing catheter ablation is lacking. Attempts to find whether duration of the procedure used, number of RF applications, or anticoagulation protocols might be associated with a reduction in the frequency of thromboembolic events have proved fruitless [8–15].

A previous study [12] revealed that the anticoagulation applied during the catheter ablation procedure is not sufficient to avoid embolic complications. Our data showed that even thought an aggressive anticoagulation regimen was not enough to abolish scarring formation, it was related to a significant reduction of embolic events.

Monitoring catheter-tip temperature is the method most commonly used to limit excess energy delivery. However, its efficacy has not been proven. In a study by Calkins comparing different RF energy delivery modes, catheter coagulum formation was lower with temperature monitoring, but Epstein et al. showed that this strategy is not accurate [8].

Fundamentals of Scar Formation

The tissue temperature depends mainly on the amount of energy delivered, the cooling effect of the blood, and the tissue contact of the ablation electrode. Coagulation of the tissue arises when the temperature exceeds approximately 50°C. If the temperature at the catheter tip–tissue interface increases quickly, a sudden rise in impedance is observed.

Furthermore, when there is blood between the electrode and the tissue during energy delivery, a rapid increase in temperature can produce charring formation on the metallic surface of the electrode. This coagulum formation could cause a rapid rise in voltage, resulting in raised impedance and more tissue scarring.

RF energy is conventionally delivered by limiting the catheter-tip temperature, and each application is maintained for a programmed time and stopped when a rise in impedance is observed. This approach may have limitations, however. Imai et al. reported the formation of a "soft thrombus" with poor adherence to the ablation electrode, which was not associated with a rise in impedance during the delivery of RF energy [16]. This thrombus is probably due to denaturation and aggregation of plasma proteins, which may occur at blood temperatures between 50°C and 80°C.

Thus, a better strategy for titration of power delivery during RF ablation is very necessary, especially for left-side procedures, in which the consequences of thrombus formation can be serious.

Study Findings

The rationale for microbubble-guided power titration is based on the premise that adequate tissue heating cannot be reliably predicted simply by monitoring impedance and temperature. The formation of only a few scattered microbubbles is believed to be an early manifestation of overheating. When this occurs, energy has to be gradually decreased until the generation of microbubbles subsides. However, if this phenomenon cannot be controlled and progresses, tissue desiccation will result, creating the milieu favorable to coagulum formation and PV stenosis. Our data show a clear correlation between ineffective power titration owing to poor visualization of bubbles and charring. In addition, the presence of type-2 bubbles seem to be an early predictor of a rise in impedance.

When an optimal power titration protocol has been followed no charring has been observed in any of the patients, even when power has been increased up to 70 W or more.

These data confirm the previous experimental model of Kalman et al. [17], who report that showers of microbubbles (type-2 bubbles) precede the development of a shaggy echo-dense thickening on the catheter tip, which was suggestive of coagulum formation. Kongsgaard et al. also reported that in vitro, intramyocardial superheating resulting in steam formation and popping may occur even with a relatively low catheter-tip temperature; and in our experience too, bubbles are visible over a wide temperature range: 20–50°C [18]. Therefore, the use of ICE is crucially important for adequate power titration, and the goal of this energy delivery strategy is to prevent the generation of microbubbles, which usually precedes a rise in impedance and scar formation.

Another very important finding in this study was the ability of ICE to allow direct visualization of scar formation when it cannot be prevented. The need for an imaging technique that would make RF ablation procedures safer has already been indicated [19].

Demolin et al. reported that a soft thrombus could form at the site with the highest temperature, which in clinical situations may not be the ablation electrode itself but the surface of the heated tissue or another catheter, with no change in any of the RF monitoring parameters [20].

In 5 patients in group 6, char developed on the mapping or ablation catheter owing to ineffective monitoring of the energy delivery.

In all these patients ICE was able to show charring early after its formation. The catheter was immediately removed from the left side, avoiding a possible cerebrovascular accident.

Study Limitation

The current study is a retrospective, nonrandomized analysis of consecutive patients undergoing PV isolation procedure for AF ablation. On the other hand, owing to the small number of patients showing char formation and embolic events it may be difficult to design a prospective study.

Conclusions

More aggressive anticoagulation with heparin reduced the incidence of periprocedural embolic events. Platelet inhibition does not have an incremental beneficial effect. None of the anticoagulation protocols abolished scar formation.

Whether alternative energy sources, such as cryoablation or open cooling with saline, might reduce scarring and/or embolic events must be examined in further studies.

References

1. Haissaguerre M, Jais P, Shah DC et al (1998) Spontaneous initiation of atrial fibrillation by ectopic beats originating in the pulmonary veins. N Engl J Med 339:659–666
2. Chen SA, Hsieh MH, Tai CT et al (1999) Initiation of atrial fibrillation by ectopic beats originating from the pulmonary veins: electrophysiological characteristics, pharmacological responses, and effects of radiofrequency ablation. Circulation 100:1879–1886
3. Marrouche NF, Martin DO, Wazni O et al (2003) Phased array intracardiac echocardiography monitoring during pulmonary vein isolation in patients with atrial fibrillation: impact on outcome and complications. Circulation 107:2710–2716
4. Zhou L, Keane D, Reed G, Ruskin J (1999) Thromboembolic complications of cardiac radiofrequency catheter ablation: a review of the reported incidence, pathogenesis and current research directions (review). J Cardiovasc Electrophysiol 10:611–620
5. Khairy P, Chauvet P, Lehmann J et al (2003) Lower incidence of thrombus formation with cryoenergy versus radiofrequency catheter ablation. Circulation 107:2045–2050
6. Natale A, Pisano E, Shewchik J et al (2000) First human experience with pulmonary vein isolation using a through-the-balloon circumferential ultrasound ablation system for recurrent atrial fibrillation. Circulation 102:1879–1882
7. Marrouche NF, Dresing T, Cole C et al (2002) Circular mapping and ablation of the pulmonary vein for treatment of atrial fibrillation: impact of different catheter technologies. J Am Coll Cardiol 40:464–474
8. Epstein MR, Knapp LD, Martindill M et al (1996) Embolic complications associated with radiofrequency catheter ablation. Atakr Investigator Group. Am J Cardiol 77:655–658
9. Cannon BC, Kertesz NJ, Friedman RA, Fenrich AL (2001) Use of tissue plasminogen activator in a stroke after radiofrequency ablation of a left-sided accessory pathway. J Cardiovasc Electrophysiol 12:723–725

10. Chen SA, Chiang CE, Tai CT et al (1996) Complications of diagnostic electrophysiologic studies and radiofrequency catheter ablation in patients with tachyarrhythmias: an eight-year survey of 3,966 consecutive procedures in a tertiary referral center. Am J Cardiol 77:41–46
11. Hindricks G, for the Multicentre European Radiofrequency Survey (MERFS) investigators of the Working Group on Arrhythmias of the European Society of Cardiology (1993) The Multicentre European Radiofrequency Survey (MERFS): complications of radiofrequency catheter ablation of arrhythmias. Eur Heart J 14:1644–1653
12. Thakur RK, Klein GJ, Yee R, Zardini M (1994) Embolic complications after radiofrequency catheter ablation. Am J Cardiol 74:278–279
13. Hockstad E, Gornick CC (1994) Mildly symptomatic pulmonary emboli associated with electrophysiologic procedures. Indications for anticoagulant use. Chest 106:1908–1911
14. Hope EJ, Haigney MC, Calkins H, Resar JR (1995) Left main coronary thrombosis after radiofrequency ablation: successful treatment with percutaneous transluminal angioplasty. Am Heart J 129:1217–1219
15. Farah A, Khan F, Machado C (2000) Thrombus formation at the site of radiofrequency catheter ablation. Pacing Clin Electrophysiol 23:538–540
16. Imai S, Nakagawa H, Yamanashi W et al (1997) Soft thrombus formation around ablation electrode without impedance rise during radiofrequency ablation using temperature control (abstract). Pacing Clin Electrophysiol 20:1204
17. Kalman JM, Fitzpatrick AP, Olgin JE et al (1997) Biophysical characteristics of radiofrequency lesion formation in vivo: dynamics of catheter tip–tissue contact evaluated by intracardiac echocardiography. Am Heart J 133:8–18
18. Kongsgaard E, Steen T, Jensen O, Aass H, Amlie JP (1997) Temperature guided radiofrequency catheter ablation of myocardium: comparison of catheter tip and tissue temperatures in vitro. Pacing Clin Electrophysiol 20:1252–1260
19. Kantoch MJ, Frost GF, Robertson MA (1998) Use of transesophageal echocardiography in radiofrequency catheter ablation in children and adolescents. Can J Cardiol 14:519–523
20. Demolin JM, Eick OJ, Munch K et al (2002) Soft thrombus formation in radiofrequency catheter ablation. Pacing Clin Electrophysiol 25:1219–1222

Radiofrequency and Microwave Ablation of Atrial Fibrillation During Open Heart Surgery: What Are the Long-Term Results?

A. Venturini, V. Cutaia, A. Asta, D. Mangino, R. Moretti, E. Polesel, A. Terrini, C. Zussa

Introduction

Atrial fibrillation (AF) is the most common cardiac arrhythmia and is characterized by disorganized atrial activity. AF is fairly common in patients with mitral valve disease and a markedly dilated left atrium. These patients rarely return to sinus rhythm spontaneously even after a successful mitral valve operation [1].

James L. Cox designed the maze procedure to cure AF [2–4]. However, most surgeons are reluctant to expose their patients to the risks of the surgical maze because of the significantly increased aortic cross-clamping time and morbidity risk including postoperative bleeding and possible lifelong pacemaker dependence. To simplify the maze procedure, different types of energy are used at present to eliminate AF in patients undergoing heart surgery, in order to create ablation lines in the left and right atrium avoiding the "cut and sew" technique. Three methods–radiofrequency, microwave, and cryoablation–have been put into practice and applied in open heart surgery for curative treatment of AF [5, 6]. However, long-term results for a large number of patients are not yet available.

Materials and Methods

Patient Characteristics

Between November 1999 and January 2003, 115 patients with AF underwent operations at our institution for valve disease (Table 1). Radiofrequency energy was used for 66 ablations, while 49 patients underwent microwave ablation. The study population consisted of 28 men (24.3%) and 87 women (75.7%)

Cardiovascular Department, Umberto I Hospital, Mestre-Venice, Italy

whose age ranged from 45 to 79 years (mean: 61 years). Most of the patients (76%) were in NYHA class II. Concomitant cardiac pathologies were (Table 2): mitral regurgitation (29 patients, 25.2%), mitral stenosis (34 patients, 29.6%), and combined aortic and mitral valve disease (52 patients, 45.2%). Forty-four patients (38.2%) had associated tricuspid valve regurgitation. AF was permanent in 84 patients (73%) and paroxysmal in 31 (27%). The median duration of AF was 24 months (range: 6–324 months). Most of the patients were on oral digoxin before the operation.

Table. 1. Patient characteristics (n=115)

Gender distribution (M/F)	28/87
Mean age (range)	61 years (45–79 years)
Type of AF:	
Permanent	84 patients (73%)
Paroxysmal	31 patients (27%)
Median duration of AF (range)	24 months (6–324 months)

Table 2. Concomitant cardiac pathologies

	No. of patients (%)
Mitral valve regurgitation	29 (25.2)
Mitral valve stenosis	34 (29.6)
Mitral and aortic valve disease	52 (45.2)

Surgical Procedure

Microwave ablations were performed using the Flex catheter (AFX Inc.). An endocardial bilateral encircling isolation of the ostia of the pulmonary veins was created after the heart was arrested: we started from the right and then moved to the left side (Fig. 1). Ablation of the right pulmonary veins usually requires one or two applications, while three to four applications are necessary to complete the left side.

Radiofrequency ablations were performed using a temperature-controlled multipolar radiofrequency catheter (Thermaline, Boston Scientific, USA). An epicardial bilateral encircling isolation of the ostia of the pulmonary veins was created. The right epicardial lesion was performed without cardiopulmonary bypass (CPB), the left lesion with CPB and beating heart, the endocardial lesions with aortic cross-clamping and cardioplegic cardiac arrest.

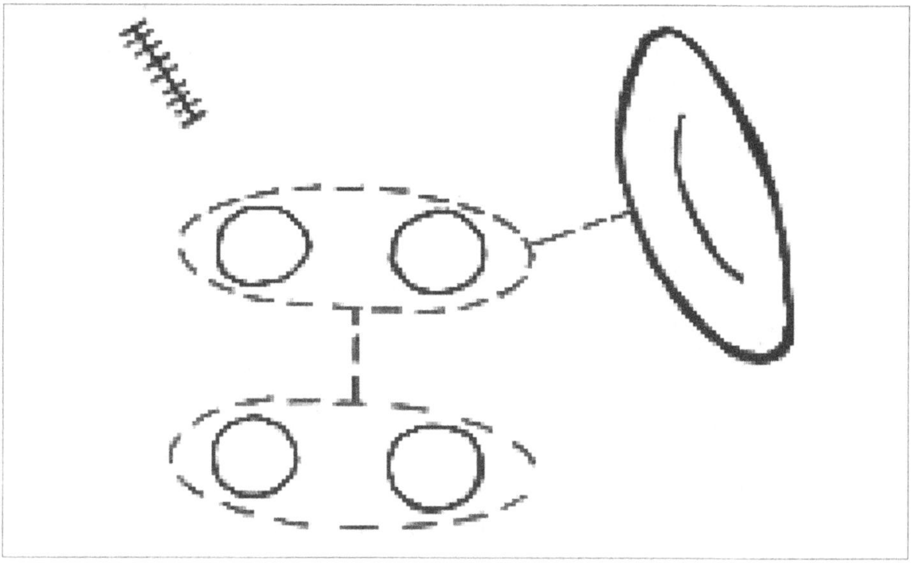

Fig. 1. Surgical procedure

Concomitant cardiac procedures (Table 3) were mitral valve repair using Gore-Tex neochordae implantation and autologous pericardium annuloplasty (29 patients, 25.2%), mitral valve replacement (34 patients, 29.6%), and mitral and aortic valve replacement (52 patients, 45.2%). Tricuspid valve repair according to de Vega was performed in 44 patients (38.2%).

Table 3. Associated cardiac procedures

	No. of patients (%)
Mitral valve repair	29 (25.2)
Mitral valve replacement	34 (29.6)
Mitral and aortic valve replacement	52 (45.2)
Tricuspid valve repair	44 (38.2)

Follow-Up

Early postoperative care was similar to that for routine heart surgery. Amiodarone infusion (900 mg in 24 h) was started in the intensive care unit in most of the patients. Postoperative early atrial arrhythmias were treated with intravenous amiodarone (300 mg in 30 min plus 900 mg in 24 h), sometimes combined with low-dose (25 mg) oral atenolol. At discharge the majority of patients (n=105; 91.3%) were on oral amiodarone therapy. DC cardioversion, if necessary, was planned 1 month after operation and performed in 47 patients (40.9%). Patients were seen in the outpatient clinic 3 and 12 months after surgery. ECG and Doppler echocardiography were performed 2 and 12 months after surgery.

Results

There were no in-hospital deaths. No patients required re-exploration for bleeding. Two patients (1.7%) underwent permanent pacemaker insertion: both of them had a severely calcified mitral valve annulus.

Mean follow-up was 19.8 months (range: 4–43 months). At discharge 49 patients (42.6 %) were in AF: all of them were on oral amiodarone, and DC cardioversion (DCS) was performed 1 month after operation in 47 patients. Fifteen patients in the AF group did not need a DCS because they were found to be in sinus rhythm at the ECG performed before the scheduled electric cardioversion. Among the 66 patients discharged in sinus rhythm, 13 required a DCS because of AF recurrence.

One patient with dilated cardiomyopathy died suddenly 8 months after operation.

At final follow-up, presence of stable sinus rhythm was found in 86 patients (74.8%; Table 4).

Table 4. Presence of sinus rhythm

At discharge	66 patients (57.4%)
At final follow-up	86 patients (74.8%)

Doppler echocardiography (Hewlett Packard, Sonos 5500) was performed in all patients at follow-up; a thrombus in the left atrial appendage was found in one patient only. The atrial filling fraction (AFF, percentage of the diastolic ventricular filling given by the atrial contraction: Vti_a/Vti_a+Vti_e) was measured in 34 patients in sinus rhythm at follow-up. Left atrial function impairment was severe (AFF<20%) in 5 patients (14.7%) and mild to moderate (AFF=20%–29%) in 9 patients (26.5%). Left atrial transport function was normal (AFF>30%) in 20 patients (58.8%).

Discussion

Various alternative methods of creating lesions have been discussed: ultrasound, laser, radiofrequency, microwave, and cryoablation. Three methods (radiofrequency, microwave, and cryoablation) have been put into practice and applied in open heart surgery for curative treatment of AF. An important point for discussion is: where should we apply the energy? Do we need to follow design of the Cox maze procedure?

The rationale of the surgical maze procedure is the following: AF is the consequence of multiple circling wavelets of activity. To perpetuate the fibrillatory activity, it is now established that a critical area of atrial musculature must remain in electrical continuity. If the atrial walls can be compartmented so that the area of each unit thus isolated is insufficient to support the circling wavelets, fibrillation ceases. "Mazes" of this kind can be created by constructing linear lesions by means of catheter ablation, and many authors have designed their own modified maze procedure–it is quite difficult to find two authors who use the same design. This has led to some degree of confusion caused by incomplete knowledge of the pathophysiology of AF. The lesions that are now most commonly used on the left side include:

- Separate encircling of the left and right pulmonary veins
- A line connecting the two encirclings that should be made more cranially or caudally according to different opinions
- Excision of the left atrial appendage
- A line connecting the left pulmonary island with the left atrial appendage
- A line connecting the left pulmonary veins with the mitral valve annulus
- A line between the pulmonary vein islands
- A line going 1 cm inside the ostia of the pulmonary vein.

The most commonly used right atrial lesions include:

- A line connecting the superior and inferior vena cava
- Excision of the right atrial appendage
- A line connecting the tricuspid valve annulus to the right atrial appendage
- A line connecting the tricuspid valve annulus to the caudal end of the posterior longitudinal atriotomy at the AV groove.

Recently Dr. Michel Haïssaguerre [7] discovered that the pulmonary veins are an important source (up to 94%) of ectopic beats initiating frequent paroxysms of AF. He demonstrated that these foci respond to treatment with radiofrequency ablation. In order to simplify the maze procedure and to try to understand a little bit about AF we decided, following Dr. Haïssaguerre's experience, to perform a separate encircling of the left and right pulmonary veins only. Our high percentage of sinus rhythm at final follow-up (74.8%) is similar to what has been found by the other authors previously mentioned who use different ablation lines. Although a larger number of patients in the long run has to be awaited for more precise conclusions, we think that there is no need for the use of additional lines. Moreover, our experience, which includes many patients with permanent AF, shows how the pulmonary veins play a key role not only in paroxysmal but also in permanent AF.

Another important point for discussion is how left atrial function changes after microwave ablation. Dr. Itoh and colleagues [8] demonstrated that after the surgical maze procedure the AFF was significantly reduced (17.6±8.8% versus 36.8±6.4% in the control group). Another study from St Louis [9] showed similar findings indicating a moderate to severe reduction in the left atrial contribution to ventricular filling. We found that in our patients left atrial activity was normal in 20 patients (58.8%). Only 5 patients (14.7%) showed severe impairment of the left atrial function (AFF<20%).

It is not widely agreed whether there is a cut-off level of the left atrial function below which we should continue oral anticoagulation. Further investigations are required to draw precise conclusions.

References

1. Flugelman MY, Hasin Y, Katnelson N et al (1984) Restoration and maintenance of sinus rhythm after mitral valve surgery for mitral stenosis. Am J Cardiol 54:617–619
2. Cox JL, Schuessler RB, D'Agostino Jr HJ et al (1991) The surgical treatment of atrial fibrillation. (III) Development of a definitive surgical procedure. J Thorac Cardiovasc Surg 101:569–583
3. Cox JL, Boineau JP, Schuessler RB, Kater KM, Lappas DG (1993) Five year experience with the Maze procedure for atrial fibrillation. Ann Thorac Surg 56:814–824
4. Cox JL, Jaquiss RDB, Schuessler RB, Boineau JP (1995) Modification of the Maze procedure for atrial flutter and atrial fibrillation. II. Surgical technique of the Maze III procedure. J Thorac Cardiovasc Surg 110:485–495
5. Chen MC, Guo GB, Chang JP et al (1998) Radiofrequency and cryoablation of atrial fibrillation in patients undergoing valvular operations. Ann Thorac Surg 65:1666–1672
6. Knaut M, Spitzer FG, Karolyi L et al (1999) Intraoperative microwave ablation for curative treatment of atrial fibrillation in open heart surgry: the MICRO-STAF and MICRO-PASS trial. Thorac Cardiovasc Surg 47(Suppl):379–384
7. Haïssaguerre M, Jais P, Shah DC et al (1998) Spontaneous initiation of atrial fibrillation by ectopic beats originating in the pulmonary veins. N Engl J Med 339:659-666
8. Itoh T, Okamoto H, Nimi T et al (1995) Left atrial function after Cox's Maze operation concomitant with mitral valve operation. Ann Thorac Surg 60:354–360
9. Feinberg MS, Waggoner AD, Kater KM et al (1994) Restoration of atrial function after the Maze procedure for patients with atrial fibrillation. Circulation 90: II-285–II-292

Minimally Invasive Surgical Approach to Radiofrequency Ablation of Atrial Fibrillation: Is the Game Worth the Candle?

C. Piorkowski, G. Hindricks, H. Kottkamp

Introduction

Atrial fibrillation (AF) is an arrhythmia that has been shown to be associated with an elevated mortality rate and with an indipendent excess risk of stroke [1]. Long-term anticoagulation and regulation of the heart rate can only partly solve the problem, owing to the risks of major bleeding [2]. In addition, many patients suffer greatly from the symptoms of AF.

Several pathophysiological mechanisms for the initiation and maintenance of AF have been suggested. In 1914 Garrey conceptualized AF as ring-like circuits of electrical activation given a critical mass of tissue [3]. During the 1920s Sir Thomas Lewis proposed the idea that one single stable re-entrant circuit was responsible for the occurrence of AF [4]. In contrast, in 1959 Moe and Abildskov presented a computer model in which AF was sustained by functional re-entrant wavelets circulating around refractory tissue rather than anatomical obstacles [5]. This hypothesis received far-reaching support from the experimental work published by Allessie during the 1970s [6]. In recent years new pathophysiological details of AF have been revealed. On one hand, the relevance of pulmonary vein triggers for the initiation of AF was described by Haissaguerre et al. [7]. On the other, Jalife et al. and other groups experimentally described a source, a stable mother re-entry, regularly generating electrical activity and in this way maintaining AF [8, 9]. Further experimental work indicated that this arrhythmogenic substrate was located around the pulmonary veins (PV) [9].

According to a particular pathophysiological approach is favored, different ablation strategies for the curative treatment of AF can be attempted. Both surgical procedures and catheter ablation techniques have been described for this purpose. Each of them provides a certain rate of success, but also carries a specific risk of typical complications.

Heart Center, Department of Electrophysiology, University of Leipzig, Germany

Surgical Procedures for the Treatment of AF

Cox et al. were the first to design a surgical concept for the curative treatment of AF, the Maze procedure, which is a cut-and-suture technique fragmenting both atria [10]. Retrospectively, and seen from the pathophysiological point of view, the Maze lesions dealt with several features of AF. The development of functional re-entrant circuits was prevented; no stable macro-reentrant circuit could form; the PV area was isolated and PV triggers eliminated; and, finally, the critical atrial tissue mass was reduced. The results in terms of restoration and maintenance of SR were excellent in patients with lone AF and in those with AF and additional mitral valve surgery [10, 11]. Nevertheless, the procedure was too complex, technically demanding, and time consuming for it ever to be widely used.

Later on the Maze concept was modified, for several reasons. Kosakai et al. used extensive cryoablation and eliminated the right atrial longitudinal incision connecting the venae cavae to shorten the procedure time. With 169 patients, this procedure covered the largest cohort among all Maze modifications, but neither the outcome nor the operating time was shown to be superior [12, 13]. Sueda et al. and Lee et al. later introduced mainly left-atrial (LA) procedures with isolation of the PV, excision of the left atrial appendage (LAA), and additional linear lesions using cryoenergy together with cut-and-suture techniques [14, 15]. To preserve the secretion of atrial natriuretic peptide and to improve the atrial transport function, Isobe et al. suggested the original Maze III without the amputation of both atrial appendages [16]. However, comparison of the outcome between Cox's Maze procedure and the Maze modifications remains difficult because of different patient characteristics. The patients from the Japanese groups tended to be more seriously ill, owing to advanced cardiac valvular disease. Furthermore, among the largest American groups only 14% of the patients were suffering from rheumatic valvular disease, whereas in the Japanese groups the corresponding figure was well above 75% [12].

Targeting the role of the PV triggers for the initiation of AF, Sueda et al. described an intraoperative PV isolation procedure using cut-and-suture techniques and cryoablation in combination [17].

In 1997 Patwardhan et al. tried to induce the lines of the original Maze III concept using a radiofrequency energy source [18]. Melo et al. performed intraoperative radiofrequency PV isolation in 1999 [19]. Pasic et al. added two linear lesions at the roof of the left atrium and from the left PV to the mitral annulus in 2001 [20]. Small patient numbers and a short follow-up time do not allow a very thorough assessment of the value of radiofrequency energy or of the individual lesion concepts for AF ablation in these three studies (Fig. 1).

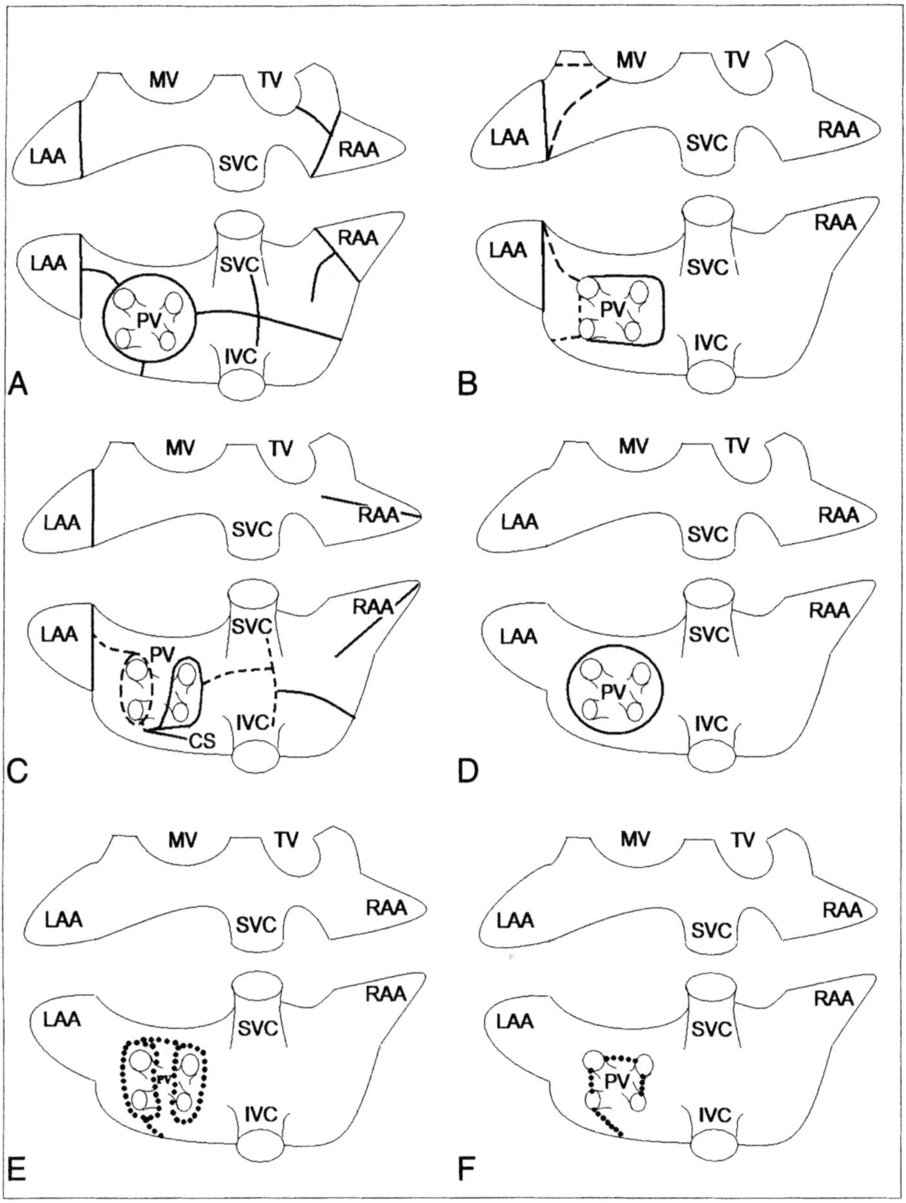

Fig. 1 A-F. Schematic showing different surgical concepts for the treatment of AF. *Continuous lines* represent cut-and-suture, *dashed lines* represent cryolesions, and *dotted lines* illustrate use of RF energy. **A** Cox's MAZE III procedure. **B** Sueda's modification with sole LA ablations. **C** Lee's modified MAZE using cryolesions and surgical incisions. **D** Surgical PV isolation suggested by Melo, who later performed the same procedure using RF energy. **E** RF PV Isolation and additional linear lesions suggested by Pasic et al. **F** The IRAAF concept by Mohr, Hindricks and Kottkamp. *LAA*, left atrial appendage; *RAA*, right atrial appendage; *SVC*, superior vena cava; *IVC*, inferior vena cava; *PV*, pulmonary veins; *CS*, coronary sinus; *MV*, mitral valve; *TV*, tricuspid valve

Intraoperative Radiofrequency Ablation of AF Using Linear Lesions (IRAAF)

With knowledge of stable re-entrant circuits around the PV orifices maintaining AF, a new curative ablation concept was published in 1998 [21]. Left-atrial linear lesions induced by radiofrequency (RF) energy were utilized to interrupt those re-entrant circuits. The lesions extended from the mitral annulus to the left lower, left upper, right upper, and right lower PV. LAA was intentionally not excised, in order to prevent a mass reduction of LA and to maintain the transport function and the secretion of natriuretic peptide. The right atrium was not treated at all. The ablation was done intraoperatively under direct vision, while the heart was not beating. Later, with minimally invasive surgical techniques, a large proportion of the patients included in the study, and all those suffering from lone AF were operated through a right lateral minithoracotomy [22, 23].

In summary 387 patients were treated between 1998 and 2001, 129 of whom were suffering from lone AF, 163 underwent the ablation together with a mitral valve operation and 95 underwent other additional cardiac surgical procedures. The follow-up is very close, almost all these patients are still being seen regularly. Regarding the 129 patients with lone AF, almost two-thirds have now completed the 2-year follow-up until now. The results in terms of restoration and maintenance of SR are excellent for the patients with paroxysmal and permanent AF. About 95% of the patients have had a continuously stable SR. The percentage of patients taking antiarrhythmic drugs for the maintenance of their SR is steadily declining. Among the patients with additional cardiac surgery the outcome was also satisfactory [22, 23] (Fig. 2).

As a major complication, 1 case of a perforation of the esophagus occurred within days after the operation. A thermal injury to the esophagus was considered a possible mechanism. Therefore, the transesophageal echoprobe was withdrawn during the ablation, and for several days after the ablation no transesophageal echo was done. Secondly, isolating material was placed between the LA and the esophagus during the ablation. Despite these precautions, the complication recurred. In summary, about 1% of the patients (4 out of 387) suffered a perforation. That risk was regarded as too high, and this specific variant of the procedure was discontinued [22, 23].

Currently cryoenergy is being investigated in respect of safety and efficacy for the intraoperative left atrial linear ablation. No esophageal perforations have been reported with this energy source so far.

Discussion

AF is an arrhythmia that is not adequately treated by conventional regimens in some patients. Therefore curative ablation strategies have been developed. The surgical concepts range from major cardiac operations such as the Maze procedure, through attempted trigger elimination by PV isolation, to the modifica-

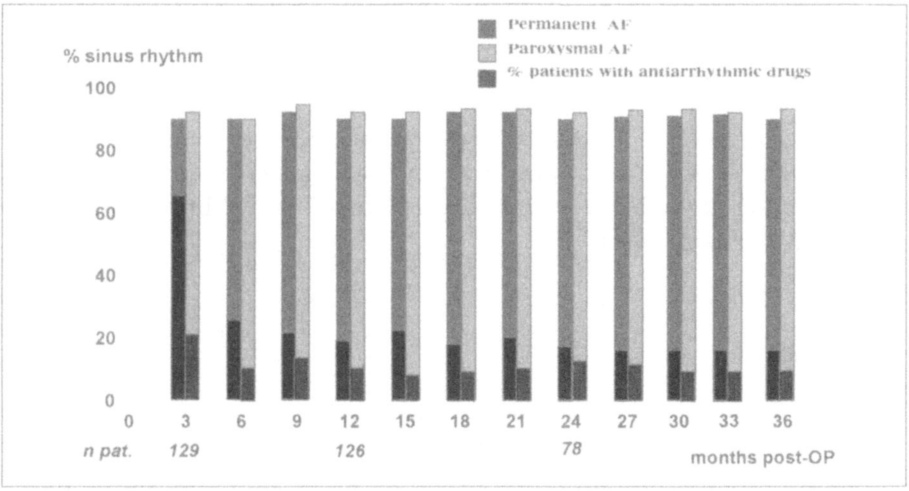

Fig. 2. Diagram illustrating the results of the IRAAF procedure for patients with lone AF. The percentage of patients in sinus rhythm is shown along the vertical axis, on the longitudinal axis the month of follow-up is also shown. In summary, 129 patients with lone AF underwent the ablation. Until now the 2-year follow-up has been completed by 78 of them. The results are shown in two separate bars, for patients with lone paroxysmal AF and with lone permanent AF. The *dark stained lower area* of each bar represents the percentage of patients taking antiarrhythmic drugs for the maintenance of their SR

tion of the AF substrate suggested by IRAAF. On the other hand, percutaneous catheter ablation techniques have been introduced. In this field most experience has been gained with trigger elimination by PV isolation.

The therapeutic value of a therapy depends on the need for the treatment, the success rate, the risk of complications, and the availability of alternative concepts. None of the procedures described above can be seen as an established standard therapy. The early surgical procedures were major operations, were performed only in small patient cohorts, and, despite the original Maze, were never used to treat patients with lone AF. The percutaneous concepts directed at the elimination of PV triggers with catheter techniques have not shown convincing success rates either. Furthermore, complications that are severe and currently not adequately treatable, such as PV stenosis, have occurred in a substantial percentage of patients [24]. With a reported high number of triggers found outside the PVs the pathophysiological basis of the whole concept could fail [25].

This is the background against which the IRAAF study has to be judged. In one of the largest patient cohorts treated for AF, with a substantial number of patients with lone AF, the results in terms of the restoration of SR were excellent. A simple concept of a few linear lesions within LA has proved to be highly effective in the curative ablation of paroxysmal and permanent AF. The procedure carries a risk of esophageal perforation of about 1%. A minimally invasive approach through a right lateral minithoracotomy has made the procedure more feasible and also more acceptable for patients with lone AF. The use of a heart-lung pump was still necessary. However, the direct vision of the endocardium gives an enormous benefit regard of the continuity of the lesions, compared to the currently available percutaneous catheter approaches.

Overall, the IRAAF study provides impressive support for the pathophysiological concept of stable re-entrant circuits around the PV bring the substrate for the maintenance of AF.

References

1. Laupacis A, Cuddy TE (1996) Prognosis of individuals with atrial fibrillation. Can J Cardiol 12 [Suppl A]:14 A -16 A
2. Taylor FC, Cohen H, Ebrahim S (2001) Systematic review of long term anticoagulation or antiplatelet treatment in patients with non-rheumatic atrial fibrillation. BMJ 322:321-326
3. Waldo AL, Van Wagoner DR (2001) Atrial fibrillation. In: Spooner PM, Rosen MR (eds) Foundations of cardiac arrhythmias. Marcel Dekker, New York, pp 479-512
4. Lewis T (1925) The mechanism and graphical registration of the heart beat, 3rd edn. Shaw and Sons, London, pp 340-342
5. Moe GK, Abildskov JA (1959) Atrial fibrillation as a self-sustained arrhytmia independent of focal discharge. Am Heart J 58:59-70
6. Allessie MA, Lammers WJEP, Bonke FIM et al (1985) Experimental evaluation of Moe's multiple wavelet hypothesis of atrial fibrillation. In: Zipes DP, Jalife J (eds) Cardiac electrophysiology and arrhythmias. Grune & Stratton, Orlando, pp 265–267
7. Haissaguerre M, Jais P, Shah DC et al (1998) Spontaneous initiation of atrial fibrillation by ectopic beats originating in the pulmonary veins. N Engl J Med 339:659-666
8. Skane AC, Mandapati R, Berenfeld O et al (1998) Spatiotemporal periodicity during atrial fibrillation in the isolated sheep heart. Circulation 98:1236-1248
9. Kumagai K, Khrestian C, Waldo AL (1997) Simultaneous multisite mapping studies during induced atrial fibrillation in the sterile pericarditis model. Circulation 95:511-521
10. Cox JL, Schuessler RB, D'Agostino HJ Jr et al (1991) The surgical treatment of atrial fibrillation. III Development of a definite surgical procedure. J Thorac Cardiovasc Surg 101:569-583
11. Isobe F, Kawashima Y (1998) The outcome and indications of the Cox Maze III procedure for chronic atrial fibrillation with mitral valve disease. J Thorac Cardiovasc Surg 116:220-227
12. Arcidi JM, Millar RC (1999) Evolution of the MAZE III procedure: are modifications necessary? Thorac Cardiovasc Surg 47 [Suppl]:362-364
13. Kobayashi J, Kosakai Y, Nakano K et al (1998) Improved success rate of the maze procedure in mitral valve disease by new criteria for patients' selection. Eur J Cardiothorac Surg 13:247-252
14. Sueda T, Nagata H, Shikata H et al (1996) Simple left atrial procedure for chronic atrial fibrillation in patients with isolated mitral valve disease. Ann Thorac Surg 62:1796-1800
15. Lee JW, Choo SJ, Kim KI et al (2001) Atrial fibrillation surgery simplified with cryoablation to improve left atrial function. Ann Thorac Surg 72:1479-1483

16. Isobe F, Kumano H, Ishikawa T et al (2001) A new procedure for chronic atrial fibrillation: bilateral appendage-preserving MAZE procedure. Ann Thorac Surg 72:1473-1478
17. Sueda T, Imai K, Ishii O et al (2001) Efficacy of pulmonary vein isolation for the elimination of chronic atrial fibrillation in cardiac valvular surgery. Ann Thorac Surg 71:1189-1193
18. Patwardhan AM, Dave HH, Tumhane AA et al (1997) Intraoperative radiofrequency microbipolar coagulation to replace incisions of maze III procedure for correcting atrial fibrillation in patients with rheumatic valvular disease. Eur J Cardiothorac Surg 12:627-633
19. Melo J, Adragao PR, Neves J et al (1999) Electrosurgical treatment of atrial fibrillation with a new intraoperative radiofrequency ablation catheter. Thorac Cardiovasc Surg 47:370-372
20. Pasic M, Bergs P, Müller P et al (2001) Intraoperative radiofrequency maze ablation for atrial fibrillation: the Berlin modification. Ann Thorac Surg 72:1484-1491
21. Kottkamp H, Hindricks G, Hammel D et al (1999) Intraoperative radiofrequency ablation of chronic atrial fibrillation: A left atrial curative approach by elimination of anatomic "anchor" reentrant circuits. J Cardiovasc Electrophysiol 10:772-80
22. Kottkamp H, Hindricks G, Autschbach R et al (2002) Specific linear left atrial lesions in atrial fibrillation: intraoperative radiofrequency ablation using minimally invasive surgical techniques. J Am Coll Cardiol 40:475-480
23. Mohr FW, Fabricius AM, Falk V et al [2002] Curative treatment of atrial fibrillation with intraoperative radiofrequency ablation: short-term and midterm results. J Thorac Cardiovasc Surg 123:919-927
24. Yu WC, Hsu TL, Tai CT et al (2001) Acquired pulmonary vein stenosis after radiofrequency ablation of paroxysmal atrial fibrillation. J Cardiovasc Electrophysiol 12:887-892
25. Schmitt C, Ndrepepa G, Weber S et al (2002) Biatrial multisite mapping of atrial premature complexes triggering onset of atrial fibrillation. Am J Cardiol 89:1381-1387

ATRIAL FIBRILLATION: PREVENTION OF THROMBOEMBOLIC COMPLICATIONS

What Is the Best Practical Scheme for Initiating Oral Anticoagulant Treatment in Outpatients with Atrial Fibrillation?

R. Cazzin, P. Serra, C. Fusilli

Atrial Fibrillation and Thromboembolism

Patients with atrial fibrillation (AF) have an approximately four-fold increased risk of stroke and systemic embolism [1]. Generally thrombus forms in the left atrial appendage because of the relative inactivity of the atria during AF [2]. The risk of stroke exists in all patients with AF, but the incidence of stroke is related to coexistent cardiovascular disease, hypertension, diabetes, or previous stroke [3, 4]. Advancing age is associated with increased stroke risk, probably due to the effect of left atrium enlargement and left ventricular diastolic dysfunction, frequently observed in elderly patients [5, 6]. Nearly half of AF-associated strokes occur in patients older than 75 years.

Antithrombotic strategy for prevention of stroke and systemic embolism is based on the results of large randomized trials which showed that adjusted-dose oral anticoagulation with warfarin is highly efficacious in preventing stroke, with a risk reduction of 68% versus placebo [7]. This reduction is similar for both primary and secondary prevention.

Antithrombotic Therapy

Currently warfarin is commonly used to decrease risk of systemic arterial thromboembolism. It is a difficult drug to use because of its narrow therapeutic index, but it is still the mainstay of oral anticoagulant treatment. Aspirin offers only a modest protection against stroke for patients with AF.

The target intensity of anticoagulation involves a balance between prevention of thromboembolism and avoidance of hemorrhagic complications. The commonly accepted therapeutic international normalized ratio (INR) should be between 2.0 and 3.0 for patients with nonrheumatic AF. The INR range of

Department of Cardiology, Hospital of Portogruaro, Portogruaro, Venice, Italy

1.6–2.5, proposed to reduce risk of hemorrhage in patients aged over 75 years, appears to be associated with a lower efficacy than that achieved with higher-intensity anticoagulation [8].

Ischemic strokes occurring during anticoagulant therapy would be concomitant with discontinuation of warfarin or inadequate INR (<2.0 IU).

Prevention Strategies

When starting anticoagulation therapy it is important to review the risks and benefits with the patient and consider the medical, social, dietary and medication history, the patient's level of education, and his or her understanding and likely adherence to the therapy [9].

In outpatients warfarin should be started at a dose of 4–5 mg per day. Randomized trials [10, 11] have shown that patients are more likely to have an INR in the therapeutic range 3–5 days after starting warfarin with a 5-mg dose than with a 10-mg dose, because 10 mg more frequently results in a supertherapeutic INR [12]. A lower starting dose and gradually raising the INR are recommended in the guidelines for antithrombotic therapy in patients with AF, especially the elderly or those with low body weight, congestive heart failure, or liver disease [13].

The INR response after initiation of warfarin treatment is dependent on the half-lives of vitamin K coagulation factors. The initial increase in the INR is primarily a response to decreased levels of circulating factor VII and IX, factors with a shorter half-life. The first consequence will be an *anticoagulant effect* [14]. The real *antithrombotic effect* may be achieved in up to 5 days, depending on the clearance of circulating prothrombin (elimination half-life of about 60 h). Therefore, higher starting doses of warfarin (above 5 mg) may lead to a rapid increase in the INR that should not necessarily be considered as a good response, since this is simply a phase of anticoagulant effect. The goal should be to gradually increase the INR to achieve the antithrombotic effect. In this way the risk of inducing a paradoxical hypercoagulable state should be less [15].

The College of American Pathologists recommends the INR be checked at least four times during the 1st week of therapy and then less frequently, depending on the stability of the INR [16]. Recently, an easy scheme has been published for rapid prediction of the warfarin maintenance dose in outpatients after few days of 5 mg/day of warfarin administration [17].

In older age, excess of anticoagulation is associated with increased bleeding complications [12]. Apart from this, elderly people have a very high prevalence in the population of patients with AF and are those appearing to benefit particularly from the anticoagulant therapy.

Because of aging in the general population and the results of a recent clinical trial [18] indicating that rhythm control is no better than rate control for preventing morbidity and mortality in many patients with AF, the impact of patients undergoing anticoagulation is likely to became relevant in the near future.

Conclusions

Many patients with AF will probably start anticoagulant treatment as outpatients, and the recent recommendations state that patients should start treatment at a dosage near to the maintenance dosage [19]. With this simple prescription scheme and brief monitoring of INR, physicians working in outpatient departments can improve their own performance and their patients' compliance. New antithrombotic agents are also being developed. Some direct thrombin inhibitors with no need for anticoagulation monitoring and fewer drug interactions are currently being compared with warfarin. If trials show similar efficacy and safety in preventing thromboembolism in patients with AF, these drugs may ultimately start to replace warfarin because of their advantages.

References

1. Miller VT, Rothrock JF, Pearce LA et al (1993) Ischemic stroke in patients with atrial fibrillation: effect of aspirin acccording to stroke mechanism. Stroke prevention in Atrial Fibrillation Investigators. Neurology 43:32–36
2 Manning WJ, Leeman DE, Gotch PJ et al (1989) Pulsed Doppler evaluation of atrial mechanical function after electrical cardioversion of atrial fibrillation. J Am Coll Cardiol 13:617–623
3. Anonymous (1992) Predictors of thromboembolism in atrial fibrillation: I. Clinical features of patients at risk. The Stroke Prevention in Atrial Fibrillation Investigators. Ann Intern Med 116:1–5
4. Anonymous (1992) Predictors of thromboembolism in atrial fibrillation: II. Clinical features of patients at risk. The Stroke Prevention in Atrial Fibrillation Investigators. Ann Intern Med 116:6–12
5. Dittrich HC, Pearce LA, Asinger LW et al (1999) Left atrial diameter in nonvalvular atrial fibrillation: an echocardiographic study. Stroke Prevention in Atrial Fibrillation Investigators. Am Heart J 137:494–499
6. Dreslinski GR, Frohlich ED, Dunn FG et al (1981) Echocardiographic diastolic ventricular abnormality in hypertensive heart disease: atrial emptying index. Am J Cardiol 47:1087–1090
7. Hart RG, Benavente O, McBride R, Pearce LA (1999) Antithrombotic therapy to prevent stroke in patients with atrial fibrillation: a meta-analysis. Ann Intern Med 131:492–501
8. Hylck EM, Skates SJ, Sheehan MA, Singer DE (1996) An analysis of the lowest effective intensity of prophylactic anticoagulation for patients with nonrheumatic atrial fibrillation. N Engl J Med 335:540–546

9. Brandjes DP, Hejjboer H, Buller HR et al (1992) Acenocoumarol and heparin compared with acenocoumarol alone in the initial treatment of proximal vein thrombosis. N Engl J Med 327:1485–1489
10. Harrison L, Johnston M, Massicotte MP et al (1997) Comparison of 5 mg and 10 mg loading doses in initiation of warfarin therapy. Ann Intern Med 126:133–136
11. Crowter MA, Ginsberg JB, Kearon C et al (1999) A randomized trial comparing 5 mg and 10 mg warfarin loading doses. Ann Intern Med 159:46–48
12. Palareti G, Coccheri S, Poggi M et al (1996) Bleeding complications of oral anticoagulant treatment: an inception-cohort, prospective collaboratory study (ISCOAT). Lancet 348:423–428
13. Fuster V, Ryden LE, Asinger RW et al (2001) ACC/AHA/ESC Guidelines for the management of patients with atrial fibrillation: executive summary. Circulation 104:2118–2150
14. Ansell J, Hirsh J, Dalen J et al (2001) Managing oral anticoagulant therapy. Chest 119:225–285
15. Hirsh J, Dalen JE, Anderson DR et al (2001) A simple scheme to initiate oral anticoagulant treatment in outpatients with nonrheumatic atrial fibrillation. Am J Cardiol 88:1214–1216
16 Fairweather RB, Ansell J, Van den Besselaar AM et al (1998) College of American Pathologists Conference XXXI on laboratory monitoring of anticoagulant therapy. Laboratory monitoring of oral anticoagulant therapy. Arch Pathol Lab Med 122:768–781
17. Pengo V, Biasiolo A, Pegoraro C (2001) A simple scheme to initiate oral anticoagulant treatment in outpatients with nonrheumatic atrial fibrillation. Am J Cardiol 88:1214-1216
18. Wyse DG, Waldo AL, DiMarco JP et al for the Atrial Fibrillation Follow-up Investigation of Rhythm Management (AFFIRM) Investigators (2002) A comparison of the rate control and rhythm control in patients with atrial fibrillation. N Engl J Med 347:1825–1833
19. Cooper MW, Hendra TJ (1998) Prospective evaluation of a modified Fennerty regimen for anticoagulating elderly people. Age Ageing 27:655–656

How Intense Should Anticoagulation Be at the Time of Cardioversion to Reduce the Risk of Thromboembolism?

N. Baldi, V.A. Russo, V. Morrone, L. Di Gregorio, L. Liconso, G. Polimeni

Background

For patients undergoing cardioversion of atrial fibrillation (AF) or atrial flutter (AFl) the risk of thromboembolism ranged from 1.6% up to 7% in case-control series [1–4]. In uncontrolled and nonrandomized studies, anticoagulation decreases the risk of an embolic event after cardioversion to less than 1.6% [3–5].

The conventional strategy for anticoagulation in patients with AF longer than 2 days requires that warfarin therapy (prothrombin time to an INR of 2.0–3.0) should be given for 3 weeks before elective cardioversion and be continued, after normal sinus rhythm has been restored, for at least 4 weeks [6]. This approach must be adopted both for electrical and for pharmacological cardioversion. On the other hand, the introduction of transesophageal echocardiography into clinical practice has allowed the detection of thrombi in the left appendage with a high degree of accuracy [7, 8]. This technique has also been proposed as a safe means of expediting cardioversion with short-term anticoagulant therapy. The results of a randomized multicenter prospective study comparing the two techniques of anticoagulation have recently been published [9].

In this chapter we consider four points concerning anticoagulant treatment before cardioversion:

1. What is the likeliest mechanism of action of warfarin?
2. How intense should anticoagulation be at the time of cardioversion to reduce the risk of thromboembolism?
3. What is the role of heparin in the prevention of thromboembolism?
4. What approach should be adopted in cardioversion of AFl?

Department of Cardiology, S. Annunziata Hospital, Taranto, Italy

Mechanism of Action of Warfarin

Warfarin, a coumarin derivative, produces an anticoagulant effect by interfering with the cyclic interconversion of vitamin K and its 2,3 epoxide. The antithrombotic effect of warfarin has been conventionally attributed to its anticoagulant effect, which in turn is mediated by the reduction of four vitamin K-dependent coagulation factors. More recent evidence, however, suggests that the anticoagulant and the antithrombotic effect can be dissociated, and that the reduction of prothrombin and possibly factor X is more important than the reduction of factors VII and IX for the antithrombotic effect [10]. In the prophylaxis of thromboembolism the action of warfarin consists not only in the organization and in the adhesion of the thrombus to the atrial wall [11], but also in the resolution of thrombi [12].

The mechanism of thromboembolism is debated. According to common opinion, an embolism is caused by detachment of a "preformed" thrombus during the phase of passage from AF to the sinus rhythm due to a renewed atrial contraction. This hypothesis should imply that the exclusion of atrial thrombus by transesophageal echocardiography could allow cardioversion without anticoagulation. Actually, just using transesophageal echocardiography, it was possible to verify that the exclusion of thrombus does not avoid the risk of thromboembolism when the anticoagulation therapy is omitted [13].

How Intense Should Anticoagulation Be at the Time of Cardioversion?

In the recent ACC/AHA/ESC Guidelines for the management of patients with AF [14], in the "Recommendations for antithrombotic therapy to prevent ischemic stroke and systemic embolism in patients with AF undergoing cardioversion," in class I indications the prescription is to anticoagulate patients with AF lasting more than 48 h or of unknown duration for at least 3–4 weeks before and after cardioversion (INR 2–3; level of evidence: B). The suitability of keeping the INR between 2 and 3 is determined by the values recommended in the prophylaxis of thromboembolism in chronic AF. Is this a correct extrapolation?

Recently Gallagher et al. [15] have opposed this argument. Briefly, they have reviewed the case records of 1950 patients who underwent 2639 attempts at DC cardioversion. Cardioversion was preceded by warfarin therapy for at least 3 weeks in 1932 instances. No embolic complications occurred in 779 attempts performed with an INR of at least 2.5 (95% confidence limits 0%–0.48%), compared with 7/754 (0.9%) in those with an INR below 2.5 and 2/339 (0.5%) in those in which INR was not recorded.

From the analysis of data presented by these authors it is possible to extrapolate the following points: in 2 of 9 patients with embolism the INR was unknown; 3 of the remaining 7 patients at the time of cardioversion had an INR between 1.4 and 1.7–and the risk of embolism with an INR below 2 is widely known [16]-1 had an INR of 2, and 3 had an INR of 2.2. Moreover, at the time of embolic complication (the embolic events occurred between 6 h and 22 days after cardioversion, median 1.9 days, mean 5.1 days), the INR was known in only five cases and ranged between 1.7 and 2.5 (mean 2.1). No median value is presented. As Olshansky has said [17], the entire case recommending an INR of 2.5 or more as a condition for stroke prevention could hinge on two people with an INR greater than 2.0, with the remainder having an INR below 2.0. An INR of 2.5 at the time of cardioversion may ensure that recent INR values before cardioversion have remained over 2.0, considering daily fluctuations. It is difficult to ascertain what the INR values were in the 3 weeks before cardioversion in the study of Gallagher et al. Basing a sweeping recommendation on such a small subset is fraught with the danger of error. These few patients may not be enough to mount a case to maintain an INR at the level of 2.5.

On the other hand, other authors have confirmed the validity of ACC/AHA/ESC recommendations if the INR values in the previous 3 weeks are carefully observed, provided that the value taken into consideration each week, for 3 consecutive weeks, is at least 2.0 [17].

What is the disadvantage of "constantly keeping" an INR of 2.5 or above? Keeping this value, fluctuations of the index could frequently take the INR value up to 3 or more in the individual patient.

The intensity of anticoagulation is the major risk factor of bleeding. This factor becomes more relevant in the presence of other factors such as underlying clinical disorders, concomitant administration of nonsteroidal anti-inflammatory drugs, age over 65 years, and comorbid conditions such as renal insufficiency or anemia [10]. Considering that the risk of thromboembolism concomitant with an elective cardioversion of an AF is achievable for less than 1%, whereas the risk of hemorrhage is low, and considering that the data of the work carried out by Gallagher et al. [15] are not conclusive, in our opinion it is still good medical practice to keep the INR between 2 and 3, ensuring that such values are consecutively present each week during the 3 weeks before cardioversion.

To conclude this section, however, it must be remembered that, at least in certain conditions, the recent results of the AFFIRM study [18], which have shown a similar prognosis in patients in whom the sinus rhythm has been controlled and in those with AF in whom only the frequency has been controlled, are very likely to reduce the number of cardioversions for AF.

What Is the Role of Heparin in the Prevention of Thromboembolism?

The ACC/AHA/ESC Guidelines prior to immediate cardioversion in patients with recent-onset AF accompanied by symptoms or signs of hemodynamic instability, suggest, if not contraindicated, administering heparin concurrently by continuous infusion in a dose adjusted so as to prolong the activated partial thromboplastin time up to 1.5–2 times the reference value and next to provide oral anticoagulation (INR 2–3) for a period of at least 3–4 weeks, as for patients undergoing elective cardioversion (level of evidence: C). In circumstances other than this the use of heparin is not advisable since the risk/benefit ratio has not been explored.

What Approach Should Be Adopted in Cardioversion of AFl?

It is by now accepted that chronic AFl is associated with long-term risk of thromboembolism similar to AF, and that the risk is reduced by maintaining effective warfarin anticoagulation [19–21]. On the other hand, an episode of thromboembolism has been described after cardioversion of this arrhythmia too [22–24]. Gallagher et al. [15] also describe an episode of thromboembolism after cardioversion of atrial flutter–tachycardia. In total, five episodes of ascertained thromboembolism are reported: 3 among 323 cardioversions of patients pretreated with warfarin (in one of them the INR value at the time of cardioversion was unknown; the others had an INR of 1.5 and 2 respectively) and 2 among 396 cardioversions of patients not given anticoagulation treatment. The overall rate of embolism in those with AFl receiving anticoagulants was similar to that in patients not receiving anticoagulants. On the basis of these data, however, and considering the poor quality of the casuistics as well, it is not possible to argue either that anticoagulation should not be carried out or what the efficacious level of anticoagulation would be. Therefore, it is good medical practice to give anticoagulation treatment to these patients as well before cardioversion, maintaining the INR between 2 and 3.

References

1. Lown B, Perlroth MG, Kapddbey S et al (1963) Cardioversion of atrial fibrillation: a report on the treatment of 65 episodes in 50 patients. N Engl J Med 269:325–331
2. Resnekov L, Mc Donald L (1967) Complications in 220 patients with cardiac dysrhythmias treated by phased direct current shock and indications for electroconversion. Br Heart J 29:926–935
3. Weinberg DM, Mancini GBJ (1989) Anticoagulation for cardioversion of atrial fibrillation. Am J Cardiol 63:745–746
4. Arnold AZ, Mick MJ, Mazurek RP et al (1992) Role of prophylactic anticoagulation for direct current cardioversion in patients with atrial fibrillation or atrial flutter. J Am Coll Cardiol 19:851–855
5. Bjerkelund CJ, Orning OM (1969) The efficacy of anticoagulant therapy in preventing embolism related to DC electrical cardioversion of atrial fibrillation. Am J Cardiol 23: 208–216
6. Laupacis A, Alberg G, Dalen J et al (1998) Antithrombotic therapy in atrial fibrillation. Chest 114(Suppl):579S–589S
7. Aschenberg W, Schluter M, Kremer P et al (1986) Transesophageal two-dimensional

echocardiography for the detection of left atrial appendage thrombus. J Am Coll Cardiol 7:163–166
8. Fatkin D, Scalia G, Jacobs N et al (1996) Accuracy of biplane transesophageal echocardiography in detecting left atrial thrombus. Am J Cardiol 77:321–323
9. Klein AL, Grimm RA, Murray RD et al (2001) Use of transesophageal echocardiography to guide cardioversion in patients with atrial fibrillation. N Engl J Med 344:1411–1420
10. Hirsh J, Fuster V, Ansell J et al (2003) American Heart Association/American College of Cardiology foundation guide to warfarin therapy. Circulation 107:1692–1711
11. Goldman MJ (1959) The management of chronic atrial fibrillation: indications and method of conversion to sinus rhythm. Progr Cardiovasc Dis 2:465–479
12. Corrado G, Tadeo G, Beretta S et al (1999) Atrial thrombi resolution after prolonged anticoagulation in patients with atrial fibrillation: a transesophageal echocardiographic study. Chest 115:140–143
13. Black IW, Fatkin D, Sager KB et al (1994) Exclusion of atrial thombus by transesophageal echocardiography does not preclude embolism after cardioversion of atrial fibrillation: a multicenter study. Circulation 89:2509–2513
14. Fuster V, Ryden LE, Asinger RW et al (2001) ACC/AHA/ESC Guidelines for the management of patients with atrial fibrillation: executive summary. Circulation 104:2118–2150
15. Gallagher MM, Hennessy BJ, Edvarsson N et al (2002) Embolic complications of direct current cardioversion of atrial arrhythmias: association with low intensity of anticoagulation at the time of cardioversion. J Am Coll Cardiol 40:926–933
16. Hylek EM, Skates SJ, Sheehan MA et al (1996) An analysis of the lowest effective intensity of prophylactic anticoagulation for patients with non-rheumatic atrial fibrillation. N Engl J Med 335:540–546
17. Olshansky B (2002) High intensity anticoagulation for cardioversion of atrial arrhythmias? The shocking truth. J Am Coll Cardiol 40:934–936
18. The Atrial Fibrillation Follow-up Investigation of Rhythm Management (AFFIRM) Investigators (2002) A comparison of rate control and rhythm control in patients with atrial fibrillation. N Engl J Med 347:1825–1833
19. Lanzarotti CJ, Olshansky B (1997) Thromboembolism in chronic atrial flutter: is the risk understimated? J Am Coll Cardiol 30:1506–1511
20. Seidl K, Hauer B, Schwick NG et al (1998) Thromboembolic events in patients with atrial flutter. Am J Cardiol 82:580–583
21. Biblo LA, Yuan Z, Quan KJ et al (2001) Risk of stroke in patients with atrial flutter. Am J Cardiol 87:346–349
22. Mehta D, Baruch L (1996) Thromboembolism following cardioversion of "common" atrial flutter: risk factors and limitations of transesophageal echocardiography. Chest 110:1001–1003
23. Liaudet L, Mehtari R, Enrico JF (1997) Cerebral thromboembolism after direct curent cardioversion for pure atrial flutter. Intensive Care Med 23:196–197
24. Wood KA, Eisenberg SJ, Kalman JM et al (1997) Risk of thromboembolism in chronic atrial flutter. Am J Cardiol 79:1043–1047

Warfarin Underuse for Nonvalvular Atrial Fibrillation: How to Adjust Our Aims?

G. Di Pasquale, E. Cerè, A. Lombardi, B. Sassone, S. Biancoli, R. Vandelli

Epidemiology

Atrial fibrillation (AF) is the most common arrhythmia in clinical practice; its prevalence increases substantially with age, representing a growing epidemic with substantial effects on mortality and morbidity [1]. The more recent epidemiological data come from a large cross-sectional study in adults in California involving a population of 1.89 million [2]. The prevalence of AF was 0.95%, increasing from 0.1% among adults younger than 55 years to 9.0% in persons aged 80 years or older. The authors estimate that approximately 2.3 million adults in the USA currently have AF and project that this will increase to more than 5.6 million by the year 2050, with more than 50% of affected individuals aged 80 years or older. In Italy it is estimated that there are about 500,000 cases of AF at present, with 60,000 new cases per year.

However, the real prevalence of AF is difficult to establish, because the arrhythmia is often silent or paroxysmal. In 45% of patients in the SPAF III study [3], AF was detected as an incidental finding by routine standard ECG. In patients with symptomatic paroxysmal AF, the asymptomatic episodes are more frequent (12:1) than symptomatic ones [4]; in many cases 24-h Holter recording is negative, and some authors suggest prolonged automatic event monitoring [5].

Thromboembolic Risk

In the absence of any antithrombotic therapy the annual risk of stroke and systemic thromboembolism is 4.5%, rising to 8% in subjects older than 75 years. When the risk of transient ischemic attack (TIA) and silent cerebral infarction are also taken into account, the cerebral embolic risk exceeds 7% per year [6,

Unità Operativa di Cardiologia, Ospedale di Bentivoglio, Bentivoglio (BO), Italy

7]. Clinical features independently associated with a high risk of stroke in AF patients have been defined and integrated into several risk stratification schemes. High risk factors include age >75 years, prior stroke/TIA or systemic embolism, a history of hypertension, congestive heart failure or poor left-ventricular systolic function, rheumatic mitral valve disease, and prosthetic heart valves. Moderate risk factors include age 65–75 years, diabetes mellitus, and coronary artery disease with preserved left-ventricular function.

It is evident from thromboembolic risk stratification that older age (>75 years) per se is a high risk factor for thromboembolism, and all patients older than 75 years should receive oral anticoagulant treatment (OAT) for effective prophylaxis. This represents a therapeutic dilemma because of the higher risk of life-threatenig hemorrhages, in particular cerebral hemorrhage, in these patients during OAT.

Transesophageal echocardiography (TEE), which is the most sensitive clinical tool for the evaluation of left atrium, left atrial appendage, and aorta, provides further markers of thromboembolic risk. The presence of spontaneous echo-contrast, low flow velocities within the left atrial appendage, and complex aortic plaques is associated with a risk of stroke 2- to 4-fold that in subjects with none of these [8].

Oral Anticoagulant Treatment

Indications for OAT

The effectiveness of OAT for the prevention of thromboembolism and stroke has been definitively assessed by a number of randomized clinical trials [9, 10]. Six trials (AFASAK, SPAF, BAATAF, CAFA, SPINAF, and EAFT) compared adjusted-dose warfarin with placebo. Overall, adjusted-dose warfarin reduced the incidence of stroke by 62% (95% CI, 48–72%); absolute risk reductions were 2.7% per year for primary prevention [number needed to treat (NNT) for 1 year to prevent one stroke = 37] and 8.4% per year (NNT = 12) for secondary prevention.

The efficacy of aspirin for stroke prevention in AF patients is unclear and more controversial [9, 10]. Six trials (AFASAK, SPAF I, EAFT, ESPS II, LASAF, and UK TIA) compared antiplatelet therapy with placebo. Meta-analysis of all six trials showed that aspirin reduced the incidence of stroke by 22% (CI, 2–38%). On the basis of these six trials, the absolute risk reduction was 1.5% per year (NNT=67) for primary prevention and 2.5% per year (NNT=40) for secondary prevention. Although all six trials showed trends toward reduced stroke with aspirin, this result was statistically significant only in the SPAF I Study.

Recommendations for treatment based on the evidence from clinical trials and thromboembolic risk stratification were reconfirmed at the Sixth 2001 Consensus Conference on Antithrombotic Therapy of the American College of

Chest Physicians [10] and in the 2001 ACC/AHA/ESC Guidelines for the Management of Patients with AF [11].

OAT is mandatory in patients at high risk of AF (those with any high risk factor or with more than one moderate-risk factor), providing that high-quality monitoring of OAT is possible and no risk factors for bleeding are present. These two last requirements are particularly important when decisions on OAT in patients older than 75 years are made.

Aspirin is a possible and acceptable alternative to OAT in moderate-risk patients (those without high risk factors and with only one moderate risk factor). In this group of patients the choice between aspirin and OAT is based on the assessment of the risk/benefit ratio of OAT and also on the patient's preference [12].

Finally, aspirin is the treatment of choice in low-risk patients (those without any high risk or moderate risk factors). This group is made up of patients with no clinical or echocardiographic evidence of cardiovascular disease.

Underuse

Despite the strong evidence for the efficacy of OAT, warfarin is still little used for stroke prevention in patients with AF in general clinical practice [13, 14].

In a large, contemporary cohort of ambulatory patients with nonvalvular AF and no known contraindications, only 55% received warfarin [14]. Only 59% of patients with one or more risk factors for stroke and no contraindications were receiving warfarin. Among a subset of "ideal" candidates for warfarin (persons 65–74 years of age who had no contraindications and had had a previous stroke or had hypertension, or both), only 62% had evidence of warfarin use.

Underutilization of OAT is especially evident among elderly people with AF, in whom, paradoxically, the thromboembolic risk is higher. Major reasons for the underuse of OAT are the difficulty of high-quality monitoring of OAT, especially in older patients, and the fear of bleeding. Therefore, new and safer and effective thromboprophylactic strategies for AF are warranted, particularly for older patients, who represent a substantial proportion of the AF population.

Difficulties in Management

The management of OAT must include regular monitoring of INR, which should be kept in the narrow therapeutic range of 2.0–3.0 most of the time by means of adjustments to the dose. Many factors can influence INR stability: interacting drugs or illnesses, dietary habits (change in vitamin K intake), poor patient compliance with the therapeutic schedule, physician's ability to calculate the appropriate dosage. Risk factors for bleeding during OAT include advanced age, intensity of anticoagulation, recent initiation of warfarin therapy, patient characteristics, and drug interactions.

The relationship between advanced age and OAT-associated bleeding is controversial. In a prospective Italian collaborative study (ISCOAT), the frequency of bleeding complications was studied in outpatients followed up in anticoagulation clinics [15]. The rates of fatal, major, and minor bleeding events were quite low: 0.25, 1.1 and 6.2 per 100 patients-years of follow-up, respectively. However, the rate was higher in older patients and during the first 90 days of treatment than later. A previous study also showed that the risk of major bleeding was highest during the first month of therapy (3% during that month) and decreased to approximately one-third that rate after the first 3 months of therapy [16]. Several factors may contribute to the increased risk of bleeding within the first months of each OAT course. First, OAT can unmask a cryptic, often neoplastic, lesion. Secondly, dose adjustment may be less well controlled at the start of treatment.

A clear correlation has been reported between the intensity of OAT and the risk of bleeding. In the ISCOAT study in patients aged ≥75 years the risk of bleeding increased with INR ≥3.0 and became disproportionally high for INR >4.5 [17]. However, about one-fifth of all bleeding events occurred at INR <2.0, indicating that INR lower than 2.0 neither precludes bleeding in the elderly nor offers adequate protection from thrombotic events.

Multiple-drug therapy or polypharmacy is quite common in the elderly, with the consequent risk of adverse drug interactions. In a recent large study in patients undergoing OAT for AF, patients taking three or more drugs had more bleeding or thromboembolic complications than patients who took fewer than three drugs (24.4% / 100 patient-years versus 4.3%) [18].

Finally, in the elderly the decline in cognitive function also reduces compliance with OAT; unsuspected reduction of mental ability or attention levels was found in a significant number of elderly patients receiving OAT, with poor quality control of the therapy [19].

For all these reasons, when OAT is prescribed for elderly patients, careful and continuing evaluation of the patients is necessary to ensure that the risk of bleeding does not outweigh the benefits expected from anticoagulation.

Keeping the Risk of Bleeding to a Minimum

High-quality monitoring of OAT is the key to a lower risk of bleeding. The Sixth ACCP Consensus Conference on Antithrombotic Therapy recommends that clinicians employ a systematic process to manage oral anticoagulation dosing, involving a well-informed provider, reliable PT monitoring, and an organized system of follow-up, patient communication, and education [10].

A systematic approach to anticoagulation management such as is offered in anticoagulation clinics can improve the safety and effectiveness of warfarin therapy by reducing the incidence of related and unrelated complications. In most cases coordinated care can be defined as a specialized program of patient management focused predominantly, if not exclusively, on managing OAT. A program is often directed by a single physician and the actual management is usually conducted by nurses, pharmacists, or physician assistants. This care can be contrasted with that provided by a patient's own physician, without systematic coordination (routine medical care).

The data available indicate that the type of coordinated care offered by anticoagulation clinics will reduce the incidence of adverse outcomes and also use financial resources more economically. A meta-analysis of six studies comparing coordinated versus routine anticoagulation revealed that roughly five episodes of bleeding events per 100 patient-years were averted by coordinated care [20]. Chiquette et al. [21] also demonstrated that compared with conventional medical care, anticoagulation clinics improved anticoagulation control, reduced the rates of bleeding and thromboembolic events and saved $ 162,058 per 100 patients annually by reducing the numbers of admissions to hospital and visits to emergency departments.

Moreover, the quality of OAT can be improved by using a computerized system that includes algorithms with the capability to suggest OAT dosing and to schedule appointments [22, 23].

Recommendations

In the management of older patients with permanent AF, a risk-to-benefit assessment is warranted before OAT is initiated. Major considerations should include:

- AF electrical cardioversion, which could obviate the need of long-term OAT at least in some cases.
- Thromboembolic risk stratification in the individual patient; the prevalence of additional risk factors for thromboembolism besides advanced age (i.e., hypertension, prior stroke or TIA, heart failure or left-ventricular dysfunction, diabetes mellitus) should reinforce the decision for OAT.
- Patient's inherent risk of bleeding with OAT.
- Ability to provide high-quality monitoring of OAT through coordinated medical care (e.g., in an anticoagulation clinic).
- Patient information about OAT.

References

1. Tsang TSM, Gersh BJ (2002) Atrial fibrillation: an old disease, a new epidemic. Am J Med 113:432-435
2. Go AS, Hylek EM, Phillips KA et al (2001) Prevalence of diagnosed atrial fibrillation in adults. National implications for rhythm management and stroke prevention: the Anticoagulation and Risk Factors In Atrial Fibrillation (ATRIA) Study. JAMA 285:2370-2375
3. Blackshear JL, Kopecky SL, Litin SC, Safford RE, Hammil SC (1996) Management of atrial fibrillation in adults: prevention of thromboembolism and symptomatic treatment. Mayo Clin Proc 71:150-160

4. Page RL, Wilkinson WE, Clair WK, McCarthy EA, Pritchett EL (1994) Asymptomatic arrhythmias in patients with paroxysmal atrial fibrillation and paroxysmal supraventricular tachycardia. Circulation 89:224-227
5. Roche F, Gaspoz JM, Da Costa A et al (2002) Frequent and prolonged asymptomatic episodes of paroxysmal atrial fibrillation revealed by automatic long-term event recorders in patients with a negative 24-hour Holter. Pacing Clin Electrophysiol 25:1587-1593
6. Atrial Fibrillation Investigators (1994) Risk factors for stroke and efficacy of antithrombotic therapy in atrial fibrillation: analysis of pooled data from five randomized controlled trials. Arch Intern Med 154:1449-1457
7. Hart RG, Pearce LA, McBride R et al, on behalf of the Stroke Prevention in Atrial Fibrillation (SPAF) Investigators (1999) Factors associated with ischemic stroke during aspirin therapy in atrial fibrillation. Analysis of 2012 participants in the SPAF I-III clinical trials. Stroke 30:1223-1229
8. Di Pasquale G, Urbinati S, Pinelli G (1995) New echocardiographic markers of embolic risk in atrial fibrillation. Cerebrovasc Dis 5:315-322
9. Hart RG, Benavente O, McBride R, Pearce LA (1999) Antithrombotic therapy to prevent stroke in patients with atrial fibrillation: a meta-analysis. Ann Intern Med 131:492-501
10. Albers GW, Dalen JE, Laupacis A, Manning WJ, Petersen P, Singer DE (2001) Antithrombotic therapy in atrial fibrillation. Sixth ACCP Consensus Conference on Antithrombotic Therapy. Chest 119 [Suppl]:194S-206S
11. Fuster V, Ryden L et al (2001) ACC/AHA/ESC guidelines for the management of patients with atrial fibrillation: executive summary. Am J Cardiol 38:1231-1265
12. Di Pasquale G, Cerè E, Biancoli S et al (2002) Antiplatelet agents for prevention of thromboembolism in atrial fibrillation : when, why, and which one? In: Raviele A (ed) Cardiac arrhythmias 2001. Springer-Verlag Italia, Milan, pp 422-435
13. Bungard TJ, Ghali WA, Teo KK, Mc Alister FA, Tsuyuki RT (2000) Why do patients with atrial fibrillation not receive warfarin? Arch Intern Med 160:41-46
14. Go AS, Hylek EM, Borowsky LH, Phillips KA, Selby JV, Singer DE (1999) Warfarin use among ambulatory patients with nonvalvular atrial fibrillation: the anticoagulation and risk factors in atrial fibrillation (ATRIA) study. Ann Intern Med 131: 927-934
15. Palareti G, Leali N, Coccheri S et al, on behalf of the Italian Study on Complications of Oral Anticoagulant Therapy (1996) Bleeding complications of oral anticoagulant treatment: an inception-cohort, prospective collaborative study (ISCOAT). Lancet 348:423-428
16. Landefeld CS, Goldman L (1989) Major bleeding in outpatients treated with warfarin. Incidence and prediction by factors known at the start of outpatient therapy. Am J Med 87:144-152
17. Palareti G, Hirsh J, Legnani C et al (2000) Oral anticoagulation treatment in the elderly: a nested prospective, case-control study. Arch Intern Med 160:470-478
18. Wehinger C, Stollberger C, Langer T, Schneider B, Finsterer J (2001) Evaluation of risk factors for stroke/embolism and of complications due to anticoagulant therapy in atrial fibrillation. Stroke 32:2246-2252
19. Palareti G, Poggi M, Guazzaloca G et al (1997) Assessment of mental ability in elderly anticoagulated patients: its reduction is associated with a less satisfactory quality of treatment. Blood Coagul Fibrinolysis 8:411-417
20. Ansell JE, Hughes R (1996) Evolving models of warfarin management: anticoagulation clinics, patient self-monitoring, and patient self-management. Am Heart J 132:1095-1100

21. Chiquette E, Amato MG, Bussey HI (1998) Comparison of an anticoagulation clinic with usual medical care: anticoagulation control, patient outcomes, and health care costs. Arch Intern Med 158:1641-1647
22. Fitmaurice DA, Hobbs FD, Delaney BC, Wilson S, McManus R (1998) Review of computerized decision support system for oral anticoagulation management. Br J Haematol 102:907-909
23. Manotti C, Moia M, Palareti G, Pengo V, Ria L, Dettori AG (2001) Effect of computer-aided management on the quality of treatment in anticoagulated patients: a prospective, randomized, multicenter trial of APROAT (Automated Program for Oral Anticoagulated Treatment). Haematologica 86:1060-1070

SUPRAVENTRICULAR TACHYARRHYTHMIAS: DIAGNOSIS AND TREATMENT

Palpitations of Unknown Origin: How Frequent Are Supraventricular Arrhythmias?

F. Giada, A. Raviele

Initial Diagnostic Evaluation of Patients with Palpitations

In patients with palpitations it is essential to ascertain whether there is a structural heart disease and/or heart disease at risk of arrhythmias, and to obtain an electrocardiographic recording during the episodes of palpitation. Thus, in all subjects with palpitations, the initial evaluation will involve a thorough clinical history, a careful objective examination, and 12-lead ECG at the baseline and, if possible, during an episode of palpitations [1].

Twelve-lead electrocardiographic recording during the course of spontaneous symptoms constitutes the gold standard for the diagnostic evaluation of palpitations. Indeed, electrocardiographic recording is able to establish whether or not the palpitations are associated with a cardiac rhythm disorder and, in the majority of cases, leads to the correct diagnosis of the arrhythmia responsible [2, 3]. However, in normal clinical practice it is not always possible to perform a 12-lead ECG during a spontaneous episode of palpitations. The ECG does, of course, yield valuable information even when not performed during an episode of palpitations, especially with regard to the presence of heart disease or conduction abnormalities.

In some particular situations it may be useful to perform blood chemistry examinations, such as hemochrome, electrolytes, blood glucose, and thyroid function tests [3]. Effort stress testing is indicated in case of palpitations associated with physical effort. The need for further investigations (echocardiogram, coronary angiography, etc.) will depend on the nature of the heart disease suspected or ascertained.

In a good proportion of patients, initial evaluation yields a definitive diagnosis of the cause of the palpitations, or at least excludes the presence of major arrhythmic disorders with reasonable certainty [3]. However, the lack of an electrocardiographic recording during the episode of palpitation permits only a presumptive diagnosis of the etiology of the palpitations [4].

Cardiovascular Department, Umberto I Hospital, Mestre-Venice, Italy

When the initial diagnostic evaluation fails to elucidate the cause of symptoms, the palpitations are considered to be of unexplained origin. In this case, if the palpitations are frequent, sustained, poorly tolerated, and accompanied by other symptoms, or if the patient is suffering from heart disease, second-line diagnostic investigations, i.e., prolonged electrocardiographic monitoring and electrophysiological study, should be undertaken [1].

Prolonged Electrocardiographic Monitoring

Prolonged electrocardiographic monitoring includes the following devices: Holter monitoring, telemetry, event recorders, external loop recorders, and implantable loop recorders (ILRs). The United States Food and Drug Administration has recently approved the following indications for the use of ILRs: patients with clinical syndromes or conditions at high risk of arrhythmia, and patients with transitory symptoms that may suggest a cardiac rhythm disorder. These devices have been used successfully in the study of syncope [5], in which they have shown a better cost/efficacy ratio than conventional tests, and could also prove useful in the study of palpitations of unknown origin [6–9].

Indications

According to the ACC/AHA and Italian Guidelines for ambulatory electrocardiography (AECG) [7], recurrent palpitations whose origin remains unknown after initial evaluation represent a class I indication for prolonged electrocardiographic monitoring. Holter monitoring is useful when symptoms occur daily or in patients who are unable to activate a device for prolonged electrocardiographic monitoring. Event recorders may prove useful in very compliant patients with infrequent palpitations that are fairly long-lasting and unaccompanied by hemodynamic impairment that is likely to hinder their use. Indeed, it is essential that the patient be able to activate the device correctly. External loop recorders are recommended in cases of infrequent, short-lasting palpitations associated with hemodynamic impairment in very compliant patients. Finally, ILRs could be recommended in poorly compliant patients with rare (i.e., monthly/annual frequency), short-lasting palpitations associated with hemodynamic impairment.

Diagnostic Yield

Prolonged electrocardiographic monitoring is regarded as diagnostic only when it is possible to establish a certain correlation between the palpitations and the electrocardiographic recording. Therefore, in patients who do not develop clinical symptoms during prolonged electrocardiographic monitoring, these investigations are deemed nondiagnostic. Holter and loop recorders–devices also able to record arrhythmic events automatically–are regarded as probably diagnostic also if the patients have evidence of asymptomatic sustained supraventricular tachycardia (>1 min), or ventricular tachycardia (>10 beats).

Whenever it is possible to establish a relationship between patients' symptoms and an ECG trace, the specificity of the test, at least in respect of formulating the diagnosis of arrhythmic or nonarrhythmic palpitations, is 100%. The sensitivity of the test, by contrast, is extremely variable and depends upon the type of device employed, the duration of the monitoring period, the patient's compliance, and the frequency of symptoms.

In patients with palpitations of unknown origin, Holter monitoring has been shown to have a rather low sensitivity (33%–35%) [10]. In a meta-analysis of seven studies conducted in patients with syncope and/or palpitations of unknown origin, the sensitivity of Holter monitoring has been reported to be only 22% [11]. External loop recorders have displayed a sensitivity of 66%–73% in the study of palpitations of unknown origin [10]. No definitive data are currently available about the diagnostic yield of event recorders or of ILRs.

Electrophysiological Studies

The electrophysiological study (EPS) is a provocative test. It is performed by means of the transesophageal technique (at rest and during effort) or the endocavitary technique (under pharmacological stress, if deemed necessary), in accordance with standard protocols [12]. In addition to being costly and invasive, this provocative test has a low sensitivity in the case of palpitations of unknown origin [6, 12–14]. Moreover, the correspondence between the induced arrhythmia and the arrhythmia responsible for the patient's clinical symptoms is unproven. EPS positivity only reveals the presence of a pathological substrate, which may (or may not) be responsible for the palpitations. It is therefore essential to establish the association between the induced arrhythmia and reproduction of the patient's spontaneous symptoms. EPS has a low positive predictive value. EPS does, however, offer the advantage not only of enabling the type of arrhythmia responsible for the palpitations to be correctly identified, but also of enabling ablation therapy of the arrhythmia itself to be undertaken during the same session.

Indications

According to ACC/AHA guidelines for clinical intracardiac electrophysiological and catheter ablation procedures [12]," long-term ambulatory recording is the most useful procedure for documenting cardiac rhythm associated with palpitations," and "EPS are used if recording attempts fail to provide an answer." EPS is an ACC/AHA class I indication in patients with unexplained palpitations in whom a high pulse rate has been documented by a qualified person, and in patients with palpitations preceding syncope. EPS is a class II indication in patients with clinically significant palpitations, suspected to be of cardiac origin, in whom symptoms are sporadic and cannot be documented. In patients with heart disease who suffer from sustained palpitations with hemodynamic impairment, EPS is generally carried out by means of the intracavitary method and should precede the use of electrocardiographic monitoring. In patients without heart disease, or with mild heart disease, EPS normally follows the use of electrocardiographic monitoring, and may be also performed by means of the transesophageal technique.

Diagnostic Yield

EPS is regarded as diagnostic if it induces any tachycardia accompanied by reproduction of the spontaneous symptoms, or if it induces sustained supraventricular tachycardia (>1 min) or sustained ventricular tachycardia (>30 s or requiring urgent interruption), even without reproduction of the spontaneous symptoms. It is considered negative if it does not induce the above-mentioned tachycardias.

The specificity and sensitivity of EPS depend on the stimulation protocol employed, the type of arrhythmias induced, and the patients studied. Aggressive protocols increase the sensitivity of the test at the expense of its specificity. The specificity of EPS is high (95%–100%) when the induced arrhythmia is sustained atrioventricular node re-entrant tachycardia (AVNRT) and atrioventricular re-entrant tachycardia (AVRT), or monomorphic ventricular tachycardia (100%), whereas it is lower, especially in patients with structural heart disease, when the induced arrhythmia is atrial fibrillation and atrial flutter (60%–83%), nonsustained ventricular tachycardia (45%–75%), or ventricular fibrillation (50%–96%) [6, 12–14].

While the sensitivity of EPS in patients with documented tachycardia is quite good (67%–100% for AVNRT/AVRT, and 60%–85% for atrial fibrillation and atrial flutter), data about the sensitivity of EPS in the study of palpitations of unknown origin are scant and incomplete, and it is probably quite low. In young patients with palpitations of unexplained origin, and without structural heart disease, EPS has displayed a variable sensitivity ranging between 58% and 87%. In older patients and in patients with severe structural heart disease its sensitivity is probably considerably lower [6, 12–14].

Diagnosed Conditions in Patients with Unexplained Palpitations

Most patients with palpitations of unexplained origin who undergo prolonged electrocardiographic monitoring are found to have benign atrial premature beats (0%–13%), ventricular premature beats (12%–36%), normal sinus rhythm (18%–39%), or sinus tachycardia (5%–29%). Supraventricular tachycardia accounts for a high percentage of the diagnosed conditions in patients with palpitations of unexplained origin (4%–18%), both in patients with and those without heart disease. Atrial fibrillation and atrial flutter are also frequent findings in these patients (2%–17%), whereas ventricular tachycardia is much less frequent (0%–2%), and it is typical of patients with severe structural or arrhythmogenic heart disease [6, 12–14].

Future Studies

In spite of all these extensive, costly, and time-consuming instrumental examinations (prolonged electrocardiographic monitoring and EPS), it is still sometimes impossible to establish the cause of palpitations, thus leaving the patient in apprehension and the physician in doubt as to the diagnosis. In the study of Weber and Kapoor [3] the etiology of palpitations could not be determined in 16% of patients. Indeed, currently available investigative techniques have been shown to be of somewhat variable diagnostic value, especially in patients with fairly infrequent palpitations. Moreover, there are no specific guidelines that distinguish patients in whom it is appropriate to perform continuous monitoring from those for whom intermittent AECG is adequate, and we do not know what is the most cost-effective diagnostic approach to the investigation of patients with relatively frequent palpitations. To solve these issues, we designed an ongoing multicenter, prospective, randomized clinical trial, the Recurrent Unexplained Palpitations (RUP) Study. The main aim of this study is to assess the diagnostic yield and the cost-effectiveness of the ILR in patients with palpitations of unknown origin. To this end, the diagnostic yield of the ILR will be compared with that of the traditional diagnostic strategy.

References

1. Zimetbaum P, Josephson ME (1998) Evaluation of patients with palpitations. N Engl J Med 338:1369–1373
2. Brugada P, Gursoy S, Brugada J, Andriess E (1993) Investigation of palpitations. Lancet 341:1254–1258
3. Weber BE, Kapoor WH (1996) Evaluations and outcomes of patients with palpitations. Am J Med 100:138–148
4. Lessmeier TJ, Gamperling D, Johnson-Liddon V et al (1997) Unrecognized paroxysmal supraventricular tachycardia: potential for misdiagnosis as panic disorders. Arch Intern Med 157:537–543
5. Krahn AD, Klein GJ Raymond Y, Norris C (1998) Final results from a pilot study with an implantable loop recorder to determine the etiology of syncope in patients with negative noninvasive and invasive testing. Am J Cardiol 82:117–119
6. Zipes DP, Miles WM, Klein LS (1995) Assesment of patient with cardiac arrhythmia. In. Zipes DP, Jalife J (eds) Cardiac electrophysiology: from cell to bedside. Saunders, Philadelphia, pp 1009–1012
7. Crawford MH, Bernstein SJ, Deedwania PC et al (1999) Guidelines for ambulatory

electrocardiography: executive summary and recommendations. A report of the American College of Cardiology/American Heart Association task force on practice guidelines (committee to revise the guidelines for ambulatory electrocardiography. Circulation 100:886–893

8. Waktare JEP, Camm AJ (2001) Holter and event recordings for arrhythmia detection. In: Zareba W, Maison-Blanche P, Locati EH (eds) Noninvasive electrocardiology in clinical practice. Futura, Armonk, NY, pp 3–30
9. Zimtbaum PJ, Josephson ME (1999) The evolving role of ambulatory arrhythmia monitoring in general practice. Ann Intern Med 150:848–856
10. Di Marco JP, Philbrick JT (1990) Use of ambulatory electrocardiographic (Holter) monitoring. Ann Intern Med 113:53–68
11. Kinlay S, Leitch JW, Neil A et al (1996) Cardiac event recorders yield more diagnoses and are more cost-effective than 48-hour Holter monitoring in patients with palpitations. Ann Intern Med 124:16–20
12. Zipes DP, DiMarco JP, Gillette PC et al (1995) Guidelines for clinical intracardiac electrophysiological and catheter ablation procedures: a report of the American College of Cardiology/American Heart Association task force on practice guidelines (Committee on Clinical Intracardiac Electrophysiologic and Catheter Ablation Procedures). J Am Coll Cardiol 26:555–573
13. Ross DL, Farre J, Bar FWHM et al (1980) Comprehensive clinical electrophysiologic studies in the investigation of documented or suspected tachycardias. Circulation 61:1010–1016
14. Bonso A, Delise P, Corò L et al (1991) Palpitazioni d'origine sconosciuta: qual'è l'utilità della stimolazione atriale transesofagea? In: Piccolo E, Raviele A (eds) Aritmie cardiache. Milan, Centro Scientifico Editore, pp 229–236

Acute Termination of Atrial Flutter: Class III Drugs or Transesophageal Pacing?

A. Bonso, S. Themistoclakis, A. Rossillo, A. Raviele

Introduction

Atrial flutter (AFL) is an arrhythmia which occurs frequently. Epidemiological data show an incidence of 88/100 000 new cases per year in the general population in USA, with 200 000 new cases every year [1]. The main predictors of this arrhythmia are heart failure and chronic obstructive pulmonary disease. It often coexists with atrial fibrillation (AF); moreover, it is not unusual that patients undergoing antiarrhythmic treatment with class IC drugs or amiodarone for the treatment of AF develop episodes of AFL. Often AFL is poorly tolerated due to the high ventricular response. This happens even in patients with good control of ventricular rate at rest, who do not tolerate AFL during effort, since ventricular rate increases suddenly.

Today radiofrequency ablation is the first-line therapy in selected patients with AFL [2]. However, immediate treatment is often necessary for the patient who comes to hospital with AFL. Sinus rhythm can be obtained through various techniques: external direct current cardioversion-defibrillation (DC shock), transesophageal pacing (TEP), or drug-based reconversion. The first is certainly the most efficient and is the first choice in an emergency. TEP has been proved to be a valid alternative to DC shock, since no general anesthesia is required. Reconversion with class IA and IC [3–5] drugs or amiodarone and sotalol has low efficacy. The class III drugs dofetilide and ibutilide [6–17] have proved to be so highly effective in AFL reconversion that they have become a valid alternative to other therapies.

Transesophageal Pacing

The possibility of interrupting AFL by means of atrial stimulation was demon-

Division of Cardiology, Cardiovascular Department, Umberto I Hospital, Mestre–Venice, Italy

strated in 1967 [18]. The TEP technique takes advantage of the anatomical proximity of left atrium and esophagus to stimulate the atria appropriately. Endocavitary studies of mapping and stimulation through the entrainment technique made it possible to reconstruct the electroanatomical circuit of AFL around a tricuspid valve annulus [19]. The presence of a well-defined macrocircuit with an excitable gap (depending on the velocity of conduction and the refractory period) allows the electric stimulus to enter the circuit and then interrupt it. The size of the excitable gap is one of the factors which influences success rate of TEP. In fact, AFL often has a rate of nearly 300 cycles per minute and so it has a small excitable gap. By stimulating from the left atrium, the difficulty of entering the circuit increases the aggressiveness of the protocol. This fact together with the relative distance from the target circuit may explain the percentage of failure with this technique as compared to direct endocavitary stimulation of the right atrium. To reach the AFL circuit located in the right atrium the electric impulse activates the left atrium passively. This is probably one of the reasons for the frequent transformation of AFL into AF with the most aggressive protocols. In this case it is often necessary to treat the AF afterwards.

In order to facilitate the reconversion of AFL through TEP, pretreatment with antiarrhythmic drugs has been suggested, also to avoid later AF. The purpose of the antiarrhythmic pretreatment is to increase the excitable gap of AFL by slowing conduction velocity or lengthening the refractory period. Several works have reported a higher efficacy in reconverting AFL after drugs pretreatment either orally or intravenously, in particular with class IA (disopyramide, procainamide) [20, 21], class IC (propafenone, flecainide) [22–24], and class III drugs (ibutilide) [25], although some authors have not reported significant differences between pretreated and nonpretreated patients, or even greater difficulty in the reconversion after pretreatment. In particular with amiodarone, greater efficacy has been reported with acute pretreatment and lower efficacy with chronic pretreatment. The explanation of this apparent paradox lies in the fact that chronic treatment, unlike acute treatment, acts mainly by lengthening the atrial refractory period, shortening the excitable gap [26].

The protocols of stimulation establish a stimulus from 10 to 20 ms duration with an intensity ranging from 15 to 20 mA and an interelectrode distance of 3 cm. TEP is performed with a stimulation protocol beginning from a cycle length (CL) 10% shorter than the AFL CL, decreasing in steps of 10 ms to a pacing CL of 100 ms; then bursts of 100- and 70-ms CL lasting at least 10 s are delivered. The best position for stimulating can be reached when the bipolar stimulation poles record a clear diphasic atrial activation.

The percentages of reconversion seem to be affected by both the aggressivity of the protocol, the pacing duration, and the operator's skill. Usually with this technique the success rate of reconversion aiming at sinus rhythm ranges from 43% to 90% [26–29]. This wide variability depends mainly on the criteria for efficacy. In fact, the lowest values are achieved when only restoring sinus rhythm or a very short period of AF is taken into account. The highest values are achieved when transformation into AF and its persistence are taken into account.

Several other variables can also influence therapeutic success [26, 29], e.g., the arrhythmia duration. Arrhythmia onset within less than 24 h seems to be related to a higher percentage of reconversion (97%), but these results have not been reported by all authors. An increase in left atrial diameter seems to be another factor which diminishes TEP efficacy. Atrioventricular ratio deflection recording at the site of stimulation is another important factor for TEP efficacy.

Class III Antiarrhythmic Agents: Ibutilide and Dofetilide

Ibutilide is a methanesulfonamide derivative with structural similarities to the antiarrhythmic agent sotalol. The drug increases action potential duration by blocking the rapid component of the delayed-rectifier outward potassium current (I_{Kr}) and, uniquely among available class III drugs, by activating the slow inward sodium plateau current ($I_{Na\text{-}s}$). Over a limited range of stimulation rates, ibutilide increases action potential duration without significant reverse use dependence or loss of effect at rapid pacing rates [30].

The prolongation of action potential by ibutilide leads to an increase in atrial and ventricular effective refractory period–the essential component of ibutilide's antiarrhythmic and proarrhythmic activities. In patients with AFL, ibutilide causes greater prolongation of refractoriness than slowing conduction; this effect tends to reduce the excitable gap in the re-entry circuit and contributes to arrhythmia termination [31]. Ibutilide has no direct effect on conduction velocity and does not alter PR or QRS intervals, and causes only a mild decrease in sinus rate and ventricular response during AF and AFL. Ibutilide administration is not associated with clinically important adverse effects on contractility, cardiac output, or arterial and pulmonary pressure, even in patients with ventricular dysfunction or congestive heart failure. The drug is not available for long-term oral use because of extensive first-pass metabolism in the liver. Our effect and potential complication declines after 1 h [11–17].

Three clinical trials have demonstrated that ibutilide [11, 13, 17] is superior to placebo in terminating AFL, with most patients converting within 30 min. The success rate ranged from 58% to 70%. The main dosage administered of ibutilide is 1 mg over 10 min (in patients weighing over 60 kg; it is 0.01 mg/kg in patients weighing less than 60 kg). If the arrhythmia does not terminate within 10 min after the end of the initial dose, a second 10-min infusion of 1 mg is administered. Predictors of successful arrhythmia conversion include the duration of arrhythmia before treatment and left atrial size. It is noteworthy that ibutilide, even when ineffective, enhances termination of AFL by overdrive atrial pacing [25]. Comparative trials with procainamide and sotalol have shown superior efficacy of ibutilide [14–16].

Polymorphic ventricular tachycardia is the most worrying adverse event associated with ibutilide. In clinical trials this side effect appears within 1 h in 4.4%–12.5% of patients. Predictors of increased risk were female gender, non-white race, a lower heart rate, and a history of heart failure.

Dofetilide has similar properties to ibutilide. Therefore dofetilide has large proven by oral administration. Dofetilide has a success rate of 54% when used intravenously to reconvert AFL [6–10].

Ibutilide Compared to TEP

Two randomized studies have investigated the efficacy and safety of TEP in comparison with ibutilide infusion [32, 33]. The first evaluated 33 patients (mean age 58 years) with AFL onset less than 30 days previously and without antiarrhythmic pretreatment. The end-point was sinus rhythm reconversion within 1 h after the procedure. AFL was reconverted in 50% of patients treated with TEP as compared with 66% of patients treated with ibutilide; the difference was not statistically significant. Seventy-eight percent of the patients had structural heart disease and all were hemodynamically stable. Among the variables, the only one that influenced the success of therapy was arrhythmia duration. In particular, ibutilide proved to be more efficient than TEP in reconverting AFL of longer duration.

The second study enrolled 52 consecutive patients (mean age 56 years) coming from the emergency ward because of typical AFL (30 patients), atypical AFL (8 patients), and atrial tachycardia (14 patients). Mean duration of arrhythmia was 10 days. Seventy-three percent of patients were undergoing antiarrhythmic pretreatment with class IC or III drugs (22/29 of the TEP group and 16/23 of the ibutilide group). Sixty-five percent of patients had structural heart disease,with a mean ejection fraction of 59%. Patients with heart failure, long QT, severe bradycardia, left bundle branch block, or quinidine treatment were not included in the study (6 patients). End-point was sinus rhythm reconversion within 1 h after the procedure. Sinus rhythm was achieved in 41% of the TEP group and 91% of the ibutilide group. In particular, sinus rhythm was achieved in 36% (8/22) of the pretreated and 57% (4/7) of the nonpretreated TEP group, while in the ibutilide group sinus rhythm was obtained in 87% (14/16) of pretreated and 100% (6/6) of nonpretreated patients. The study showed a higher efficacy of ibutilide than TEP in patients already undergoing antiarrhythmic treatment and referred to the emergency ward for synchronization of atrial arrhythmias such as typical and atypical AFL and atrial tachycardia.

In conclusion, both reports showed that ibutilide is more efficient than TEP in reconverting AFL and demonstrated its safety and tolerability in a selected group of patients. No adverse events were reported in the two studies, but the benefits and risks of ibutilide should be carefully considered for each patient to minimize the occurrence of proarrhythmic adverse events. For this reason, patients treated with ibutilide should be monitored for at least 2 or 3 h. TEP is less effective than ibutilide but can be used in reconverting almost all patients with AFL, with the exception of the rare subjects who do not tolerate the procedure and of real emergency conditions. It is also performed in patients not using ibutilide because of the great risk of ventricular arrhythmia complications, e.g., patients with heart failure or severe bradycardia. TEP has a lower probability of reconversion in long-term AFL in patients with heart disease with enlarged atria who easily develop AF.

References

1. Granada J, Uribe W, Cyhou PH et al (2000) Incidence and predictors of atrial flutter in the general population. J Am Coll Cardiol 36:2242–2246
2. Natale A, Newby KH, Pisanò E et al (2000) Prospective randomized comparison of antiarrhythmic therapy versus first-line radiofrequency ablation in patients with atrial flutter. J Am Coll Cardiol 35:1898–1904
3. Bianconi L, Boccadamo R, Pappalardo A et al (1989) Effectiveness of intravenous propafenone for conversion of paroxysmal atrial fibrillation or flutter to sinus rhythm. Am J Cardiol 64:335–338
4. Suttorp MJ, Kingma JH, Lie-A-Huen L et al (1989) Intravenous flecainide versus verapamil for conversion of paroxysmal atrial fibrillation or flutter to sinus rhythm. Am J Cardiol 63:693–696
5. Antman EM, Beamer Ad, Cantillon C et al (1990) Therapy of refractory symptomatic atrial fibrillation and atrial flutter: a staged care approach with new antiarrhythmic drugs. J Am Coll Cardiol 15:698–707
6. Olshansky B (1996) Dofetilide versus quinidine for atrial flutter: vive la difference. J Cardiovasc Electrophysiol 7:809–827
7. Falk RH, Pollak A, Singh SN et al (1997) Intravenous dofetilide, a class III antiarrhythmic agent, for the termination of sustained atrial fibrillation or flutter. J Am Coll Cardiol 29:385–390
8. Suttorp MJ, Polak PE, Van't-Hof A et al (1992) Efficacy and safety of a new selective class III antiarrhythmic agent dofetilide in paroxysmal atrial fibrillation or atrial flutter. Am J Cardiol 69:417–418
9. Bianconi L, Dinelli L, Papalardo A et al (1995) Comparison of intravenously-administered dofetilide vs amiodarone in the acute termination of atrial fibrillation and flutter: a multi-centered randomized, double-blind placebo-controlled study. Circulation 92 (Suppl I):I–775
10. Singh S, Berk M, Zoble R et al (1998) Oral dofetilide for conversion of patients with chronic atrial fibrillation or atrial flutter to normal sinus rhythm: a multicenter study. J Am Coll Cardiol 31(Suppl A):369A–370A
11. Ellenbogen KA, Stambler BS, Wood MA et al (1996) Efficacy of intravenous ibutilide for rapid termination of atrial fibrillation and atrial flutter: a dose-response study. J Am Coll Cardiol 28:130–136
12. Naccarelli GV, Lee KS, Gibson GK, VanderLugt J (1996) Electrophysiology and pharmacology of ibutilide. Am J Cardiol 78(suppl 8A):12–16
13. Stambler BS, Wood MA, Ellenbogen KA et al (1996) Efficacy and safety of repeated intravenous doses of ibutilide for rapid conversion of atrial flutter or fibrillation. Circulation 94:1613–1621

14. Murray KT (1998) Ibutilide. Circulation 97:493–497
15. Kowey PR, VanderLugt JT, Luderer JR (1996) Safety and risk/benefit analysis of ibutilide for acute conversion of atrial fibrillation/flutter. Am J Cardiol 78(Suppl 8A):46–52
16. Kowey PR (1997) Use of ibutilide following cardiac surgery. J Am Coll Cardiol 98:633
17. Abi-Mansour P, Carberry PA, McCowan RJ et al (1998) Conversion efficacy and safety of repeated doses of ibutilide in patients with atrial flutter and atrial fibrillation. Study investigator. Am Heart J 136:632–642
18. Haft JL, Kosowsky BD, Lau SH et al (1967) Termination of atrial flutter by electrical pacing of the atrium. Am J Cardiol 20:229
19. Feld GK, Fleck, Chen PS et al (1992) Radiofrequency catheter ablation for the treatment of human type I atrial flutter: identification of a critical zone in the reentrant circuit by endocardial mapping technique. Circulation 86:1233
20. Della Bella P, Marenzi G, Tondo C et al (1989) Effects of disopyramide on cycle length, effective refractory period and excitable gap of atrial flutter, and relation to arrhythmia termination by overdrive pacing. Am J Cardiol 63:812–816
21. Olshansky B, Okomura K, Hess PG et al (1988) Use of procainamide with rapid atrial pacing for successful conversion of atrial flutter to sinus rhythm. J Am Coll Cardiol 11:359–364
22. Doni F, Della Bella P, Kheir A et al (1995) Atrial flutter termination by overdrive transesophageal pacing and the facilitating effect of oral propafenone. Am J Cardiol 76:1243–1246
23. D'Este D, Bertaglia M, Mantovan R et al (1997) Efficacy of intravenous propafenone in termination of atrial flutter by overdrive transesophageal pacing previously ineffective. Am J Cardiol 79:500–502
24. Heldal M, Orning OM (1993) Effects of flecainide on termination of atrial flutter by rapid atrial pacing. Eur Heart J 14:421–424
25. Stambler BS, Wood MA, Ellenbogen KA (1996) Comparative efficacy of intravenous ibutilide versus procainamide for enhancing termination of atrial flutter by atrial overdrive pacing. Am J Cardiol 77:960–966
26. Vincenti A, Cirò A, De Ceglia S et al (2001) Predictors of failure of transoesophageal cardioversion of common atrial flutter. Europace 3:10–15
27. Chung DC, Kerr CR, Cooper J (1987) Termination of spontaneous atrial flutter by transesophageal pacing. Pacing Clin Electrophysiol 10:1147
28. Guarnerio M, Furlanello F, Del Greco M et al (1989) Transesophageal atrial pacing: a first choice technique in atrial flutter therapy. Am Heart J 117:1241
29. Kantharia BK, Mookherjee S (1995) Clinical utility and the predictors of outcome of overdrive atrial transesophageal atrial pacing in the treatment of the atrial flutter. Am J Cardiol 76:144–147
30. Raviele A, Bonso A, Gasparini G et al (1999) Ibutilide for cardioversion of atrial fibrillation: how effective and safe is it? In: Raviele A (ed) Cardiac arrhythmias. Springer, Milan, pp 186–190
31. Tai CT, Chen SA, Feng AN et al (1998) Electropharmacologic effects of class I and class III antiarrhythmia drugs on typical atrial flutter: insights into the mechanism of termination. Circulation 19:1935–1945
32. Fera MS, Mazza A, Bettiol F et al (2001) Ibutilide versus transesophageal atrial pacing for atrial flutter treatment. Europace 2(suppl):A17
33. Rossillo A, Bonso A Themistoclakis S et al (2002) Confronto tra studio elettrofisiologico transesofageo e ibutilide nella riconversione delle aritmie atriali sincronizzate. Ital Heart J 3(suppl): 173S

Atrial Flutter Induced by Class IC Drugs/Amiodarone: What Are the Long-term Results of Cavo-tricuspidal Isthmus Ablation?

P. Delise, N. Sitta, L. Corò, L. Sciarra, E. Marras

Introduction

Many patients present with both atrial fibrillation (AFib) and atrial flutter (AFL) [1–8]. For example, 5–22% of patients with AFib also have AFL [4–8] and at least 10–35% of patients with clinically predominant AFL also suffer from AFib [1–4]. Association of the two arrhythmias in the same patient is related to multiple factors. First, the same atrial anatomic substrate can facilitate both multiple wavelet re-entry of AFib and right-atrial macro-re-entry of AFL. Second, AFib can trigger AFL [1, 2]. Third, AFL, like other supraventricular arrhythmias (focal atrial tachycardia, atrioventricular re-entrant tachycardia related to an overt or a concealed Kent bundle, and atrioventricular nodal re-entrant tachycardia) [9–12] can trigger AFib, a phenomenon that has been described by Pristowsky [13] as "tachycardia-induced tachycardia." Finally, the two arrhythmias may have a common trigger constituted by automatic foci of pulmonary veins [12].

The occurrence of AFL in patients with AFib is facilitated by antiarrhyhmic drugs. This has been observed by several authors, who have demonstrated the occurrence of AFL in 5–22% of patients with AFib after treatment with class 1C drugs or amiodarone [5–8].

In some of these patients, class 1C or III antiarrhythmic drugs are effective in preventing AFib, so that while AFL recurs during treatment, AFib is totally prevented or its recurrence is prevented to a greater degree [5–8].

Some authors [7, 14–18] have suggested a hybrid therapy in patients presenting with both AFL and AFib: ablation of the cavo-tricuspid isthmus (CTI) associated with the chronic administration of antiarrhythmic drugs. The rationale of hybrid therapy is that AFL can be eliminated by CTI ablation while AFib is prevented by means of antiarrhythmic drugs. CTI ablation in AFL currently has a >90% acute success rate and it is rare for it to cause complications or be followed by recurrences [19]; antiarrhythmic drugs prevent AF in at least 50% of cases.

Operative Unit of Cardiology, Hospital of Conegliano, Treviso, Italy

Efficacy of Hybrid Therapy (CTI Ablation+Antiarrhythmic Drugs) in Patients with Both Atrial Flutter and Fibrillation

Many authors [14-18, 20-24] suggest that hybrid therapy can eliminate AFL and prevent or significantly reduce the frequency of AFib episodes in 73–90% of cases during a mean follow-up ranging from 4 to 14 months.

Schumacher et al. [7], in a small observational study performed in patients with both AFL and AFib during follow-up periods of 11±4 months, observed that after CTI ablation 37% of patients remained free of all arrhythmias and an additional 42% of patients had a significantly lowered recurrence of AFib recurrence, while only 15% had no clinical benefit.

Nabar et al. [15], in another small observational study in mean follow-up times of 4 months, observed a clinical benefit in 85% of cases (disappearance of AFib in 70% and fewer recurrent episodes of AFib in 15%).

Bonso et al. [23], in a large multicenter retrospective study involving 101 patients with both AFL and AFib treated by this therapy, achieved the elimination of recurrent AFL/AFib in 54% of patients at 6 months and in 50.5% at 1, 2, 3, and 4 years.

Stabile et al. [24] performed a randomized prospective study in patients in whom flecainide acutely converted AFib into AFL and demonstrated that patients treated with the hybrid therapy had a significantly lower incidence of recurrence of AFib/AFL (42%) during a follow-up period of 24±7 months than did patients treated with oral flecainide only (78%) or with CTI only (92%). In the same study a control group of patients in whom flecainide was not able to convert AFib into AFL after a hybrid therapy had a 92% recurrence rate of AFib.

Lee et al. [21] compared the effect of CTI ablation on quality of life in two groups of patients with documented AFL in isolation and in patients with both AFL and AFib; the former group in each case discontinued drug therapy, while the latter continued with it. During a follow-up of 6 months CTI ablation eliminated AFib in 44% of patients with both arrhythmias before ablation. Quality of life significantly improved in both groups, although the improvement was greater in patients with AFL in isolation before ablation.

Personal Experience with Hybrid Therapy in Patients with Both Atrial Flutter and Fibrillation

In a previous paper [18], we reported our results in a limited series of patients successfully treated with CTI ablation for AFL. In accordance with previous studies, in patients presenting with both AFL and AFib, during a mean follow-up of about 1 year we observed the prevention of both AFL and AFib in about half the patients. Furthermore, a significant improvement in quality of life was found both in patients with AFL alone and in patients with both AFL and AFib, although the improvement was slightly greater in the former group. In any case, in about two-thirds of patients in the group with both arrhythmias CTI had a clinical benefit (> 50% reduction in symptom score).

Our present series involves 79 consecutive patients who have undergone successful CTI ablation for AFL.

The patients are divided into two groups. The 26 patients in group A had documented AFL only before ablation; the 53 patients in group B had both paroxysmal or persistent AFL and AFib before ablation. In group B, 28 patients had AFL alone during antiarrhythmic therapy (group B1), while 25 (group B2) continued to experience both AFL and AFib during antiarrhythmic therapy. After ablation, group A patients discontinued their antiarrhythmic therapy, while group B patients continued theirs.

The clinical characteristics were similar in both groups, except for the duration of symptoms, which was longer in group B (Table 1).

In all patients, CTI ablation was performed according to standard criteria [20]. Electrophysiologically successful CTI was defined by the achievement of a bidirectional CTI block.

Before ablation, quality of life was evaluated in all patients by administering the Minnesota Living with Heart Failure Questionnaire (LHFQ) [15] and calculating an SSS (Specific Symptom Scale) score. The Minnesota LHFQ [25] consists of 21 questions, each with a score from 0 (well) to 5 (unwell). The SSS consists of 6 questions about symptoms: palpitations, rest and effort dyspnea, effort intolerance, asthenia, and angina. The score ranges from 0 (well) to 10 (unwell).

On discharge, patients were instructed to return to hospital promptly in the event of sustained palpitations or of sustained symptoms that could possibly be related to arrhythmia relapse, in order to undergo electrocardiography. In the case of unsustained symptoms, patients underwent 24-h Holter monitoring. In any case, patients were asked to keep a diary of the number and duration of episodes of recurrent palpitations.

Table 1. Patient characteristics

	Group A (AFL)	Group B (AFL+AF)	P
N	26	53	
Age (years)	62 ± 9	63 ± 10	NS
M / F	24 / 2	43 / 10	NS
Symptoms (months)	30 ± 34	86 ± 87	<0.01
Palpitations	84%	92%	NS
Heart disease	16 / 13	27 / 26	NS
EF (%)	53 ± 11	58 ± 9	NS
Left atrium (mm)	42 ± 7	43 ± 5	NS

Patients were recalled 3 months after ablation and at the end of follow-up (18 ± 12 months). During follow-up examinations, they underwent an interview focusing particularly on arrhythmia relapses, a clinical evaluation, and electrocardiography. In addition, Minnesota LHFQ and SSS questionnaires were administered.

Before ablation and during follow-up, the number of episodes of presumed AFib (or AFL before CTI ablation) per month was calculated on the basis of the subjective episodes of palpitations reported by patients.

During follow-up, 5 (13%) of the 26 patients in group A and 20 (38%) of the 53 in group B had documented AFib. AFib recurred in 7 (25%) of the 28 group B1 and 13 (52%) of the 25 group B2 patients ($p = 0.04$, Table 2). In the 20 group B patients who had documented recurrent AFib, the number of AFib episodes per month during the 12 months preceding ablation was 0.4 ± 0.24. During follow-up, the number of AFib episodes per month fell to 0.15 ± 0.15 (–60%, $P < 0.001$).

Before ablation, Minnesota LHFQ scores were similar in groups A and B (Table 3). After ablation, at the end of follow-up the LHFQ score had fallen significantly in both group A and group B [from 32 ± 7 to 7 ± 6; –77%; $P < 0.001$ and from 28 ± 13 to 8 ± 6; –71%; $P < 0.001$; the difference between groups A and B in the reduction in LHFQ score was not significant (NS)]. Similarly, before ablation the SSS scores were similar in groups A and B (Table 4). After ablation, at the end of follow-up, SSS scores had significantly decreased in both group A and group B (from 24 ± 11 to 5 ± 5; –77%; $P < 0.001$ and from 21 ± 10 to 8 ± 7; –62%; $P < 0.001$; the difference between group A and group B was NS). The reductions in both LHFQ and SSS scores during follow-up were significantly greater in patients without documented recurrent AFib than in those who had documented recurrent AFib (Tables 3, 4).

Quality of life significantly improved (>50% reduction in LFHQ or SSS score) in 100% of group A and in 75.5% of group B patients in terms of LHFQ, and in 93% of group A and 63.5% of group B patients in terms of SSS (P=NS).

Table 2. Documented recurrences of atrial fibrillation (AF) during follow-up (18 ± 12 months)

	No. of patients *n*	With recurrent AF %
Group A (AFL only)	26	5 (13%)*
Group B (AFL+AFib)	53	20 (37.7%)
*B1 (AFL only)[a]	28	7 (25%)**
*B2 (AFL+AFib)[a]	25	13 (52%)

*For comparison of group A vs group B $p = 0.09$; **for comparison of group B1 vs group B2 $p = 0.04$

[a]After antiarrhythmic therapy

Table 3. Quality of life as reflected in score on the Minnesota Living with Heart Failure Questionnaire (LHFQ)

	Before ablation	FU	Δ	*p*
Group A (AFL only) (N=26)	32 ± 7	7 ± 6	–77%	0.001
Group B (AFL+AFib) (N=53)	28 ± 13	8 ± 6	–71%	0.001
No recurrent AFib	25 ± 12*	5 ± 3**	–80%	0.01
Recurrent AFib	31 ± 10*	15 ± 12**	–53%	0.01

*No recurrent vs recurrent AFib: $p = 0.16$; **No recurrent vs recurrent AFib: $p = 0.002$

Table 4. Quality of life as reflected in score on the Specific Symptom Scale (SSS)

	Before ablation	FU	Δ	*p*
Group A (AFL only) (N=26)	24 ± 11	5 ± 5	–77%	0.001
Group B (AFL+AFib) (N=53)	21 ± 10	8 ± 7	–63%	0.001
No recurrent AFib	20 ± 11*	5 ± 5**	–75%	0.001
Recurrent AFib	24 ± 10*	13 ± 7**	–45%	0.001

*No recurrent vs recurrent AFib: $p = 0.33$; **No recurrent vs recurrent AFib: $p = 0.003$

Table 5. Reduction of > 50% in LHFQ and SSS scores

	LHFQ	SSS
Group A (N=26)	100%*	93%•
Group B (N=53)	75.5%*	63.5%•
No recurrent AFib	100%♦	84%**
Recurrent AFib	50%♦	33%**

*Group A vs group B $p = 0.01$; • Group A vs group B $p = 0.013$; ♦ no reccurent AFib vs recurrent AFib $p = 0.5$; **no recurrent AFib vs recurrent AFib $p = 0.7$

In group B patients without documented recurrent AFib, quality of life significantly improved (> 50% reduction in LFHQ or SSS score) in 100% of cases according to LHFQ scores and in 84% according to SSS scores. Among the group B patients with documented recurrences quality of life improved in a lower proportion of cases (50% and 30%, respectively, for LHFQ and SSS).

Conclusions

Many studies, including ours, have demonstrated that hybrid therapy can eliminate AFib in about half the patients who present with both AFL and AFib before CTI ablation. Better results than this can be obtained in the subgroup of patients who present with AFL alone during antiarrhythmic drug therapy, as the result of prevention of AFib and its conversion to AFL. In such cases our study shows that both types of arrhythmia were prevented in 75% of cases during a mean follow-up of 18 months. In the remainder of patients symptomatic AFib continues to recur after hybrid therapy, but the number of symptomatic episodes significantly decreases.

According to some authors [21, 22], our own study shows that quality of life improves after CTI ablation in patients with only AFL before ablation. However, there is also some improvement in quality of life in patients in whom the hybrid therapy is performed for both AFL and AFib. Specifically, a significant improvement in quality of life (> 50% reduction of LHFQ or SSS score) can be obtained in 93–100% of patients with only AFL and in 63.5–75.5% of patients with both AFL and AFib. The reason why about two-thirds of the latter patients experience a significant improvement in the quality of life though symptomatic documented AFib is eliminated in only half of them, is very probably related to the marked reduction in symptomatic episodes of AFib after ablation.

In conclusion, hybrid therapy is effective in patients with both AFL and AFib. Indeed, it can eliminate both types of arrhythmia in about 50% of such cases, and significantly improves quality of life in about two-thirds of cases.

Unlike pulmonary vein isolation [12], hybrid therapy is not curative; as it eliminates AFL it cannot eliminate the cause of AFib. However, pulmonary vein isolation is a complex and risky procedure, which should be undertaken only in carefully selected patients. As AFL ablation is a safe technique [19], hybrid therapy should therefore be regarded as the first-line therapy in patients with both AFL and AFib.

References

1. Philippon F, Plumb VJ, Epstein AE, Kay GN (1995) The risk of atrial fibrillation following radiofrequency catheter ablation of atrial flutter. Circulation 92:430–435
2. Rothinger FX, Karch MR, Steiner PR, Sippens-Gronewegen A, Lesh M (1997) Relationship between atrial fibrillation and typical atrial flutter in humans. Activation sequence changes during spontaneous conversion. Circulation 96:3484–3491
3. Kalman JM, Olgin JE, Saxon LA et al (1997) Electrocardiographic and electrophysiologic characterization of atypical atrial flutter in man. Use of activation and entrainment mapping and implications for catheter ablation. J Cardiovasc Electrophysiol 8:121–144

4. Levy S, Breithard G, Campbell WF et al (1998) Atrial fibrillation: current knowledge and recommendations for management. Eur Heart J 19:1294–1320
5. Bianconi L, Mennuni M, Lukic V et al (1996) Effect of oral propafenone administered before electrical cardioversion of chronic atrial fibrillation: a placebo-controlled study. J Am Coll Cardiol 28:700–706
6. Riva S, Tondo C, Carbucicchio C et al (1999) Incidence and clinical significance of transformation of atrial fibrillation to atrial flutter in patients undergoing long-term antiarrhythmic drug treatment. Europace 1:242–247
7. Schumaker B, Jung W, Lewalter T, Vahlhaus C, Wolpert C, Luderitz B (1999) Radiofrequency ablation of atrial flutter due to administration of class 1C antiarrhythmic drugs for atrial fibrillation. Am J Cardiol 83:710–713
8. Natale A, Tomassoni F, Fanelli R et al (1997) Occurrence of atrial flutter after initiation of amiodarone therapy of paroxysmal atrial fibrillation. Circulation 96:I–385
9. Sung RJ, Castellanos A, Mallon SM, Bloom MG, Gelband H, Myerburg RJ (1977) Mechanisms of spontaneous alternation between reciprocating tachycardia and atrial flutter-fibrillation in the Wolff-Parkinson-White syndrome. Circulation 56:409–416
10. Delise P, Themistoclakis S, Gianfranchi L et al (1996) Clinical usefulness of slow pathway ablation in patients with both atrioventricular node reentrant tachycardia and atrial fibrillation. Eur Heart J 17 [Abstr Suppl]:271
11. Delise P, Gianfranchi L, Paparella N et al (1997) Clinical usefulness of slow pathway ablation in patients with both paroxysmal AV nodal reentrant tachycardia and atrial fibrillation. Am J Cardiol 79:1421–1423
12. Jais P, Haissaguerre M, Shah DC et al (1997) A focal source of atrial fibrillation treated by discrete radiofrequency ablation. Circulation 95:572–576
13. Pristowsky EN (1995) Tachycardia-induced tachycardia: a mechanism of initiation of atrial fibrillation. In: Di Marco JP, Prystowsky EN (eds) Atrial arrhythmias: state of the art. Futura, Armonk, NY, pp 81–95
14. Bonso A, Gasparini S, Themistoclakis S, Delise P et al (1998) Atrial flutter radiofrequency catheter ablation modifies the recurrence of atrial fibrillation. G Ital Cardiol 28 [Suppl 1]:375–377
15. Nabar A, Rodriguez LM, Timmermans C et al (1999) Effect of right atrium isthmus ablation on the occurrence of atrial fibrillation. Circulation 99:1441–1445
16. Nabar A, Rodriguez LM, Timmermans C et al (2001) Class IC antiarrhythmic drug-induced atrial flutter: electrocardiographic and electrophysiologic findings and their importance for long-term outcome after right atrial isthmus ablation. Heart 85:424–429
17. Sitta N, Delise P, Corò L, Fantinel M (2001) Utilità clinica della terapia ibrida in pazienti con flutter e fibrillazione atriale. Ital Heart J 2 [Suppl 2]:67
18. Delise P, Sitta N, Corò L, Fantinel M, Cannarozzo P (2002) Clinical usefulness of hybrid therapy in patients with both atrial flutter and fibrillation. In: Proceedings of the Symposium on "The New Frontiers" of Arrhythmias, Marilleva, 6-13 April 2002, pp 266–269
19. Fisher B, Haissaguerre M, Garrigues Poquet F et al (1995) Radiofrequency catheter ablation of common atrial flutter in 80 patients. J Am Coll Cardiol 25:1365–1373
20. Lee H, Tai CT, Yu WC et al (1999) Effects of radiofrequency catheter ablation on quality of life in patients with atrial flutter. Am J Cardiol 84:278–283
21. Huang DT, Monaham KM, Zimetbaum P et al (1998) Hybrid pharmacological and ablative therapy: a novel and effective approach for the management of atrial fibrillation. J Cardiovasc Electrophysiol 9:462–469

22. Anselme F, Saudi MD, Poty MD et al (1999) Radiofrequency catheter ablation of common atrial flutter. Significance of palpitations and quality-of-life evaluation in patients with proven isthmus block. Circulation 99:534–540
23. Bonso A, Rossillo A, Zoppo F et al (2002) Class IC or amiodarone induced atrial flutter during chronic treatment of atrial fibrillation. Long term follow up of hybrid pharmacological and ablative therapy. Pacing Clin Electrophysiol 24(II):614
24. Stabile G, De Simone A, Turco P et al (2001) Response to flecainide infusion predicts long-term success of hybrid pharmacologic and ablation therapy in patients with atrial fibrillation. J Am Coll Cardiol 37:1639–1644
25. Rector TS, Kubo SH, Cohn JN (1987) Patients' self-assessment of their congestive heart failure. II. Content, reliability and validity of a new measure, the Minnesota Living with Heart Failure Questionnaire. Heart Failure 3:198–209

Non-Isthmus-Dependent Atrial Flutter: How to Locate and Ablate the Re-entry Circuit

I. Mangat[1], M. M. Scheinman[2]

Atrial flutter (AFL) is a generic term for rapid macroreentrant atrial arrhythmias, presenting a surface ECG with little or no isoelectric interval between flutter waves. Originally, AFL was described as a macroreentrant arrhythmia which propagated in a counterclockwise direction around the tricuspid annulus (when viewed in the left anterior oblique projection). However, with the discovery of new forms of AFL and curative ablative techniques, terminology has become ever-important in the description and definition of these arrhythmias. The goal of this chapter is to establish a systematic approach to recognizing the various forms of AFL, with an emphasis on the role of ablation therapy.

Because the majority of AFLs in clinical practice require the cavotricuspid isthmus (CTI) as a critical part of the arrhythmia circuit, we have categorized AFLs into those that are isthmus-dependent and those that are not. We feel that the more precise anatomic designation is preferable to so-called typical or atypical forms (Fig. 1).

Although multiple papers from various different centres have been published on the mechanisms and treatment of non-CTI dependent AFL, it is difficult to appreciate its true incidence. Importantly, the incidence of various forms of non-CTI dependent AFL may also be misrepresented in the published literature because not all patients with these arrhythmias are referred to electrophysiologists, and of those that are, not all patients with non-CTI-dependent forms of AFL will be taken to the laboratory.

ECG Manifestation of CTI-Dependent Atrial Flutter

CTI dependent AFL is a macroreentrant circuit which propagates around the tricuspid annulus in either a clockwise (CW) or counterclockwise (CCW) fashion (when viewing the tricuspid annulus in a left anterior oblique (LAO) pro-

[1]Department of Medicine, Division of Cardiology, St. Michael's Hospital, University of Toronto, Toronto, Ontario, Canada; [2]Department of Medicine, Division of Cardiology, University of California San Francisco, San Francisco, California, USA

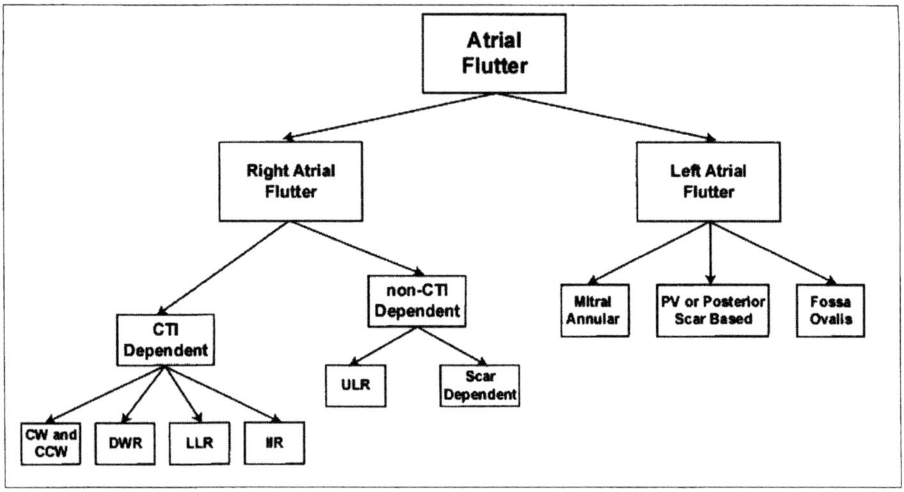

Fig. 1. This diagram represents a useful mechanism-based schematic for the classification of AFL. *CTI*, cavotricuspid isthmus; *DWR*, double wave re-entry; *LLR*, lower loop re-entry; *IIR*, intra-isthmus reentry; *ULR*, upper loop re-entry; *PV*, pulmonary vein

jection). The cycle length of the tachycardia is equal to the time taken for the flutter circuit to complete one cycle around the tricuspid annulus. Thus, typically the ECG shows regular consistent depolarization of the atrium without any true isoelectric period. Additionally, because flutter is consistent from one beat to the next, one finds beat to beat consistency of the flutter wave morphology and cycle length. In general, CCW AFL generates flutter waves that are predominantly negative in the inferior leads, positive in V1, and negative in V6. As expected, CW AFL is the exact opposite, with predominantly positive flutter waves inferiorly, negative flutter waves in V1, and positive flutter waves in V6. This ECG pattern is explained by the sequence of activation of the left atrium, with CCW AFL producing a caudo-cranial activation, while CW AFL is the opposite. Interestingly, though this ECG pattern is relatively consistent, rare patients with CW or CCW AFL will exhibit the opposite polarity of flutter waves in the inferior leads to what is expected [1].

The cycle length of typical CTI-dependent AFL ranges from 200-300 ms, though it may be slower in patients with enlarged or abnormal atria, or those on medications which prolong conduction. Faster forms of AFL should alert one to the possibility of a non-CTI-dependent form of AFL.

ECG Manifestation of Non-CTI-Dependent Atrial Flutter

ECG manifestations of non-CTI-dependent forms of AFL are less well documented. Forms of AFL that involve the free wall of the right atrium, may have

ECG manifestations that are very similar to that of CW or CCW AFL. During left AFL circuits, the inferior leads tend to have diminished amplitude with dominant positive or multiphasic flutter waves in V1 and V2. A negative flutter wave in lead I has also been described in some patients with left AFL circuits [2].

Atrial Flutter vs. "Coarse Atrial Fibrillation"

It is very important to be able to differentiate between AFL and so-called coarse atrial fibrillation. Atrial flutter, regardless of type, usually has consistent beat to beat morphology of the flutter waves, with a regular interval from one flutter wave to the next. It is true, that during transition phases between one type of AFL and the next (especially during unstable flutters, such as double wave re-entry), variability in flutter wave morphology and beat to beat flutter cycle length can be seen. However, atrial fibrillation typically has a much more unstable pattern, and cannot be reproduced in multiple leads. Despite these important differences, the electrocardiographic pattern does not always correspond to the intracardiac signals: occasionally intracardiac atrial fibrillation can have the appearance of AFL on the electrocardiogram, and vice versa, especially if the atrium is diseased and prone to fibrillatory conduction [3, 4].

Mapping Techniques

Before detailing the various forms of AFL, it is important to note that many different mapping techniques are currently available for accurate identification of these circuits. Conventionally, these arrhythmias have been mapped by positioning several multipolar catheters in the chamber of interest to get a general understanding of the arrhythmia circuit. Subsequently, pace mapping is performed to assess for the presence of concealed entrainment (entrainment mapping), which then defines the presence of a critical isthmus of conduction which is part of the arrhythmia circuit [5]. This technique has various limitations, including the need for a stable, easily inducible arrhythmia which does not degenerate upon various pacing manoeuvres which are required for entrainment mapping. Currently, although entrainment mapping is still a critical tool for mapping atrial and ventricular arrhythmias, the utility of multipolar catheters for identification of complex atrial arrhythmias has largely been replaced by various advanced mapping techniques. The ideal mapping technique is one which provides both anatomic and electrical information about the chamber of interest, and is thus able to accurately identify the flutter circuit and the critical isthmus which can then be targeted for ablation. Because detailed examination of various mapping techniques is beyond the scope of this chapter, we have not made an effort to examine individual techniques, but will address the relative merits of certain techniques while highlighting examples.

CTI-Dependent Flutters

CW and CCW Atrial Flutter

Clockwise and CCW AFL utilize the same circuit and critical isthmus, but propagate around the atrium in opposite directions. Together, they represent the most common form of AFL that is seen in clinical practice, encompassing the vast majority of all AFLs. The schematic for the CCW form of AFL, along with representative intracardiac electrograms is noted in Fig. 2. Although both CW and CCW AFL utilize the same right atrial circuit, the CCW form is seen more often in clinical practice.

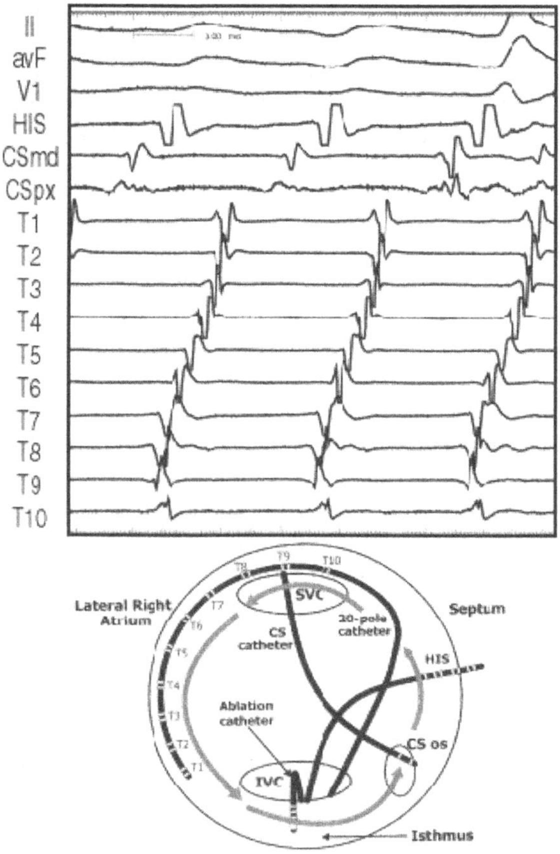

Fig. 2. Simultaneous ECG leads II, avF, and V1 with intracardiac electrograms from the anterior septum (*HIS*), mid and proximal coronary sinus (*CSmd*, *CSpx*), and multiple electrograms from a multipolar catheter around the tricuspid annulus as shown in the schematic. Activation proceeds in a CCW direction around the tricuspid annulus when viewed in the LAO projection as in the schematic, with the *light grey arrows* indicating the flutter course

It is important to understand the anatomic and functional boundaries that allow this macroreentrant tachycardia to persist. It is a very stable rhythm, and can be very difficult to manage with conventional antiarrhythmic medications [6]. The anterior anatomic boundary for the circuit is the tricuspid annulus, while the superior vena cava (SVC) and inferior vena cava (IVC) form the postero-superior and infero-posterior boundaries. The posterolateral boundary is a functional boundary created by the crista terminalis, a ridge of atrial tissue which separates the smooth from trabeculated right atrium, and extends from the region of the sinus node, along the lateral aspect of the right atrium, and continues along the floor of the right atrium as the eustachian ridge.

This form of AFL is readily terminated and cured by creating a line of block (usually by radiofrequency catheter ablation) in the CTI between the inferior aspect of the tricuspid annulus and the IVC. Long-term success of this procedure is dependent on the creation of a complete line of block which does not allow conduction in either direction (bidirectional block) [7-10]. Although multiple methods for detection of bidirectional block are available, no one method will suffice for every case, and it is worthwhile to be familiar with the various techniques.

Lower Loop Re-entry

Lower loop re-entry (LLR) is a CTI-dependent form of AFL, which usually occurs in association with CCW AFL. It involves a breakdown in the functional block which normally occurs along the crista terminalis during CCW flutter. This breakdown allows for the presence of transcristal conduction, such that activation can proceed around the posterior aspect of the right atrium, and reach the lateral wall of the right atrium earlier than would be expected (Fig. 3) [11]. Although lower loop re-entry is readily terminated and cured by the same lesion set that is necessary for CW and CCW AFL, it is important to recognize for several reasons. First, the activation sequence of the intracardiac electrograms can be very different from typical AFL, and can be variable from one beat to the next as changes in transcristal conduction occur. These changes in activation can occasionally lead one to mistakenly identify LLR as a non-CTI-dependent arrhythmia and prematurely abandon the procedure, especially if advanced mapping technologies are not available. Second, after completion of a lesion in the CTI, the presence of persistent transcristal conduction can give the appearance of "pseudoisthmus conduction" during coronary sinus (CS) pacing. Thus, in this circumstance, it can be extremely useful to position a multipolar catheter in such a way as to straddle the CTI, and assess electrogram characteristics immediately medial and lateral to the isthmus lesion (Fig. 4a, b), and thus eliminate the confusion that can be created by transcristal conduction.

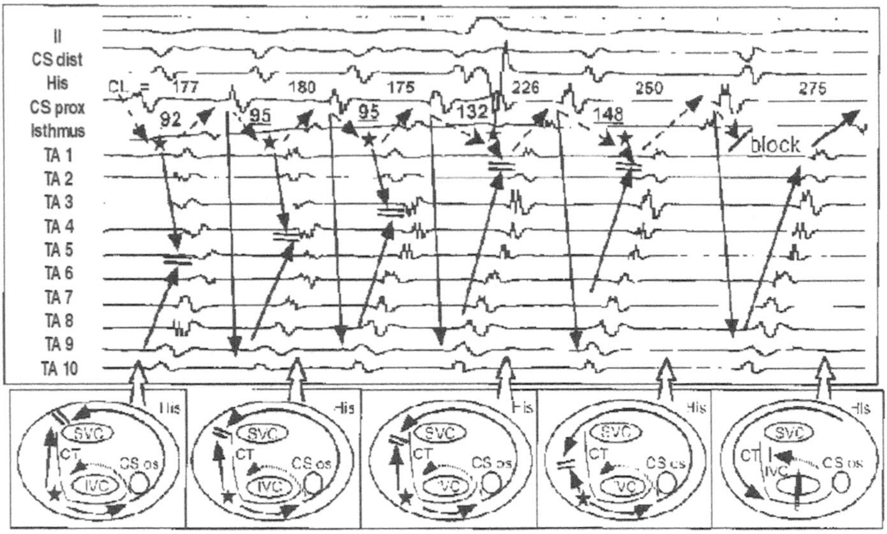

Fig. 3. Simultaneous recordings from surface lead II, proximal and distal coronary sinus (CS prox and CS dist), anterior septum (His), cavotricuspid isthmus (Isthmus), and 10 bipolar recording sites along the tricuspid annulus – TA1 through TA10 (as in Figure 2). Spontaneous reversion of induced LLR to typical CCW AFL. This figure depicts spontaneous conversion of LLR to CCW AFL. Note significant variability of cycle length that was associated with progressive prolongation of conduction time in posterior limb (*dashed arrows*) of LLR (from CS os to TA 1 and Isthmus) before conversion to typical CCW AFL. This progressive delay shifted site of collision (*double bars*) caudally and may represent increasing functional conduction block along the crista terminalis that led to conversion. Difference in local activation times between TA1 and Isthmus was also increased. This can be explained by a breakthrough site across the crista terminalis during LLR between TA1 and Isthmus that led to simultaneous activation wave fronts, orthodromically to Isthmus and antidromically to TA1. On conversion to CCW AFL, Isthmus was activated sequentially by a wave front propagating from TA1, resulting in an increased difference in local activation time. *Stars* indicate site of breakthrough. (From [11], with permission)

Intra-Isthmus Re-entry

More recently our group has described a novel flutter circuit with re-entry confined to the medial aspect of the CTI. During this arrhythmia, entrainment mapping identifies the lateral CTI as being outside the circuit, while the medial CTI and CS os are in the circuit. The CS os appears to act as a pivot point for this circuit. Ablation of the medial but not lateral CTI is curative.

Double Wave Re-entry

Double wave re-entry (DWR) is an entity which occurs during CTI-dependent AFL, and is usually identified by an acceleration of the tachycardia cycle length

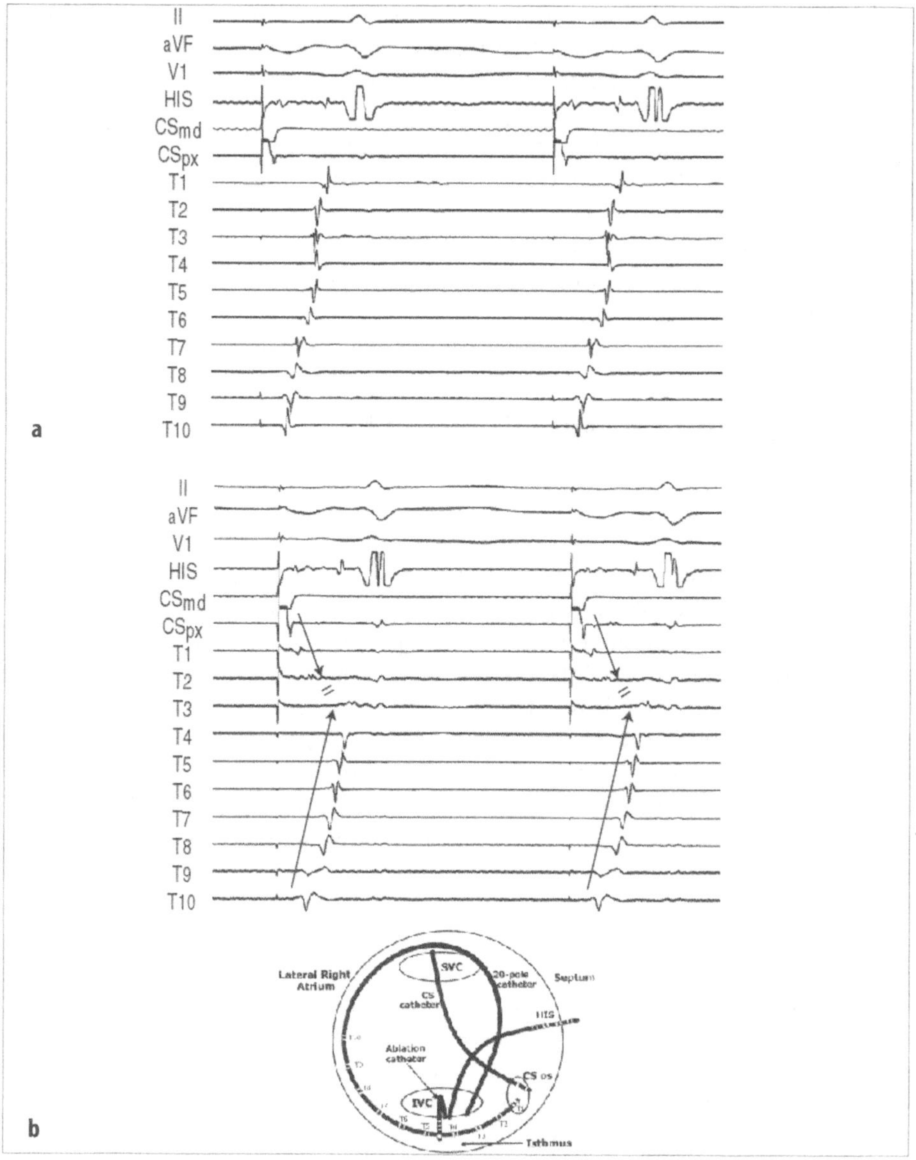

Fig. 4a,b. **a.** Recordings as in Figure 2. With catheters positioned as in Figure 2, after ablation, CS pacing shows that the earliest electrogram in the multipolar catheter is occurring at T3, which is unexpected and may be confused for incomplete isthmus block. Likely, what is occurring in this case is a posterior breakthrough around the IVC and across the crista terminalis, leading to earlier activation of T3 than would be expected if activation were to go all the way around the annulus. **b.** Recordings as in Figure 4a. Now, with the catheter positioned as in the schematic shown, one notes that when pacing from the coronary sinus, activation stops at T2, and lateral to the ablation line (likely at T3), endocardial activation proceeds lateral to medial, suggesting that isthmus conduction is not present, and true block (in the CW direction) exists without a significant change in the electrogram activation patterns around the tricuspid annulus [12]. It is usually initiated by a critically timed atrial impulse which finds the CTI refractory in one direction only, and then allows for two waves of re-entry: one from the original ongoing activation, and one from the new stimulus, until refractoriness is reached and the second wave is blocked, allowing for resumption of the CTI-dependent flutter. This form of tachycardia is usually transient, and may be a precursor of atrial fibrillation [13]. Importantly, because DWR utilizes the same re-entrant circuit as CTI-dependent AFL, the creation of a linear lesion in the CTI to cure the initial arrhythmia will also abolish the DWR.

Non-CTI-Dependent Right Atrial Flutter Circuits

Upper Loop Re-entry

Upper loop re-entry (URL) is a non-CTI-dependent circuit in the upper right atrium, which usually occurs in conjunction with CW AFL or LLR (Figure 5) [14]. During ULR, activation proceeds from the atrial septum, posteriorly towards the lateral right atrium, and then superiorly around the SVC and back to the atrial septum. Meanwhile, the low lateral right atrium and CTI are activated passively, with a collision of wavefronts in the low lateral right atrium or CTI region. During ULR, pacing from the CTI demonstrates a lack of concealed entrainment, proving that the CTI is no longer a critical part of the circuit. If ULR persists after ablation of an associated CW form of AFL, 3-dimensional mapping techniques may be needed to delineate the exact nature of the circuit to allow for ablation.

Right Atrial Scar

The presence of scar in the right atrium, either idiopathic or from an atriotomy during cardiac surgery, may be a responsible substrate for the development of non-CTI-dependent forms of AFL. Usually, these forms of AFL involve re-entry around the scar, usually being found at the lateral or posterolateral region of the right atrium. Recognition of this type of re-entry usually requires advanced mapping techniques, as conventional catheter placement may not readily be able to differentiate this arrhythmia from typical CTI-dependent AFL (depending on the exact location of the re-entrant circuit) (Fig. 6) [14]. These forms of AFL are readily treated by identification of the extent of scar in the right atrium, followed by the creation of a linear lesion extending from one area of scar to another, or extension of the scar to either the SVC, IVC, or tricuspid annulus, thus preventing a re-entrant loop.

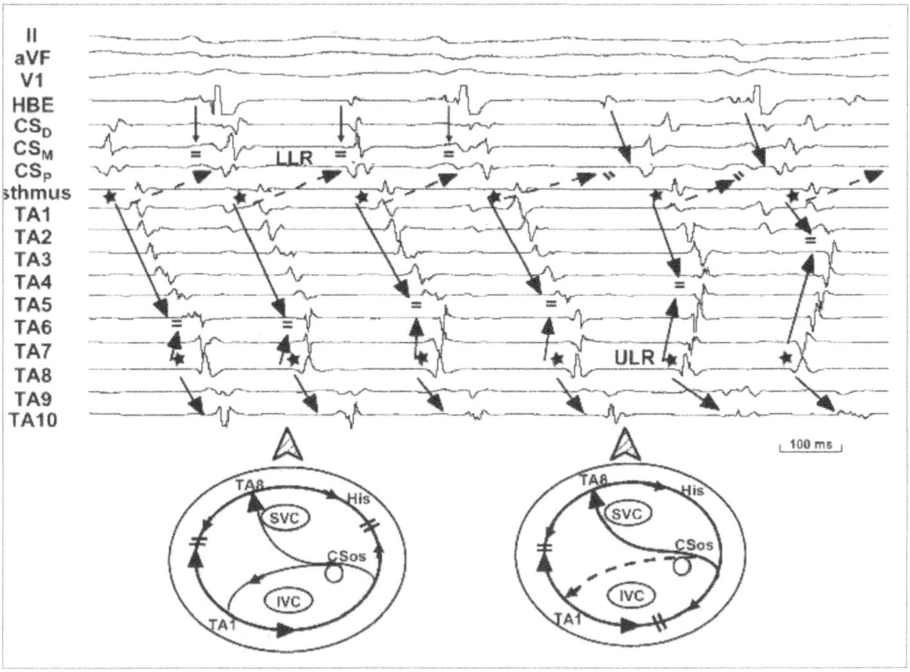

Fig. 5. Simultaneous recordings from ECG leads II, aVF and V1, intracardiac recordings from anterior septum (HBE), coronary sinus - distal, mid, and proximal (CSD, CSM, CSP), cavotricuspid isthmus, and lateral tricuspid annulus (TA1 to TA10). First 4 beats show evidence of LLR with breakthrough at TA1 and TA8. Evidence that LLR is "driver" is shown by increase in tachycardia cycle length (TCL) from isthmus, CS, and TA1 to TA8 as conduction time through isthmus increases (dashed line from TA1 to CSOS). Septum is captured from TA8 breakthrough and is associated with less change in TCL compared with TA1 to TA8. The latter is interpreted as being due to early breakthrough over TA8, producing conduction slowing over upper septum. Note near simultaneous activation of HBE and CSOS during those first 4 beats. After spontaneous conduction block in isthmus (after beat 4), HBE electrogram clearly precedes that from CS, and point of collision moves to area of proximal isthmus. Schematic diagram below, beats 5 and 6, shows ULR pattern with same 2 early breakthrough sites. *Arrows* indicate wavefront propagation, short double lines indicate wavefront collision, and *stars* denote sites of early breakthrough over the lateral tricuspid annulus. (From [14] with permission)

Left Atrial Flutter Circuits

Left AFL circuits are becoming more and more important to recognize, as procedures which involve changes to left atrial anatomic and electrical substrate increase. Such procedures include left atrial surgery for valve replacement or atrial septal defect repair, left atrial ablation for pulmonary vein isolation, and cardiac transplantation.

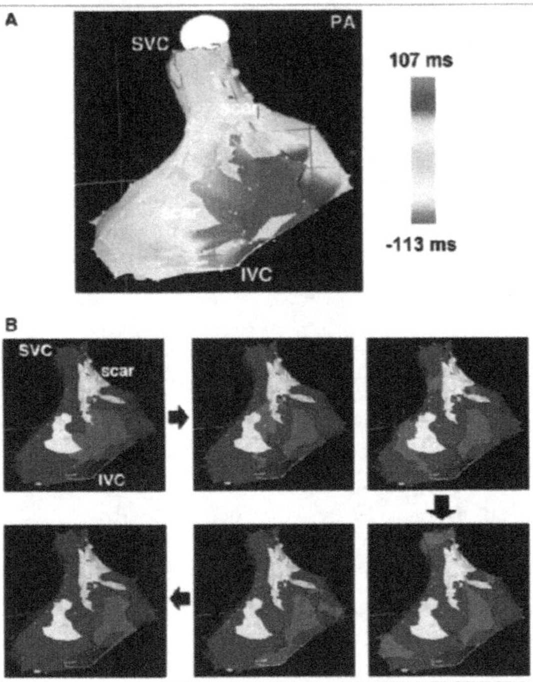

Fig. 6a, b. a. Biosense-Webster CARTO activation map in posteroanterior (PA) projection view shows macroreentrant circuit involving 2 low-voltage areas (scars) along the posterolateral wall of RA. Time scale on right shows that map contains 220 ms of data that were similar to TCL. **b.** CARTO Biosense propagation map (figure arranged in CW order) shows that reentrant wave front goes through channel between 2 scars and spreads over posterolateral wall in figure-8 pattern. Linear ablation between scars terminated tachycardia, and ablative lesion was extended from lower scar to IVC to prevent use of this area as channel for separate tachycardia. (From [14] with permission)

Mitral Annular

A re-entrant circuit around the mitral annulus, in either a CW or CCW fashion is a common form of left AFL, but represents less than 50% of all left AFLs. This arrhythmia may be more common in patients who have structural heart disease, especially mitral regurgitation, although it has been described in patients with an absence of structural heart disease. Electroanatomic mapping using a system such as the CARTO (Biosense Webster Inc., Diamond Bar, CA, USA) mapping system, has allowed accurate identification of such arrhythmias, and is useful for guiding ablation. In the example shown in Figure 7, the electroanatomic map allowed identification of an anterior silent area, or scar, which allowed for termination and cure of the arrhythmia by an ablation line which connected this scar to the mitral annulus [15]. In the absence of such a region of scar in the atrium, the arrhythmia may be treated by extension of an ablation line from the mitral annulus to the left lower pulmonary vein (so called mitral isthmus).

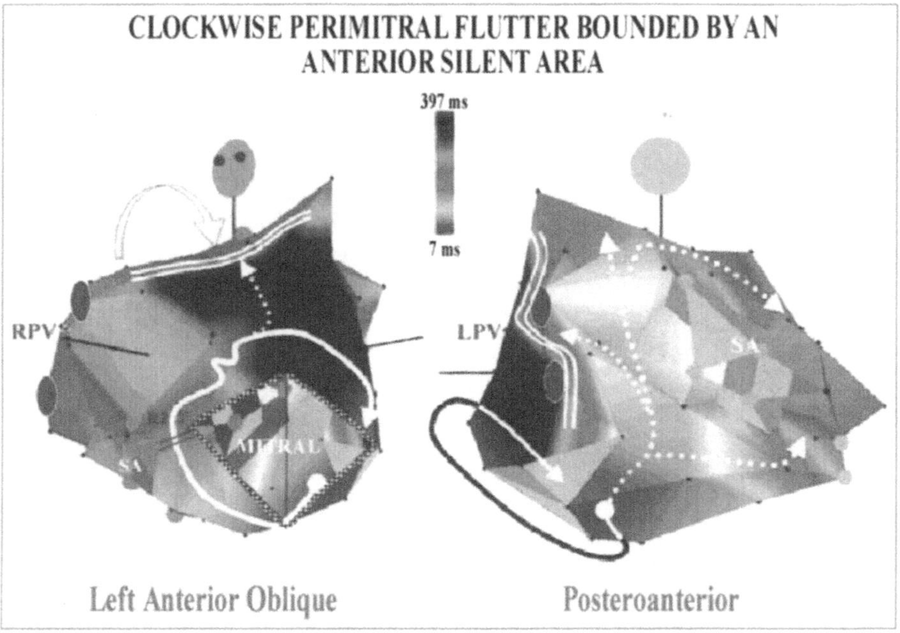

Fig. 7. Two views of the left atrium. In this patient, CW perimitral flutter (cycle length, 400 ms) was diagnosed by 3D mapping system. In this example, the re-entrant circuit was bound laterally by a silent area (*SA*), in gray. Posteroanterior view shows zone of block anchored in left pulmonary vein (LPV) and posterior silent area with bystander activation proceeding superiorly and inferiorly, colliding on its right lateral aspect. Ablation was achieved with a 2-minute RF application to connect mitral annulus to anterior silent area. *Solid arrows* indicate circuit loop(s); *dotted arrows*, passive activation; *double line*, zone of block; and *RPV*, right pulmonary vein. (From [15] with permission)

Pulmonary Vein With or Without Left Atrial Scar Circuits

Several different forms of re-entrant arrhythmias may be noted to involve the pulmonary veins. These circuits commonly occur in patients who are also burdened with atrial fibrillation, although they may also occur as a sole arrhythmia, especially in association with mitral disease. Generally, it is unusual for such a circuit to involve only one pulmonary vein, and typically involves two or more pulmonary veins in association with a region around the posterior left atrium which may be electrically silent. These are often complex circuits requiring advanced mapping techniques to identify and ablate. A schematic representation of the various types of AFL that can exist in the left atrium and involve the pulmonary veins is shown in Figure 8 [15]. Treatment of these arrhythmias generally requires the extension of a line of ablation from a pulmonary vein boundary to another area of scar or anatomic boundary, such as the mitral annulus. Occasionally, depending on the left atrial substrate and

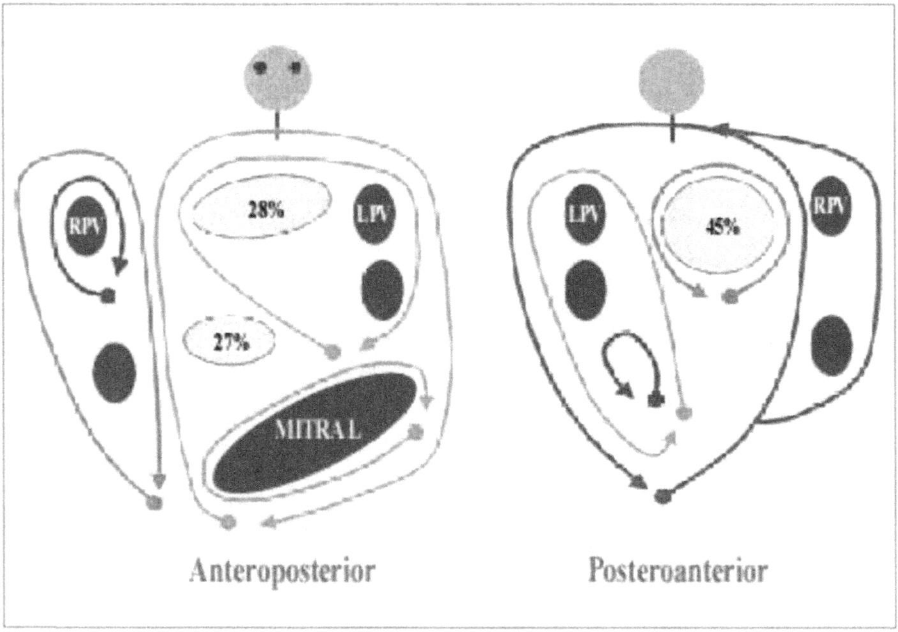

Fig. 8. Schematic representation of locations of silent areas (*light ovals*) and their percentage with various different forms of atypical flutter circuits encountered in the left atrium. *RPV*, right pulmonary vein; *LPV*, left pulmonary vein; *MITRAL*, mitral valve annulus. (From [15] with permission)

presence or absence of previous atrial lesions, termination of the arrhythmia may require electrical circumferential isolation of one or more pulmonary veins. Thus, in these types of arrhythmias, it is also very important to be able to identify regions of scar or electrically silent areas, which allow for development of a successful ablation strategy. This is usually accomplished with detailed activation and voltage mapping of the left atrium using a 3-dimensional electroanatomic mapping system.

Fossa Ovalis

The fossa ovalis is a specialized structure, which consists of a median collagenous raphe separating orthogonal muscle bundles. Re-entrant left AFLs have been described to circuit around the fossa ovalis on the left side of the septum, with the right pulmonary veins serving as the posterior barrier [16]. The region between the pulmonary veins and the fossa serves as a critical isthmus. Additionally, in patients who have undergone correction of atrial septal defects, scars in the region of the fossa ovalis may also be responsible for arrhythmia substrate. Mapping and ablation of these complex AFLs is best accomplished using detailed advanced mapping techniques.

Ablation Procedures and Efficacy

Overall, the efficacy of radiofrequency ablation for AFL depends on the type(s) of AFL, and the rigor with which one pursues detailed mapping. A North American Registry suggests that the long-term recurrence rate for ablation of typical AFL approaches 15 %. However, with newer techniques and more stringent identification of bidirectional block in the CTI, recurrence rates may be as low as 4 % [17]. For non-CTI-dependent AFL, however, the average success rate is unknown, as published papers are typically from highly experienced centres, and may overestimate success relative to general application. In such highly experienced centres, using 3-dimensional mapping techniques for left AFLs, for example, ablation efforts may be associated with as high as a 73 % success rate [15, 18].

Conclusions

Clearly, the most important types of AFL are those that are cavotricuspid isthmus-dependent. These arrhythmias have characteristic patterns that can easily be recognized with conventional electrogram-based mapping techniques, and readily abolished with ablation in the CTI. Non-CTI-dependent flutters, however, are more complex, and typically require the use of 3-dimensional mapping techniques to accurately identify the arrhythmia circuit. Despite their complexity, rigorous mapping still makes these arrhythmias amenable to ablation.

References

1. Oshikawa N, Watanabe I, Masaki R et al (2002) Relationship between polarity of the flutter wave in the surface ECG and endocardial atrial activation sequence in patients with typical counterclockwise and clockwise atrial flutter. J Interv Card Electrophysiol 7:215-223
2. Bochoeyer A, Yang Y, Cheng J et al (2003) Surface electrocardiographic characteristics of right and left atrial flutter. Circulation 108:60-66
3. Leier CV, Schaal SF (1980) Biatrial electrograms during coarse atrial fibrillation and flutter-fibrillation. Am Heart J 99:331-341
4. Knight BP, Michaud GF, Strickberger SA, Morady F (1999) Electrocardiographic differentiation of atrial flutter from atrial fibrillation by physicians. J Electrocardiol 32:315-319
5. Olgin JE, Kalman JM, Fitzpatrick AP, Lesh MD (1995) Role of right atrial endocardial structures as barriers to conduction during human type I atrial flutter. Activation and entrainment mapping guided by intracardiac echocardiography. Circulation 92:1839-1848
6. Natale A, Newby KH, Pisano E et al (2000) Prospective randomized comparison of antiarrhythmic therapy versus first-line radiofrequency ablation in patients with atrial flutter. J Am Coll Cardiol 35:1898-1904

7. Cauchemez B, Haissaguerre M, Fischer B et al (1996) Electrophysiological effects of catheter ablation of inferior vena cava-tricuspid annulus isthmus in common atrial flutter. Circulation 93:284-294
8. Poty H, Saoudi N, Abdel AA, Nair M, Letac B (1995) Radiofrequency catheter ablation of type 1 atrial flutter. Prediction of late success by electrophysiological criteria. Circulation 92:1389-1392
9. Poty H, Saoudi N, Nair M, Anselme F, Letac B (1996) Radiofrequency catheter ablation of atrial flutter. Further insights into the various types of isthmus block: application to ablation during sinus rhythm. Circulation 94:3204-3213
10. Schwartzman D, Callans DJ, Gottlieb CD et al (1996) Conduction block in the inferior vena caval-tricuspid valve isthmus: association with outcome of radiofrequency ablation of type I atrial flutter. J Am Coll Cardiol 28:1519-1531
11. Cheng J, Cabeen WR, Jr, Scheinman MM (1999) Right atrial flutter due to lower loop reentry: mechanism and anatomic substrates. Circulation 99:1700-1705
12. Cheng J, Scheinman MM (1998) Acceleration of typical atrial flutter due to double-wave reentry induced by programmed electrical stimulation. Circulation 97:1589-1596
13. Yang Y, Mangat I, Glatter KA, Cheng J, Scheinman MM (2003) Mechanism of conversion of atypical right atrial flutter to atrial fibrillation. Am J Cardiol 91:46-52
14. Yang Y, Cheng J, Bochoeyer A et al (2001) Atypical right atrial flutter patterns. Circulation 103:3092-3098
15. Jais P, Shah DC, Haissaguerre M et al (2000) Mapping and ablation of left atrial flutters. Circulation 101:2928-2934
16. Cheng J, Steiner PR, Lee RJ, Scheinman MM (1999) Unusual form of atrial flutter utilizing the isthmus between the right pulmonary veins and fossa ovalis (Abstract). Pacing Clin Electrophysiol 22:704
17. Mangat I, Yang Y, Cheng J, Keung EC, Scheinman MM (2003) Optimizing the detection of bidirectional block across the flutter isthmus for patients with typical isthmus-dependent atrial flutter. Am J Cardiol 91:559-564
18. Ouyang F, Ernst S, Vogtmann T et al (2002) Characterization of reentrant circuits in left atrial macroreentrant tachycardia: critical isthmus block can prevent atrial tachycardia recurrence. Circulation 105:1934-1942

Complex Supraventricular Tachycardia Ablation: What Is the Role of Alternative Technology?

M. Tritto[1], R. De Ponti[2], G. Spadacini[1], M. Lanzotti[2], P. Moretti[1], B. Molinari[2], R. Marazzi[2], J. A. Salerno-Uriarte[2]

Radiofrequency catheter ablation is a safe and effective treatment for curing supraventricular tachycardias (SVT), including those related to different forms of atrioventricular (AV) nodal reentry and to the Wolff–Parkinson–White syndrome. Although this treatment is largely considered as a first-line therapy for these tachycardias, under some circumstances the safety and/or the effectiveness of the procedure might be endangered. This review will focus on the difficulties that can be met during SVT catheter ablations, and on the role of special tools and new technologies in improving the success rate and reducing the complications.

Complex SVT Ablations

SVT catheter ablation procedures may be hampered by several factors, including difficult anatomy, complex or resistant arrhythmia substrates, and risky target sites. Early studies reported a 9%–17% cumulative incidence of lengthy or failed catheter ablation procedures in the setting of Wolff–Parkinson–White syndrome [1, 2]. Problems related to catheter manipulation have been reported in nearly 40%–50% of these cases, and they often occur in the presence of distorted anatomy caused by congenital malformations or acquired heart disease. In particular, Ebstein's anomaly [3] and coronary sinus abnormalities [4, 5] are frequently associated with right-sided and posteromedial accessory pathways (APs), respectively. Broad, multicomponent or epicardial APs, often located in the posteromedial region, also represent a challenging situation and account for a large number of complex SVT ablations. Finally, unusual accessory fibers connecting the right or left appendage with the ipsilateral ventricle have been occasionally reported [6, 7].

University of Insubria, Varese: [1]Cardiology Department "Mater Domini", Castellanza (VA), and [2]Department of Cardiovascular Sciences, Ospedale di Circolo and Fondazione Macchi, Varese, Italy

Ablation of some SVT substrates located in the septal area is associated with a higher risk of complications due to their proximity to the normal AV conduction system. In particular, an incidence of inadvertent AV block as high as 10%–20% is reported when the "fast pathway" is targeted during catheter ablation of AV nodal re-entrant tachycardias [8]. Likewise, incidences of AV block and right bundle branch block up to 20% and 57%, respectively, have been reported in early, small series of patients with anteroseptal or midseptal APs [9]. On the other hand, a minimally aggressive approach including low-energy delivery and power titration is nonetheless associated with a high recurrence rate, which can be as high as 26% in patients with parahisian bypass tracts [10].

Role of Alternative Approaches

In order to improve the success rate and reduce the risks associated with some complex SVT ablations, special approaches and or/alternative technologies can be utilized. Provided that the procedure is performed by an experienced operator [1], problems related to catheter positioning and/or stability can be successfully overcome using long guiding sheaths (e.g., in cases of right free wall APs, especially when associated with Ebstein anomaly), or a superior vena cava approach (e.g., in cases of anterior or anteroseptal substrates). The latter approach is also crucial when femoral vein catheterization or catheter advancement through the inferior vena cava is impracticable due to vessel thrombosis or congenital malformations [11]. Posteromedial APs are associated with a coronary sinus diverticulum in 9%-17% of cases [4, 5]. Retrograde coronary sinus angiography allows definition of the anatomy of the posteromedial region and hence could be useful to guide the ablation of these APs. In addition, due to the distinctive anatomical characteristics of the pyramidal space, posteromedial APs are often broad or multicomponent. Therefore, in these cases, a combined approach including right-sided, left-sided, and coronary sinus radiofrequency current applications might be required to completely eliminate the components of the AP. Finally, in selected APs (i.e., those that are epicardial and/or connect the appendage with the ventricle), a transpericardial approach might be considered [6, 12].

Role of Alternative Technologies

Despite optimal catheter position and stability, and detailed knowledge of the anatomical landmarks, some SVT substrates may still be resistant to conventional energies or are associated with an increased risk of complications. Broad, epicardial, or unusual APs might be unresponsive to standard radiofrequency energy delivery. High-power settings and multiple applications may increase the rate of complications (charcoal or clot formation, vessel narrowing, etc.). Experimental and clinical studies have demonstrated that radiofrequency energy delivery through irrigated-tip catheters permits deeper and wider lesions without significantly affecting the safety [13, 14]. In fact, catheter tip cooling (by means of saline flowing through an open or closed circuit) artificially increases the local convective cooling and, hence, the amount of power delivered. A recent study has reported a 5.7% prevalence of APs (most frequently located within the coronary sinus) resistant to conventional radiofrequency current delivery which were successfully ablated by means of an irrigated-tip catheter [14]. However, complications due to vascular injury (narrowing of coronary sinus tributaries) were occasionally noted [14]. In addition, early experimental studies revealed a potential risk of damage of nearby coronary arteries [15]. Hence, this type of energy delivery should be used cautiously and reserved only for selected cases.

On the other hand, some SVT substrates are located in very risky areas or occur in growing young patients. In these cases, a more discrete lesion capable of being modulated or, within certain limits, even reversed is highly desirable. A lesional energy that has these characteristics is cryothermy, which was introduced in the early 1980s for closed-heart surgical treatment of Wolff–Parkinson–White patients [16]. In fact, histological studies have demonstrated that a lesion produced by cryothermal energy is well demarcated and shows preservation of the underlying tissue architecture without thrombus formation [17–19]. In addition, clinical experience has revealed that within certain degrees of cooling the lesion is completely reversible (i.e., no functional damage occurs), thus allowing the operator to monitor the effects (whether desired or undesired) on the target substrate ("cryo-mapping"). Finally, the borders of the lesion are well defined because of the tight adherence of the probe to the tissue due to ice formation.

Recently, cryothermal energy systems allowing percutaneous transcatheter energy delivery have become available for clinical application. These systems have been tested in several arrhythmic substrates with encouraging results in terms of safety and effectiveness, as demonstrated by preliminary reports [20–25]. When the septal area is targeted for ablation (i.e., anteroseptal or midseptal APs, "fast" AV nodal pathway), a very careful approach must be considered, including: (1) accurate mapping on both sinus rhythm and orthodromic AV re-entrant tachycardia (in the presence of APs) to correctly define the area of His bundle potential recording; (2) optimization of the catheter/tissue contact, especially in cases of abrupt changes of the cardiac rhythm (e.g., tachycardia interruption); (3) energy modulation. Regarding the latter two points, when cryothermal ablation is employed, optimal tissue contact is allowed by catheter adherence, while energy titration permits the safety and effectiveness of the application to be monitored before an irreversible lesion is obtained. Our step-by-step energy titration protocol includes a first test application at −30 °C (Fig. 1). As soon as this value is reached, the temperature is maintained for 30 s, during which its effect is continuously monitored. If an interruption of conduction over the target substrate occurs, the same temperature is kept

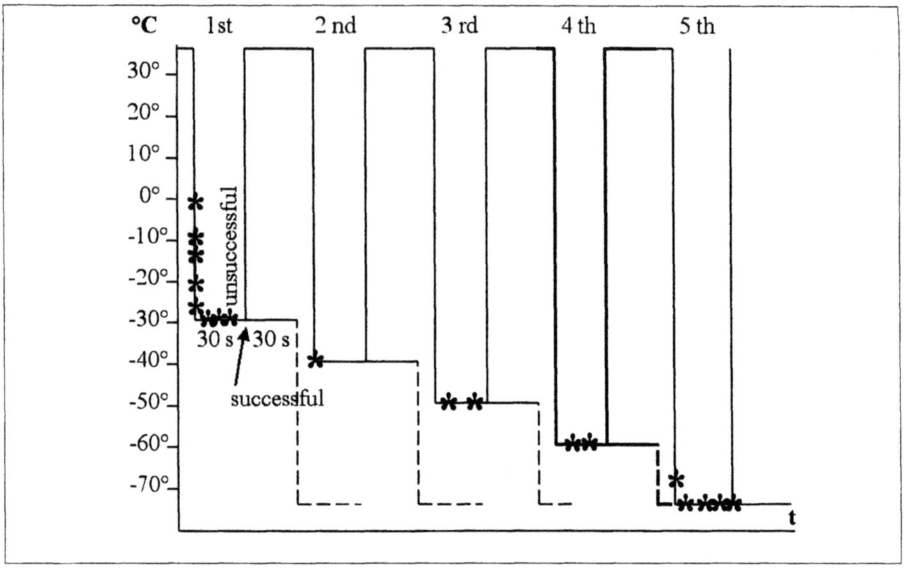

Fig. 1. Scheme for test applications prior to cryoablation. Test applications are made at progressively lower temperatures; if an application is unsuccessful it is interrupted after 30 s, if successful it is continued for another 30 s. Subsequently, transition to ablation at –75°C is made if no adverse effect is noted. Asterisks identify the effective temperature in each patient. *t*, time

for another 30 s in order to evaluate, by pacing maneuvers (permitted by the catheter adherence), the effects on the accessory and normal conduction pathways. If no change in normal conduction system properties is observed over this additional time, the system is switched to ablation mode by reducing the temperature to –75 °C for a maximum of 120–240 s depending on the target substrate (parahisian or anterior paraseptal and midseptal APs, respectively). Conversely, if the first 30-s application is not effective, it is discontinued and, after rewarming, other test applications are performed with a step-by-step drop in temperature from –40 °C to –75 °C and an identical strategy in the case of conduction interruption over the AP. At any time during the protocol, if modification of the normal conduction properties is suspected or observed (Fig. 2), the application must be promptly interrupted and the normal AV conduction system properties tested. Over the last 12 months, 18 patients (10 males, mean age 34±19 years, range 9–66 years) with septal APs (n=11) or typical AV nodal reentrant tachycardia (n=7) underwent catheter ablation with cryothermal energy. In the latter group, five patients had previously undergone failed radiofrequency catheter ablation attempts, and in two of them a "fast" AV nodal pathway ablation was planned. The remaining two patients were of pediatric age. Cryothermal ablation was performed through a 7F, 4-mm-tip catheter (Freezor, Cryocath Technologies Inc., Montreal, Canada) using the

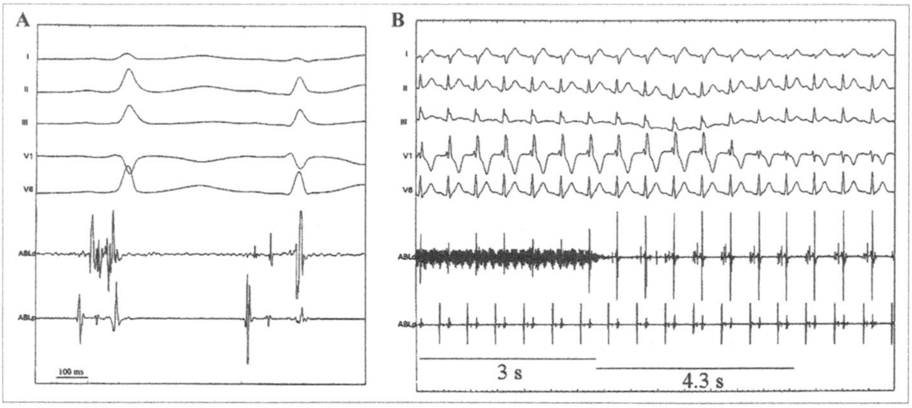

Fig. 2. Surface and intracavitary recordings of cryoablation of a parahisian accessory pathway. From top to bottom leads I, II, III, V1, and V6 and bipolar recordings from the distal (ABLd) and proximal (ABLp) electrode pairs of the ablation catheter are shown. In panel A loss of preexcitation is observed at -20°C; the application is then interrupted early (panel B) because of the appearance of right bundle branch block, which reverts soon after discontinuation of the application

above described energy titration protocol. Seventeen out of 18 patients were successfully treated; during test applications the mean effective temperature was −40±25 °C (with the majority of test applications effective at temperatures ranging between 0 °C and −30 °C), while the mean delivery time at −75 °C was 860±1511 s. In three cases, inadvertent transient damage of the normal AV conduction system was observed (A–H interval prolongation during "slow pathway" ablation in two cases and right bundle branch block during anteroseptal AP ablation in the other), with complete recovery after cryothermal energy discontinuation. At a 9±3-month follow-up, one patient had AP conduction recurrence and was successfully retreated. No significant complications were observed acutely or during the follow-up, thus confirming that this type of energy is safe and effective especially for use in high-risk substrates.

In conclusion, standard catheter ablation approaches and technologies are usually effective in curing the vast majority of SVTs. Nonetheless, in selected cases, the use of alternative approaches and/or technologies are of paramount importance to enhance the success rate of the procedures and significantly reduce the associated risks.

References

1. Morady F, Strickberger A, Ching Man K et al (1996) Reasons for prolonged or failed attempts at radiofrequecy catheter ablation of accessory pathways. J Am Coll Cardiol 27:683–689

2. Salerno JA, De Ponti R, Storti C, Zardini M, Longobardi M (1997) Prolonged or failed attempts at RF ablation of accessory pathways: what are the causes? In: Raviele A (ed) Cardiac arrhythmias 1997. Springer, Milan, pp 166–171
3. Pressley JC, Wharton JM, Tang ASL et al (1992) Effect of Ebstein's anomaly on short- and long-term outcome of surgically treated patients with Wolff–Parkinson–White syndrome. Circulation 86:1147–1155
4. Guiraudon GM, Guiraudon CM, Klein GJ, Sharma AD, Yee R. (1988) The coronary sinus diverticulum: a pathologic entity associated with the Wolff–Parkinson–White syndrome. Am J Cardiol 62:733–735
5. Tebbenjohanns J, Pfeiffer D, Shumacher B et al (1996) Direct angiography of the coronary sinus: impact on left posteroseptal accessory pathway ablation. Pacing Clin Electrophysiol 19:1075–1081
6. Lam C, Schweikert R, Kanagarantam L, Natale A (2000) Radiofrequency ablation of a right atrial appendage–ventricular accessory pathway by transcutaneous epicardial instrumentation. J Cardiovasc Electrophysiol 11:1170–1173
7. Shah MJ, Garabedian H, Garoutte MC, Cecchin F (2001) Catheter ablation of a right atrial appendage to the right ventricle connection in a neonate. Pacing Clin Electrophysiol 24(No 9, PtI):1427–1429
8. Zhu DWX, Maloney JD (1997) Radiofrequency catheter ablative therapy for atrioventricular nodal reentrant tachycardia. In: Singer I (ed) Interventional electrophysiology. Williams & Wilkins, Baltimore, pp 275–313
9. Zhu DWX (1997) Radiofrequency cathether ablative therapy for anteroseptal and midseptal accessory atrioventricular pathways. In: Singer I (ed) Interventional electrophysiology. Williams & Wilkins, Baltimore, pp 253–273
10. De Ponti R, Storti C, Zardini M et al (1999) Ablation of antero-septal and intermediate septal accessory pathways: how safe is it? How can one minimize the risk of A-V block? In: Raviele A (ed) Cardiac arrhythmias 1999. Springer, Milan, pp 185–192
11. Avella A, De Ponti R, Tritto M et al (2001) Radiofrequency catheter ablation of atrioventricular nodal reentry tachycardia: selective approach to the slow pathway via the superior vena cava. Ital Heart J 2:142–146
12. Sapp J, Soejima K, Couper GS, Stevenson WG (2001) Electrophysiology and anatomic characterization of an epicardial accessory pathway. J Cardiovasc Electrophysiol 12:1411–1414
13. Nakagawa H, Yamanashi WS, Pitha JV et al (1995) Comparison of in vivo tissue temperature profile and lesion geometry for radiofrequency ablation with a saline-irrigated electrode versus temperature control in a canine thigh muscle preparation. Circulation 91:2264–2273
14. Yamane T, Jais P, Shah DC et al (2000) Efficacy and safety of an irrigated-tip catheter for the ablation of accessory pathways resistant to conventional radiofrequency ablation. Circulation 102:2565–2568
15. Nakagawa H, Yamanashi WS, Pitha JV (1995) Effective delivery of radiofrequency energy through the coronary sinus without impedance rise using a saline irrigated electrode (Abstract). J Am Coll Cardiol 777–1
16. Klein GJ, Guiraudon GM, Perkins DG et al (1984) Surgical correction of the Wolff–Parkinson–White syndrome in the closed heart using cryosurgery: a simplified approach. J Am Coll Cardiol 3:405–409
17. Fujino H, Thompson RP, Germroth PG et al (1993) Histologic study of chronic catheter cryoablation of atrioventricular conduction in swine. Am Heart J 125:1632–1637
18. Rodriguez LM, Leunissen J, Hoekstra A et al (1998) Transvenous cold mapping and cryoablation of the atrioventricular node in dogs: observation of chronic lesions and

comparison to those obteined using radiofrequency ablation. J Cardiovasc Electrophysiol 9:1055–1061
19. Lustgarten LD, Keane D, Ruskin J (1999) Cryothermal ablation: mechanism of tissue injury and current experience in the treatment of tachyarrythmias. Prog Cardiovasc Dis 41:1488–1498
20. Skanes AC, Dubuc M, Klein GJ et al (2000) Cryothermal ablation of the slow pathway for the elimination of atrioventricular nodal reentrant tachycardia. Circulation 102: 2856–2860
21. Dubuc M, Khairy P, Rodriguez-Santiago A et al (2001) Catheter cryoablation of the atrioventricular node in patients with atrial fibrillation: a novel technology for ablation of cardiac arrythmias. J Cardiovasc Electrophysiol 12:439–444
22. Kimman GJP, Szili-Torok T, Theuns DAMJ, Jordaens LJ (2001) Transvenous cryothermal catheter ablation of a right anteroseptal accessory pathway. J Cardiovasc Electrophysiol 12:1415–1417
23. Lanzotti ME, De Ponti R, Tritto M, Spadacini G, Salerno-Uriarte JA (2002) Successful treatment of anteroseptal accessory pathways by transvenous cryomapping and cryoablation. Ital Heart J 3:128–132
24. Rodriguez LM, Geller C, Tse HF et al (2002) Acute results of transvenous cryoablation of supraventricular tachycardia (atrial fibrillation, atrial flutter, Wolff–Parkinson–White syndrome, atrioventricular nodal reentry tachycardia). J Cardiovasc Electrophysiol 13:1082–1089
25. Riccardi R, Gaita F, Caponi D et al (2003) Percutaneous catheter cryothermal ablation of atrioventricular nodal reentrant tachycardia: efficacy and safety of a new ablation technique. Ital Heart J 4:35–43

Late Atrial Tachyarrhythmias After Repair of Congenital Heart Disease
What is the Mechanism and How Can They Be Localized and Ablated?

R. Mantovan

Supraventricular arrhythmias are often seen in patients who have undergone corrective surgery for congenital heart disease, and they are associated with elevated morbidity. Although atrial fibrillation is a common finding in such patients, many supraventricular arrhythmias take the form of reentrant atrial tachycardia and/or flutter [1–4]. Several recent papers have focused on the mechanisms and the characteristics of these arrhythmias. Because of the clear relationship between atrial reentrant tachycardias and the presence of scars or prosthetic materials they are called 'incisional' atrial tachycardias [5–13]. These arrhythmias can occur more frequently after correction of atrial septal defect, tetralogy of Fallot, Mustard and Senning or Fontan procedures [1–4].

The real prevalence of these arrhythmias is not really known. In small retrospective series prevalences of 32–57% after Fontan procedures [4, 13] and about 15% after Mustard [2, 13] procedures are reported, while in a recent paper an incidence of only 2.9% was reported for incisional atrial tachycardias after atrial septal defect repair [1]. However, owing to the greater prevalence of this pathology, many incisional atrial tachycardia could be expected secondary to atrial septal defect closure.

Mechanism

A reentrant arrhythmia can arise when several conditions are present [14]: first of all a unidirectional block of an impulse, then the presence of a slow-conducting path, and finally the presence of a circuit. Recent papers have shown the crucial role of anatomical conduction barriers (tricuspid annulus, eustachian ridge, crista terminalis) in the flutter mechanism [15]. Barriers are often surgically created in patients who undergo surgical repair of congenital heart disease, and especially in those in whom right atrial incisions are need-

Divisione di Cardiologia, Ospedale Regionale "Ca' Foncello", Treviso, Italy

ed. Experimental models [16] provide evidence of the need for two barriers to stabilize a reentry. Moreover, enlarged and fibrotic atria such as are seen in patients subjected to surgery for congenital heart disease can show several area of slow conduction. All these findings can account for the high incidence of reentrant atrial arrhythmia in such patients.

According to the different scars and anatomical barriers present, several incisional atrial reentrant tachycardias can occur in the same patient; this is the main reason why ablation is difficult and the recurrence rate of these arrhythmias is high.

However, some reentrant circuit patterns are rather recurrent in different diseases [13]. First of all, the majority of arrhythmia circuits are localized in the right atrium. In patients with a history of atrial septal defect closure peritricuspid valve reentry (common flutter) and periatriotomy reentry in the right later atrial free wall are predominantly present. However, a figure-of-eight dual-loop intra-atrial reentry with a loop around the tricuspid valve sharing a common anterior channel with a loop around the lateral atriotomy scar has been described [17] (Fig. 1). In patients, when a Mustard or Senning operation has been performed earlier the isthmus between the tricuspid annulus and the insertion of the baffle is often part of the circuit. After a Fontan procedure, apart from the reentrant tachycardia around the atriotomy a reentry with an isthmus located at the junction of the atrium and the pulmonary artery is often found.

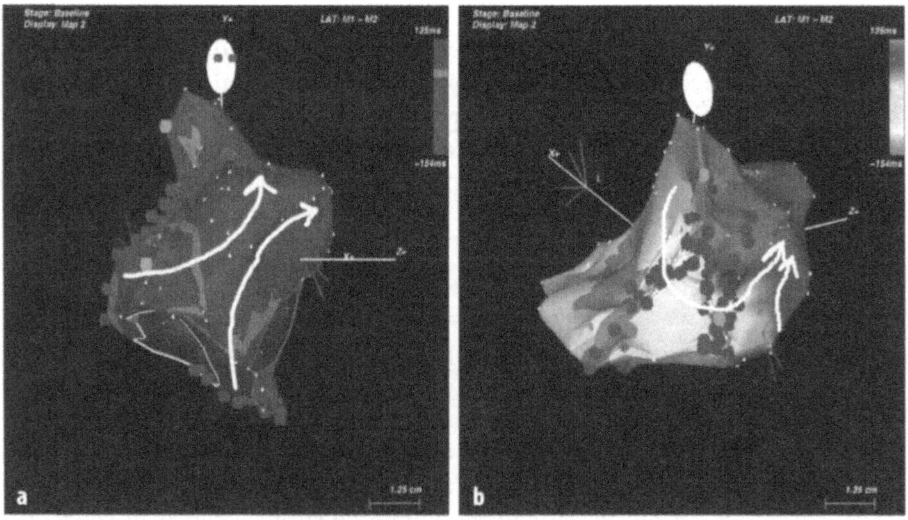

Fig. 1. a Electroanatomical mapping (Carto system) of a reentrant atrial tachycardia after atrial septal defect closure. Propagation map in right oblique view showing two activation fronts creating a figure-of-eight double-loop tachycardia. Ablation of the cavo-tricuspidal isthmus is shown. **b** Activation map of the same patient in a more posterior view, showing the scars and the radiofrequency ablations creating connections between scars and between scars and inferior vena cava

Mapping and Ablative Strategies

Two approaches have been proposed for mapping and ablation of postsurgical incisional tachycardias: electrophysiological and anatomical [5–13]. In the first approach the ablation target is identified by searching for isolated diastolic atrial potential during tachycardia and entrainment pacing is then used to confirm participation within the reentrant circuit. The second approach is based on the concept that incisional tachycardia results from reentry around the atriotomy scar; a linear lesion is created between the atriotomy and an anatomical barrier. This approach is often integrated by the use of a nonfluoroscopic mapping system [18, 19]. Nevertheless, it is common practice for the two approaches to be integrated.

First of all careful and extensive cardiac mapping is necessary to identify the critical components of the reentry circuit. An initial attempt to localize areas of anatomical or functional block and scarring has to be made. These areas are usually characterized by the presence of split atrial electrograms (Fig. 2) or very low or absent signal.

Subsequently endocardial atrial activation is performed during tachycardia, usually by means of several multielectrode catheters (Fig. 2). Recently the use of electroanatomical mapping using Carto system has been developed (Fig. 1) [10–12]. This technique allows reconstruction of 3D atrial anatomy with a nonfluoroscopic system; meanwhile an activation map is constructed.

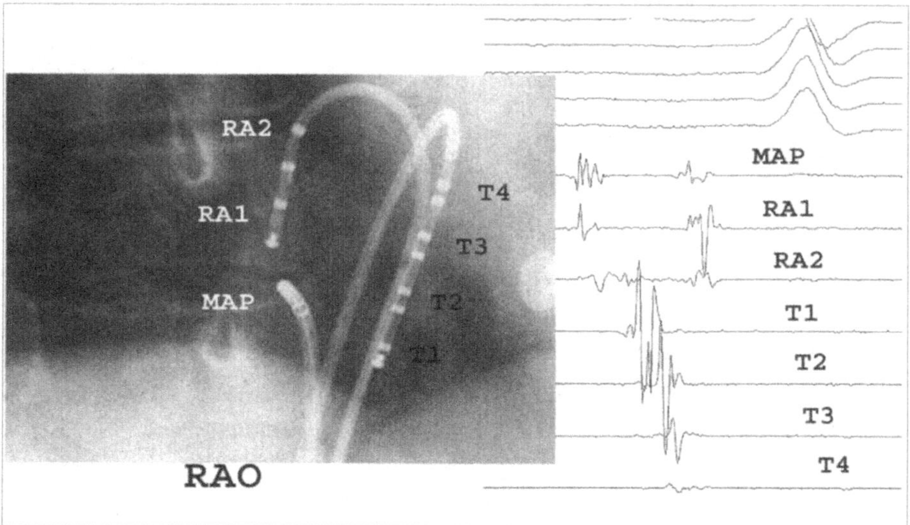

Fig. 2. Mapping of the scar during electrophysiological study. The *first panel* shows the catheter position in right anterior oblique view: T1–T4 catheter lies along lateral tricuspid valve ring, RA catheter and mapping catheter (*MAP*) lie on right lateral atrial free wall. The endocardial bipolar electrograms from RA1, RA2 and the tip of the mapping catheter during low atrial rhythm (*second panel*) show a clear split potential at the point of the surgical scar

The electrophysiological approach requires identification of the critical slow-conducting isthmus of the reentrant circuit. In this area fragmented, low-amplitude, mid-diastolic or presystolic atrial potentials are often recorded. However, the identification of a critical isthmus can be achieved by using the entrainment technique [7]. All reentrant tachycardia can be transiently entrained by fixed-rate overdrive stimulation. If pacing has occurred in an unprotected area of the circuit (outer loop) or outside of the circuit the surface ECG shows a progressive fusion with incremental pacing (manifested entrainment); fusion occurs as a result of atrial activation that occurs in part from the stimulus site and in part from the previous paced wavefront exiting the zone of slow conduction. In case of pacing from a protected area inside the reentrant circuit, the paced rhythm orthodromically propagates to the exit site of the reentry circuit in the same manner as during tachycardia. Therefore, no surface ECG or intracardiac recording fusion will occur (concealed entrainment).

The critical isthmus is characterized by the presence of concealed entrainment and by a difference between the postpacing interval (PPI) and the tachycardia cycle length (TCL) that is less than 30 ms (Fig. 3). The PPI is defined as the time from the last stimulus artifact to the first recorded electrogram at the pacing site. Pacing demonstrating concealed entrainment but a PPI 30 ms longer than TCL can occur in bystander area.

When a critical isthmus is identified, radiofrequency current should be delivered across it to create a complete line of block at that level. This is successful when tachycardia terminates during the application of radiofrequency and is no longer inducible (Fig. 3). Sometimes a successful outcome can be

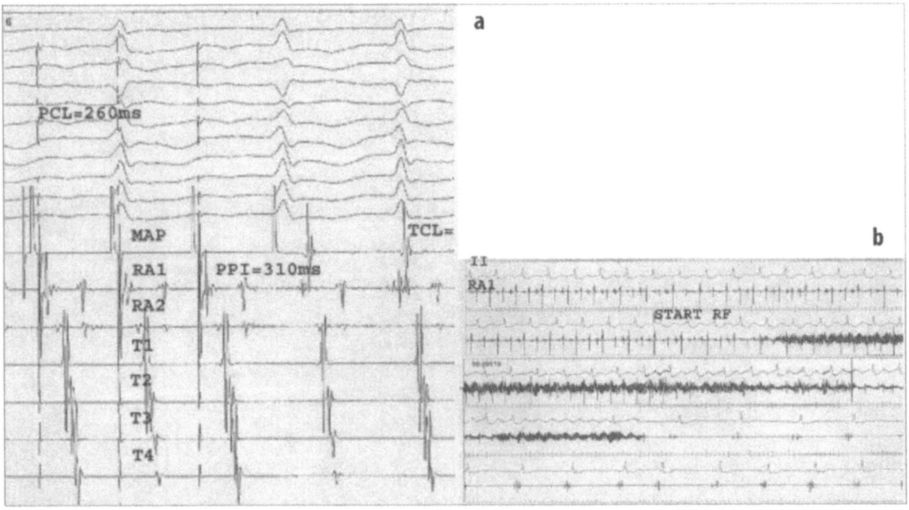

Fig. 3a,b. Same case as in Fig. 2. a) Concealed entrainment from the tip of mapping catheter positioned between the scar (split potential) and the inferior vena cava (PCL pacing cycle length, PPI postpacing cycle length, TCL tachycardia cycle length). b) Radiofrequency applied to the same site terminated the tachycardia. The lesion extended from scar to inferior vena cava

obtained with only a few radiofrequency pulses, but it has been suggested [13] that lesions connecting the surgical incision to an appropriate boundary or linking two anatomical boundaries be created (Fig 1).

Although this approach is often effective, it has several limitations, which should be addressed. First of all, more reentrant tachycardia circuits can be present in the same patient after surgical repair of congenital disease. It can be that during the electrophysiological study some clinical atrial tachycardias are not inducible or not sustained and cannot therefore be mapped with conventional tools. Moreover, entrainment pacing can also terminate or change the tachycardia. Recently Nakagawa et al. [12] proposed an anatomical approach by way of an electroanatomical mapping system (Carto) used to localize all components of reentrant circuit. These authors identified 29 narrow channels between scars in 15 patients. All 15 reentrant tachycardias mapped were propagated through narrow channels. All but one of these channels were ablated in order to eliminate other potential reentrant circuits. They achieved 100% acute success, and during the follow-up only 1 patient had recurrent atrial reentrant tachycardia. Moreover, the authors showed during entrainment pacing that many sites within the circuit, but outside the isolated channel, exhibited a diastolic potential, concealed entrainment, and PPI equal to the TCL. These data suggest extending the role of an electroanatomical mapping system and of an anatomical approach to treatment of incisional atrial arrhythmias.

Acute and Long-term Outcome

Ablative techniques achieve the acute elimination of at least one tachycardia in 73–100% of patients. However, tachycardia recurs after acute success in 7–53% of patients [5–13].

The wide variation in success rates is due to many variables: first of all the selection of patients, who have anatomical differences and different types of arrhythmias, and then the individual experience of each cardiology center. In addiction, the introduction of new ablative and mapping tools could increase the success rate.

Recently Triedman et al. [20] analyzed the factors associated with the result of radiofrequency catheter ablation for intra-atrial reentrant tachycardia. On the basis of a multivariate analysis they showed that independent predictors of acute procedural success were the use of an irrigated-tip catheter and observation of atrial fibrillation before the ablation (negative predictor). The favorable effect of catheter irrigation may reflect the difficulties in creating transmural ablative lesions [21], while atrial fibrillation is likely to represent a marker for a complex arrhythmia substrate and/or more severe hemodynamic derangement. Positive factors contributing to long-term outcome were complete procedural success, use of electroanatomical mapping, and higher right atrial saturation, while the likelihood of recurrent arrhythmias increases with the number of circuits found during the initial procedure. This finding has been confirmed by other authors [13].

Therefore, the long-term outcome of patients affected by postsurgical atrial reentrant tachycardia seems to be connected with the availability of advanced mapping and ablative technology, the underlying severity of illness, and the complexity of the arrhythmias.

In addition to transcatheter ablation techniques, the preventive and curative role of surgery must be focused. Surgical techniques may have a role in arrhythmogenesis. Ebels [22] reported an increased incidence of supraventricular arrhythmias in patients in whom lesions to the crista terminalis were created [23] or two incisions were made close to each other [24]. Bink-Boeskens et al. [25] showed a significant decrease in postoperative arrhythmias after changing the cannulation technique. Moreover, in selected cases supraventricular arrhythmias can be treated during surgery by using endocardial radiofrequency ablation [26].

Conclusions

Incisional atrial reentrant tachycardias after surgical repair of congenital disease are relatively rare and severe arrhythmias. Treatment is often a challenge for the electrophysiologist. A careful knowledge of the anatomy and of the arrhythmia mechanisms is always required. However, the increasing ablative experience and the availability of new mapping and ablative tools can improve the success rate. Moreover, preventive surgical techniques and new intraoperative ablations tools could reduce the incidence of new incisional arrhythmias.

References

1. Mantovan R, Gatzoulis MA, Pedrocco A et al (2003) Supraventricular arrhythmia before and after surgical closure of atrial septal defects: spectrum, prognosis and management. Europace 5:133–138
2. Van Hare GF, Lesh MD, Ross BA, Perry JC, Dorostkar PC (1996) Mapping and radiofrequency ablation of intraatrial reentrant tachycardia after the Senning or Mustard procedure for transposition of the great arteries. Am J Cardiol 77:985–991
3. Kirsh JA, Walsh EP, Triedman JK (2002) Prevalence of and risk factors for atrial fibrillation and intra-atrial reentrant tachycardia among patients with congenital heart disease. Am J Cardiol 90:338–340
4. Durongpisitkul K, Porter CJ, Cetta F et al (1998) Predictors of early- and late-onset supraventricular tachyarrhythmias after Fontan operation. Circulation 98:1099–1107
5. Triedman JK, Saul P, Weindling SN et al (1995) Radiofrequency ablation of intra-atrial reentrant tachycardia after surgical palliation of congenital heart disease. Circulation 91:707–714
6. Baker BM, Lindsay BD, Bromberg B et al (1996) Catheter ablation of intra-atrial reentrant tachycardias resulting from previous atrial surgery: locating and transecting the critical isthmus. J Am Coll Cardiol 28:411–417
7. Kalman JM, VanHare GF, Olgin JE et al (1996) Ablation of "incisional" re-entrant atrial tachycardia complicating surgery for congenital heart disease: use of entrain-

ment to define a critical isthmus of conduction. Circulation 93:502–512
8. Collins KK, Love BA, Walsh EP et al (2000) Location of acutely successful radiofrequency catheter ablation of intra-atrial re-entrant tachycardia in patients with congenital heart disease. Am J Cardiol 86:969–974
9. Triedman JK, Bergau DM, Saul JP, Epstein MR, Walsh EP (1997) Efficacy of radiofrequency ablation for control of intra-atrial re-entrant tachycardia in patients with congenital heart disease. J Am Coll Cardiol 30:1032–1038
10. Dorostkar PC, Cheng J, Scheinman MM (1998) Electroanatomical mapping and ablation of the substrate supporting intra-atrial re-entrant tachycardia after palliation for complex congenital heart disease. Pacing Clin Electrophysiol 21:1810–1819
11. Love BA, Collins KK, Walsh EP, Triedman JK (2001) Electroanatomic characterization of conduction barriers in sinus/atrially paced rhythm and association with intra-atrial re-entrant tachycardia circuits following congenital heart disease surgery. J Cardiovasc Electrophysiol 12:17–25
12. Nakagawa H, Shah N, Matsudaira K et al (2001) Characterization of reentrant circuit in macroreentrant right atrial tachycardia after surgical repair of congenital heart disease: isolated channels between scars allow "focal" ablation. Circulation 103:699–709
13. Anne W, van Rensburg H, Adams J et al (2002) Ablation of post-surgical intra-atrial reentrant tachycardia. Predilection target sites and mapping approach. Eur Heart J 23:1609–1616
14. Mines G (1913) On dynamic equilibrium in the heart. J Physiol 46:349–383
15. Olgin JE, Kalman JM, Lesh MD (1996) Conduction barriers in human atrial flutter: correlation of electrophysiology and anatomy. J Cardiovasc Electrophysiol 7:1112–1126
16. Frame LH, Page RL, Boyden PA, Fenoglio JJ Jr, Hoffman BF (1987) Circus movement in the canine atrium around the tricuspid ring during experimental atrial flutter and during reentry in vitro. Circulation 76:1155–1175
17. Shah D, Jais P, Takahashi A et al (2000) Dual-loop intra-atrial reentry in humans. Circulation 101:631–639
18. Ben-Haim SA, Osadchy D, Schuster I et al (1996) Nonfluoroscopic, in vivo navigation and mapping technology. Nat Med 2:1393–1395
19. Molenschot M, Ramanna H, Hoorntje T et al (2001) Catheter ablation of incisional atrial tachycardia using a novel mapping system: LocaLisa. Pacing Clin Electrophysiol 24:1616–1622
20. Triedman JK, Alexander ME, Love BA et al (2002) Influence of patient factors and ablative technologies on outcomes of radiofrequency ablation of intra-atrial re-entrant tachycardia in patients with congenital heart disease. J Am Coll Cardiol 39:1827–1835
21. Blaufox AD, Numan MT, Laohakunakorn P et al (2002) Catheter tip cooling during radiofrequency ablation of intra-atrial reentry: effects on power, temperature, and impedance. J Cardiovasc Electrophysiol 13:783–787
22. Ebels T (1997) Can intraatrial reentry be prevented by changes in surgical technique? Pacing Clin Electrophysiol 20 [Pt II]:2118–2120
23. Gandhi SK, Bromberg BI, Rodefeld MD et al (1996) Lateral tunnel suture line variation reduces atrial flutter after the modified Fontan operation. Ann Thorac Surg 61:1299–1309
24. Ebels T, Elzenga NJ, Brenken U (1992) Right atrial auricle as inter-caval tunnel in the cavopulmonary connexion: method to avoid the sinus node and its blood supply. In: Minami K, Körfer R, Wada J (eds) Cardiothoracic surgery. What's new in current

practice. Elsevier–Excerpta Medica, Amsterdam, pp 9–16
25. Bink-Boelkens MTE, Meuzelaar KS, Eygelaar A (1988) Arrhythmias after repair of secundum atrial septal defect: the influence of surgical modification. Am Heart J 115:629–633
26. Mantovan R, Pedrocco A, Buià G et al (2002) Radiofrequency ablation during atrial septal defect repair surgery: a new treatment of atrial fibrillation (abstract). Europace 3 [Suppl] abs 238

Late Atrial Arrhythmias as a Complication After Valvular Heart Surgery: Is There A Place for Prevention?

D. Mangino, A. Asta, A. Venturini, E. Polesel, R. Moretti, A. Terrini, C. Zussa

Introduction and Background

Atrial arrhythmias, mostly atrial fibrillation (AF), are the most frequent complication after cardiac surgery. The incidence of postoperative AF (pAF) is 11–40% after coronary artery bypass grafting (CABG) [1–10] and over 50% after valve surgery [11, 12]. Technical advances in surgery and anesthesia and changing methods of myocardial protection have not decreased the incidence of postoperative atrial tachyarrhythmias. While the consequences of this arrhythmia are generally not life threatening (pAF), it can result in stroke, ventricular arrhythmia, pneumonia, and hemodynamic deterioration, especially in patients with depressed cardiac function. In addition, increased length and cost of hospital stay are observed. The underlying mechanism of recurrent AF in patients who are not undergoing surgery appears to be multiple, simultaneously propagating reentrant electrical impulses, or wavefronts, that circulate inside the atria. Less is known about the cause of pAF, for which other arrhythmogenic factors exist. Many factors have been tested as independent variables predictive of pAF, from systemic hypertension to postoperative bleeding, atrial manipulation, myocardial protection, cross-clamping time, excessive production of catecholamines, and respiratory or renal parameters [4, 7, 13, 14], but most have proved to be poorly correlated with the onset of pAF.

Meta-analysis of these clinical reports has shown that age, valvular heart disease, and preoperative AF episodes are the only independent factors that are mildly correlated with an increased risk of pAF [4, 7, 14, 15].

As an estimate, less than 5% of surgical patients under 40 years of age, but more than one-third of those of 70 or older, have postoperative atrial arrhythmias. Age-associated changes in the atria, such as dilatation, muscle atrophy, and decreased conduction, may explain the strong association.

Concomitant valvular heart disease is also associated with pAF. It is not

Cardiovascular Department, Umberto I Hospital, Mestre-Venice, Italy

clear whether this is because of the additional complexity of the surgical procedure required or has something to do with the valvular disease itself.

Some authors have tried to identify the subgroups of patients who are more predisposed to pAF and to treat them prophylactically with such drugs as β–blockers, verapamil, and digoxin [14]. Their results showed only a slight reduction in the incidence of pAF, which was not statistically significant.

Good results were obtained with prophylactic use of amiodarone given i.v. or per OD [16, 17]. We have used oral amiodarone to prevent pAF earlier only in patients undergoing CABG and aortic valve replacement (AVR), in whom it was effective in reducing the incidence of atrial fibrillation. The purpose of this study was to assess the use of short-term oral preoperative amiodarone as prophylaxis against pAF in patients undergoing valvular heart surgery.

Materials and Methods

From December 2001 to February 2003, 128 consecutive patients scheduled for valvular heart surgery were enrolled in the study. The operations performed were AVR (aortic valve replacement), MVR (mitral valve replacement), and mitral valve repair. Exclusion criteria were current AF, previous episodes of paroxysmal AF, treatment with anti-arrhythmic drugs during the year before operation, and any contraindication to the use of amiodarone.

The patients were randomly divided in two groups. Group A consisted of 68 patients (14 MVR, 18 mitral valve repair; 36 AVR) prophylactically treated with amiodarone, 600 mg per day, for 7 days before operation, then 200 mg per day until discharge from hospital. Group B contained 60 patients (17 MVR, 16 mitral valve repair; 27 AVR), who were studied as controls (Table 1). Informed consent was obtained from each patient in group A.

The mean preoperative total dose of amiodarone was 4.8±0.96 g over a period of 13±7 days. All the patients underwent cardiac surgery with a moderately hypothermic cardiopulmonary bypass and cardioplegic blood flow arrest. After surgery each patient was monitored with three-lead telemetry monitoring until discharged from hospital. Patients were checked once a week in the out-patient clinic for cardiac rhythm for 1 month after surgery.

Table 1. Clinical characteristics of the patients groups

	Group A (N=68)	Group B (N=60)
Age (years; ±SD)	57.4±8.4	64.5±7.6
Sex (M/F)	39/29	36/24
NYHA class (mean±SD)	2.6±0.7	2.5±0.6
LVEF (mean±SD)	0.49±0.14	0.51±0.10
CPB time (min; mean±SD)	135±31	119±24
Aortic XC time (min; mean±SD)	89±32	78±36

Results

Clinical results are summarized in Table 2. No significant differences in 30-day mortality and morbidity were found between the two groups.

Postoperative AF occurred in 17 of the 68 patients in group A (25%) and 31 of the 60 patients in group B (51.6%) (P=0.003). In the case of pAF amiodarone was infused to restore sinus rhythm with an i.v. bolus of 5 mg/kg followed by continuous infusion of 900 mg during a 24-h period and oral administration of one 200-mg tablet a day for a month thereafter.

Regarding the type of surgery, pAF occurred at a higher rate in patients who had undergone mitral valve procedures. A higher incidence of pAF was found in patients with mitral stenosis and left atrial enlargement (10 patients in group A and 12 in group B). All these patients underwent MVR.

Table 2. Clinical results

	Group A (N=68)	Group B (N=60)
30-day mortality	1	1
Temporary bradyarrhythmias	4	2
Complete atrioventricular block	2	4
Ventricular arrhythmias	0	1
Low output syndrome	2	3
Prolonged ventilatory support	4	5

Amiodarone prophylaxis resulted in a lower ventricular rate at pAF onset. The duration of pAF was 12.2±7.1 h in group A and 18.2±24.4 h in group B.

Patients in the amiodarone group were hospitalized for significantly fewer days than were patients in the control group (6.5±2.6 vs 8.4±4.2 days, p=0.04). None of the patients discharged from hospital in sinus rhythm showed AF during the month of follow-up after discharge. No side effects of amiodarone were observed, whether the prophylactic or the therapeutic protocol was used.

Discussion

Postoperative AF is the most frequent complication after cardiac surgery, and it has clinical and economic implications. Prophylactic treatment with many agents has failed to demonstrate efficacy in most cases [7]. Only β–blockers (sotalol) and amiodarone seem to have had some positive results.

The administration of sotalol in dosages ranging from 80 to 120 mg is associated with a decrease in the occurrence of pAF [18]. However, pAF still occurred in 26% of the patients treated with sotalol. Moreover, β–blockers may be contraindicated in patients with severe LV dysfunction, chronic obstructive pulmonary disease, and peripheral vascular disease, who make up the population more predisposed to developing pAF.

Intravenous infusion of amiodarone during the perioperative period yielded positive results in preventing pAF, but the side effects, mostly severe bradycardia, warranted discontinuation of treatment in 10–20% of cases [14, 18]. Oral administration of amiodarone allowed good prevention of pAF without significant side effects.

Our earlier experience after coronary artery bypass surgery and aortic valve replacement confirms the efficacy of this approach.

Oral administration of amiodarone also seems to be effective in preventing pAF after heart valve surgery. The difference in the incidence of pAF between the patients who received this prophylactic treatment and the control group was significant (P=0.003), and no adverse effects were observed.

Our results confirm that the incidence of pAF is higher in patients undergoing mitral valve procedures than after aortic valve replacement. The subpopulation with mitral stenosis and left atrial enlargement is more predisposed to pAF.

Prophylactic oral administration of amiodarone also reduced the duration of hospitalization and consequently the cost.

In light of these results we suggest the adoption of short-term oral prophylaxis with amiodarone not only in patients scheduled for coronary artery bypass surgery but also in patients undergoing valve procedures. In patients with a history of mitral stenosis and left atrial enlargement the Maze procedure may be justified to prevent atrial fibrillation even though sinus rhythm is present preoperatively [19, 20].

References

1. Ormerod OJM, McGregor CGA, Stone DL, Wisbey C, Petch MC (1984) Arrhythmias after coronary by-pass surgery. Br Heart J 51:618–621
2. Rubin DA, Niemiski KE, Reed GE, Hermann MV (1987) Predictors, prevention and long term prognosis of atrial fibrillation after by-pass graft operation. J Thorac Cardiovasc Surg 94:331–335
3. Lauer MS, Eagle KA, Buckley MJ, De Sanctis RW (1989) Atrial fibrillation following coronary bypass surgery. Prog Cardiovasc Dis 31:367–378
4. Fuller JA, Adams GG, Buxton B (1989) Atrial fibrillation after coronary artery grafting: is it a disease of elderly? J Thorac Cardiovasc Surg 97:821–825
5. Yousif H, Davies G, Oakley CM (1990) Peri-operative supraventricular arrhythmias in coronary artery bypass surgery. Int J Cardiol 26:313–318
6. Crosby LH, Woll KR, Wood KL, Pifalo WB (1990) Effect of activity on supraventricular tachyarrhythmias after coronary bypass surgery. Heart Lung 19:666–670
7. Frost L, Molgaard H, Christiansen EH et al (1992) Atrial fibrillation and flutter after coronary artery bypass surgery: epidemiology, risk factors and preventive trials. Int J Cardiol 36:253–261

8. Cox JL (1993) A perspective of postoperative atrial fibrillation in cardiac operations. Ann Thorac Surg 56:405–409
9. Pires LA, Wagshal AB, Lancey R, Huang S (1995) Arrhythmias and conduction disturbances after coronary artery bypass graft surgery: epidemiology, management and prognosis. Am Heart J 129:799–808
10. Gaylord E (1996) Changing incidence of atrial fibrillation following coronary artery bypass grafting: a retrospective analysis. Br J Clin Pract 50:164–165
11. Ommen SR, Odell JA, Stanton MS (1997) Atrial arrhythmias after cardiothoracic surgery. N Engl J Med 336:1429–1434
12. Asher CR, Miller DP, Grimm RA, Cosgrove DM, Chung MK (1998) Analysis of risk factors for development of atrial fibrillation early after cardiac valvular surgery. Am J Cardiol 87: 892–895
13. Crosby LH, Pifalo WB, Woll KR, Burkholder JA (1990) Risk factor for atrial fibrillation after coronary artery coronary artery bypass grafting. Am J Cardiol 66:1520–1522
14. Leitch JW, Thompson D, Baird DK, Harris PJ (1990) The importance of age as a predictor of atrial fibrillation and flutter after coronary bypass grafting. J Thorac Cardiovasc Surg 100:338–342
15. Andrews TC, Reimond SC, Berlin JA, Antman EM (1991) Prevention of supraventricular arrhythmias after coronary bypass surgery: a meta-analysis of randomized control trials. Circulation 84 [Suppl III]:236–244
16. Guarnieri T, Nolan S, Gottlieb SO, Dudek A, Lowry DR (1999) intravenous amiodarone for the prevention of atrial fibrillation after open heart surgery: the Amiodarone Reduction in Coronary Heart (ARCH) Trial. J Am Coll Cardiol 34:343–347
17. Daud EG, Strickberger SA, Man KC et al (1997) Preoperative amiodarone as prophylaxis against atrial fibrillation after heart surgery. N Engl J Med 337:1785–1791
18. Pfisterer MB, Kloter-Weber UCD, Huber M et al (1997) prevention of supraventricular tachyarrhythmias after open heart operation by low-dose sotalol: a prospective, double blind, randomized, placebo-controlled study. Ann Thorac Surg 64:1113–1119
19. Jessurun ER, van Hemel NM, Kelder JC et al (2000) Mitral valve surgery and atrial fibrillation: is atrial fibrillation surgery also needed? Eur J Cardiothorac Surg 17:530–537
20. Vogt PR, Brunner-La Rocca HP, Rist M et al (1998) Preoperative predictors of recurrent atrial fibrillation late after successful mitral valve reconstruction. Eur J Cardiothorac Surg 13:619–624

VENTRICULAR ARRHYTHMIAS AND SUDDEN DEATH

Coffee Enhances Sympathetic Activity and Induces Cardiac Arrhythmias: True or False?

G. Zuin, E. Piccolo, F. Di Pede, M. Celestre, A. Raviele

Coffee and Its Pharmacological Properties

Coffee, the most important source of caffeine, is extracted from the fruit of *Coffea arabica*. The basis of the popularity of all the caffeine-containing beverages has been the ancient belief that these beverages have stimulant and anti-soporific actions that elevate mood, decrease fatigue, and increase capacity for work. Caffeine, a methylated xanthine, possesses several pharmacological actions of therapeutic interest: relaxation of smooth muscle, notably bronchial muscle, stimulation of the central nervous system and cardiac muscle, and induction of diuresis. A cup of coffee contains about 85 mg of caffeine and is used as unfiltered (espresso), filtered ("American coffee"), or decaffeinated. The administration of moderate doses of caffeine (500 mg) in healthy, non-smoking, habitual coffee drinkers significantly raises average ambulatory blood pressure during the working day and evening and reduces average heart rate by 2 bpm [1]. Caffeine also increases by 32% the levels of free epinephrine excreted during the working day and evening. In addition, caffeine amplifies the increase in blood pressure and heart rate associated with higher levels of self-reported stress during the daily activities [1]. Acutely caffeine induces an increase in muscle sympathetic nervous activity and blood pressure in non-habitual coffee drinkers, whereas habitual coffee drinkers exhibit lack of blood pressure increase despite sympathetic activation [2]. Because decaffeinated coffee also increases blood pressure and muscle sympathetic activity in non-habitual drinkers, ingredients other than caffeine may be responsible for cardiovascular activation [2]. The consumption of very high doses of unfiltered and filtered coffee increases plasma homocysteine and total cholesterol levels [3]. Hyperhomocysteinemia promotes the atherosclerotic process through endothelial cell damage and interfering with the vasodilatory effect of endothelial-derived nitric oxide. Christensen et al. [3] showed that abstention

Department of Cardiology, Umberto I Hospital, Mestre–Venice, Italy

from filtered coffee reduces the concentrations of plasma homocysteine and cholesterol. The hyperhomocysteinemia is caused by compounds that are not removed in the filtering process. Decaffeinated coffee increases levels of low-density lipoprotein cholesterol [4].

Coffee and Incidence of Coronary Heart Disease

Blood pressure, cholesterol, homocysteine, and stress reactivity elevation caused by caffeine consumption could contribute to an increase risk of coronary heart disease in the adult population. In a study at the John Hopkins School of Medicine, systolic and diastolic blood pressure were marginally higher in those who drank five or more cups a day, but when the authors took into account factors such as smoking, alcohol drinking, weight, and exercise, coffee had little impact on chronic high blood pressure [5].

Some studies have shown that both filtered and unfiltered coffee lead to an increase in cardiovascular morbidity and mortality [6], but others have not [7]. Furthermore, high consumption of decaffeinated coffee (>4 cups/day) is associated with a marginally significant increase in the risk of coronary heart disease [7].

In the Italian population the risk of nonfatal acute myocardial infarction was around unity for coffee intake up to three cups per day (espresso and mocha), but rose to 1.9 for six cups or more per day [8].

Coffee and Cardiac Arrhythmias

In normal subjects a high dose of caffeine (approximately 500 mg) during a 24-h Holter test does not affect cardiac rhythm and rate and does not cause clinically significant ventricular or supraventricular dysrhythmia [9]. Graboys and Bedell [10] suggest that a small proportion of lone atrial fibrillation patients (<20%) is related to coffee intake, whereas alcohol consumption was more frequently associated with atrial fibrillation in this population (47%) [11].

Donnerstein et al. [12] observed a small prolongation of the duration of the QRS (signal averaged) and no change in P wave duration after moderate caffeine ingestion, suggesting that the prolongation of QRS may be a factor in the arrhythmias associated with caffeine. From a clinical point of view, patients with recent myocardial infarction do not appear to exhibit increased ventricular premature beats after three to five cups of coffee [13–15]. In the paper by Myers et al. [13] 300 mg of caffeine was administered to 70 patients 7 days after acute myocardial infarction and continuous ECG recording was performed. Caffeine increased mean blood pressure and plasma epinephrine significantly, but did not increase the occurrence or severity of ventricular arrhythmias. In patients with pre-existing malignant ventricular arrhythmias,

Graboys et al. [16] reported no significant difference in ventricular premature beats or complex arrhythmias. Others authors confirmed these data. Chelsky et al. [17] showed that patients with a history of symptomatic nonsustained ventricular tachycardia, ventricular tachycardia,or ventricular fibrillation, plasma catecholamine and inducibility or severity of arrhythmias evaluated with electrophysiological testing after ingestion of 275 mg of caffeine were not altered significantly. Other authors examined the effect of a high dose of caffeine (900 mg) and reported an increase in pre-existing ventricular arrhythmias in patients with organic heart disease and low ejection fraction [18]. Moreover, in a retrospective case-control study, heavy coffee consumption (>10 cups per day) was an independent risk indicator for sudden cardiac arrest in patients with coronary artery disease [19].

Conclusions

Coffee generally increases the sympathetic activity, particularly in nonhabitual coffee drinkers. Mild or moderate (<3–6 cups/day) consumption of coffee has no significant effect on the risk of coronary artery disease and cardiac arrhythmias. Heavy coffee drinkers (>6 cups/day) have an increased risk of coronary artery disease, ventricular arrhythmias, and sudden cardiac arrest.

The American Heart Association and American Medical Association agree that drinking a few cups of coffee a day will not harm most people. Thomas Graboys and Susanna Bedell [10] in an editorial in *American Heart Journal* concluded that some people are more sensitive to caffeine than others and may feel that it "affects" their hearts, and suggest that "common sense once again dictates that if coffee bothers you, don't drink it; otherwise why should we physicians, as we all too often do, modify life's pleasures without a sound basis of scientific accuracy to do so?"

References

1. Lane JD, Pieper CF, Phillips-Bute BG, Bryant E, Kuhn CM (2002) Caffeine affects cardiovascular and neuroendocrine activation at work and home. Psychosom Med 64:595–603
2. Corti R , Binggeli C, Sudano I et al (2002) Coffee acutely increases sympathetic nerve activity and blood pressure independently of caffeine content. Role of habitual versus nonhabitual drinking. Circulation 106:2935–2940
3. Christensen B, Mosdol A, Retterstol L, Landaas S, Thelle DS (2001) Abstention from filtered coffee reduces the concentrations of plasma homocysteine and serum cholesterol–a randomized controlled trial. Am Clin Nutr 74:302–307
4. Bak A, Grobbee DE (1989) The effect on serum cholesterol levels of coffee brewed by filtering or boiling. N Engl J Med 321:1432–1437
5. Klag MJ, Wang NY, Meoni LA et al (2002) Coffee intake and risk of hypertension. Arch Intern Med 162:657–662

6. LaCroix A, Mead LA, Liang KY, Bedell C, Pearson TA (1986) Coffee consumption and the incidence of coronary heart disease. N Engl J Med 315:977–982
7. Grobbee DE, Rimm EB, Giovannucci E et al (1990) Coffee, caffeine, and cardiovascular disease in men. N Engl J Med 323:1026–1032
8. Tavani A, Bertuzzi M, Negri E, Sorbara L, La Vecchia C (2001) Alcohol, smoking, coffee and risk of non-fatal acute myocardial infarction in Italy. Eur J Epidemiol 17:1131–1137
9. Newcombe PF, Renton KW, Rautaharju PM, Spencer CA, Montague TJ (1988) High-dose caffeine and cardiac rate and rhythm in normal subjects. Chest 94:90–94
10. Graboys TB, Bedell SE (1998) Caffeine ingestion: yet another wake-up call? Am Heart J 136:574–575
11. Wilhelmsen L, Rosengren A, Lappas G (2001) Hospitalizations for atrial fibrillation in the general male population: morbidity and risk factors. J Intern Med 250:382–389
12. Donnerstein RL,Zhu D, Samson R et al (1998) Acute effects of caffeine ingestion upon signal averaged electrocardiograms. Am Heart J 136:643–646
13. Myers MG, Harris L, Leenen FHH, Grant DM (1987) Caffeine as a possible cause of ventricular arrhythmias during the healing phase of acute myocardial infarction. Am J Cardiol 59:1024–1028
14. Myers MG, Harris L (1990) High dose caffeine and ventricular arrhythmias. Can J Cardiol 6:95–98
15. Lynn LA, Kissinger JF (1992) Coronary precautions: should caffeine be restricted in patients after myocardial infarction? Heart Lung 21:365–371
16. Graboys TB, Blatt CM, Lown B (1989) The effect of caffeine on ventricular ectopic activity in patients with malignant ventricular arrhythmia. Arch Intern Med 149:637–639
17. Chelsky LB, Cutler JE, Griffith K et al (1990) Caffeine and ventricular arrhythmias. An electrophysiological approach. JAMA 264:2236–2240
18. Harris S, Hill R, Varaghese A et al (1989) Caffeine is proarrhythmic in patients with organic heart disease. J Am Coll Cardiol 13:32A
19. de Vreede-Swagemakers JJ, Gorgels AP, Weijenberg MP et al (1999) Risk indicators for out of hospital cardiac arrest in patients with coronary artery disease. J Clin Epidemiol 52:601–607

Is the Cause of Arrhythmogenic Right Ventricular Cardiomyopathy Congenital or Acquired?

C. Basso[1], A. Rampazzo[2], B. Bauce[3], F. Calabrese[1], G. Danieli[2], A. Nava[3], M. Valente[1], G. Thiene[1]

Arrhythmogenic right ventricular cardiomyopathy/dysplasia (ARVC/D) is a myocardial disease in which the myocardium of the right ventricular free wall is partially or almost entirely replaced by fatty or fibrofatty tissue [1–3]. The process begins at the epicardium and gradually extends through the myocardium towards the subendocardium. The anterior right ventricular outflow tract, the apex, and the inferoposterior wall are the most frequently affected sites, constituting the so-called "triangle of dysplasia" [4]. Histological examination of affected myocardial tissue demonstrates residual myocytes interspersed among adipocytes and fibrous tissue, providing a substrate for ventricular arrhythmias that may range from asymptomatic premature ventricular beats to ventricular tachycardia, which is typically of left bundle branch block morphology, merging into ventricular fibrillation. Sudden cardiac death may be the first manifestation of the disease, particularly during effort [2]. The left ventricle may be involved with disease progression accounting for heart failure [3–5].

Despite the advances in our knowledge of the morphological substrates, natural history, clinical diagnosis, antiarrhythmic therapy and preventive strategies, the etiopathogenesis of ARVC/D remains a matter of debate. In other words it is still a source of controversy whether the absence of the right ventricular myocardium is a congenital or an acquired phenomenon. In the past 10 years, progress in molecular genetics has helped to refine our understanding of this disorder.

Nomenclature and Nosology

The different etiopathogenetic hypotheses are reflected in the many eponyms and misnomers which have been used in the past to denote this disease.

Institutes of [1]Pathology, [2]Biology, and [3]Cardiology, University of Padua Medical School, Italy

ARVC/D is an old morbid entity known under various terminologies, such as, among others, parchment heart, Uhl's disease, right ventricular hypoplasia or aplasia, and auricularization of the right ventricular pressure curve [6–9]. The term "right ventricular dysplasia" was introduced by Frank et al. in late 1970s [10]. In 1982 Marcus et al. [4] demonstrated the peculiar fatty histological composition of the right ventricular free wall due to a nonischemic myocardial disease. In the 1980s Nava et al. [11] started observing familial cases of ARVC/D and showed that the condition was consistent with a genetic pattern of autosomal dominance with variable penetrance and polymorphic clinical presentation, from occult forms to overt congestive heart failure. A familial occurrence is now reported in up to 30–50% of cases in different series. Since the first pathology report of sudden death in the young and athletes due to ARVC/D by Thiene and coworkers [2], it appeared evident that the morbid process of fibrofatty replacement confined to the right ventricle was more consistent with an acquired myocardial atrophy than with a congenital absence of the myocardium, and thus the term "right ventricular cardiomyopathy" was introduced [2]. Finally ARVC/D was included in the revised WHO classification of cardiomyopathies [12].

Etiopathogenesis

Insights from Morphological Studies

Myocardial absence in the right ventricular free wall, with or without left ventricular involvement, is the key histopathological feature of ARVC/D [2, 3]. Morphological investigations have clearly demonstrated that the morphological substrate is in keeping with a dynamic, acquired, and progressive process, with evidence of ongoing myocyte death and inflammation as well as various stages of healing (i.e., active and replacement-type fibrosis) [3, 5, 13].

Congenital absence of the right ventricular myocardium, like that observed in Uhl's disease, was first postulated, thus justifying the use of the term "aplasia" or "hypoplasia" (anomalous cell composition of an organ or tissue due to, respectively, absent or defective development) and "dysplasia" (anomalous cell composition of an organ or tissue due to maldevelopment) [14]. However, clinical and pathological findings indicate that the pathobiology of ARVC/D consists of acquired progressive loss of the right ventricular myocardium with fatty or fibrofatty replacement, as a consequence of an unknown myocardial injury and repair process [3, 5]. In particular, study of a large number of family members demonstrated that onset of the disease in infancy is exceptional, the peak being in the age group of 16–35 years [15]. At the same time, in the experience of juvenile sudden death collected over a 30-year period, only one case of ARVC/D occurred below the age of 10 [16].

Genetically determined atrophy (dystrophy) is in keeping with the familial occurrence, which has been reported in up to 30–50% of cases in different

ARVC/D series. In almost all families, ARVC/D is transmitted with an autosomal dominant pattern [16]. Potential candidates included cytoskeleton protein encoding genes, ion channels encoding protein genes, apoptosis, and viral receptor genes. Nine genetic loci associated with this disease have been ascertained so far by genetic linkage or candidate gene analysis [17–25], and mutations in genes at three loci have now been discovered [25–27] (Table 1). In accordance with the genetic background, the term "myocardial dystrophy" appears more appropriate as indicating the pathogenetic process that is implicated in ARVC/D, like Duchenne's or Becker's skeletal muscle dystrophies, which are also characterized by peripheral muscle atrophy with fatty infiltration. The recent discovery of the involvement of desmosomal protein mutations (see below) in both a recessive and a dominant variant of ARVC/D suggests that at least some forms of ARVC/D might result from cytoskeletal protein defects with cell-to-cell signaling abnormalities, intercellular disruption, cell death, and fibrofatty replacement.

Myocarditis and programmed cell death (apoptosis) are frequent observations in ARVC/D. However, it is not clear whether these processes are primary or reactive phenomena.

Table 1. Genetics of ARVC/D

Author	Year	ARVC type	Mode of transmission	Chromosome locus	Gene defect
Rampazzo et al. [17]	1994	ARVD1	Autosomal dominant	14q23–q24	Unknown
Rampazzo et al. [18] Tiso et al. [27]	1995 2001	ARVD2	Autosomal dominant	1q42–q43	Ryr2
Severini et al. [19]	1996	ARVD3	Autosomal dominant	14q12–q22	Unknown
Rampazzo et al. [20]	1997	ARVD4	Autosomal dominant	2q32.1–q32.2	Unknown
Ahmad et al. [21]	1998	ARVD5	Autosomal dominant	3p23	Unknown
Li et al. [22]	1999	ARVD6	Autosomal dominant	10p12–p14	Unknown
Melberg et al. [23]	1999	ARVD7 + myopathy	Autosomal dominant	10q22.3	Unknown
Coonar et al. [24]	1998	Naxos disease, ARVC + palmoplantar	Autosomal recessive	17q21	Plakoglobin
McKoy et al. [26]	2000	keratosis			
Rampazzo et al. [25]	2003	ARVD8	Autosomal dominant	6p24	Desmoplakin

As for inflammatory infiltrates, they have been demonstrated at post mortem in up to two-thirds of cases, especially in the fibrofatty variant, and mainly consist of T-lymphocytes and macrophages [3, 13]. The availability of a spontaneous animal model is also contributing to improvements in insights into the etiopathogenesis of the disease. Evidence of myocardial injury and repair in the setting of myocarditis and apoptosis was recently found at histology in a feline spontaneous animal model of ARVC/D [28], all features in keeping with an inflammatory pathogenesis.

Several inflammatory hypotheses have been advanced: infective, toxic, and immunological. The role of humoral autoimmunity was ruled out by assessment using indirect immunofluorescence of the circulating organ antibodies [29]. In contrast to this, the experiments of Matsumori and Kawai on viral myocarditis in mice, demonstrating the development of right ventricular aneurysms, suggested a pathogenetic role for viral infection in ARVC/D [30].

The role of infectious agents was first advanced in the setting of sporadic cases, suggesting that ARVC/D is a sequela of myocarditis, like some forms of nonfamilial dilated cardiomyopathy. This hypothesis prompted several authors to test the role of cardiotropic viruses as potential etiological agents (Table 2). After the first evidence in 1998 of coxsackievirus B3 in the myocardium of some ARVC/D patients [31], Calabrese et al. did not find any positivity for enteroviral genome in a consecutive series of 20 ARVC/D patients investigated by endomyocardial biopsy [32]. On the contrary, more recently Bowles et al. [33] reported a 59% positivity for cardiotropic viruses, including both enterovirus and adenovirus, among 12 patients with sporadic ARVC/D. At all events, it is unclear whether the detection of viruses represents a cause and effect relationship or whether the diseased myocardium is more prone to virus infection. In the latter instance, the detection of viruses may simply be a marker of the pathological changes occurring in the underlying damaged myocardium which explain an increased susceptibility to infection with cardiotropic viruses. The theory of a superimposed infection upon a diseased myocardium is supported by the work of Diong and Knowlton [34], who demonstrated that dystrophin-deficient mice with increased disruption of the sarcolemma are more susceptible to enterovirus infection of the myocardium and the onset of virus-induced cardiomyopathy.

Table 2. Viral detection in ARVC/D series

Author	Year	No. of ARVC patients	Percentage with viral myocarditis	Virus type
Grumbach et al. [31]	1998	8	37	Entero
Calabrese et al. [32]	2000	20	0	–
Bowles et al. [33]	2002	12	59	Entero, adeno

However, since myocarditis has been found in members of the same family with ARVC/D [35, 36], the hypothesis of a genetic predisposition to viral infection in familial ARVC/D must be considered. Viral infection may act as an external trigger, and a genetic defect of viral receptor protein, which many viruses share, may result in increased susceptibility to viral infection and inflammation with myocardial injury and fibrofatty replacement.

Myocardial apoptosis has been discussed as another potential mechanism of myocardial atrophy and subsequent replacement by fatty or fibrofatty tissue in ARVC/D. Following initial findings by James [37] apoptosis was reported either in postmortem specimens [38] or in endomyocardial biopsy samples of ARVC/D patients [39]. In the latter investigation, a particularly high apoptotic index was found in those with a recent onset or acute bursts of symptoms or signs.

Because inflammation and apoptosis may be triggered by several factors which have been implicated in the ARVC/D etiopathogenesis (e.g., catecholamine stress, mechanical stretch, viruses, disruption of cell adhesion, or intracellular calcium overload), it is possible that they could be regarded as secondary phenomena rather than as primary disease mechanisms.

Insights from Molecular Genetics

Nine genetic loci associated with this disease have been ascertained and mutations in genes at three loci have now been discovered [17–27]. These genetic studies have shed light on some of the pathogenetic mechanisms. Mutations in genes encoding desmoplakin (DSP) and junctional plakoglobin (JUP) suggest that structural abnormalities at cell–cell junctions may promote cardiac myocyte death (injury), with the repair process consisting of replacement by adipose and fibrous tissue [25, 26]. On the other hand, mutations in the gene encoding the cardiac ryanodine receptor (Ryr2) suggest that cytoplasmic calcium overload may lead not only to arrhythmias characteristic of ARVC/D, but also to structural changes [27]. Many of the unanswered questions concerning the pathogenesis of ARVC/D will be clarified only by the identification of other genes associated with this disease.

One potential mechanism of ARVC/D, myocyte loss secondary to metabolic or ultrastructural defects (genetically determined atrophy or dystrophy), would be analogous to that implicated in many inherited forms of dilated cardiomyopathy. The identification of genetic mutations in DSP and JUP, in patients with the typical autosomal dominant ARVC/D (ARVD8) and in the recessive variant of ARVC/D associated with nonepidermolytic palmoplantar keratoderma and woolly hair (Naxos disease), respectively, is consistent with this mechanism [25, 26]. JUP is a cytoplasmic protein which is a submembranous constituent of cell–cell adhering junctions (i.e., desmosomal and adherent junctions) and participates in bridging the intermediate filament and the intracellular actin to the transmembrane complexes which connect adjacent cells.

DSP is also a constituent of the desmosome, anchoring intermediate filaments to the plasma membrane. Therefore, both proteins are essential for maintaining tissue integrity and have a structural function similar to other proteins implicated in dilated cardiomyopathy.

A homozygous two-base pair deletion (TG) in the gene encoding JUP was identified on chromosome 17q21 in the recessive ARVC/D variant of Naxos disease, resulting in a frameshift and premature termination of the protein [26]. More recently, an S299R mutation in exon 7 of DSP was demonstrated in a family with typical autosomal dominant ARVC/D (ARVD8); as a consequence, a protein kinase C phosphorylation site involved in plakoglobin binding and in clustering of desmosomal cadherin–plakoglobin complexes is disrupted [25]. To further emphasize the parallels between ARVC/D and dilated cardiomyopathy, a single base pair deletion in DSP was found in a family with autosomal recessive dilated cardiomyopathy, associated with keratoderma and woolly hair (so-called "Carvajal syndrome") [40]. Thus, at least in some variants of ARVC/D, a degenerative mechanism similar to that observed in dilated cardiomyopathy appears to be involved. The pathogenetic cascade of events should start with the altered integrity of cell–cell junctions, followed by myocyte death and a repair process consisting of replacement of dead myocytes by fatty and fibrous tissue.

A second step forwards in the understanding of the etiopathogenesis of the disease occurred with the identification of mutations in the cardiac Ryr2 gene leading to ARVD2, a variant of ARVC/D which is associated with effort-dependent polymorphic ventricular arrhythmias [27]. This polypeptide monomer is part of a homotetrameric membrane-spanning calcium channel on the sarcoplasmic reticulum and interacts with four regulatory 12-kDa FK-506 binding proteins (FKBP12.6). This channel plays a key role in excitation–contraction coupling and intracellular calcium homeostasis within the cardiac myocyte. Six distinct missense mutations in different families have been identified so far [41]. Interestingly, mutations in the Ryr2 gene have been identified in families with isolated catecholaminergic polymorphic ventricular tachycardia transmitted in an autosomal dominant pattern and no evidence of structural heart disease [42–44]. In other words, it is thus clear that two disorders, ARVC/D and catecholaminergic polymorphic ventricular tachycardia, can result from mutations in the same gene. An intriguing question is why different mutations in the Ryr2 gene lead to two distinct phenotypes. At present, mutations in the amino cluster have been reported only in families demonstrating ARVC/D, and, conversely, mutations in the carboxyl cluster have been reported only in families demonstrating catecholaminergic polymorphic ventricular tachycardia. It is possible that each group of amino acids, when mutated, alters the function or structure of the polypeptide in a distinct manner, so that both groups of mutations produce the catecholaminergic polymorphic ventricular tachycardia phenotype, but only one group in addition is associated with the structural changes characteristic of ARVC/D. An alternative hypothesis is that mutations in the same gene produce different phenotypes because of differing genetic backgrounds, i.e., the presence of different alleles of modifier genes.

As to the pathogenetic cascade of events whereby the mutations identified in the Ryr2 gene lead to ARVC/D, Ryr2 missense mutations might first alter the ability of the calcium channel to remain closed, thus promoting massive calcium release from the sarcoplasmic reticulum, impairing excitation–contraction coupling and inducing cell death.

Despite the identification of three causative mutations in ARVC/D at the level of the Ryr2, plakoglobin, and desmoplakin genes, respectively, the early predilection of the disease for the right ventricle remains a mystery. Both plakoglobin and desmoplakin as well as Ryr2 are widely expressed in many tissues, and are not specific to one cardiac ventricle. This observation is even more puzzling when considering cytoskeletal cell-to-cell proteins, since another mutation in desmoplakin has been demonstrated to cause a clinical phenotype of dilated cardiomyopathy [40]. As possible explanations of the selective right chamber involvement, a greater role for plakoglobin and desmoplakin in maintaining the structural integrity of the right ventricle, and the relative thinness of the right ventricular free wall, which makes it more susceptible to mechanical stress, have been advocated.

Acknowledgements. This study was supported by ARVC/D Project, QLG1-CT-2000-01091 5th Framework Programme European Commission, Brussels, the Ministry of Health, Rome, and Telethon no. 1288, Rome, Italy.

References

1. Nava A, Rossi L, Thiene G (eds) (1997) Arrhythmogenic right ventricular cardiomyopathy/dysplasia. Elsevier, Amsterdam
2. Thiene G, Nava A, Corrado D, Rossi L, Pennelli N (1988) Right ventricular cardiomyopathy and sudden death in young people. N Engl J Med 318:129-133
3. Basso C, Thiene G, Corrado D, Angelini A, Nava A, Valente M (1996) Arrhythmogenic right ventricular cardiomyopathy. Dysplasia, dystrophy or myocarditis? Circulation 94:983-991
4. Marcus FI, Fontaine G, Guiraudon G, Frank R, Laurenceau JL, Malergue S, Grosgogeat Y (1982) Right ventricular dysplasia. A report of 24 adult cases. Circulation 65:384-398
5. Corrado D, Basso C, Thiene G, McKenna WJ, Davies MJ, Fontaliran F, Nava A, Silvestri F, Blomstrom-Lundqvist C, Wlodarska EK, Fontaine G, Camerini F (1997) Spectrum of clinicopathologic manifestations of arrhythmogenic right ventricular cardiomyopathy/dysplasia: a multicenter study. J Am Coll Cardiol 30:1512-1520
6. Osler WM (1905) The principles and practice of medicine, 6th edn. New York, Appleton, p 820
7. Segall HN (1950) Parchment heart. Am Heart J 40:948-950
8. Uhl HSM (1952) A previously undescribed congenital malformation of the heart: almost total absence of the myocardium of the right ventricle. Bull Johns Hopkins Hosp 91:197-209
9. Dalla Volta S, Battaglia G, Zerbini E (1961) Auricularization of right ventricular pres-

sure curve. Am Heart J 61:25-33

10. Frank R, Fontaine G, Vedel J, Mialet G, Sol C, Guiraudon G, Grosgogeat Y (1978) Electrocardiology of 4 cases of right ventricular dysplasia inducing arrhythmia. Arch Mal Coeur Vaiss 71:963-72
11. Nava A, Scognamiglio R, Thiene G, Canciani B, Daliento L, GF, Martini B, Stritoni P, Fasoli G (1988) Familial occurrence of right ventricular displasia: a study involving nine families. J Am Coll Cardiol 12:1222-1228
12. Richardson P, McKenna WJ, Bristow M, Maisch B, Mautner B, O'Connel J, Olsen E, Thiene G, Goodwin J, Gyarfas I, Martin I, Nordet P (1996) Report of the 1995 WHO/ISFC Task Force on the definition and classification of cardiomyopathies. Circulation 93:841-842
13. Thiene G, Corrado D, Nava A, Rossi L, Poletti A, Boffa GM, Daliento L, Pennelli N (1991) Right ventricular cardiomyopathy: is there evidence of an inflammatory aetiology? Eur Heart J 12:22-25
14. Robbins SL, Cotran RS, Kumar V (1984) Pathologic basis of disease, 3rd edn. Saunders, Philadelphia
15. Nava A, Bauce B, Basso C, Muriago M, Rampazzo A, Villanova C, Daliento L, Buja GF, Corrado D, Danieli GA, Thiene G (2000) Clinical profile and long-term follow-up of 37 families with arrhythmogenic right ventricular cardiomyopathy. J Am Coll Cardiol 36:2226—2233
16. Basso C, Calabrese F, Corrado D, Thiene G (2001) Postmortem diagnosis in sudden cardiac death victims: macroscopic, microscopic and molecular findings. Cardiovasc Res 50:290-330
17. Rampazzo A, Nava A, Danieli GA, Buja GF, Daliento L, Fasoli G, Scognamiglio R, Corrado D, Thiene G (1994) The gene for arrhythmogenic right ventricular cardiomyopathy maps to chromosome 14q23-q24. Hum Mol Genet 3:959-962
18. Rampazzo A, Nava A, Erne P, Eberhard M, Vian E, Slomp P, Tiso N, Thiene G, Danieli GA (1995) A new locus for arrhythmogenic right ventricular cardiomyopathy (ARVD2) maps to chromosome 1q42-q43. Hum Mol Genet 4:2151-2154
19. Severini GM, Kraijnovic M, Pinamonti B, Sinagra GF, Fioretti P, Brunazzi MC, Falaschi A, Camerini F, Giacca M, Mestroni L (1996) A new locus for arrhythmogenic right ventricular dysplasia on the long arm of chromosome 14. Genomics 31:193-200
20. Rampazzo A, Nava A, Miorin M, Fonderico P, Popa B, Tiso N, Livolsi B, Zimbello R, Thiene G, Danieli GA (1997) ARVD4 a new locus for ARVC maps to chromosome 2 long arm. Genomics 45:259-263
21. Ahmad F, Li D, Karibe A, Gonzalez O, Tapscott T, Hill R, Weilbaecher D, Blackie P, Furey M, Gardner M, Bachinsky LL, Roberts R (1998) Localization of a gene responsible for arrhythmogenic right ventricular dysplasia to chromosome 3p23. Circulation 98:2791-2795
22. Li D, Ahmad F, Gardener MJ, Weilbaecher D, Hill R, Karibe A, Gonzalez O, Tapscott T, Sharratt GP, Bachinsky LL, Roberts R (2000) The locus of a novel gene responsible for arrhythmogenic right ventricular dysplasia characterized by early onset and high penetrance maps to chromosome 10p12-p14. Am J Hum Genet 66:148-156
23. Melberg A, Oldfors A, Blomstrom-Lundquist C, Stalberg E, Carlsson B, Larsson E, Lidell C, Eeg-Olofsson KE, Wikstrom G, Henriksson KG, Dahl N (1999) Autosomal dominant myofibrillar myopathy with arrhythmogenic right ventricular cardioyopathy. Ann Neurol 46:684-692
24. Coonar AS, Protonotarios N, Tsatsopoulou A, Needham EWA, Houlston RS, Cliff S, Otter AI, Murday VA, Mattu RK, McKenna WJ (1998) Gene for arrhythmogenic right ventricular cardiomyopathy with diffuse nonepidermolytic palmoplantar keratoder-

ma and woolly hair (Naxos disease) maps to 17q21. Circulation 97:2049-2058

25. Rampazzo A, Nava A, Malacrida S, Beffagna G, Bauce B, Rossi V, Zimbello R, Simionati B, Basso C, Thiene G, Towbin JA, Danieli GA (2002) Mutation in human desmoplakin domain binding to plakoglobin causes a dominant form of arrhythmogenic right ventricular cardiomyopathy. Am J Hum Genet 71:1200-1206
26. McKoy G, Protonotarios N, Crosby A, Tsatsopoulou A, Anastasakis A, Coonar A, Norman M, Babooonian C, Jeffrey S, McKenna WJ (2000) Identification of a deletion in plakoglobin in arrhythmogenic right ventricular cardiomyopathy with palmoplantar keratoderma and woolly hair (Naxos disease). Lancet 355:2119-2124.
27. Tiso N, Stephan DA, Nava A, Bagattin A, Devaney J, Stanchi F, Larderet G, Brahmbhatt B, Brown K, Bauce B, Muriago M, Basso C, Thiene G, Danieli GA, Rampazzo A (2001) Identification of mutations in the cardiac ryanodine receptor gene in families affected with arrhythmogenic right ventricular cardiomyopathy type 2 (ARVD2). Hum Mol Genet 10:189-194
28. Fox PR, Maron BJ, Basso C, Liu SK, Thiene G (2000) Spontaneous occurrence of arrhythmogenic right ventricular cardiomyopathy in the domestic cat: a new animal model of human disease. Circulation 102:1863-1870
29. Valente M, Calabrese F, Angelini A, Caforio ALP, Basso C, Thiene G (1997) Pathobiology. In: Nava A, Rossi L, Thiene G (eds) Arrhythmogenic right ventricular cardiomyopathy/dysplasia. Elsevier, Amsterdam, pp 147-158
30. Matsumori A, Kawai C (1980) Coxsackievirus B3 perimyocarditis in BALB/c mice: experimental model of chronic perimyocarditis in the right ventricle. J Pathol 131:97-106
31. Grumbach IM, Heim A, Vonhof S, Stille-Siegener M, Mall G, Gonska BD, Kreuzer H, Andreas S, Figulla HR (1998) Coxsackievirus genome in myocardium of patients with arrhythmogenic right ventricular dysplasia/cardiomyopathy. Cardiology 89:241-245
32. Calabrese F, Angelini A, Thiene G, Basso C, Nava A, Valente M (2000) No detection of enteroviral genome in the myocardium of patients with arrhythmogenic right ventricular cardiomyopathy. J Clin Pathol 53:382-387
33. Bowles NE, Ni J, Marcus F, Towbin J (2002) The detection of cardiotropic viruses in the myocardium of patients with arrhythmogenic right ventricular dysplasia/cardiomyopathy. J Am Coll Cardiol 39:892-895
34. Diong D, Knowlton KU (2001) Dystrophin deficiency markedly increases enteroviral cardiomyopathy: genetic predisposition to viral heart disease. Circulation 104(II):82
35. Sabel KG, Blomstrom-Lundqvist C, Olsson SB, Enestrom S (1990) Arrhythmogenic right ventricular dysplasia in brother and sister: is it related to myocarditis? Pediatr Cardiol 11:113-116
36. D'Amati G, Fiore F, Giordano C, De Biase L, Laurenti A, Gallo P (1998) Pathologic evidence of arrhythmogenic cardiomyopathy and myocarditis in two siblings. Cardiovasc Pathol 7:39-46
37. James TN (1994) Normal and abnormal consequence of apoptosis in the human heart. From postnatal morphogenesis to paroxysmal arrhythmias. Circulation 90:556-573
38. Mallat Z, Tedgui A, Fontaliran F, Frank R, Durigon M, Fontaine G (1996) Evidence of apoptosis in arrhythmogenic right ventricular dysplasia. N Engl J Med 335:1190-1196
39. Valente M, Calabrese F, Thiene G, Angelini A, Basso C, Nava A, Rossi L (1998) In vivo evidence of apoptosis in arrhythmogenic right ventricular cardiomyopathy. Am J Pathol 152:479-484
40. Norgett EE, Hatsell SJ, Carvajal-Huerta L, Cabezas JC, Common J, Purkis PE et al

(2000) Recessive mutation in desmoplakin disrupts desmoplakin-intermediate filament interactions and causes dilated cardiomyopathy, woolly hair and keratoderma. Hum Mol Genet 9:2761-2766

41. Bauce B, Rampazzo A, Basso C, Bagattin A, Daliento L, Tiso N, Turrini P, Thiene G, Danieli GA, Nava A (2002) Screening for ryanodine receptor type 2 mutations in families with effort-induced polymorphic ventricular arrhythmias and sudden death. Early diagnosis of asymptomatic carriers. J Am Coll Cardiol 40:341-349
42. Laitinen PJ, Brown KM, Piippo K, Swan H, Devaney JM, Brahmbhatt B et al (2001) Mutations of the cardiac ryanodine receptor (RyR2) gene in familial polymorphic ventricular tachycardia. Circulation 103:485-490
43. Priori SG, Napolitano C, Tiso N, Memmi M, Vignati G, Bloise R et al (2001) Mutations in the cardiac ryanodine receptor gene (hRyR2) underlie catecholaminergic polymorphic ventricular tachycardia. Circulation 103:196-200
44. Swan H, Piippo K, Viitasalo M, Heikkila P, Paavonen T, Kainulainen K et al (1999) Arrhythmic disorder mapped to chromosome 1q42-q43 causes malignant polymorphic ventricular tachycardia in structurally normal hearts. J Am Coll Cardiol 34:2035-2042

Is ICD Implantation Useful in Patients with Arrhythmogenic Right-ventricular Cardiomyopathy?

D. Corrado[1], L. Leoni[1], G. Buja[1], G. Thiene[2], on behalf of the Investigators of the Defibrillator in Arrhythmogenic Right Ventricular Cardiomyopathy/Dysplasia in North Italy (DARVIN) Study

Introduction

The natural history of arrhythmogenic right-ventricular cardiomyopathy / dysplasia (ARVC/D) is closely related to ventricular electrical instability, which can precipitate sudden arrhythmic death, mostly in adolescents and young adults [1–4]. Heart failure is rare, and occurs later during the disease course as a result of progression of the right-ventricular disease and left-ventricular involvement [4]. ARVC/D has become an emerging indication for implantable-cardioverter defibrillator (ICD) to prevent sudden arrhythmic death in the setting of cardiomyopathy [5]. Although there is definitive clinical evidence that ICD is the most effective therapy for both primary and secondary prevention of sudden death in patients with coronary artery disease [6–8], there are very few published data on the efficacy and safety of such a therapy in patients with ARVC/D, mostly because of the relatively low prevalence of the disease in the general population and the relatively low event rate [9–11]. Current indications for ICD implantation in patients with arrhythmogenic right-ventricular cardiomyopathy / dysplasia are empiric, being based widely on the experience gained by different centers using analogies with other conditions requiring antiarrhythmic therapy [12]. Since the identification of clinical findings that predict clinical outcome has remained elusive, there is a gathering tendency to implant a ICD indiscriminately once the disease has been diagnosed, regardless of risk stratification [12].

Further, major concerns have been raised about the risk of perforation due to implantation of the lead into a thin right-ventricular free and the difficulty of maintaining adequate sensing and pacing thresholds during follow-up because of the progressive loss of right-ventricular myocardium [10, 12].

In this chapter we review the available studies addressing the efficacy and safety of ICD therapy in patients with ARVC/D, with particular reference to the

Departments of [1]Cardiology and [2]Cardiovascular Pathology, University of Padua Medical School, Italy

DARVIN study [13], which is the first to address the clinical impact of ICD therapy applied to change the natural history of ARVC/D in a relatively large patient population treated for both secondary and primary prevention of sudden death.

Previous Studies

Breithard et al. [9] reported in 1991 on 18 patients with ARVC/D who received an ICD because of drug-refractory ventricular tachycardia or ventricular fibrillation or previous cardiac arrest without reproducible induction of ventricular tachycardia or ventricular fibrillation. Only the first patient received an epicardial lead system, a transvenous approach being used in the subsequent 17 patients. Among these patients, 12 received a transvenous subcutaneous system and the remaining 5, a purely transvenous lead system. Thirteen of the devices implanted had antitachycardia pacing capabilities. Although there were no serious perioperative complications, a major problem was encountered with placement of the tranvenous lead, which required testing of two or more positions (range 2–9; median 4) in 10 of 17 patients (59%) to achieve satisfactory sensing and pacing results. During a follow-up of 17±11 months, 9 of the 18 patients (50%) experienced a total of 130 episodes of appropriate ICD therapies, ranging in frequency from 1 to 40 episodes per patient (median 11 episodes). Because of the high rate of tachycardia or the inability of the device to perform antitachycardia pacing, 59 of these 130 episodes (45%) were terminated by shock therapy, whereas the remaining 71 episodes (55%) were effectively terminated by antitachycardia pacing.

Link et al. [10] reported on 12 patients with ARVC/D who were treated with ICD. Their mean age was 31±9 years (range 15-48). Patients presented with presyncope [5], syncope [4], or cardiac arrest [3]. During programmed electrical stimulation 9 patients had sustained VT, while 3 patients had no inducible arrhythmia. Transvenous leads were placed in 9 patients. In these patients the pacing thresholds were significantly higher, R-wave amplitudes were significantly lower, and defibrillation thresholds were not significantly different than in a cohort of patients without ARVC/D. There were no acute or chronic complications of right-ventricular lead placement. Follow-up averaged 22±13 months (range 1–45). There was one sudden death after 1 month of follow-up. Of the 12 patients, 8 have had appropriate therapy delivered by the ICD. Six patients received sotalol to reduce the frequency of ICD discharges.

Tavernier et al. [11] described 9 consecutive patients (8 male and 1 female; mean age 36 years) with ARVC/D presenting with ventricular tachycardia and hemodynamic collapse (n=6) or ventricular fibrillation (n=3) treated with an ICD. After a mean follow-up of 32±24 months, all patients were alive. Six patients underwent a median of 19 (range 2–306) appropriate ICD interventions for events detected in the ventricular tachycardia window; 4 received a median of 2 (range 1–19) appropriate ICD interventions for events detected in the VF window. Inappropriate interventions were recorded for sinus tachycardia (18 episodes in 3 patients), atrial fibrillation (3 episodes in 1 patient), and for nonsustained polymorphic ventricular tachycardia (1 episode in 1 patient).

The DARVIN Study

The DARVIN Study is an observational, multicenter study aimed at determining the efficacy and safety of defibrillation therapy based exclusively on electrograms stored by the device in a large patient population with ARVC/D and at high risk for sudden death [13]. The study population consisted of 132 patients (93 males, 39 females, age 40±15 years) who were recruited at 22 institutions in North Italy and at 1 in the US (see Appendix 1). In 95 patients (78%), indications for an ICD implant were a history of either cardiac arrest or sustained ventricular tachycardia (secondary-prevention group); the other 37 (22%) had one or more risk factors for sudden death in the absence of spontaneous ventricular tachyarrhythmias (primary-prevention group). During a mean follow-up of 39±25 months, there were 4 deaths: 2 sudden, 1 due to infective endocarditis and 1 to congestive heart failure. Sixty-four patients (48%) had at least 1 appropriate ICD intervention; 15 (12%) had inappropriate interventions; and 21 (16%) had ICD-related complications. Fifty-three of the 64 patients (83%) were receiving antiarrhythmic drugs at the time of the first appropriate discharges: 28 received sotalol, 13, β-blockers, 11, amiodarone (alone in 5 and in association with β-blockers in 6), and 1, flecainide. Analysis of the stored electrograms showed that 32 patients (24%) experienced ventricular fibrillation or flutter, which in all likelihood would have been fatal had it not been for the device. The ventricular fibrillation-/flutter-free survival rate was 72% at 36 months, compared with the actual patient survival of 96% ($P <$ 0.001). The incidence of ventricular fibrillation/flutter was similar in both primary and secondary prevention groups (7.0% vs 7.4% per year). Patients who received ICD devices because of hemodynamically stable VT had a significantly lower incidence of ventricular fibrillation/flutter (log rank = 0.017). A history of cardiac arrest or hemodynamically unstable ventricular tachycardia, young age, and left-ventricular involvement were independent predictors of ventricular fibrillation/flutter.

Therefore, one of the major findings of the DARVIN Study was that during a mean of 3.3 years' follow-up, approximately 50% of the 132 patients had at least one appropriate ICD intervention, despite antiarrhythmic therapy. Furthermore, 24% of the total patient population experienced one or more episodes of ventricular fibrillation/flutter documented by stored intracardiac ECG data that in all likelihood would have been fatal in the absence of the treatment with the device. Analysis of risk factors showed that younger age, a history of cardiac arrest, hemodynamically unstable ventricular tachycardia, and left-ventricular involvement were independent clinical variables associated with the occurrence of such life-threatening arrhythmias. Treatment with a

ICD did not, however, improve survival in the subgroup of patients presenting with hemodynamically stable monomorphic ventricular tachycardia.

The high incidence of ICD interventions in the DARVIN Study is in agreement with data from the small series of patients with ARVC/D previously reported by Breithard et al. (9 of 18 patients; 50%) [9], Link et al. (8 of 12 patients, 67%) [10], and Tavernier et al. (7 of 9 patients, 78%) [11]. Precise data on the efficacy of ICD as opposed to antiarrhythmic therapy cannot be derived from this nonrandomized study. However, the majority of appropriate interventions and 53% of shocks on ventricular fibrillation/flutter occurred despite concomitant antiarrhythmic therapy with β-blockers and/or class III antiarrhythmic drugs. This finding highlights the impression that the protection provided by ICD against sudden death is by far superior.

Analysis of the incidence of ICD interventions that were triggered by ventricular fibrillation/flutter suggests a significant improvement in survival throughout the follow-up period, with an actual patient survival rate of 98%, compared with a ventricular fibrillation/flutter-free survival rate of 72% at 36 months.

In the DARVIN Study, patients who received prophylactic ICD for primary prevention (i.e., patients with one or more risk factors but without spontaneous sustained ventricular tachyarrhythmias) had a similar incidence of appropriate interventions triggered by ventricular fibrillation/flutter to patients with a history of aborted sudden death or sustained VT (7.0% vs 7.4% per year, respectively). Although no definitive recommendation on ICD implantation can be made with regard to primary prevention of sudden death, the finding that appropriate ICD therapy characteristically occurred in patients who underwent implantation because two or more risk factors were present is relevant for risk stratification.

It is noteworthy that the DARVIN patient population is a high-risk subgroup of ARVC/D patients who are not comparable with most patients with the disease, who can be either left untreated or treated effectively with antiarrhythmic drugs because of their low arrhythmic risk [14, 15].

In the DARVIN study there was a lower rate of both inappropriate ICD interventions and complications than previously reported. Inappropriate therapy was administered to 16% of patients in the present study, compared with 33% of those reported by Link et al. [10] and 44% of patients in the study of Tavernier et al. [11]. This discrepancy may be explained by the wider use of beta-blockers and sotalol, which reduced the number of inappropriate interventions for both sinus tachycardia and supraventricular tachyarrhythmias. Moreover, nearly one fourth of the DARVIN study patients had dual-chamber detection algorithms that improved discrimination of ventricular from supraventricular arrhythmias. With regard to complications, it is interesting to note that during follow-up 5 patients required an additional septal lead because of lost ventricular sensing/pacing functions, most probably because of progressive replacement of right-ventricular myocardium by fibrofatty tissue.

The DARVIN study design was that of a retrospective survey involving 22 collaborative medical centers with possible limitations in patient selection. This suggests the need for a prospective controlled study with total mortality as the primary end-point in order to define the survival benefit of ICD implantation conclusively in patients with ARVC/D and its superiority over other therapeutic modalities. However, for any inheritable cardiac diseases, such as hypertrophic cardiomyopathy [16], cardiac ion channel diseases [17, 18], and ARVC/D, a prospective-randomized study design is difficult for ethical reasons and practical limitations predominantly linked to the relatively low disease prevalence and low event rate. In this regard a 10-year interval was required to generate the data on 132 patients. Since many years will be required for completion of a prospective evaluation in the use of ICD in patients with ARVC/D, the DARVIN data will be the best available for some time regarding the efficacy/safety of ICD in this disease.

Conclusions

ICD provides life-saving protection by effectively terminating ventricular tachycardia or fibrillation in high-risk patients with ARVD/C. The available data support the prophylactic use of ICD in ARVD/C patients for both primary and secondary prevention of sudden death.

Acknowledgements. This work was supported in part by a research grant from Guidant Corporation, St. Paul, Minn., USA. Participating centers and investigators are listed in Appendix 1.

Appendix 1. Centers and Investigators that Took Part in the DARVIN Study

Divisione di Cardiologia, Università di Padova, Italy: D. Corrado, L. Leoni, G. Buja, A. Ramondo, A. Nava, B. Bauce, L. Daliento, S. Iliceto, C. Basso, F. Maddalena, G. Thiene; New England Medical Center and Tufts University School of Medicine, Boston: M. Link, M. Estes III; Divisione di Cardiologia, Cliniche Gavazzeni, Bergamo, Italy: M. Zardini; Cardiologia, Azienda USL, Bologna, Italy: F. Naccarella; Divisione di Cardiologia, Bolzano, Italy: W. Rauhe; Divisione di Cardiologia, Spedali Riuniti, Brescia, Italy: A. Curnis; Divisione di Cardiologia, Ospedale "P. Cosma", Camposampiero, Italy: P. Turrini, R. Verlato; Divisione di Cardiologia, Ospedale Civile di Conegliano, Italy: L. Corò, P. Delise; Divisione di Cardiologia, Ospedale Civile di Legnago, Italy: I. Diran; Divisione di Cardiologia, Ospedale "Umberto I", Mestre, Italy: A. Corrado, G. Gasparini, A. Raviele; Centro Cardiologico Monzino, Milan, Italy: P. Della Bella, C. Carbucicchio; Istituto Clinico Humanitas, Milan, Italy: M. Gasparini; Divisione di Cardiologia, Ospedale Niguarda, Milano, Italy: M. Lunati; Divisione di Cardiologia, Ospedale "Santa Maria degli Angeli", Pordenone, Italy: E. Dametto, F. Zardo; Divisione di Cardiologia, Ospedale "Santa Maria del Carmine", Rovereto, Italy: M. Maines, G. Vergara; Divisione di Cardiologia, Divisione di Cardiologia, Ospedale Civile di Rovigo, Italy: F. Zanon; Divisione di Cardiologia, Ospedale Mauriziano, Torino, Italy: F. Gaita; Ospedale "S. Chiara", Trento, Italy: M. Del Greco, M. Disertori; Divisione di Cardiologia, Ospedale Maggiore, Trieste, Italy – E. Pez, G. Sinagra; Divisione di Cardiologia, Ospedale "Santa

Maria Misericordia", Udine, Italy: A. Proclemer; Divisione di Cardiologia, Università di Insubria, Varese, Italy: J.A. Salerno Uriarte; Divisione di Cardiologia, Ospedale Civile Maggiore di Verona, Italy: G. Zanotto; Divisione di Cardiologia, Ospedale Civile di Vicenza, Italy: R. Ometto.

References

1. Marcus FI, Fontaine G, Guiraudon G et al (1982) Right ventricular dysplasia. A report of 24 adult cases. Circulation 1982;65:384–398
2. Thiene G, Nava A, Corrado D et al (1988) Right ventricular cardiomyopathy and sudden death in young people. N Engl J Med 318:129–133
3. Basso C, Thiene G, Corrado D et al (1996) Arrhythmogenic right ventricular cardiomyopathy. Dysplasia, dystrophy, or myocarditis? Circulation 94:983–991
4. Corrado D, Basso C, Thiene G et al (1997) Spectrum of clinicopathologic manifestations of arrhythmogenic right ventricular cardiomyopathy/dysplasia: a multicenter study. J Am Coll Cardiol 30:1512–1520
5. Corrado D, Basso C, Thiene G (2000) Arrhythmogenic right ventricular cardiomyopathy: diagnosis, prognosis, and treatment. Heart 83:588–595
6. Moss AJ, Hall WJ, Cannom DS et al (1996) Improved survival with an implanted defibrillator in patients with coronary disease at high risk for ventricular arrhythmia. N Engl J Med 335:1933–1940
7. The Antiarrhythmics versus Implantable Defibrillators (AVID) Investigators (1997) A comparison of antiarrhythmic-drug therapy with implantable defibrillators in patients resuscitated from near-fatal ventricular arrhythmias. N Engl J Med 337:1576–1583
8. Buxton AE, Lee KL, Fisher JD, Josephson ME, Prystowsky EN, Hafley G (2000) A randomized study of the prevention of sudden death in patients with coronary artery disease. N Engl J Med 341:1882–1890 (erratum) N Engl J Med 342:1300
9. Breithard G, Wichter T, Haverkamp W et al (1994) Implantable cardioverter defibrillator therapy in patients with arrhythmogenic right ventricular cardiomyopathy, long QT syndrome, or no structural heart disease. Am Heart J 127:1151–1158
10. Link M, Wang PJ, Haugh CJ, Homoud MK, Foote CB, Costeas XB, Estes III NAM (1997) Arrhythmogenic right ventricular dysplasia: clinical results with implantable cardioverter defibrillator. J Interv Card Electrophysiol 1:41–48
11. Tavernier R, Gevaert S, de Sutter J et al (2001) Long term results of cardioverter defibrillator in patients with right ventricular dysplasia and malignant ventricular tachyarrhythmias. Heart 85:53–56
12. Corrado D, Fontaine G, Marcus FI, McKenna WJ, Nava A, Thiene G, Wichter T (2000) Arrhythmogenic right ventricular dysplasia/cardiomyopathy. Need for an international registry. Circulation 101:e101-e106
13. Corrado D, Leoni L, Link M et al (2003) Implantable cardioverter-defibrillator therapy for primary and secondary prevention of sudden death in patients with arrhythmogenic right ventricular cardiomyopathy/dysplasia (abstract). Eur Heart J 24: (in press)
14. Blomstrom-Lundqvist C, Sabel CG, Olsson SB (1987) Long term follow-up of 15 patients with arrhythmogenic right ventricular dysplasia. Br Heart J 58:477–488
15. Nava A, Bauce B, Basso C, Muriago M, Rampazzo A, Villanova C, Daliento L, Buja G, Corrado D, Danieli GA, Thiene G (2000) Clinical profile and long-term follow-up of

37 families with arrhythmogenic right ventricular cardiomyopathy. J Am Coll Cardiol 36:2226–2233
16. Maron BJ, Shen WK, Link MS et al (2000) Efficacy of implantable cardioverter-ICDs for the prevention of sudden death in patients with hypertrophic cardiomyopathy. N Engl J Med 342:365–373
17. Silka MJ, Kron J, Dunningam A et al (1993) Sudden cardiac death and the use of implantable cardioverter defibrillator in pediatric patients. Circulation 87:800–807
18. Brugada J, Brugada R, Antzelevitch C et al (2002) Long-term follow-up of individuals with the electrocardiographic pattern of right bundle-branch block and ST-segment elevation in precordial leads V1 to V3. Circulation 105:73–78

What is the Prevalence, Incidence and Prognostic Value of Brugada-type Electrocardiogram in the General Population?

H. SAKURADA, H. OKAZAKI, T. TEJIMA

Patients who have no structural heart disease but whose ECGs are characterized by unique changes in the ST segment elevation on leads V1–V3, with or without a right bundle branch block (RBBB) pattern, occasionally develop ventricular fibrillation (VF). Such patients are recognized as having Brugada syndrome and are at high risk for sudden cardiac death. Although more than 10 years have passed since the first report by Brugada and Brugada [1], there is still no pharmacological treatment that can reliably prevent VF. Therefore, patients who have a Brugada-type ECG pattern (ST elevation in V1–V3 with or without RBBB; "Brugada-type ECG patterns") and have experienced an episode of syncope and/or aborted sudden cardiac death are strongly advised to receive an implantable cardioverter-defibrillator (ICD). On the other hand, there are substantial numbers of individuals who exhibit the Brugada-type ECG patterns without clinical symptoms, arrhythmia, or a family history of sudden cardiac death. These individuals may be found on ECG examinations performed at health check-ups or for other medical reasons than monitoring for cardiac diseases. Therefore, an emphasis has been put on individuals who exhibit ECG patterns compatible with the Brugada syndrome while showing no clinical symptoms or family history of sudden cardiac death. However, the prognosis of these asymptomatic individuals with Brugada-type ECG patterns has not been clarified.

To understand the natural history of Brugada syndrome, with or without symptoms, it is necessary to evaluate the prevalence, incidence, and prognostic value of Brugada-type ECG patterns for individuals in the general population. In this article, we review these with reference to the specific literature.

Several studies [2–8] have been performed to examine the prevalence of Brugada-type ECG patterns in the general population (Table 1); five of these studies were conducted in Japan. Tohyou et al. [2] reported a 0.07% prevalence of ECG patterns with the coved-type ST elevation in V1–V3 among 4,092

Department of Cardiology, Tokyo Metropolitan Hiroo General Hospital, Tokyo, Japan

Table 1. Comparison of the prevalence of the typical coved-type ECG in the general population

Reference	Total no. of subjects	Mean age (years)	No. of men	Prevalence		
				Total	Men	Women
[2]	4,092	46.3	3,198	0.07%	0.09%	0.00%
[3]	3,300			0.21%		
[4]	10,000	42±19	8,913	0.16%	0.18%	0.00%
[5]	13,929	58±10	3,691	0.12%	0.38%	0.03%
[6]	4,788	<50 at first exam	1,956	0.15%	0.36%	0.00%
[7]	1,000	39±10	632	0.10%	0.16%	0.00%
[8]	12,000			0.02%		
[9]	592	36±10	346	0.00%	0.00%	0.00%

healthy Japanese adults (average age 46.3 years). All the subjects exhibiting a typical coved-type ST elevation were men, and this feature had a prevalence of 0.09% in healthy middle-aged men. Takenaka et al. [3] examined the prevalence of coved-type ST segment elevation in leads V1 and V2, finding it in 0.21% of 3,300 individuals undergoing routine health check-ups. In this study, none of the individuals experienced syncope or succumbed to sudden death during a follow-up of 42.5±21.6 months. Atarashi et al. [4] collected ECGs from 10,000 working adults (8,913 men, mean age 42±9 years) and found 16 men (0.16%) with a coved-type ST elevation. Miyasaka et al. [5] reviewed 13,929 individuals in whom an ECG was recorded during routine health examinations in a medium-sized Japanese city. The saddleback type of ST segment elevation was present in 61 and the coved type in 37 patients (0.26%). In those with the coved type of ST elevation, 17 cases had an rsR' pattern (defined as typical by the authors) and 20 had an Rsr' pattern. The prevalence of all types was 0.7%; that of the coved type was 0.26%; and that of the coved rSR' pattern was 0.12%. Among males, the prevalence of all types was 2.14% and that of the coved rsR' pattern was 0.38%. After 2.6±0.3 years of follow-up there had been 1 death in a subject who showed the saddleback-type ST elevation, and 139 deaths among 13,831 subjects without Brugada-type ECG patterns. There was no significant difference in the incidence of sudden cardiac death between individuals with and without Brugada-type ECG patterns. Matsuo et al. [6] investigated 4,788 subjects (1,956 men and 2,832 women) who had suffered from fallout from the atomic bombs dropped on the cities of Hiroshima and Nagasaki in 1945. They were <50 years old in 1958 and had undergone biennial health examinations including ECG. The investigators calculated the prevalence of Brugada-type patterns at the time of the first examination and the 40-year incidence. There were a total of 32 Brugada-type ECG cases (27 men). At the first examination, 7 men (0.15%) already had the typical ECG patterns (146.2 per 100,000 persons;

these were called prevalence cases). The remaining 25 cases, referred to as incident cases, manifested the coved-type ST elevation during subsequent examinations. The annual incidence was 14.2 per 100,000. This is the only report that specifies the annual incidence. The authors also studied the long-term prognoses of subjects showing Brugada-type ECG patterns and found 7 subjects who had died unexpectedly during a follow-up of 40 years. Only 0.4% of the individuals without Brugada-type ECG patterns had died unexpectedly.

Hermida et al. [7] showed that 1 out of 1,000 subjects (0.1%) had coved-type ST elevation, and 60 (6%) had the saddleback type. Among these 61 individuals, cardiovascular mortality was zero during a mean follow-up period of 49±30 months. Monroe and Littman [8] obtained ECGs from 12,000 unselected noncardiac patients and showed that 50 had saddleback-type ST elevation, while only 2 (0.017%) had the coved type. Viskins et al. [9] examined 592 patients who had been referred for electrophysiological evaluation of supraventricular arrhythmias (excluding Wolff-Parkinson-White syndrome) or referred to one of the surgical services. The coved-type ST elevation typical for Brugada syndrome was not seen in any of these patients. However, RsR' and some elevation of the ST segment in leads V1 and V2 (which the authors defined as a possible Brugada sign) were seen in 5 cases (1%).

From all these reports, the prevalence of typical coved-type ECG is calculated as 0.1% in all healthy subjects and 0.22% in men. The data also show that the prevalence is much higher in Japan than in Europe. This higher prevalence may support the idea that idiopathic VF is more frequent in Southeast Asia than in Europe. Although ECG abnormalities constitute the hallmark of the syndrome, the ST segment changes are dynamic, varying over time, and can normalize transiently, as shown in Fig. 1. This means that the prevalence rates

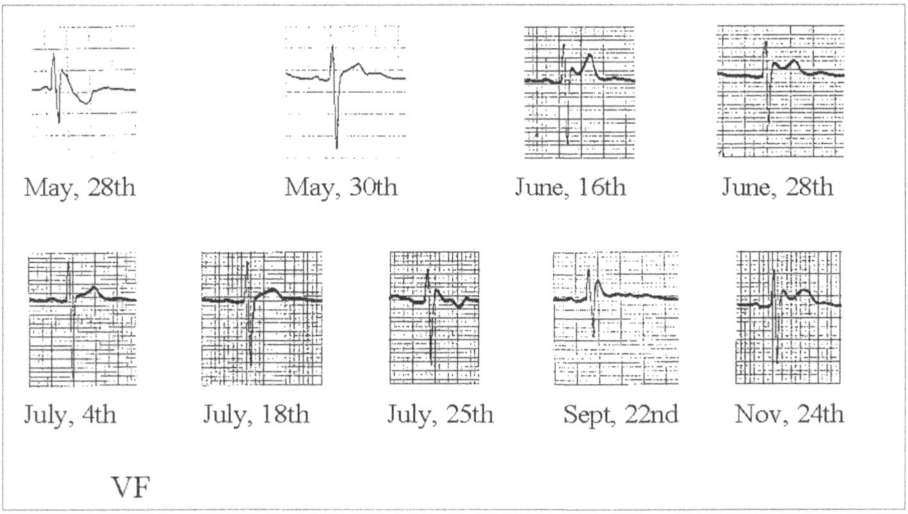

Fig. 1. Day-to-day variation in ST segment in V2 lead in a symptomatic patient with Brugada syndrome. VF, ventricular fibrillation

might be underestimated, depending on the frequency of ECG examinations and the types and characteristics of the study subjects. Further study is necessary, with long-term follow-up in large populations.

References

1. Brugada P, Brugada J (1992) Right bundle branch block, persistent ST segment elevation and sudden cardiac death: a distinct clinical and electrocardiographic syndrome. A multicenter report. J Am Coll Cardiol 20:1391–1396
2. Tohyou Y, Nakazawa K, Ozawa A et al (1995) A survey in the incidence of right bundle branch block with ST segment elevation among normal population (in Japanese). Jpn J Electrocardiol 15:223–226
3. Tkenaka S, Kusano KF, Hisamatsu K et al (2001) Relatively benign clinical course in asymptomatic patients with Brugada-type electrocardiogram without family history of sudden death. J Cardiovasc Electrophysiol 12:2–6
4. Atarashi H, Ogawa S, Harumi K et al (2001) Three-year follow-up of patients with right bundle branch block and ST segment elevation in the right precordial leads. J Am Coll Cardiol 37:1916–1920
5. Miyasaka Y, Tsuji H, Yamada K et al (2001) Prevalence and mortality of the Brugada-type electrocardiogram in one city in Japan. J Am Coll Cardiol 38:771–774
6. Matuso K, Akahoshi M, Nakashima E et al (2001) The prevalence, incidence and prognostic value of the Brugada-type electrocardiogram. J Am Coll Cardiol 38:765–770
7. Hermida JS, Lemoine JL, Aoun FB et al (2000) Prevalence of the Brugada syndrome in an apparently healthy population. Am J Cardiol 86:91–94
8. Monroe MH, Littmann L (2000) Two-year case collection of the Brugada syndrome electrocardiogram pattern at a large teaching hospital. Clin Cardiol 23:849–851
9. Viskin S, Fish R, Zeltser D et al (2000) Prevalence of the Brugada sign in idiopathic ventricular fibrillation and healthy controls. Heart 84:31–36

Brugada Syndrome or Brugada Mimicry?

R.N.W. Hauer

Introduction

The vast majority of patients dying suddenly within 1 h after the onset of their symptoms have cardiac arrest in the setting of structural heart disease. Such events are most frequently due to ventricular tachyarrhythmias, such as rapid ventricular tachycardia (VT) and ventricular fibrillation (VF). In a minority of patients these arrhythmias occur in the apparently normal heart. A patient with an "apparently normal" heart can fall in either of two categories: (1) patients with no evidence at all of structural heart disease and (2) those with a minor disorder and/or not easy detectable structural disorder (Table 1).

Although the electrocardiographic (ECG) features of Brugada syndrome and catecholaminergic polymorphic VT (CPVT) were first reported as early as 1953 and 1978, respectively [1, 2], these diagnoses were not accepted as specific entities until they were described in detail by Brugada and Brugada in 1992 [3] and by Leenhardt et al. in 1995 [4]. Because of their recent recognition and

Table 1. Life-threatening ventricular arrhythmias in the apparently normal heart

Without structural disease	Disorder that is minor and/or difficult to detect
Long-QT syndromes	Wolff-Parkinson-White syndrome
Brugada syndrome	Hypertrophic cardiomyopathy (troponin T mutation)
Catecholaminergic polymorphic VT	Arrhythmogenic right-ventricular dysplasia
Idiopathic VF	Mitral valve prolapse

Heart Lung Center Utrecht, University Medical Center, Utrecht, The Netherlands

controversial diagnostic criteria, both conditions are frequently subcategorized as specific forms of idiopathic VF. In the absence of signs of Brugada syndrome and CPVT in the ECG and of long-QT syndrome, the diagnosis may remain as unspecific idiopathic VF. In a recent study of 37 patients with idiopathic VF, the diagnosis of Brugada syndrome was recognized in 3-24% of the patients, depending on the criteria used [5]. As a discrepancy of this magnitude would obviously give rise to conflicting results in present and future studies, the need for a consensus statement was recognized, and such a statement was published in 2002 [6]. This report from the Study Group on the Molecular Basis of Arrhythmias of the European Society of Cardiology reflects our present knowledge about the diagnosis of Brugada syndrome. It is no more than the agreed opinion of experts in the field, and further refinement is expected as our knowledge expands. With these limitations in mind, the Brugada ECG pattern, Brugada syndrome, and Brugada mimicry may be distinguished.

The Brugada ECG Pattern

When the Brugada ECG pattern is found in symptomatic patients, their condition is defined as Brugada syndrome. The Brugada ECG pattern is characterized by ST-segment elevation in at least two right precordial leads in the absence of identifiable structural heart disease (Fig.1). Only a coved ST-segment elevation with J-wave amplitude ≥2 mm (0.2 mV) combined with a gradually descending ST-segment followed by a negative T-wave is accepted as the

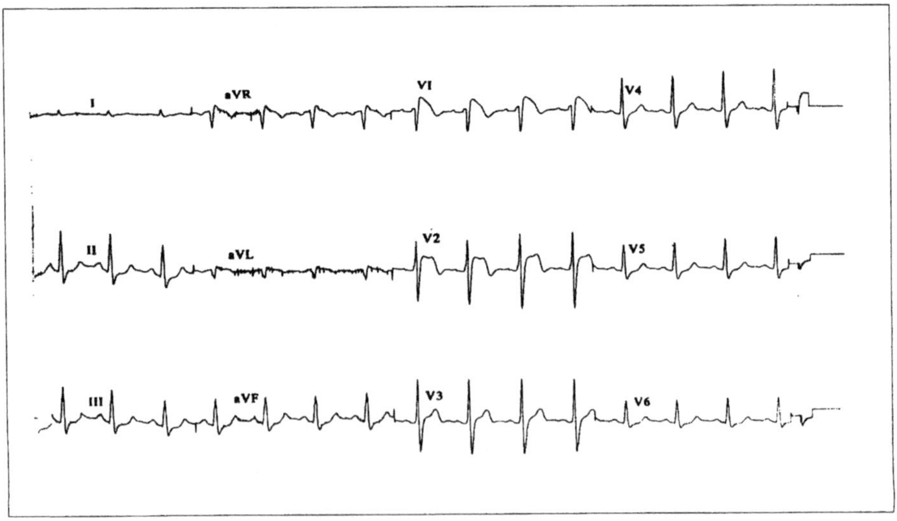

Fig. 1. Brugada ECG pattern in a patient without structural heart disease who had previously been resuscitated because of ventricular fibrillation. This ECG pattern was recorded exclusively while on flecainide therapy

typical Brugada ECG pattern, which is also referred to as a type-1 repolarization pattern. Type-2 and type-3 repolarization patterns are also characterized by right precordial ST-segment elevation and a J-wave amplitude ≥2 mm; however, in both these types a saddleback configuration of the ST-segment is typical, the T-wave will be positive or biphasic, and the latter half of the ST-segment will be elevated ≥1 mm (type 2) or <1 mm (type 3). Repolarization of types 2 and 3 is not typical for the Brugada pattern [6].

Repolarization is not static. Sequential ECGs may show no abnormality, minor ST-segment elevation, saddleback ST-segment shift and the typical Brugada ECG pattern (type-1 repolarization). In addition, the Brugada ECG pattern can be obtained by means of a drug challenge, specifically with ajmaline, flecainide (Fig. 1) and, to a lesser degree, procainamide.

Brugada Syndrome and Brugada Mimicry

The diagnostic criteria for the Brugada syndrome are summarized in Table 2. The Brugada ECG pattern should be recorded in at least one of a series of sequentially obtained ECGs. Alternatively, a Brugada ECG pattern may be obtained by drug challenge. In the absence of type-1 repolarization the diagnosis of Brugada syndrome should be rejected.

Syncopal VT and VF are the typical symptoms of Brugada syndrome. In our series of 37 patients with unspecific idiopathic VF [5] we identified only 3 patients (8%) with Brugada syndrome when the consensus criteria for the Brugada ECG pattern were applied. Since the Brugada syndrome is a familial disease that has been linked to mutations in the *SCN5A* gene, the diagnosis of Brugada syndrome is accepted in asymptomatic individuals with both a Brugada ECG pattern and a positive family history, as mentioned in Table 2 [6].

Finally, absence of any evidence of structural heart disease is considered mandatory for this diagnosis. The exclusion of structural heart disease can be difficult. As an example, hypertrophic cardiomyopathy with muscular disarray may be present without hypertrophy detectable on the echocardiogram. Thus,

Table 2. Diagnostic criteria for Brugada syndrome

Brugada ECG pattern
Syncopal VT/VF
No evidence of structural heart disease
Family history - Sudden cardiac death (age < 45 years) - Brugada ECG pattern

ECG, electrocardiogram

a thorough cardiological evaluation following a predefined protocol is required. The diagnostic tests should include at least: clinical history and physical examination, blood chemistry and haematology, resting ECG, exercise ECG, 24-h Holter recording, echocardiography, coronary angiography, left- and right-ventricular ciné-angiography, an electrophysiological study, ergonovine provocation, and perhaps magnetic resonance imaging and ventricular biopsies.

In the presence of less pronounced ECG abnormalities than would qualify as the Brugada ECG pattern (type-1 repolarization) and in the absence of a positive drug challenge, the ECG pattern may mimic the configuration observed in Brugada syndrome. If the Brugada ECG pattern occurs in patients with structural heart disease it will also be regarded as Brugada mimicry. It can occur in acute ischemia and myocardial infarction, arrhythmogenic right-ventricular dysplasia, cardiomyopathies, cocaine intoxication, and even in normal subjects. Thus, for a diagnosis of Brugada syndrome, the findings should include not only the Brugada ECG pattern and absence of structural heart disease, but also VT or VF, and/or a positive family history.

References

1. Osher HL, Wolff L (1953) Electrocardiographic pattern simulating acute myocardial injury. Am J Med Sci 226:541-545
2. Coumel P, Fidelle J, Lucet V, Attuel P, Bouvrain Y (1978) Catecholaminergic-induced severe ventricular arrhythmias with Adams-Stokes syndrome in children: report of four cases. Br Heart J 40:28-37
3. Brugada P, Brugada J (1992) Right bundle branch block, persistent ST segment elevation and sudden cardiac death: a distinct clinical and electrocardiographic syndrome: a multicenter report. J Am Coll Cardiol 20:1391-1396
4. Leenhardt A, Lucet V, Denjoy I, Grau F, Ngoc DD, Coumel P (1995) Catecholaminergic polymorphic ventricular tachycardia in children. A 7-year follow-up of 21 patients. Circulation 91:1512-1519
5. Remme CA, Wever EFD, Wilde AAM, Derksen R, Hauer RNW (2001) Diagnosis and long-term follow-up of the Brugada syndrome in patients with idiopathic ventricular fibrillation. Eur Heart J 22:400-409
6. Wilde AAM, Antzelevitch Ch, Borggrefe M, Brugada J, Brugada R, Brugada P, Corrado D, Hauer RNW, Kass RS, Nademanee K, Priori SG, Towbin JA (2002) Proposed diagnostic criteria for the Brugada syndrome. Circulation 106:2514-2519

Ventricular Tachycardia or Conduction Disease: What Is the Mechanism of Death in Brugada Syndrome?

G. Buja[1], L. Leoni[1], D. Corrado[1], C. Basso[2], B. Bauce[1], A. Nava[1], S. Iliceto[1], G. Thiene[2]

Introduction

A distinct electrocardiographic (ECG) pattern of right bundle branch block with ST-segment elevation in V1-V2-V3 was first described in 1989 in patients who suddenly died affected by subclinical right ventricular cardiomyopathy [1]. In the late 1990s, Brugada et al. [2] reported on eight patients with the same ECG configuration and sudden death and suggested that this new clinical entity was secondary to a primary "functional" disorder but not a structural abnormality. They advanced the hypothesis that "marked dispersion of refractoriness of cardiac tissue or extreme anisotropic conduction properties of the conduction system and the ventricular muscle" was the underlying pathophysiologic substrate of the syndrome. The findings of right bundle branch block, ST-segment elevation, and sudden death were then recognized in different clinical entities, both structural and functional (Table 1) [3].

The Brugada syndrome (BS) is today classified as: syncope or sudden cardiac death secondary to inherited, idiopathic polymorphic ventricular tachycardia/idiopathic ventricular fibrillation without demonstrable structural heart disease and a characteristic ECG pattern resembling right bundle branch block with persistent J-point and ST-segment elevation, usually convex upward from V1 to V3 and a normal QTc interval [4-6]. Therefore, the occurrence of ventricular tachyarrhythmias is the main mechanism leading to sudden death in patients affected by BS. Complete AV block or asystole has never been-recorded at the time of death. However, the observation of prolonged PR or HV interval in nearly 50% of BS patients [2, 4, 5], the presence of a true right bundle branch block or a superior axis deviation with S1-S2-S3 (S wave in L1-L2-L3) pattern reflecting a parietal delay of conduction in the anterior wall and the outflow tract of right ventricle [7, 8]. The demonstration that mutations in the gene encoding the Na-channel SCN5A are linked to three forms of primary

Departments of [1]Cardiology and [2]Pathology, University of Padua, Italy

Table 1. Classification of the syndrome of right bundle branch block, right precordial st-segment elevation, and sudden death

Structural Heart Disease
Arrhythmogenic Right Ventricular Cardiomyopathy
Familial right ventricular conduction and myocardial disease
Infiltrative cardiomyopathy
Functional Heart Disease
Brugada Syndrome
Sudden unexplained death syndrome
Vagally induced ventricular fibrillation

electrical diseases: the long QT syndrome, BS, and cardiac conduction defects [9]. The description of members of the same family showing either isolated progressive cardiac conduction defect (ICCD) and BS [10], and the evidence at autopsy of pathologic alterations of conduction system after sudden death of patients showing right bundle branch block and ST-segment elevation [7, 8], all raise the question of the role of conduction defects in determining sudden death. Moreover, the frequent detection of abnormal late potentials (LP), a marker of conduction but not repolarization abnormality, in BS patients and the reported evidence that signal-averaged electrocardiography (SAEG) may be useful for risk stratification of patients with BS [11] support the idea that conduction disturbance per se is arrhythmogenic and challenge the prevailing opinion that early repolarization abnormalities and not conduction disturbances could determine the arrhythmogenic substrate in the BS population [12].

Mechanisms of Arrhythmia: Delayed Conduction vs Early Repolarization Abnormalities

The reentry of cardiac impulse is one of the major mechanisms involved in cardiac arrhythmias at any level. Unidirectional block and conduction delay are two properties promoting the initiation of *anatomical* reentry characterized by anatomically defined separate pathways. *Functional* reentry lacks confining anatomical boundaries and occurs in contiguous fibers exhibiting functionally different electrophysiologic properties. Leading circle reentry, random reentry, anisotropic reentry, and figure-of-eight reentry are example of these complex mechanisms [13, 14].

Epicardial cells display a pronounced phase 1, the so-called spike-and-dome morphology, secondary to the presence of the transient outward current, *Ito*. This morphology is the result of three different currents: *INa, Ito*, and L-type calcium current, *ICa*. A reduction in *INa* or L-type *ICa* or an increase in *Ito* provokes loss of the action potential dome with abbreviation of the epicardial action potential while the endocardial action remains unchanged, resulting in epicardial-endocardial heterogeneity of repolarization [15, 16]. Studies by Antzelevitch et al. [17] provided experimental evidence that heterogeneous distribution of action potential duration across the right ventricular wall may be the basis for both a right precordial ST-segment elevation and rapid polymorphic ventricular tachycardia or fibrillation. An inherited channelopathy with marked reduction or blockade of the sodium channel may result in the loss of the action potential dome in the epicardium but not in the endocardium and provoke a transmural current flow that accounts for ST-segment elevation. Propagation of the action potential dome from sites at which it is maintained to sites at which it is abolished may result in isolated local reexcitation (phase-2 reentry or functional reentry), triggering polymorphic ventricular tachycardia or fibrillation favored by transmural dispersion of refractoriness.

Conduction Disturbance in Brugada Syndrome

Since the original study by Brugada et al., prolongation of the HV interval has been recorded in as many as 50% of BS patients [4, 5]. It usually reflects a conduction defect in the His-Purkinje system. No significant differences were found in the duration of the HV interval between symptomatic or asymptomatic BS patients [18], and a prolonged HV interval was not found to be correlated to the presence of LP [11]. However, the HV interval was significantly longer in the asymptomatic individuals who became symptomatic during follow-up than in those who did not develop symptoms [18].

The percentage of BS patients showing abnormal LP is about 80% [11]. It is noteworthy that univariate and multivariate analysis reveals the presence of LP as an independent predictor of life-threatening events [11]. Kasanuki et al. [19] confirmed the presence of abnormal LP in four patients with right precordial ST-segment elevation associated with vagus-induced ventricular fibrillation and demonstrated, by means of body surface mapping, conduction abnormalities localized predominantly between the anterior right ventricular wall and the outflow tract.

Kirschner et al. [20] performed autopsy studies in 18 South Asian victims of sudden unexplained death syndrome, a clinical entity similar to BS, and found structural changes in specialized conduction system in 14 of them. In 8 members of a family with cardiomyopathy mainly involving the right ventricular myocardium and the specialized conduction system, right bundle branch block, ST-segment elevation, inducible monomorphic ventricular tachycardia (1 patient) and sudden death (1 patient) were documented [7].

In a prospective clinicopathologic study of sudden cardiac death in young people, an ECG was available in 96 of 273 victims, and 13 out of 96 (14%) showed right precordial ST-segment elevation, isolated (9 cases) or associated with right bundle branch block (4 cases). At autopsy, all but 1 of these patients were found to have right ventricular cardiomyopathy, predominantly located in the right ventricular anterior wall in patients with right precordial ST-segment elevation. In 3 of 4 patients with the ECG pattern of true right bundle branch block the histological examination of the conduction system showed involvement of the branching bundle and proximal right bundle branch [8]. These findings confirm that a structural His-Purkinje system disease may underlie the finding of prolonged HV interval in some patients with right bundle branch block and ST-segment elevation. Intracardiac conduction degeneration (ICCD), also called Lev-Lenegre disease, is characterized by progressive alteration of cardiac conduction through the His-Purkinje system with right or left bundle branch block. It may lead to complete AV block, causing syncope and sudden death, and it is the most frequent reason for pacemaker implantation in the world as a whole [21]. Interestingly, Kyndt et al. [10] in 2001, reported a large French family in which a single mutation in the *SCN5A* gene led to either BS (2 brothers and their descendants) or to ICCD (3 sisters and their descendants). The same gene mutation can lead, then, to different ECG phenotypes, to different syndromes, and to different risks, such as tachyarrhythmias or inversely complete AV block. The pathophysiologic sequence of the BS and ICCD may possibly result from the same defect: a loss of function of the mutated sodium channel protein. To explain how the same gene mutation can lead to such different ECG phenotypes and opposite electrophysiological alterations, would require postulation of a role for as-yet unidentified modifier gene(s) and/or environmental factors. The reported male preponderance of BS and female-preponderance of ICCD suggest that sex difference may be related to genetic factors influencing the phenotype and sex hormones can impact cardiac electrophysiology.

In summary, the demonstration of conduction defects in BS patients may well explain the ECG changes and electrical instability secondary to reentry in these patients. In addition, different phenotypes (BS or ICCD) in members of the same family might lead to syncope or sudden death through tachyarrhythmias or asystole/AV block.

Repolarization Abnormalities in BS

Both theoretical considerations and in vivo experiments support the idea that the aforementioned inherited repolarization abnormality underlies BS [5]. The high inducibility and reproducibility of VT/VF during electrophysiologic testing favor reentry as the arrhythmogenic mechanism [22]. Moreover, both the recording during spontaneous episodes, and the induction with programmed electrical stimulation of polymorphic ventricular tachyarrhythmias with short-coupled extrasystoles or extrastimuli, respectively, as initiating beats, reinforce this mechanism.

Macroscopic T wave alternans (TWA) associated with premature ventricular contractions was described in a BS patient during febrile illness [23]. By contrast, Ikeda et al. [11] found that microvolt TWA and corrected QT-interval dispersion (QTD), noninvasive markers reflecting repolarization abnormalities, were not independent predictors of life-threatening events in BS patients and did not differ from those of normal individuals, despite the presence of ST-segment elevation at the time of the tests. Eckardt et al. [24] found the body surface area of ST elevation, or area of inhomogeneous repolarization, correlated to the inducibility of ventricular arrhythmias during ventricular stimulation in patients with BS. In a case report, Shimizu et al. [25] measured, epicardial and endocardial activation-recovery intervals in the right ventricular outflow tract in a BS patient simultaneously, by recording a unipolar electrogram. The paradoxic abbreviation of repolarization in epicardium during increasing of ST-segment elevation supports the hypothesis that heterogeneous repolarization across the ventricular wall in the RVOT is responible for accentuation the of ST segment. Nagase et al. [26] recorded epicardial and endocardial unipolar electrograms in six BS patients before and after class IC antiarrhythmic drug administration. The duration of the local electrograms was also correlated with SAEG. The investigators conclude that an "epicardial abnormality" in the RVOT, characterized by delayed potentials coinciding with late potentials, is detectable in these patients.

In this review, we have described the data on the underlying mechanism responsible for the ECG features of and the pathophysiologic substrate for tachyarrhythmias in BS. ECG manifestations of the syndrome have been attributed to one of two basic mechanisms: (1) conduction delay in the right-ventricular epicardial-free wall in the outflow tract, and (2) premature repolarization of the right-ventricular epicardial action potential secondary to loss of the dome. On the basis of reported data, these two theories remain a debatable issue. Finally, experimental and clinical studies favor reentry as the mechanism underlying the arrhythmogenic potential in BS patients. Whether it is initiated and maintaned by the same mechanism and whether it is due to delayed conduction or dispersion of repolarization has not yet been clearly explained.

References

1. Martini B, Nava A, Thiene G, Buja G, Canciani B, Scognamiglio R, Daliento L, Dalla Volta S (1989) Ventricular fibrillation without apparent heart disease: description of 6 cases. Am Heart J 118:1203-1209
2. Brugada P, Brugada J (1992) Right bundle branch block, persistent ST-segment elevation and sudden cardiac death: a distinct clinical and electrocardiographic syndrome. J Am Coll Cardiol 20:1391-1396
3. Corrado D, Buja G, Basso C, Nava A, Thiene G (1999) What is the Brugada syndrome? Cardiol Rev 7:191-195
4. Gussak I, Antzelevitch C, Bjerregaard P, Towbin JA, Chaitman BR (1999) The Brugada syndrome: clinical, electrophysiologic and genetic aspects. J Am Coll Cardiol 33:5-15
5. Alings M, Wilde A (1999) "Brugada" syndrome. Clinical data and suggested pathophysiologic mechanism. Circulation 99:666-673
6. Wilde A, Antzelevitch C, Borggrefe M et al (2002) Proposed diagnostic criteria for the Brugada syndrome. Consensus report. Circulation 106:2514-2519

7. Corrado D, Nava A, Buja G, Martini B, Fasoli G, Oselladore L, Turrini P, Thiene G (1996) Familial cardiomyopathy underlies syndrome of right bundle branch block, ST segment elevation and sudden death. J Am Coll Cardiol 27:443-448
8. Corrado D, Basso C, Buja G, Nava A, Rossi L, Thiene G (2001) Right bundle branch block, right precordial ST-segment elevation, and sudden death in young people. Circulation 103:710-717
9. Bezzina CR, Rook MB, Wilde A (2001) Cardiac sodium channel and inherited arrhythmia syndromes. Cardiovasc Res 49:257-271
10. Kyndt F, Probst V, Potet F, Demolombe S, Chevallier J, Baro I, Moisan J, Boisseau P, Schott J, Escande D, Le Marec H (2001) Novel SCN5A mutation leading either to isolated cardiac conduction defect or Brugada syndrome in a large French family. Circulation 104:3081-3086
11. Ikeda T, Sakurada H, Sakabe K, Sakata T, Takami M, Tezuka N, Nakae T, Noro M, Enjoji Y, Tejima T, Sugi K, Yamaguchi T (2001) Assessment of non-invasive markers in identifying patients at risk in the Brugada syndrome: insight into risk stratification. J Am Coll Cardiol 37:1628-3164
12. Gussak I, Bierregard P, Hammil SC. (2001) Clinical diagnosis and risk stratification in patients with Brugada syndrome. J Am Coll Cardiol 37:1635-1638
13. Rubart M, Zipes DP (2001) Genesis of cardiac arrhythmias: electrophysiological considerations. In: Braunwald E, Zipes DP, Libby P (eds) Heart disease. A textbook of cardiovascular medicine, vol 22. Saunders Company; Philadelphia, pp 659-699
14. Spach MS, Heidlage JF, Dolber PC (2000) The dual nature of anisotropic discontinuous conduction in the heart. In: Zipes DP, Jalife J, (eds) Cardiac electrophysiology. From cell to bedside, vol. 25. Saunders Company; Philadelphia, pp 213-222
15. Yan GX, Antzelevitch C (1996) Cellular basis for the electrocardiographic J wave. Circulation 93:372-379
16. Yan GX, Antzelevitch C (1999) Cellular basis for the Brugada syndrome and other mechanisms of arrhythmogenesis associated with ST-segment elevation. Circulation 100:1660-1666
17. Antzelevitch C (1998) The Brugada syndrome. J Cardiovasc Electrophysiol 9:513-516
18. Brugada P, Geelen P, Brugada R, Mont L, Brugada J (2001) Prognostic value of electrophysiologic investigations in Brugada syndrome. J Cardiovasc Electrophysiol 12:1004-1007
19. Kasanuki H, Ohnoshi S, Ohtuka M, Matsuda N, Nirei T, Isogai R, Shoda M, Toyoshima Y, Hosoda S (1997) Idiopathic ventricular fibrillation induced with vagal activity in patients without obvious heart disease. Circulation 95:2277-2285
20. Kirschner RH, Echner FAO, Baron RC (1986) The cardiac pathology of sudden unexpected nocturnal death in southeast Asian refugees. JAMA 256:2700
21. Probst V, Hoorntje TM, Hulsbeek M, Wilde A, Escande D, Mannens M, Le Marec H (1999) Cardiac conduction defects associate with mutations in SCN5A. Nat Genet 23:20-21
22. Gasparini M, Priori SG, Mantica M, Coltorti F, Napolitano C, Galimberti P, Bloise R, Ceriotti C (2002) Programmed electrical stimulation in Brugada Syndrome: how reproducible are the results? J Cardiovasc Electrophysiol 13:880-887
23. Morita H, Nagase S, Kusano K, Ohe T (2002) Spontaneous T wave alternans and premature ventricular contractions during febrile illness in a patient with Brugada syndrome. J Cardiovasc Electrophysiol 13:816-818
24. Eckardt L, Bruns HJ, Paul M et al (2002) Body surface area of ST elevation and presence of late potentials correlate to the inducibility of ventricular tachyarrhythmias in Brugada syndrome. J Cardiovasc Electrophysiol 13:742-749

25. Shimizu W, Aiba T, Kurita T, Kamakura S (2001) Paradoxic abbreviation of repolarization in epicardium of the right ventricular outflow tract during augmentation of Brugada-type ST segment elevation. J Cardiovasc Electrophysiol 12:1418-1421
26. Nagase S, Kusano KF, Morita H et al (2002) Epicardial electrogram in the right ventricular outflow tract in patients with the Brugada syndrome. Using the epicardial lead. J Am Coll Cardiol 39:1992-1995

Idiopathic Ventricular Tachycardia: Is Radiofrequency Ablation the First Line Therapy?

D. J. CALLANS

Introduction

The development and refinement of catheter based ablative techniques has had a remarkable effect on the treatment of many types of arrhythmias. The impact of catheter ablation has been favorably compared to that of penicillin for the treatment of pneumococcal pneumonia [1]. Advances in these techniques have essentially eliminated the need for arrhythmia surgery (except for atrial fibrillation), a field that was vigorous only 15 years ago. At the same time, confidence in the use of antiarrhythmic drugs has suffered as our awareness of the cardiac and non-cardiac side effects of such therapy has grown. Clinical trial experience in treating arrhythmias ranging from ventricular tachycardia (VT) in structural heart disease (such as the Cardiac Arrhythmia Suppression Trial [2]) to atrial fibrillation in patients largely without structural heart disease (such as the AFFIRM Trial [3]) has consistently demonstrated the potential survival disadvantage conferred by antiarrhythmic drug therapy. These considerations, coupled with the lack of complete efficacy of drug therapy, have led to a further increase in enthusiasm for nonpharmacologic treatment strategies.

Despite these general considerations, it is important to acknowledge that the relative merit of pharmacologic and ablation therapy depends on the specific arrhythmia syndrome and the patient. Only limited data are available directly comparing these treatment strategies. Catheter ablation therapy has been demonstrated to be superior to pharmacologic therapy in patients with frequent symptomatic episodes of atrioventricular nodal reentry tachycardia [4] and patients with recurrent atrial flutter [5]. The ablation strategies used to approach these arrhythmia syndromes are well developed; contemporary studies in experienced laboratories demonstrate success rates are > 95 %, and procedural risks are low.

Division of Cardiovascular Medicine, Department of Medicine, University of Pennsylvania School of Medicine, Philadelphia, Pennsylvania, USA

Comparative data of catheter ablation and pharmacologic therapy is not available for idiopathic VT. Pharmacologic therapy for this syndrome is not as likely to be harmful as it is for atrial fibrillation or patients with structural heart disease, particularly as beta-adrenergic blockers are the mainstay. In addition, ablation strategies are not as well developed as they are for supraventricular arrhythmias. Furthermore, we are just discovering unusual idiopathic VT syndromes, arising from regions with complex anatomic relationships that require a great deal of experience and often a substantial tolerance for risk, to successfully treat with catheter ablation. Nonetheless, largely by analogy to the points developed above, I will discuss the concept that catheter ablation represents first line therapy for a variety of idiopathic VT syndromes, superior in efficacy and safety to pharmacologic therapy. Central to this argument is the assumption that catheter ablation is performed by experienced operators. Recent survey information attests to less uniform success rates with complex as opposed to routine catheter ablation [6].

Catheter Ablation of Idiopathic Ventricular Tachycardia

There are several distinctive syndromes of VT that occur in patients without structural heart disease, recognized by their clinical and electrocardiographic characteristics. Although VT can arise from any location in either ventricle, the majority of idiopathic VT comes from well-recognized areas. The following discussion of the primacy of catheter ablation will be arranged by VT site of origin. Success rates may be expected to vary widely by anatomic location, as does the relative procedural risk. In addition, for the purposes of this discussion, only symptomatic patients will be considered. Idiopathic VT is known to have a benign prognosis; in the absence of symptoms, neither pharmacologic nor nonpharmacologic therapy is warranted. Finally, because nonsustained VT (or even frequent PVCs) commonly cause symptoms in these syndromes, and because the ablation strategies for nonsustained and sustained arrhythmias in this setting are largely identical, they will be considered together.

Right Ventricular Outflow Tract Tachycardia

Right ventricular outflow tract (RVOT) tachycardia is the most common form of idiopathic VT and comprises 70-80 % of all idiopathic VT [7]. RVOT VT is also called repetitive monomorphic VT, which refers to its frequent existence as isolated repetitive PVCs or salvos of nonsustained VT. Symptoms are classically exercised induced, although there are differences in VT provocation between men and women [8]. RVOT VT has a characteristic ECG morphology, a narrow left bundle branch block pattern and tall positive forces in the inferior leads. The syndrome has a benign prognosis, and although syncope can occur in sustained forms of tachycardia, sudden death is rare [9], if arrhythmogenic RV dysplasia is excluded. Drug therapy typically commences with beta-adrenergic blocking agents, which is effective in only 25-50 % [10, 11]. Beta-blockers are often difficult for young patients to tolerate, and their favorable effects can be overcome by exercise or emotional stress. Calcium antagonists and type IC antiarrhythmic agents are also commonly used [12, 13].

Success rates for catheter ablation of RVOT VT have ranged from 83-100 % [14-20]. However, it is important to consider that these results precede recent improvements in our understanding of this syndrome. First, strategies for mapping RVOT VT and PVCs have improved since these initial series. The primary mapping strategy for idiopathic VT is pace mapping; attention to matching the exact components of the paced and VT QRS morphology in all 12 leads is essential for success [21]. We have found that pace map morphologies have predictable relationships to anatomic location on a 9-site map of the RVOT [22]. This proves helpful in "fine tuning" pace map matches: moving from posterior to anterior results in a more negative complex in lead I and a later precordial R wave transition. Second, initial attempts at catheter ablation in the RVOT failed to recognize the nearly uniform anatomic relationship to the superior "septal" aspect of the RVOT[1]. This confusion led to difficulties in catheter mapping and occasional severe complications [16], presumably related to catheter manipulation and ablation on the thin RV free wall. A recent study from our group used electroanatomic mapping to precisely delineate anatomic relationships in the RV outflow tract area [23]. Pace map and VT morphologies from the superior RVOT demonstrate unique site dependent ECG morphologies that effectively distinguish free wall from septal and posterior versus anterior locations (Fig. 1). Finally, arrhythmia syndromes that mimic RVOT VT that cannot be successfully ablated from the right ventricle are now recognized. Precordial R wave transitions earlier than V3 [19], or a broad R wave in V1 despite predominant negative forces [20] are important signs of LVOT or LV epicardial VT, which will be considered below. Inability to duplicate the VT morphology with pace mapping from the RVOT should prompt consideration of these variants.

Left Ventricular Outflow Tract Tachycardia

Recently, several syndromes of LV outflow tract VT have been described [11, 19, 20, 24, 25]. These tachycardias present clinically in an identical fashion to RVOT, with both repetitive monomorphic NSVT and sustained varieties. Although idiopathic VT can arise from multiple locations from the LV, important variations to recognize include VT that arises from the right and left

[1] Although commonly referred to as septal, the posterior aspect of the RVOT abuts the ascending aorta, as the pulmonic valve is superior and anterior to the aortic valve.

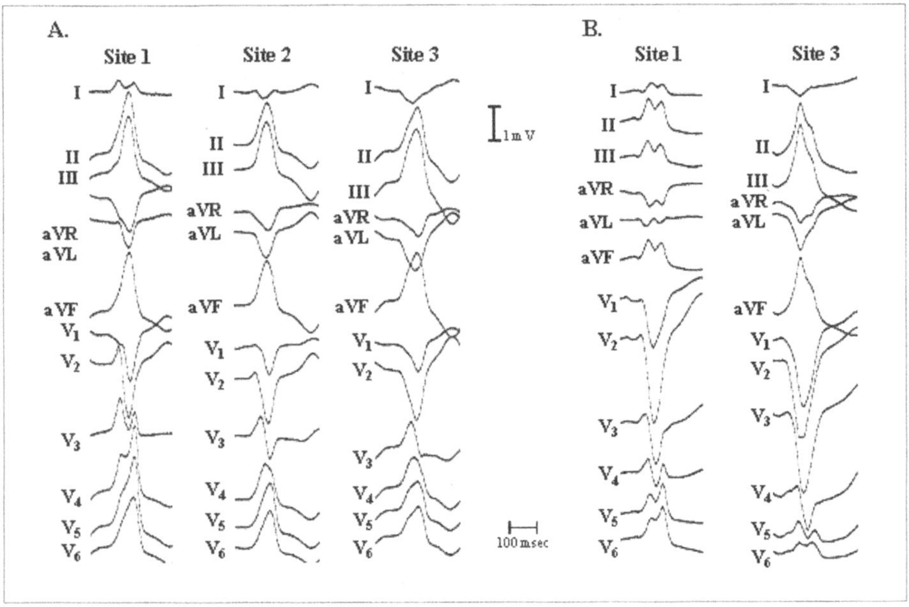

Fig. 1. ECG morphologies of spontaneous arrhythmias originating from superior septal and free-wall sites. In our mapping scheme of the RVOT, septal sites 1, 2 and 3 are just proximal to the pulmonic valve arranged in a posterior to anterior relationship; free-wall sites 1 and 3 are across from their corresponding septal sites. VTs from septal sites have tall monophasic R waves in the inferior leads and an R wave transition at approximately V3. Moving from site 1 to site 3 results in a change from a positive to a negative complex in lead I. Free-wall sites have a similar pattern in lead I, but show later R wave transition and notching in the inferior leads. (Reprinted from Dixit S. et al., J Cardiovasc Electrophysiol 2002;14:1-7, with permission)

sinuses of Valsalva [24, 25] and from the LV epicardium. As discussed above, there are electrocardiographic clues that can help differentiate RVOT and LVOT sites of origin. The most important difference is an earlier precordial R wave transition owing to the posterior (rather than "leftward") relationship of the LVOT and anterior LV epicardium to the RVOT (Fig. 2). Several investigators have demonstrated that ablation can be safely and effectively performed within the sinus of Valsalva [24, 25], although spectacular complications have been observed [26]. Monitoring the relationship of the ablation electrode and the coronary ostium with angiography or intracardiac echocardiography may be helpful in preventing complications [24, 25]. VT arising from the anterior LV epicardium apical to the aortic root, often closely related to the course of the left anterior descending coronary artery, has also been demonstrated and ablated with coronary venous [27] and transcutaneous pericardial approaches [24, 28]. Although VT from this site of origin does not have a characteristic morphology, there are several clues. As this anatomic location is posterior and

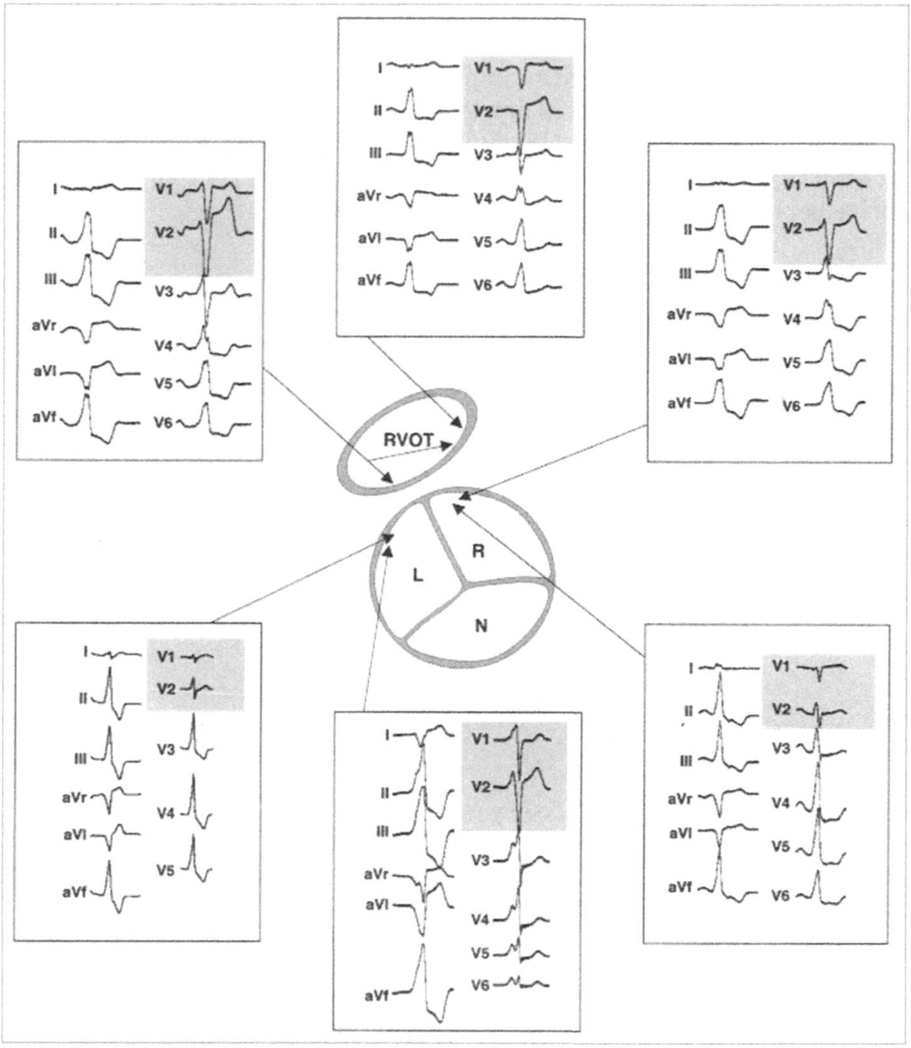

Fig. 2. Typical 12-lead ECG morphologies observed at superior septal sites in the RVOT and the coronary cusps. From the RVOT, qS or rS morphologies are recorded in leads V1 and V2. From the left coronary cusp, there is a taller, broader R wave in V1 and or V2. From the right coronary cusp, V1 has a narrow qS morphology, and V2 has a broad R wave. (Reprinted from Ouyang F. et al., J Am Coll Cardiol 39:500-508, with permission)

inferior to the RV (and the majority of the LV) outflow tract, the precordial R wave transition is earlier, and the inferior leads are not as positive. The QRS duration is typically broader, as the access to the Purkinje network is delayed relative to endocardial sites. Occasionally, there is a "pattern break" in the precordial leads, with an R wave in V1 and V3, but a qS complex in V2. This seems to occur because the site of origin is directly under the location of V2, producing an entirely negative complex in a fashion analogous to the unipolar intracardiac signal recorded at the site of origin. More often, the epicardial nature of a specific VT morphology is determined when satisfactory pace maps or activation times cannot be achieved despite extensive endocardial mapping.

Obviously, although favorable results have been reported, given the increase in difficulty and risk involved, catheter ablation for LVOT VT should be performed only in laboratories with extensive experience.

Left Ventricular Septal Tachycardia

Another well-characterized VT that occurs in patients without structural heart disease is idiopathic left ventricular tachycardia (verapamil-sensitive VT). This VT has a right bundle morphology that is usually fairly narrow and typically a left superior frontal plane axis (Fig. 3). The site of origin is usually the inferior septum, and the posterior fascicle is thought to be an integral part of the cir-

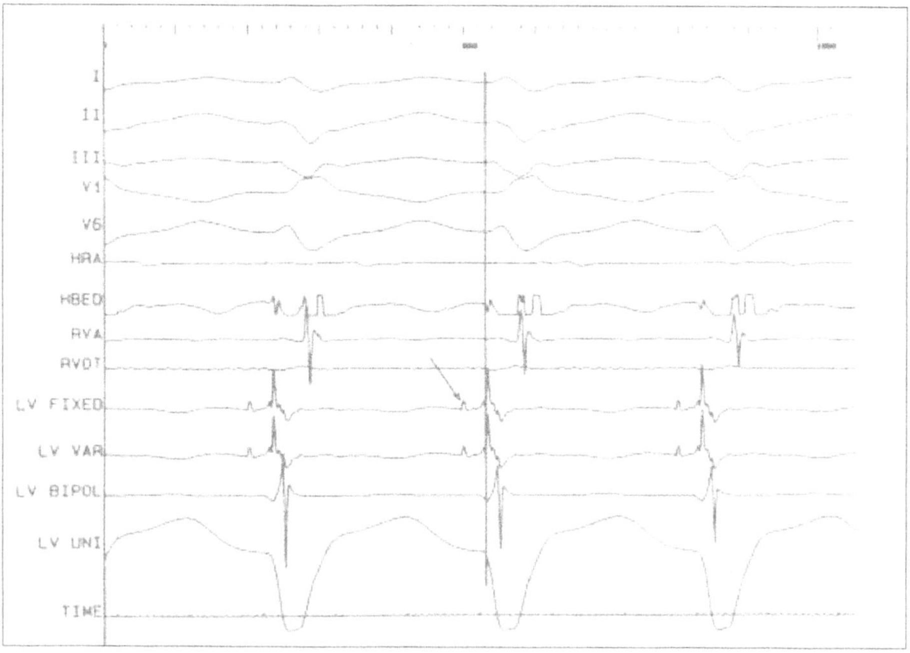

Fig. 3. Idiopathic LV septal VT. Surface leads and intracardiac recordings from the high right atrium (HRA), His bundle region (HBE), RV apex and outflow tract (RVA, RVOT), and multiple bipolar and unipolar recordings at the site of successful ablation (LV fixed, LV var, LV bipolar, LV uni) are shown. Note the sharp potential (arrow) in the bipolar LV recordings, consistent with activation of the Purkinje system. This potential precedes the onset of the QRS by 40 msec. (Reprinted from Callans D. et al., J Cardiovasc Electrophysiol 1994;5:877-894, with permission)

cuit. Syncope and sudden death are rare in this syndrome [29, 30]. Verapamil is effective in termination of acute episodes and prevention of recurrent VT [30-32]. Several small series have demonstrated that catheter ablation is safe and effective in treatment of this form of VT, with success rates greater than 90 % [16, 33-35]. Most investigators believe that ablation targets should be directed by the earliest Purkinje potential during VT (Fig. 3), although pace mapping strategies have also been used successfully. This small difference in opinion has been recently explained by several detailed mapping studies which have demonstrated that the circuit in idiopathic LV VT is larger than just a focal "exit point," involving fairly extensive portions of the Purkinje network [35].

Conclusions

Catheter ablation is safe and effective in the majority of idiopathic VT syndromes and plays an important role in the treatment of patients with important symptoms. Although there have been no direct comparisons of the efficacy of catheter ablation and pharmacologic therapy, many feel that catheter ablation is the correct first line therapy. The response to antiarrhythmic drugs in these syndromes is variable and unpredictable. The risks incurred by unsuccessful therapy are small, but so are the risks of curative ablation. The typical patient with symptomatic idiopathic VT is young and active, unlikely to be taking other medications, and susceptible to the side effects of beta-blockers. Catheter ablation provides curative therapy and should be offered the initial strategy in patients with symptoms that require any type of treatment.

References

1. Plumb VJ (1995) Catheter ablation of the accessory pathways of the Wolff-Parkinson-White syndrome and its variants. Prog Cardiovasc Dis 37:295-306
2. CAST Investigators (1989) Preliminary report: Effect of encainide and flecainide on mortality in a randomized trial of arrhythmia suppression after myocardial infarction. N Engl J Med 321:406-412
3. Wyse DG, Waldo AL, DiMarco JP et al (2002) A comparison of rate control and rhythm control in patients with atrial fibrillation. N Engl J Med 347:1825-1833
4. Cheng CH, Sanders GD, Hlatky MA et al (2000) Cost-effectiveness of radiofrequency ablation for supraventricular tachycardia. Ann Intern Med 133:864-876
5. Natale A, Newby KH, Pisano E et al (2000) Prospective randomized comparison of antiarrhythmic therapy versus first-line radiofrequency ablation in patients with atrial flutter. J Am Coll Cardiol 35:1898-9104
6. Scheinman MM, Huang S (2000) The 1998 NASPE prospective catheter ablation registry. Pacing Clin Electrophysiol 23:1020-1028
7. Brooks R, Burgess JH (1998) Idiopathic ventricular tachycardia: A review. Medicine 67:271-294
8. Marchlinski FE, Deely MP, Zado ES (2000) Sex-specific triggers for right ventricular

outflow tract tachycardia. Am Heart J 139:1009-1013
9. Altemose GT, Buxton AE (1999) Idiopathic ventricular tachycardia. Annu Rev Med 50:159-177
10. Buxton AE, Waxman HL, Marchlinski FE et al (1983) Right ventricular tachycardia: clinical and electrophysiologic characteristics. Circulation 68:917-927
11. Mont L, Seixas T, Brugada P et al (1992) The electrocardiographic, clinical, and electrophysiologic spectrum of idiopathic monomorphic ventricular tachycardia. Am Heart J 124:746-753
12. Gill JS, Blaszyk K, Ward DE et al (1993) Verapamil for suppression of idiopathic ventricular tachycardia of left bundle branch-like morphology. Am Heart J 126:1126-1133
13. Ritchie AH, Kerr CR, Qi A et al (1989) Nonsustained ventricular tachycardia arising from the right ventricular outflow tract. Am J Cardiol 64:594-598
14. Klein LS, Shih HT, Hackett F et al (1992) Radiofrequency catheter ablation of ventricular tachycardia in patients without structural heart disease. Circulation 85:1666-1674
15. Calkins H, Kalbfleisch SJ, El-Atassi R et al (1993) Relation between efficacy of radiofrequency catheter ablation and site of origin of idiopathic ventricular tachycardia. Am J Cardiol 71:827-833
16. Coggins DL, Lee RJ, Sweeney J et al (1994) Radiofrequency catheter ablation as a cure for idiopathic ventricular tachycardia of both left and right ventricular origin. J Am Coll Cardiol 23:1333-1341
17. Wilber DJ, Baerman J, Olshansky B et al (1993) Adenosine sensitive ventricular tachycardia: clinical characteristics and response to catheter ablation. Circulation 87:126-134
18. Movsowitz C, Schwartzman D, Callans DJ et al (1996) Idiopathic right ventricular outflow tract tachycardia: narrowing the anatomic location for successful ablation. Am Heart J 131:930-936
19. Callans DJ, Menz V, Schwartzman D et al (1997) Repetitive monomorphic tachycardia from the left ventricular outflow tract: electrocardiographic patterns consistent with a left ventricular site of origin. J Am Coll Cardiol 29:1023-1027
20. Krebs ME, Krause PC, Engelstein ED et al (2000) Ventricular tachycardia mimicking those arising from the right ventricular outflow tract. J Cardiovasc Electrophysiol 11:45-51
21. Gerstenfeld E, Dixit S, Patel V et al (2002) Quantitative comparison of spontaneous and paced 12-lead ECG during outflow tract ventricular tachycardia. Pacing Clin Electrophysiol 25:634 (abstract)
22. Jadonath RL, Schwartzman DS, Preminger MW et al (1995) Utility of the 12-lead electrocardiogram in localizing the origin of right ventricular outflow tract tachycardia. Am Heart J 130:1107-1113
23. Dixit S, Gerstenfeld EP, Callans DJ, Marchlinski FE (2003) Electrocardiographic patterns of superior right ventricular outflow tract tachycardias: Distinguishing septal and free-wall sites of origin. J Cardiovasc Electrophysiol 14:1-7
24. Kanagaratnam L, Tomassoni G, Schweikert R et al (2001) Ventricular tachycardias arising from the aortic sinus of valsalva: an under-recognized variant of left outflow tract ventricular tachycardia. J Am Coll Cardiol 37:1408-1414
25. Ouyang F FP, Ho SY, Hebe J et al (2002) Repetitive monomorphic ventricular tachycardia originating from the aortic sinus cusp: electrocardiographic characterization for guiding catheter ablation. J Am Coll Cardiol 39:500-508
26. Friedman PL, Stevenson WG, Bittl JA et al (1997) Left main coronary artery occlusion

during radiofrequency ablation of idiopathic outflow tract ventricular tachycardia. Pacing Clin Electrophysiol 20:1185 (abstract)
27. Stellbrink C, Diem D, Schauerte P et al (1997) Transcoronary venous catheter ablation of ventricular tachycardia. J Cardiovasc Electrophysiol 8:916-921
28. Sosa E, Scanavacca M, d'Avila A, Pilleggi F (1996) A new technique to perform epicardial mapping in the electrophysiology laboratory. J Cardiovasc Electrophysiol 7:531-536
29. Ohe T, Aihara N, Kamakura S et al (1995) Long-term outcome of verapamil-sensitive sustained left ventricular tachycardia in patients without structural heart disease. J Am Coll Cardiol 25:54-58
30. German LD, Packer DL, Bardy GH, Gallagher JJ (1983) Ventricular tachycardia induced by atrial stimulation in patients without symptomatic cardiac disease. Am J Cardiol 52:1202-1207
31. Klein GJ, Millman PJ, Yee R (1987) Recurrent ventricular tachycardia sensitive to verapamil. Pacing Clin Electrophysiol 7:938-948
32. Ohe T, Shimomura K, Aihara N et al (1988) Idiopathic sustained left ventricular tachycardia: clinical and electrophysiological characteristics. Circulation 77:560-568
33. Nakagawa H, Beckman KJ, McClelland JH et al (1993) Radiofrequency catheter ablation of idiopathic left ventricular tachycardia guided by a Purkinje potential. Circulation 88:2607-2617
34. Wen M-S, Yeh S-J, Wang C-C et al (1994) Radiofrequency ablation therapy in idiopathic left ventricular tachycardia with no obvious structural heart disease. Circulation 89:1690-1696
35. Ouyang F, Cappato R, Ernst S et al (2002) Electroanatomic substrate of idiopathic left ventricular tachycardia: unidirectional block and macroreentry within the purkinje network. Circulation 105:462-469

Ventricular Tachycardia from the Aortic Cusps: Localization and Ablation

F. E. Marchlinski, D. Lin, S. Dixit, J. Jacobson, W. Sauer, M. McKernan, J. F. Ren

Repetitive monomorphic VT occurring in the absence of structural heart disease typically originates in the outflow tract regions of the right and less commonly the left ventricles [1-8]. An unusual origin for this tachycardia in the outflow tract region is the cusps of the aortic valve. Importantly, this site of origin may be more common than previously recognized [9, 10]. This review will 1) characterize the anatomic relationship of the pulmonic and aortic valves, 2) identify surface electrocardiographic clues that suggest an origin from the aortic cusps and 3) describe the use of magnetic electroanatomic recording and intracardiac echo for identifying precise catheter position when mapping and ablating in the aortic cusp region and finally 4) describe an ablation and energy delivery strategy at these sites which are in close proximity to the ostium of the coronary arteries.

Anatomic Considerations and Arrhythmia Mechanism

Most outflow tract tachycardias originate from the superior and anterior aspect of the septal region just below the pulmonic valve. The pulmonic valve typically is positioned superiorly, rightward and commonly anterior to the aortic valve region (Fig. 1). Importantly, we have previously shown that the septal aspect of the area just below the pulmonic valve tends to demonstrate a flat or actually convex shape [1, 8]. This convexity of the superior and septal aspect of the RVOT allows for the aortic valve cusps to sit squarely within the crescent shaped septal region (Fig. 1). The posterior septal side of the RVOT just inferior to the pulmonic valve typically abuts the right coronary cusp while the anterior septal surface abuts the junction of the right and left cusps or actually may be located directly anterior to the medial aspect of the left

Electrophysiology Section, Division of Cardiology, University of Pennsylvania Health System, Philadelphia, Pennsylvania, USA

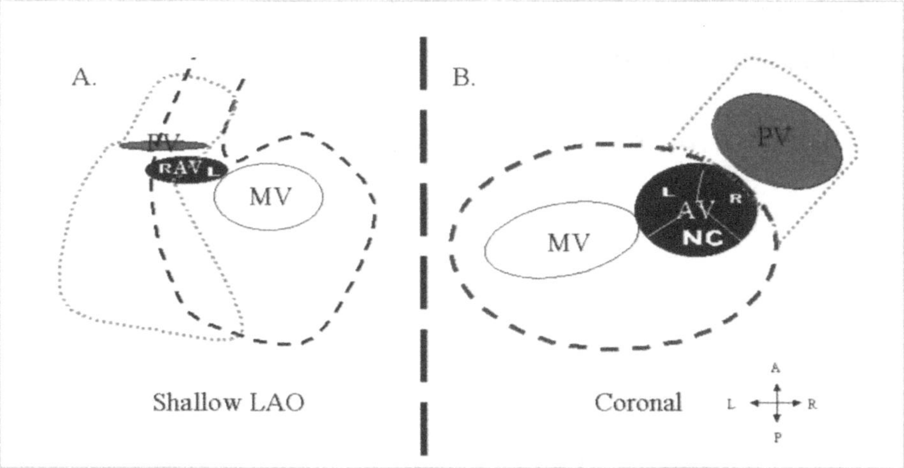

Fig. 1. Relationship of aortic valve (*AV*) and aortic cusps to anatomy of right ventricular outflow tract and mitral valve (*MV*) schematically represented in the shallow left anterior oblique (*LAO*) view and coronal view. The latter view shows a cross section at the level of the aortic and pulmonic valves. Of note, represented are the typical anatomic positions. In many patients the aortic valve will not parallel the pulmonic valve (*PV*) but will have a more vertical tilt and parallel the mitral valve (see Fig. 6) . Although the typical relationship of the left aortic cusp will be in proximity to the anterior septal right ventricular outflow tract and the right coronary cusp the posterior margin there is considerable variability from patient to patient. In **B** one also notes the concave nature of the septal region of the superior RVOT. *R*, right coronary cusp; *L*, left coronary cusp; *NC*, noncoronary cusp

coronary cusp. An extreme convexity of the superior RVOT septal region, which is occasionally seen, can actually create a leftward direction for the most posterior and anterior aspects of the superior RVOT septal border and result in a negative QRS complex in lead 1.

In most young patients the aortic valve is positioned horizontally in the frontal plane and typically parallels the pulmonic valve and is somewhat perpendicular to the mitral valve (Figs. 1, 2). Unlike the pulmonic valve, which tends to be positioned horizontally in the frontal plane, the aortic valve may assume more of a vertical orientation (see below) with the noncoronary cusp frequently positioned at the level of the superior aspect of the tricuspid valve. These anatomic considerations are critical when analyzing the 12 lead ECG patterns of spontaneous arrhythmias and locating the site of origin of these outflow tract tachycardias.

The arrhythmia mechanism most consistent with the cause of repetitive monomorphic VT seen in the outflow tract region appears to be calcium dependent triggered activity [11]. Of note, no discrete anatomic abnormalities are associated with these arrhythmias. Voltage maps have identified bipolar electrograms with normal amplitude in this region. It is thought that perhaps

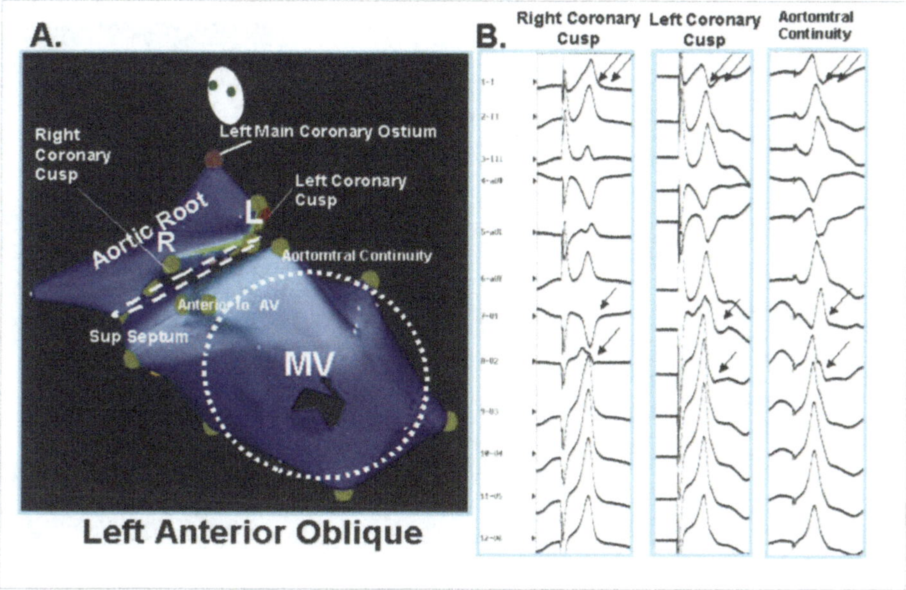

Fig. 2. Relationship of right and left aortic cusps to subaortic endocardial anatomy and their associated ECG patterns. **A** Coronal left anterior oblique view of an electroanatomic map of the aortic root and endocardial left ventricular outflow tract with tagged sites of pacemapping. The view mimics **A** in Fig. 1. Note the ostium of the left main coronary artery has also been tagged and anatomic distance of the left main coronary ostium to the left coronary cusp can be identified. The approximate aortic and mitral valve locations are highlighted. **B** 12 lead ECGs at sites of pacemaps in the aortic cusps and at the aortomitral continuity. Leads V1 and V2 are highlighted by the single arrows. Note the negative QRS in V1 and the transition by V2 when pacing the right coronary cusp and the QRS in V1 and positive QRS in V2 when pacing the left coronary cusp. When pacing the aortomitral continuity on the endocardium a QR complex is noted in V1. The QRS complex in lead 1 (*double arrow*) changed from all R to RS with catheter transition from right coronary cusp to left coronary cusp

the right and left ventricular perivalvular region may have ventricularization with limited or strand like muscle bundles identified. These isolated muscle fibers may be more prone to demonstrate either abnormal automaticity or triggered activity. This is the same mechanism thought to be responsible for the repetitive triggers associated with atrial fibrillation initiation from the isolated muscle bundles entering the pulmonary veins [12]. Such triggered activity has been described in muscle fibers originating from the atrial aspect of the mitral valve region [13, 14]. This hypothesis helps to explain why these tachycardias are almost exclusively seen to originate in an arc-like pattern beginning at the superior aspect of the tricuspid valve and extending superiorly and more commonly septally along the right ventricle just under the pulmonic valve. Activation continues leftward to include the cusp of the aortic valve and

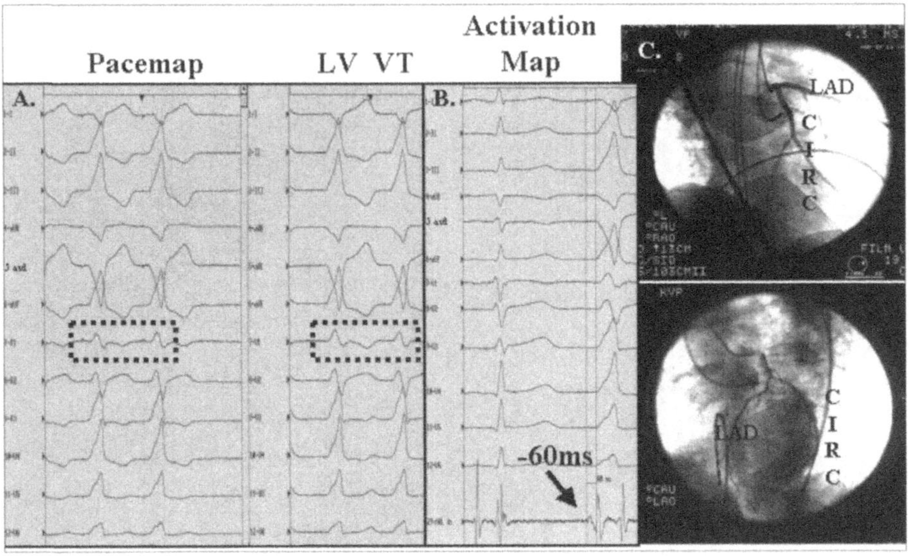

Fig. 3. VT originating from the left coronary cusp. **A** The ECG pattern for the spontaneous VT and the pacemap shows the typical early precordial R wave transition and the typical w pattern in V1 (broken boxes) associated with an origin from the left coronary cusp. **B** Activation map with catheter placed at the left coronary cusp. The recording shows a discrete low amplitude potential at -60 ms before the onset of the QRS. **C** Catheter position in the left aortic cusp coupled with angiographic images of the left coronary system in the RAO and LAO views identifying the ablation catheter tip position approximately 2 cm below the left main coronary orifice. The catheter location was associated with the pace and activation maps shown and was the site of effective and safe catheter ablation

the anterior left ventricle both endocardially and epicardially just in front of the aortic valve and finally ending at the anterior margin of the mitral valve. As will be described below, ventricular pacing can be performed from the cusp of the aortic valve and activation during VT from this area appears to be associated with a local electrogram that tends to be isolated and is frequently associated with an electrogram to QRS interval that ranges from 30 to 80 ms before the QRS onset (Fig. 3). The electrogram characteristics are consistent with an isolated discrete muscle bundle that is located on the cusp.

Surface ECG Clues to Localization of VT to the Aortic Cusps

The location, rotation and horizontal positioning of the heart in the chest, as well as the body habitus, influence surface ECG characteristics. Despite these limitations, the surface ECG provides important clues regarding arrhythmia localization in the setting of outflow tract tachycardias. The ECG is probably particularly helpful in this setting because of 1) the absence of structural heart disease which can further alter ECG patterns of activation, 2) the focal nature of the arrhythmia source and 3) the tendency for these arrhythmias to occur in younger patients which probably limits the anatomic variability in cardiac positioning that is associated with aging. A recognition of the changes in the ECG patterns that occur when one moves along the arc of origin of these arrhythmias from the top of the tricuspid annulus to the lateral mitral annulus is helpful for localizing the optimum site for catheter ablation.

R Wave Progression

RVOT tachycardias tend to have an R wave progression that is positive by V3 or V4 (Fig. 4). In contrast, as we move leftward across the septum to the aortic cusp region, we typically see an R wave progression that is positive by V2 or V3 for the right coronary cusp and by V1 or V2 for the left coronary cusp. Characteristically, even though the net vector for the QRS complex may be

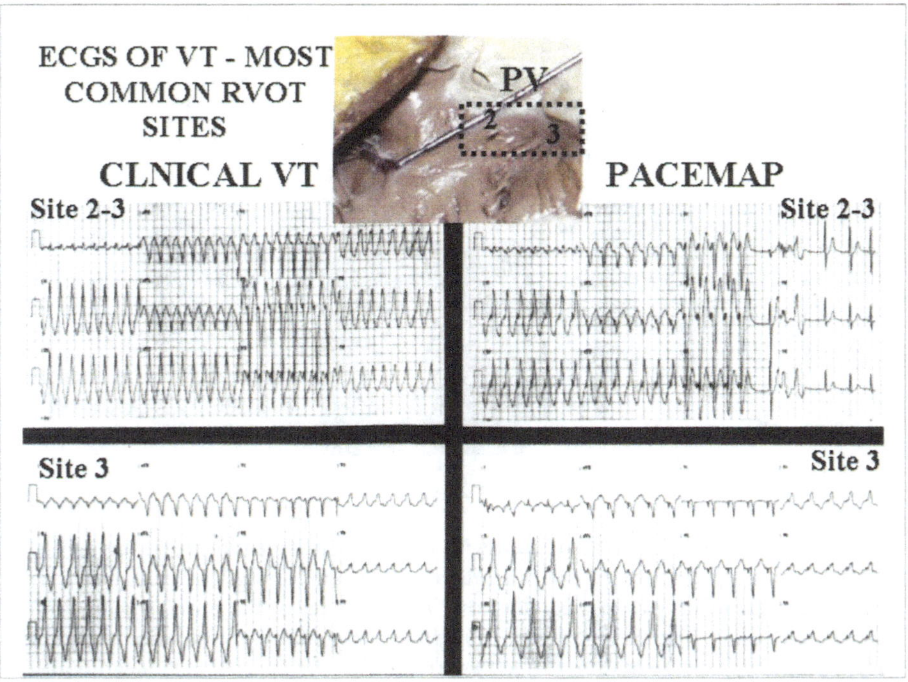

Fig. 4. VT from the most common RV outflow tract sites of origin on the septal and anterior margin of the right ventricle just under the pulmonic valve. The 12 lead ECGs show a precordial transition by V4. The precordial transition is never before V3 from VT originating from the RVOT. The pacemaps from the sites shown in the insert mimic the spontaneous arrhythmia. The insert shows the septal anatomy of the RVOT just below the pulmonic valve. The most anterior and leftward site 3 will characteristically show a negative QRS in lead 1

positive in V1 with a tachycardia originating from the left coronary cusp, flat or negative components to the QRS complex in this precordial lead (W pattern) are characteristic (Fig. 3). This ECG feature is important because as we continue leftward with triggers from the superior mitral annulus, the QRS complex becomes uniformly positive in lead V1 (Fig. 5). Ouyang and colleagues noted that the R wave duration in V1 and V2 tended to be broader when VT originated from the aortic valve cusps than the RVOT septum. An R wave duration >50% of the total QRS duration or an R/S ratio greater than 30% in V1 or V2 were uniformly associated with an aortic cusp origin in their small series of 7 patients.

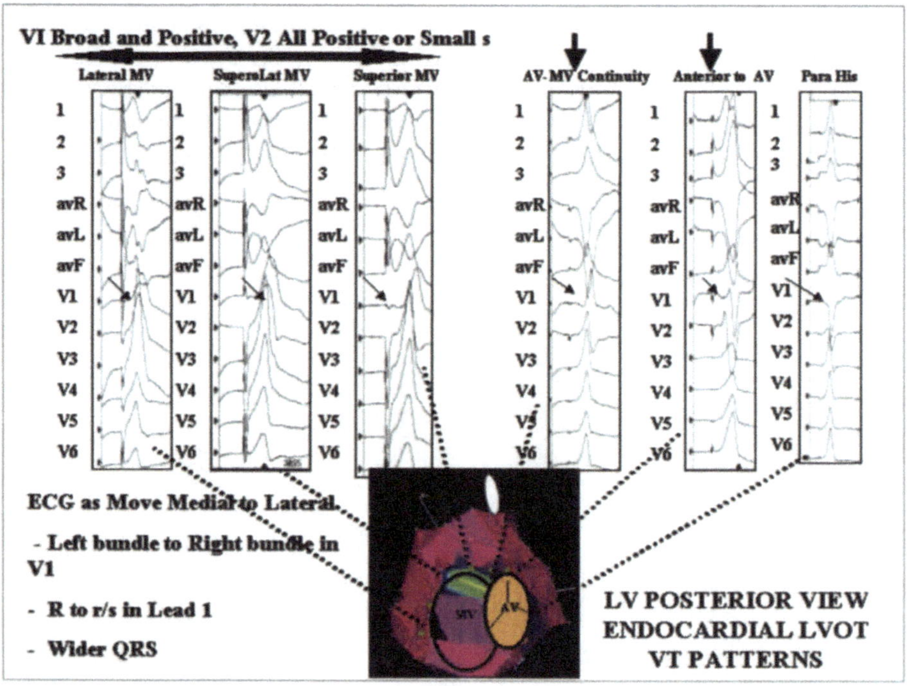

Fig. 5. 12 Lead ECG patterns associated with origin form the endocardial region of the LVOT adjacent to the aortic and mitral valves. Pacemapping was performed from perivalvular sites laterally to medially from lateral border of the mitral annulus to the paraHisian region. The sites of pacemapping were tagged on the posterior view of the electroanatomic voltage map of the left ventricle with the approximate location of the aortic and mitral valves noted on the insert. The characteristic ECG features in V1 and V2 associated with a position above the mitral annulus are highlighted (broad horizontal arrow at top of figure). V1 records broad positive deflection. The ECG morphologies just apical to the aortic valve are also shown (vertical arrows on top of figure). These patterns closely mimic those noted from the cusps of the aortic valve, which also tend to show a multiphasic QRS pattern in lead V1 (W pattern). Although the QRS in lead 1 tends to have a more positive force from the endocardium, sufficient overlap exists from patient to patient that detailed pace and activation mapping is warranted

Amplitude of the QRS in the Inferior Leads

The tallest R waves seen in the inferior ECG leads (II, III, avF) tend to be associated with a VT origin from the superior and anterior RV outflow tract septum, which is the commonest site of origin for the majority of these VTs. Importantly, although the cusps of the aortic valve sit inferior to the RVOT septal surface, nevertheless, the R wave amplitude will be similarly tall if the aortic valve sits perpendicular to the frontal plane and remains parallel to the pulmonic valve. This is probably because the muscular septum will be anatomically located below both valve structures and will be activated in a similar fashion from either right or left perivalvular structures. As the aortic valve assumes a more vertical tilt in the frontal plane, VT from the aortic cusp will tend to have smaller amplitude than the typical RVOT tachycardia originating from the anterior septum just under the pulmonic valve. When the tilt is vertical, the right coronary cusp will actually be positioned fairly inferiorly and VT originating from the right coronary cusp may have an isoelectric to slightly negative QRS complex in limb lead 3 (Fig. 6). Even if the aortic valve has a ver-

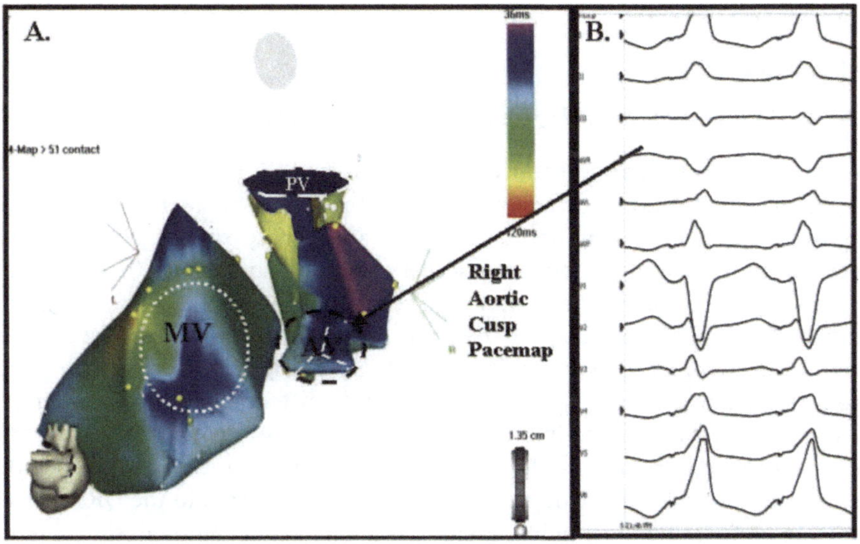

Fig. 6. 12 lead ECG morphology associated with origin from the right aortic cusp. **A** Electroanatomic map of the outflow tract of the left ventricle (LV), the right ventricle (RV) and the aortic cusp region. The approximate anatomic location of the valve structures can be identified and are superimposed on the electroanatomic map. Note the vertical tilt to the aortic valve, which more closely parallels the mitral valve (contrast to Figs. 1 and 2). **B** Pacemap from the right coronary cusp shows a frontal plane axis consistent with the inferior and posterior displacement of the aortic valve with the QRS in lead 3 isoelectric. Variations in the anatomic location of the aortic valve will cause anticipated changes in the electrocardiographic patterns associated with VT from the associated aortic cusps. The broad r in V1 and V2 with the QRS transition in V3 is typical of an aortic cusp origin

tical tilt in the frontal plane, the left coronary cusp will still remain superior and VT originating from the left coronary cusp will continue to demonstrate a positive QRS frontal plane axis.

QRS Morphology in Lead I

The QRS morphology in lead I may vary in tachycardias originating from the aortic cusps. VT from the left cusp will tend to have a QS or RS complex; whereas VT from the right coronary cusp may have a significant R wave in lead 1 depending upon how posterior and inferior the right coronary cusp is positioned. In young patients with vertically positioned hearts the QRS in lead 1 may be negative from VT originating from a sizeable area surrounding the aortic valve. Of note, in the patients with a horizontally positioned heart the entire area surrounding the aortic valve will have a rightward position relative to the LV apex and lateral wall and a positive QRS in limb lead 1 can be seen. The QRS morphology can also be influenced dramatically by ECG lead placement. Care must be given to confirming placement of the limb leads on the shoulders and not the back or chest.

Aortic Cusp VT

12-Lead ECG Distinction from VT to Endocardium or Epicardium in Aortic Valve Region

As might be anticipated, the ECG morphology of VT originating from the superior LV septum and free wall just anterior to the aortic valve closely approximates the VT originating from the aortic cusp region. We have documented the ECG morphology in a series of patients by pacing the endocardium just inside the aortic valve area and compared the QRS morphology to that noted when pacing the cusp of the aortic valve. Patterns were indeed similar with an early precordial transition and "W" pattern in V1 noted with pacing from the endocardium (Fig. 5). The only subtle difference in the QRS complex tended to be identified in limb lead 1. In the patients in whom the aortic valve was positioned horizontally the QRS complex in lead 1 during aortic cusp pacing tended to have a more negative vector when contrasted to the QRS generated from endocardial pacing just inside the aortic valve. Although this clue may be helpful for excluding an endocardial origin, detailed pacemapping and if possible activation mapping are still recommended.

Importantly, the pattern associated with epicardial VT sites of origin just anterior to the aortic valve may mimic the pattern associated with the aortic cusp (Figs. 7, 8). If the QRS pattern is predominantly negative in lead I and the QRS during aortic cusp pacemap has a net positive vector in lead 1, then an epicardial location for the site of origin must be anticipated and epicardial mapping via pericardial puncture should be considered.

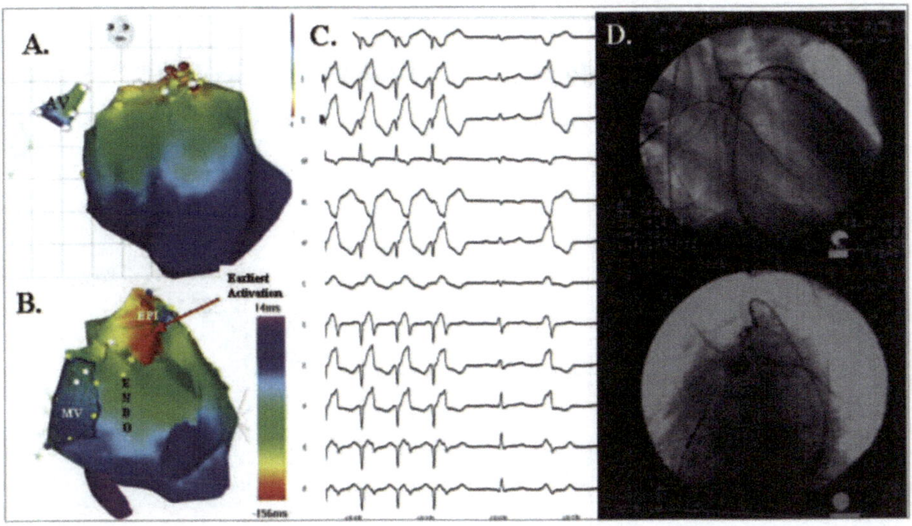

Fig. 7. Ventricular tachycardia from the epicardium anteror and lateral to the aortic valve. **A** Electroanatomic map in a shallow LAO view of the aortic cusps and the LV endocardium. The earliest endocardial activation was displaced laterally on the endocardium. **B** Activation map of the LV epicardium is superimposed on the endocardium and a right posterior view of the LV is shown with the location of the MV identified and the earliest site of activation from the LV epicardium identified by arrow and the red color on the activation map. The site was anterior and slightly lateral to the left aortic cusp. **C** Pacemap from epicardial site showing earliest activation mimicked the VT morphology. Note how negative the QRS complex is in lead 1 which is consistent with an epicardial origin. **D** Fluoroscopic images showing the catheter tip location along the left anterior descending coronary artery with access to the epicardium gained via pericardial puncture

Activation and Pacemapping

Based on surface ECG analysis, a decision can be made early during a planned ablation procedure on the need for more detailed activation and pacemapping from the region of the aortic cusps. Of note, activation mapping in reported series have identified local electrograms preceding the QRS by 30 to 80 ms when VT is localized to the aortic cusps [9, 10]. Not uncommonly, a distinct bipolar electrogram signal is identified that does not correlate with the onset of a sharply negative unipolar signal [10]. This finding may reflect the small amount of muscle activated from this origin on the cusp. Pacemapping may also be used to confirm a QRS morphology that mimics the VT (Fig. 3). Importantly, Ouyang and colleagues have suggested, based on their experience in two patients, that pacemapping at sites demonstrating early bipolar electrogram may not identify a good 12 lead ECG match. No mention was made regarding the stimulus output in that report. Nevertheless, it is possible that strand like muscle fibers producing the characteristic bipolar signal potential

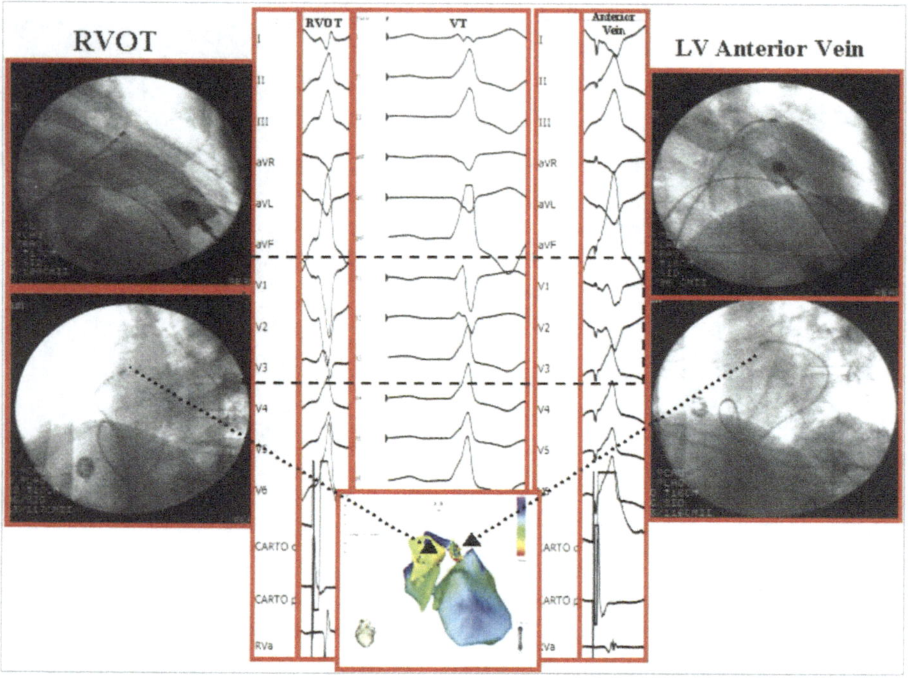

Fig. 8. Epicardial origin for LV VT identified by pacemapping via the coronary sinus. The QRS pattern in V1-V3 (broken lined box) during VT suggested an origin from the aortic cusp with a broad R wave in V2 and transition by V3. However pacemapping from the cusps failed to identify a pattern that approximated the VT and activation mapping failed to identify early activity. The QRS pattern was not mimicked by RVOT or LVOT endocardial pacing and was most closely mimicked by pacing in an anterior vein of the CS. The activation was also the earliest recorded in the vein and is identified on the electroanatomic activation map (insert). These findings would suggest an origin from the epicardium anterior to the left coronary cusp and would require access via the pericardium for more detailed mapping. The fluoroscopic location of the catheter at the sites of RVOT and anterior vein producing the pacemap ECG morphologies are shown

and causing VT may not be activated with current delivery during attempted pacemapping in selected patients. The exact role of pacemapping will require confirmation with careful attention paid to the stimulus strength used. If the timing of the electrogram recorded from the aortic cusps during VT is not early and if pacemapping produces an RS in lead one or a more leftward frontal plane axis, then careful mapping must be performed on both the endocardium and epicardium just in front of the aortic valve regions to identify a non-cusp origin in the vicinity of the aortic valve.

In performing pacemapping from the aortic cusps in a consecutive series of patients using electroanatomic mapping or intracardiac echo to confirm the catheter tip location, we have noted that pacing from the non coronary cusp always results in atrial and not ventricular capture. Kanagaratnum et al. have suggested that VT from the noncoronary cusp can occur [9]. To resolve this discrepancy of observations, we suggest the confirmation of a noncoronary cusp origin of VT accompanied by imaging of catheter position during activation and pacemapping.

Imaging to Identify Catheter Tip Location in the Aortic Cusps

Although catheter tip position can be identified with a reasonable degree of accuracy with careful catheter manipulation using fluoroscopic guidance, imaging tools are available which allow for more reliable catheter tip tracking. Electroanatomic mapping allows for documentation of the catheter tip positioning in each of the cusps at the time of activation and or pacemapping. A separate anatomic shell can be established which can pinpoint the catheter tip location at the time of activation mapping or with pacemapping (Figs. 2, 9).

Intracardiac echo can also be used to identify the catheter tip position. Visualization of the tricuspid aortic valve is easily achieved. Catheter tip position marked by increased echogenicity allows for confirmation of location in the aortic cusp (Fig. 10).

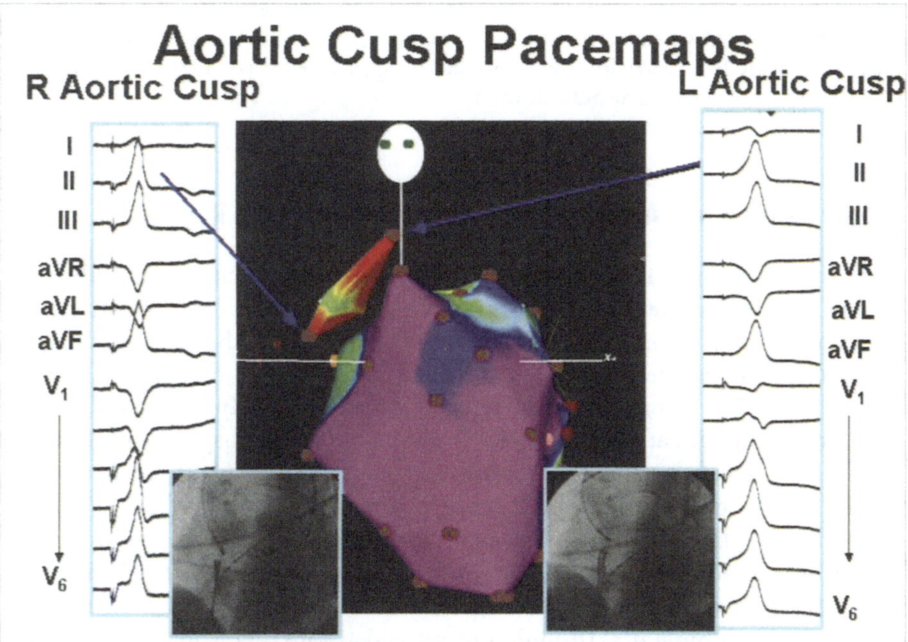

Fig. 9. Anatomic location of the right and left aortic cusp identified on left anterior oblique fluoroscopic and electroanatomic imaging. The electroanatomic imaging allows for detailed definition of the cusps relative to the LV endocardial anatomy. Pacemaps from cusps identify typical patterns of QRS morphology. Note the broad R and transition by V3 from the right coronary cusp and the QR in V1 with the transition by V2 noted with pacemapping from the left coronary cusp

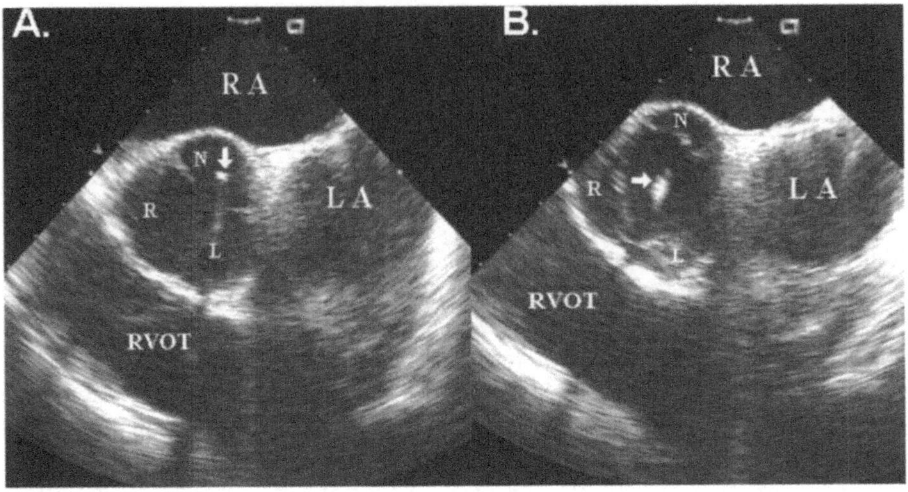

Fig. 10. Image of the aortic cusps using intracardiac echo. Ultrasound catheter transducer placed in the right atrium showing the short-axis view of the aortic root (sinus of Valsalva). **A** The mapping/ablation catheter tip located in the noncoronary (N) cusp can be readily identified during end diastole (arrow). **B** The catheter shaft is identified during end systole (arrow) and can be seen between the cusps consistent with the tip placement within the left ventricle. *L*, left coronary cusp; *LA*, left atrium; *R*, right coronary cusp; *RVOT*, right ventricular outflow tract

Energy Delivery and Ablation Strategy in the Aortic Cusp Region

Once activation and pacemapping has confirmed an aortic cusp origin, ablation can be performed. Because of proximity to the coronary artery ostium, an assessment of the coronary ostial location relative to the catheter tip in the aortic sinuses has been recommended. Typically, the left main coronary ostium is located more than 10 mm above the left aortic cusp (Fig. 3). In contrast, the right coronary ostium lies at a distance of 5 to 10mm above the cusp. As a routine, we tag the ostial location using electroanatomic mapping and only if the distance is within 10 mm do we routinely perform coronary angiography (Fig. 2).

Despite confirmation of a safe anatomic distance, a cautious approach to energy application is warranted. We use temperature regulated energy delivery to achieve a maximum 50-degree target. Of note, energy application is titrated cautiously, beginning at a 10-Joule output and titrated by 5-Joule increments until a maximum output of 30 Watts is achieved. If the tachycardia terminates during energy titration and a temperature of 45 degrees has been achieved, no further increment in power will be made. Energy application duration is limited to 60 seconds. Our experience has confirmed the absence of coronary spasm and preserved aortic valve structure using this approach.

Conclusions

Ventricular tachycardia originating from the cusps of the aortic valve may be more common than previously recognized. The origin from aortic valve cusps is strongly suggested by the early precordial QRS transition pattern during VT in leads V1 or V2 and broad R wave representing at least 50% of the QRS complex in these leads. A "W" pattern in lead V1 suggests an origin from or in close proximity to the left coronary cusp. Activation mapping and pacemapping can be used to accurately confirm the location. Imaging using electroanatomic mapping or intracardiac echo can be used to confirm an aortic cusp location and pinpoint the relationship of the ablation catheter tip position and coronary artery ostium. A cautious approach to energy delivery is appropriate with successful elimination of symptomatic tachycardia anticipated in most patients.

References

1. Morady F, Kadish AH, DiCarlo L et al (1990) Long-term results of catheter ablation of idiopathic right ventricular tachycardia. Circulation 82:2093-2099
2. Jadonath RL, Schwartzman D, Preminger MW et al (1995) The utility of the 12-lead electrocardiogram in localizing the site of origin of right ventricular outflow tract tachycardia. Am Heart J 130:1107-1113
3. Coggins DL, Lee RJ, Sweeney J et al (1994) Radiofrequency catheter ablation as a cure for idiopathic tachycardia of both left and right ventricular origin. J Am Coll Cardiol 23:1333-1341
4. Movsowitz C, Gottlieb CD, Callans DJ et al (1996) Idiopathic right ventricular outflow tract tachycardia: narrowing the anatomic location for successful ablation. Am Heart J 131:930-936
5. Callans DJ, Menz V, Schwartzman D et al (1997) Repetitive monomorphic tachycardia from the left ventricular outflow tract: electrocardiographic patterns consistent with a left ventricular site of origin. J Am Coll Cardiol 29:1023-1027
6. Marchlinski FE, Deely MP, Zado ES (2000) Gender specific triggers for right ventricular outflow tract tachycardia. Am Heart Journal 139:1009-1013
7. Dixit S, Marchlinski FE (2001) Clinical characteristics and catheter ablation of left ventricular outflow tract tachycardia. Curr Cardiol Reports 3:305-313
8. Dixit S, Gerstenfeld EP, Callans DJ, Marchlinski FE (2003) Electrocardiographic patterns of superior right ventricular outflow tract tachycardias: Distinguishing septal and free wall sites of origin. J Cardiovasc Electrophysiol 14:1-7
9. Kanagaratnum L, Tomassoni G, Scweiker R et al (2001) Ventricular tachycardias arising from the aortic sinus of valsalva: an under-recognized variant of left ventricular outflow tract tachycardia. J Am Coll Cardiol 37:1408-1414
10. Ouyang F, Fotuhi P, Hebe J et al (2002) Rerpetitive monomorphic ventricular tachycardia originating from the aortic sinus cusp: electrocardiographic characterization for guiding catheter ablation. J Am Coll Cardiol 39:500-508
11. Lerman BB, Kenneth SM, Markovitz SM (1997) Mechanisms of idiopathic left ventricular tachycardia. J Cardiovasc Electrophysiol 8:571-583

12. Chen SA, Hsieh MH, Tai CT et al (1999) Initiation of atrial fibrillation by ectopic beats originating from the pulmonary veins. Circulation 100:1879-1886
13. Mallavarapu C, Callans DJ, Schwartzman D et al (1996) Radiofrequency catheter ablation of atrial tachycardia with unusual left atrial sites of origin: report of two cases. Pacing Clin Electrophysiol 19(6): 988-992
14. Wit AL, Rosen MR, Hoffman BF (1974) Electrophysiology and pharmacology of cardiac arrhythmias II. Relationship of normal and abnormal electrical activity of cardiac fibers to genesis of arrhythmias. Am Heart J 88:515-524

Extreme Left Vetricular Hypertrophy: An Indicator of Increased Risk of Sudden Death in Hypertrophic Cardiomyopathy

P. Bernabò[1], C. Autore[2], P. Spirito[1]

Since the first modern descriptions of hypertrophic cardiomyopathy (HCM) in 1958, sudden and unexpected cardiac death has been recognized as the most devastating feature in the natural history of this disease [1–3]. The fact that sudden death most often occurs in young patients in the absence of previous symptoms makes this event particularly dramatic [4]. However, despite several decades of research, the heterogeneous clinical spectrum and diverse natural history of HCM continue to represent a major obstacle to the identification of those patients at high risk of dying suddenly. Recent observations indicating that the implantable cardioverter-defibrillator (ICD) is highly effective in preventing sudden death in patients with HCM have further increased the need for accurate indicators of risk [5].

At present, the ICD is regarded as definitely justified for secondary prevention of sudden death in HCM patients who have survived a cardiac arrest or have experienced one or more episodes of sustained ventricular tachycardia [2, 3, 5]. The indications to the ICD for prophylactic primary prevention of sudden death remain more uncertain. Several features are considered markers of increased risk, including a history of sudden death in young family members, nonsustained ventricular tachycardia on Holter monitoring, abnormal blood pressure response during exercise, and unexplained syncope, particularly when exertional or in young patients [2, 3, 6]. None of these markers, however, is associated with a high relative risk of sudden death. Therefore, the decision to implant an ICD must usually be based on a careful evaluation of the overall risk profile of the individual patient.

Extreme Left Ventricular Hypertrophy as a Risk Factor for Sudden Death

In the early 1990s, patients with HCM and extreme left ventricular hypertro-

[1]Divisione di Cardiologia, Ente Ospedaliero Ospedali Galliera, Genoa; [2]Dipartimento di Scienze Cardiovascolari e Respiratorie, Università di Roma “La Sapienza”, Policlinico Sant’Andrea, Rome, Italy

phy ($\geq$30 mm) were first reported to have a substantially higher risk of sudden death than patients with mild hypertrophy [7]. More recently, two independent investigations in large and consecutively enrolled HCM populations reported an increased risk associated with greater magnitude of left ventricular hypertrophy [8, 9]. One of these studies, performed in about 500 patients with HCM, showed that the risk of sudden death increased progressively in direct relation to maximal left ventricular wall thickness (measured by echocardiography as the greatest thickness at any site in the left ventricular wall) [8]. At the extremes of the morphologic spectrum, patients with a wall thickness $\geq$30 mm were predominantly adolescents or young adults with no or only mild symptoms and had a substantial long-term risk of sudden death (about 20% at 10 years and 40% at 20 years), while those with mild hypertrophy (<20 mm wall thickness) and without other generally accepted risk factors appeared to be at low risk.

The second study, which included more than 600 patients, confirmed the results of the first investigation and showed that patients with extreme hypertrophy ($\geq$30 mm) had the highest risk of sudden death [9]. In both investigations, patients with extreme hypertrophy had an estimated long-term risk of sudden death of about 20% at 10 years and represented about 10% of the study population, but accounted for more than 25% of the sudden deaths [8, 9].

More recently, the relation between left ventricular wall thickness and age was investigated in more than 800 patients with HCM. Extreme left ventricular hypertrophy ($\geq$30 mm) was relatively frequent in young patients, but uncommon in older patients [10]. In particular, extreme hypertrophy was present in about 15% of the patients younger than 30 years, and in fewer than 5% of those older than 60; furthermore, a wall thickness of 35 mm or greater was present in about 7% of the younger but in none of the older patients. This body of evidence from particularly large HCM populations indicates that extreme hypertrophy is associated with an unfavorable prognosis and a high long-term risk of sudden death (Fig. 1). Consistent with these conclusions are also previous observations showing a direct association between magnitude of hypertrophy and occurrence of nonsustained ventricular tachycardia in HCM [11]. Therefore, we believe that serious consideration should be given to primary prophylactic prevention of sudden death with the ICD in those young patients with HCM who have extreme forms of left ventricular hypertrophy.

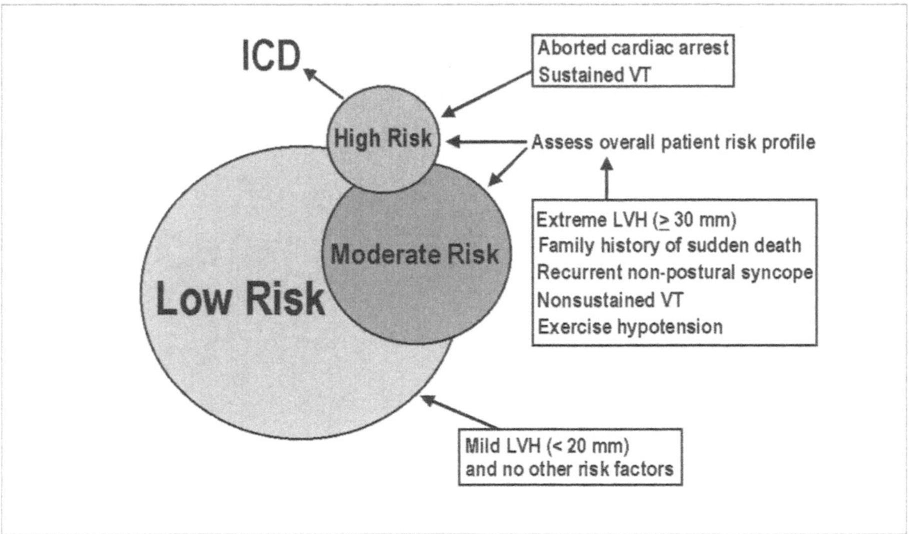

Fig. 1. Strategy for risk stratification and prevention of sudden death in hypertrophic cardiomyopathy (see text for details). *ICD*, implantable cardioverter defibrillator; *LVH*, left ventricular hypertrophy; *VT*, ventricular tachycardia

References

1. Teare D (1958) Asymmetrical hypertrophy of the heart in young adults. Br Heart J 20:1–8
2. Spirito P, Seidman CE, McKenna WJ et al (1997) The management of hypertrophic cardiomyopathy. N Engl J Med 336:775–785
3. Maron BJ (2002) Hypertrophic cardiomyopathy. A systematic review. JAMA 287:1308–1320
4. Maron BJ, Olivotto I, Spirito P et al (2000) Epidemiology of hypertrophic cardiomyopathy-related death revisited in a large non-referral-based patient population. Circulation 102:858–864
5. Maron BJ, Shen WK, Link MS et al (2000) Efficacy of the implantable cardioverter-defibrillator for the prevention of sudden death in hypertrophic cardiomyopathy. N Engl J Med 342:365–373
6. Elliott PM, Poloniecki J, Dickie S et al (2000) Sudden death in hypertrophic cardiomyopathy: identification of high risk patients. J Am Coll Cardiol 36:2212–2218
7. Spirito P, Maron BJ (1990) Relation between extent of left ventricular hypertrophy and occurrence of sudden cardiac death in hypertrophic cardiomyopathy. J Am Coll Cardiol 15:1521–1526
8. Spirito P, Bellone P, Harris KM et al (2000) Magnitude of left ventricular hypertrophy and risk of sudden death in hypertrophic cardiomyopathy. N Engl J Med 342:1778–1785
9. Elliot PM, Gimeno Blanes JR, Mahon et al (2001) Relation between severity of left ventricular hypertrophy and prognosis in patients with hypertrophic cardiomyopathy. Lancet 357: 420–424

10. Maron BJ, Piccininno M, Bernabò P et al (2003) Relation of extreme left ventricular hypertrophy to age in hypertrophic cardiomyopathy. Am J Cardiol 91:626–628
11. Spirito P, Watson RM, Maron BJ (1987) Relation between extent of left ventricular hypertrophy and occurrence of ventricular tachycardia in hypertrophic cardiomyopathy. Am J Cardiol 60:1137–1142

Does a Maximum Left Ventricular Thickness Greater than 30 mm Identify Patients with Hypertrophic Cardiomyopathy at Risk of Sudden Death?

I. Olivotto, F. Cecchi

Despite very significant advances in the understanding of hypertrophic cardiomyopathy (HCM), the identification of patients at high risk of sudden death remains challenging [1, 2]. The possibility of achieving primary prevention of sudden death following the introduction of the implantable cardioverter-defibrillator in clinical practice has further highlighted the need for reliable indicators of risk. Unfortunately, all markers of risk identified to date have shown a disappointingly low positive predictive value [2].

In the last two decades, the debate as to whether the magnitude of left ventricular (LV) hypertrophy has an influence on prognosis in HCM patients has produced conflicting results [3–8]. Recently, two large studies have reported a direct relationship between maximum LV wall thickness and risk of HCM-related mortality, mostly due to an excess in sudden and unexpected death [3, 5]. In both studies, risk appeared to be particularly high in the small subsets of patients with maximum LV thickness of 30 mm or greater, although the positive predictive value was consistently low. In the study by Elliott et al., however, the number of additional established risk factors for sudden death was a better predictor than wall thickness [5]. Therefore, the authors conclude that the risk of sudden death associated with a LV wall thickness of 30 mm or greater in patients without other risk factors is insufficient to justify aggressive prophylactic therapy [5].

In our experience, the severity of hypertrophy expressed as maximum LV wall thickness did not represent a significant prognostic indicator in patients with HCM [8]. Indeed, with the exception of the small subset with thickness values of 15 mm or less, with a consistently benign clinical course, the distribution of sudden death and overall cardiovascular mortality was not significantly different among four other classes of increasing thickness ranging from 16–19 mm to 30 mm or greater. In our patient population, a maximum LV wall thickness of 30 mm or greater was not incompatible with a normal life

Regional Referral Center for Myocardial Diseases, Azienda Ospedaliera Careggi, Florence, Italy

expectancy, nor associated with an increase in disease-related complications. Moreover, none of the most relevant markers of electrical or hemodynamic instability, including syncope, nonsustained ventricular tachycardia, abnormal blood pressure response to exercise, and atrial fibrillation, were significantly associated with the degree of maximum LV thickness [8].

Our findings, however, are not necessarily in disagreement with the other two studies with regard to patients with extreme LV hypertrophy (≥30 mm): indeed, the combined analysis of the three studies consistently showed that the increase in risk among patients with extreme LV hypertrophy was consistently confined to the subgroup below 18 years of age, whereas mortality among adult patients was relatively low (7%) and comparable to that among patients with only mild hypertrophy [8]. Thus, existing evidence suggests that extreme LV thickness may represent a marker of risk *per se* only in those patients diagnosed at a very young age, and it should not prompt aggressive management in the absence of other documented risk factors in adult patients [5, 8]. Indeed, the most appropriate approach to risk stratification based on current knowledge is necessarily multifactorial. A comprehensive evaluation should include the known predictors of risk, which include, besides maximum LV wall thickness, a family history of sudden death, abnormal blood pressure response to exercise, nonsustained ventricular tachycardia, and unexplained syncope [2]. Moreover, recent studies have shown that the presence of atrial fibrillation, resting LV outflow obstruction, and microvascular dysfunction also have an important impact on outcome in HCM patients [9–11].

Finally, it is to be remembered that a single measurement of maximum LV thickness, although reproducible and practical for clinical purposes, does not accurately reflect the total burden of hypertrophy in individual patients, and thus represents only a crude estimate of the morphological severity of HCM. Moreover, a quantitative approach to hypertrophy is necessarily limited in that it overlooks individual differences in the LV wall structure. Indeed, several pathophysiological substrates coexisting in the hypertrophic myocardium, including disarray, fibrosis and ischemia, are possibly more relevant than the extent of hypertrophy itself in determining HCM-related risk, and ideally require a comprehensive assessment in each patient [12].

In conclusion, the maximum LV wall thickness should be considered in the context of a multifactorial approach to risk stratification. Extreme LV hypertrophy does not justify aggressive prophylactic treatment in the absence of additional established markers of risk; only in those patients diagnosed at very young age might the presence of a maximum LV wall thickness of 30 mm or greater represent *per se* a potential marker of risk of sudden death.

Acknowledgements. This work was supported by grants from the Italian Ministry for Scientific and Technologic Research (Grant COFIN 2002).

References

1. Maron BJ (2002) Hypertrophic cardiomyopathy: a systematic review. JAMA 287:1308–1320
2. Elliott PM, Poloniecki J, Dickie S et al (2000) Sudden death in hypertrophic cardiomyopathy: identification of high risk patients. J Am Coll Cardiol 36:2212–2218
3. Spirito P, Bellone P, Harris KM et al (2000) Magnitude of left ventricular hypertrophy and risk of sudden death in hypertrophic cardiomyopathy. N Engl J Med 342:1778–1785
4. Spirito P, Maron BJ (1990) Relation between extent of left ventricular hypertrophy and occurrence of sudden cardiac death in hypertrophic cardiomyopathy. J Am Coll Cardiol 15:1521–1526
5. Elliott PM, Gimeno B Jr, Mahon NG et al (2001) Relation between severity of left-ventricular hypertrophy and prognosis in patients with hypertrophic cardiomyopathy. Lancet 357:420–424
6. Maron BJ, Roberts WC, Epstein SE (1982) Sudden death in hypertrophic cardiomyopathy: a profile of 78 patients. Circulation 65:1388–1394
7. Louie EK, Maron BJ (1986) Hypertrophic cardiomyopathy with extreme increase in left ventricular wall thickness: functional and morphologic features and clinical significance. J Am Coll Cardiol 8:57–65
8. Olivotto I, Gistri R, Petrone P et al (2003) Maximum left ventricular thickness and risk of sudden death in patients with hypertrophic cardiomyopathy. J Am Coll Cardiol 41:315–321
9. Olivotto I, Cecchi F, Casey SA et al (2001) Impact of atrial fibrillation on the clinical course of hypertrophic cardiomyopathy. Circulation 104:2517–2524
10. Maron MS, Olivotto I, Betocchi S et al (2003) Effect of left ventricular outflow tract obstruction on clinical outcome in hypertrophic cardiomyopathy. N Engl J Med 348:295–303
11. Cecchi F, Olivotto I, Gistri R et al (2001) Coronary microvascular dysnfunction and prognosis in hypertrophic cardiomyopathy. New Engl J Med (in press)
12. Shirani J, Pick R, Roberts WC, Maron BJ (2000) Morphology and significance of the left ventricular collagen network in young patients with hypertrophic cardiomyopathy and sudden cardiac death. J Am Coll Cardiol 35:36–44

Drug-Induced Torsade de Pointes. Role of Genetic Factors

N. El-Sherif, G. Turitto

Introduction

Inherited long QT syndrome (LQTS) is an uncommon cardiac electrophysiologic abnormality that predisposes to a malignant polymorphic ventricular tachyarrhythmia, commonly known as Torsade de Pointes (TdP) [1]. Mutations in several cardiac ion channels genes have been identified that cause the hereditary LQTS/TdP [2]. During the past several years, a number of approved and marketed drugs, both cardiovascular and non-cardiovascular agents, have been associated with QT interval prolongation, TdP, and sudden cardiac death [3]. Several of these drugs have been removed from the market or have had restrictive labeling. This has caused significant concern among the regulatory agencies, the pharmaceutical industry, the medical profession, and the public. The mechanisms of drug-induced LQTS/TdP are not fully understood. It has been suggested that a forme fruste of the congenital LQTS may play a key role in the acquired LQTS/TdP. A better understanding of the factors involved in drug-induced LQTS/TdP will help to implement effective preventive and therapeutic measures.

Ionic Basis of Congenital LQTS and TdP

Congenital LQTS is caused by mutations in potassium (K^+) and sodium (Na^+) cardiac ion channel genes, with specific genetic types of the syndrome identified, as shown in Table 1 [2]. It is estimated that LQT1, caused by KVLQT1 IKs potassium channel gene mutations, and LQT2, caused by HERG IKr potassium channel gene mutations, account for the majority (87 %) of cases of LQTS with known genotype [4]. LQT3 accounts for 8 %, whereas LQT5 and LQT6 are extremely rare accounting for less than 5 % of LQTS cases. Homozygous

Cardiology Division, Department of Medicine, State University of New York, Downstate Medical Center and New York Harbor Health Care Center, Brooklyn, New York, USA

Table 1. Genetic background of inherited forms of LQTS

LQTS Type	Chromosomal Locus	Mutated Gene	Ion Current Affected
Romano-Ward Syndrome			
LQT1	Chr. 11p15.5	KVLQT1 (KCNQ1) (heterozygotes)	Potassium current (I_{Ks})
LQT2	Chr. 7q35-36	HERG	Potassium current (I_{Kr})
LQT3	Chr. 3p21-24	SCN5A	Sodium current (I_{Na})
LQT4	Chr. 4q25-27	?	?
LQT5	Chr. 21q22.1-22.2	KCNE1 (heterozygotes)	Potassium current (I_{Ks})
LQT6	Chr. 21q22.1-22.2	MiRP1	Potassium current (I_{Kr})
Jervell and Lang-Nielsen Syndrome			
JLN1	Chr. 11q15.5	KVLQT1 (KCNQ1) (homozygotes)	Potassium current (I_{Ks})
JLN2	Chr. 21q22.1-22.2	KCNE1 (homozygotes)	Potassium current (I_{Ks})

KVLQT1 and KCNE1 mutations are associated with congenital deafness (Jervell and Lange-Nielsen syndrome) and account for less than 1 % of LQTS. Around 200 different mutations of these genes have been found so far [4]. There is significant phenotypic variation of the electrocardiographic findings (T-wave morphology), factors triggering cardiac events and risk of cardiac events, depending on which gene and which mutations are involved. Because not all known incidents of LQTS are caused by mutations of the above genes, other genes causing this disorder are expected to be identified.

Drug-induced LQTS and TdP

The ionic mechanisms of pharmacologically-induced prolonged repolarization and early afterdepolarization (EAD) formation can be complex. Several pharmacological agents act by affecting more than one ionic current either in a synergistic or opposing direction. More important, the synergistic effects of other interventions are frequently required for critical lengthening of repolarization and the generation of EADs. A slow driving rate, as well as low extracellular K^+, usually play a significant synergistic effect. The slow driving rate probably acts by reducing the I_p. Low extracellular K^+ will decrease K^+ conductance, which in turn will affect a number of currents, including I_k, I_{k1} and I_f.

The list of drugs causing LQTS and TdP is continuously increasing [3] (Table 2). Literally any pharmacologic agent that can result in prolonged QT can induce LQTS [5]. The incidence of TdP has not been correlated with the plasma concentrations of drugs known to precipitate this arrhythmia. However, high plasma concentrations, resulting from excessive dose or reduced

Table 2. Abbreviated list of drugs reported to cause prolongation of the QT interval or Torsade de Pointes

Category of drug	Drugs
Antiarrhythmic	
Class IA	Disopyramide, procainamide, quinidine
Class III	Amiodarone, bretylium, sotalol, dofetilide,ibutilide
Antimicrobial	Erythromycin, trimethoprim-sulfamethoxazole, Clarithromycin
Antifungal	Fluconazole, ketoconazole, itraconazole
Antimalarial or antiprotozoal	Chloroquine, halofantrine, mefloquine, pentamidine, quinine
Antihistamine	Astemizole, terfenadine, diphenydramine
Gastrointestinal prokinetic	Cisapride
Psychoactive	Chloral hydrate, haloperidol, lithium, phenothiazines, pimozide, tricyclic antidepressants
Anti-HIV	Efavirenz
Miscellaneous	Amantidine, indapamide, probucol, tacrolimus, vasopressin

metabolism of some of these drugs, may increase the risk of precipitating TdP. Such reduced metabolism may result from the concomitant use of other drugs that interfere with cytochrome P_{450} enzymes. Medications reported to interfere with the metabolism of some drugs associated with TdP include systemic ketoconazole and structurally similar drugs (fluconazole, itraconazole, metronidazole); serotonin re-uptake inhibitors (fluoxetine, fluvoxamine, sertraline) and other antidepressants (nefazodone); HIV protease inhibitors (indinavir, ritonavir, saquinavir); dihydropyridine calcium-channel blockers (felodipine, nicardipine, nifedipine), and erythromycin and other macrolide antibiotics. Grapefruit and grapefruit juice may also interact with some drugs by interfering with cytochrome P_{450} enzymes. TdP may also result from the use of drugs causing QT prolongation in patients with medical conditions, such as hepatic dysfunction or congenital LQTS, or in those with electrolyte disturbances (particularly hypokalemia and hypomagnesemia). Electrolyte disturbances may be induced by corticosteroids, diuretic therapy, liquid protein diet, severe diarrhea or vomiting.

The Electrophysiologic Mechanism of Drug-Induced LQTS and TdP

Both the congenital and acquired LQTS are due to abnormalities (intrinsic and/or acquired) of the ionic currents underlying ventricular repolarization. Prolongation of the repolarization phase acts as a primary step for the generation of early EADs. EAD-induced triggered beats arise predominantly from the Purkinje network [6]. In LQTS, prolonged repolarization is associated with increased spatial dispersion of repolarization [6, 7]. The focal EAD-induced triggered beat(s) can infringe on the underlying substrate of inhomogeneous repolarization to initiate reentrant excitation in the form of rotating scrolls. The mechanism of the characteristic twisting morphology of TdP was explained on the basis of transient bifurcation of a predominantly single rotating scroll into two simultaneous scrolls, involving both the right and left ventricles separately [7].

Recently, the electrophysiologic mechanism of acquired LQTS was investigated in a canine model of cardiac hypertrophy, in which dogs with chronic atrio-ventricular (AV) block develop ventricular hypertrophy secondary to chronic volume overload [8]. The study demonstrated that volume overload hypertrophy in dog was associated with prolonged ventricular repolarization and increased tridimensional dispersion of repolarization (TDR) compared to non-hypertrophied heart. Furthermore, the hypertrophied heart was more susceptible to the repolarization prolonging effects of a class III antiarrhythmic agent, dofetilide, a selective blocker of I_{Kr}. Dofetilide resulted in significantly more prolongation of ventricular repolarization of the hypertrophied heart. More importantly, the drug resulted in differentially greater prolongation of repolarization at endocardial/mid-myocardial regions, compared to epicardial regions resulting in increased TDR. The increased TDR at contiguous myocardial sites represented the primary electrophysiologic substrate for the development of functional conduction block and reentrant tachyarrhythmias, such as TdP. The study demonstrated that a high dose of dofetilide resulted in prolongation of repolarization, increased TDR, and uncommonly in TdP in normal heart. On the other hand, the hypertrophied heart was more susceptible to the proarrhythmic consequences of dofetilide at doses that are considered within the clinical range. The study provided the electrophysiologic basis for the reported dose-related incidence of dofetilide-induced TdP in patients [9]. It also justified the current recommendations for dose-titration and close monitoring of the effects of the drug in the clinical setting [10].

Drug-Induced LQTS/TdP. Environmental and Genetic Factors

The susceptibility of certain individuals to drug-induced LQTS/TdP can be related to both environmental and genetic factors that modulate key cardiac ion channels and currents involved in the syndrome. These factors include electrolytes and acid-base abnormalities, specially hypokalemia and hypomagnesemia, as well as bradycardia. Certain cardiac pathologic states like hypertrophy, post-infarction remodeling and heart failure, are known to be associated with downregulation of key K^+ channel genes and currents that result in prolongation of action potential duration (APD). Furthermore, in addition to the downregulation of K^+ genes and currents [11], in the post-infarction remodeled heart there are alterations of Na^+ channel kinetics and gene expression that result in increase of late Na^+ currents and contribute to prolongation of the APD [12].

The majority of drug-induced LQTS/TdP is associated with block of the cardiac HERG K^+ channels and depressed I_{Kr} [2]. A recent study provides a structure-function basis for the promiscuous character of the HERG channels [13]. There is a high-affinity drug block of HERG channels by a number of different compounds that interact with amino acids located on the S6 transmembrane domain and pore helix of the HERG channel subunit that face the cavity of the channel. The aromatic residues of the S6 domain that interact with these drugs are unique to eag/erg K^+ channels but not to other Kv channels. The authors suggested that a model based on structure-activity correlation could be used to develop a virtual screening tool to eliminate compounds that are likely to block HERG channels from further development.

Genetic risk factors for drug-induced LQTS/TdP include, besides the increased susceptibility of post-pubertal women, the so-called "repolarization reserve" [14]. This concept emphasizes the occurrence of TdP secondary to repolarization-prolonging drugs as a patient-specific response. This is supported by reports of patients who developed additional episodes of LQTS/TdP during subsequent exposure to a repolarization-prolonging drug different from the one that initially caused their arrhythmia. In one study, in patients who developed TdP secondary to the class III drug, Almokalant, the drug-induced QTc prolongation was more marked compared to patients who did not develop TdP. This difference was not related to the dose of the drug but rather to individual susceptibility [15].

Is Drug-Induced LQTS/TdP a Forme-Fruste of Congenital LQTS?

It has been suggested that the presence of a forme-fruste of congenital LQTS could play a key role in patient-specific drug-induced LQTS/TdP. However, the data so far have shown that a minority of patients with drug-induced LQTS/TdP have mutations in one of the genes known to cause congenital LQTS. The KCNE 2 encoded Mink-related peptide 1 (MiRP1), a subunit of the cardiac K^+ channel I_{Kr}, has been associated with inherited LQTS. A study of 98 patients with drug-induced LQTS, identified four patients with missense variants: three mutations decreased K^+ flux at baseline, and a single-nucleotide polymorphism (SNP) that is present in 1.6 % of healthy individuals [16]. The patient with SNP had a normal electrocardiogram at rest but developed a very long QT interval on Bactrim due to inhibition of the channel by the sulfamethoxazole component of the drug [16]. In another study of 16 consecutive patients with drug-induced LQTS/TdP, one patient was identified with a missense mutation on HERG [17]. On the other hand, a recent study identified a common variant of the cardiac Na^+ channel gene, SCN5A (Y1102), present in 19.2 % of West African and Caribbean patients and 13.2 % of African American patients [18]. The variant allele accelerated channel activation, increasing the likelihood of channel bursting activity and abnormal cardiac repolarization. These patients may have an increased susceptibility to drug-induced LQTS/TdP.

Drug-Induced LQTS/TdP: Role of Modifier Genes

In the past several years, a large number of gene mutations have been associated with congenital LQTS [4]. Not all mutations have the same phenotypic expression. Several family numbers of patients with congenital LQTS/TdP may be silent gene carriers. The penetrance of a particular mutation does not depend solely on the specific mutation, but can be modified by the individual genetic background [19]. In general, genotype-phenotype correlation studies show significant variability in the phenotype expression of the disease among affected individuals with identical causal mutations. Overall, causal mutations account for a fraction of the variability of phenotypes and genetic background, referred to as the modifier genes, but play a significant role. Modifier genes are genes that are not involved in the genesis of the disease but modify the severity of the phenotypic expression. The final phenotype is the result of interactions between the causal genes, genetic background (modifier genes), as well as environmental factors. Modifier genes have been investigated in other cardiac diseases like hypertrophic cardiomyopathy [20] and heart failure [21]. Identification of the modifier genes will complement the results of studies of causative genes and could enhance genetic-based diagnosis, risk stratification, and implementation of preventive and therapeutic measures in patients with drug-induced LQTS/TdP.

Drug-Induced LQTS/TdP: Regulatory Response

Drug regulatory agencies, such as the Food and Drug Administration (FDA) in the United States and the Committee for Proprietary Medicinal Products (CPMP) of the European Agency for the Evaluation of Medicinal Products, now scrutinize the potential QT prolonging effects of all new drugs undergoing regulatory approval, as well as marketed drugs with QT prolongation observed during postmarketing surveillance. The CPMP has published a document, "Points to Consider: The Assessment of the Potential for QT Interval Prolongation by Non-Cardiovascular Medicinal Products," that is already influencing the way electrocardiographic data are collected and analyzed during clinical trials related to regulatory approval [22]. Recently, a task force of the International Society for Holter and Noninvasive Electrocardiology has suggested guidelines for EKG evaluation of drug-related QT prolongation and other alterations in ventricular repolarization [23]. Similar standardization activity is now underway on the North American continent under the collaborative umbrella of the Canadian agency and the FDA. From the regulatory perspective, it is vitally important that the distinction between drug-induced and spontaneous QT interval prolongation is carefully made. If this is not done, a harmless drug may be inappropriately labeled and denied to needy patients. On the other hand, when repolarization abnormalities go unrecognized, the public may be placed at unnecessary risk.

Conclusions

There is not always a direct correlation between the degree of drug-induced QT interval prolongation and the propensity to induce TdP. Although, at present, it is difficult to predict which patients are at risk for TdP, careful assessment of the risk to benefit ratio is important before prescribing drugs known to be able to cause QT interval prolongation.

Acknowledgements. Supported in part by NES Veterans Administration Cardiovascular REAP program.

References

1. El-Sherif N, Turitto G (2003) Torsade de Pointes. Curr Opin Cardiol 18:6-13
2. Zareba W, Moss AJ (2001) Long QT syndrome in children. J Electrocardiol 34:167-171
3. Haverkamp W, Breithardt G, Camm AJ et al (2000) The potential for QT prolongation and pro-arrhythmia by non-anti-arrhythmic drugs: Clinical and regulatory implications. Report on a policy conference of the European Society of Cardiology, Cardiovasc Res 47:219-233
4. Splawski I, Shen J, Timothy KW et al (2000) Spectrum of mutations in long QT syndrome genes. KVLQT1, HERG, SCN5A, KCNE1, and KCNE2. Circulation 102:1178-1184
5. Castillo R, Pedalino RP, El-Sherif N, Turitto G (2002) Efavirenz-associated QT prolongation and Torsade de pointes arrhythmia. Ann Pharmacother 36:1006-1008
6. El-Sherif N, Caref EB, Yin H, Restivo M (1996) The electrophysiological mechanism of ventricular tachyarrhythmias in the long QT syndrome: tridimensional mapping of activation and recovery patterns. Circ Res 79:474-492
7. El-Sherif N, Chinushi M, Caref EB, Restivo M (1997) Electrophysiological mechanism of the characteristic electrocardiographic morphology of torsade de pointes tachyarrhythmias in the long QT syndrome. Detailed analysis of ventricular tridimensional activation patterns. Circulation 96:4392-4399
8. Kozhevnikov DO, Yamamoto K, Robotis D et al (2002) Electrophysiological mechanisms of enhanced susceptibility of hypertrophied heart to acquired torsade de pointes

arrhythmias. Tridimensional mapping of activation and recovery patterns. Circulation 105:1128-1134
9. Mazur A, Anderson ME, Bonney S et al (2001) Pause-dependent polymorphic ventricular tachycardia during long-term treatment with dofetilide: a placebo-controlled, implantable cardioverter-defibrillator-based evaluation. J Am Coll Cardiol 37:1100-1105
10. Torpe-Pedersen C, Molar M, Bloch-Thomsen PE et al (1999) Dofetilide in patients with congestive heart failure and left ventricular dysfunction. Danish Investigations of Arrhythmia and Mortality in Dofetilide Study Group. N Engl J Med 341:857-865
11. Huang B, Qin D, El-Sherif N (2000) Early down-regulation of K^+ channel genes and currents in the post infarction heart. J Cardiovasc Electrophysiol 11:1252-1261
12. Huang B, El-Sherif T, Gidh-Jain M et al (2001) Alterations of sodium channel kinetics and gene expression in the post infarction remodeled myocardium. J Cardiovasc Electrophysiol 12:218-225
13. Mitcheson JS, Chen J, Lin M et al (2000) A structural basis for drug-induced long QT syndrome. Proc Natl Acad Sci 97:12329-12333
14. Roden DM (1998) Taking the 'idio' out of idiosyncratic: Predicting torsades de pointes. PACE 21:1029-1034
15. Houltz B, Darpo B, Edvardsson N et al (1998) Electrocardiographic and clinical predictors of torsade de pointes induced by almokalant infusion in patients with chronic atrial fibrillation or flutter. A prospective study. PACE 21:1044-1057
16. Sesti F, Abbott GW, Wei J et al (2000) A common polymorphism associated with antibiotic-induced cardiac arrhythmia. Proc Natl Acad Sci USA 97:10613-10618
17. Chevalier P, Rodriquez C, Bontemps L (2001) Non-invasive testing of acquired long QT syndrome: Evidence of or multiple arrhythmogenic substrates. Cardiovasc Res 50:386-398
18. Splawski I, Timothy KW, Tateyama M (2002) Variant of SCNSA sodium channel implicated in risk of cardiac arrhythmias. Science 297:1333-1336
19. Priori SG, Napolitano C, Schwartz PJ (1999) Low penetrance in the long-QT syndrome: Clinical impact. Circulation 99:529-533
20. Marian J (2002) Modifier genes for hypertrophic cardiomyopathy. Curr Opin Cardi0l 17:242-252
21. Le Corvoisier P, Park HY, Carlson KM et al (2003) Impact of genetic polymorphism in heart failure prognosis. Arch Mol Coeur Vaiss 96:197-206
22. Committee for Proprietary Medicinal Products. Points to Consider: The Assessment of the Potential for QT Interval Prolongation by Non-Cardiovascular Medicinal Products. The European agency for the Evaluation of Medicinal products. December 1997
23. Moss AJ, Zareba W, Benhorin J et al (2001) ISHNE guidelines for electrocardiographic evaluation of drug-related QT prolongation and other alterations in ventricular repolarization: Task Force summary. A report of the Task Force of the International Society for Holter and Noninvasive Electrocardiology (ISHNE), Committee on Ventricular Repolarization. Ann Noninvasive Electrocardiol 6:333-341

Identifying Patients at High Risk for Sudden Cardiac Death: Is Low Ejection Fraction Alone Enough, or Do We Need Additional Testing?

S.M. NARAYAN,[1] M.E. CAIN[2]

Introduction

Sudden cardiac death (SCD) from ventricular tachycardia (VT) or ventricular fibrillation (VF) remains a major cause of mortality in the U.S. and Western Europe, and claims 2-3 lives per 100,000 per year [1, 2]. The incidence of SCD has not declined in tandem with significant advances in the management of acute coronary syndromes, congestive heart failure (CHF) and cardiovascular disease in general, further highlighting the importance of identifying and treating patients at high risk for VT/VF.

Reduced left ventricular ejection fraction (LVEF) has consistently been shown to predict first episodes of sustained VT or VF in patients with [3, 4] and without [5] coronary artery disease (CAD), recurrent VT or VF [6] and to predict the anti-arrhythmic benefits of revascularization [7].

However, LVEF alone does not optimally predict VT or VF. Death due to VT or VF represents a smaller proportion of total mortality with progressive reductions in LVEF (in the Multicenter Unsustained Tachycardia Trial (MUSTT) among patients with CAD, unsustained VT and LVEF ≤ 40% [3]) (Fig. 1), and with worsening CHF class [8].

To more specifically identify the risk of VT or VF in patients with low LVEF, additional indices of electrical vulnerability are required. In MUSTT, programmed ventricular stimulation (PVS) successfully identified a high risk of arrhythmic SCD for patients in all LVEF ranges; non-inducibility combined with LVEF ≥ 30 % identified a particularly low risk group (Fig. 2) [3].

However, the role of PVS has been questioned in patients without CAD [5] and with CAD but LVEF ≤ 30 % [9]. Mechanistically, reduced LVEF may simply be a marker for arrhythmic substrates, or it may contribute to arrhythmias via mechano-electric feedback – the interaction of stretch with electrical depolarization, repolarization and conduction.

[1]Division of Cardiology, University of California and VAMC, San Diego, California;
[2]Division of Cardiology, Washington University, St. Louis, Missouri, USA

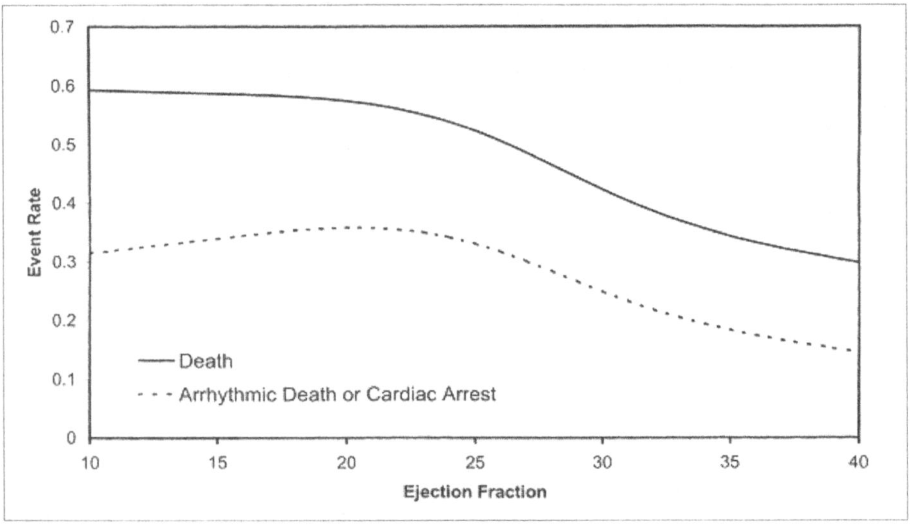

Fig. 1. Reduced LVEF alone sub-optimally predicts ventricular arrhythmias in MUSTT [3], since patients with the lowest LVEF die proportionally less often from ventricular arrhythmias. Reproduced with permission [3]

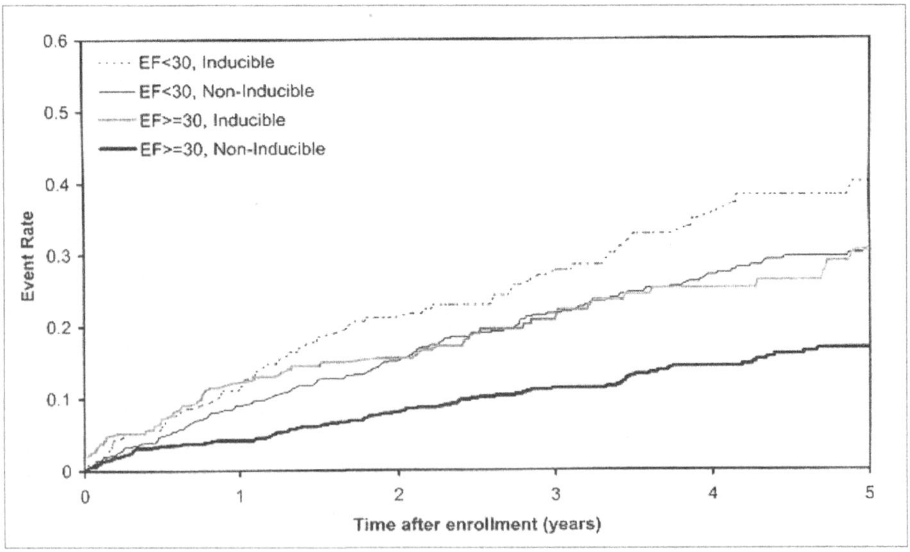

Fig. 2. Ventricular arrhythmias/cardiac arrest events in MUSTT. Although LVEF > 30 % predict lower event rates, PVS non-inducibility indicates an even lower risk group. Reproduced with permission [3]

Structural Uniformities and Arrhythmias

Scar or fibrosis can result in non-uniform repolarization and slow conduction that, in turn, are required for unidirectional conduction block and the initiation or maintenance of reentry [10]. Post-myocardial infarction (MI), a reduced LVEF reflects the presence of this scar, explaining the heightened tendency towards induced and spontaneous VT [3]. Conversely, the absence of scar is likely to explain the lower risk of VT/VF in patients with comparably reduced LVEF from both non-ischemic etiologies [11], and ischemic cardiomyopathy without documented MI [12].

It is increasingly appreciated that anisotropies in conduction and repolarization may result in reentry even without structural pathology. Myocytes show strong axial preferences for anisotropic conduction, repolarization and gap junctional conduction. By exaggerating steep repolarization gradients, such anisotropy has been shown to contribute to reentry in guinea-pig ventricle with [13] or without [14] conventional structural barriers.

Mechano-Electric Feedback: Ventricular Stretch and Arrhythmias

Reduced LVEF and concomitant ventricular stretch may directly exaggerate anisotropies in conduction and repolarization, and thus contribute to reentry, with or without structural pathology. This phenomenon may explain why decompensated heart failure is associated clinically with ventricular arrhythmias [8], as well as with a reduced electrical threshold for VF induced in experimental animals [15].

Stretch promotes the formation of after-depolarizations [16], that may initiate triggered arrhythmias and may also facilitate reentry. Sustained stretch has been shown to unfavorably alter ventricular refractoriness and action potential duration [16, 17] and reduce conduction velocity [17, 18] in experimental animals. Non-uniformities in stretch, or more precisely fiber strain, throughout the heart may exaggerate non-uniformities in conduction and repolarization and facilitate reentry. Fibers have a complex apicobasal and endo-to-epicardial arrangement in the intact heart, complicating quantifications of strain. However, using optical imaging in intact rabbit heart together with a three-dimensional digital model of rabbit ventricular fiber orientation, we recently demonstrated that conduction velocity slowing and action potential changes were greatest in regions of maximal fiber strain [18].

Indices of Non-uniform Repolarization: T-Wave Alternans

Indices of non-uniform repolarization appear to detect a propensity for ventricular arrhythmias. T-wave alternans (TWA) is one such promising index that detects fluctuations on the ECG of T-wave shape, duration or timing that occur every-other-beat. TWA reflects spatial non-uniformity in ventricular repolarization, since changes in the recovery sequence induce corresponding changes in T-wave shape, as well as temporal non-uniformity. This is because myocytes with prolonged repolarization may be able to repolarize fully only every-other-cycle. A substantial body of literature that spans 'bench to bedside' now links repolarization alternans with substrates for ventricular arrhythmias in myocytes, numerical simulations, *in vitro* [14] and *in vivo* animal hearts and patients at PVS [19, 20] and on long-term follow up for arrhythmia-free survival [20].

TWA Magnitude Predicts Ventricular Arrhythmias

Although TWA was first noted visually, it is usually more subtle and most often detected using spectral analysis [19]. A TWA magnitude ≥ 1.9 μV is abnormal. In patients with CAD and LVEF ≤ 40 %, such TWA predicts inducible VT or VF with high sensitivity (≥ 90 %) and specificity (≥ 85 %). TWA is independent of PVS and, in a recent multicenter study, was more predictive for spontaneous arrhythmias or cardiac arrest than PVS (relative risks 10.9 versus 7.9) [20]. Preliminary data suggest that TWA predicts VT/VF in patients with CAD and LVEF ≤ 30 % (similar to patients enrolled in MADIT-II [4]), and in patients with non-ischemic cardiomyopathy [21].

Temporal Dynamics of TWA Improve its Specificity

The dynamics of repolarization following perturbations in rate or rhythm may be central in the initiation of reentry. We hypothesized that exaggerated TWA following ventricular premature depolarizations (VPDs), that frequently initiate VT, would indicate a greater risk for arrhythmic SCD. We analyzed TWA magnitude, its distribution (early or late) within the T-wave, and TWA phase before and after VPDs introduced at PVS. TWA phase reflects the continuity of alternation of successive T-waves that, following a VPD, may remain unchanged or reverse (Fig. 3).

We discovered that VPDs augmented TWA magnitude, displaced TWA later in the T-wave and caused TWA phase reversal more significantly in inducible than non-inducible patients with CAD, reduced LVEF and non-sustained VT [19]. On mean follow-up of 36.0±12.0 months, TWA phase reversal was a more specific indicator for all-cause mortality and arrhythmic SCD than PVS or TWA magnitude [22]. In non-inducible patients, post-VPD TWA magnitude augmentation predicted arrhythmic SCD [23]. TWA in the late T-wave may more specifically indicate non-uniform repolarization and, by interfering with the next activation wavefront, initiate reentry [24]. Data acquired from *in vitro* studies suggest that TWA phase reversal may represent discordant alternans (spatially juxtaposed islands of alternans of opposite phase) and its presence indicates a high risk for conduction block and reentry [14].

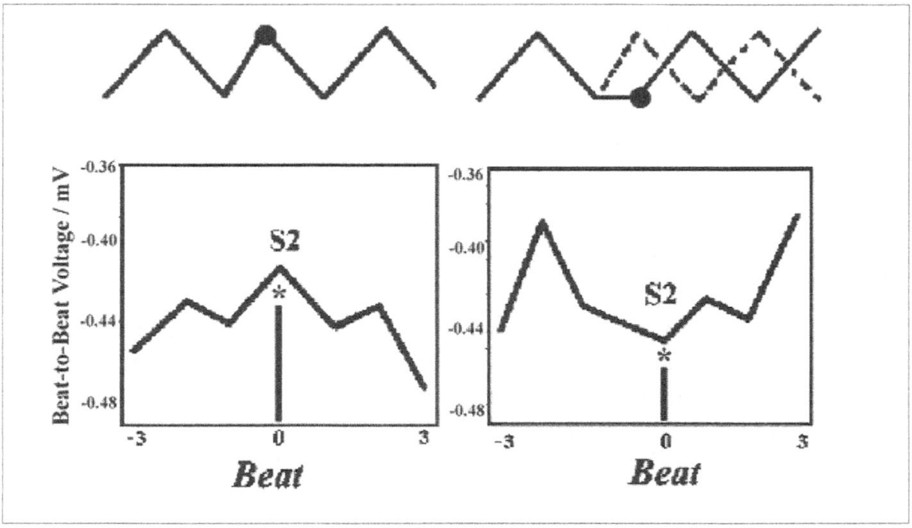

Fig. 3. TWA phase consistency (*left*) and reversal (*right, solid line*) in the alternating pattern of voltage at one T-wave point (*vertical*), for successive beats (*horizontal*) before and after a VPD (*beat 0, filled circle, S2*). Lower panels show actual data [19]

TWA May Reflect the Spatial Distribution of Structural Disease

Repolarization non-uniformity [10], and therefore TWA, may be most linked with ventricular arrhythmias when measured in regions of structural pathology. Among patients with CAD and eccentric left ventricular hypertrophy, TWA magnitude consistently increases with left ventricular mass index. However, the slope of this relationship was steeper in inducible patients, supporting the notion that non-uniform repolarization contributes to the excess incidence of SCD in patients with left ventricular hypertrophy. Significant TWA also correlated spatially with echocardiographic wall motion abnormalities. TWA predicted death or arrhythmic SCD in these patients over a mean follow-up of 34.5±13.0 months [25].

Slow Conduction and Arrhythmias

Although the contribution of slow conduction to reentrant arrhythmias has long been recognized [10], recent data from MADIT-II suggest that, in patients with CAD and reduced LVEF, prolongation of QRS duration and risk of VT/VF may go hand in hand.

Hemodynamically, the sequelae of overtly slow conduction (QRS prolongation) are partially reversed by cardiac resynchronization therapy, which improves heart failure class and LVEF [26] in tandem with improving ventricular synergy. However, these benefits occur whether or not QRS narrowing is seen [27], and are of greater magnitude in patients without MI scar [26]. Furthermore, the reduction in risk for VT/VF with cardiac resynchronization is more modest than improvements in heart failure. Therefore, QRS prolongation *per se* may not reflect those aspects of slow conduction contributing to a high risk for VT/VF. More sensitive indices of slow conduction are required for this purpose.

Occult Slow Conduction: Signal-Averaged ECG

Slowed conduction through structural substrates for ventricular arrhythmias, such as inflammation, edema, fibrosis or scar, results in electrical potentials that may be too small for detection on the surface ECG. The signal-averaged ECG (SAECG) uses computerized averaging of ECG complexes recorded during sinus rhythm to facilitate the detection of these microvolt-level signals in the time or frequency domain.

Time Domain Abnormalities

Late potentials are low-amplitude, high frequency signals recorded during sinus rhythm that reflect slow and fragmented myocardial conduction through scar that may form a substrate for re entrant VT. Data acquired from patients enrolled in MUSTT with CAD, reduced LVEF and normal QRS duration demonstrated that an abnormal SAECG identified patients at high risk of SCD, particularly in combination with LVEF < 30 % (Fig. 4), and was more predictive than PVS [28].

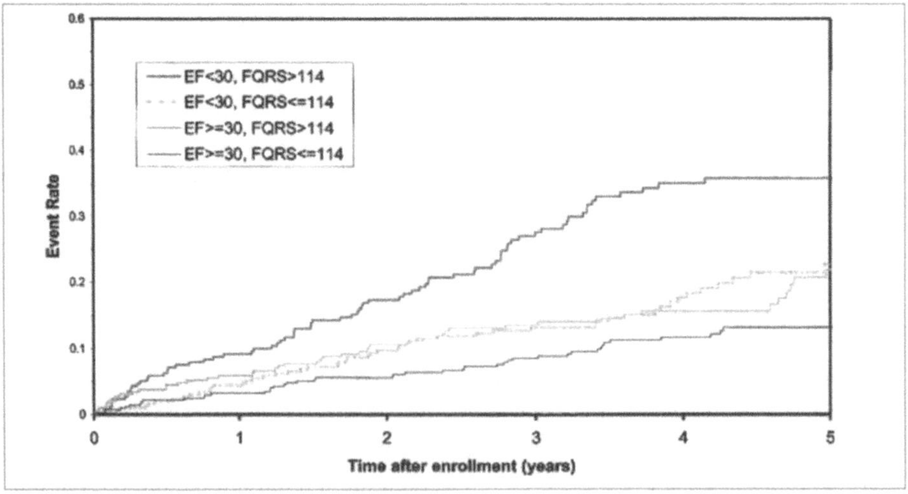

Fig. 4. Kaplan-Meier estimates of arrhythmic death or cardiac arrest by SAECG and LVEF for abnormal (fQRS > 114) and normal (fQRS ≤ 114) SAECG, and EF stratified at 30%; from MUSTT [28]. Abnormal SAECG indicates a high event rate for for all patients, but particularly in combination with LVEF < 30 %

Mechanistically, although late potentials indicate myocardial scar, we have shown that they may not represent the fingerprint of conduction through myocardium culpable in initiating reentrant VT [29].

Frequency Domain Abnormalities

Pro-arrhythmic conduction abnormalities through scar during sinus rhythm may leave a 'fingerprint' that is easier to detect in the frequency domain. Fourier analysis of the SAECG shows that spectra from 20-100 Hz differ between patients with and without VT [30]. This signature persists throughout the cardiac cycle rather than just the QRS terminus [31]. The predictive accuracy of SAECG spectral abnormalities for VT is unchanged by bundle branch delay [30], implying that their substrate may contribute to re-entrant arrhythmias independent of the sequence or total duration of ventricular activation.

Localizing Regions of Pro-Arrhythmic Slow Conduction Using Spectral Analysis of Body Surface Potential Maps

The *spatial selection* of ECG leads, optimized to detect the spectral 'fingerprint' of pro-arrhythmic scar, may further improve the identification and localization of such tissue over the use of stereotypical leads. To address this hypothesis, we computed isoharmonic maps of the body surface during sinus rhythm in patients with CAD and normal subjects. We found that a broadened bandwidth of ECG spectra at the maximum or minimum of each patient's isoharmonic map of 1-7 Hz significantly separated patients with VT from those without. Spatially selected ECGs performed significantly better than analyses using stereotypical Frank leads [32].

The epicardial region responsible for generating the spectral 'fingerprint' may be inferred, theoretically, from optimally placed patient-specific ECG leads using inverse solution mathematics. This approach is a major focus of our current work. First, we record body surface potential maps (BSPMs) of electrograms from 192 unipolar leads covering the entire torso. Second, we reconstruct a digital torso surface by databasing the position of these electrodes using a computer-linked robotic stylus in each recumbent patient. Electrode positions are joined in software using polygons then smoothed to yield the torso surface. Third, epicardial contours, obtained from transthoracic echocardiography at the time of BSPM or magnetic resonance imaging (MRI), are registered to the torso model. Preliminary data suggests that the BSPM spectral 'fingerprint' corresponds to epicardium within 1 cm of echocardiographic or MRI-verified scar. We are currently using intracardiac electroanatomic mapping at PVS to verify that induced VT arises from these regions.

Autonomic Tone and Identifiers of High Risk Patients

A detailed discussion of additional indices that predict risk for arrhythmic SCD is beyond the scope of this review. However, elevated sympathetic tone facilitates the initiation and maintenance of ventricular arrhythmias, and can be measured indirectly from current-generation pacemakers and defibrillators by a reduced standard deviation of R-R intervals [33] or by the failure of R-R intervals to shorten after a spontaneous VPD [34]. These indices predict cardiac mortality in patients post-MI and may add to the predictive ability of reduced LVEF and the (time-domain) SAECG [33]. Baroreflex sensitivity, which reflects autonomic tone by quantifying sinus rate slowing after blood pressure increases, also predicts arrhythmic SCD risk in patients with reduced post-MI LVEF [35]. Finally, although other indices exist for slow conduction or non-uniform repolarization, most are either less effective (such as QT dispersion) or less well validated (such as the QT variability index).

Conclusions

Reduced LVEF may contribute to ventricular arrhythmias directly via stretch or indirectly by indicating pro-arrhythmic substrates. However, reduced LVEF alone suboptimally identifies high risk patients. Identification is improved by the use of TWA, metrics of slow conduction, or of elevated sympathetic tone. Furthermore, these indices are synergistic. The SAECG is more predictive when combined with assessments of LVEF and autonomic tone [33], and TWA is more predictive when combined with PVS [20] or assessments of LVEF. Future improvements in identifying high risk patients will come from further understanding of the pathophysiology of ventricular arrhythmogenesis.

Acknowledgements. Supported by grants K23-HL-70529 (SMN) and R01-HL-50295 (MEC) from the National Heart, Lung and Blood Institute, and Grant-in-Aid 0265120Y (SMN) from the American Heart Association, Western Regional Affiliate.

References

1. BayesdeLuna A, Coumel P, Leclerq JF (1989) Ambulatory sudden cardiac death: Mechanisms of production of fatal arrhythmia on the basis of data from 157 cases. American Heart Journal 117:151-159
2. Zheng Z-J, Croft JB, Giles WH et al (2001) Sudden Cardiac Death in the United States, 1989 to 1998. Circulation 104:2158-2163
3. Buxton AE, Lee KL, Hafley GE et al (2002) Relation of Ejection Fraction and Inducible Ventricular Tachycardia to Mode of Death in Patients With Coronary Artery Disease: An Analysis of Patients Enrolled in the Multicenter Unsustained Tachycardia Trial. Circulation 106:2466-2472

4. Moss AJ, Zareba W, Hall WJ et al (2002a) Prophylactic Implantation of a Defibrillator in Patients with Myocardial Infarction and Reduced Ejection Fraction. N Engl J Med 346:877-883
5. Grimm W, Hoffmann J, Menz V et al (1998b) Programmed ventricular stimulation for arrhythmia risk prediction in patients with idiopathic dilated cardiomyopathy and nonsustained ventricular tachycardia. J Am Coll Cardiol 32:739-745
6. Hallstrom AP, McAnulty JH, Wilkoff BL et al (2001) Patients at lower risk of Arrhythmia Recurrence: A subgroup in Whom Implantable Defibrillators may not offer benefit. J Am Coll Cardiol 37:1093-1099
7. Veenhuyzen GD, Singh SN, McAreavey D et al (2001) Prior Coronary Artery Bypass Surgery and Risk of Death Among Patients With Ischemic Left Ventricular Dysfunction. Circulation 104:1489-1493
8. Stevenson WG, Stevenson LW (2001) Prevention of Sudden Death in Heart Failure. J Cardiovascular Electrophysiol 12:112-114
9. Moss A, Daubert J, Zareba W (2002b) MADIT-II: Clinical Implications. Card Electrophysiol Rev 6:463-465
10. Kuo C-S, Munakata K, Reddy CP et al (1983) Characteristics and possible mechanism of ventricular arrhythmia dependent on the dispersion of action potential durations. Circulation 67:1356-1367
11. Bansch D, Antz M, Boczor S et al (2002) Primary Prevention of Sudden Cardiac Death in Idiopathic Dilated Cardiomyopathy: The Cardiomyopathy Trial (CAT). Circulation 105:1453-1458
12. Buxton AE, Hafley GE, Lehmann MH et al (1999a) Prediction of Sustained Ventricular Tachycardia Inducible by Programmed Stimulation in Patients With Coronary Artery Disease: Utility of Clinical Variables. Circulation 99:1843-1850
13. Laurita KR, Rosenbaum DS (2000) Interdependence of Modulated Dispersion and Tissue structure in the Mechanism of Unidirectional Block. Circulation Research 87:922-928
14. Pastore JM, Girouard SD, Laurita KR et al (1999) Mechanism Linking T-wave Alternans to the Genesis of Cardiac Fibrillation. Circulation 99:1385-1394
15. Jalal S, Williams GR, Mann DE et al (1992) Effect of acute ventricular dilatation on fibrillation thresholds in the isolated rabbit heart. Am J Physiol 263:1306-1310
16. Franz MR, Cima R, Wang D et al (1992) Electrophysiological Effects of Myocardial stretch and Mechanical Determinants of Stretch-Activated Arrhythmias. Circulation 86:968-978
17. Zabel M, Portnoy S, Franz MR (1996b) Effect of sustained load on dispersion of ventricular repolarization and conduction time in the isolated intact rabbit heart. J Cardiovasc Electrophysiol 7:9-16
18. Sung D, Mills RW, Narayan SM et al (2003) Ventricular Filling Slows Epicardial Conduction and Increases Action Potential Duration in an Optical Mapping Study of the Isolated Rabbit Heart. J Cardiovasc Electrophys 14:739-749
19. Narayan SM, Lindsay BD, Smith JM (1999d) Demonstrating the Pro-arrhythmic Preconditioning of Single Premature Extrastimuli Using the Magnitude, Phase and Temporal Distribution of Repolarization Alternans. Circulation 100:1887-1893
20. Gold MR, Bloomfield DM, Anderson KP et al (2000a) A Comparison of T Wave Alternans, Signal Averaged Electrocardiography and Programmed Ventricular Stimulation for Arrhythmia Risk Stratification. J Am Coll Cardiol 36:2247-2253
21. Kitamura H, Ohnishi Y, Okajima K et al (2002) Onset Heart Rate of Microvolt-Level T-Wave Alternans Provides Clinical and Prognostic Value in Nonischemic Dilated Cardiomyopathy. J Am Coll Cardiol 39:295-300

22. Narayan SM, Lindsay BD, Cain ME et al (2001) Phase Reversal and Magnitude of T-Wave Alternans Predict Spontaneous Ventricular Arrhythmias and Long-Term Survival [abstract]. PACE 24 (4 part 2)
23. Narayan SM, Smith JM, Cain ME (2002a) Augmentation of T-Wave Alternans after Ventricular Extrasystoles Predicts Survival in Patients Non-Inducible for Ventricular Arrhythmias [abstract]. Pacing and Clinical Electrophysiology 25 (4 Part II):165
24. Narayan SM, Smith JM (2000c) Exploiting Rate Hysteresis in Repolarization Alternans to Optimize the Sensitivity and Specificity for Ventricular Tachycardia. J Am Coll Cardiol 35:1485-1492
25. Narayan SM, Davila-Roman VG, Gropler RJ et al (2000g) Performance of Repolarization Alternans Determines Arrhythmic Susceptibility in Patients with Left Ventricular Hypertrophy [abstract]. Pacing and Clinical Electrophysiology (PACE) 23 (4 part II):157
26. St John Sutton MG, Plappert T, Abraham WT et al (2003) Effect of Cardiac Resynchronization Therapy on Left Ventricular Size and Function in Chronic Heart Failure. Circulation 107:1985
27. Gasparini M, Mantica M, Galimberti P et al (2003a) Beneficial effects of biventricular pacing in patients with a "narrow" QRS. Pacing Clin Electrophysiol 26:169-174
28. Gomes JA, Cain ME, Buxton AE et al (2001) Prediction of Long-Term Outcomes by Signal-Averaged Electrocardiography in Patients With Unsustained Ventricular Tachycardia, Coronary Artery Disease, and Left Ventricular Dysfunction. Circulation 104:436-441
29. Hood MA, Pogwizd SM, Peirick J et al (1992b) Contribution of Myocardium Responsible for Ventricular Tachycardia to Abnormalities Detected by Analysis of Signal-Averaged ECGs. Circulation 86:1888-1901
30. Lindsay BD, Markham J, Schechtman KB et al (1988) Identification of patients with sustained ventricular tachycardia by frequency analysis of signal-averaged electrocardiograms despite the presence of bundle branch block. Circulation 77:122-130
31. Cain ME, Ambos HD, Markham J et al (1991) Diagnostic Implications of Spectral and Temporal Analysis of the Entire Cardiac Cycle in patients with ventricular tachycardia. Circulation 83:1637-1648
32. Kavesh NG, Cain ME, Ambos HD et al (1994) Enhanced detection of distinguishing features in signal-averaged electrocardiograms from patients with ventricular tachycardia by combined spatial and spectral analyses of entire cardiac cycle. Circulation 90:254-263
33. Farrell TG, Bashir Y, Cripps T et al (1991a) Risk stratification for arrhythmic events in postinfarction patients based on heart rate variability, ambulatory electrocardiographic variables and the signal-averaged electrocardiogram. J Am Coll Cardiol 18:687-697
34. Schmidt G, Malik M, Barthel P et al (1999) Heart-rate turbulence after ventricular premature beats as a predictor of mortality after acute myocardial infarction. Lancet 353:1390-1396
35. La Rovere MT, Jr JTB, Marcus FI et al (1998) Baroreflex sensitivity and heart-rate variability in prediction of total cardiac mortality after myocardial infarction. ATRAMI (Autonomic Tone and Reflexes After Myocardial Infarction) Investigators [see comments]. Lancet 351:478-484

What Is The Prognostic Value of Non-Sustained Ventricular Tachycardia in Patients Without Severely Depressed Ejection Fraction After Myocardial Infarction?

G. Turitto, N. El-Sherif

Complex Ventricular Ectopy (CVE)/Non-Sustained Ventricular Tachycardia (NS-VT) in the Post-Myocardial Infarction (MI) Period: Background

The predictive accuracy of CVE/NS-VT for serious arrhythmic events/sudden cardiac death (SCD) in the post-MI period has undergone radical evaluation in the last 2 decades. In 1981, Bigger et al reported on 430 patients who sustained acute MI and underwent a 24-hour Holter electrocardiogram (ECG) prior to hospital discharge [1]. Fifty patients (11.6%) had NS-VT, in the form of ≥ 3 ventricular premature complexes. This group of patients had 38% 1-year mortality rate, compared with a rate of 11.6% in the group without NS-VT. NS-VT had a significant association with many other post-MI risk factors. However, VT was still significantly related to mortality when other variables, including left ventricular ejection fraction (LVEF) were controlled statistically using a multiple logistic regression model. Similar conclusions were later published by Bigger et al. from 820 patients in the Multicenter Post-Infarction Program, of whom 11% had NS-VT recorded on Holter ECG 11±3 days post-MI [2]. NS-VT had a strong and statistically significant association with all-cause and arrhythmic mortality, independent of other risk stratifiers, including depressed LVEF.

Since the advent of current management strategies of acute MI that emphasize prompt revascularization, a majority of patients who survive their first MI tend to have a relatively preserved LVEF [3, 4]. In 1999, Hohnloser et al reported a study on 325 consecutive acute MI survivors in whom a Holter ECG was performed 10±6 day after acute MI [5]. There was a low prevalence of NS-VT (9%), and in only 2.4% of patients it was found together with depressed LVEF. During a 30±12-month follow-up, 25 patients had serious arrhythmic events/SCD. On multivariate analysis, only LVEF, heart rate variability (HRV), and status of the infarct-related artery, but not NS-VT were independent risk

Cardiac Electrophysiology Section, State University of New York, Downstate Medical Center, Brooklyn, New York, USA factors. Similar conclusions were repeatedly reported in the last several years [6-8]. For example, in a report of the MITRA Trial (Maximal Individual Therapy in patients with acute MI), a multicenter registry of 54 Hospitals in Germany, 2420 patients had a Holter ECG [8]. In multivariate analysis, none of the complex ventricular arrhythmias/NS-VT alone correlated with mortality. It should be emphasized again that the incidence of serious arrhythmic events/SCD in the post-MI revascularization era has decreased significantly in line with improved preservation of LVEF. In the European Infarct Study, a secondary prevention study of acute MI, a Holter ECG was obtained 14-31 days post-MI [9]. There was a rather low 2-year mortality of 6.9%. CVE/NS-VT and LV dysfunction alone were associated with a low mortality of 4.0% and 3.6%, respectively. However, the combination of both defined a high-risk group with a 2-year mortality of 16.7%.

The Need For New Innovative Strategies For Risk Stratification In Post-MI Patients

The lack of predictive accuracy of CVE/NS-VT in post-MI patients with relatively preserved LVEF equally applies to other conventional post-MI risk stratifiers. For example, in a recent study by Klingenheben et al., HRV and baroreflex sensitivity, both markers of autonomic dysfunction, did not have predictive power in infarct survivors with preserved LVEF [4]. In spite of the above literature, all recently completed as well as ongoing SCD primary implantable cardioverter-defibrillator (ICD) prophylaxis trials included post-MI patients with one or more of the conventional risk stratifiers for SCD [3]. The electrophysiological surrogates for SCD included, besides CVE/NS-VT, measures of myocardial conduction disorder, dispersion of cardiac repolarization, and autonomic imbalance (Table 1). Although all these measures are based on

Table 1. Risk stratification for sudden cardiac death

Conventional Risk Stratifiers of Sudden Cardiac Death	
Electrophysiologic surrogates	Functional contractile surrogates
* Measures of myocardial conduction disorder	* NYHA Class
- Signal averaged ECG	* Left ventricular ejection fraction
- Electrophysiologic study	* Left ventricular mass
* Measures of dispersion of repolarization	* Peak oxygen consumption
- QT dispersion	* Brain natriuretic peptide
- T-wave alternans	
* Measures of autonomic imbalance	
- Resting heart rate	
- Heart rate variability	
- Baroreflex sensitivity	

sound scientific evidence, unfortunately most of them have a low positive predictive power. This would preclude their wide application as guidelines for ICD implantation in patients known to be at risk for SCD and explains why a depressed LVEF (≤ 35%) was universally adopted as a primary entry criterion in all these trials. In fact, one of the recently completed trials, MADIT II, has dispensed with electrophysiologic risk stratifiers altogether and entered patients based only on LVEF ≤ 30% [10]. The effectiveness of ICD prophylaxis in post-MI patients based primarily on a low LVEF remains controversial and the cost to the health care system of promulgating this approach would be substantial [11]. For the immediate future, attempts to optimize the selection process for primary ICD prophylaxis in post-MI patients that go beyond depressed LVEF must continue. Some of the "novel" risk factors that are currently under investigation are discussed in the following paragraphs.

Family Clustering of SCD

Population studies have reported that "familial clustering of SCD events" is an important independent factor in multifactorial analyses of SCD risk. Evidence favoring a focus on genetic factors was presented in recent epidemiological studies that suggested not only that familial risks for SCD appear substantial, but that they are statistically distinct and separable from familial risks of MI [12-14]. In one study, parental history of SCD increased the relative risk of SCD to 1.8 after adjustment for conventional coronary artery disease (CAD) risk factors [13]. In a small subset in which there was a history of both maternal and parental SCD events, the relative risk for SCD in offsprings was up to 9.4.

The Autonomic System and Enhanced Susceptibility to SCD

Autonomic neural influences, especially increased adrenergic and decreased cholinergic activity, can modulate the susceptibility to SCD [15]. Resting heart rate has been shown to be an independent risk factor for SCD in middle aged men [16]. There are data showing the heritability of heart rate variation [17]. Adrenergic agonists are known to trigger ventricular arrhythmias, and their circulating levels have similar diurnal patterns as SCD events [18].

Cardiac Gene Mutations and Enhanced Susceptibility to SCD

The discovery of literally hundreds of different mutations in the genes causing the phenotypic long QT syndrome raised the possibility that silent polymorphism or mutations of cardiac genes may be more prevalent in the asymptomatic general public. This may contribute to enhanced susceptibility to arrhythmogenesis and SCD under specific circumstances [15, 19]. The interaction of silent genetic alterations with pathological states like acute ischemia remains to be determined.

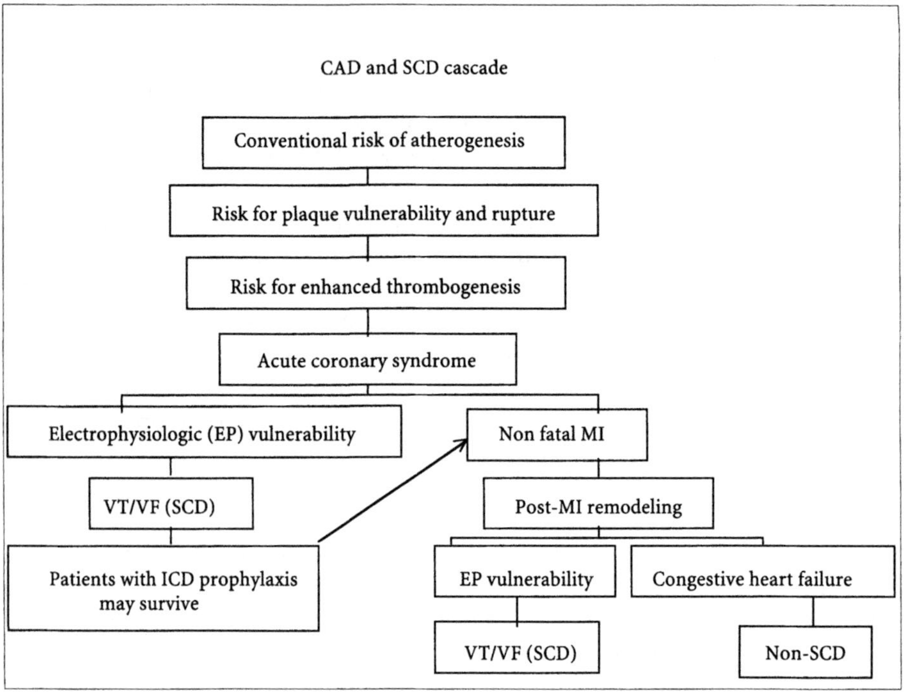

Fig. 1. Coronary artery disease and sudden cardiac death cascade

CAD and SCD Cascade (Fig. 1)

Patients with similar degrees of CAD may suffer from SCD or nonfatal ischemic events. The reason for this difference is currently not clear. There is a new understanding of the cascade that relates the distal events of atherosclerosis to the proximal event of SCD. New risk markers for SCD in CAD are likely to cluster under factors that may directly facilitate the development of acute coronary syndromes, specifically those factors that may facilitate transient triggering events, including plaque rupture, enhanced thrombogenesis and coronary artery spasm [15,19]. There are significant new data that show correlation between SCD and: 1) markers of plaque vulnerability such as heritable alterations of specific matrix metalloproteinases; 2) markers of enhanced thrombogenesis, such as increased D-dimer, increased apo-B, and decreased apo-A1, polymorphism in platelet glycoprotein receptors, etc.; 3) genetic variations that predispose to vasospasm, such as variations in vascular endothelial nitric oxide synthetase (eNOS) system; 4) markers of inflammatory response, such as C-reactive protein (CRP) [15,19].

Diabetes, CAD and Risk of SCD

The prevalence of impaired glucose tolerance and diabetes may be as high as 39% and 31% respectively, in patients admitted with acute MI [20]. Conversely, cardiovascular disease is the leading cause of death in individuals with type 2-diabetes [21]. This is compatible with the "common soil' hypothesis, which postulates that both diabetes and cardiovascular disease have common genetic and environmental antecedents, i.e. "they spring from the same soil" [22]. There is evidence that diabetes is a significant risk factor for SCD [23].

Left Ventricular Hypertrophy (LVH) and SCD

In patients with hypertension, there is a statistically significant relationship between LVH and CVE/NS-VT, however, the prognostic value of this marker is also poor in this setting [24]. In the Framingham study, the presence of asymptomatic ventricular arrhythmias in 1-hour ECG recordings obtained in subjects with LVH was associated with a statistically significant increase in mortality, which became marginally significant after adjusting for covariates [25].

SCD and Improving Systolic Function

Although the exact mechanisms involved in the strong correlation between decreased LVEF and increased incidence of SCD are not clearly defined, it is now recognized that one way to combat SCD is to try to halt or improve the deterioration in LV function. Recent years have seen significant advances in the treatment of ventricular systolic dysfunction and heart failure. The therapeutic armamentarium includes not only pharmacological agents, but also electrical devices, like biventricular pacemakers in selected patients [26].

Conclusions

Management of SCD in post-MI patients is undergoing a radical change in direction. It is becoming increasingly appreciated that besides depressed LV systolic function, new markers for plaque vulnerability, enhanced thrombogenesis, specific genetic alterations of the autonomic nervous system, cardiac sarcolemmal and contractile proteins may better segregate patients with atherosclerotic CAD who are at high risk of SCD from those who may suffer from nonfatal ischemic events. The rapidly developing fields of microchips technology, and proteomics may allow rapid and cost-effective mass screening of multiple risk factors for SCD. The ultimate goal is not only to change the current direction of management strategy of SCD in the post-MI patients away from increased ICD utilization, but to identify novel methods for risk stratification, risk modification and prevention of SCD that could be applied to the general public at large.

References

1. Bigger JT Jr, Weld FM, Rolnitzky LM (1981) Prevalence, characteristics and significance of ventricular tachycardia (three or more complexes) detected with ambulatory electrocardiographic recording in the late hospital phase of acute myocardial infarction. Am J Cardiol 48:815-823
2. Bigger JT, Fleiss JL, Rolnitzky LM, and the Multicenter Post-Infarction Research Group (1986) Prevalence, characteristics and significance of ventricular tachycardia detected by 24-hour continuous electrocardiographic recordings in the late hospital phase of acute myocardial infarction. Am J Cardiol 58:1151-1160
3. Hohnloser SH, Gersh BJ (2003) Changing late prognosis of acute myocardial infarction. Impact on management of ventricular arrhythmias in the era of reperfusion and the implantable cardioverter-defibrillator. Circulation 107:941-946
4. Klingenheben T, Hohnloser SH (2003) Usefulness of risk stratification for future cardiac events in infarct survivors with severely depressed versus near-normal left ventricular function: results from a prospective long-term follow-up study. Ann Noninv Electrocardiol 8:68-74
5. Hohnloser SH, Klingenheben T, Zabel M et al (1999) Prevalence, characteristics and prognostic value during long-term follow-up of nonsustained ventricular tachycardia after myocardial infarction in the thrombolytic era. J Am Coll Cardiol 33:1895-1902
6. Maggioni AP, Zuanetti G, Franzosi MG et al, on behalf of the GISSI Investigators (1993) Prevalence and prognostic significance of ventricular arrhythmias after acute myocardial infarction in the fibrinolytic era. GISSI-2 results. Circulation 87:312-322
7. de Chillou C, Sadoul N, Bizeau O et al (1997) Prognostic value of thrombolysis, coronary artery patency, signal-averaged electrocardiography, left ventricular ejection fraction, and Holter electrocardiographic monitoring for life-threatening ventricular arrhythmias after a first acute myocardial infarction. Am J Cardiol 80:852-858
8. Drogemuller A, Seidl K, Schiele R et al (2003) Prognostic value of non-sustained ventricular tachycardias after acute myocardial infarction in the thrombolytic era: importance of combination with ventricular premature beats. Z Kardiol 92:164-172
9. Andresen D, Bethge KP, Boissel JP et al (1990) Importance of quantitative analysis of ventricular arrhythmias for predicting the prognosis in low-risk postmyocardial infarction patients. European Infarction Study Group. Eur Heart J 11:529-536
10. Moss AJ, Zareba W, Hall J et al (2002) Prophylactic implantation of a defibrillator in patients with myocardial infarction and reduced ejection fraction. New Engl J Med 346:877-883
11. Bigger JT (2002) Expanding indications for implantable cardiac defibrillators. New Engl J Med 364:931-933
12. Friedlander Y, Siscovick DS, Weinmann S et al (1998) Family history as a risk factor for primary cardiac arrest. Circulation 97:155-160
13. Jouven X, Desnos M, Guerot C, Ducimetiere P (1999) Predicting sudden death in the population: The Paris Prospective Study I. Circulation 99:1978-1983
14. Friedlander Y, Siscovick DS, Arbogast P et al (2002) Sudden cardiac death and myocardial infarction in first degree relatives as predictors of primary cardiac arrest. Atherosclerosis 162:211-216
15. Spooner PM, Albert C, Benjamin EL et al (2001) Sudden cardiac death, genes, and arrhythmogenesis: Consideration of new population and mechanistic approaches from a National Heart, Lung, and Blood Institute Workshop, Part II. Circulation 103:2447-2452

16. Jouven X, Zureik M, Desnos M et al (2001) Resting heart rate as a predictive risk factor for sudden death in middle aged men. Cardiovasc Res 50:373-378
17. Singh JP, Larson MG, O'Donnell CJ et al (1999) Heritability of heart rate variability: The Framingham Heart Study. Circulation 99:2251-2254
18. Muller JE (1999) Circadian variation and triggering of acute coronary events. Am Heart J 137(pt 2):51-58
19. Spooner PM, Albert C, Benjamin EL et al (2001) Sudden cardiac death, genes, and arrhythmogenesis: Consideration of new population and mechanistic approaches from a National Heart Lung, and Blood Institute Workshop, Part I. Circulation 103:2361-2364
20. Haffner SM (2002) Glucose-intolerance testing in acute myocardial infarction. Lancet 359:2127-2128
21. American Diabetes Association: diabetes facts and figures, (2000) Available from http://www.diabetes.org
22. Stern MP (1995) Diabetes and cardiovascular disease: "the "common soil" hypothesis (review). Diabetes 44:396-374
23. Balkau B, Jouven X, Ducimetiere P et al (1999) Diabetes as a risk of factor for sudden death. Lancet 354:1968-1969
24. Zehender M, Faber T, Koscheck U, Meinertz T, Just H (1995) Ventricular tachyarrhythmias, myocardial ischemia, and sudden cardiac death in patients with hypertensive heart disease. Clin Cardiol 18:377-383
25. Bikkina M, Larson MG, Levy D (1993) Asymptomatic left ventricular arrhythmias and mortality risk in subjects with left ventricular hypertrophy. J Am Coll Cardiol 22:1111-1116
26. Bradley DJ, Bradley EA, Baughman KL et al (2003) Cardiac resynchronization and death from progressive heart failure: a meta-analysis of randomized controlled trials. JAMA 289:754-756

Mechanical/Surgical Revascularization in Patients with Ventricular Fibrillation and Coronary Artery Disease: Is It Enough, or Do We Also Need an Implantable Cardioverter Defibrillator?

M. Lunati, M. Paolucci, G. Magenta, G. Cattafi, R. Vecchi, M. Schirru, T. Di Camillo

Sudden cardiac death (SCD) affects around 300,000–450,000 people annually in the USA, representing around 50% of all cardiac deaths. Patients with a medical history of ventricular tachycardia (VT) or ventricular fibrillation (VF) run a high risk of death in the short term, and studies dating back to the 1970s have shown a 45% mortality rate at 2 years. SCD accounts for at least 50% of patient deaths from heart failure and ischemia. From 1980 onward the positive effects of automatic implantable cardiac defibrillators (ICD) in secondary prevention of SCD began to be recognized, but the suspicion that the ICD was only able to change death from sudden to expected in those patients who were too compromised to benefit from therapies other than chemotherapy caused a certain skepticism.

More recent controlled studies (CASH [1], AVID [2], CIDS [3], MADIT [4]) have, however, confirmed the superiority of ICD over pharmacological therapy both for primary prevention of SCD and in reducing overall mortality in patients resuscitated after VT/VF (secondary prevention), and this superiority is even more evident in the more compromised patients.

In subjects who have survived out-of-hospital cardiac arrest (CA), ischemic cardiomyopathy is without doubt the most frequent underlying pathology (70–80%). SCD caused by VF, often preceded by VT, is the first sign of cardiomyopathy in 50% of cases.

The high incidence of significant coronary disease in patients who have survived CA and the direct evidence that transitory myocardial ischemia can generate fatal ventricular arrhythmias have given rise to the hypothesis that ischemia is a trigger mechanism for fatal ventricular arrhythmias and that revascularization is a suitable therapy for reducing overall and arrhythmic mortality in this type of patient. Because there are no randomized studies dealing specifically with this area, the effects of myocardial revascularization [coronary artery bypass grafting (CABG) or percutaneous transluminal coro-

S.C. Elettrofisiologia, Dipartimento Cardio-Toraco-Vascolare "A. De Gasperis", A.O. Niguarda-Cà Granda, Milano, Italy

nary angioplasty (PTCA)] on the electrophysiological substrate and its role in preventing recurrences of malignant ventricular arrhythmias in patients with ischemic cardiomyopathy remain unclear.

We can identify two groups of patients affected by ischemic cardiomyopathy who can suffer SCD: (1) patients with infarction scars producing malignant re-entry tachyarrhythmias and (2) patients experiencing a first or new coronary thrombotic event.

While there seems to be a well-defined diagnostic approach to identifying patients in the first group, the identification of patients at risk from SCD as a result of a coronary thrombotic event is definitely more difficult. The facts that the development of coronary disease can be unpredictable and that the thrombotic events often occur in lesions that have hitherto been noncritical cast doubt on the idea of a direct causal relationship between the presence of critical stenosis and the risk of a coronary event.

Because we are not yet able to detect potentially unstable coronary lesions, the only possible clinical approach is based on defining the site and the extension of the ischemic area.

Coumel [5] observed that the coexistence of anatomical substrate, myocardial ischemia and neuro-vegetative influences was a fundamental precondition for the onset of disturbances of the cardiac rhythm which, from an electrophysiological standpoint, are based on a defined re-entrant circuit, sustained ventricular tachycardia (VT) or multiple micro-re-entrants (VF). The correction of one of these factors could theoretically prevent the onset of the arrhythmic event.

Despite the high probability that an acute ischemic event is the root cause of a significant proportion of arrhythmic events, the role of myocardial ischemia as a trigger of malignant arrhythmias in postacute myocardial infarction (AMI) is hard to quantify. It is difficult to assess the relative importance of ischemia and structural anomalies, such as ventricular aneurysm and previous infarction.

In addition, it must not be forgotten that malignant ventricular arrhythmias can appear without any clear clinical or instrumental signs of myocardial ischemia. In some studies with patients affected by sustained VT and/or VF according to Holter recordings, the ventricular tachyarrhythmia was not generally preceded by ischemic-type changes in the ECG, at least in the ECG lead traces examined. In addition, the majority of patients who survived the event show a clear arrhythmogenic substrate [lower ejection fraction (EF), ventricular late potential (VLP), and induction of clinical ventricular tachyarrhythmia on electrophysiological study).

In reality we do not know how many patients have suffered cardiac arrest as a result of a primary ischemic event in the absence of clinical evidence of ischemia. In patients with a history of CA or VT and acute ischemia in whom myocardial revascularization is considered to be indicated, revascularization could in theory modify or eliminate the arrhythmogenic substrate and so suppress the sustained ventricular arrhythmias in patients in whom myocardial ischemia is the only or the principal cause of electrical instability.

It is reasonable to assume that myocardial ischemia is the only determining factor for malignant arrhythmia in patients who are at a low risk of arrhythmic events because of an absence of a definite arrhythmogenic substrate, while the arrhythmogenesis exerts a modulating influence in patients with previous infarction with one or more indicators of arrhythmic risk. Even though there are limits imposed by the fact that plaque development is unpredictable, the exploration and correction of residual ischemia is an essential part of the treatment and indicative of the prognosis for patients with recent AMI.

Three mechanisms have been proposed to explain the positive role of myocardial revascularization in reducing SCD: (1) prevention of reversible acute ischemia, (2) electrical stabilization of the peripheral zone of any previous necrosis, (3) reduction of the possibility of infarction recurrence and extension of the scar tissue.

The effect of revascularization on the incidence of SCD was examined in 13,476 patients in the CASS register [6] who exhibited significant coronary stenosis: the incidence of SCD at 5 years was 2% and 6%, respectively, in revascularized and nonrevascularized patients, and this difference was even more significant (9% vs 21%) in the high-risk groups (three-vessel disease with heart failure).

The CASS data also indicate that revascularization has a considerable benefit, above all in high-risk patients, with an overall mortality rate of 12%, as against 25% in patients treated with drug therapy. It should be noted that the follow-up mortality is 50% due to SCD.

In the CABG Patch Trial [7, 8] (patients with indications for CABG, EF <36% and VLP), the overall mortality at 3 years was similar in patients who did not receive an ICD and in those who did have one implanted (24% against 27%), while the incidence of SCD was extremely low, but significantly higher in the group without ICDs than in the group with such implants (6.2% versus 4%). It must be said that the significance of this study is conditioned by the fact that the population studied was likely to be at low risk.

Myocardial revascularization as a sole solution appears to be useful only in patients with VT and/or VF that is clearly caused by ischemia (during a stress test or physical activity) and with proximal critical stenosis that will respond positively to revascularization [9], while in cases where the arrhythmic event cannot be ascribed to the presence of transitory ischemia its role does not appear to be well defined.

In patients with clinical VT and previous myocardial infarction the inducibility of ventricular arrhythmia remains high (70–80%) despite revascularization, with lesser effects of revascularization itself on the arrhythmogenic substrate.

The electrophysiological study is of no use in identifying patients with VT/VF who could benefit from revascularization as a sole therapy, because it can reveal an arrhythmic substrate but cannot take account of reversible factors that could lead to an arrhythmic event (low positive and negative predictive accuracy).

There is some clinical evidence that seems to confirm these considerations: in the studies conducted by Lessmeier et al. [10] (300 patients with ischemic cardiomyopathy and history of VT/VF) and Geleen et al. [11] (18 patients with sustained VT and signs of ischemia) the ICD-appropriate shocks delivered were similar in the revascularized and the nonrevascularized groups. These data have also been confirmed by other studies (Link [12], 1999: 29 patients with CA from VF who had undergone CABG and ICD implant) in which appropriate shocks were observed despite revascularization in a significant percentage of patients (37–43%); in these studies the electrophysiological study appeared unable to predict the arrhythmic recurrence, since the inducibility of the ventricular arrhythmias during programmed ventricular stimulation did not correlate significantly with the postoperative arrhythmic recurrence.

It seems, then, that although it improves survival rates, myocardial revascularization cannot be regarded as the sole therapy in patients with ischemic cardiomyopathy and sustained ventricular arrhythmia not clearly related to ischemia.

Scar tissue from previous infarction behaves as a stable arrhythmogenic substrate, which, in the presence of ischemia, can undergo significant electrophysiological changes leading to the onset of sustained clinical arrhythmia or the formation of a new re-entrant circuit, creating sustained VTs that are morphologically different. The annual incidence of monomorphic VT recurrence is 3–5% in the 15 years following the first event [13]; the arrhythmia is inducible during electrophysiological studies in 65–75% of patients with previous infarction and is reproducible in more than 90% of cases after 6 years.

In ischemic cardiomyopathy with previous necrosis there are many electrophysiological mechanisms that can determine the onset of malignant ventricular arrhythmias. For most patients with previous infarction, an ischemia-related trigger mechanism for the arrhythmias can be neither demonstrated nor excluded. If the ischemia is really the trigger for the arrhythmias, the correction of the coronary lesions, especially in the case of documented pre-revascularization reversible ischemia, would be a predictive indicator of arrhythmic recurrence.

In a group of 58 patients with previous myocardial infarction, ventricular arrhythmias uncorrelated with acute ischemic events and with coronary disease needing revascularization, Brugada et al. [14] reported that following revascularization a high proportion of ventricular arrhythmias were inducible (in only 9 patients out of 61 did the arrhythmia become noninducible) and arrhythmic recurrences were more frequent in the follow-up (in 32 out of 61 patients). In a high number of patients the underlying arrhythmic substrate was unaltered. The recurrence of arrhythmic events correlated with the low EF fraction but not with the ischemia prior to revascularization, indicating that the presence of reversible ischemia is not a marker of an ischemia-related mechanism for arrhythmias. In addition, cardiac mortality in the enrolled patients was 3% at 3 years, compared with the 5–10% at 2–5 years reported in the literature, which confirms the efficacy of a combined therapy with both revascularization and antiarrhythmic treatment (drug or ICD).

Left-ventricular function is a powerful independent predictive factor of overall cardiac mortality and is now well known as a reliable tool in the prognostic stratification of cardiomyopathic patients. The results of the MADIT 2 study provide further support for this notion, which in reality goes back a long way (as long ago as in 1982 the results of the Multicentric Post Infarction Research Group [15] showed how overall mortality in the 1st year after AMI increased exponentially if the EF was below 35%).

Consequently, in this group of patients (with ischemic cardiomyopathy and severely depressed EF) primary rather than secondary prevention is needed, and whether the mechanism triggering the arrhythmias is related to ischemia or not is no longer relevant, unless we hold that revascularization can improve the systolic function of the left ventricle (hibernating and stunned myocardium).

The fact that the arrhythmias are not often inducible under electrophysiological study confirms the importance of transitory and functional factors in the genesis of VF (50% of patients in the CASH study had no inducible arrhythmias at the baseline electrophysiological study, and only 20% of these were induced by polymorphic VF or TV; when the AVID register [16] is examined, it emerges that VT/FV was inducible only in 26% of patients with episodes of VT/VF). In the literature, VF inducibility in patients with clinical VF varies between 10% and 40%, according to the population selected (with or without previous infarction, with or without systolic dysfunction, with or without previous VT) [17].

As already highlighted, myocardial ischemia, as with electrolytic imbalance and the pro-arrhythmic effect of the drugs, is a transitory and correctable condition that can precipitate ventricular arrhythmia. The identification of a reversible cause has always suggested a low risk of arrhythmic event recurrence should the cause be eliminated, so that in this case the guidelines do not suggest ICD implant for secondary prevention.

Evidence of correctable ischemia during VT/VF, in the absence of scar tissue from previous necrosis, therefore identifies patients at low risk of recurrence, while patients with VT/VF and myocardial scarring could be at higher risk of arrhythmic recurrence, since it is impossible to remove the arrhythmic substrate (scar) in these patients.

In this regard the observational data from the AVID register appear interesting: they suggest that in patients with episodes of CA attributable to transitory and correctable causes the risk of future arrhythmic events remains high even after correction of the transitory precipitating factors. In these patients the arrhythmic recurrences and the SCD are probably more frequent than is generally thought. The underlying reason for this paradox could be a misunderstanding of the correctable and transitory causes, failure in correcting the reversible cause, failure to identify other underlying causes, which may not diminish on treatment of the transitory and reversible cause, or the successive reappearance of the reversible cause, which has been only temporarily corrected. It is possible that in these patients there is a high intrinsic risk despite elimination of the correctable cause.

The ideal therapy for these patients is not known, but they probably need more aggressive evaluation, treatment, and follow-up than is currently practiced. Further research appears necessary to study the causes of VT/VF that are truly reversible.

Even though no prospective randomized studies on large numbers of patients are available that would enable us to define the most appropriate treatment for coronary disease patients and those who have undergone CA reanimation (revascularization only? revascularization plus ICD? revascularization and prophylactic antiarrhythmic therapy?), we believe that a re-examination of smaller studies published some years ago could prove interesting.

In 1993 Manolis et al. [18] hypothesized a possible beneficial, though non-decisive, effect of myocardial revascularization as sole therapy in patients with sustained ventricular arrhythmias (53 patients). After CABG, under electrophysiological study the inducibility of a major ventricular arrhythmia decreased from 89% to 55% and survival was also good (94% at 1 year and 91% at 2–3 years).

On the other hand, Natale et al. [19] (1994) concluded that in their 58 patients with spontaneous episodes of polymorphic VF or VT and severe operable coronary disease (40 with previous acute myocardial infarction), CABG myocardial revascularization provided no protection against the recurrence of malignant ventricular arrhythmia. Only the implant of an ICD, carried out in all the patients enrolled, had a significant impact in terms of reducing overall mortality, with survival rates of 81% at 2 years, 76% at 3 years, and 71% at 4 years (58% at 4 years was predicted). Natale concluded that ischemia does not represent the predominant trigger mechanism for arrhythmic episodes, but goes further, saying that even if the cause is ischemia, since this can recur unpredictably following revascularization (inadequate revascularization, progression of the disease of the native vessels, and occlusion of the grafts, phenomena that generally appear 5–10 years after revascularization), implantation of an ICD should be considered at least in patients with a low EF, in order to modify the otherwise negative prognosis of this subgroup of patients.

Multivariate analysis showed that an EF below 30% and the induction of arrhythmia on electrophysiological study were independent indications for ICD implantation. No other variable (age, sex, number of bypasses, history of infarction, type of induced arrhythmia) was predictive of death or of shock delivery frequency. As a means of predicting a favorable outcome after revascularization, postoperative electrophysiological study has had good positive but low negative prediction rates.

One limitation of this study is that real overall mortality was compared with the theoretical expected rate calculated on the assumption that ICD intervention preceded by syncope or presycope was comparable to an episode of SCD. The use of "appropriate intervention of the ICD" as a surrogate survival end-point cannot be accepted, for a variety of reasons.

The type of arrhythmia has an important role in predicting the efficacy of revascularization. In 1990 Kelly et al. [20] observed how patients who exhibited VT in the preoperative electrophysiological study benefited less from correction of the ischemia than did patients in whom VF was induced, irrespective of the EF.

The severity of the cardiomyopathy also seems to have an important role. In 1995 Wiesfeld et al. [21] studied 85 patients with previous acute myocardial infarction and spontaneous episodes of SVT/VF and found that the outcome of revascularization was positive in only a small subgroup of patients with severe coronary disease and with a clear causal role of ischemia in the arrhythmia. In patients in whom ischemia was only a concomitant cause revascularization did not adequately prevent severe arrhythmic events.

It is interesting to compare the studies of Kelly (revascularization and antiarrhythmic drugs in patients with inducible persistent ventricular arrhythmia), Natale (revascularization and ICD in all patients), and Manolis (revascularization and ICD in selected patients with postoperative inducible and insuppressible ventricular arrhythmia). The overall survival at 2 years in these studies was, respectively, 95%, 81.6%, and 88%. The survival data in the Natale study were no better than in the other two, when in reality we would have expected higher survival. Why? Maybe because of the different degree of severity of the underlying cardiomyopathy: the average EF, for example, was 46%, 37%, and 36%, respectively. Nonetheless, even this cannot explain why survival at 3 years was 76.6% in the Natale study and 84% in the Manolis study, even though the EFs were almost identical. There must be other important and unknown influences that affect outcome in these patients, and this consideration can only reinforce the previously highlighted necessity for prospective and randomized clinical trials.

References

1. Kuck KH, Cappato R, Siebels J, Ruppel R (2000) Randomized comparison of antiarrhythmic drug therapy with implantable defibrillator in patients resuscitated from cardiac arrest: the Cardiac Arrest Study Hamburg (CASH). Circulation 102:748
2. The AVID Investigators (1997) A comparison of antiarrhythmic drug therapy with implantable defibrillators in patients resuscitated from near fatal ventricular arrhythmias. N Engl J Med 337:1576–1583
3. Connolly SJ, Gent M, Roberts RS et al (2000) Canadian Implantable Defibrillator Study (CIDS): a randomized trial of the implantable cardioverter against amiodarone. Circulation 101:1297–1302
4. Moss AJ, Hall WJ, Cannom DS et al (1997) Improved survival with an implanted defibrillator in patients with coronary artery disease at high risk for ventricular arrhythmia. N Engl J Med 337:1933–1940
5. Coumel P (1987) The management of clinical arrhythmias. An overview on invasive versus non invasive electrophysiology. Eur Heart J 8:92–99
6. Holmes DR Jr, Davis KB, Mock MB et al (1986) The effect of medical and surgical treatment on subsequent sudden cardiac death in patients with coronary artery disease: a report from the Coronary Artery Surgery Study. Circulation 73:1254–1263

7. Bigger JT Jr (1997) Prophylactic use of implanted cardiac defibrillators in patients at high risk for ventricular arrhythmias after coronary artery by-pass graft surgery. N Engl J Med 337:1569
8. Bigger JT, Whang W, Rottman JN et al (1999) Mechanism of death in the CABG Patch Trial: a randomized trial of implantable cardiac defibrillator prophylaxis in patients at high risk of death after coronary artery bypass graft surgery. Circulation 99:1416–1421
9. Berntsen RF, Gunnes P. Lie M, Rasmussen K (1993) Surgical revascularization in the treatment of ventricular tachycardia and fibrillation exposed by exercise-induced ischaemia. Eur Heart J 14:1297
10. Lessmeier TJ, Lehmann MH, Steinman RT et al (1994) Implantable cardioverter-defibrillator therapy in 300 patients with coronary artery disease presenting exclusively with ventricular fibrillation. Am Heart J 128:211–218
11. Geelen P, Primo J, Wellens F, Brugada P (1999) Coronary artery by-pass grafting and defibrillator implantation in patients with ventricular tachyarrhythmias and ischemic heart disease. Pacing Clin Electrophysiol 22:1132–1139
12. Link MS, Cesarz CA, Griffith JL et al (1999) Evaluation of coronary revascularization to prevent tachycardia recurrences in survivors of ventricular fibrillation. Am J Cardiol 83:960–962
13. Josephson ME (1993) Clinical cardiac electrophysiology: techniques and interpretations, 2nd edn. Lea & Febiger, Philadelphia London
14. Brugada J, Aguinaga L, Mont L et al (2001) Coronary artery revascularization in patients with sustained ventricular arrhythmias in the chronic phase of a myocardial infarction: effects on the electrophysiologic substrate and outcome. J Am Coll Cardiol 37:529–533
15. The Multicenter Post-Infarction Research Group (1983) Risk stratification and survival after myocardial infarction. N Engl J Med 309:331–336
16. Brodsky MA, Mitchell LB, Halperin BD et al (2002) AVID Investigators. Prognostic value of baseline electrophysiologic studies in patients with sustained ventricular tachyarrhythmia: the Antiarrhythmic versus Implantable Defibrillators (AVID) Trial. Am Heart J 144:478
17. Morady F, DiCarlo L, Winston S et al (1984) Clinical features and prognosis of patients with out of hospital cardiac arrest and a normal electrophysiologic study. J Am Coll Cardiol 4:39–44
18. Manolis AS, Rastegar H, Estes M (1993) Effects of coronary artery by pass grafting on ventricular arrhythmias: results with electrophysiological testing and long-term follow up. Pacing Clin Electrophysiol 16:984–991
19. Natale A, Sra J, Axtell K et al (1994) Ventricular fibrillation and polymorphic ventricular tachycardia with critical coronary artery stenosis: does by-pass surgery suffice? J Cardiovasc Electrophysiol 5:988–994
20. Kelly P, Ruskin JN, Vlahakes GJ et al (1990) Surgical coronary revascularization in survivors of prehospital cardiac arrest: its effect on inducible ventricular arrhythmias and long-term survival. J Am Coll Cardiol 15:267–273
21. Wiesfeld AC, Crijns HJ, Hillege HL et al (1995) The clinical significance of coronary anatomy in post-infarct patients with late sustained ventricular tachycardia or ventricular fibrillation. Eur Heart J 16:818–824

Surgical Revascularization in Patients with "Ischemia-related" Ventricular Fibrillation: Is It Sufficient to Prevent Sudden Death?

R.N.W. Hauer

Acute ischemia is a major contributing factor in sudden cardiac death attributable to ventricular fibrillation [1, 2]. Surgical revascularization is a generally accepted treatment for acute ischemia. However, the role of revascularization in secondary prevention for the survivors of cardiac death is controversial [3, 4]. In the presence of acute ischemia as the only causative factor in the arrhythmia, revascularization has proved very effective in the case of critical narrowing of at least one coronary artery [5]. If narrowing is due to coronary spasm, however, calcium blockers and ICD implantation are the preferred therapies. Polymorphic ventricular tachycardia and ventricular fibrillation are the typical arrhythmias caused by acute ischemia.

In the presence of other arrhythmogenic factors, such as a scar from a previous myocardial infarction, it is less likely that revascularization will provide complete protection [6, 7]. Frequently, these patients have spontaneous and inducible monomorphic ventricular tachycardia, although polymorphic arrhythmias may also occur. If such patients have signs of acute ischemia, revascularization should be combined with ICD implantation or with map-guided surgery. However, even in patients with a myocardial scar, acute ischemia may be more important as arrhythmogenic factor. This may explain the absence of an additional benefit of ICD implantation in patients undergoing aorto-coronary bypass grafting in the CABG patch trial [8]. Other patients may have ischemia, but surviving bundles embedded within the scar tissue are the electrophysiological substrate for the arrhythmia. Careful cardiologic evaluation is needed for selection of the appropriate therapeutic strategy.

Heart Lung Center Utrecht, University Medical Center, Utrecht, The Netherlands

References

1. O'Rourke RA (1992) Role of myocardial revascularization in sudden cardiac death. Circulation 85 [Suppl I]:I-112–I-117
2. DiMarco JP, Haines DE (1990) Sudden cardiac death. Curr Prob Cardiol 15:185–232
3. Every NR, Fahrenbruch CE, Hallstrom AP, Weaver WD, Cobb LA (1992) Influence of coronary bypass surgery on subsequent outcome of patients resuscitated from out of hospital cardiac arrest. J Am Coll Cardiol 19:1435–1439
4. Wyse DG, Friedman PL, Brodsky MA, Beckman KJ, Carlson MD, Curtis AB, Hallstrom AP, Raitt MH, Wilkoff BL, Greene HL, for the AVID investigators (2001) Life-threatening ventricular arrhythmias due to transient or correctable causes: high risk for death in follow-up. J Am Coll Cardiol 38:1718–1724
5. Kron IL, Lerman BB, Haines DE, Flanagan TL, DiMarco JP (1989) Coronary bypass grafting in patients with ventricular fibrillation. Ann Thorac Surg 48:85–89
6. Ruskin JN, McGovern B, Garan H (1990) Sudden death. In: Stein JH (ed) Internal medicine, 3rd edn. Little, Brown, Boston, pp 108–112
7. Wilber DJ, Garan H, Finkelstein D et al (1998) Out-of-hospital cardiac arrest: use of electrophysiologic testing in the prediction of long-term outcomes. N Engl J Med 318:19–24
8. Bigger JT Jr (1997) Prophylactic use of implanted cardiac defibrillators in patients at high risk for ventricular arrhythmias after coronary-artery bypass graft surgery. N Engl J Med 337:1569–1575

New-onset Ventricular Tachyarrhythmias After Cardiac Surgery: Significance and Treatment

G. Crescenzi, S. Benussi, G. Landoni, O. Alfieri

Definition and Incidence

Many cases of sudden death are caused by sustained ventricular tachyarrhythmias: new-onset ventricular tachycardia (VT) and ventricular fibrillation (VF) are infrequent but dreaded postoperative complications after cardiac surgery.

Ventricular arrhythmias, such as isolated ventricular premature beats or non-sustained VT, occur commonly after cardiac surgery and do not seem to have an adverse effect on prognosis [1]. In contrast, sustained VT and VF are life-threatening events, bearing quite a high postoperative mortality [2]. VT is defined by the occurrence of three or more consecutive premature ventricular complexes. A VT is termed 'sustained' when it lasts more than 30s or when it causes cardiovascular collapse. Two principal types of VTs have been described after cardiac surgery: monomorphic VT, with uniform QRS morphology, and polymorphic VT, with a typical beat-to-beat variability in QRS morphology. VF is defined as a ventricular rhythm with no discernable QRS complexes.

Life-threatening ventricular arrhythmias most commonly occur as a result of ischemic heart disease: their incidence in the recovery phase of cardiac surgery is very low, but reaches 0.7-3.1% after coronary artery bypass grafting (CABG) [3]. In fact, there is a well-defined anatomical substrate in patients with coronary artery disease: areas of myocardial necrosis and scarring constitute a real barrier for the propagation of an electrical impulse, which encounters pathways of slow conduction; as a result, single or multiple reentrant circuits may become established generating VT/VF. Predisposing factors include myocardial ischemia, low cardiac output, metabolic disturbances, drug interactions, and severe left-ventricular dysfunction (ejection fraction below 35%) [4].

Department of Cardiac Surgery and Cardiovascular Anesthesia, Vita-Salute University of Milan, IRCCS San Raffaele Hospital, Milan, Italy

Underlying Mechanisms

The electrophysiological mechanisms underlying perioperative arrhythmias are not completely understood. They can be ascribed to a combination of transient perioperative factors, such as circulating catecholamines, alterations in the autonomic nervous system tone, electrolyte imbalance (potassium, magnesium), periprocedural myocardial ischemia or infarction, and residual ischemia resulting from incomplete revascularization. Nonetheless, ventricular tachyarrhythmias can also be the expression of a chronic arrhythmogenic substrate [5, 6].

Recent studies have indicated that monomorphic and polymorphic VT are generated by different electrophysiological mechanisms.

Sustained polymorphic VT, which is more often due to acute ischemia than to chronic infarct scarring, is the presenting morphology in one-third of the subjects. Polymorphic VT is usually associated with acute ischemia. Two-thirds of the cases present with perioperative myocardial infarction (MI). Recent MI and acute ischemia may trigger VT in combination with multiple perioperative risk factors, such as hemodynamic instability, catecholaminergic stimulation, and metabolic abnormalities.

Sustained monomorphic VT generally involves re-entry through myocyte bands surviving in the infarct and is the presenting VT morphology in two-thirds of subjects. The majority of them have no evidence of perioperative MI, but almost invariably these patients have an old MI, a lower ejection fraction than patients with polymorphic VT, and clinical evidence of congestive heart failure: when all three of these risk factors (prior MI, ejection fraction <35%, and severe congestive heart failure) are present simultaneously, the risk of VT is extremely high (30%).

These features add credence to the idea that an underlying arrhythmogenic substrate is involved. This substrate, silent before surgery, may become functional after reperfusion of nonviable areas of prior necrosis and scar tissue. The hypothesis has been proposed that resumption of blood flow to previously poorly perfused infarcted areas can potentially restore electrophysiological function to surviving cells within the myocardial scar and create the possibility of re-entrant circuits after a state of "electrical hibernation." A recent paper [2] showed that one particular factor is strongly associated with the development of monomorphic VT: placement of a bypass graft across a non-collateralized, totally occluded artery supplying a chronic infarct zone. When present, this factor was associated with a 22-fold increase in the risk of postoperative VT.

Prognosis

Patients with ischemic heart disease remain at constant risk of sudden cardiac death from a refractory episode of ventricular tachyarrhythmia. This risk is usually higher in patients with a poor left-ventricular function and clinical evidence of severe congestive heart failure [4].

It is well known that surgical revascularization controls these unexpected terminal events more effectively than conventional medical therapy and that it also decreases the expected mortality among patients with left-ventricular dysfunction [7].

Patients who develop VT/VF experience hospital mortality rates as high as 25%; however, a difference in prognosis can be identified between the two previously identified groups: polymorphic VT, usually a complication in the setting of perioperative MI, has a high mortality rate during the acute phase but it is associated with a good long-term outcome; monomorphic VT carries a high in-hospital and long-term mortality [5, 6].

Treatment

With the development of pulseless VT or VF, standard advanced life support interventions (defibrillation and cardiopulmonary resuscitation) are started to terminate the arrhythmia and support vital functions. Amiodarone (300-mg bolus) has replaced lidocaine as the antiarrhythmic drug of first choice for VT/VF refractory to electrical shocks; lidocaine should be used if amiodarone is not available. Amiodarone by continuous perfusion can also prevent further arrhythmic events.

After successful advanced life support, appropriate therapy to stabilize the patient consists in correction of any underlying electrolyte imbalance, acid-base abnormalities and hypoxemia, discontinuation of type-1 antiarrhythmic agents, and the implementation of temporary pacing at rates of 80-100 beats/min to prevent bradycardia and minimize QT-prolongation.

Emergency cardiopulmonary support in the intensive care unit is a life-saving maneuver in patients suffering postoperative cardiac arrest as a result of refractory VF. Examinations for risk stratification of patients experiencing VT or VF postoperatively should include coronary arteriogram if graft malfunction is suspected, especially if monomorphic VT is observed.

Prophylactic use of class I antiarrhythmic drugs in patients at high risk for death from ventricular arrhythmia after CABG is ineffective and can worsen cardiac failure in patients with ejection fraction <35% [4].

In patients with reduced left-ventricular ejection fraction and clinical evidence of severe heart failure, it is reasonable to consider implantation of an internal cardioverter defibrillator (ICD). The Coronary Artery Bypass Graft Patch Trial [8] found that late survival was not inproved by prophylactic implantation of an ICD at the time of elective CABG in patients at high risk for sudden cardiac death (SCD): this finding can be explained by the preventive effect of CABG per se (this antiarrhythmic benefit has been shown to operate within the first postoperative year and to last for up to 6 years [7]). Although prophylactic use is not indicated, the implantation of an ICD is advisable in patients with severe congestive heart failure or low ejection fraction who have had an episode of postoperative VF or hemodynamically unstable VT [9].

Conclusions

Knowledge of the different morphological presentations (polymorphic vs monomorphic) and the clinical context (history of a prior MI, site of coronary graft placement, perioperative ischemia or MI) makes it easier to understand the causes of VT/VF and to select the appropriate therapeutic and preventive measures.

The better outcome of patients with low ejection fraction after CABG when compared to that of medical treatment alone is due to the revascularization of hibernating myocardium. The future challenge in this setting is to restore blood flow to hibernating myocardium without performing a bypass graft across an artery supplying a potentially arrhythmogenic myocardial scar.

References

1. Pinto RP, Romerill DB, Nasser WK et al (1996) Prognosis of patients with frequent premature ventricular complexes and nonsustained ventricular tachycardia after coronary artery bypass graft surgery. Clin Cardiol 19:321-324
2. Ducceschi V, D'Andrea A, Liccardo B et al (2000) Ventricular tachyarrhythmias following coronary surgery: predisposing factors. Int J Cardiol 73:43-48
3. Steinberg JS, Gaur A, Sciacca R et al (1999) New-onset sustained ventricular tachycardia after cardiac surgery. Circulation 99:903-908
4. Pires LA, Wagshal AB, Lancey R et al (1995) Arrhythmias and conduction disturbances after coronary artery bypass graft surgery: epidemiology, management, and prognosis. Am Heart J 129:799-808
5. Azar RR, Berns E, Seecharran B et al (1997) De novo monomorphic and polymorphic ventricular tachycardia following coronary artery bypass grafting. Am J Cardiol 80:76-78
6. Saxon AL, Wiener I, Natterson PD et al (1995) Monomorphic versus polymorphic ventricular tachycardia after coronary artery bypass grafting. Am J Cardiol 75:403-405
7. Kaul TK, Barry LF, Lee SR et al (1998) Ventricular arrhythmia following successful myocardial revascularization: incidence, predictors and prevention. Eur J Cardiothorac Surg 13:629-636
8. Bigger JT (1997) Prophylactic use of implanted cardiac defibrillators in patients at high risk for ventricular arrhythmias after coronary artery bypass graft surgery. N Engl J Med 337:1569-1575
9. Cook JR, Rizo-Patron C, Curtis AB et al (2002) Effect of surgical revascularization in patients with coronary artery disease and ventricular tachycardia or fibrillation in the Antiarrhythmics Versus Implantable Defibrillators (AVID) Registry. Am Heart J 143:821-826

Electrophysiologically Guided Antiarrhythmic Surgery for Treatment of Frequently Recurrent Ventricular Tachycardia: What Role Does It Have Today?

R. De Ponti, J. A. Salerno-Uriarte

Antiarrhythmic Surgery for Ventricular Tachycardia: A Historical Overview

At the end of the 1970s, direct surgical operations [1] targeting the arrhythmogenic area proved better than "blind" aneurysmectomy for the treatment of drug-refractory, life-threatening ventricular arrhythmias [2-4]. Several surgical techniques, e.g., encircling or partial endocardial ventriculotomy [1, 5], endocardial resection [6], cryoablation [7], and laser ablation [8], also used in combination [9], were developed for the surgical treatment of ventricular tachycardias refractory to medical therapy.

Soon it was clear that, in order to be as effective as possible and to limit the extent of surgery, which in turn may affect ventricular function in the long term, the surgical approaches had to be guided by intraoperative mapping to locate the arrhythmogenic substrate [10-15]. Starting as a sequential point-by-point manual technique, intraoperative mapping became more and more sophisticated with the use of computerized mapping systems. These allowed fast acquisition and interpretation of signals during ventricular tachycardia as well as during sinus rhythm, and even during nonsustained arrhythmias, by using multielectrode arrays placed on the epicardial surface (Fig. 1a) and in the ventricular cavity (Fig. 1b). On the basis of the isochronal (Fig. 2) or the isopotential (Fig. 3) maps obtained, the electrophysiologist was able to locate and define the arrhythmogenic substrate of each morphology of ventricular tachycardia induced during the intraoperative electrophysiologic study. Close and fruitful cooperation between electrophysiologist and cardiac surgeon made mapping-guided antiarrhythmic surgery not only possible, but also effective. Myocardial revascularization and mitral valve surgery were often combined.

During the 1980s, antiarrhythmic surgery was mainly performed in patients with ischemic heart disease, drug-refractory ventricular tachycardias

Department of Cardiovascular Sciences, Ospedale di Circolo e Fondazione Macchi-University of Insubria, Varese, Italy

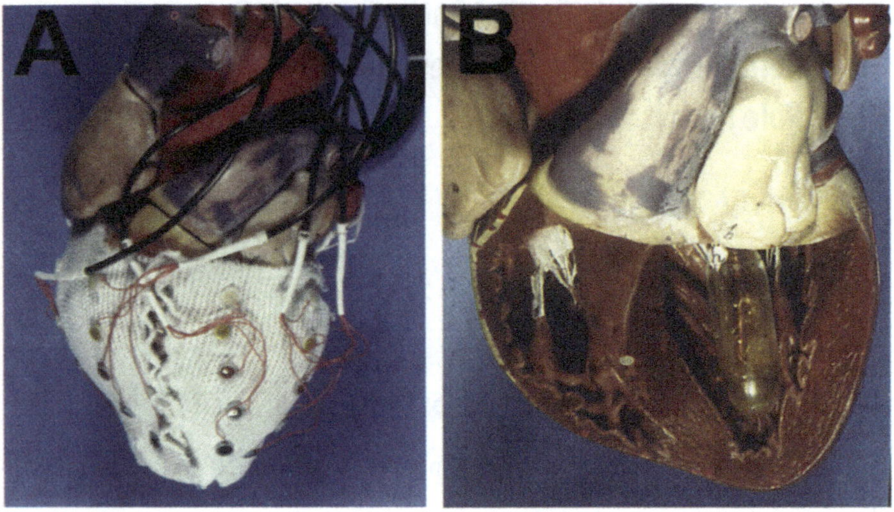

Fig. 1A, B. Multielectrode arrays for computerized systems to record epicardial (**A**) or endocardial (**B**) potentials. In **A**, electrodes are mounted on an expandable mesh and disposed by the surgeon in a standardized position on the ventricular epicardium. The olive-shaped catheter shown in **B** was introduced into the left ventricular cavity transmitrally to record unipolar potentials in a noncontact way, through the blood pool

and, for technical surgical reasons, a well-defined ventricular aneurysm. At that time, no further patient selection was made in respect of the time of onset of the ventricular arrhythmias after the acute myocardial infarction and the presence of poor left ventricular function. In any case, the results, reported in a collaborative study [16], were more than acceptable, with relatively low intraoperative mortality (12% on average, but around 20% in some series) and long-term (5-year) survival and recurrence rates of 57% and 10%, respectively. With regard to the long-term survival, it is noteworthy that, while sudden cardiac death accounted for 5%, most deaths were reported as nonsudden cardiac death, in an era when pharmacologic and nonpharmacologic therapies for congestive heart failure were not as well developed as they are today.

Antiarrhythmic Surgery in the Era of Implantable Devices and Catheter Ablation

During the 1990s, a decade of intensive development of implantable devices and catheter ablation, several centers continued the use of antiarrhythmic surgery for ventricular tachycardia. During this period, improvement in the aforementioned results was mainly due to two factors: (1) patient selection and (2) modification of the surgical technique, which now consisted of remodeling

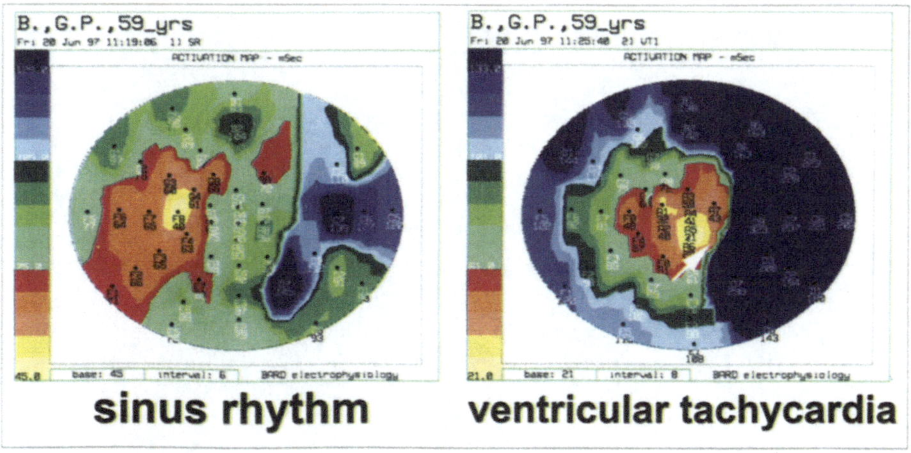

Fig. 2. Isochronal maps of the epicardium generated by a computerized mapping system, recorded during sinus rhythm and ventricular tachycardia in the same patient. The map shows a polar view of the ventricular mass, with the apex in the center and the basal segments along the outer perimeter; the *left* part represents the left ventricle, the *right* one the right ventricle. The color-coded scale indicates the activation time, from *yellow* (earliest activation) to *blue* (latest activation). In sinus rhythm, the free wall of the right ventricle is activated early and the epicardial breakthrough of the activation over the right bundle is evident (*yellow* spot); the large area of late activation (*blue*) is related to an old inferolateral myocardial infarction. During ventricular tachycardia, the earliest activated epicardial site is located in the posterior area of the left ventricular apex, with a left-to-right-to-left activation sequence, which results in a left bundle branch block morphology and superior axis deviation on the surface electrocardiogram. The area between the earliest and latest activation site (*arrow*), where maximum compression of isochronal lines is observed, indicates the area of slow conduction, which is of particular interest when planning the surgical ablation strategy

the left ventricle. Most deaths after antiarrhythmic surgery, both perioperative and in the long-term follow-up, occurred in patients with marked depression of left ventricular function (left ventricular ejection fraction <25-30%) [17]. The conclusion was drawn from this that patients with poor left ventricular function were not ideal candidates for antiarrhythmic surgery and, therefore, they had to be excluded from this treatment option. Importantly, it was acknowledged that the global ejection fraction value was not a reliable parameter for this preoperative evaluation, especially when a large aneurysm was present. Conversely, left ventricular wall motion score, which allowed better evaluation of the residual left ventricular function, was used as a criterion to select patients who, having preserved function of the nonaneurysmal segments, would most benefit from antiarrhythmic surgery [18, 19]. In addition, the operative technique developed in such a way that surgery was no longer merely aneurysmectomy and aneurysmorrhaphy: the left ventricular geometry was carefully reconstructed by using autologous pericardial tissue or a pros-

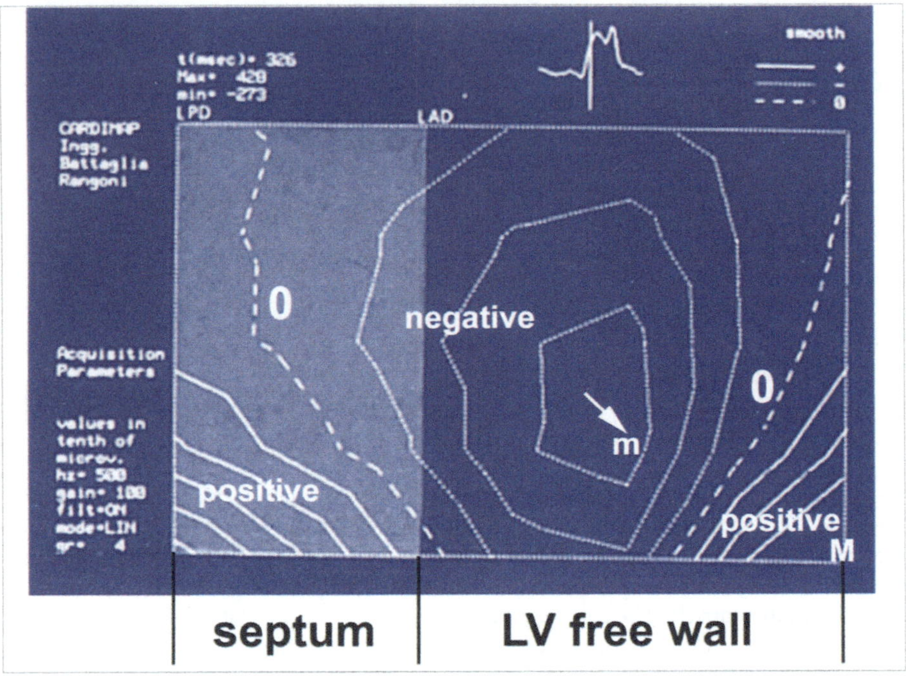

Fig. 3. Isopotential endocardial map of the left ventricle at the QRS onset during ventricular tachycardia, recorded by the device shown in Fig. 1b. In this two-dimensional rectangular map, from *left* to *right*, the septum (from posterior to anterior) and the left free wall (from anterior to posterior) are represented. The *dashed lines* (lines of 0 potential) distinguish the negative from the positive areas, identifying the border of the activation wavefront. In this postinfarction ventricular tachycardia, the most negative area, indicated by the "m" (*arrow*), identifies the exit point from the slow conduction area in the anterolateral wall of the left ventricle, close to the apex. Point *M* indicates the most positive area

thetic patch [20-22]. These factors, together with avoidance of concomitant mitral valve surgery [23, 24] and early surgery after acute myocardial infarction [25], not only contributed to the reduction of perioperative mortality (now stably well below 10%) and fatal congestive heart failure during long-term follow-up, but also led to better patient outcome. Actually, consistent data show that surgery for ventricular tachycardia improves both systolic and diastolic left ventricular function [26], and that this improvement can be clinically relevant with a consistent change in NYHA functional class, especially in patients with an old anterior myocardial infarction [23].

One issue is still controversial: whether intraoperative mapping is still mandatory or not. Several authors [27-29] suggest that intraoperative mapping is obsolete and can be replaced by the extensive use of cryoablation, whereas others [30, 31] are strongly of the opinion that better results can be achieved by mapping-guided surgery. This “to map or not to map” dilemma can be moderated by considering that in some centers earlier experience of mapping-guided procedures contributed to refining the technique, so that now mapping in these centers is less essential, although still useful to orient and limit surgery.

Antiarrhythmic Surgery for Ventricular Tachycardia: What Is Its role Today?

At present, antiarrhythmic surgery: (1) is able to cure both tolerated and untolerated postinfarction ventricular tachycardia; (2) may provide favorable ventricular remodeling with a clinically relevant long-lasting improvement of left ventricular function; (3) is associated with very low operative mortality; and (4) can be combined with surgical revascularization when required. On the basis of these considerations, a young patient with postinfarction ventricular arrhythmias, a well-defined anteroapical aneurysm, and preserved contractility of the nonaneurysmal segments can be considered an ideal candidate for antiarrhythmic surgery, especially if surgical revascularization is deemed necessary. This therapeutic option applied in this subset of patients in a well-experienced center not only has a high success rate in abolishing ventricular arrhythmias, but also provides functional improvement, being able to prevent congestive heart failure, a “leitmotiv” in the long-term follow-up of these patients [32]. For this reason, in some patients with well-tolerated ventricular tachycardia associated with a large and well-defined anteroapical aneurysm, antiarrhythmic surgery may be preferable to catheter ablation, since it also prevents progressive deterioration of left ventricular function. Finally, a careful postoperative assessment, which should include invasive electrophysiologic testing, should be able to identify patients requiring adjunctive therapy such as an implantable cardioverter-defibrillator, catheter ablation, or antiarrhythmic drug therapy. However, prospective randomized studies are required to assess the best treatment strategy after surgery in this patient population.

References

1. Guiraudon G, Fontaine G, Frank R et al (1978) Encircling endocardial ventriculotomy: a new surgical treatment for life-threatening ventricular tachycardias, resistant to medical treatment following myocardial infarction. Ann Thorac Surg 26:438-444
2. Harken AH, Horowitz LN, Josephson ME (1980) Comparison of standard aneurysmectomy and aneurysmectomy with direct endocardial resection for the treatment of recurrent sustained ventricular tachycardia. J Thorac Cardiovasc Surg 80:527-534
3. Ostermeyer J, Breithardt G, Kolvenbach R, Borggrefe M (1982) The surgical treatment of ventricular tachycardias: simple aneurysmectomy versus electrophysiologically guided procedures. J Thorac Cardiovasc Surg 84:701-715
4. Boineau JP, Cox JL (1982) Rationale for a direct surgical approach to control ventricular arrhythmias: relation of specific intraoperative techniques to mechanism and location of arrhythmic circuit. Am J Cardiol 49:381-396

5. Ostermeyer J, Breithardt G, Borggrefe M et al (1984) Surgical treatment of ventricular tachycardias. Complete versus partial encircling endocardial ventriculotomy. J Thorac Cardiovasc Surg 87:517-525
6. Josephson ME, Harken AH, Horowitz LN (1979) Endocardial excision: a new surgical technique for the treatment of recurrent ventricular tachycardia. Circulation 60:1430-1439
7. Camm J, Ward DE, Spurrel RAJ, Rees GM (1980) Cryothermal mapping and cryoablation in the treatment of refractory cardiac arrhythmias. Circulation 63:67-74
8. Svenson RH, Gallagher JJ, Selle JG et al (1987) Neodymium-YAG laser photocoagulation: a successful new map-guided technique for the intraoperative ablation of ventricular tachycardia. Circulation 76:1319-1328
9. Viganò M, Martinelli L, Salerno JA et al (1986) Ventricular tachycardia in post-myocardial infarction patients. Results of surgical therapy. Eur Heart J 7(suppl A):165-168
10. Gallagher JJ, Kasell JH, Cox JL et al (1982) Techniques of intraoperative electrophysiologic mapping. Am J Cardiol 49:221-240
11. De Bakker JM, Janse MJ, Van Capelle FJ, Durrer D (1983) Endocardial mapping by simultaneous recording of endocardial electrograms during cardiac surgery for ventricular aneurysm. J Am Coll Cardiol 2:947-953
12. Miller JM, Harken AH, Hargrove WC, Josephson ME (1985) Pattern of endocardial activation during sustained ventricular tachycardia. J Am Coll Cardiol 6:1280-1287
13. Salerno JA, Klersy C, Viganò M et al (1986) Ventricular tachycardia in postmyocardial infarction patients. Preoperative and intraoperative mapping. Eur Heart J (suppl A):157-163
14. Frank G, Lowes D, Baumgart D et al (1988) Surgical alternatives in the treatment of life-threatening ventricular arrhythmias. Eur J Cardiothorac Surg 2:207-216
15. Mickleborough L, Harris L, Downar E et al (1988) A new intraoperative approach for endocardial mapping of ventricular tachycardia. J Thorac Cardiovasc Surg 95:271-280
16. Borggrefe M, Podczeck A, Ostermeyer J, Breithardt G and the Surgical Ablation Registry (1988) Long-term results of electrophysiologically guided antitachycardia surgery for ventricular tachyarrhythmias: a collaborative report on 665 patients. In: Breithardt G, Borggrefe M, Zipes DP (eds) Nonpharmacological therapy of tachyarrhythmias. Futura, Mount Kisko, NY, pp 109-132
17. Lawrie GM, Pacifico A, Kaushik R et al (1991) Factors predictive of results of direct ablative operations for drug-refractory ventricular tachycardia. Analysis of 80 patients. J Thorac Cardiovasc Surg 101:44-55
18. Van Hemel NM, Kingma JH, Defauw JAM, Vermeulen FEE (1989) Left ventricular wall motion score as a criterion for selecting patients for direct surgery in the treatment of post-infarction ventricular tachycardia. Eur Heart J 10:304-315
19. Nath S, Haines DE, Kron IL et al (1993) Regional wall motion analysis predicts survival and functional outcome after subendocardial resection in patients with prior anterior myocardial infarction. Circulation 88:70-76
20. Viganò M, Graffigna A, Salerno JA (1992) La chirurgia delle aritmie ischemiche intrattabili. G Ital Cardiol 22:373-380
21. Cooley DA, Frazier OH, Duncan JM et al (1992) Intracavitary repair of ventricular aenurysm and regional dyskinesia. Ann Surg 215:417-424
22. Dor V, Sabatier M, Di Donato M et al (1998) Efficacy of endoventricular patch plasty in large postinfarction akynetic scar and severe left ventricular dysfunction: comparison with a series of large dyskinetic scars. J Thorac Cardiovasc Surg 116:50-59
23. Salerno JA, De Ponti R, Angoli L et al (1992) Comparative outcomes of electrical and surgical treatments in patients with inducible ventricular tachycardia. In: Santini M,

Pistolese M, Alliegro A (eds) Progress in clinical pacing. Futura, Mount Kisko, NY, pp 343-350
24. Von Oppel UO, Milne D, Okreglicki A, Scott Millar RN (2002) Surgery for ventricular tachycardia of left ventricular origin: risk factors for success and long-term outcome. Eur J Cardiothorac Surg 22:762-770
25. Bourke JP, Campbell RW, McComb JM et al (1999) Surgery for postinfarction ventricular tachycardia in the pre-implantable cardioverter defibrillator era: early and long term outcomes in 100 consecutive patients. Heart 82:156-162
26. Bourke JP, Hawkins T, Hilton CJ et al (2000) Effects of surgery for postinfarction ventricular tachycardia on parameters of left ventricular function. Am J Cardiol 85:703-709
27. Guiraudon GM, Thakur RK, Klein GJ et al (1994) Encircling endocardial cryoablation for ventricular tachycardia after myocardial infarction: experience with 33 patients. Am Heart J 128:982-989
28. Frapier JM, Hubaut JJ, Pasqiue JL, Chaptal PA (1998) Large encircling cryoablation without mapping for ventricular tachycardia after anterior myocardial infarction: long-term outcome. J Thorac Cardiovasc Surg 116:578-583
29. Wellens F, Geelen P, Demirsoy E et al (2002) Surgical treatment of tachyarrhythmias due to postinfarction left ventricualr aneurysm with endoaneurysmorrhaphy and cryoablation. Eur J Cardiothorac Surg 22:771-776
30. Bakker PFA, de Lange F, Hauer RNW et al (2001) Sequential map-guided endocardial resection for ventricular tachycardia improves outcome. Eur J Cardiothorac Surg 19:448-454
31. Nitta T, Mitsuno M, Rokkas CK et al (2001) Cryoablation of ventricular tachycardia guided by return cycle mapping after entrainment. J Thorac Cardiovasc Surg 121:249-258
32. Hallstrom AP, Greene HL, Wilkoff BL et al and the AVID investigators (2001) Relationship between rehospitalization and future death in patients treated for potentially lethal arrhythmias. J Cardiovasc Electrophysiol 12:990-995

Heart Transplantation in Frequently Recurrent Drug-Refractory Tachyarrhythmias: is it Worthwhile?

D. G. Benditt[1], V. Tholakahalli[1], S. Sakaguchi[1], C. Ermis[1], M.-T. Olivari[2], F. Lü[1]

Introduction

Despite the fact that many cardiac transplantation candidates manifest potentially worrisome rhythm disturbances, refractory life-threatening cardiac arrhythmias (specifically ventricular tachyarrhythmias) are rarely the primary indication for cardiac transplantation. As a result, available clinical experience with this potential transplant indication is small. Nevertheless, as methods for stabilizing hemodynamics in the sickest heart failure patients progress (e.g., left ventricular assist devices (LVADs), ACORN left ventricular (LV) stenting, intractable cardiac arrhythmias may increasingly play a role in transplantation decision making. This communication examines the current status of cardiac arrhythmias as an indication for heart transplantation.

Etiologic Basis of Refractory Ventricular Arrhythmias

Life-threatening cardiac arrhythmias may occur in the setting of relatively normal ventricular function (e.g., hypertrophic cardiomyopathy [HOCM], arrhythmogenic right ventricular dysplasia [ARVD], Brugada syndrome, long QT syndromes, and primary idiopathic ventricular tachycardia). However, the vast majority of tachyarrhythmias refractory to conventional treatment occur in conjunction with severe LV dysfunction and congestive heart failure (CHF). In this latter circumstance, mechanical-electrical feedback, scar related reentry, and neurohumoral factors may play important roles in establishing the milieu for arrhythmogenesis. Furthermore, the presence of elevated circulating catecholamines, particularly the extreme norepinephrine levels associated with progressive severe heart failure, would be anticipated to increase the risk for arrhythmias of any mechanism to become sustained and life threatening.

[1]Cardiac Arrhythmia Center, Department of Medicine, Cardiovascular Division, University of Minnesota Medical School; [2]Minneapolis Heart Institute, Minneapolis, Minnesota, USA

Mode of Death in Patients with Ventricular Arrhythmias and Severe LV Dysfunction

Patients with CHF are at high risk for ventricular arrhythmias and death from cardiac cause. In fact, most CHF patients have frequent and often complex ventricular arrhythmias (i.e., runs, polymorphous forms); approximately 50 % to 70% of these individuals have episodes of non-sustained ventricular tachycardia (VT) during ambulatory electrocardiographic monitoring. However, available evidence suggests that while ventricular arrhythmias are an important source of mortality in these high risk patients, a substantial number of deaths (including many in which an arrhythmia may have been the apparent initiating event) are not reversible by conventional treatment techniques, including appropriately functioning implantable cardioverter-defibrillators (ICDs). In this regard, in a review of 320 patient deaths observed during trials of several Medtronic (Medtronic Inc., Minneapolis, Minnesota) transvenous ICD systems [1], a mode of death could be ascribed for 317 patients. Ninety deaths (28 %) were classified as sudden, 156 (49 %) were considered non-sudden but of cardiac cause, and 71 (22 %) were attributed to non-cardiac factors. In 68 patients in whom sufficient information was available for the independent death review committee to make a determination, deaths were further categorized according to the presumed mechanism. Not surprisingly, the most common arrhythmia associated with sudden death in these ICD patients was ventricular tachycardia/ventricular fibrillation (VT/VF) that had proved irreversible despite treatment with appropriate shocks. However, even though the study population comprised a select group of ventricular arrhythmia prone individuals (i.e., the patients had been treated with ICDs for conventional indications), death due to electromechanical dissociation (EMD) was surprisingly frequent (29 %). Furthermore, the occurrence of EMD deaths appeared to correlate with severity of New York Heart Association (NYHA) functional class.

Prevention of Life-Threatening Ventricular Tachyarrhythmias in Severe LV Dysfunction Patients

LV dysfunction patients with CHF of severity sufficient to warrant screening for cardiac transplantation are prone to high annual mortality (currently averaging 20% or higher per year). In these cases, current pharmacological intervention is directed primarily towards attempting to ameliorate the underlying disease state as much as possible; the principal available agents are angiotensin inhibitors, angiotensin II receptor blockers, and beta-adrenergic blockers. In regard to the latter, beta-adrenergic blocking drugs are important in patients with CHF and ventricular arrhythmias. Clinical trials with beta-blockers have shown a reduction in sudden cardiac death, as well as in all-cause mortality, in both post-infarction patients and patients with CHF regardless of origin. As a result, patients with LV systolic dysfunction should routinely undergo long-term treatment with beta-blockers, unless contraindicated or not tolerated. The optimum dosing is however quite variable, and typically may take several months to achieve [2].

With the possible exception of amiodarone, antiarrhythmic drugs are no longer deemed to be useful for improving survival. In essence, suppression of ventricular ectopic rhythms in patients with heart disease did not reduce mortality risk in controlled clinical trials. In fact several such drugs (e.g., flecainide, encainide, and propafenone in the CAST and CASH trials) were associated with a worse mortality outcome. Other drugs (e.g., sotalol, dofetilide and azimilde) have exhibited neutral mortality outcomes; these latter agents have found a role in treatment of co-morbidities such as atrial fibrillation, but are of no real importance for diminishing life-threatening arrhythmia risk.

For the most part, antiarrhythmic drug therapy has been superceded (where economic factors permit) by ICD treatment. ICDs have been shown to be effective for enhancing survival in patients with refractory ventricular arrhythmias, even in the presence of severely impaired left ventricular dysfunction. In the specific instance of patients awaiting heart transplantation, a recent study from this center reported a substantial total mortality benefit in ICD treated patients on the waiting list compared to similar patients treated with comparable medications (including beta-blockers and amiodarone) but who had not received an ICD [3]. Data comprised findings from consecutive patients considered suitable for cardiac transplantation and placed on the waiting list. Of the 310 patients, 111 (36%) underwent successful cardiac transplantation and 164 (53%) died while waiting; 35 patients remain on the waiting list. Twenty-nine (49%) ICD patients survived until cardiac transplantation, 13 (22%) patients died, and 17 (28.9%) remain on the waiting list. By contrast, among non-ICD patients, 82 (33%) received transplants, 151 (60%) died, and 18 (7.1%) remain on the waiting list. Survival rates at the 6th month and 1st, 2nd, 3rd and 4th year were better for all ICD patients compared to non-ICD patients ($p=0.0001$). Furthermore, ICD treatment was associated with improved survival, independent of concomitant treatment with beta-blocker or amiodarone. Among ICD and non-ICD patients treated with a beta-blocker or amiodarone, survivals at the 1st and 4th years were; 93% vs. 69%, and 57% vs. 32%, respectively ($p=0.003$). In essence, ICD therapy is helpful in this very high-risk patient subset, but total mortality rates still average in excess of 10% per year.

It is unlikely that ablation or conventional surgical approaches to arrhythmia management will substantially diminish the mortality risk beyond that achieved by ICD therapy to date. Ablation of ventricular tachyarrhythmias (VT) in patients with poor LV function is limited by the hemodynamic instability often encountered during mapping and the multicentric nature of arrhythmias in very sick hearts. Surgical techniques of necessity further compromise residual (and already marginal) ventricular function and are associated with high intra-operative mortality. Thus, in the setting of very poor LV function the survival benefit likely to accompany ablation techniques is at best questionable; an *ICD would still* be recommended by most electrophysiologists.

Current Role of Cardiac Transplantation for Refractory Ventricular Arrhythmias

Cardiac transplantation may reasonably be considered when patients have frequently recurrent appropriate ICD shocks due to frequent or incessant drug refractory ventricular arrhythmias (VT storms) and when ablation fails or is impracticable. The incidence of heart transplantation for VT storms seems to be low because either the VT storm subsides or patients die before they have a chance to receive a heart. In an unpublished review of over 300 heart transplantations undertaken at the University of Minnesota and Minneapolis Heart Institute during a 22 year period, only 5 were undertaken primarily for arrhythmia indications. In each case the ventricular arrhythmias were incessant and, in several instances, resulted in multiple ineffective ICD shocks.

In recent years, LVAD support has proved invaluable to sustain the circulation in the face of refractory ventricular tachyarrhythmias until a heart could be obtained [4]. In this setting, LVADs may be used as a bridge to recovery, or to transplantation, or less desirably as permanent treatment (so-called 'destination' therapy). In regard to potential recovery, these devices may provide the time and environment for the ventricle to 'reverse' ventricular dysfunction and may thereby help to diminish the impact of key structural abnormalities that exacerbate arrhythmic risk (see earlier). In brief, it is reasonable that LVAD use be aggressively studied as a means of perhaps averting progression to transplantation in some instances. For example, acute lymphocytic myocarditis can present as intractable ventricular tachyarrhythmias. There is evidence that these patients seem to do well with ventricular assist device providing sufficient "rest" to the heart for recovery.

Current Status of Heart Transplantation for Ventricular Arrhythmias

End-stage heart disease with refractory heart failure is by far the most common reason for heart transplantation. The typical candidates are usually in NYHA functional class IV with an anticipated survival of less than one year. As indicated earlier, many of these patients with end-stage cardiac disease have life threatening ventricular arrhythmias. However, only in a very small proportion of cases (approximately 1.5% in our center) is arrhythmia denoted the principal indication for transplantation although it is listed among appropriate indications for heart transplantation [5] (Table 1).

Data on intractable arrhythmias requiring heart transplantation is scarce. Most of the data available is before ICD and ventricular assist device era. The exact number of these patients undergoing heart transplantation for this indication is not known, but the estimated incidence is less than 1%. In one published series of 400 hearts transplants over 13 years, there were 3 (0.75%) patients in whom life threatening arrhythmias required heart transplantation [6].

Table 1. Indications for heart transplantation as recommended by United Network of Organ Sharing (UNOS), American Society of Transplant Physicians and the National Institutes of Health

Refractory end-stage CHF on maximal medical therapy
Intractable, recurrent malignant ventricular arrhythmias
Disabling angina pectoris without surgically correctable lesions
Congenital uncorrectable cardiac lesions or tumors

Bourke et al [7] studied the role of heart transplantation in the management of recurrent ventricular tachyarrhythmias in 22 patients following myocardial infarction divided into 2 groups. Group A, with both CHF and ventricular tachyarrhythmias, comprised 17 consecutive patients for whom transplantation was considered the best primary non-pharmacological treatment. Group B, with progressive CHF following antiarrhythmic surgery for ventricular tachyarrhythmias, comprised five consecutive patients assessed and planned for transplantation after antiarrhythmic surgery. In group A, 8 patients underwent transplantation and all survived the first 30 day period. At median follow up of 55 months (range 11 to 109 months) seven of this subgroup were still alive. Five patients died of recurrent ventricular tachyarrhythmias before transplantation, despite circulatory support. In the face of uncontrollable ventricular tachyarrhythmias, four of these underwent "high risk" antiarrhythmic surgery while awaiting transplantation: three died of CHF within 30 days and one was saved by heart transplantation two days after arrhythmia surgery. Mortality for the transplantation strategy in group A patients was 47% by intention to treat analysis. Quality of life in the 8 who did receive transplants, however, was good and only one died during median follow up of 56 months. The 5 patients in group B were accepted for transplantation for progressive CHF at a median of 21 months (range 12 to 28 months) after antiarrhythmic surgery. One died of CHF before transplantation, 22 months after initial surgery; another died of high output CHF 3 days after transplantation. Thus mortality of the intended strategy was 40%. The 3 transplanted patients are alive and well at 8-86 months. The authors conclude that although the short and medium term outcome in category A or B patients who undergo transplantation is good, the overall success of the transplantation strategy in category A patients is limited by lack of donors in the short time frame in which they are required.

Conclusions

The incidence of patients with intractable arrhythmias who might benefit from heart transplantation is unknown. The current number of heart transplants for that indication (about 1% of all transplants) probably markedly understates the actual number of potential cases. Furthermore, most published data pre-dates ICD and ventricular assist device era. In the era of increasingly available circulatory support, the number of these otherwise irretrievable patients who can be kept alive until a donor heart becomes available could increase substantially. In the interim, guidelines established by the Bethesda conference on cardiac transplantation and subsequently adopted by UNOS [5], provide a basis for heart transplantation for patients with refractory arrhythmias when there are:

a) Recurrent symptomatic life-threatening arrhythmias, which cannot be controlled by all appropriate conventional medical and surgical modalities,
b) Prolonged periods of documented electromechanical dissociation following electrical cardioversion of VT or VF to normal sinus rhythm.

References

1. Mitchell LB, Pineda EA, Titus JL et al (2002) Sudden death in patients with implantable cardioverter defibrillators: the importance of post-shock electromechanical dissociation. J Am Coll Cardiol 39:1323-1328
2. Hunt SA, Baker DW, Chin M H et al (2001) ACC/AHA Guidelines for the Evaluation and Management of Chronic Heart Failure in the Adult: Executive Summary A Report of the American College of Cardiology/American Heart Association Task Force on Practice Guidelines. Circulation 104:2996-3007
3. Ermis C, Zadeii G, Zhu AX et al (2003) Improved Survival of Cardiac Transplantation Candidates with Implantable Cardioverter Defibrillator Therapy: Role of Beta-Blocker or Amiodarone Treatment. J Cardiovasc Electrophysiol 14:1-6
4. Koerner MM, Durand JB, Lafuente JA et al (2000) Cardiac transplantation: the final therapeutic option for the treatment of heart failure. Curr Opin Cardiol 15:178-182
5. United Network of Organ Sharing (1996) Listing criteria approved for public comment. Update. UNOS: Washington DC p 8
6. Olivari MT, Windle JR (2000) Cardiac transplantation in patients with refractory ventricular arrhythmias. J Heart Lung Transplant 19:S38-S42
7. Bourke JP, Loaiza A, Parry G et al (1998) Role of orthotopic heart transplantation in the management of patients with recurrent ventricular tachyarrhythmias following myocardial infarction. Heart 80:473-478

Ablation of Unstable Ventricular Tachycardia

F.E. Marchlinski, D. Lin, H. Nayak, A.M. Russo, H. Hsia, S. Dixit, E. Gerstenfeld, D. Callans, W. Pulliam, S. Siddique, S. Del Castillo, E. Zado

Introduction

It is critical to begin any discussion on ablation of unstable ventricular tachycardia with background information supporting the importance of the effort. First, stable, mappable ventricular tachycardias represent the tip of the arrhythmia iceberg. In order for any arrhythmia to be mappable it must be reliably inducible and hemodynamically tolerable. The ventricular tachycardia must also be stable in response to the catheter manipulation and pacing required to identify the appropriate site for ablative therapy during activation and entrainment mapping [1–4]. In a consecutive series of "ideal" patients presenting with hemodynamically tolerated ventricular tachycardia and referred for catheter ablation, 30% had only unmappable VT at the time of electrophysiological evaluation [5]. Secondly, ICD event monitoring after device implantation has documented rapid unmappable VT in most patients regardless of the clinical indication for initial device therapy [6–8]. Finally, in looking to the future, a strategy for prevention of sudden cardiac death that uses ablative therapy must target the substrate for unmappable ventricular tachycardia [9].

General Strategies for Mapping Unstable Ventricular Tachycardia

Until recently, all mapping and ablation strategies were directed at hemodynamically tolerated ventricular tachycardia and required point-by-point data acquisition. Mapping and successful ablation required ventricular tachycardia induction with an attempt to identify activation during electrical diastole that represented a necessary part of the arrhythmia circuit by pacing during induced arrhythmia. One approach to unstable ventricular tachycardia was to slow the tachycardia with antiarrhythmic drug therapy to allow for hemody-

Electrophysiology Section, Division of Cardiology, University of Pennsylvania Health System, Philadelphia, Pennsylvania, USA

namic stability and application of standard mapping techniques. Intravenous procainamide or intravenous amiodarone was characteristically administered. Following a gram of procainamide the rate of ventricular tachycardia slowed, typically by 60–100 ms [10, 11]. In many patients, drug administration resulted in an arrhythmia that was better tolerated hemodynamically and permitted more detailed mapping. Unfortunately, the administration of antiarrhythmic drugs frequently resulted in different and/or new morphologies of ventricular tachycardia (VT) and occasional noninducibility of the arrhythmia. In addition, the direct hemodynamic effects of acute intravenous drug administration frequently precluded hemodynamic tolerance of the ventricular tachycardia despite slowing the rate. Thus, this approach to mapping unstable VT has been in large part abandoned.

An alternative strategy to rate slowing of unstable VT is to attempt to maintain hemodynamic stability during VT with the infusion of intravenous pressor support and/or mechanical measures, such as intra-aortic balloon counter pulsation, and more recently peripheral cardiopulmonary bypass. Although these techniques may be helpful and even advisable in selected patients, the institution of such measures may not always result in uniform success in maintaining hemodynamic stability. In addition, these measures frequently require an incredible investment in terms of resources and manpower and have their own associated morbidity.

A third approach to unmappable, rapid VT is that of simultaneous multisite rapid mapping using either real-time electrogram recordings from a multipolar basket catheter or virtual unipolar electrograms using the EnSite mapping system (Endocardial Solutions Inc.) [12–14]. Because of the concern related to *chordal* disruption with a multipolar splined basket catheter, this mapping tool has largely been abandoned for VT. However, the EnSite mapping system continues to represent an important mapping tool used at many centers. Self-limited VT and VT with changing morphologies can be assessed by means of this system. Limitations of the system related to its field of view and the accuracy of virtual recordings when the recording balloon is located at a distance in dilated hearts have recently been described [15]. Importantly, Schilling et al. have had substantial success in using the system for ablation of mappable and unmappable/unstable VT [14]. A detailed discussion of this technology is beyond the scope of this report, and the reader is directed to the references provided for additional information. The rest of the report will focus on our experience using substrate mapping to create an anatomically driven strategy for ablation of unstable VT [16, 17].

Surgical Experience with Ventricular Tachycardia Ablation

In designing an ablation strategy we wanted to target the anatomic substrate and limit the need for activation mapping and pacing stimulation during VT. In attempting to develop an ablation strategy for unstable VT, we referred to the extensive surgical ventricular tachycardia ablation experience [18–22]. Targeting the anatomy for surgical ablation had been a reasonably successful approach for eliminating VT in the setting of chronic coronary artery disease. Successful VT elimination was achieved in 70–85% of the patients. Importantly, the anatomic target was not an aneurysmectomy alone; an aneurysmectomy alone was associated with a high arrhythmia recurrence rate [19]. Successful surgical ablation required removal of the visually distinct scarred endocardial border zone that extended from the transmurally scarred aneurysm to the normal myocardium. This "subendocardial resection" pioneered by Josephson and Harken [21] and Moran et al. [22] dramatically improved the outcome of the surgical approach to VT therapy. As indicated, this surgical approach was guided by a direct visual assessment of normal and abnormal or scarred endocardium. After entering the left ventricle via an incision into the densely scarred aneurysm and performing a small aneurysmectomy, the surgeon was able to visually identify the scarred endocardium that extended between the dense scar and the normal myocardium. Surgical ablative therapy "peeled off" or resected the endocardial and subendocardial fibrotic tissue, which is characterized microscopically by dense areas of fibrosis coupled with islands of viable muscle. It was thought that the surgeon, by resecting the subendocardium extending from the densely scarred aneurysm to the normal tissue, successfully interrupted the endocardial components of (a) sizable VT circuit(s) [18].

Voltage Mapping to Define the Endocardial Substrate

In attempting to develop a catheter-based approach to ablation that would mimic the surgical technique, the first goal was to demonstrate the ability to define the endocardial anatomy with catheters in sufficient detail for it to mimic the surgeon's direct visualization of the border zone. Identification of the border zone would allow for a catheter-based anatomic approach to the ablation of unstable VT. The use of electroanatomic voltage mapping has been shown to provide the requisite detailed depiction of the endocardial anatomy [16, 17, 23–25]. When the color range for the display of the voltage is adjusted to between 0.5 mV and 1.5 mV, the display does indeed mimic the visual assessment of the scar made in the operating theater. A densely scarred central area consistent with thickened aneurysm formation will characteristically have a signal amplitude less than 0.5 mV and will be represented by a red color on the computer-generated images of the endocardium (Fig. 1). This densely scarred endocardium will characteristically be surrounded by a sizable border zone extending from the dense scar towards normal myocardium. This border zone area will typically have bipolar electrogram signal amplitudes between 0.5 mV and 1.5 mV. Some additional adjustment is made to the slightly higher voltage cutoff value of 2.0 mV when there is evidence of left ventricular (LV) hypertrophy. In size, the border zone mimics the extensive area of endocardial

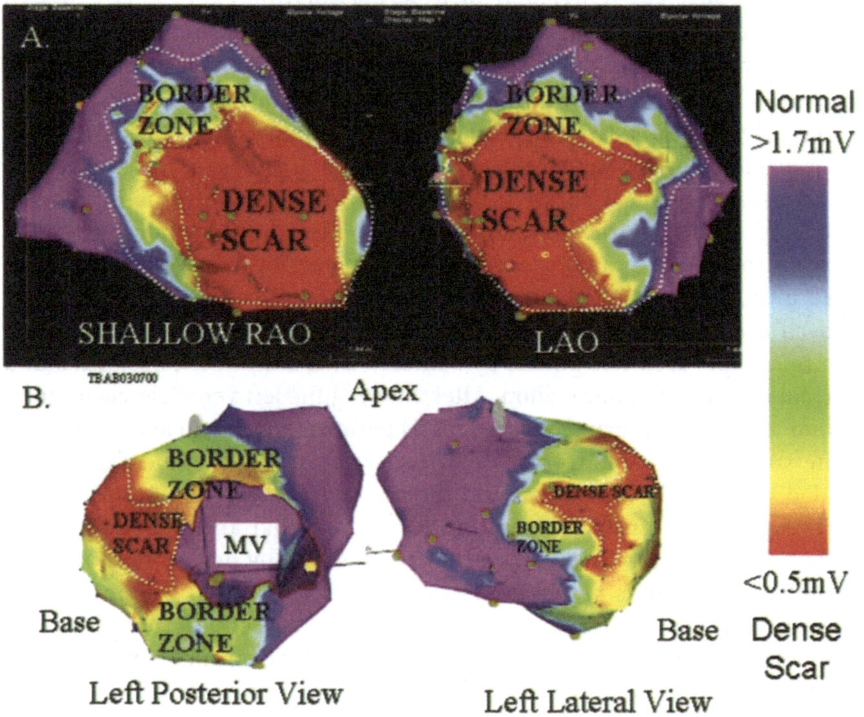

Fig. 1A, B. Bipolar endocardial voltage maps in patient with chronic coronary artery disease and VT. A Voltage map with large apical septal infarction with densely infarcted myocardium represented by an area with signal amplitude <0.5 mV surrounded by a sizeable border zone with signal amplitude between 0.5 mV and 1.7 mV. B Voltage map from patient with posterior myocardial infarction with densely infarcted zone with signal amplitude <0.5 mV, surrounded by a border zone until normal myocardium is approached near the apical region

scarring that is characteristically resected with surgical VT ablative therapy. The border zone is contiguous with an area represented by the color purple and indicates normal endocardium. It is noteworthy that we have confirmed that normal bipolar signal amplitude is larger in the left than the right ventricle and that 95% of all signals in the left ventricle are >1.62 mV and 95% of those in the right ventricle, >1.42 mV [26]. It is of interest that even in the nonhypertrophied normal left ventricle only 92% of the signals have an amplitude >2.0 mV. This indicates that the distinction between normal and abnormal bipolar electrogram signals is marked and that if sufficient sampling is performed there is little difference between them in the bipolar voltage map images when the color range is varied between 0.5–1.5 mV and 0.5–2.0 mV (Fig. 2).

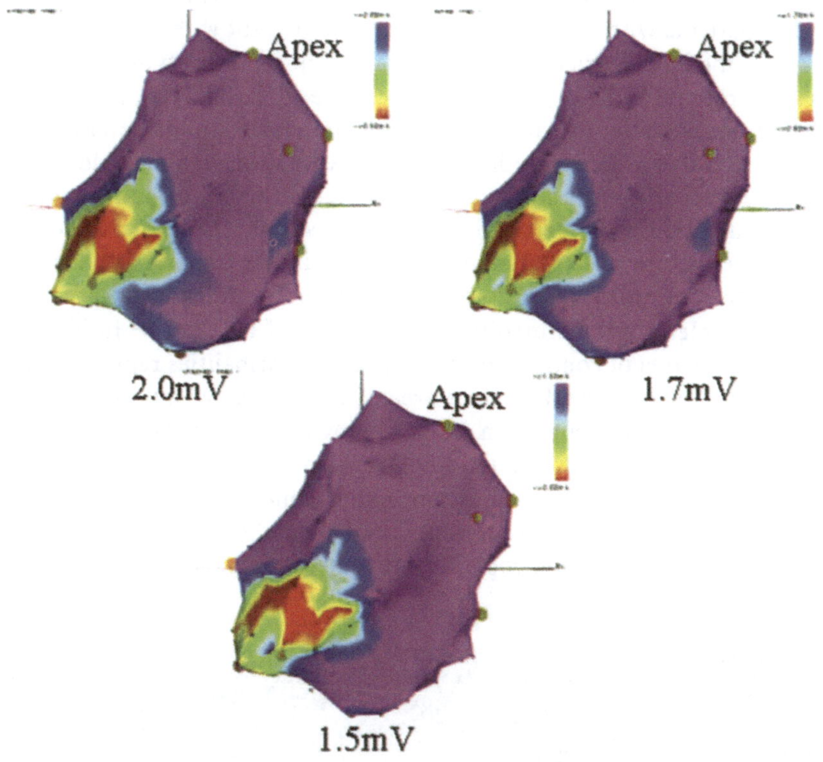

Fig. 2. Effect of modifying the color range of bipolar voltage map on the characteristics of region of abnormal electrograms in patient with inferoseptal infarct and ventricular tachycardia (VT). The voltage map is displayed showing the bottom of the left ventricle with the upper limit of the voltage range identified by the color purple highlighted beneath each figure. The lower limit is maintained at 0.5 mV in all views. The average voltage recorded from normal left ventricular (LV) endocardium is 4.8 mV and 90% of normal bipolar electrograms have an amplitude >2.0 mV. As a result there is little change in the size of the region showing abnormal bipolar electrograms when the upper limit of the color range is increased from 1.5 to 2.0 mV

Importantly, our ability to define endocardial anatomy using bipolar voltage maps has not only proven to be of value in patients with the substrate of chronic coronary artery disease with prior myocardial infarction, but also in patients with left ventricular or right ventricular (RV) cardiomyopathy and VT. In all three settings, sizable areas of endocardial scarring are defined as having areas of abnormal voltage with a signal amplitude <1.5 mV. In all settings, characteristic areas of dense scarring with signal amplitude <0.5 mV are surrounded by a variably sized border zone with a signal amplitude between 0.5 and 1.5 mV and represented by the color range between red and purple. Notably, we have documented a unique distribution of endocardial bipolar electrogram voltage abnormalities both in patients with LV cardiomyopathy and in patients with RV cardiomyopathy who present with sustained VT (Figs. 3, 4). In the left ventricle the electrogram abnormalities typically involve the base surrounding the mitral and aortic valve [27]. Similarly, in patients with RV cardiomyopathy the area with abnormal electrograms extends from the pulmonic valve area, involving a large cone-shaped area of endocardium on the free wall and septum, or in some patients the abnormality involves the region surrounding the tricuspid valve. Interestingly, the intracardiac substrate for VT defined by voltage mapping is quite similar in patients with coronary artery disease and RV cardiomyopathy, with an endocardial area showing abnormal electrograms involving an average of 60–65 cm^2 in both patient groups. This area of contiguous electrogram abnormalities represents approximately 40% of the overall surface area of the respective left and right ventricles. In contrast, patients with LV cardiomyopathy and VT have endocardial electrogram abnormalities extending over a much smaller area. On average an area of only 21 cm^2 gives rise to contiguous abnormal electrograms. The area of abnormal electrograms represents only about 12% of the total endocardial surface area of the cardiomyopathic left ventricle (Fig. 3).

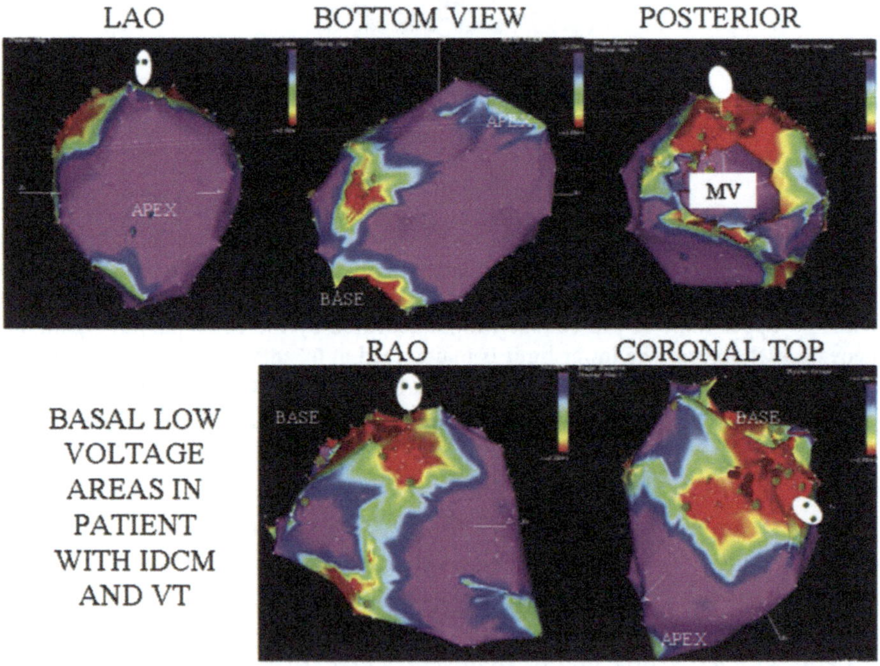

Fig. 3. Endocardial bipolar voltage map in patient with LV dilated cardiomyopathy and VT. Each panel shows bipolar voltage maps of the LV in a different projection. Areas of low voltage surround the mitral and aortic valve regions near the base of the left ventricle. Area with marked voltage abnormality (<0.5 mV) is surrounded by a border zone before endocardium with normal voltage is encountered at the base (MV mitral valve)

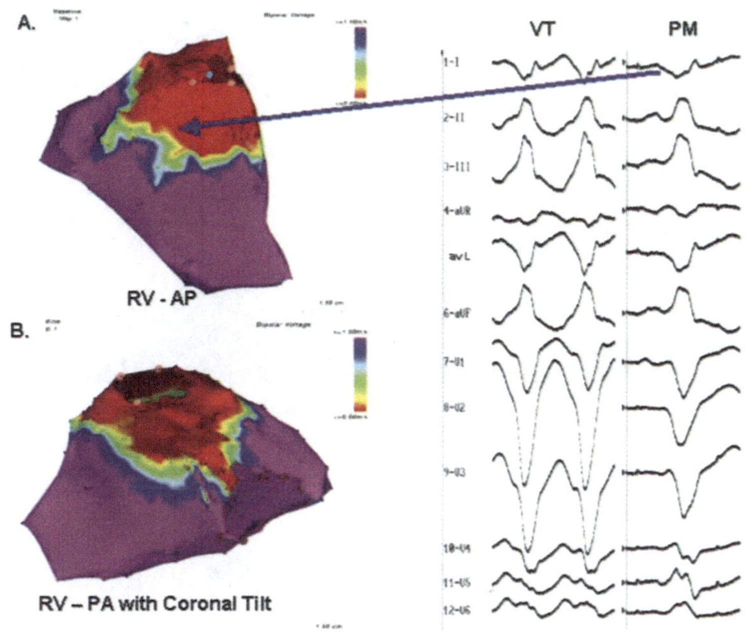

Fig. 4A, B. Bipolar voltage map and VT in patient with right-ventricular (*RV*) cardiomyopathy. The bipolar voltage map is shown in the AP (**A**) and PA (**B**) views. A cone-shaped area of low voltage is identified which extends from the pulmonic valve over the free wall and septum. The rapid VT was localized to the free wall only according to the pacemap. Linear lesions would extend from the area of dense scarring represented by the red color to the normal myocardium. Only the free wall was targeted for linear lesions based on the pacemap information. The distribution of abnormal myocardium surrounding the pulmonic and/or tricuspid valves is typical of the anatomic substrate associated with VT in the setting of RV cardiomyopathy

Ablation Strategy Coupled with Voltage Mapping

On recognizing that the voltage maps mimic the surgeon's view of the endocardium, we attempted to design an ablation strategy that might mimic the surgical ablation of the endocardium and subendocardium. Recognizing the limited tissue destruction resulting from point ablation lesion deployment, we felt that it was critical to identify a strategy for regionalizing a specific area of the border zone to target with repeated point lesions. Once an area of interest was regionalized, these point lesions could then mimic the surgeon's blade in targeting the border zone between the densely scarred aneurysm and the edge of normal myocardium (Fig. 5). We felt that the site of the best pace map would approximate the site of the exit site of the VT circuit [28, 29]. Pacemapping could be used as an appropriate tool for regionalizing the site for deployment of the individual point lesions along the border zone.

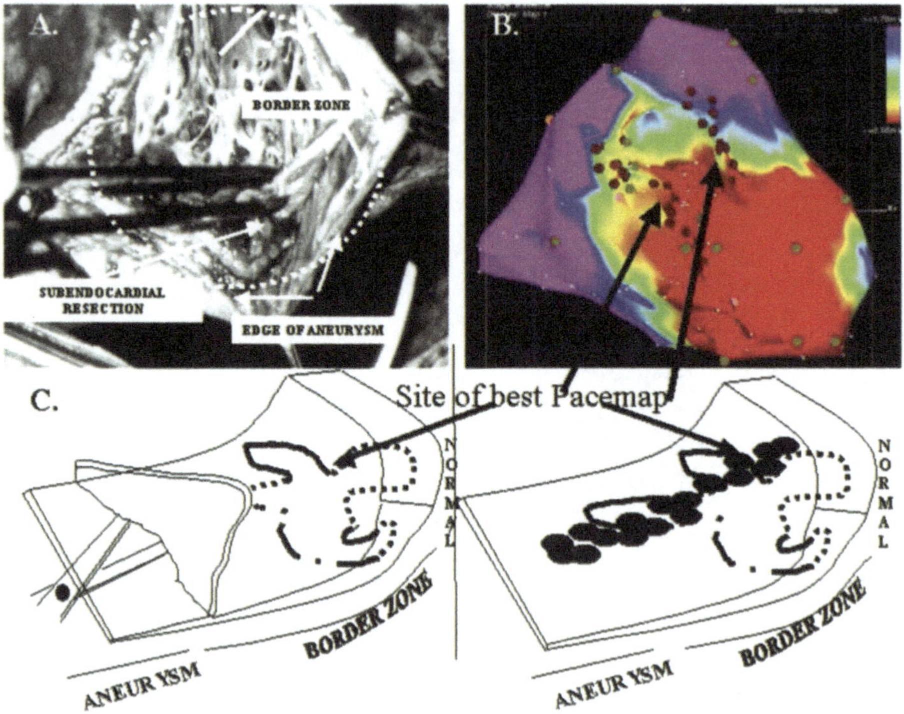

Fig. 5A–C. Comparison of surgical versus catheter-based ablation for unstable VT. A Surgeon's view of the scarred endocardium through an apical ventriculotomy. The surgical procedure removes the visually distinct abnormal endocardium and subendocardium in the attempt to interrupt the VT circuit. B Bipolar endocardial voltage map in a patient with large apical infarction and VT, with linear ablation lesions placement guided by pacemapping along the edge of the dense scar (red). C Surgical ablation contrasted with catheter-based linear lesions targeting the border zone. Both techniques target the endocardial aspect of the border zone in attempting to interrupt the endocardial aspect of the VT circuit

The ablation strategy for unstable VT now consists of a four-step process:

1. A bipolar voltage map is created to characterize the anatomic substrate.
2. The 12-lead ECGs during all induced and spontaneous VTs are assessed to identify the region of the borderzone that lies adjacent to or just within the dense scar to perform more detailed pacing.
3. Pacing is then performed along the edge of the dense scar and border zone in an attempt to identify the best 12-lead ECG match of the induced and spontaneous VTs. The sites identifying the best 12-lead ECG match of the paced maps to the VT are then tagged on the three-dimensional voltage map.
4. Point radiofrequency lesions are then introduced with the lesions extend-

ing 1-2 cm into the densely scarred endocardium and crossing over a 2- to 8-cm length through the border zone until normal endocardium or an anatomic boundary is reached. Each point lesion is placed on the voltage map to confirm the contiguous linear nature of the lesion application (Figs. 5, 6). Linear lesions are placed through all sites demonstrating the best-paced map match. Caution is used to avoid significant tissue destruction during the approaches to areas demonstrating contiguous normal-amplitude electrograms.

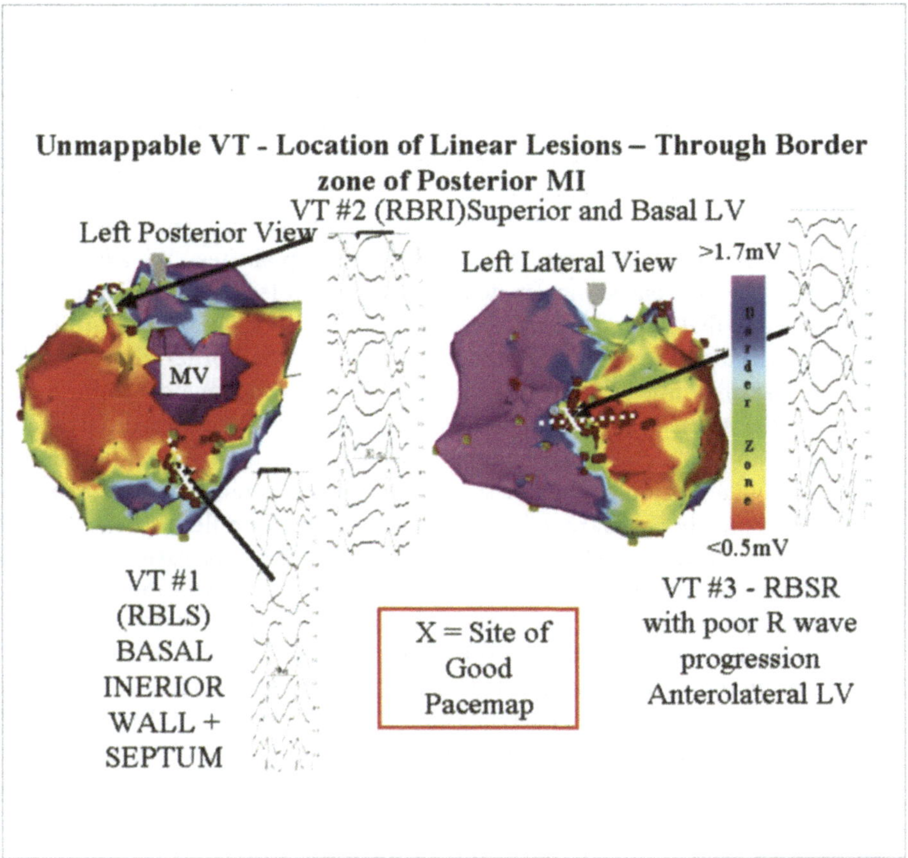

Fig. 6. Process for localizing and ablation of unmappable VT in setting of ischemic cardiomyopathy. Voltage map consistent with large posterior infarction is shown along with three distinct VTs with QRS morphology consistent with a site from the LV base and apical portion of posterior infarction are shown. After the site showing the best pacemap match of induced VT has been identified and tagged on the voltage maps, linear lesions are created by applying repeated point lesions from dense scar through the border zone to normal myocardium or the anatomic boundary of the mitral annulus. The location of the lesions through the border zone is guided by the analysis of the 12-lead ECG during VT and the pacemap match, which is indicated by the white X along the border zone

Application of Endocardial Linear Lesion Technique in Patients with Right- or Left-ventricular Cardiomyopathy

Our initial success in arrhythmia control in patients with ischemic heart disease was encouraging [17]. After demonstrating that the endocardial anatomy in patients with RV cardiomyopathy, and to lesser extent LV cardiomyopathy, and VT mimics the anatomy of patients with coronary artery disease, we attempted a similar ablation strategy in these two disease settings. In patients with RV cardiomyopathy and VT, areas of abnormal endocardium are usually identified extending from the tricuspid and/or pulmonic valves and involving both the septum and the free wall. Similar to the steps taken in patients with chronic coronary artery disease and VT, the edge of the densely scarred myocardium (signal amplitude <0.5 mV) abutting the border zone is then paced after a careful analysis of the 12-lead ECG of induced and spontaneous VTs to help identify the region of interest for the more detailed pacing (Fig. 4). The 12-lead ECG analysis of VT in the setting of RV cardiomyopathy allows for regionalization to the appropriate free wall or septal sites [30]. After identification of the best paced map match, repeated point lesion application creates linear lesions that extend from the densely scarred thickened myocardium in close proximity to the valvular structures through the border zone to either the valvular anatomic boundary or the edge of the normal myocardium.

A similar strategy has also been used in patients with LV cardiomyopathy in this setting. The abnormal endocardium appears to be concentrated near the perivalvular region of the left ventricle. Ventricular tachycardia morphologies will typically be characterized by either a left bundle branch block or right bundle branch block pattern with early R-wave progression across the precordium consistent with the basal origin. Linear lesions will then characteristically be placed through the sites of the best paced map match and extend from the normal endocardium through the border zone and densely scarred myocardium to the edge of the mitral and/or aortic valves (Fig. 7).

Most of our reported experience in ablating unstable VT has been with energy application using the standard RF energy system and the standard 4-mm-tip electromagnetic mapping catheter [17, 18]. Lesion application typically targets a temperature of 55° for 60–90 s. In our experience, in order to target all induced and spontaneous ventricular arrhythmias, an average of 45 radiofrequency energy applications are applied per patient, with the median number of linear lesions equal to 3 and the average length of the linear lesion equal to 3.2 cm, with a range of 1.0–8.6 cm. Because of limitations in power delivery using standard RF energy application, we now typically supplement standard radiofrequency energy application with a cooled-tip or irrigated RF energy delivery system [31]. Because the irrigated electromagnetic mapping catheter is still investigational in the US, we frequently use a two-catheter approach. The electromagnetic voltage map information guides placement of the cooled tip catheter adjacent to the tip of the Carto catheter. A different color tag is used in attempts to identify the location of the cool-tipped lesions.

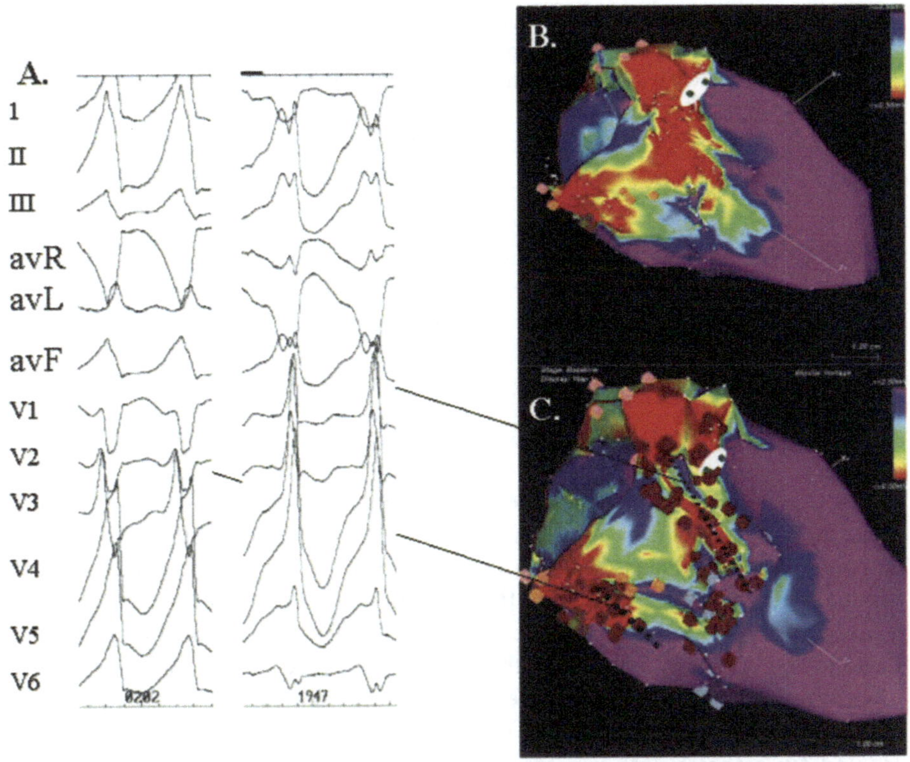

Fig. 7A–C. Process for localizing and ablation of unmappable VT in setting of nonischemic cardiomyopathy. A Two distinct VTs with QRS morphology consistent with a site from the left ventricular base with early R-wave progression. B Bipolar endocardial voltage map of the left ventricle. An abnormal low-voltage area is identified over the superior base in proximity to the mitral and aortic valves. This pattern of abnormality is common in patients with LV cardiomyopathy and VT. C Linear lesions that extend through the sites of the best pacemap match. The lesions extend from the normal voltage areas defined by the color purple to the valvular structures

Ablation Outcome for Frequent Unmappable Ventricular Tachycardia

We now have extensive experience using our ablation approach as described above in patients with frequent recurrent unmappable VT against the different disease substrates, including coronary disease, RV cardiomyopathy, and LV cardiomyopathy [32]. In a series of 61 patients with frequent (median greater than 30 VTs per month), unmappable VT, we observed no recurrence of VTs in 62%, and an additional 15 patients, or 25%, had satisfactory arrhythmia control with only infrequent VT episodes (less than 1 every 3 months) during long-term follow-up (Table 1). The best outcome with respect to arrhythmia control appears to be achieved in patients with coronary disease or RV cardiomyopathy. Satisfactory arrhythmia control can be anticipated in over 85% of patients.

Table 1. Outcome of ablation for frequent (median >30 VT/3 months), unmappable VT in 61 patients during a median follow-up of 14 months (1–56 months) (AD coronary artery disease, LVCM left-ventricular cardiomyopathy, RVCM right ventricular cardiomyopathy

	No recurrence		Infrequent VT (<1/3months)		Frequent VT (>1/3months)*	
	n	%	n	%	n	%
Overall (N = 61)	37	61	15	25	9	14
CAD (N=36	23	64	9	25	4	11
RVCM (N=13)	10	77	3	23	0	-
LVCM (N=12)	4	33	3	25	5	42

A good clinical outcome with the deployment of linear lesions has also been documented by Soejima et al. in patients with unstable VT in the setting of coronary artery disease [33]. In contrast, 30–40% of patients with LV cardiomyopathy have frequent arrhythmia recurrence during long-term follow-up requiring repeated ablation procedures or consideration for cardiac transplantation. The difficulty with arrhythmia control in the setting of LV cardiomyopathy may be multifactorial. We have documented thick perivalvular endocardial fibrosis with difficulty in creating ablation lesions despite the use of a cooled-tip catheter with radiofrequency energy delivery (Fig. 8). In selected

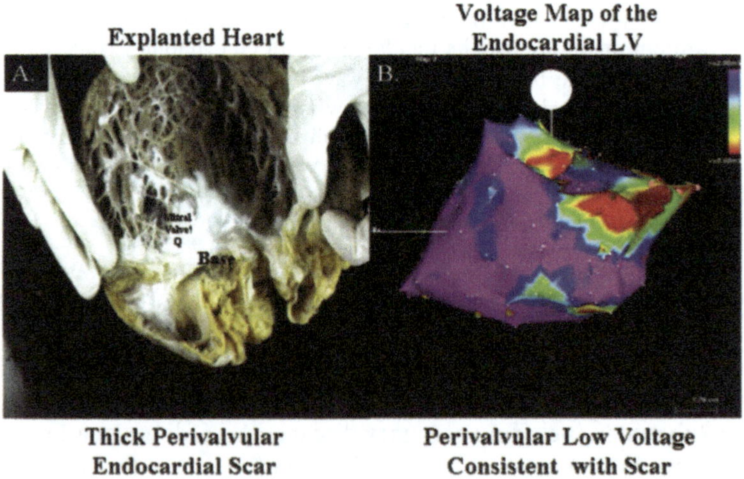

Fig. 8A, B. Thick endocardial scar surrounding the mitral valve in patient with nonischemic cardiomyopathy and VT. A Endocardium from explanted heart, with thick white scar that was resistant to standard and cooled-tipped radiofrequency energy. B Display of endocardial bipolar voltage characteristics and documentation of the low-voltage signals surrounding the inferior base of the left ventricle. These figures confirm the value of the voltage map for documenting the endocardial pathology

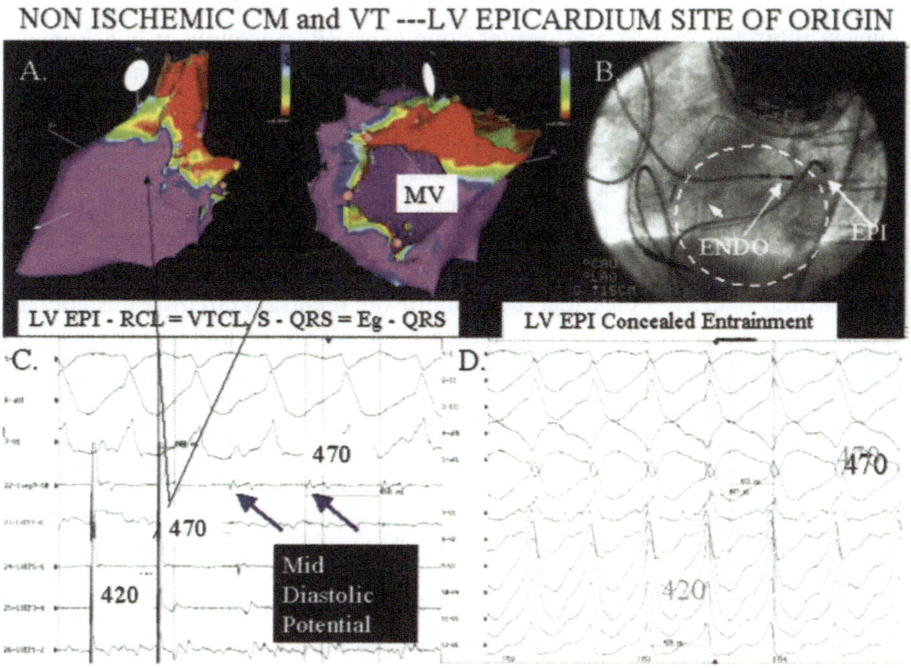

Fig. 9A–D. Epicardial VT in patient with nonischemic cardiomyopathy. A Bipolar endocardial voltage map showing perivalvular region of low voltage surrounding the mitral and aortic valves. B Left anterior oblique fluoroscopic image showing endocardial and epicardial catheter positioning near the lateral wall of the left ventricle. The broken line circle represents the silhouette of the left ventricle. C Pacing during VT from the LV epicardium at site demonstrating mid diastolic activity. D Evidence, produced by pacing, of concealed entrainment with a stimulus to QRS equal to the electrogram to QRS, the paced QRS matching the QRS of the VT and the return cycle after pacing equal to the VT cycle length

patients we have also documented an epicardial origin of VT in the setting of LV cardiomyopathy and in fact suspect that this finding may be more common than previously recognized (Fig. 9) [34, 35].

Current Limitations and Future Directions

It is worth considering the current limitations of our ablation approach to unstable ventricular tachycardia described above, and also the potential future developments. First, it is acknowledged that pacemapping has limitations in identifying the exit site for any origin of the VT circuit. Acknowledging this limitation of pacemapping, we currently create a second linear lesion perpendicular to the first in selected patients who have persistent inducible VTs after the first linear lesion attempt that is oriented perpendicular to the edge of the densely infarcted muscle and border zone (Fig. 10). Secondly, it is acknowledged that we currently have a limited understanding of the relationship of the components and size of the VT circuit to the anatomic substrate. Much work is under way with detailed endocardial mapping and stimulation during mappable VT to characterize the size and transmural extent of the VT circuit. We are hopeful that with the detailed characterization of the size and the extent of the circuit of mappable VT a more uniformly successful anatomic approach to ablation of unstable VT can be developed. Thirdly, in recognition of the potential intramural and or epicardial location for the reentrant circuit, especially in the setting of LV cardiomyopathy, we have also pursued an aggressive approach in attempting to define the epicardial anatomic substrate for VT in this disease setting. It is noteworthy that in our preliminary experience using the epicardial access techniques pioneered by Sosa et al. we have found a new wrinkle in the ability to assess epicardial scar [36, 37]. This wrinkle is the presence of epicardial fat and epicardial vasculature. In one of our patients with recurrent ventricular tachycardia and nonischemic cardiomyopathy, our voltage map defined extensive areas of epicardial low-voltage regions consistent with epicardial scarring (Fig. 11). However, the pathological analysis of the

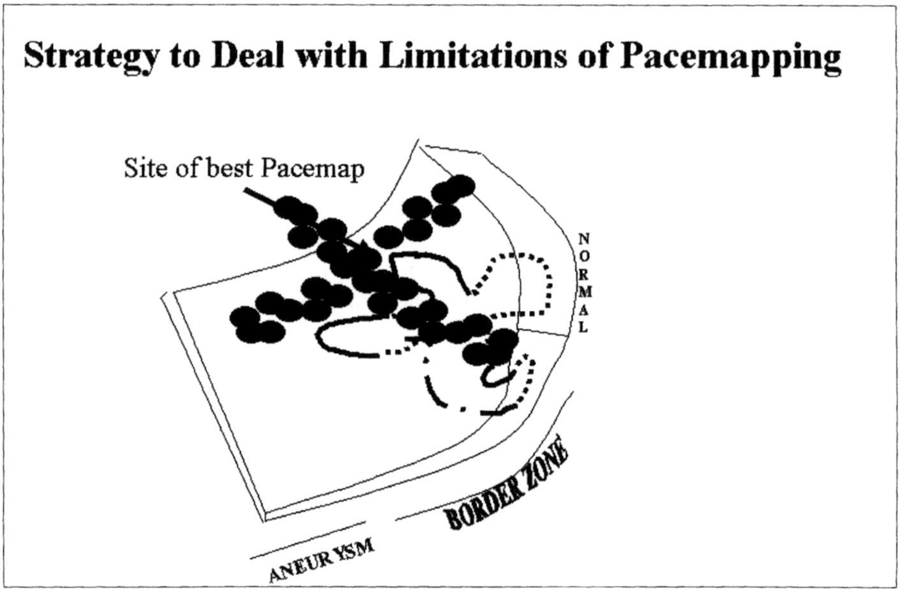

Fig. 10. Ablation strategy to deal with persistent VT inducibility after initial linear lesion. The first linear lesion is typically placed perpendicular to the dense scar and extends from the normal myocardium or an anatomic barrier through the border zone until densely scarred myocardium is reached. The pacemap match may only approximate the exit and may represent activation from a dead end pathway at a significant distance. A single linear lesion may fail to pass through the reentrant circuit. A second linear lesion running perpendicular to the first will increase the likelihood of interrupting a circuit that involves the endocardium

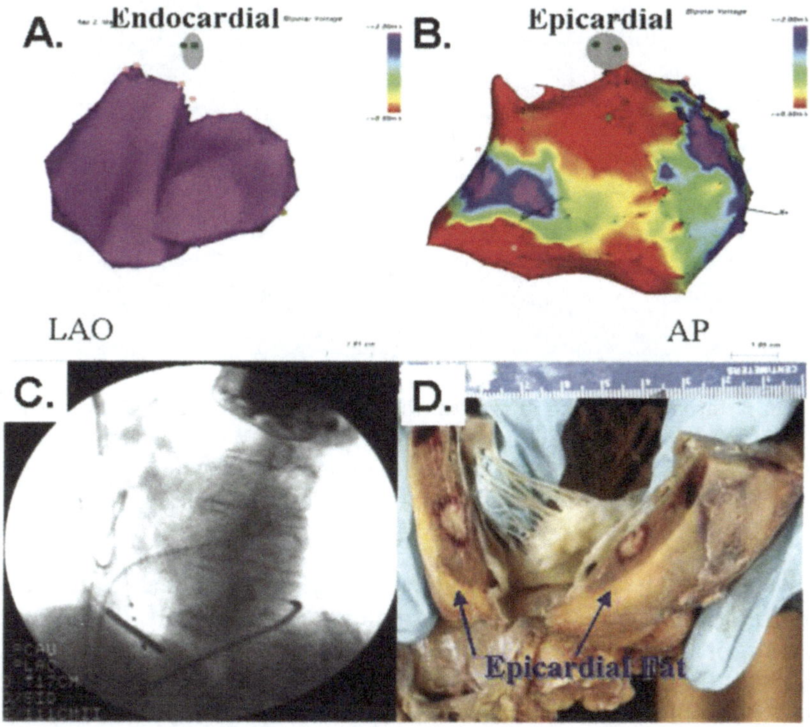

Fig. 11A–D. Endocardial and epicardial substrate in patient with VT. **A** Normal endocardial voltage maps of the right and left ventricles in the left anterior oblique view. All of the endocardium is represented by the purple color indicating a signal amplitude >2.0 mV. **B** Epicardial voltage maps in the shallow left anterior oblique projection. The voltage map was created after gaining access to the LV epicardium via pericardial puncture (**C**). **D** Explanted heart from the same patient, who received a heart transplant for recurrent VT and refractory heart failure. It is of note that no gross epicardial or endocardial scarring was evident. Epicardial low voltage was due to the thick layer of epicardial fat present over most of the epicardial surface. This patient shows how epicardial fat, in addition to the coronary vasculature, can influence epicardial voltage mapping and ablation

myocardium at the time of cardiac transplantation documented no visible endocardial or epicardial scarring, but rather a thickened and quite extensive layer of epicardial fat [38]. This epicardial fat and the coronary vasculature can alter the signal amplitude recorded from the epicardium and make the interpretation of voltage maps using standard criteria limited at best. Finally, the success of linear ablation lesions will be critically dependent on our ability to create lesions in scarred myocardium. The use of cooled-tip, large-tip and other types of energy delivery need to be considered, as does the use of techniques allowing better assessment of lesion formation. We have been investigating the value of intracardiac echo and have found this tool useful in characterizing acute lesion development (Fig. 12).

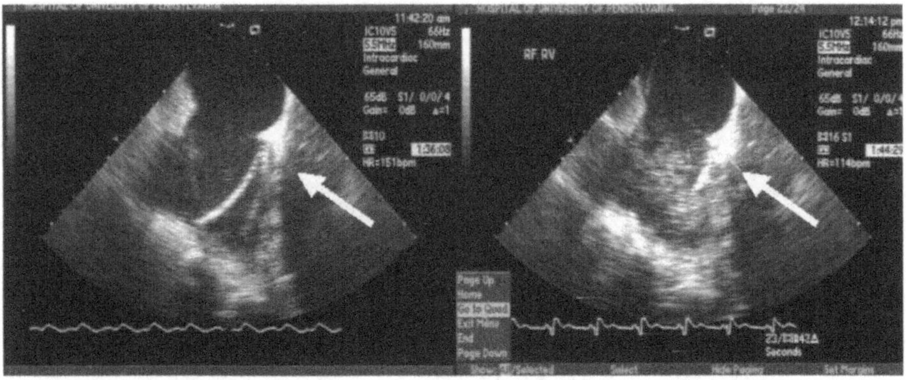

Fig. 12A, B. Intracardiac echo images showing lesion formation at basal segment of the RV adjacent to the tricuspid annulus in patient with RV cardiomyopathy and VT. **A** Before RF energy application, with catheter tip location shown (arrow). **B** During RF energy application bubble formation and tissue swelling are seen

We hope that with a better understanding of (1) the characteristics of the arrhythmia substrate, both endocardially and epicardially, (2) the size and location of the arrhythmia circuit and how it relates to this substrate, and finally (3) the capability for more effective creation and monitoring of lesions, we will extend the use of ablative therapy. Ablative therapy will then be used not only in the treatment of stable and unstable VT, but also to target the anatomy in patients at high risk for life-threatening arrhythmias to reduce the risk of sudden death [9].

References

1. El-Shalakany A, Hadjis T, Papageorgiou P et al (1999) Entrainment/mapping criteria for the prediction of termination of ventricular tachycardia by single radiofrequency lesion in patients with coronary artery disease. Circulation 99:2283–2289
2. Stevenson WG, Khan H, Sager P et al (1993) Identification of reentry circuit sites during catheter mapping and radiofrequency ablation of VT late after myocardial infarction. Circulation 88:1647–1670
3. Marchlinski FE, Gottlieb CD, Callans DJ et al (1997) Ablative therapy for VT in the setting of chronic coronary artery disease. In: Ellenbogen K, Epstein A (eds) Sudden cardiac death: past, present and future. Futura, Armonk, pp 199–224
4. Rothman SA, Hsia HH, Cossú SF et al (1997) Radiofrequency catheter ablation of postinfarction VT. Long term success and the significance of inducible nonclinical arrhythmias. Circulation 96:3499–3508
5. Callans DJ, Zado E, Sarter BH, Schwartzman D, Gottlieb CD, Marchlinski FE (1998) Procedural efficacy of radiofrequency ablation for ventricular tachycardia in patients with healed myocardial infarction: an intention to treat analysis. Am J Cardiol 82:429–432.
6. Marchlinski FE, Saligan JRP, Reddy T, Movsowitz C, Menz V (1994) Stored diagnostic

information in implantable cardioverter defibrillators: optimum recording techniques and duration. In: Santini M (ed) Progress in clinical pacing. Futura Publishing, Rome, pp 89–108
7. Marchlinski FE, Gottlieb CD Schwartzman D, Gonzalez-Zuelgaray J, Callans DJ (1995) Electrical events associated with ventricular tachycardia initiation and their prevention. In: Zipes DP, Jalife J (eds) Cardiac electrophysiology from cell to bedside, 2nd edn. Saunders, Philadelphia, 863–877
8. Russo AM, Dixit S, Verdino R et al (2003) Frequency and timing of defibrillator events in patients without documented arrhythmias: who is at highest risk? J Am Coll Cardiol 41:137A
9. Alonso C, Lin D, Poku J et al (2003) The role of transcatheter ablation in the prevention of sudden death. In: Santini M (ed) Sudden death – nonpharmacological treatment. Arianna Editrice, France (in press)
10. Marchlinski FE, Buxton AE, Kindwall KE et al (1988) Comparison of individual and combined effects of procainamide and amiodarone in patients with sustained ventricular tachyarrhythmias. Circulation 78:583–591
11. Grimm W, Cho JG, Marchlinski FE (1994) Effects of incremental doses of procainamide in patients with sustained uniform ventricular tachycardia. J Card Electrophysiol 5:313–322
12. Schalij MK, Van Rugge FP, Siezenga M et al (1998) Endocardial activation mapping of ventricular tachycardia in patients: first application of a 32-site bipolar mapping electrode catheter. Circulation 98:2168–2179
13. Strickberger SA, Knight BP, Michaud GF et al (2000) Mapping and ablation of ventricular tachycardia guided by virtual electrograms using a noncontact, computerized mapping system. J Am Coll Cardiol 35:414–421
14. Shilling RJ, Peters NS, Davies DW (1999) Feasibility of a noncontact catheter for endocardial mapping of human ventricular tachycardia. Circulation 99:2543–2552
15. Aoyama H, Nakagawa H, Baltazar de Castro J et al (2003) Accuracy of noncontact mapping in identifying lines of conduction block as a function of distance (abstract). J Am Coll Cardiol 41:19A abs 1042
16. Marchlinski FE, Callans DJ, Gottlieb CD, Zado E (2000) Linear ablation lesions for control of unmappable ventricular tachycardia in patients with ischemic and nonischemic cardiomyopathy. Circulation 101:1288–1296
17. Marchlinski FE, Callans DJ, Zado ES et al (2002) Approach to unstable ventricular tachycardia. In: Schalij MJ, Janse MJ, van Oosterom A, Wellens HJJ, van der Wall EE (eds) Einthoven 2002: 100 years of electrocardiography. The Einthoven Foundation, Leiden, pp 75–85
18. Marchlinski FE, Josephson ME (1987) Surgical treatment of ventricular tachyarrhythmias. In: Platia EV (ed) Non-pharmacologic management of cardiac arrhythmias, chap 15. Lippincott, Philadelphia, pp 340–363
19. Couch OA (1959) Cardiac aneurysm with VT and subsequent excision of aneurysm. Circulation 20:251–253
20. Horowitz LN, Harken AH, Kastor JA, Josephson ME (1980) Ventricular resection guided by epicardial and endocardial mapping for treatment of recurrent VT. N Engl J Med 302:589–593
21. Moran JM, Kehoe RH, Loeb JM et al (1982) Extended endocardial resection for the treatment of VT and ventricular fibrillation. Ann Thorac Surg 34:538–552
22. Hargrove WC, Miller JM, Vassallo JA, Josephson ME (1986) Improved results in the operative management of VT related to inferior wall infarction: importance of the annular isthmus. J Thorac Cardiovasc Surg 92:726–732

23. Shpun S, Gepstein L, Hayam G, Ben-Haim SA (1997) Guidance of radiofrequency endocardial ablation with real-time three-dimensional magnetic navigation system. Circulation 96:2016–2021
24. Gepstein L, Hayam G, Ben-Haim SA (1997) A novel method for nonfluoroscopic catheter-based electroanatomical mapping of the heart. In vitro and in vivo accuracy results. Circulation 95:1611–1622
25. Marchlinski F, Callans D, Gottlieb C et al (1998) Magnetic electroanatomical mapping for ablation of focal atrial tachycardias. Pacing Clin Electrophysiol 21:1621–1635
26. Marchlinski FE, Callans DJ, Russo AM et al (2000) Normal ventricular electrogram signal amplitude using magnetic electroanatomic mapping influence of recording polarity and mapped chamber (abstract). J Am Coll Cardiol 35:120A
27. Hsia HH, Callans DJ, Marchlinski FE (2003) Characterization of endocardial electrophysiologic substrate in patients presenting with non-ischemic cardiomyopathy and monomorphic ventricular tachycardia. Circulation (in press)
28. Josephson ME, Waxman HL, Cain ME, Gardner MJ, Buxton AE (1982) Ventricular activation during ventricular endocardial pacing. II. Role of pace-mapping to localize the origin of VT. Am J Cardiol 50:11–22
29. Miller JM, Marchlinski FE, Buxton AE, Josephson ME (1988) Relationship between the 12-lead electrocardiogram during VT and endocardial site of origin inpatients with coronary artery disease. Circulation 77:759–766
30. Dixit S, Gerstenfeld EP, Callans DJ, Marchlinski FE (2003) Electrocardiographic patterns of superior right ventricular outflow tract tachycardias: distinguishing septal and free wall sites of origin. J Cardiovasc Electrophysiol 14:1–7
31. Calkins H, Epstein A, Packer D et al (2000) Catheter ablation of ventricular tachycardia in patients with structural heart disease using cooled radiofrequency energy. Results of a prospective multicenter study. J Am Coll Cardiol 35:1905–1914
32. Marchlinski FE, Callans DJ, Hsia HH et al (2001) Late outcome after linear radiofrequency ablation for unmappable ventricular tachycardia: influence of type of heart disease. Circulation 104(17):II-621
33. Soejima K, Suzuki M, Maisel WH et al (2001) Catheter ablation in patients with multiple and unstable ventricular tachycardias after myocardial infarction: short ablation lines guided by reentry circuit isthmuses and sinus rhythm mapping. Circulation 104:664–669
34. Marchlinski FE, Rose G, Kleiman R, Callans D, Hanna M (1993) Sudden death in nonischemic cardiomyopathy. In: Josephson ME (ed) Sudden cardiac death. Blackwell Scientific, Cambridge Mass, pp 383–396
35. Hsia HH, Marchlinski FE (2002) Characterization of the electroanatomic substrate for monomorphic ventricular tachycardia in patients with nonischemic cardiomyopathy. Pacing Clin Electrophysiol 25:1114–1127
36. Sosa E, Scanavacca M, D'Avila A, Pilleggi F (1996) A new technique to perform epicardial mapping in the in the electrophysiology laboratory. J Cardiovasc Electrophysiol 7:531–536
37. Sosa E, Scanavacca M, D'Avila et al (2000) Nonsurgical transthoracic epicardial catheter ablation to treat recurrent ventricular tachycardia occurring late after myocardial infarction. J Am Coll Cardiol 35:1442–1449
38. Dixit S, Narula N, Callans DJ, Marchlinski FE (2003) Electro-anatomic mapping of human heart: epicardial fat masquerading as scar. J Cardiovasc Electrophysiol (in press)

Ablation of Ventricular Tachycardia: Can the Current Results be Improved Using Intracardiac Echocardiography?

D. J. Callans, J.-F. Ren

Introduction

Intracardiac echocardiography (ICE) offers many conceptual advantages in ventricular tachycardia (VT) ablation, although presently it is not routinely used. This discussion will focus on the potential application of ICE imaging to ablation procedures for idiopathic and post-infarction VT, as well as the remaining obstacles preventing more wide-scale implementation.

ICE Imaging in Interventional Electrophysiology

Interventional electrophysiology is in the midst of a sea change in the way that arrhythmia substrates are targeted. The previous viewpoint focused on electrophysiologic data solely, and mapping was performed during arrhythmias to localize a singular "vulnerable parameter" related to the zone of slow conduction. In theory, a single ablation lesion delivered to this critical site would abolish the tachycardia. The evolving viewpoint emphasizes identification of ablation targets by their relationship to anatomic structures. The first example was ablation of the tricuspid - IVC isthmus for cure of typical atrial flutter [1, 2]; similar strategies have developed for atrial fibrillation (pulmonary vein) and VT (infarct border zone). The focus is on ablation of the anatomic structures necessary for arrhythmia maintenance, often using complex lesion sets.

The degree of anatomic resolution provided by fluoroscopic imaging is not optimal to guide anatomic ablation procedures. Anatomic structures cannot be directly observed, but must be inferred from catheter position and intracardiac recordings. Ablation catheter contact with the myocardium cannot be assessed, unless this contact is very poor. Fluoroscopic imaging offers no feedback as to whether a lesion was actually created at the intended site. ICE imaging is capa-

Division of Cardiovascular Medicine, Department of Medicine, University of Pennsylvania School of Medicine, Philadelphia, Pennsylvania, USA

ble of resolving all of these inherent limitations in fluoroscopic imaging. Most importantly, ICE imaging allows positioning of the ablation catheter with reference to anatomic structures, and provides real time monitoring of catheter tissue contact and lesion creation.

There are two different commercially available platforms for ICE imaging, mechanical (radial) and phased array (sector) imaging. The reader is referred to extensive reviews detailing the aspects of the respective imaging strategies [3, 4]. Briefly, radial imaging uses a mechanically rotating single ultrasound transducer operating at 9 MHz (Boston Scientific, Watertown MA, USA). This technique supplies a radial "cross sectional" (relative to the long axis of the catheter) image; the catheter is in the center of the circular image (Fig. 1). Single plane phased array imaging (Acuson, Mountain View, CA, USA) involves integrated scanning of 64 ultrasound crystals arranged longitudinally along the access of the ICE catheter. This technique provides images at a range of frequencies (5.5-10 MHz) with a 90 degree sector that resembles transesophageal echocardiographic images (Fig. 2). One of the most important advantages of phased array imaging is the consistent ability to image left heart structures with right heart catheterization.

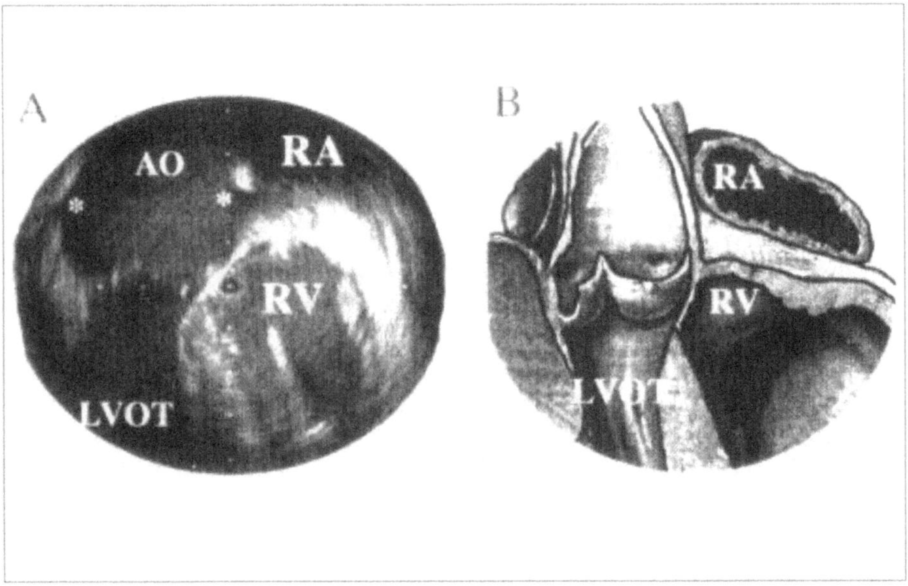

Fig. 1. Radial ICE imaging in ablation of left ventricle (LV) outflow tract VT. The imaging catheter is positioned adjacent to the right atrial septum, near the His bundle recording site circular artifact at the center of the image in panel A). The image demonstrates the complex anatomic relationships between the aortic root, sinuses of Valsalva and the coronary ostia (*asterisks*). Panel B is a schematic representation of the anatomic structures demonstrated in Panel A. (Reprinted from Lamberti et al., J Cardiac Electrophys 2001;12:529-535, with permission)

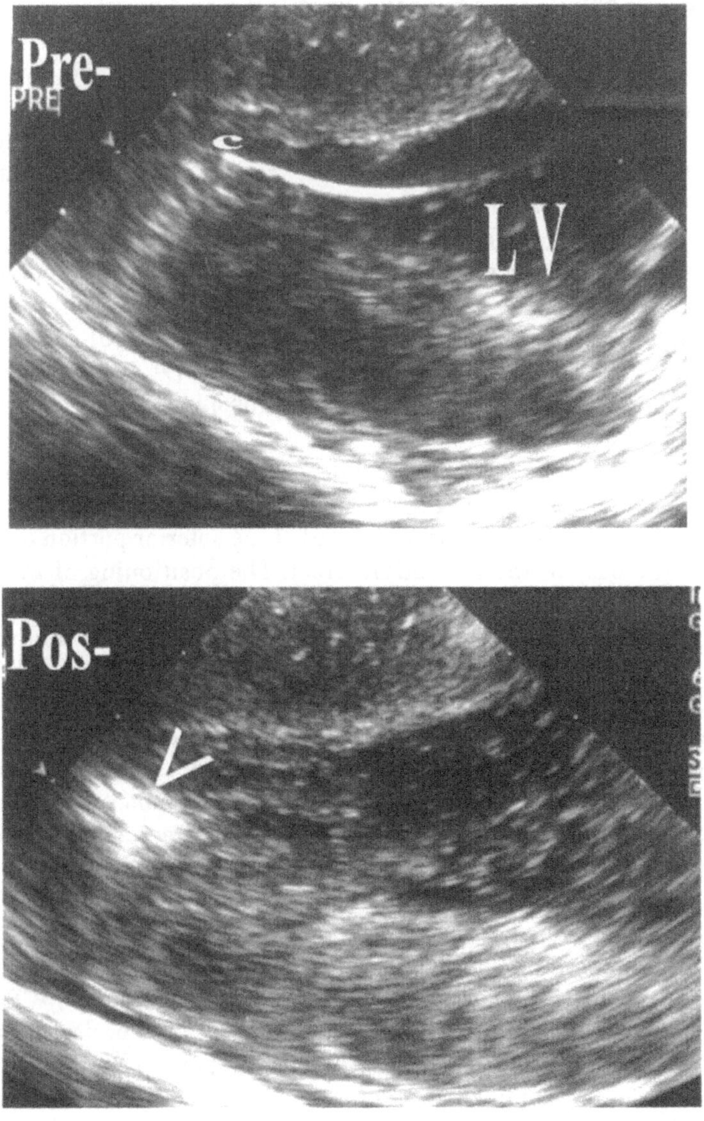

A

B

Fig. 2. Phased array imaging in ablation of LV idiopathic VT from near the LV apex. The imaging catheter is positioned in the right atrium and deflected downward to produce a long axis view of the LV apex left, septum top, free wall bottom. Although LV hypertrophy is evident, this patient had no associated structural heart disease. In panel A, the ablation catheter and the tip electrode (*c*) can be seen and catheter contact assessed in real time. Panel B demonstrates the imaging characteristics observed after lesion delivery (*arrow*). The increase in echo density and corresponding decrease in contractile function correspond to tissue changes induced by energy delivery, probably secondary to interstitial edema

ICE Imaging in Ablation of Idiopathic Ventricular Tachycardia

Although idiopathic VT can arise from any location within the myocardium, many of the most common sites of origin are closely related to identifiable anatomic structures. Right ventricular (RV) outflow tract VT is typically located just beneath the pulmonic valve [5]; anecdotally, many procedural failures seem due to initial ablation considerably below the valve annulus resulting in tissue swelling closing the entrance to this narrow inlet. LV outflow tract VT is often located in/near the sinuses of Valsalva [6, 7]; failure to appreciate the anatomic relationship of the ablation site and the proximal coronary arteries is fraught with considerable peril [8]. The relationship of LV idiopathic (Belhassen) VT to "false tendons" has been proposed [9]. ICE imaging may be useful in demonstrating these anatomic relationships, adding to procedural efficacy and safety.

Lamberti and coworkers (2001) demonstrated the utility of ICE imaging in a series of 5 patients with LV outflow tract VT [10]. The ICE imaging catheter (9 Fr. 9 MHz, Boston Scientific), was positioned at the anterior portion of the atrial septum or the base of the RV outflow tract. The positioning of the ablation catheter relative to the aortic root, coronary cusps and coronary ostia was demonstrated in all patients, and catheter–tissue contact was confirmed and monitored (Fig. 1). Ablation procedures were acutely successful in all patients, and recurrent VT was not observed during a 9 month follow up. No procedural complications occurred and both intracardiac and standard chest wall echocardiography demonstrated no damage to the aortic root or surrounding structures. This experience represents an important "proof of concept" demonstrating how ICE imaging can assist mapping in LV outflow tract ablation procedures and potentially replace adjunctive coronary angiography in demonstrating a safe distance between the ablation target and the coronary arteries.

In our own laboratory, we have used phased array ICE imaging to guide ablation of idiopathic VT arising from the LV outflow tract, the LV endocardium (Fig. 2) and the LV epicardium. For LV epicardial ablations, ICE imaging provides assistance in guiding percutaneous access to the pericardium as well as real-time monitoring to exclude pericardial tamponade. In this application, ICE imaging cannot completely replace adjunctive coronary angiography as imaging of the arteries distal to the aortic root is not as reliable at present. Furthermore, as demonstrated in Figure 2, ICE imaging provides a clear demonstration of lesion development with RF energy delivery, particularly in normal myocardium.

ICE Imaging in Ablation of VT in the Setting of Healed Myocardial Infarction

Using traditional electrophysiologic mapping techniques, ablation of VT in the setting of healed myocardial infarction is modestly successful in highly selected patients with relatively slow, well tolerated tachycardias [11, 12]. The majority of patients with coronary disease VT have tachycardias that are not sufficiently well tolerated to allow the prolonged mapping during VT necessary for successful focal ablation. Similar limitations are frequently observed in patients with arrhythmogenic RV dysplasia and VT in the setting of dilated cardiomyopathy. Anatomically based ablation of the VT substrate obviates this difficulty by linear ablation of the infarct border zone. Our group, and others have demonstrated the utility of an anatomic approach to VT ablation guided by electroanatomic voltage mapping of the infarct during sinus rhythm. Electroanatomic mapping is performed to demonstrate the three dimensional relationships of the infarct anatomy; bipolar electrogram amplitude is used to distinguish normal (> 2.0 mV), border zone (0.5–2.0 mV) and infarct tissue (< 0.5 mV). Pace mapping during sinus rhythm is used to approximate the VT circuit exit site for each specific VT morphology. Using the site of the best pace map as an "anchor," a linear lesion is delivered in a radial fashion from the dense scar through the exit site and out to either normal myocardium or to an anatomic barrier, such as the mitral annulus. An initial series of 16 patients with RV cardiomyopathy and healed infarction and frequent episodes of drug refractory unmappable VT (6–55 episodes/month) demonstrated excellent arrhythmia control in all but 1 patient during intermediate term follow up [13]. Subsequent experience showed that linear ablation in 53 patients with advanced structural heart disease and a median arrhythmia burden of 30 episodes/month resulted in no further VT in 60 % of patients, with infrequent VT episodes (1 episode per 3 month period) in an additional 25 % [14].

The potential application for ICE imaging in substrate-based ablation should be obvious. In fact, an important validation of electroanatomic voltage mapping as a reliable technique in characterizing the infarct anatomy involved direct comparison of this technique to ICE and pathologic analysis in a porcine model of anterior infarction [15]. The infarct anatomy and adjacent wall motion characteristics are well demonstrated by ICE, and the position of the ablation catheter with reference to the infarct can be monitored (Figure 3). Although the echodensity changes in the infarct and infarct border are not as marked as those observed in normal tissue, ICE imaging can verify lesion delivery, particularly when using irrigated RF energy [16]. One disadvantage of ICE imaging is the difficulty in relating individual lesions in three-dimensional space along the intended linear lesion; the relationship of individual lesions in the construction of a linear lesion is easier to manage with electroanatomic mapping.

The sudden development of cardiogenic shock is a recognized complication of VT ablation, particularly with irrigated RF delivery [17]. In the porcine model of anterior infarction, we performed ICE imaging during linear lesion delivery using irrigated RF energy at the infarct border zone [18]. ICE imaging demonstrated that lesion delivery resulted in acutely increased echodensity and local wall thickness at the RF site. In addition, despite the fact that lesions were delivered to poorly functioning areas within the infarct border zone, transient

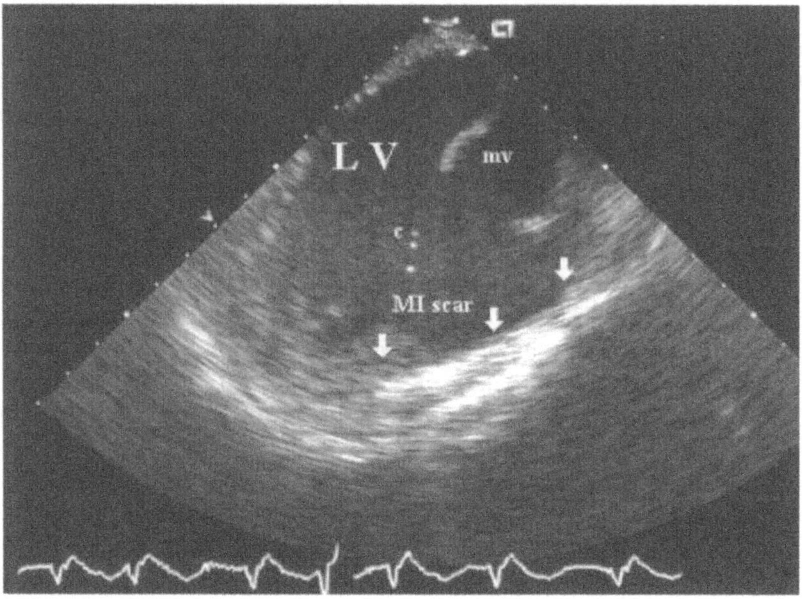

Fig. 3. Phased array imaging for VT ablation in the setting of healed posterior lateral infarction. A long axis view of the LV is shown; the infarct (*arrows*) is characterized by increased echodensity, thinning and akinesis in real time imaging. An ablation catheter (c) including the individual distal electrodes, is seen in the LV cavity

systolic dysfunction was observed in adjacent areas (1 cm from ablation site) of normal myocardium fractional shortening (-38 ± 34 %, $p < 0.01$). Importantly, systolic dysfunction recovered at each individual site within 30 minutes, and global LV function pre- and post-ablation was not effected. These data led us to speculate that cardiogenic shock observed in clinical VT ablation procedures may result from "stunning" of working myocardium adjacent to ablation lesions in patients with advanced structural heart disease and limited reserve. Real-time ICE imaging monitoring of global and regional LV systolic performance may improve the safety of complex anatomic VT ablation procedures.

Obstacles Preventing Wide Spread Use of ICE Imaging in VT Ablation Procedures

Despite the potential advantages of ICE imaging in VT ablation discussed above, ICE imaging is not used in the majority of laboratories for VT procedures. Furthermore, to date there have been no studies comparing the efficacy and safety of ICE guided procedures to conventional techniques. Some of the present barriers preventing more wide scale application of ICE imaging in this application are listed in Table 1. Although technically feasible, operators are somewhat reluctant to position the imaging catheter within the left heart. The limited depth of field available with radial ICE imaging restricts its application in left heart imaging to the LV outflow tract area. Far field imaging of the entire LV from venous catheter positions is possible with phased array ICE imaging even in patients with enlarged ventricles. The imaging windows for LV visualization are more difficult than those used for atrial ablation and some degree of struggling with the learning curve will be required, even for operators with considerable ICE imaging experience. The additional catheter cost is a consideration, particularly in the absence of studies firmly establishing improved efficacy and safety. Finally, as discussed above, although ICE imaging provides excellent two-dimensional imaging of each individual lesion, it provides no framework to organize the relationship of each lesion point target within the three-dimensional linear lesion set. The development of real-time three-dimensional ICE imaging or a "marriage" of data generated from two-dimensional ICE imaging and electroanatomic mapping may eventually provide this important imaging information.

Table 1. Factors limiting wide scale application of ICE imaging in VT ablation procedures

Requirement of LV imaging from venous catheterization
Comfort level with LV imaging windows
Probable need for additional operator for manipulation of the ICE catheter
Difficulty establishing 3D relationship of individual RF targets to the linear lesion as a whole
Additional cost of imaging catheters

Conclusions

ICE imaging is an emerging strategy for ablation of idiopathic VT as well as VT that arises in the setting of advanced structural heart disease. Important advantages of ICE imaging (Table 2) include the ability to direct the ablation catheter with reference to important anatomic landmarks (particularly for substrate-based ablation), the ability to identify and avoid adjacent structures (such as the proximal coronary arteries), real-time monitoring of catheter-tissue contact and visualization of lesion creation. In addition, ICE imaging provides real-time monitoring that can result in prompt detection and treatment of procedural complications, such as thrombus formation, pericardial effusion and decreases in LV function. ICE imaging for VT ablation will increase in importance as operator experience with ICE imaging in general increases.

Table 2. Advantages provided by ICE imaging during VT ablation procedures

Ability to direct the ablation catheter to important anatomic landmarks
Ability to visualize and avoid, adjacent structures coronary arteries)
Real-time monitoring of catheter–tissue contact
Visualization of lesion creation
Monitoring of LV function and procedural complications (thrombus, pericardial effusion)

References

1. Poty H, Saoudi N, Abdel Aziz A et al (1995) Radiofrequency catheter ablation of type 1 atrial flutter. Prediction of late success by electrophysiological criteria. Circulation 92:1389-1392
2. Schwartzman D, Callans DJ, Gottlieb CD et al (1996) Conduction block in the inferior vena caval-tricuspid valve isthmus: association with outcome of radiofrequency ablation of type I atrial flutter. J Am Coll Cardiol 28:1519-1531
3. Ren JF, Schwartzman D, Callans DJ et al (1999) Intracardiac echocardiography (9 MHz) in humans: methods, imaging views and clinical utility. Ultrasound Med Biol 25:1077-1086
4. Ren J-F, Marchlinski FE, Callans DJ, Herrmann HC (2002) Clinical use of AcuNav diagnostic ultrasound catheter imaging during left heart radiofrequency ablation and transcatheter closure procedures. J Am Soc Echocardiogr 15:1301-1308
5. Movsowitz C, Schwartzman D, Callans DJ et al (1996) Idiopathic right ventricular outflow tract tachycardia: narrowing the anatomic location for successful ablation. Am Heart J 131:930-936
6. Ouyang F FP, Ho SY, Hebe J et al (2002) Repetitive monomorphic ventricular tachycardia originating from the aortic sinus cusp: electrocardiographic characterization for guiding catheter ablation. J Am Coll Cardiol 39:500-508
7. Kanagaratnam L, Tomassoni G, Schweikert R et al (2001) Ventricular tachycardias arising from the aortic sinus of valsalva: an under-recognized variant of left outflow tract ventricular tachycardia. J Am Coll Cardiol 37:1408-1414
8. Friedman PL, Stevenson WG, Bittl JA et al (1997) Left main coronary artery occlusion during radiofrequency ablation of idiopathic outflow tract ventricular tachycardia. Pacing Clin Electrophysiol 20:1185 (abstract)
9. Thakur RK, Klein GJ, Sivaram CA et al (1996) Anatomic substrate for idiopathic left ventricular tachycardia. Circulation 93:497-501
10. Lamberti F, Calo L, Pandozi C et al (2001) Radiofrequency catheter ablation of idiopathic left ventricular outflow tract tachycardia: Utility of intracardiac echocardiography. J Cardiovasc Electrophysiol. 12:529-535
11. Kim YH, Sosa-Suarez G, Trouton TG et al (1994) Treatment of ventricular tachycardia by transcatheter radiofrequency ablation in patients with ischemic heart disease. Circulation 89:1094-1102
12. Callans DJ, Zado E, Sarter BH et al (1998) Efficacy of radiofrequency catheter ablation for ventricular tachycardia in healed myocardial infarction. Am J Cardiol 82:429-432

13. Marchlinski FE, Callans DJ, Gottlieb CD, Zado E (2000) Linear ablation lesions for control of unmappable ventricular tachycardia in patients with ischemic and nonischemic cardiomyopathy. Circulation 101:1288-1296
14. Marchlinski FE, Callans DJ, Hsia HH et al (2001) Late outcome after linear radiofrequency ablation for unmappable ventricular tachycardia: Influence of type of heart disease. Circulation 104:II-621 (abstract)
15. Callans DJ, Ren JF, Michele J et al (1999) Electroanatomic left ventricular mapping in the porcine model of healed anterior myocardial infarction. Correlation with intracardiac echocardiography and pathological analysis. Circulation 100:1744-1750
16. Ren JF, Callans DJ, Michele JJ et al (2001) Intracardiac echocardiographic evaluation of ventricular mural swelling from radiofrequency ablation in chronic myocardial infarction: irrigated-tip versus standard catheter. J Interv Card Electrophysiol 5:27-32
17. Calkins H, Epstein A, Packer D et al (2000) Catheter ablation of ventricular tachycardia in patients with structural heart disease using cooled radiofrequency energy: results of a prospective multicenter study. Cooled RF Multi Center Investigators Group. J Am Coll Cardiol 35:1905-1914
18. Callans DJ, Ren JF, Narula N et al (2001) Effects of linear, irrigated-tip radiofrequency ablation in porcine healed anterior infarction. J Cardiovasc Electrophysiol 12:1037-1042

IMPLANTABLE CARDIOVERTER DEFIBRILLATOR: PRACTICAL ASPECTS, INDICATIONS AND COST-EFFECTIVENESS

Left Ventricular Dysfunction and Electrophysiologic Study in the Primary and Secondary ICD Trials

D. S. Cannom

During the last 20 years the utility of electrophysiologic study (EPS) for risk stratification in patients with coronary artery disease has been studied without reaching consensus. During the 1980s this procedure was the mainstay of risk stratification for patients with sustained ventricular tachycardia (VT) or sudden death.

The need for effective tools to risk stratify coronary artery patients is obvious. Sudden death from cardiac causes accounts for 50 % of all deaths from cardiovascular causes [1]. During the late 1980s, clinical trials showed that antiarrhythmic drug therapy was not effective in reducing mortality in high risk patients [2]. A series of recent clinical trials have proven the implantable cardioverter defibrillator (ICD) effective in reducing mortality in high risk patients–both post- and pre-event–but the number of patients treated as a result of these indications is relatively small. The majority of sudden deaths occur among patients who are not candidates for inclusion in such trials as AVID, MADIT I and MADIT II.

A variety of clinical measures to identify risk for serious arrhythmias has been established and includes measures of cardiovascular function, ambient ventricular rhythms, electrocardiographic features suggesting risk and electrophysiologic testing [3]. Electrophysiologic testing, the ability to induce a sustained ventricular tachyarrhythmia by programmed stimulation, has been employed for twenty years as a way to identify a patient at increased risk of a clinical arrhythmia [4]. The sensitivity, positive predictive value and reproducibility of the technique has been high for patients with a previous myocardial infarction, but not for those with nonischemic cardiomyopathy [5]. The technique has been useful in deciding whether an episode of significant syncope is due to an arrhythmia, especially in the patient with decreased left ventricular function.

In the late 1980s, clinicians attempted to suppress induced ventricular arrhythmias with medication. However, after many sudden death survivors were treated, it became clear that there was an unacceptably high incidence of

Department of Cardiology, Good Samaritan Hospital, Los Angeles, California, USA

recurrent arrhythmias. In one study of 331 sudden cardiac death (SCD) survivors treated with drugs (with ICDs used in those patients whose arrhythmias could not be suppressed with drugs), the predictors of total cardiac mortality were 1) an ejection fraction (EF) of less than 0.40, 2) the absence of an ICD and 3) persistence of inducible sustained VT [6]. The marked survival benefit of the ICD group over those patients treated with antiarrhythmic drug regimens predicted to be "successful" was realized in patients with EFs both over and under 40 %. The worst results were those patients with EFs under 40 % treated with drugs; they had a three year survival of 52 % and a 5 year survival of only 28 % [6]. Such data effectively ended the era of EPS as a predictor of risk and drug suppression as a measure of clinical protection.

The AVID study further changed clinical approach to sudden death. In this randomized clinical trial of post-SCD/sustained VT high risk patients, EPS was not used as a risk stratifier [7]. Even so, in the AVID trial, a number of patients underwent EPS and in those patients the results had no value in predicting the outcome of patients without an ICD [8].

In the mid 1990s there still remained uncertainty about the benefits of electrophysiologic study in patients who had not experienced a clinical arrhythmia. Wilber and colleagues (1990) studied a population of coronary artery patients with EF < 40 % and nonsustained VT who underwent electrophysiologic study and serial drug testing. In this era, patients who had not experienced a lethal arrhythmia were not treated with ICDs. The patients who were either noninducible, or inducible and suppressed, experienced much better survival in followup than those patients who were inducible and not suppressed. There remained a need for a prospective, randomized trial, as opposed to the retrospective analysis of the type used in the Wilber study [9], to compare the benefits of the ICD versus aggressive medical therapy.

The MADIT I study addressed this question. Inclusion criteria for MADIT I had similarities to those of the Wilber study (i.e. the presence of coronary artery disease, an EF < 36 %, nonsustained VT on Holter, with inducibility and nonsuppression at EPS). The enrolled patient group was randomized to either an ICD or to what was considered "best medical therapy," usually amiodarone. The results of this small study were striking; there was a 54 % reduction in total mortality in the ICD group. MADIT I first showed the value of the prophylactic use of the ICD in a population identified as high risk by the use of EPS.

A post hoc analysis of the MADIT I data showed that all of the survival benefit in the trial occurred in patients with an ejection fraction under 26 % [10]. The MADIT II study design was similar to MADIT I but with some important differences. Again, the study population were patients with coronary artery disease (CAD) and a prior infarction, but the EF level for inclusion was lowered to 30 % and there was no requirement for an EP study or any Holter data showing ambient ectopy. (EP studies were routinely performed in many centers but did not effect randomization.) Patients were randomized to either a prophylactic ICD or best medical therapy [11]. Again, the ICD showed a striking benefit of 31 % reduction in total mortality, and the study was terminated prematurely.

From 593 patients, EP data was obtained incidently (rather than per protocol). Of these patients, 211 (36 %) were inducible and 382 (64 %) were noninducible using standard techniques. Over time, inducibility was associated with use of ICD for episodes of VT (often using the antitachycardia feature of the ICD), while patients who were noninducible had more frequent ICD therapy for ventricular fibrillation (VF) [12] (Fig. 1). Noninducible patients tended to be sicker with a higher NYHA heart failure class, less beta blocker use and higher BUN (Fig. 2). Of particular interest is that of the 29 patients in MADIT II who had a post-randomization cardiac arrest aborted by the ICD, 24 were noninducible. Thus, in this high risk population who actually had life saving shocks in the MADIT II trial, the enrollment EP study was not predictive of the patient who would receive benefit from the ICD. This data argues against the commonly held belief that noninducible patients with a low EF die due to heart failure or electromechanical dissociation rather than arrhythmias. In the MADIT II study, the low EF population utilizes their ICD at a high rate but is not predicted by EPS.

Surprisingly, MADIT II demonstrated the poor reproducibility of EPS. Of the EP positive group, 27 % were not inducible on repeat testing at one year. Of the EP negative group, 18 % were inducible on repeat testing at one year. To date, this and all the EP data from MADIT II has been presented only at scientific sessions of NASPE. The final manuscripts have not been published in a peer reviewed journal.

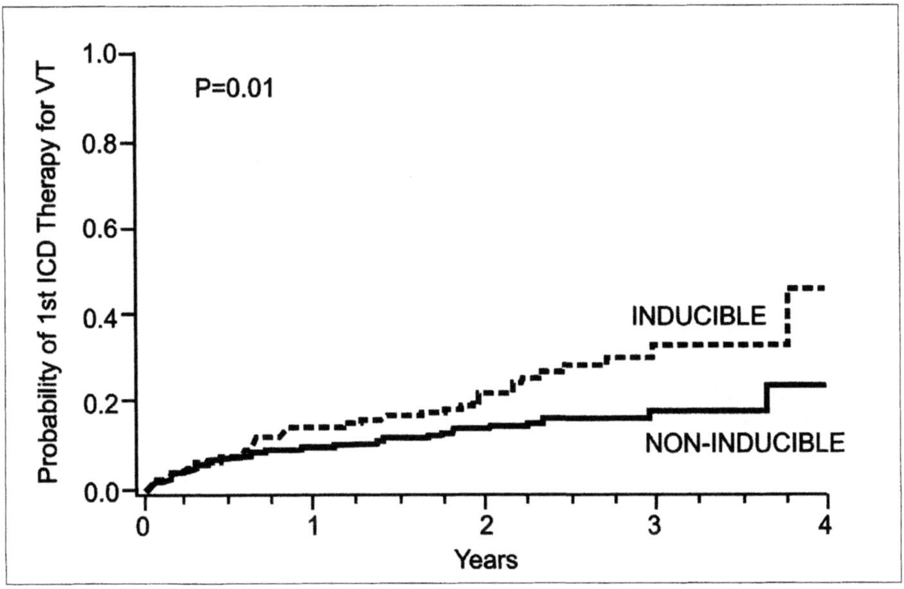

Fig. 1. MADIT II Inducibility. Shown is data from the MADIT II study comparing the effect of inducibility on therapy for VT or the ICD. Patients who were inducible had a higher likelihood of using their device for VT using the antitachycardia pacing function of their ICD [12]

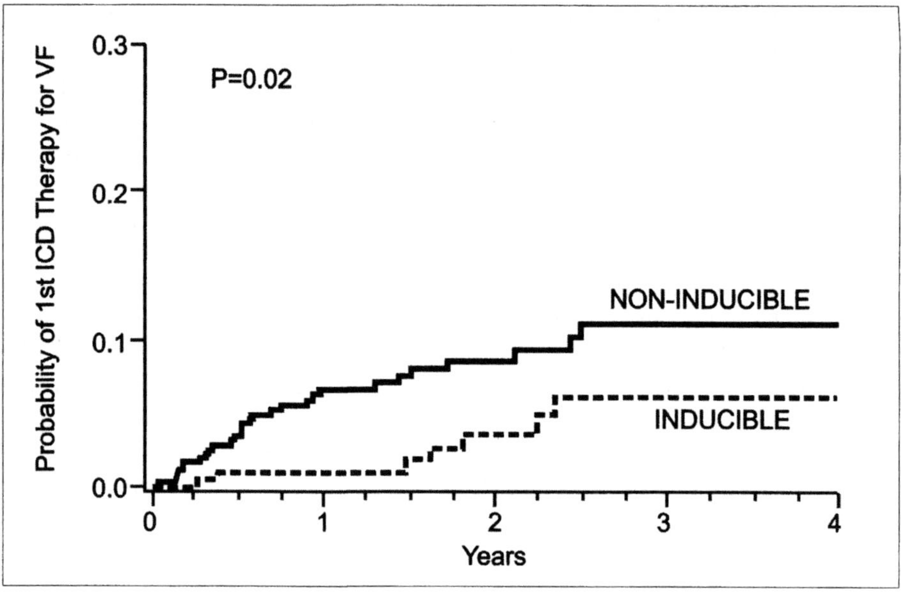

Fig. 2. MADIT II Inducibility. This figure compares the inducibility status with first ICD therapy for ventricular fibrillation. The noninducible patients had a higher use of their device or shocks due to VF. Thus, inducibility did not predict the patients who were most likely to use their device for probable life-saving shock (see text) [12]

The MUSTT trial has recently been published with significant concurrence with the MADIT II data. The MUSTT trial was specifically designed to study patients with CAD, an EF < 40 % and unsustained VT on Holter. A positive EP study was required for inclusion in the trial and patients were randomized to either EP-guided therapy (which could result in an ICD if antiarrthymics failed to suppress induction) or placebo [13]. This trial was very large and carefully done. A total of 2202 patients were studied, of whom 767 were inducible. The noninducible patients were followed in a registry and untreated. Including the patients in the placebo arm of the main trial, there were 1791 patients on no antiarrhythmic drugs available for analysis.

A subsequent study [13] found that both EF and inducibility predicted subsequent mortality in a multivariate analysis. The 5 year total mortality of patients with an EF < 30 % was high (54 %) and significantly higher than patients having an EF > 30 % (36 %) (p 0.0001). The risk of death from an arrhythmic event over a 5 year period was also higher with an EF < 30 % (33 %) in contrast to those with an EF > 30 % (20 %) (p 0. 0001). Low EF alone predicts both total mortality and arrhythmic mortality irrespective of EP induction status. This observation was maintained throughout the duration of the study. However, programmed stimulation has greater prognostic utility in coronary patients with a higher EF, between 30 and 40 %, rather than under 30 % (Fig. 3).

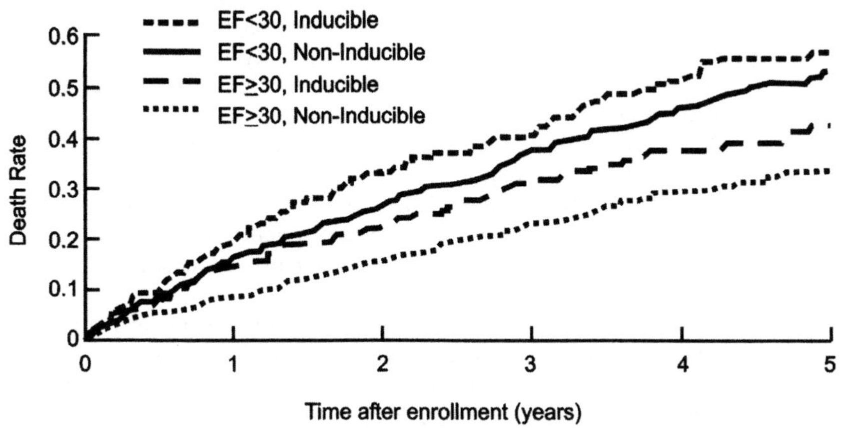

Fig. 3. MUSTT Inducibility. This figure shows the relationship between EF and inducible VT and total mortality in the MUSTT trial. Patients with an EF under 30 % did poorly, irrespective of their inducibility status. Survival was better in those patients with an EF over 30 % and was best in patients who had an EF over 30 % and were noninducible [13]

There is concordance between findings from the MUSTT study (above) and the preliminary EP data from the MADIT II trial. The highest risk patients in both MADIT II and MUSTT were best identified by low EF alone. The EP study added nothing in terms of predicting risk. Other populations, especially coronary artery disease patients with an EF between 30 and 40 %, have a better likelihood of having arrhythmic risk predicted by a positive EPS. This was confirmed in both MADIT I and MUSTT.

There is uncertainty among clinicians about the best way to identify and treat patients with moderate and low risk for sudden death (e.g., coronary artery patients with EF > 40 %). A recent surge of interest in resuscitative strategies for the patient experiencing a cardiac arrest out of hospital, whether in an airport or at home, suggests that some investigators are shifting emphasis to the event itself (cardiac arrest) rather than its identification pre-event [14, 15].

The clinical implication of these data seems clear. CAD patients with an EF < 30 % are ICD candidates without the need for an EP study. This, of course, implies that there are no serious comorbidities and each referral for an ICD must be made on a case by case basis. For the CAD patient with an EF between 30 and 40 %, an EP study is useful in deciding about ICD implantation. Those findings are so clear that I doubt whether any future clinical studies will substantially change these recommendations. The recent ACC/AHA guidelines for *ICD implantation* are consistent with these findings [16].

References

1. Myerburg RJ, Kessler KM, Castellanos A (1993) Sudden cardiac death: epidemiology, transient risk and intervention assessment. Ann Intern Med 119:1187-1197
2. Echt DS, Liebson PR, Mitchell LR et al (1991) Mortality and morbidity in patients receiving encainide, flecainide, or placebo: the Cardiac Arrhythmia Suppression Trial. N Engl J Med 324:781-788
3. Hukuri HV, Castellanos A, Myerburg RJ (2001) Sudden death due to cardiac arrhythmias. N Engl J Med 345:1473-1482
4. Brugada P, Green AL, Abdullah H, Wellens HJJ (1984) Significance of ventricular arrhythmias induced by programmed ventricular stimulation: the importance of the type of ventricular arrhythmia induced and the number of premature stimuli required. Circulation 69:87-92
5. Prystowsky EN (1988) Electrophysiologic-electropharmacologic testing in patients with ventricular arrhythmias. Pacing Clin Electrophysiol 11:225-251
6. Powell AC, Fuchs T, Finkelstein DM et al (1993) Influence of implantable cardioverter-defibrillators on the long-term prognosis of survivors of out-of-hospital cardiac arrest. Circulation 88:1083-1092
7. The Antiarrhythmics Versus Implantable Defibrillators (AVID) Investigators (1997) A comparison of antiarrhythmic drug therapy with implantable defibrillators in patients resuscitated from near-fatal ventricular arrhythmias. N Engl J Med 337:1576-1583
8. Brodsky MA, Mitchell B, Halperin BD et al (2002) Prognostic value of baseline electrophysiology studies in patients with sustained ventricular tachyarrhythmia: the Antiarrhythmics Versus Implantable Defibrillator (AVID) trial. Am Heart J 144:178-484
9. Wilber DJ, Olshansky B, Moran JF, Scanlon PJ (1990) Electrophysiological testing and nonsustained ventricular tachycardia. Use and limitations in patients with coronary artery disease and impaired ventricular function. Circulation 82:350-358
10. Moss AJ, Hall WJ, Cannom DS et al (1996) Improved survival with an implanted defibrillator in patients with coronary disease at high risk for ventricular arrhythmia. N Engl J Med 335:1933-1940
11. Moss AJ, Fadl Y, Zareba W et al (2001) Survival benefit with an implanted defibrillator in relation to mortality risk in chronic coronary heart disease. Am J Cardiol 88:516-520
12. From Late Breaking Trials Conference presented at NASPE's 23rd Annual Scientific Sessions (2002) held in San Diego, California. NASPE late breaking trials
13. Buxton AE, Lee KL, Hafley GE et al (2002) Relation of ejection fraction and inducible ventricular tachycardia to mode of death in patients with coronary artery disease. Circulation 106:24660-2472
14. Page RL, Joglar JA, Kowal RC et al (2000) Use of automated external defibrillators by a U.S. airline. N Engl J Med 343:1210-1216
15. Wellens HJJ, Gorgels AP, deMunter H (2003) Cardiac arrest outside of a hospital: how can we improve results of resuscitation? Circulation 107:1948-1950
16. Gregoratos G, Abrams J, Epstein AE et al (2002) ACC/AHA/NASPE 2002 guideline update for implanation of cardiac pacemakers and antiarrhythmia devices: a report of the American College of Cardiology/American Heart Association task force on practice guidelines. Circulation 106:1-17

New Evidence from the Secondary Endpoints of the MADIT II Study

S. L. Higgins

Introduction

The landmark Multicenter Automatic Defibrillator Implantation Trial II (MADIT II) demonstrated that the implantable defibrillator (ICD) improved survival in post-infarction patients with left ventricular ejection fractions of 30 or lower [1]. Despite rigorous scrutiny, the study has resulted in acceptance of this recommendation by numerous regulatory agencies, both in the United States and Europe. MADIT II has been heralded as one of the most important research studies in cardiology in the past 20 years.

In addition to the primary endpoint of mortality, the MADIT II trial collected detailed information on the enrolled patients until study conclusion, with data available from over 8000 follow-up visits. This data has resulted in numerous sub-studies utilizing retrospective analysis. While none of these sub-studies are published in other than abstract format, a review of the available information is of interest.

Background

Published in March 2002, the MADIT II study presented information on 1232 enrolled patients from July 1997 until the trial was stopped by the data and safety monitoring board on November 20, 2001. Follow-up averaged 20 months (range 6 days to 53 months). The inclusion and exclusion criteria are well-reviewed in the primary manuscript [1]. Briefly, the enrollment criteria included a prior myocardial infarction (MI) and a left ventricular ejection fraction of 0.30 or less. Patients were not required to have an electrophysiology study and were randomly assigned to receive either an implantable defibrillator (ICD) (742 patients), or conventional medical therapy (490 patients) which was

Regional Cardiac Arrhythmia Center, Scripps Memorial Hospital, La Jolla, California, USA

encouraged to not include anti-arrhythmic therapy unless required for another problem, such as atrial arrhythmias. After initial randomization in a 3:2 ratio respectively, each of the two treatment groups was followed at the same frequency, every three months.

As well publicized the patients in the ICD arm had a 14.2 % mortality as compared to the 19.8 % mortality in the conventional therapy group. This difference was highly significant statistically, with a hazard ratio of 0.69 for the ICD group risk (p=0.016). A limited analysis of subgroup stratified for age, sex, ejection fraction, New York Heart Association (NYHA) class and QRS duration showed no differences between the two treatment groups. As a result, prophylactic ICD implantation was recommended for all patients meeting the enrollment criteria.

The sub-studies performed to date can be classified into 4 major areas of interest

- Value of electrophysiologic study
- Factors influencing mortality
- Time-dependence of mortality risk
- Non-invasive markers predicting risk

Sub-studies on Inducibility at EP Study

Inducibility at electrophysiologic study (EPS) was not an enrollment criterion in MADIT II, unlike the original MADIT study. However, studies were done at enrollment on some of the patients randomized to ICD therapy and their outcome was monitored. Daubert et al presented this data in abstract format in May, 2003 [2]. EPS was performed in 583 of the 742 patients randomized to the ICD arm. Inducibility was conservatively defined as in the original MADIT study: sustained ventricular fibrillation (VF) only if induced with single or double extrastimuli, sustained ventricular tachycardia (VT) with single, double or triple stimuli. Most of the studies were performed with a catheter prior to surgery, though a minority were device-based tests. The outcome of the inducibility played no role in the subsequent implantation. Of the 593 who underwent EPS, 211 (36 %) had inducible ventricular tachyarrhythmias. Results are reproduced in Table 1.

Table 1. Inducibility Status and Ventricular Tachyarrhythmia Occurrence (adapted from Daubert et al [2])

	Inducible (%)	Noninducible (%)	Unadj p	Hazard ratio
2-yr VT incidence	29	19.3	0.023	1.57
2-yr VF incidence	2.2	8.1	0.028	0.46
2-yr. VT/VF incidence	31.2	27.4	0.28	1.28

The data shows a strong trend ($p = 0.07$) that EPS inducibility is predictive of the subsequent occurrence of VT. Surprisingly, an equally strong trend was noted regarding the finding that lack of EPS inducibility was more likely associated with a clinical ICD shock for VF. Those who had an inducible VT or VF were less likely to receive a shock for VF. The authors conclude that EPS is not useful as a risk stratifier in the selection of patients for prophylactic ICD implantation.

In a related presentation, Reek et al. looked at reproducibility of VT/VF induction in patients enrolled from their two high enrolling MADIT II centers [3]. In 56 patients, they performed EPS at implantation and in selected patients annually, as shown in Table 2. They conclude that results of repeated EPS in MADIT II patients demonstrate poor predictability of inducibility, at least with device based testing. This data provides an explanation for the findings of Daubert et al. as it suggests that EPS is not a reliable predictor of either repeat EPS over time or clinical need for device therapy.

Table 2. Serial EPS data (adapted from Reek et al [3]). Data listed include those inducible at subsequent EPS stratified by baseline EPS

INDUCIBILITY	implant	1 year	2 years	3 years
N	56	34	23	21
inducible	13	10	4	NA
non-inducible	0	18	11	NA

Factors Influencing Mortality

The primary endpoint in MADIT II was total mortality, as it was in the original MADIT trial. While this resolves any issues regarding bias regarding mortality classification, it does not provide detailed data regarding the presumed mode of death. With that in mind, Greenberg et al. analyzed details of deaths in the MADIT II study [4]. The End Point Review committee obtained detailed reports from hospital records and witnesses regarding the terminal event and classified them according to pre-determined categories [5]. As expected, they found that primary arrhythmic deaths and sudden death (≤ one hour) were greatly reduced in the ICD group. Figure 1 shows device usage relating to mortality. When the curve of device usage is superimposed upon the device mortality arm, the combined curve approximates that of the control arm.

Concern has been raised that beta-blocker usage diminishes the need for ICD therapy in the MADIT II population. Interestingly, the original manuscript included a table that showed the hazard ratios of patients regarding beta-blocker therapy but it was eliminated in editorial review. Brodine confirms that beta-blocker usage was similar in the two arms, 64 % in ICD patients and 61 % in conventional patients [6]. As expected, beta-blockers were

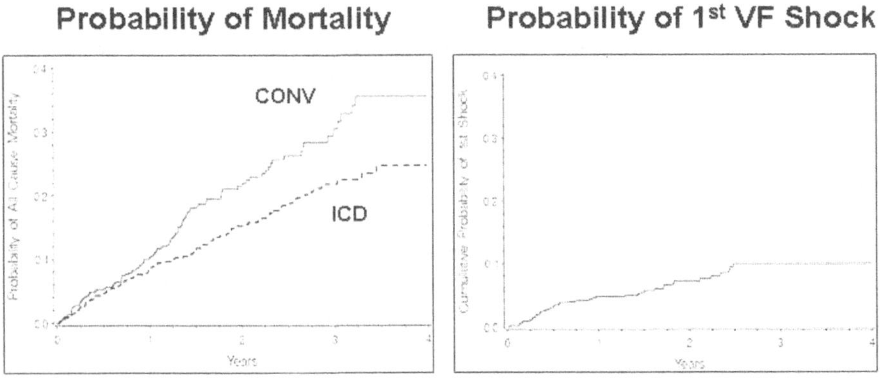

Fig. 1. The graph on the left shows the probability of mortality over time for the two arms in the trial. On the right is the probability of first shock over the same time period

associated with better survival ($p<0.0004$) but equal distribution of the therapy did not influence the results. It was noted that in follow-up, beta-blockers were associated with a weak trend towards a delay in first appropriate ICD therapy ($p=0.16$).

Time Dependence of Mortality Risk

After reviewing the CABG-Patch data, Wilber and colleagues hypothesized that the impact of coronary revascularization (CR) may play a role in the MADIT II results [7]. If so, they presumed that a greater ICD benefit would be seen in those patients farther from revascularization. As is seen with many other variables in MADIT II, the incidence of CR was evenly distributed among the two arms as well as the type of CR, CABG only in 401 patients, percutaneous CR only in 244 and both in 306 for a total of 951 of the 1232 enrolled patients. In both treatment groups, mortality from CR significantly increased as a function of time ($p=0.036$ conventional, $p=0.0003$ ICD). However, ICD survival benefit was similar across all time periods reviewed. The authors conclude that prophylactic ICDs may be beneficial post-MI, even in the setting of recent CR.

Similarly, these same authors looked at time-dependence of mortality risk and defibrillator benefit following MI [8]. Concern has been raised that newer treatments for coronary disease may alter the epidemiology of post-MI risk making ICDs of lesser benefit. In an editorial on the MADIT II study, Buxton suggested that the benefit from an ICD may diminish the longer a patient is post-MI [9]. Interestingly, in the MADIT II sub-study analysis, investigators found that the mortality benefit *increased* as a function of time from last MI. For example, in the quartile from 1-17 months post-MI, the conventional mortality was 15.6 % and ICD mortality 13.8 %. In the fourth quartile, those with an MI greater than 10 years prior to enrollment, conventional mortality was 26.7 % and ICD mortality 16.9 %. They conclude that aggressive use of prophylactic ICDs in MADIT II patients in the very late phase after MI is warranted.

Non-Invasive Markers Predicting Risk

As part of the MADIT II data evaluation, patients had several non-invasive tests performed for subsequent analysis. Zareba and colleagues analyzed these tests to determine potential predictors of ICD therapy and mortality risk. With signal-averaged EKGs, late potentials were not associated with the risk of ventricular arrhythmias requiring ICD therapy except for filtered QRS duration [10, 13]. In another analysis, frequent premature ventricular contractions on a ten minute Holter EKG were associated with mortality in the conventional group and ICD therapy for VT/VF in the ICD group [11]. Heart rate turbulence was not predictive of outcome.

In the ten minute resting high-resolution EKG recordings of MADIT II enrollees, a QT variability index was calculated in the ICD recipients [12]. Increased QT variability, considered a marker for repolarization lability, was found to be associated with a significantly (hazard ratio 1.69, p=0.018) greater risk for ventricular tachyarrhythmias requiring ICD therapy.

Conclusions

The Multicenter Automatic Defibrillator Implantation Trial II (MADIT II) demonstrated that the implantable defibrillator (ICD) improved survival in post-infarction patients with left ventricular ejection fractions of .30 or lower. In addition, detailed data was collected for all patients enrolled in both the ICD and conventional therapy arms. Preliminary analysis of this data has yielded several very interesting findings which substantiate findings of several other previously published studies, including DAVID, MADIT, MUSTT, and CABG-Patch. Other interesting findings reviewed include inducibility at EP study, both at baseline and annually after implant, mechanism of death, beta-blocker usage, time-dependence of mortality, and non-invasive markers of sudden death risk. Additional evaluation of this valuable data set should result in further advances in the management of life-threatening cardiac arrhythmias.

References

1. Moss AJ, Zareba W, Hall WJ et al (2002) Prophylactic implantation of a defibrillator in patients with myocardial infarction and reduced ejection fraction. N Engl J Med 346:877-883
2. Daubert JP, Zareba W, Schuger CD et al, for the MADIT II Investigators (2003) Does

EPS inducibility in MADIT II patients predict subsequent VT and/or VF events? PACE 26:960

3. Reek S, Klein HU, Erdogan A et al, for the MADIT II Investigators (2003) Reproducibility of electrophysiological testing in patients with remote myocardial infarction and severe LV-dysfunction: MADIT II substudy. PACE 26:960
4. Greenberg HM, Case RB, Brown MW et al, for the MADIT II Investigators (2003) Mechanisms of mortality in the multicenter automatic defibrillator implantation trial (MADIT-II). PACE 26:961
5. Epstein A, Carlson M, Fogoros R et al (1996) Classification of death in antiarrhythmia trials. J Am Coll Cardiol 27:433-442
6. Brodine WN, Tung RT, Lee JK et al (2003) Beta blocker use and appropriate ICD therapy in the MADIT-II study. PACE 26:961
7. Wilber DJ, Klein HU, Zareba W et al (2003) Does time from coronary revascularization influence the survival benefit of prophylactic implantable defibrillators in patients with impaired ventricular function following myocardial infarction? PACE 26:972
8. Wilber DJ, Zareba W, Hall WJ et al (2003) Time-dependence of mortality risk and defibrillator benefit following myocardial infarction: lessons from the multicenter automatic defibrillator implantation trial II. PACE 26:961
9. Zareba W, Steinberg J, Moss AJ et al, for MADIT II investigators (2003) Signal-averaged ECG and outcome in MADIT II patients. PACE 26:943
10. Buxton AE (2003) The clinical use of implantable cardioverter defibrillators: Where are we now? Where should we go? Ann Intern Med 138:512–514
11. Berkowitsch A, Neumann T, Erdogan A et al (2003). Prognostic significance of heart rate turbulence and frequency of ventricular premature beats in MADIT II patients. PACE 26:1027
12. Haigney MC, Zareba W, Gentlesk P et al (2003) QT variability and appropriate ICD therapy in MADIT-II patients. PACE 26:942
13. Perkiomaki JS, Zareba W, Steinberg JS et al (2003) Relationship of heart rate variability and signal averaged electrocardiographic parameters to inducibility of ventricular tachyarrhythmias in postinfarction patients with reduced left ventricular function. PACE 26:1091

The Real Economic Impact of the MADIT-II Study on the European Medical Community

G. Boriani, M. Biffi, C. Martignani, C. Camanini, C. Valzania, I. Diemberger, C. Greco, A. Branzi

The Problem of High-cost Treatments in Europe

One of the most relevant problems in current cardiological practice is the possibility of implementing, in patients who have a specific indication, a series of treatments of proven efficacy but of high cost. This problem involves percutaneous transluminal coronary angioplasty (PTCA) and cardioverter-defibrillators (CDs) [1]. Table 1 shows the number of procedures performed in the year 2000 in the European Union (15 countries) and in the whole of Europe (33 countries). As the table shows, the increase in population obtained by adding

Table 1. Overall population and high cost cardiological procedures performed in the year 2000 in the European Union (15 countries: Austria, Belgium, Denmark, Finland, France, Germany, Greece, Ireland, Italy, Luxembourg, The Netherlands, Portugal, Spain, Sweden, and the United Kingdom) and in the whole of Europe (the European Union plus the following 18 countries: Bulgaria, Croatia, Czech Republic, Estonia, Hungary, Iceland, Israel, Latvia, Lithuania, Macedonia, Norway, Poland, Romania, San Marino, Slovak Republic, Slovenia, Switzerland, and Turkey). Modified from [1]

	European Union	Whole of Europe	Increment in Europe vs European Union
Inhabitants	370 million	580 million	+57%
Percutaneous coronary angioplasty	430 000	520 000	+21%
Coronary artery bypass graft	280 000	330 000	+18%
Pacemakers	160 000	185 000	+16%
CDs	12 500	13 500	+8%

Institute of Cardiology, University of Bologna, Policlinico S. Orsola–Malpighi, Bologna, Italy

18 countries to those within the European Union is not followed by a parallel increase in the number of high-cost procedures, suggesting marked difficulties due to economic reasons in using these treatments in routine daily practice.

Moreover, taking a more general view, the issue of increasing costs for health care systems due to high-cost devices or treatments such as CDs, stents, or devices for cardiac resynchronization or left ventricular assistance prompts some considerations: (1) health care systems are more sensitive to financial crisis in the case of treatments such as devices with high implant costs, than they are in the case of treatments with continuous, diluted costs (such as drugs); (2) health care systems where a part of medical costs are covered by thirty payers may be reset at a level with increased costs much more easily than health care systems with a fixed national budget; (3) health care systems usually perform financial evaluations of new therapies (based on costs), rather than economic evaluations (based on cost-effectiveness, cost-benefit, or cost-utility).

Clinical Use of CDs: the Cost Issue

Since its introduction in clinical practice, the CD has been considered an expensive type of treatment, with a large amount of the costs due to the device itself and the implantation, followed in time by the costs of device replacement. The possibility of implanting a CD system by the transvenous technique has markedly reduced the costs of hospitalization and contributed to widespread use of CD systems, although important differences remain between implantation rates in the United States and in Europe, with implantation rates in the former generally five times higher than in Western European countries in the year 2000 [2]. Moreover, marked differences in implantation rates exist between different countries within Europe [2–4]. In the year 2000, the implantation rates per million inhabitants varied from 67 in Germany to 19 and 13 in the United Kingdom and France, respectively [4].

A series of randomized, prospective, controlled clinical trials has validated the use of CDs in specific subsets of patients, for both primary and secondary prevention of sudden cardiac death. The results of these trials have suggested the definition of appropriate guidelines for CD use [5, 6]. It is difficult to assess whether the above-mentioned guidelines are applied in daily practice, but a series of indirect findings suggest that even in the United States the actual rate of CD implantation may be lower than what would be expected by a projection based on current guidelines for CD implantation [7]. On the other hand, it must be stressed that strict application of definite criteria for CD implantation in the field of secondary prevention of sudden death (e.g., AVID criteria) may result in an impressive increase in CD implantations and consequent related costs, in comparison to current implantation rate in the UK [8]. It appears clear that despite the reduction in device price seen in recent years, the problem of CD cost remains a major determinant of full acceptance and application of CD therapy.

In recent years the possibility of primary prevention of sudden death by using CDs in selected groups of high-risk patients has aroused great interest, and a series of prospective controlled studies have been planned. The MADIT II study [9] has highlighted the possibility of effective primary prevention of sudden death in patients with coronary artery disease selected by means of a few clinical data and without expensive screenings (i.e., electrophysiological study). Patients with a previous myocardial infarction and low left ventricular ejection fraction (≤30%) may benefit from implantation of a CD, with a reduction of the mortality risk of about 31% in the following 2 years. In light of these data, implantation of a CD should be proposed in this kind of patient, even if the problem of limited economic resources to afford the cost of the devices has to be faced. Indeed, apart from the scientific result, the problems raised by the MADIT-II study relate to the effective possibility of adopting this therapeutic strategy in clinical practice, and this question is still open.

MADIT-II and the Cost Issue: the Difficulties in Applying MADIT-II Indications in Europe

The results of the MADIT-II study should potentially increase the number of CD implantations markedly; however, the key point is to assess what financial resources are available to afford the increasing costs for health care systems. Although the MADIT-II study has the advantage over MADIT-I and MUSTT of avoiding a complex, time-consuming, and expensive process of screening for the candidates, it is clear that the trial raises a series of questions centering on how to translate it into clinical practice in the context of limited economic resources. As reported in the MADIT-II study [9], approximately 400 000 new patients per year present with coronary artery disease and advanced heart failure in the United States, and if a substantial proportion of these patients are proposed to undergo implantation of a CD, the costs to the health care system will be significantly higher than in the past.

The European countries have a broad range of economic status, and CD implantation rates per million inhabitants seem to be even more profoundly affected by the variability in countries' wealth than are other procedures, especially if the utilization of CDs is compared with other invasive procedures such as coronary angioplasty [1, 2]. Moreover, the differences among European countries in the utilization of high-cost cardiological procedures are marked, not only in a comparison among the 15 countries of the European Union, but, even more, when the other 18 countries included geographically in the European region and included in the European Society of Cardiology are taken into consideration [1]. As shown in Table 1, an analysis that takes into account all of the 33 countries of the European region showed a percentage increase in use of CDs in the year 2000 that was much lower than the increase in the number of inhabitants included in the analysis, suggesting a marked underuse of CDs in the second group of countries.

The differences among the European countries involve both the general economic status and the characteristics of the respective health care systems. Health expenditure taken as a percentage of gross domestic product varies within a series of European countries, from 2.2% in the Russian Federation to 5.8% in Greece and 8.2% in Italy and up to 10.4 % in Germany [10]. In this view, it is clear that the European situation will vary from countries where the general situation and the application of MADIT-II are close to those seen in the United States (e.g., Germany) to other economic realities where, in view of economic constraints, prevention of sudden death by costly devices does not at present appear to be a strategy to be considered as suitable in a substantial proportion of patients (Eastern Europe).

Potential Solutions to the Problem of MADIT-II Costs

Various approaches to the problem of applying MADIT-II in clinical practice may be proposed. The authors of MADIT-II expressed their hope that market forces will drive down the cost of CDs, and this may represent one of the potential answers to the economic problems raised by this trial. An alternative approach, however, was proposed by J.T. Bigger in an editorial commenting on the MADIT-II trial [11]. He proposed that more careful screening of candidates, with identification within the MADIT-II patients of those likely to obtain the highest benefit, may contribute to better identification of potential candidates for preventive CDs, thus improving cost-effectiveness. Data from a subgroup analysis of the MADIT-II study [12] showing that patients with a wide QRS complex at baseline (>120 ms) had a greater reduction in total mortality than did the whole population suggest a subgroup that may obtain the highest benefit in survival from CD implantation.

It is clear that a reduction in the price of CD devices remains a key point for wider use of CDs, and probably this factor may be more crucial in Europe than in the United States. It has been proposed that simpler and less sophisticated devices ("shock-only devices with a total capability of 8–10 shocks") [13] should be offered at a lower price to reduce the cost of increasing CD use. This proposal to use a "Volkswagen instead of a Rolls-Royce" [13] has to be considered as a possible solution to limit costs for the health care system, but in our view it may have a series of clinical drawbacks, e.g., device exhaustion if arrhythmic storms occur, or loss of full protection after delivery of some shocks because of limited shock capabilities.

In the long term, further evaluation of the cost-effectiveness and cost-utility of CDs is necessary [3] in order to assess in which subgroups of patients CD implantation for primary prevention of sudden death is affordable, despite current economic constraints. Moreover, the perspective of wider use of CDs must also consider the setting of heart failure patients, in whom the impact on survival of both conventional CDs or CDs with biventricular pacing capabilities is currently being evaluated in controlled studies [14–16].

Conclusions

At present we do not know the real economic implications of MADIT-II in Europe, but we may expect great variations in the way this type of strategy is applied by the various European countries. This heterogeneity will reflect differences in the economic status of the countries, in the type of their health care systems, and in the mode of reimbursement for device costs. Moreover, different positions of medical doctors with regard to the potential legal implications of not implanting a CD in a patient with a MADIT-II indication may occur in different cultural and economic situations. Thus, it is clear that the European situation will vary between countries where the general situation and the application of MADIT-II are close to those in the United States (e.g., Germany) and other economic realities where, in view of the economic constraints, prevention of sudden death by costly devices does not appear to be at present a strategy that may be applied in a substantial proportion of patients (Eastern Europe).

References

1. Simoons ML (2003) Cardio-vascular disease in Europe: challenges for the medical profession. Eur Heart J 24:8–12
2. Camm AJ, Nisam S (2000) The utilization of the implantable defibrillator: a European enigma. Eur Heart J 21:1998–2004
3. Boriani G, Biffi M, Martignani C et al (2001) Cost-effectiveness of implantable cardioverter-defibrillators. Eur Heart J 22:990–996
4. Seidl K, Senges J (2002) Geographic differences in implantable cardioverter defibrillator usage. J Cardiovasc Electrophysiol 13(1 Suppl):S100–105
5. Gregoratos G, Abrams J, Epstein AE et al (2002) ACC/AHA/NASPE 2002 guideline update for implantation of cardiac pacemakers and antiarrhythmia devices: a report of the American College of Cardiology/American Heart Association task force on practice guidelines (ACC/AHA/NASPE committee to update the 1998 pacemaker guidelines). J Am Coll Cardiol 40:1703–1719
6. Priori SG, Aliot E, Blomstrom-Lundqvist C et al (2001) Task force on sudden cardiac death of the European Society of Cardiology. Eur Heart J 16:1374–1450
7. Ruskin JN, Camm AJ, Zipes DP et al (2002) Implantable cardioverter defibrillator utilization based on discharge diagnoses from Medicare and managed care patients. J Cardiovasc Electrophysiol 13:38–43
8. Pathmanathan RK, Lau EW, Cooper J et al (1998) Potential impact of antiarrhythmic drugs versus implantable defibrillators on the management of ventricular arrhythmias: the Midlands trial of empirical amiodarone versus electrophysiologically guided intervention and cardioverter implant registry data. Heart 80:68–70
9. Moss AJ, Hall J, Cannom DS et al (1996) Improved survival with an implantable defibrillator in patients with coronary disease at high risk for ventricular arrhythmia. Multicenter Automatic Defibrillator Implantation Trial Investigators. N Engl J Med 335:1933–1940
10. Boersma H, Doornbos G, Bloemberg BPM et al (1999) Cardiovascular diseases in Europe. European Society of Cardiology, Sophia Antipolis, France, pp 1–60

11. Bigger JT (2002) Expanding indications for implantable cardiac defibrillators. N Engl J Med 346:931–933
12. Zareba W (2002) Late breaking clinical trials: noninvasive electrocardiology and outcome in MADIT II patients. NASPE 2002, 23rd scientific session, San Diego, 8–11 May 2002, available at www.naspe.org
13. Zipes DP (2001) Implantable cardioverter-defibrillator: a Volkswagen or a Rolls Royce: how much will we pay to save a life? Circulation 103:1372–1374
14. Cleland JG, Thackray S, Goodge L et al (2002) Outcome studies with device therapy in patients with heart failure. J Cardiovasc Electrophysiol 13 (1 Suppl):S73–S91
15. Bradley DJ, Bradley EA, Baughman KL et al (2003) Cardiac resynchronization and death from progressive heart failure. A meta-analysis of randomized controlled trials. JAMA 289:730–740
16. Bristow MR (2003) Cardiac resynchronization therapy reduces hospitalizations, and cardiac resynchronization therapy and implantable defibrillator reduce mortality in chronic heart failure. Results of the COMPANION trial. Late breaking clinical trials. American College of Cardiology, 52nd Annual Scientific Session, Chicago, 30 March to 2 April 2003

Post-infarction Patients with Left Ventricular Ejection Fraction of 30%–40%, Non-sustained Ventricular Tachycardia, and without Inducible Tachyarrhythmias: Is ICD Therapy Necessary?

H. U. Klein, S. Reek, C. Geller, A. Auricchio

Introduction

Several important trials in the last few years have evaluated the use of the implantable cardioverter-defibrillator (ICD) in patients considered at high risk of sudden death [1–5]. There is little doubt that the ICD is the only approach currently available that is able to reduce the incidence of sudden unexpected arrhythmic death in patients who have survived a myocardial infarction and have a significantly reduced left ventricular (LV) function. Studies such as AVID [1], Muticenter Automatic Defibrillator Implantation Trial (MADIT) [3], and MADIT II [5] have demonstrated that patients with a very low LV ejection fraction (LV-EF, less than 26%) benefit most from the ICD. This, however, does not mean that patients with coronary artery disease with somewhat better-preserved LV function, i.e., LV-EF between 40% and 30%, have a low incidence of sudden arrhythmic death. More than 56% of patients with remote myocardial infarction who later die suddenly have a LV-EF greater than 30% [6]. As stated recently by Buxton [7], it is necessary to identify potential victims of sudden death that can be saved by ICD treatment in this large reservoir of lower-risk post myocardial infarction patients. Since 85%–90% of sudden deaths occur with the first arrhythmic event [8], and only 10%–15% with recurrent arrhythmic episodes, the role of primary prevention of sudden death becomes even more important.

Determination of who needs anti-arrhythmic treatment is a subject of appropriate risk stratification. It has long been accepted that ventricular tachyarrhythmias are associated with increased mortality, especially sudden death, in patients with recent or remote myocardial infarction. Non-invasive risk stratification techniques, such as Holter monitoring, late potential recording, and even more recently introduced approaches like heart rate variability, T-wave alternans, and heart rate turbulence have limitations. They all have rela-

Division of Cardiology, University Hospital Magdeburg, Magdeburg, Germany

tively low positive predictive accuracy, and combined together they are difficult to apply as a widespread technique for risk stratification in primary prevention.

Role of Electrophysiological Testing

Electrophysiological (EP) testing with programmed stimulation has frequently been applied to predict the efficacy of anti-arrhythmic drug treatment for the prevention of ventricular tachycardia (VT) or sudden death in patients with chronic ischemic heart disease [9]. It has been recognized, however, that anti-arrhythmic drugs are ineffective and even dangerous in patients with coronary artery disease. The remarkable success of ICD therapy for the prevention of sudden arrhythmic death has rendered EP study to predict drug efficacy unacceptable.

EP study continues to be used as a risk stratification tool in patients with chronic ischemic heart disease with remote myocardial infarction, since it has been demonstrated that patients with remote myocardial infarction who can be induced into sustained monomorphic VT have a significantly higher risk of future spontaneous VT/VF episodes than patients who cannot be induced into sustained VT [10].

There is still no generally accepted stimulation protocol, but there is agreement that at least three extra stimuli at two right ventricular sites with two driving cycles should be applied. The question of what renders a patient "non-inducible" is still unanswered. The meaning of an induced polymorophic VT is unclear, and the same is true for the induction of only non-sustained VT or short runs of repetitive ventricular responses. The type of stimulation response clearly depends upon the aggressiveness of the stimulation protocol. Therefore, the assessment of "non-inducibility" as a low-risk marker needs a clear definition, and there has to be consensus of what means reproducibility of the induced arrhythmia.

Even before studies like MADIT [3] and Multicenter Unsustained Tachycardia Trial (MUSTT) [4], it could be demonstrated that the highest risk of sudden death is found in patients with impaired LV dysfunction, assessed by a LV-EF of less than 40%, and episodes of non-sustained VT during Holter monitoring [9]. Therefore primary prevention trials studied a patient population with a high enough annual mortality in order to demonstrate improved survival with the implantable defibrillator. Patients with non-sustained VT in a post myocardial infarction setting with poor LV function (LV-EF <40%), who are inducible to sustained VT and remain inducible after administration of anti-arrhythmic drugs, were considered to have a 2-year mortality of about 40% [9]. Therefore both trials, MADIT and MUSTT, used EP testing as a risk stratification technique in order to differentiate between high- and low-risk patients, depending upon suppression of the induced VT or ventricular fibrillation (VF) episode after anti-arrhythmic drug administration. It needs to be emphasized, however, that MUSTT was not designed to be an ICD trial for primary prevention. MUSTT was designed to assess the efficacy of serial EP drug testing. Only inducible patients that remained non-suppressible with anti-arrhythmic drugs received ICD treatment. Nevertheless, both MADIT and MUSTT followed by MADIT II [5] and most likely in the future SCD-Heft set the pace for successful ICD treatment as primary prevention in post myocardial infarction patients with low LV-EF. What is the role of EP testing for risk stratification, and which LV-EF still needs an EP study prior to ICD implantation?

Multicenter Automatic Defibrillator Implantation Trial

The MADIT trial [3] investigated patients with remote myocardial infarction and LV-EF ≤35% who had non-sustained VT (≥3 beats) during Holter monitoring. Sustained VT/VF had to be induced twice and patients were enrolled if intravenous class IA anti-arrhythmic drugs (procainamide) were unable to suppress repeated induction of VT/VF. Patients were randomly assigned to receive either an ICD or conventional medical therapy. The study enrolled 196 patients that were inducible but not suppressed, but the major shortcoming of MADIT was that the participating centers did not keep consistent logs of eligible patients who were not inducible or who were suppressed by procainamide. The long-term outcome of the non-inducible patients and the suppressible patients therefore remained uncertain. Only a few centers reported a sub-study of patients that were eligible but not inducible–and therefore did not receive an ICD [11]. These patients showed a 2-year overall mortality of 8%. MADIT clearly demonstrated that patients with a reduced LV-EF of less than 35%, with non-sustained VT, and inducible non-suppressible VT/VF have a significant benefit of the ICD, being associated with a 54% reduction in overall mortality. Sudden arrhythmic death was reduced to about 75% in the ICD-treated group.

When MADIT patients were classified into a subset of patients with a more-preserved LV-EF of 26%–35% and a subset of patients with a LV-EF of <26%, the real benefit of ICD treatment was found in patients with LV-EF <26%, together with patients with a QRS duration of >120 ms and a need for heart failure treatment [12, 13].

Multicenter Automatic Defibrillator Implantation Trial II

The outcome of MADIT II [5] demonstrated that there is no need for testing VT inducibility or suppressibility of induced VT in patients submitted to ICD treatment with LV-EF ≤30%. Compared with patients that received optimal medical treatment but no ICD, there was a 31% relative reduction of overall mortality with ICD treatment. The hazard ratio for the risk of death from any cause in the ICD arm compared with the conventional arm was 0.69.

Arrhythmic mortality showed a 62 % relative reduction in the ICD group.

The two Kaplan-Meier curves of MADIT and MADIT II show a different behavior. Survival curves of MADIT separate immediately after enrollment of patients with non-sustained VT that was inducible and not suppressible, whereas the Kaplan-Meier curves of survival in MADIT II start to separate after 8 months. This suggests that patients in MADIT II without inducible non-sustained VT seem to have a somewhat lower arrhythmic risk. The benefit of ICD therapy became obvious the longer the trial went on, illustrating that even long after the acute myocardial infarction event sudden arrhythmic death is unpredictable and ICD back-up is needed.

EP Testing in MADIT II

Although EP testing was not a necessary enrollment criterion in MADIT II, 583 ICD-treated patients underwent EP testing at the time or soon after ICD implantation. Of those undergoing EP testing, 64% were non-inducible and 34% became inducible to VT/VF with up to three extra stimuli. During the follow-up period, VT requiring ICD therapy occurred more frequently in patients who were inducible than in those who were non-inducible. Most interesting, however, was the paradoxical finding that spontaneously occurring VF requiring ICD therapy occurred more often in patients who were non-inducible. Altogether, the incidence of VT or VF necessitating ICD intervention was not significantly more frequent in inducible patients [14]. From these interesting findings one can conclude that EP inducibility may be predictive of subsequent occurrence of stable sustained monomorphic VT, but not of the more life-threatening arrhythmic event of VF. Therefore, EP testing is not a very useful stratification technique for high-risk arrhythmic events in patients with remote myocardial infarction and low LV-EF (≤30%).

This conclusion can be confirmed by our own results [15]. Patients who were enrolled in MADIT II underwent repeat EP testing during the follow-up period in order to assess the reproducibility of EP test results. Programmed stimulation was repeatedly performed with device-based testing in subsequent years in 56 MADIT II patients that were randomized to ICD treatment. Of the 23% patients that were inducible during the initial EP test, 27% became non-inducible with the second stimulation. Of the 77% initially non-inducible patients, 18% were inducible with the second EP test. With a third EP test, 60% of patients who were inducible after the second EP test became non-inducible. Of the non-inducible patients after the second test, 11 % became inducible. From our results of repeat EP testing in patients with low LV-EF after myocardial infarction, we conclude that there is poor predictability of inducibility, and therefore risk stratification with EP testing for ICD indication in the MADIT II population is unnecessary.

Multicenter Unsustained Tachycardia Trial

The MUSTT trial [4] enrolled patients with coronary artery disease, remote myocardial infarction who had non-sustained VT during Holter monitoring, and LV dysfunction ≤40%. Patients who were inducible to sustained VT were randomized to receive either anti-arrhythmic therapy selected by EP testing or to remain with no specific anti-arrhythmic treatment. ICD therapy was recommended only after two or three unsuccessful drug regimens.

The primary endpoint of MUSTT was arrhythmic death or resuscitated cardiac arrest. The overall result of MUSTT showed that patients without specific anti-arrhythmic treatment have a 5-year actuarial probability of a life-threatening arrhythmic event of 32%, whereas patients with EP-guided therapy demonstrated an event rate of 25% ($p=0.04$). However, the benefit of anti-arrhythmic treatment was only true for those patients that underwent ICD implantation. The probability of an arrhythmic event was 9% when ICD therapy was used compared with 32% in untreated patients and 37% in patients who received and remained under anti-arrhythmic drug treatment. Data from the MUSTT study support that patients with LV-EF of ≤40% after myocardial infarction who have non-sustained VT that is inducible to VT/VF are best treated with an ICD in order to prevent sudden arrhythmic death.

Different from the MADIT trial, patients in MUSTT who were non-inducible were followed in a registry [16]. This allowed the comparison of non-inducible patients with those who were inducible but did not receive anti-arrhythmic treatment. The 2-year arrhythmic event rate was 12% in the non-inducible patients, but 18% in inducible patients without treatment ($p<0.005$). The 5-year incidence was 24% for the non-inducible and 32% for inducible patients without treatment ($p<0.001$). There was no significant difference in outcome between patients in whom no VT at all, only unsustained VT, or polymorphic sustained VT was induced.

These results from MUSTT emphasize that in patients with more-preserved LV function (LV-EF ≤40%) non-inducibility indicates a lower incidence of future arrhythmic events. EP testing is able to better stratify patients with lower risk of sudden death. The risk of life-threatening arrhythmic events in non-inducible patients remains, however, unacceptably high (12% within 2 years) also mandating ICD protection as primary prevention. This is even more important since only 35% of the eligible MUSTT patients were initially inducible into VT/VF.

Relationship between EF and VT Inducibility

The recently published sub-study of MUSTT patients [16] who did not receive anti-arrhythmic therapy indicates that LV-EF and VT inducibility are independent predictors of arrhythmic death and total mortality. Patients with LV-EF <30% had a significantly higher incidence of total mortality and arrhythmic death than patients with LV-EF of 30%–40%. The percentage of deaths classified as arrhythmic death within total mortality was similar in patients with poor LV-EF (<30%) and better LV-EF (30%–40%). Independent of LV-EF, the relative contribution of arrhythmic events to total mortality was significantly higher in patients with inducible VT/VF than in non-inducible patients (58% versus 46%, p=0.004). It is important to note that the effect of inducibility on the likelihood of arrhythmic death is LV-EF dependent. Patients with LV-EF >30% who were inducible had a higher percentage of arrhythmic deaths (61%) than patients who were not inducible (42%, p=0.002). In contrast, the percentage of arrhythmic deaths in patients with LV-EF <30% was not significantly different between inducible and non-inducible patients. The conclusion from the MUSTT sub-study of patients who did not receive anti-arrhythmic treatment is that both total mortality and arrhythmic mortality is higher in patients with LV-EF <30% and in patients with inducible VT/VF. However, even the non-inducible patients with LV-EF <30% have a sudden death risk of 15% within 2 years and 31% within 5 years, respectively.

Both the non-inducible MADIT patients and the untreated MUSTT patients have an unsatisfactorily high arrhythmic death risk of 8% within 2 years. This may lead to the request that patients with LV-EF between 30% and 40% who are non-inducible with EF testing are also better protected with ICD therapy. There are, however, no trial data to support this. Therefore, until different results are available, patients with a LV-EF between 30% and 40% with non-sustained VT late after myocardial infarction have to be submitted to EP testing, and if they remain non-inducible they should be left without ICD treatment.

Conclusions

The currently available results from primary prevention trials such as MADIT, MADIT II, and MUSTT clearly indicate that patients with remote myocardial infarction and reduced LV function (LV-EF <40%) are best protected against sudden arrhythmic death with implantation of an ICD. Patients with LV-EF <30% do not need further risk stratification, such as Holter monitoring or EP testing. Patients with a LV-EF between 30% and 40% should undergo Holter monitoring and EP testing. Inducibility of VT/VF needs ICD therapy, whereas non-inducible patients should not receive ICD treatment until further data from prospective trials are available showing that even those patients with significantly lower–but still unsatisfactorily high–sudden death mortality have a better outcome with implanted ICDs. So far, inducibility of polymorphic VT even with only one or two extra stimuli does not render the patient "inducible" and does not justify ICD implantation.

References

1. AVID Investigators (1997) A comparison of antiarrhythmic drug therapy with implantable defibrillators in patients resuscitated from near-fatal ventricular arrhythmias. N Engl J Med 337:1576–1583
2. Kuck K-H, Cappato R, Siebels J, Rüppel R (2000) CASH investigators. Randomized comparison of antiarrhythmic drug therapy with implantable defibrillators in patients resuscitated from cardiac arrest: The Cardiac Arrest Study Hamburg (CASH). Circulation 102:748–754
3. Moss AJ, Hall WJ, Cannom DS et al (1996) Improved survival with an implanted defibrillator in patients with coronary disease at high risk for ventricular arrhythmia. Multicenter automatic defibrillator implantation trial investigators. N Engl J Med 335:1933–1940
4. Buxton AE, Lee KL, Fisher JD et al (1999) A randomized study of the prevention of sudden death in patients with coronary artery disease. N Engl J Med 341:1882–1890
5. Moss AJ, Zareba W, Hall WJ et al, for the Multicenter Automatic Defibrillator Implantation Trial II Investigators (2002) Prophylactic implantation of a defibrillator in patients with myocardial infarction and reduced ejection fraction. N Engl J Med 346:877–883
6. Vreede-Swagemakers JJ de, Gorgels AP, Dubois-Arbouw WI et al (1997) Out-of-hospital cardiac arrest in the 1990's: a population-based study in the Maastricht area on incidence, characteristics and survival. J Am Coll Cardiol 30:1500–1505
7. Buxton AE (2003) The clinical use of implantable cardioverter defibrillators: where are we now? Where should we go (editorial). Ann Intern Med 138:512–514
8. Myerburg RJ (2002) Scientific gaps in the prediction and prevention of sudden cardiac death. J Cardiovasc Electrophysiol 13:709–723
9. Wilber DJ, Olshansky B, Moran JF, Scanlon PJ (1990) Electrophysiological testing and nonsustained ventricular tachycardia: use and limitation in patients with coronary artery disease and impaired ventricular function. Circulation 82:350–358
10. Buxton AE, Lee KL, Di Carlo L et al (2002) Electrophysiologic testing to identify patients with coronary artery disease who are at risk for sudden death. Multicenter Unsustained Tachycardia Trial investigators. N Engl J Med 342:1937–1945
11. Daubert JP, Higgins SL, Zareba W, Wilber DJ (1997) Comparative survival of MADIT-eligible but noninducible patients (abstract). J Am Coll Cardiol 25:78A
12. Moss AJ, Fadl Y, Zareba W, Cannom DS, Hall WJ (2001) Survival benefit with an implanted defibrillator in relation to mortality risk in chronic coronary heart disease. Am J Cardiol 88:516–520
13. Moss AJ (2000) Implantable cardioverter defibrillator therapy. The sickest patients benefit the most. Circulation 101:1638–1640
14. Daubert JP, Zareba W, Schuger CD et al (2003) Does EPS inducibility in MADIT II patients predict subsequent VT and/or VF events? (abstract). Pacing Clin Electrophysiol 26:960
15. Reek S, Klein HU, Neumann T et al (2003) Reproducibility of electrophysiologic testing in patients with remote myocardial infarction and severe left ventricular dysfunction: MADIT II Substudy (abstract). Pacing Clin Electrophysiol 26:960
16. Buxton AE, Lee KL, Hafley GE et al (2002) Relation of ejection fraction and inducible ventricular tachycardia to mode of death in patients with coronary artery disease. Circulation 106:2466–2472

Secondary Prevention of Sudden Death in Post-Infarction Patients: When is ICD Implantation Really Cost-Effective?

S. R. Raj[1], R. S. Sheldon[2]

Introduction

Implantable cardioverter defibrillator (ICD) use has grown rapidly due to a combination of factors, including improvements in device technology, evidence from randomized clinical trials and the intuitive appeal of an "electrical life insurance policy". Unfortunately, the ICD is quite expensive. This has led to recent efforts to determine whether and when ICD implantation is cost-effective from a societal perspective, as opposed to a patient perspective. We will briefly review the clinical trial evidence for cost-effectiveness in the secondary prevention of sudden cardiac death with an ICD in a post-myocardial infarction population.

Three large randomized trials compared the efficacy of ICDs versus antiarrhythmic drug therapy: the Antiarrhythmic Versus Defibrillator (AVID) trial [1], the Canadian Implantable Defibrillator Study (CIDS) [2], and the Cardiac Arrest Study Hamburg (CASH) [3]. AVID [1] assessed the relative benefit of antiarrhythmic drugs versus ICDs on the survival of patients who had been resuscitated from ventricular fibrillation; or who had ventricular tachycardia (VT) with syncope; or had hemodynamically significant sustained VT with a left ventricular ejection fraction ≤ 40%. The primary endpoint was total mortality using an intention to treat analysis, with a pre-specified cost-effectiveness analysis using prospectively collected data. Of the 1885 patients eligible for randomization, 1016 patients were randomized to therapy with an ICD (n=507) or antiarrhythmic drug therapy (n=509). The subjects were 80% male with a mean age of 65 ± 10 years. The 2 study groups matched well. Of the 509 patients randomized to drug therapy, 496 received empiric amiodarone therapy and 13 received sotalol.

Over a mean follow-up of 18.2 ± 12.2 months, the crude death rates were 15.8 ± 3.2% (n=80) in the ICD group and 24 ± 3.7% (n=122) in the antiarrhythmic drug group. The ICD group had a greater survival than the antiar-

[1]Departments of Medicine and Pharmacology, Vanderbilt University, Nashville, Tennessee, USA; [2]Cardiovascular Research Group, University of Calgary, Calgary, Alberta, Canada

rhythmic drug group at 1 year (89.3% vs. 82.3% survival); at 2 years (81.6% vs. 74.7%); and at 3 years (75.4% vs. 64.1%). While the results of AVID are statistically significant, the unadjusted prolongation of life by ICD therapy was only 2.7 months over the first 3 years. Furthermore, this benefit came at a cost of more rehospitalizations in the ICD group (75%) than in the drug group (65%) at 2 years.

CIDS [2] enrolled 659 patients who were eligible for randomization to either amiodarone, or an ICD if they had documented ventricular fibrillation; had out an out of hospital cardiac arrest requiring electrical shock; sustained VT causing syncope; sustained VT ≥ 150 beats per minute in patients with left ventricular ejection fraction ≤ 35% associated with symptoms of hemodynamic compromise; or had unmonitored syncope with later documentation of spontaneous VT or sustained VT induced during an electrophysiological study. The primary endpoint was total mortality. All patients were followed for at least 1 year, with a cumulative follow-up of 48 months. There was a nonsignificant trend towards a reduction in total mortality in the ICD group (8.3%/year) compared with the amiodarone group (10.2%/year). This was almost entirely due to a nonsignificant reduction in the risk of arrhythmic death with the ICD compared with amiodarone (3.0%/year vs. 4.5%/year; p=0.09). The cumulative total mortality risk in the ICD group and amiodarone group at 1 year was 9.5% vs. 11.2%; at 2 years was 14.8% vs. 21.0%; and at 3 years was 23.3% vs. 27.1%. While there was an almost 30% relative risk reduction at 2 years, it was only 15% by 3 years. With over 300 patients still being followed at 3 years, this finding may represent a true diminution of the benefit of the ICD over time.

CASH [3] was an open-label comparison of antiarrhythmic drug therapy versus ICD for survivors of cardiac arrest due to a sustained VT. There was a more restrictive enrollment criterion used than in either AVID or CIDS. CASH began randomizing patients in 1987 equally to metoprolol, propafenone, amiodarone, or ICD. The primary study endpoint was total mortality. The propafenone arm of the study was prematurely terminated after an interim analysis revealed that this group had a significantly higher mortality rate (29.3%) compared with the ICD group (11.5%; p=0.01). A total of 288 patients were recruited to the remaining 3 arms of the study: 99 to the ICD group, 92 to the amiodarone group, and 97 to the metoprolol group. For final analysis, the amiodarone and metoprolol groups were combined into one antiarrhythmic drug group. Over a mean follow-up 57 ± 34 months, the crude death rate in the antiarrhythmic drug group (44.4%) was non-significantly greater than in the ICD group (36.4%, p=0.08).

The data from AVID, CIDS and CASH were pooled and analyzed in a meta-analysis [4]. The fixed effects analysis showed that the ICD benefit was consistent throughout the 3 studies (p heterogeneity = 0.31). The risk reduction for total mortality with the ICD over amiodarone was 28% (95% CI: 13% to 40%; p=0.0006). For arrhythmic death, the relative risk reduction was 50% (95% CI: 33% to 63%; p<0.0001). Over a follow-up period of 6 years, the mean survival was extended by 4.4 months with the ICD.

Cost-Effectiveness Analysis of the ICD for Secondary Prevention of SCD

ICD therapy has been demonstrated to save lives in several patient groups [4]. However, can society afford such an expensive medical therapy? Given the numerous health care interventions competing for the same health care resources, does the increased availability of ICD therapy provide society with optimal use of its resources [5]?

Basic Principles

A cost-effectiveness analysis quantifies the cost and health outcome for various treatments for a given disorder. The primary health outcomes in these studies are differences in life expectancy. This is an incremental cost-effectiveness analysis, which is the difference in costs between the two therapies divided by the difference in life expectancy between the two therapies, expressed in dollars per life year saved [5]. By convention, therapies are considered "cost-effective" if the cost per life year saved, in US dollars, is < $40,000; are considered "borderline cost-effective" if they are between $40,001-$60,000; and are considered "expensive" or "unattractive" if they are >$60,000 [6].

Early Decision Analysis Models

In the 1990s, several cost-effectiveness analyses of ICD therapy were performed using decision analysis models [7-10]. These models considered the cost-effectiveness of ICD among patients for the secondary prevention of ventricular arrhythmias. Therapy with an ICD was compared with amiodarone in the majority of the cases.

Kuppermann et al. [7] compared costs for 203 patients treated with an ICD with historical controls from the pre-ICD era treated with conventional drug therapy. Mortality data were extracted from observational data in the contemporary published literature. Over a projected lifetime time horizon, the incremental cost-effectiveness was $7,400 per year of life saved. This was based upon an estimated gain in life of 1.9 years. Larson et al. [8] compared ICD therapy with amiodarone over a lifetime time horizon. Costs were based upon just 64 patients from the New England Medical Center (21 ICD treated patients and 43 amiodarone treated patients). The estimated gain in life from an ICD over amiodarone was 2.22 years, with a cost-effectiveness ratio of $13,800 per year of life saved.

Owens et al. [10] used a decision analysis model of ICD versus amiodarone assessed over a lifetime time horizon, with effectiveness data taken from preliminary clinical trial and ICD registry data. Their cost-effectiveness estimates were very sensitive to assumptions about the incremental benefit of the ICD over amiodarone. If the ICD reduced mortality by 40%, then the incremental cost-effectiveness was $37,300 per life year saved. However, if the mortality reduction with an ICD was only 20%, then the incremental cost-effectiveness increased to $74,400 per life year saved. The early decision analysis models all put estimates of the incremental cost-effectiveness of an ICD over amiodarone (or drug therapy) in the "cost-effective" range, but these studies greatly overestimated ICD effectiveness [5], with estimates of life-years gained from the ICD of around 2 years.

Cost-Effectiveness from Randomized Clinical Trial Data

The AVID economic analysis sub-study collected hospital and drug charges for 1008 patients and very detailed records of expenses for a subgroup of 237 patients [11]. Charges were converted to cost and data from the "detailed" subgroup was extrapolated to the overall study. Over a 3-year time horizon, the ICD group had a 0.21-year survival advantage over the antiarrhythmic drug group, and the incremental cost-effectiveness ratio was $66,677 per year of life saved by the ICD. These data suggest that the benefits of the ICD over amiodarone were moderately unattractive from a cost-effective perspective [6].

The CIDS economic analysis [12] was conducted on the first 430 patients enrolled in the Canadian Implantable Defibrillator Study (CIDS) [2], but were extrapolated to the entire study population. The CIDS analysis had the longest time horizon (6 years) of the clinical trial-based economic analyses. The ICD prolonged life by a mean of 0.23 years over this time span. Costs were calculated from a single payer (government) viewpoint, with all patients assumed to have a non-thoracotomy ICD for the purpose of the cost calculation [12]. Costs were reported in 1999 Canadian dollars, but have been converted here to US dollars (C$1~US$0.65). The mean cost per patient was $31,925 greater in the ICD group than in the amiodarone group. The incremental cost-effectiveness of the ICD over amiodarone was $138,803 per life year gained. These clearly fall into an "unattractive" cost-effectiveness range [6]. O'Brien et al. also performed cost analysis with extrapolations out to 12 years. The incremental cost-effectiveness ratios ranged from $64,623 to $97,312 per year of life saved, depending on whether the survival curves continue to diverge, or converge beyond the available data [12]. The ICD did not become cost-effective under any conditions.

Are ICDs More Cost-Effective in Certain Patient Subgroups?

It would be ideal to provide ICDs mainly to those patients who derive benefit from them. Several clinical factors have been examined.

Left Ventricular Ejection Fraction

Subgroup analysis from AVID [13] reported no mortality benefit from the ICD compared to amiodarone in patients with a left ventricular ejection fraction > 35%. Domanski et al. [13] divided the AVID population into 3 groups based on left ventricular ejection fraction. A statistically significant benefit was seen in the group with an ejection fraction between 20-35%. A similar risk reduction was seen in the group with an ejection fraction < 20%, but the confidence intervals were wide due to small numbers in this group. The incremental cost of the ICD over antiarrhythmic therapy in AVID was extremely unfavorable among patients with an ejection fraction > 35% ($536,106 per year of life saved), while it was on the margin of cost-effective among patients with an ejection fraction ≤ 35% ($60,967 per year of life saved) [11]. In patients in the CIDS study with a left ventricular ejection fraction < 35%, the cost-effectiveness becomes more attractive at $70,515 per life year saved [12].

CIDS Score

We conducted a subgroup analysis of the CIDS study with the main intention of predicting risk of death based on entry clinical criteria [14]. These were advanced age (≥ 70 years), poor left ventricular ejection fraction (≤ 35%) and poor functional status (New York Heart Association Class III or IV). This predicted a highly significant gradation in risk of death. In the highest risk quartile, the ICD provided a 50% relative risk reduction, whereas there was not a significant benefit of the ICD in the remaining 3 lower risk quartiles (Fig. 1). Therefore, the sickest patients did benefit the most. From this we created a simple score that predicted benefit from the ICD compared to amiodarone therapy. Patients received 1 point for each of: age > 70 years, left ventricular

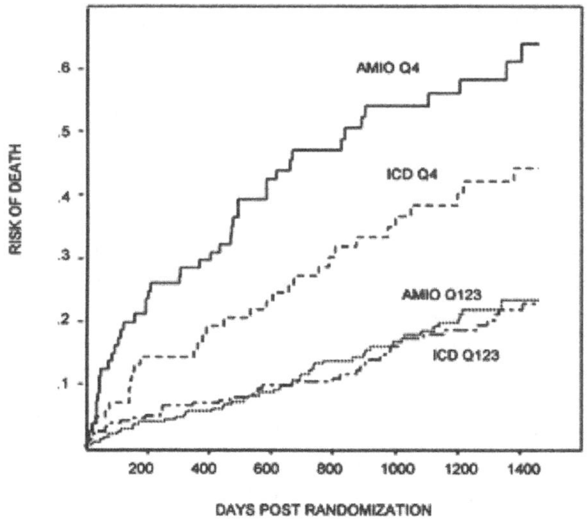

Fig. 1. Risk stratification in CIDS. The ICD decreased the risk of death compared with amiodarone, only in the quartile of patients with the highest risk (Q4). No benefit was seen in the 3 lower risk quartiles (Q123). Reproduced with permission from [14]

ejection fraction < 35%, and ≥ NYHA class III. Thirteen of the fifteen deaths prevented by the ICD occurred among patients with ≥ 2 risk factors. Use of a dichotomous score of ≥ 2 risk factors identified the patients who would benefit from ICD therapy with 87% sensitivity and 98% specificity in CIDS, and 79% sensitivity and 91% specificity in AVID [15]. The benefit of the ICD was concentrated in 25% of patients in CIDS and in 31% of patients in AVID. Patients with ≥ 2 risk factors in both the CIDS and AVID studies had approximately 50% reductions in the likelihood of death with ICD therapy, while the remaining patients were very unlikely to benefit from ICD therapy over medical therapy. If patients had ≥ 2 CIDS risk factors [14], the incremental cost of the ICD decreases to $42,377 per year of life saved, which would be cost-effective [16] by conventional standards.

Summary of Cost Effectiveness Trial Data

The early decision analysis models used overly optimistic projections of the survival benefit of ICD over antiarrhythmic drug therapy. This consequently led to incremental cost-effectiveness estimates that were significantly more favorable than has been borne from recent clinical trials. However, by using simple selection tools, such as low left ventricular ejection fraction or a high CIDS score, we can select patients in whom the ICD is cost-effective for the secondary prevention of sudden cardiac death from a societal perspective.

Acknowledgements. This work was supported in part by grant GR13914 from the Canadian Institutes of Health Research, Ottawa, Canada. Dr. Raj is a Vanderbilt Clinical Research Scholar, supported by a K12 grant from the National Institutes of Health, Bethesda, MD, USA.

References

1. The Antiarrhythmics versus Implantable Defibrillators Investigators (1997) A comparison of antiarrhythmic-drug therapy with implantable defibrillators in patients resuscitated from near-fatal ventricular arrhythmias. N Engl J Med 337:1576-1583
2. Connolly SJ, Gent M, Roberts RS et al (2000) Canadian implantable defibrillator study: a randomized trial of the implantable cardioverter defibrillator against amiodarone. Circulation 101:1297-1302
3. Kuck KH, Cappato R, Siebels J, Ruppel R (2000) Randomized comparison of antiarrhythmic drug therapy with implantable defibrillators in patients resuscitated from cardiac arrest: the Cardiac Arrest Study Hamburg (CASH). Circulation 102:748-754
4. Connolly SJ, Hallstrom AP, Cappato R et al (2000) Meta-analysis of the implantable cardioverter defibrillator secondary prevention trials. AVID, CASH and CIDS studies. Eur Heart J 21:2071-2078
5. O'Brien BJ (2000) Chapter 3. Cost effectiveness of ICD therapy: a review of published evidence. Can J Cardiol 16:1307-1312

6. Goldman L, Gordon DJ, Rifkind BM et al (1992) Cost and health implications of cholesterol lowering. Circulation 85:1960-1968
7. Kuppermann M, Luce BR, McGovern B et al (1990) An analysis of the cost effectiveness of the implantable defibrillator. Circulation 81:91-100
8. Larsen GC, Manolis AS, Sonnenberg FA et al (1992) Cost-effectiveness of the implantable cardioverter-defibrillator: effect of improved battery life and comparison with amiodarone therapy. J Am Coll Cardiol 19:1323-1334
9. Kupersmith J, Hogan A, Guerrero P et al (1995) Evaluating and improving the cost-effectiveness of the implantable cardioverter-defibrillator. Am Heart J 130:507-515
10. Owens DK, Sanders GD, Harris RA et al (1997) Cost-effectiveness of implantable cardioverter defibrillators relative to amiodarone for prevention of sudden cardiac death. Ann Intern Med 126:1-12
11. Larsen G, Hallstrom A, McAnulty J et al (2002) Cost-effectiveness of the implantable cardioverter-defibrillator versus antiarrhythmic drugs in survivors of serious ventricular tachyarrhythmias: results of the AVID economic analysis substudy. Circulation 105:2049-2057
12. O'Brien BJ, Connolly SJ, Goeree R et al (2001) Cost-effectiveness of the implantable cardioverter-defibrillator : results from the canadian implantable defibrillator study (CIDS). Circulation 103:1416-1421
13. Domanski MJ, Sakseena S, Epstein AE et al (1999) Relative effectiveness of the implantable cardioverter-defibrillator and antiarrhythmic drugs in patients with varying degrees of left ventricular dysfunction who have survived malignant ventricular arrhythmias. J Am Coll Cardiol 34:1090-1095
14. Sheldon R, Connolly S, Krahn A et al (2000) Identification of patients most likely to benefit from implantable cardioverter-defibrillator therapy: the Canadian Implantable Defibrillator Study. Circulation 101:1660-1664
15. Exner DV, Sheldon RS, Pinski SL et al (2001) Do baseline characteristics accurately discriminate between patients likely versus unlikely to benefit from implantable defibrillator therapy? Evaluation of the Canadian implantable defibrillator study implantable cardioverter defibrillatory efficacy score in the antiarrhythmics versus implantable defibrillators trial. Am Heart J 141:99-104
16. Sheldon R, O'Brien BJ, Blackhouse G et al (2001) Effect of clinical risk stratification on cost-effectiveness of the implantable cardioverter-defibrillator: the Canadian implantable defibrillator study. Circulation 104:1622-1626

Primary Prevention of Sudden Death in Post-Infarction Patients: When ICD Implantation is Really Cost-effective

S.C. Hammill

Introduction

The implantable cardioverter defibrillator (ICD) has been convincingly demonstrated to reduce mortality in randomized clinical trials that have assessed this treatment strategy for both primary and secondary prevention of sudden cardiac death [1-6]. This important advance in therapy has the potential to reduce the risk of sudden cardiac death which now affects over 400,000 persons in the United States each year. The estimated number of ICD implantations for 2003 is expected to exceed 100,000 worldwide.

Unfortunately, this effective therapy comes with a high price tag which has a negative effect on the medical system by taking money from other therapies. The recent Multicenter Unsustained Tachycardia Trial [6] (MUSTT) and Multicenter Automatic Defibrillator Implantation Trials [4, 5] (MADIT - I and II) have evaluated the large population of patients who are at risk of sudden cardiac death but have not experienced their first episode. These studies found the ICD to be effective in reducing subsequent sudden cardiac death. However, Medicare is concerned with the added financial burden to the medical system as a result of this expensive technology and has not approved reimbursement for MADIT II indications at this time. This paper will review the issues of effectiveness and cost as it relates to the ICD.

ICD Effectiveness in Randomized Clinical Trials

The ICD has been reported in six prospective randomized clinical trials to be of benefit in both primary and secondary prevention of sudden cardiac death. The three secondary prevention trials [Anti-arrhythmic vs. Implantable Defibrillators [1] (AVID), Canadian Implantable Defibrillator Study [2] (CIDS),

Department of Internal Medicine, Cardiovascular Division, Mayo Clinic, Rochester, Minnesota, USA

and Cardiac Arrest Survival Hamburg [3] (CASH)] and three primary prevention trials [4-6] (MADIT I, MADIT II, MUSTT) have demonstrated that the ICD is superior to conventional therapy in reducing overall mortality compared to the primary anti-arrhythmic drug, amiodarone. The relative risk reduction has ranged between 31 % and 55 % in primary prevention and between 20 % and 41 % in secondary prevention trials (Fig. 1). The relative risk reduction has consistently been higher in the primary as opposed to the secondary prevention trials.

The MADIT I trial [4] involved a complex protocol with enrolled patients being at least three weeks post-myocardial infarction, having nonsustained ventricular tachycardia, Class I-III congestive heart failure, and an ejection fraction under 35 %. Patients underwent electrophysiologic (EP) testing, and if they had inducible ventricular tachycardia, they were retested with intravenous procainamide. If they continued to have inducible tachycardia, they were randomized to conventional therapy or the ICD. The MUSTT [6] protocol tested the hypothesis that patients with coronary artery disease, ejection fraction less than 40 % and nonsustained ventricular tachycardia had a reduced risk for arrhythmic death and cardiac arrest with anti-arrhythmic therapy guided by EP testing in patients with inducible, sustained ventricular tachycardia. This trial reported three treatment groups: patients who underwent EP-guided therapy and a successful anti-arrhythmic was identified, patients who underwent EP guided therapy and received an ICD after failing anti-arrhythmics,

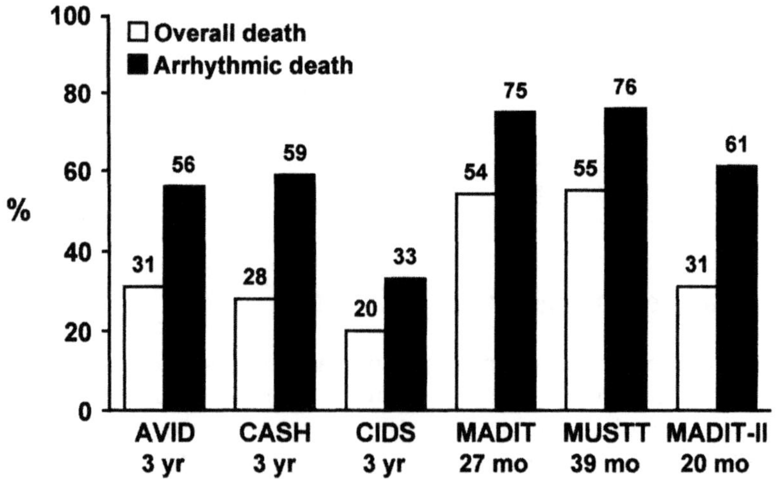

Fig. 1. Relative risk reduction associated with the ICD in the three secondary prevention trials (AVID, CASH, CIDS) and the three primary prevention trials (MADIT, MUSTT, MADIT II) [1-6]

and patients who had inducible ventricular tachycardia at EP testing and were randomized to no EP-guided anti-arrhythmic therapy. The MADIT II [5] study was much more simply designed, enrolling patients with a history of myocardial infarction at least 30 days prior to enrollment and an ejection fraction under 30 %. Patients were excluded if they had Class IV congestive heart failure, coronary bypass grafting within three months, or other significant disease. One thousand two hundred and thirty-two patients were enrolled in MADIT II and randomized using a 3:2 randomization scheme. Four hundred ninety patients underwent conventional therapy, and 742 patients ICD therapy. The study was stopped early at 20 months when a 31 % reduction in overall mortality and a 61 % reduction in arrhythmic death was observed. These three studies indicate that primary prevention of sudden cardiac death in high risk patients with coronary artery disease is successfully achieved using the ICD.

The MADIT II [5] study, if widely accepted, will significantly increase the number of ICD implantations. This study showed ICD improved survival in all sub-populations tested. However, the most effective results in reducing sudden death were observed in the following groups: under age 60, female, ejection fraction under 25 %, and QRS duration > 0.15 s. Zareba and associates evaluated the MADIT II population to determine if risk stratification tests could predict death with higher accuracy (NASPE presentation, 2002). They assessed the standard ECG, signal-averaged ECG, heart rate variability and EP testing. Only the presence of atrial fibrillation and a QRS duration > 0.12 s on the standard ECG predicted sudden death using multivariate analysis. The reduction in mortality in ICD patients ranged from 24 % in those with a QRS duration < 0.12 s to 63 % in those with a QRS duration > 0.15 seconds (Fig. 2).

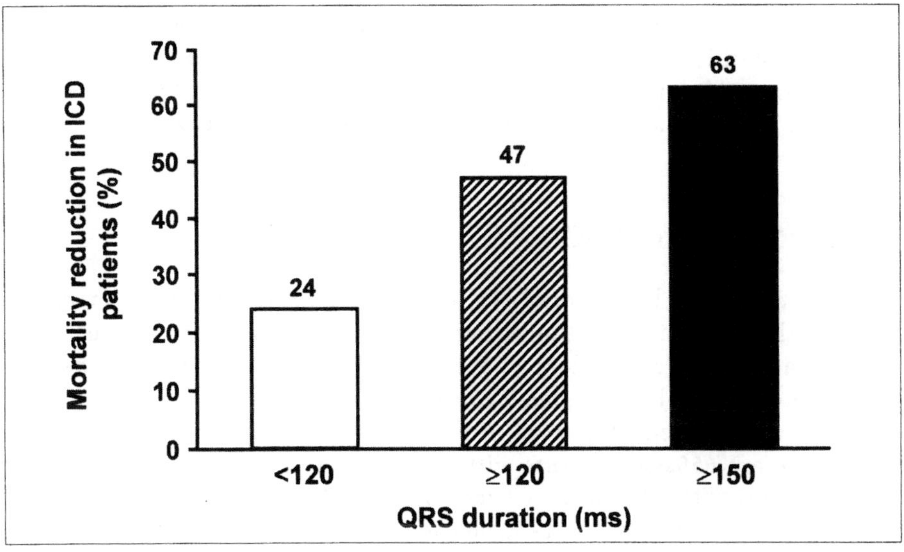

Fig. 2. Mortality reduction in ICD patients in the MADIT II trial based upon the resting ECG QRS duration (W. Zareba, NASPE Late Break Trials Presentation, San Diego, 2002)

The MADIT II study was associated with a 30 % reduction in mortality. At three years, the survival was projected to be 78 % with the ICD and 69 % with conventional therapy: a 3 % absolute survival benefit per year. This compares favorably to amiodarone which has not been demonstrated to achieve significant survival in patients following myocardial infarction. When compared with other cardiovascular trials, the ICD in the MADIT II population was associated with a similar or improved reduction in mortality [7-13].

Primary Prevention Trials in Progress

Three primary prevention studies are in progress which are anticipated to add important information to determine the proper role of ICD therapy to prevent sudden cardiac death [14]. The Beta Blocker Strategy Plus Implantation Cardioverter Defibrillator (BEST-ICD) trial began enrollment in June 1998 and evaluates whether EP guided ICD therapy will improve survival in high risk post-myocardial infarction being treated with beta blockers. Patients enrolled in this study are 5-21 days following myocardial infarction with an ejection fraction under 35 % and able to tolerate metoprolol. They are randomized to either beta blocker therapy alone, or EP guided ICD therapy. The Defibrillator in Acute Myocardial Infarction Trial (DINAMIT) assesses the use of the ICD following myocardial infarction in patients with an ejection fraction under 35 % and abnormal heart rate variability. The third trial is the Sudden Cardiac Death in Heart Failure Trial (SCD-Heft). This trial started in 1997 and tests whether amiodarone or ICD improves survival in patients with Class II or Class III congestive heart failure and ejection fraction under 36 %. All patients receive conventional therapy, with beta blockers encouraged, and are randomized to ICD, amiodarone, or placebo. Patients with ischemic and non-ischemic cardiomyopathies are enrolled in this study. The results of these trials are eagerly awaited because of the additional information they will provide to better define which patients receive the most benefit from the ICD.

Cost Effectiveness of the ICD

Dr. Bigger stated in his editorial [15] reviewing ICD therapy for primary prevention that "even the wealthiest nations cannot afford to pay to use every medical advance in any patient who might benefit". Indeed, the cost effectiveness of the ICD has been the main concern limiting its application for primary prevention of sudden cardiac death in high risk patients. It is estimated [16] that there are 650,000 patients with myocardial infarction per year in the United States with 433,300 survivors, 10 % of whom would have an ejection fraction ≤ 30 %. This results in 43,000 patients who could potentially receive an ICD at an average implantation cost of $35,000 for a total of $1.5 billion dollars to the medical system.

Cost effectiveness has been assessed in the secondary prevention trials with AVID reporting a cost of $66,677 per year of life saved by the ICD compared to anti-arrhythmics [17]. The CIDS database was evaluated to identify factors that would indicate increased risk for sudden cardiac death: advanced age, ejection fraction < 35 %, and Class II-III congestive heart failure. If no risk factors were present, the cost per year of life gained (Canadian dollars) was greater than $1 million. In contrast, if there was one risk factor, the cost was $238,388; two risk factors $96,718; and three risk factors $23,344 [18]. Clearly, the ICD is expensive therapy for secondary prevention and requires proper patient selection. Recent studies [19] have demonstrated that the ICD does not confer significant benefit compared to anti-arrhythmic drug therapy in patients who have survived a malignant ventricular arrhythmia when the ejection fraction is greater than 35 %. Cost effectiveness appears to be more favorable when the ICD is used for primary prevention. The cost effectiveness in MADIT I was $39,764 per life year gained [20]. A review of all randomized trials [21] showed a 23 % risk reduction due to the ICD and $31,500 per life year added.

A treatment is considered highly cost effective if the ratio ranges between 0 and $20,000 per year of life saved; cost effective between $20,000 and $40,000 per year of life saved; and borderline between $40,000 and $60,000 per year of life saved [13]. Therapies are considered to be expensive if they cost between $60,000 and $100,000 per year of life saved and prohibitive if greater than $100,000 per year of life saved. Therapies such as the ICD that are under $50,000 per year of life saved are considered to fall between cost effective and borderline cost effective (Fig. 3).

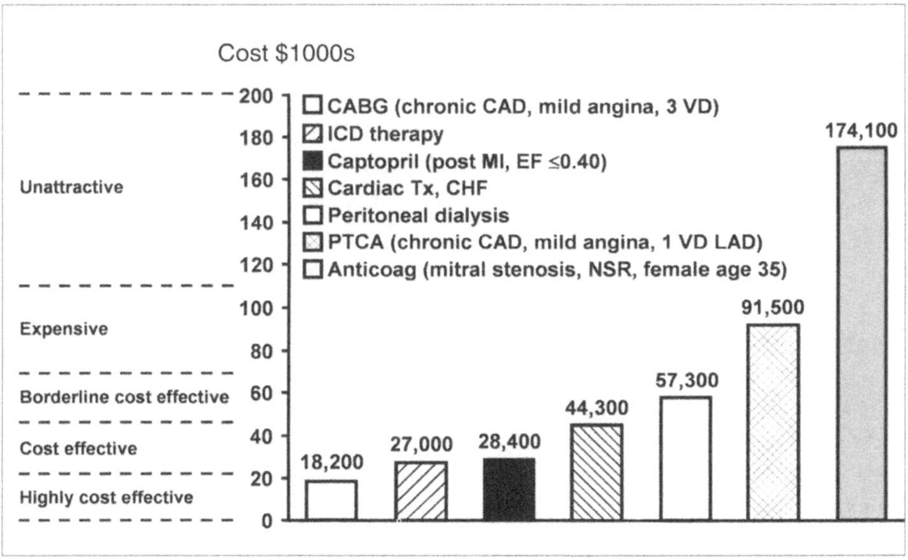

Fig. 3. Cost per year of life saved associated with various treatments used in patients with heart disease[13]

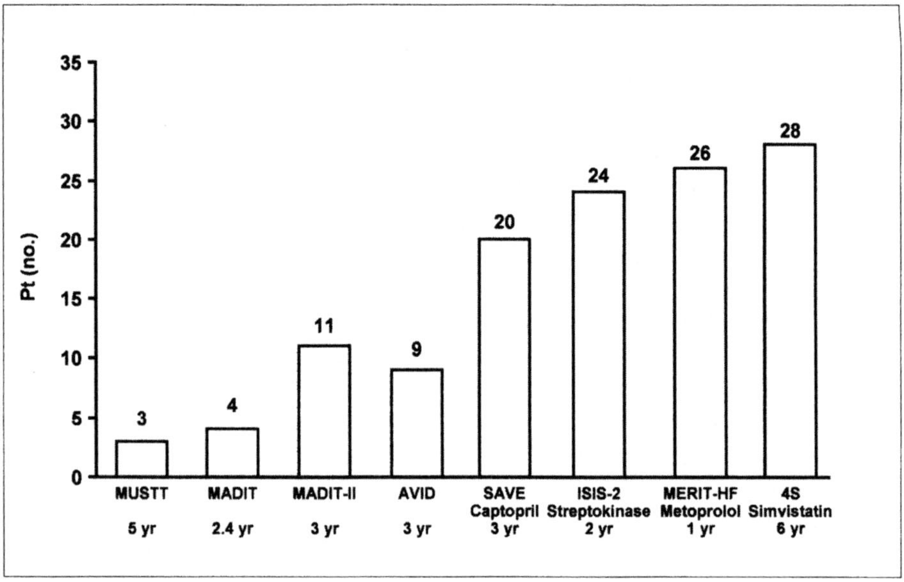

Fig. 4. Number of patients treated to prevent one death in representative primary and secondary prevention ICD trials compared with other treatments for patients with heart disease [13]

As the ICD implantation criteria become less stringent, the mortality decreases and, presumably, cost effectiveness become less appealing. In MADIT I, four ICDs had to be implanted to save one life at three years while in MADIT II, 11 ICDs had to be implanted to save one life at three years. These numbers do compare favorably with other therapies including angiotension converting enzyme (ACE) inhibitors for congestve heart failure (CHF) and statins for elevated cholesterol (Fig. 4).

MADIT II opened the ICD therapy to a much larger group of patients but, in so doing, reduced the effectiveness of the therapy [13]. It is assumed that this will also reduce the cost effectiveness of the therapy but that data has not been released.

Conclusions

The ICD does not appear to offer significant mortality benefit or cost effectiveness in patients with an ejection fraction greater than 35 % when compared to anti-arrhythmic drugs, primarily amiodarone. Prospective studies are needed to establish the effect of an ejection fraction greater than 35 % on the relative treatment effect of ICD and anti-arrhythmic drugs. At lower ejection fractions, the ICD offers improved survival when compared with anti-arrhythmic drugs. It is anticipated that the cost effectiveness of the ICD as primary prevention of sudden cardiac death in high risk patients will improve due to the following: 1) more favorable market forces decreasing the cost of the ICD, 2) improved screening of patients who might benefit from the ICD, such as the QRS duration reported in the MADIT II population, and 3) producing a simpler, less costly ICD to be used for primary prevention and then advance to more sophisticated therapy if necessary. Unfortunately, the current situation causes significant stress to the medical community when attempting to balance therapy that has been demonstrated in well-designed, randomized controlled trials to reduce mortality, with the progressively increasing cost to an already thinned and threatened medical system. The cost effectiveness of the ICD as prophylactic therapy remains a barrier to the wider use of this approach. In the future, it will be important for the physician to match the patient to the proper device by improving identification of high risk patients and for industry to make available a wider range of low cost, less sophisticated ICDs as an option to the physician.

References

1. AVID-Investigators (1997) A comparison of antiarrhythmic drug therapy with implantable defibrillator in patients resuscitated from near-fatal ventricular arrhythmias. The Antiarrhythmics Versus Implantable Defibrillators (AVID) investigators. N Engl J Med 337:1576-1583
2. Connolly SJ, Gent M, Roberts RS et al (2000) Canadian Implantable Defibrillator Study (CIDS): a randomized trial of the implantable cardioverter-defibrillator against amiodarone. Circulation 101:1297-1302
3. Kuck KH, Cappato R, Siebels J, Ruppel R (2000) Randomized comparison of antiarrhythmic drug therapy with implantable defibrillators in patients resuscitated from cardiac arrest: The Cardiac Arrest Study Group (CASH). Circulation 102(7):748-754
4. Moss AJ, Hall J, Cannom DS et al (1996) Improved survival with an implantable cardioverter-defibrillator in patients with coronary disease at high risk for ventricular arrhythmia. Multicenter automatic defibrillator implantation trial investigators. N Engl J Med 335(26):1933-1940
5. Moss AJ, Zareba W, Hall WJ et al (2002) Prophylactic implantation of a defibrillator in patients with myocardial infarction and reduced ejection fraction. N Engl J Med 346:877-883
6. Buxton AE, Lee K, Fisher JD et al (1999) A randomized study of the prevention of sudden death in patients with coronary artery disease. Multicenter unsustained tachycardia trial investigators. N Engl J Med 341:1882-1890
7. Pfeffer MA, Braunwald E, Moye LA et al (1992) Effect of captopril on mortality and morbidity in patients with left ventricular dysfunction after myocardial infarction. Results of the survival and ventricular enlargement trial. The SAVE investigators. N Engl Med 327:669-677
8. SOLVD Investigators (1991) Effect of enalapril on survival in patients with reduced left ventricular ejection fractions and congestive heart failure. The SOLVD-Investigators. N Engl J Med 325:293-302
9. CIBIS-Investigators (1999) The cardiac insufficiency bisprolol study II (CIBIS-II): a randomized trial. Lancet 353:9-13

10. ISIS-2 Collaborative Group (1988) Randomized trial of intravenous streptokinase, oral aspirin, both, or neither among ISIS-2 (Second international study of infarct survival). Lancet 2:349-360
11. Merit-HF Study Group (1999) Effect of metoprolol CR/XL in chronic heart failure: Metoprolol CR/XL randomized intervention trial in congestive heart failure (MERIT-HF). Lancet 353:2001-2007
12. 4 S Investigators (1994) Randomized trial of cholesterol lowering in 4444 patients with coronary heart disease: Scandinavian Simvastain Survival Study (4S). Lancet 344:1383-1389
13. Seidl K, Senges J (2003) Worldwide utilization of implantable cardioverter-defibrillator now and in the future. Cardiac Electrophysiology Review, In Press
14. Essebag V, Eisenberg MJ (2003) Expanding indications for defibrillators after myocardial infarction: risk stratification and cost effectiveness. Cardiac Electrophysiology Review (*in press*)
15. Bigger JT (2002) Expanding indications for implantable cardiac defibrillators. N Engl J Med 346:931-933
16. Sanders GD, Hlatky MA, Every NR et al (2001) Potential cost effectiveness of prophylactic use of the implantable cardioverter-defibrillator after myocardial infarction. Ann Int Med 135:870-883
17. Larsen G, Hallstrom A, McAnulty J et al (2002) Cost-effectiveness of the implantable cardioverter-defibrillator versus antiarrhythmic drugs in survivors of serious ventricular tachyarrhythmias. Circulation 105:2049-2057
18. Sheldon R, O'Brien BJ, Blackhouse G et al (2001) Effect of clinical risk stratification on cost-effectiveness of the implantable cardioverter-defibrillator: the Canadian implantable defibrillator study. Circulation 104(14):1622-1626
19. Domanski MJ, Sakseena S, Epstein A et al (1999) Relative effectiveness of the implantable cardioverter-defibrillator and antiarrhythmic drugs in patients with varying degrees of left ventricular dysfunction who have survived malignant ventricular arrhythmias. J Am Coll Cardiol 34:1090-1095
20. Boriani G, Biffi M, Martignani et al (2001) Cost-effectiveness of implantable cardioverter-defibrillators. Euro Hrt J 22:990-996
21. Hlatiky MA, Bigger T (2001) Cost-effectiveness of the implantable cardioverter-defibrillator. Lancet 357:1817-1818

Cost-Effectiveness of ICD Implantation in Clinical Settings Different From Ischemic Heart Disease: What Do We Know?

G. Boriani, M. Biffi, C. Martignani, C. Greco, C. Camanini, C. Valzania, I. Diemberger, F. Cecaro, A. Branzi

Clinical Effectiveness of Cardioverter Defibrillators

Sudden cardiac death is responsible for around 50% of all deaths due to cardiovascular causes [1, 2]. The implantable cardioverter defibrillator (ICD) was initially conceived by Mirowski for preventing sudden death in patients who have already experienced a life-threatening ventricular arrhythmia, such as sustained ventricular tachycardia or ventricular fibrillation. These patients are at high risk of recurrences of these malignant tachyarrhythmias, with recurrence rates around 30%–50% in a 2-year follow-up period [3]. Prospective controlled studies have demonstrated that ICDs prevent sudden death in these patients, with an improvement in overall survival in a 3- to 5-year follow-up[4–6]. The majority of patients enrolled in these trials had coronary artery disease as predominant etiology, and a wide range of ventricular function compromise was present, as well as a wide range of associated clinical conditions.

In studies evaluating ICDs, the end-point for assessing clinical efficacy was initially sudden death; however, in view of the difficulties in classifying some deaths, it was suggested that total mortality should be used as the primary end-point for studies assessing the impact of ICD on patients' prognosis. Obviously, total mortality varies significantly according to the underlying heart disease and the degree of compromise of left ventricular function. Thus, the extent of benefit from ICD implantation that may be expected and demonstrated during a follow-up of variable duration will depend on the presence or absence of concurrent potential causes of death. Although the improvement in survival is most easily demonstrated in patients with the most advanced left ventricular dysfunction in follow-ups of 3–5 years ("the sickest patients benefit the most") [7], it must be remembered that in patients without left ventricular dysfunction and with some specific types of clinical conditions (i.e., hyper-

Institute of Cardiology, University of Bologna, Italy

trophic cardiomyopathy, idiopathic ventricular fibrillation, Brugada's syndrome), prevention of sudden arrhythmic death translates into prevention of almost all the potential causes of death. It is also clear that in the above-mentioned conditions the overall impact of ICDs in prolonging overall survival should be assessed over longer follow-up times than those available to date.

Cost-Effectiveness of Cardioverter Defibrillators

There are various methods by which to assess the economic implications of a medical intervention: cost-benefit analysis, cost-effectiveness analysis, and cost-utility analysis. Moreover, economic analysis of medical interventions must also take into consideration the conditions of controlled trials and the fact that effectiveness is the actual decrease in disease achieved when the intervention is applied over a large, nonhomogeneous population.

Cost-effectiveness analysis has as its aim to assess the cost of any therapeutic intervention in relation to its possible benefits [8–11]. The cost of a treatment is the sum of direct costs (initial cost of therapy, costs of maintaining therapy, and costs caused by unfavorable effects or by complications) and indirect costs paid by the patient, the patient's family, or the community. The efficacy of a treatment is defined by the mean number of years for which the patients survives after a disease because of the treatment. Usually, incremental cost-effectiveness analysis is performed when two new therapeutic strategies are compared. The cost-effectiveness ratio is usually expressed in dollars per year of life saved ($/YLS). In the literature [8–11], a treatment is considered valid if the cost-effectiveness ratio ranges between 0 and 20 000 $/YLS, convenient if the cost-effectiveness ratio ranges between 20 000 and 40 000 $/YLS, and borderline if the cost-effectiveness ratio ranges between 40 000 and 60 000 $/YLS. It is considered unfavorable if the cost-effectiveness ratio ranges between 60 000 and 100 000 $/YLS and absolutely unfavorable above 100 000 $/YLS. Evidently, the cost-effectiveness ratio can change greatly depending on the type of population in treatment. The identification of high-risk patients ("patient targeting") seems to be the most important element in reaching a favorable cost-effectiveness ratio.

Since none of the prospective studies performed to evaluate the clinical relevance of ICD use was designed to assess cost-effectiveness as primary endpoint, what we know at present of the cost-effectiveness of ICDs derives from post-hoc analysis of major trials, and in none of these studies was the cost-effectiveness of ICDs use for cardiac disease of a definite etiology analyzed. Moreover, for those etiologies where sudden cardiac death is the leading cause of death (i.e. where there is no significant risk of death due to pump failure), the benefit of ICD and therefore the assessment of cost-effectiveness should be evaluated with follow-ups in the order of 10–15 years—a time frame difficult to apply in prospective studies. Hlatky and Bigger [12] projected the results of all the trials considering the full gain in life expectancy and reported a cost-effectiveness ratio of 31 500 $/YLS, in line with what is currently considered fully acceptable.

The etiologies different from coronary artery disease where ICDs are usually implanted to prevent sudden death are: idiopathic dilated cardiomyopathy, arrhythmogenic right ventricular dysplasia, idiopathic ventricular fibrillation, Brugada's syndrome, laminopathies, and long QT syndromes.

Although no specific data are available on cost-effectiveness, we will report some of the data supporting the use of ICDs in primary prevention of sudden death in the above-mentioned clinical conditions, making some comments on the potential implications in a cost-effectiveness evaluation.

Idiopathic Dilated Cardiomyopathy

According to the literature, this disease is traditionally considered to be associated with a high mortality rate within 2 years from diagnosis, with only a minority of patients surviving for 5 years [13]. Approximately half of the deaths are sudden and unexpected, with a proportionally higher incidence of deaths with the pattern of sudden death rather than pump failure death occurring in patients in the lower New York Heart Association functional classes. In patients with previous ventricular tachyarrhythmias, the benefits conferred by ICD treatment are probably similar to those obtainable in coronary artery disease and the cost-effectiveness should be similar. Conversely, with regard to primary prevention, at present there is no evidence of benefit to patients implanted with an ICD. Although low left ventricular ejection fraction and nonsustained ventricular tachycardia identify a subgroup of patients at higher risk of sudden death [14], no prospective study has shown that ICD alone, not associated with biventricular pacing prolongs survival when used in the setting of primary prevention of sudden death in idiopathic dilated cardiomyopathy.

The CAT study [15] failed to demonstrate a benefit of ICD implantation in patients with a recent diagnosis of dilated cardiomyopathy (<6 months) and low ejection fraction, but the result probably is greatly affected by the relatively low mortality observed in the follow-up period.

The possibility of implanting an ICD as a bridge to heart transplantation constitutes a new perspective in heart failure patients, and the impact on the outcome of patients on the transplant list has to be assessed as well as the cost-effectiveness [16].

Hypertrophic Cardiomyopathy

Hypertrophic cardiomyopathy is the leading cause of sudden death in young adults and athletes. Sudden death may be the first manifestation of the disease and an overall incidence of up to 6%–8 % per year has been reported [17]. In a series of 128 patients at high risk of sudden death because of previously sustained ventricular tachyarrhythmias or with massive left ventricular hypertrophy (wall thickness greater than 30 mm) [18] or syncope, or nonsustained ventricular tachycardia or family history of sudden death, the event rate (appropriate ICD discharge) was 5% in primary prevention and 11% in secondary prevention [19]. In patients with hypertrophic cardiomyopathy at risk of sudden death with normal or supranormal ventricular function, prevention of arrhythmic death by an ICD may imply an almost normal life expectancy. According to these considerations, the cost-effectiveness must be considered favorable in the long term, even though no evaluation has ever been done so far.

Idiopathic Ventricular Fibrillation, Brugada's Syndrome, Long QT Syndrome

These conditions are primary electrical diseases, and prognosis is dependent on the occurrence of life-threatening ventricular tachyarrhythmias. Implantation of an ICD has the potential to dramatically change the outcome of these patients, leading to a normal or almost normal life expectancy. Both patients with previous ventricular tachyarrhythmias and patients with syncope or a strong family history of sudden death are good candidates for ICD implantation [2, 3]. However, the "unnatural history" of these patients after ICD implantation must take into considerations not only the benefits conferred by the ICDs, but also the long-term complications of ICD implantation (lead-related complications including lead failure requiring reintervention, infections, etc.). No data are currently available on the long-term outcome of this kind of patients, who need to be evaluated over a follow-up of at least 10–15 years for a proper assessment of device performance and device-related costs. In these patients no cost-effectiveness evaluation has been performed hitherto.

Arrhythmogenic Right Ventricular Cardiomyopathy

This disease may share either some characteristics of primary electrical diseases or the characteristics of a cardiomyopathy that may evolve towards severe heart failure, even requiring heart transplantation [20]. The cost-effectiveness profile may therefore vary from a profile similar to dilated cadiomyopathy to a profile more similar to that of primary electrical diseases.

Laminopathies

A series of neuromuscular diseases dependent on mutations of the *LMNA* gene may have the clinical presentation of dilated cardiomyopathy with atrioventricular block, or may have a neuromuscular involvement typical of Emery–Dreifuss muscular dystrophy [21]. Families in which mutations in the *LMNA* gene carry a high risk of sudden death have been described [22], and in these cases implantation of an ICD has also been proposed for primary prevention of sudden death. The long-term prognosis of the disease, which has a wide spectrum of clinical presentations, is not fully defined and therefore the cost-benefit of ICD implantation in this subset of patients has still to be assessed.

Conclusions

The low risk of ICD implantation and the evidence that these devices provide successful termination of life-threatening ventricular tachyarrhythmias have prompted the use of ICDs in primary prevention of sudden death in specific clinical conditions associated with a substantially increased risk of sudden arrhythmic death. In conditions where sudden death has no competitive determinants of death (i.e. hypertrophic cardiomyopathy, Brugada's syndrome, idiopathic ventricular fibrillation), the use of ICDs is probably highly beneficial since it may confer an almost normal life expectancy, although this has not been proved by prospective controlled trials dedicated to these diseases. Cost-effectiveness has not been assessed in these conditions either, and remains difficult to evaluate since it needs to be carried out over long follow-up periods (at least 10–15 years) in order to obtain a substantially high number of prevented events and in order to dilute the front-load cost of the ICD implantation.

References

1. Zipes DP, Wellens HJ (1998) Sudden cardiac death. Circulation 98:2334–2351
2. Priori SG, Aliot E, Blomstrom-Lundqvist C et al (2001) Task Force on sudden cardiac death of the European Society of Cardiology. Eur Heart J 16:1374–1450
3. Gregoratos G, Abrams J, Epstein AE et al (2002) ACC/AHA/NASPE 2002 guideline update for implantation of cardiac pacemakers and antiarrhythmia devices: a report of the American College of Cardiology/American Heart Association task force on practice guidelines (ACC/AHA/NASPE committee to update the 1998 pacemaker guidelines). J Am Coll Cardiol 40:1703–1719
4. The Antiarrhythmics Versus Implantable Defibrillators (AVID) Investigators (1997) A comparison of antiarrhythmic-drug therapy with implantable defibrillators in patients resuscitated from near-fatal ventricular arrhythmias. N Engl J Med 337:1576–1583
5. Connolly SJ, Gent M, Roberts RS et al (2000) Canadian implantable defibrillator study (CIDS): a randomized trial of the implantable cardioverter defibrillator against amiodarone. Circulation 101:1297–1302
6. Ezekowitz JA, Armstrong PW, McAlister FA (2003) Implantable cardioverter defibrillators in primary and secondary prevention:a systematic review of randomized, controlled trials. Ann Intern Med 138:445–452
7. Moss AJ (2000) Implantable cardioverter defibrillator therapy: the sickest patients benefit the most. Circulation 101:1638–1640
8. Kupersmith J, Holmes-Rovner M, Rovner D et al (1995) Cost-effectiveness analysis in heart disease. Part II. Preventive therapies. Prog Cardiovasc Dis 37:243–271
9. Kupersmith J, Holmes-Rovner M, Rovner D et al (1995) Cost-effectiveness analysis in heart disease. Part III. Ischemia, congestive heart failure and arrhythmias. Prog Cardiovasc Dis 37:307–346
10. Kuppermann M, Luce BR, McGovern B et al (1990) An analysis of the cost effectiveness of the implantable defibrillator. Circulation 81:91–100
11. Boriani G, *Biffi* M, Martignani C et al (2001) Cost-effectiveness of implantable cardio-

verter-defibrillators. Eur Heart J 22:990–996
12. Hlatky MA, Bigger JT (2001) Cost-effectiveness of the implantable cardioverter defibrillator? Lancet 357:1817–1818
13. Fuster V, Gersh BJ, Giuliani ER et al (1981) The natural history of idiopathic dilated cardiomyopathy. Am J Cardiol 47:525–531
14. Follansbee WP, Michelson EL, Morganroth J (1980) Nonsustained ventricular tachycardia in ambulatory patients: characteristics and association with sudden cardiac death. Ann Intern Med 92:741–747
15. Bansch D, Antz M, Boczor S et al (2002) Primary prevention of sudden cardiac death in idiopathic dilated dilated cardiomyopathy: the Cardiomyopathy Trial (CAT). Circulation 105:1453–1458
16. Weintraub WS, Cole J, Tooley JF (2002) Cost and cost-effectiveness studies in heart failure research. Am Heart J 143:565–576
17. Spirito P, Bellone P, Harris KM et al (2000) Magnitude of left ventricular hypertrophy and risk of sudden death in hypertrophic cardiomyopathy. N Engl J Med 342:1778–1785
18. Maron BJ (2002) Hypertrophic cardiomyopathy:a systematic review. JAMA 287:1308–1320
19. Maron BJ, Shen WK, Link MS et al (2000) Efficacy of implantable cardioverter-defibrillators for the prevention of sudden death in patients with hypertrophic cardiomyopathy. N Engl J Med 10; 365–373
20. Corrado D, Basso C, Nava A et al (2001) Arrhythmogenic right ventricular cardiomyopathy: current diagnostic and management strategies. Cardiol Rev 9:259–265
21. Boriani G, Gallina M, Merlini L et al (2003) Clinical relevance of atrial fibrillation/flutter, stroke, pacemaker implant, and heart failure in Emery–Dreifuss muscular dystrophy: a long-term longitudinal study. Stroke 34:901–908
22. Becane HM, Bonne G, Varnous S et al (2000) High incidence of sudden death with conduction system and myocardial disease due to lamins A and C gene mutation. Pacing Clin Electrophysiol 11:1661–1666

Expanding ICD Indications: Can We Afford It?

M. Santini, M. Russo, R. Ricci, C. Pignalberi, B. Magris, L. Santini

Sudden cardiac death is a great health problem in Western countries, accounting for about 300 000/500 000 events per year in the United States and Europe. It is one of the most important causes of death in the adult population in the developed countries. Since coronary artery disease (CAD) is the leading cause of sudden death, its epidemiology follows the incidence and prevalence of known risk factors for coronary artery disease.

Ventricular fibrillation is the culprit arrhythmia in about 80% of cases of sudden cardiac death, while the other arrhythmias identified in witnessed sudden cardiac deaths were atrioventricular block or other bradycardias in 15% of the cases and pulseless electrical activity in only 5% of the cases.

In the great majority of cases sudden cardiac death is associated with structural heart disease, mainly CAD (about 80% of cases); other cardiac abnormalities associated with increased risk of sudden death are cardiomyopathies such as dilated or hypertrophic cardiomyopathy and heritable arrhythmogenic disorders such as the different types of long QT syndrome, Brugada's syndrome, and arrhythmogenic right ventricular dysplasia [1–5].

From the beginning in studies on risk factors for sudden cardiac death, it was clearly evident that left ventricular function plays a key role in the problem; several studies have shown that the lower the left ventricular ejection fraction (LVEF), the higher the risk of dying suddenly. However, despite the huge amount of clinical and experimental data collected in many studies, it has not been possible to identify risk factors on which to base an algorithm for clinicians to help them provide the best treatment available. Moreover, trials on pharmacological interventions with antiarrhythmic drugs produced disappointing results in terms of total mortality. Apart from amiodarone, all antiarrhythmic drugs tested in large clinical trials increased total mortality in comparison with placebo; amiodarone merely provided a null effect [6–10]. Other studies questioned the role of programmed ventricular stimulation (PVS) in

Cardiovascular Department, San Filippo Neri Hospital, Rome, Italy

choosing the best antiarrhythmic therapy and, sometimes, in identifying the patients at the highest risk [11].

The discouraging results of drug therapy prompted the development of nonpharmacological strategies to prevent sudden death, such as catheter interventions and, especially, implantable devices. As soon as technical progress gave cardiologists reliable implantable devices such as the modern automatic defibrillators (implantable cardioverter-defibrillators, ICDs), many clinical trials were planned and conducted in order to determine the relative effectiveness of ICDs compared to alternative strategies in different clinical settings: a lot of data gave us the certainty that ICDs were the best therapeutic option for the so-called secondary prevention of sudden death (that is, prevention of a fatal episode in patients who have survived a cardiac arrest or malignant ventricular tachycardias). Notwithstanding these results, some questions remain unanswered. Debated issues in secondary prevention relate to the role of ICDs compared to amiodarone in patients with relatively preserved left ventricular function; the AVID trial, because of the small sample size and the relatively short follow-up, did not show a statistically significant difference in survival curve in the subgroup of patients with LVEF higher than 32%. On the other hand, the AVID registry shed a dark light on sustained ventricular arrhythmias considered to be secondary to a correctable cause and therefore "benign." There is similar uncertainty in defining the relative effectiveness of ICDs compared to amiodarone in the CASH and CIDS trials, due to low sample power, the inclusion criteria, and the type of implantation performed (in CASH some implantations were via a thoracotomy). Despite these limitations, it is our opinion that ICD should be the first-line therapy in secondary prevention in patients with relatively preserved LVEF (in the absence of contraindications), because of the significant side effects of amiodarone, its incomplete protective action (in the CASCADE study amiodarone was unable to prevent a high number of sudden deaths) and the need to take the drug life-long [12–18].

While evidence is still lacking about the primary prevention of sudden cardiac death in special groups, such as nonischemic cardiomyopathy patients, more recent trials have explored its feasibility by means of implantation of an ICD in post-myocardial-infarction (post-MI) patients known to be at increased risk (i.e., patients with LVEF lower than 40%, complex ventricular arrhythmias during Holter monitoring, and inducibility of sustained ventricular arrhythmias during PVS); this target group of patients was very similar to those in whom a pharmacological strategy with class I antiarrhythmics and sotalol had failed to reduce risk (mortality was higher in the treated study arm). The results of these trials (MADIT I and MUSTT) showed a clear benefit (near 50% reduction of relative risk for all-cause mortality) of the implantation of an ICD in patients taking the best medical therapy too [19, 20]. The use of an ICD in this clinical setting is now considered a class I indication in the ACC/AHA/NASPE guidelines for antiarrhythmic device implantation released last year [21].

Despite the evidence discussed above, cardiologists are still dealing with some uncomfortable problems. In the MUSTT registry [22], up to 24% of patients in whom ventricular arrhythmias were not inducible at PVS experienced sudden cardiac death within 5 years, whilst the incidence of 5-year sudden death was 32% in "inducible" patients randomized to receive no antiarrhythmic therapy (a statistically significant difference).

As a matter of fact, PVS, although valuable in screening for risk in this setting, is far from optimal. The MADIT II trial [23] was conducted and recently published in an attempt to overcome these difficulties. The rationale of the trial was to consider only LVEF (the inclusion value was ≤30%) as a predictor of increased risk of sudden death in post-MI patients; trial results (a relative reduction in the risk of death from all causes of about 30% at a median follow-up of 20 months in patients who had undergone ICD implantation) led the committee to prematurely terminate enrolment. Briefly, the MADIT II trial showed a statistically significant mortality benefit of ICD compared to best medical therapy (6% of absolute risk reduction, from 20% in the control group to 14% in the ICD group). This gain in mortality reduction was obtained by a reduction in sudden death. In the control group no pharmacological antiarrhythmic therapy was provided, not even amiodarone. MADIT II gave further scientific weight to the opinion about the LVEF as a strong predictor in post-MI patients and supported the use of this technology in preventing sudden death in this special group, but, we believe, left open a large number of questions about the best way to stratify the risk.

All the above questions are very important in the light of costs: ICD technology is costly, and only a minority of patients identified as being at high risk will develop sudden death or life-threatening ventricular arrhythmias. Thus, we have to treat with a costly procedure quite a large number of patients who will never develop life-threatening cardiac arrhythmias. This issue (really important in our era of rising costs and limited resources) has been addressed in several cost-effectiveness analyses showing a favorable profile of ICD implantation in the prevention of sudden death. In the AVID cost-effectiveness substudy it was shown that the cost-effectiveness ratio is moderately favorable (about US$66 000 per life year saved in patients with LVEF≥35% and US$ 60 000 in patients with LVEF lower than 35%). In studies addressing the implantation of ICDs for the purpose of primary prevention (like MADIT I) the cost-effectiveness ratio is more favorable, being about $27 000 per life year saved overall and $23 000 in the subgroup implanted with transvenous systems [24, 25]. The cost-effectiveness ratio depends closely on the NNT (the number needed to treat, i.e., the number of patients that have to be treated in order for one life to be saved). In studies addressing primary prevention in high-risk patients the NNT is very attractive (it ranges from 3.2 in MUSTT to 11 in a preliminary and not yet published analysis of MADIT II). Only in CIDS was the cost-effectiveness ratio unattractive, mainly due to the absence of statistical significance in the superiority of ICD therapy compared to a standard pharmacological approach. In CIDS patients were enrolled not only if they had had a documented spontaneous ventricular tachyarrhythmia, but if they reported a syncope suspected to be due to ventricular tachycardia. Furthermore, the median follow-up in the CIDS was longer than that in the AVID trial (which was prematurely interrupted by the review board): these facts could explain why ICD performed worse in CIDS than in AVID, and why the former showed a less attractive cost-effectiveness ratio [14].

The above data indicate that, as a whole, defibrillator implantation is the best strategy in preventing sudden death in different high-risk patient populations. The problem is the high cost of this kind of therapy, whether real or as perceived by the medical community, although the cost-effectiveness ratio of other well accepted and extensively applied medical interventions is higher: for example, the use of ACE inhibitors, β-blockers, and statins in standard medical therapy has gained wide acceptance in spite of NNTs ranging from 20 in SAVE to 28 in 4S trials [26].

Furthermore, the publication of the MADIT II trial on primary prevention in high-risk post-MI patients has increased the controversy about the cost of primary prevention of sudden death. As mentioned above, on one hand the MADIT II trial has given further strength to the notion of the high predictive value of an easily determined parameter such as LVEF in the screening of patients at high risk of dying suddenly; on the other hand, if the results of MADIT II and of the other primary prevention trials are widely applied in routine clinical practice, the health care payment system will have to carry an extra and heavy burden.

Could the health care system bear this new burden, considering the problem of limited resources in the industrialized countries and their absence in the developing ones? At first glance, the answer must be negative – but if we take this option we shall deprive many patients of a very good therapeutic option that can effectively fight sudden death (a major health problem in our countries). How can we combine the need for the best care for patients with the economic limits of health care providers? Whilst awaiting the results of the as yet unpublished substudies of MADIT II that address the cost-effectiveness analysis, the medical community and medical devices industry should together deal with this issue. There could be several paths to follow to make the burden affordable.

The first one, as suggested by Zipes in 2001 [27], is to develop cheaper defibrillators to be implanted in patients believed to be at lower risk. To implant less sophisticated ICDs, with only basic functions, would be a reasonable choice for this class of patients. This industrial strategy needs the joint efforts of the scientific and medical communities in identifying patients at different level of risk. So far, we have several diagnostic tools available for screening patients for the risk of sudden death, as is well documented in the literature; however, none of them has shown a very reliable predictive power in detecting patients at increased risk among the totality of patients. For example, since the 24% of patients in whom ventricular arrhythmias were not inducible and who were followed up in the MUSTT registry suffered sudden cardiac death within 5 years, electrophysiological testing clearly does not so far have a reliable predictive value in the setting of MUSTT-like patients; the true value of such testing in the setting of MADIT II-like patients is still unknown and would be an interesting field to explore. Other screening parameters that have been shown to be promising (such as T wave alternans and heart rate variability) should be evaluated in this setting to obtain better characterization of the patients who will really benefit from prophylactic ICD implantation. Furthermore, we have still a lot to learn about the role of ICDs in primary prevention in patients with nonischemic cardiomyopathies, for whom consistent data are lacking at present.

To conclude, the results of all the clinical studies conducted to date have clearly established that ICD is the best therapeutic option in comparison with drugs and other strategies in preventing sudden death, especially in patients with a prior major arrhythmic event, low LVEF, and ischemic cardiomyopathy; the problem we now have to deal with is risk stratification in order to avoid pointless implantation in patients who will never develop sustained ventricular arrhythmias. This is important because of the high costs of this form of strategy: the paradox of MADIT II, conducted in order to simplify the stratification, is that oversimplification, with its attendant reduction in specificity, generated a burden for the health care system that it can no longer afford.

The combination of industrial strategies (manufacturing less expensive devices) and further research projects tailored to defining high-risk groups of patients who really will benefit from implantation is still awaited.

References

1. Santini M (2003) In: Santini M (ed) Nonpharmacological treatment of sudden death. Chapter 1. Arianna, Bologna
2. Becker LB, Smith DW, Rhodes KV(1993) Incidence of cardiac arrest: a neglected factor in evaluating survival rates. Ann Emerg Med 22:86–91
3. De Vreede-Swagemakers JJ, Gorgles AP, Dubois-Arbouw WI et al (1997) Out-OF-hospital cardiac arrest in the 1990's: a population-based study in the Maastricht area on incidence, characteristics and survival. J Am Coll Cardiol 30:1500–1505
4. Myerburg RJ, Castellanos A (2001) Cardiac arrest and sudden cardiac death. In: Braunwald E, Zipes DP, Libby P (eds) Heart disease: a textbook of cardiovascular medicine. Saunders, Philadelphia
5. Priori SG, Aliot E, Blomstrom-Lundqvist C et al (2003) European Society of Cardiology. Update of the guidelines on sudden cardiac death of the European Society of Cardiology. Eur Heart J 24:13–15
6. Echt DS, Liebson PR, Mitchell LL et al (1991) Mortality and morbidity in patients receiving encainide, flecainide or placebo. The Cardiac Arrhythmia Suppression Trial. N Engl J Med 324:781–788
7. Waldo AL, Camm AJ, deRuyter H et al (1996) Effect of d-sotalol on mortality in patients with left ventricular dysfunction after recent and remote myocardial infarction. The SWORD Investigators. Survival With Oral d-Sotalol. Lancet 348:7–12
8. Cairns JA, Connolly SJ, Roberts R, Gent M, for the CAMIAT Investigators (1997) Randomized trial of outcome after myocardial infarction in patients with frequent or

repetitive ventricular premature depolarisations: CAMIAT. Lancet 349:675–682
9. Julian DG, Camm AJ, Frangin G et al, for the EMIAT Investigators (1997) Randomized trial of effect of amiodarone on mortality in patients with left ventricular dysfunction after recent myocardial infarction: EMIAT. Lancet 349:667–674
10. Sim I, McDonald KM, Lavori PW et al (1997) Quantitative overview of randomized trials of amiodarone to prevent sudden cardiac death. Circulation 96:2823–2829
11. Mason JW for the Electrophysiologic Study versus Electrocardiographic Monitoring Investigators (1993) A comparison of electrophysiologic testing with Holter monitoring to predict antiarrhythmic-drug efficacy for ventricular tachyarrhythmias. N Engl J Med 329:445–451
12. The AVID investigators (1997) A comparison of antiarrhythmic drug therapy with implantable defibrillators in patients resuscitated from near fatal ventricular arrhythmias. N Engl J Med 337:1576–1583
13. Kuck KH, Cappato R, Siebels J, Rüppel R (2000) Randomized comparison of antiarrhythmic drug therapy with implantable defibrillators in patients resuscitated from cardiac arrest. The Cardiac Arrest Study Hamburg (CASH). Circulation 102:748–754
14. Connolly SJ, Gent M, Roberts RS et al (2000) A randomized trial of the implantable cardioverter defibrillator against amiodarone. Canadian Implantable Defibrillator Study (CIDS). Circulation 101:1297–1302
15. Epstein AE, Powell J, Yao Q et al (1999) In-hospital versus out-of-hospital presentation of life-threatening ventricular arrhythmias predicts survival: results from the AVID registry. Antiarrhythmics versus Implantable Defibrillators. J Am Coll Cardiol 34:1111–1116
16. Anderson JL, Hallström AP, Epstein AE et al (1999) Design and results of the Antiarrhythmics versus Implantable Defibrillators (AVID) registry. Circulation 99:1692–1699
17. The CASCADE Investigators (1993) Randomized antiarrhythmic drug therapy in survivors of cardiac arrest (the CASCADE study). Am J Cardiol 72:280–287
18. Greene HL (1993) The CASCADE Study: randomized antiarrhythmic drug therapy in survivors of cardiac arrest in Seattle. CASCADE Investigators. Am J Cardiol 72:70F–74F
19. Moss AJ, Hall WJ, Cannom DS et al, for the MADIT Investigators (1996) Improved survival with an implanted defibrillator in patients with coronary disease at high risk for ventricular arrhythmia. N Engl J Med 335:1933–1940
20. Buxton AE, Lee KL, Fisher JD et al, for MUSTT Investigators (1999) A randomized study of the prevention of sudden death in patients with coronary artery disease. N Engl J Med 341:1882–1890
21. Gregoratos G, Abrams J, Epstein AE, Freedman RA, Hayes DL, Hlatky MA, Kerber RE, Naccarelli GV, Schoenfeld MH, Silka MJ, Winters SL (2002) ACC/AHA/NASPE 2002 guidelines update for implantation of cardiac pace-makers and antiarrhythmia devices. A report of the American College of Cardiology/American Heart Association Task Force on Practice Guidelines (ACC/AHA/NASPE Committee to Update the 1998 Guidelines). J Am Coll Cardiol 40:1703–19
22. Buxton AE, Lee KL, DiCarlo L et al, for MUSTT Investigators (2000) Electrophysiologic testing to identify patients with coronary artery disease who are at risk for sudden death. N Engl J Med 342:1937–1945
23. Moss AJ, Zareba W, Hall WJ et al, for MADIT II Investigators (2002) Prophylactic implantation of a defibrillator in patients with myocardial infarction and reduced ejection fraction. N Engl J Med 346:877–883

24. Larsen G, Hallström A, McAnulty J et al, for the AVID Investigators (2002) Cost-effectiveness of the implantable cardioverter-defibrillator versus antiarrhythmic drugs in survivors of serious ventricular tachyarrhythmias. Results of AVID economic analysis substudy. Circulation 105:2049–2057
25. Mushlin AI, Hall J, Zwanzinger J et al, for the MADIT Investigators (1998) The cost-effectiveness of automatic implantable cardiac defibrillators: results from MADIT. Circulation 97:2129–2135
26. No Authors (1994) Randomised trial of cholesterol lowering in 4444 patients with coronary heart disease: the Scandinavian sinvastatin survival study. Lancet 344:1383-1389
27. Zipes DP (2001) Implantable cardioverter-defibrillator: a Volkswagen or a Rolls Royce. How much will we pay to save a life? Circulation 103:1372–1374

Waveform Flexibility: The Present and Future Solution for Clinically Effective Defibrillation

M. W. Kroll

A Primer on Defibrillation

Monophasic Shock

The monophasic shock defibrillates primarily by capturing cardiac myocytes regardless of their phase. Since most cells are in phases 2 and 3 during fibrillation, the shock must be strong enough to cause a new activation potential even though these cells are refractory in the usual sense of the word.

Figure 1 shows that the impact of the shock is to first charge the membrane. The cell then undergoes a nearly normal activation potential [1]. Surprisingly and fortuitously, there does not appear to be any restitution curve effect. Thus the resulting activation potentials all return to phase 4 nearly simultaneously, thus resynchronizing the ventricle and defibrillating the heart.

The quick summary of monophasic defibrillation is that it is a "super" pacing pulse. It must capture the heart in 4 dimensions, i.e. throughout its 3 spatial dimensions and its throughout its phases. The typical rheobase current is 5 amperes and a typical chronaxie is 3 milliseconds. These are respectively 1000 times and 10 times the rheobase and chronaxie for conventional pacing.

Biphasic Shock

Figure 2 is a simple schematic representation of the heart with epicardial patches on each end. This shows the state of the heart after the first phase of a biphasic shock. The myocytes in line with the electrodes are captured but not enough cells are captured to resynchronize the heart (if enough were captured, phase two would be unnecessary!)

Between the "captured" region and the "noncaptured" region is a boundary surface in which the cells will receive borderline stimulation. This is pictured

St. Jude Medical, Sylmar, California, USA

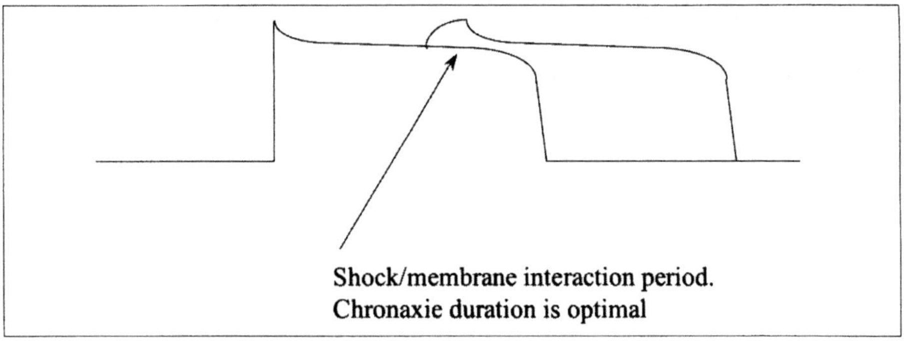

Fig. 1. Cellular response to a defibrillation shock

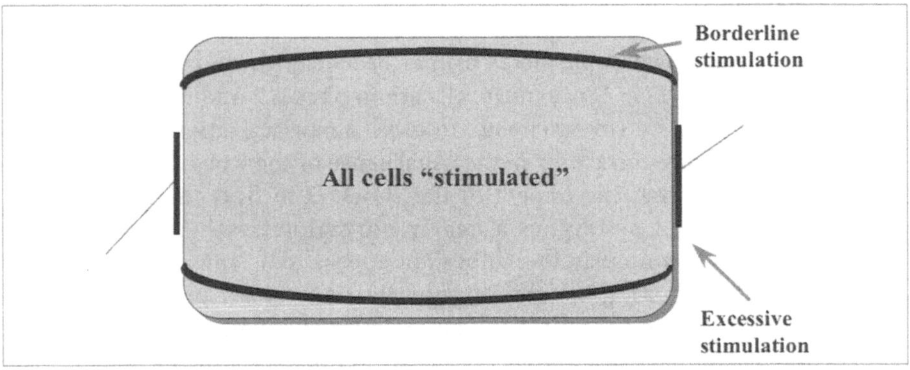

Fig. 2. Cardiac state after phase one

in Figure 3. The shock charges the cell membrane up to near its firing point but does not cause a clean capture. Hodgkin and Huxley (HH) showed that borderline stimulation leads to irregular responses [2]. These irregular responses can destroy synchronization.

A properly sized second phase of a biphasic shock will remove the residual charge from a borderline charged cell, thus preventing the irregular response. This effect is shown in Figure 4. The membrane potential is brought back down to zero. Figure 4 intentionally shows the effect of a phase two which is slightly longer than optimal. This pulls the membrane potential slightly below zero, which suggests that phase two should be shortened. In fact, using the known defibrillation capacitance and path resistance and assuming a membrane time constant, one can calculate the optimal duration for the two phases. This simple charge-burping model gives surprisingly accurate predictions for the performance of arbitrary biphasic waveforms [3]. In a retrospective analysis of published animal studies that varied biphasic phase duration, 89% of the variance in the shock performance was explained [4].

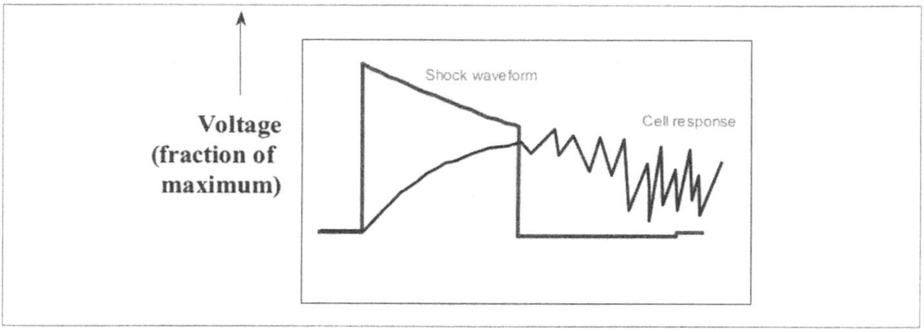

Fig. 3. Cell response to borderline stimulation

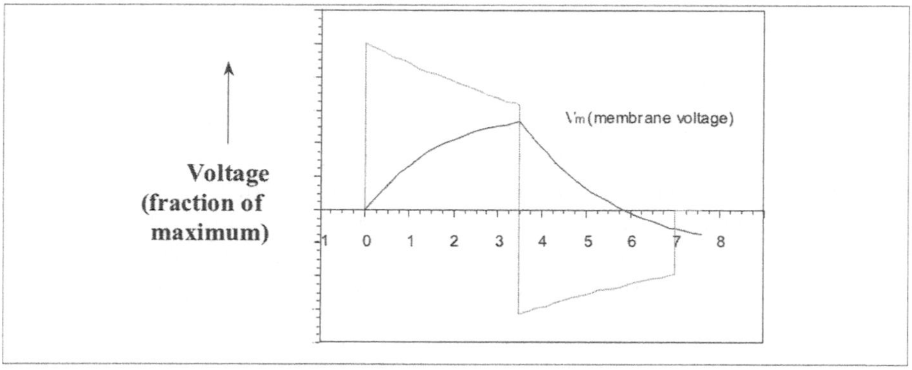

Fig. 4. Burping effect of phase two

Phase two also helps heal those cells located near the electrode which receive excessive stimulation, which can otherwise lead to desynchronizing responses. The overall action of the biphasic shock is shown in Table 1.

Table 1. Effects of the two phases

Φ1 Local Field	Cell Response	Φ 2 Effect
Excessive	Injury	Heals
Enough	"Capture"	Nothing
Borderline	Irregular	Calms
Weak	Nothing	Nothing

Effect of Cathodal Shocks

The preceding discussion of membrane charging and discharging in a linear capacitive fashion applies rather accurately to cells near the shocking anode, even at extreme electrical fields [5]. For reasons that are not yet well understood, this does not apply to cells near the cathode. Possibly for this reason, cells near the cathode tend to have an erratic response to biphasic shocks [6]. Thus, cellular data suggests that the cathode should be kept well away from the heart and the anode should be the electrode inside the heart.

Clinical Applications

Optimal Durations

The optimal duration for a biphasic waveform in a typical situation are given in Figure 5. This is based on an implantable cardioverter defibrillator (ICD) capacitance of 110 μF and assumes a membrane time constant of 3.5 ms. Note that the optimal phase one duration does increase slightly with increasing resistance to allow more charge to be delivered from the ICD capacitors. What is unexpected, is that the optimal phase two duration decreases slightly with increasing resistance. This is because the optimal phase one duration will leave more voltage on the capacitors. This higher voltage gives phase two more charge to work with and requires it to be shortened for optimal burping.

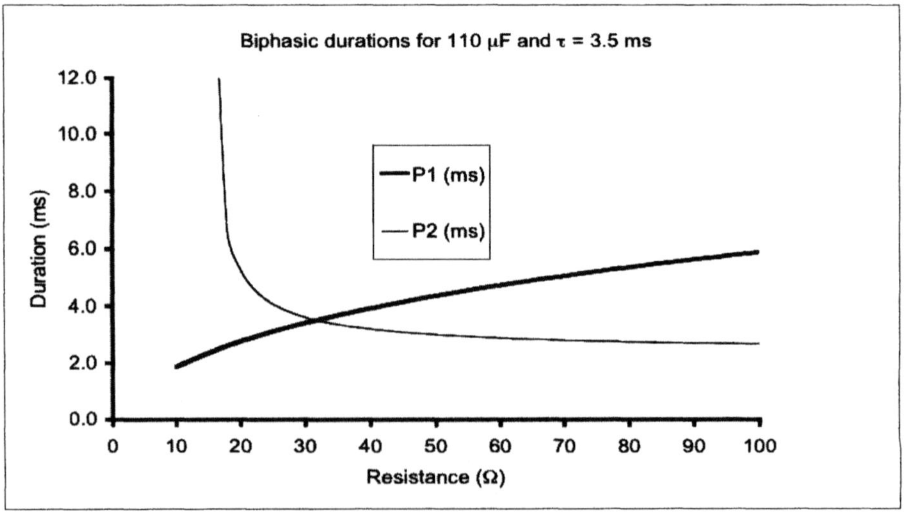

Fig. 5. Optimal phase durations

The Distraction of Tilt

Using the optimal duration we can calculate the optimal tilts for an arbitrary situation, shown in Figure 6. Note that the correct tilt for phase 1 changes with the resistance; for phase 2 the changes are dramatic and highly significant. Since a tilt setting changes the phase duration with resistance, there is a widespread misperception that this change is somehow helpful or even optimal. Tilt-based waveform programming (from major manufacturers) requires that the two phases have proportional durations (either 1:1 or 1:2/3). Figure 6 clearly shows that the optimal tilts for the two phases have no proportionality between them and the actual durations go in opposite directions with increasing resistance.

The use of tilt is an anachronism dating from the first monophasic ICDs with an approximate truncation at 1 time constant. The only justification for its use is that the delivered energy is constant with resistance - as if delivered energy was the primary determinant of defibrillation. Tilt programming gives suboptimal results, lacks any scientific modeling or cellular basis; its use is to be discouraged.

Programming Polarity

As discussed above, the right ventricular (RV) coil should be the anode (positive). This gives DFTs as good as, a better than, those from a cathodal RV coil about 90% of the time [7]. Confusion arises as anodal RV is the "reverse" setting for some brands of ICDs and thus many clinicians are in the habit of reversing the polarity for high DFT patients. There is a simple rule for polarity. At the beginning of the implant, verify that the RV coil is anodal and then ignore it. Any reversal from positive will tend to be damaging to the DFT.

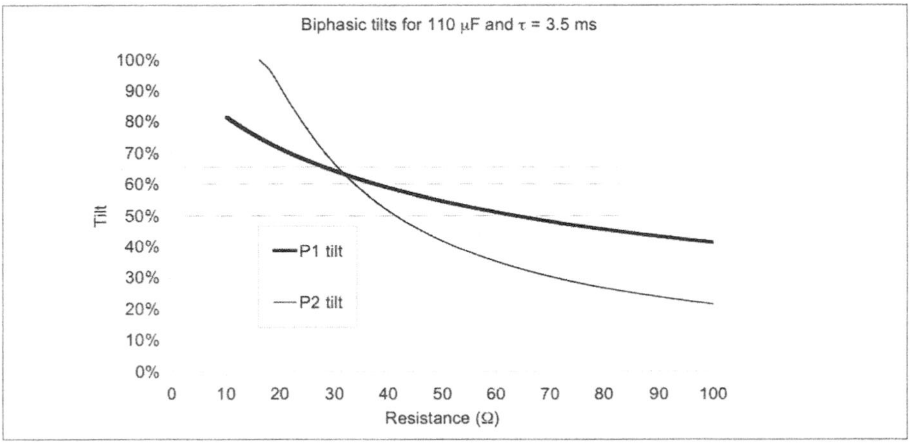

Fig. 6. Optimal phase tilts

New Waveforms

Stepped for Lower DFT

Figure 7 shows the new "stepped" biphasic waveform in the left panel and the calculated membrane response on the right. The stepped waveform may be realized by putting two shock capacitors in parallel and then in series, although there are other approaches possible. The standard biphasic initially has its peak voltage, which corresponds to the lowest membrane potential. This gives an inefficient coupling and hence wastes energy. An ascending waveform (of which the stepped is a crude approximation) will minimize this problem and hence lower the DFT. A mechanical analogy is that it is more efficient to start a car moving from first gear to second gear rather than to start in the highest gear and waste energy in the clutch.

Animal and computer modeling studies have been encouraging and human studies are in progress [8].

Rounded for Lower Pain

Present biphasic shocks almost appear to be optimized for causing maximum pain. As seen in Figure 8, the shock peaks the cardiac myocte response at the end of phase one. However, the cells involved in the pain and startle response, such as alpha motor neurons, have much smaller time constants and thus are able to respond to the leading edge of the shock. In addition, the high leading edge dV/dt may contribute to the pain perception. A rounded waveform will eliminate the leading edge derivative and reduce the peak voltage, thus possibly lowering the painfulness of the shocks. These concepts are undergoing animal and human testing.

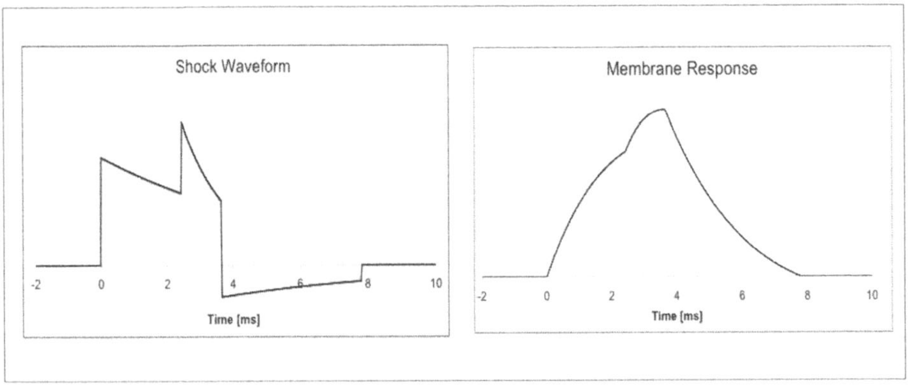

Fig. 7. Stepped waveform and membrane response

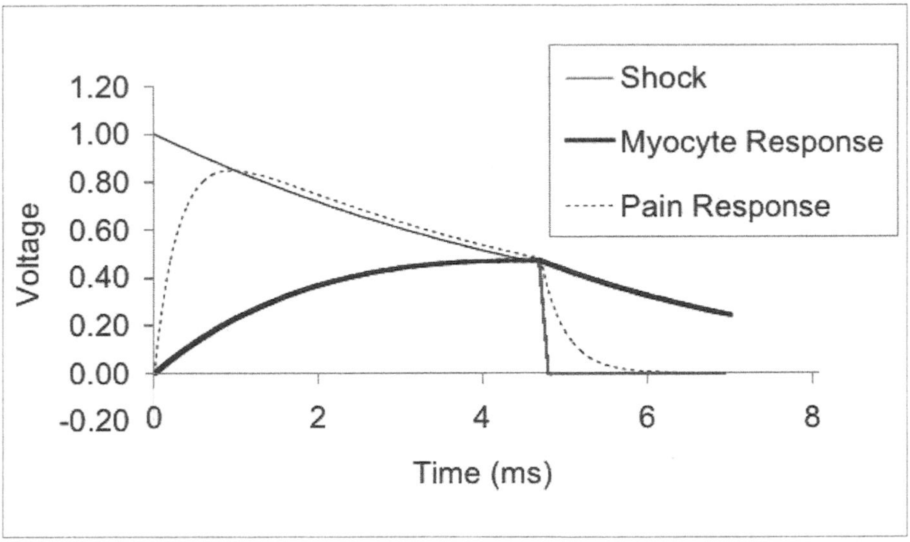

Fig. 8. Pain receptor response to standard shock

Conclusions

Within the last decade we have learned how defibrillation waveforms work and how to optimize them to reduce DFTs and increase safety margins. We are also beginning to learn how to optimize waveforms for pain control. This is very encouraging for the future of defibrillation therapy. However, it is surprising to see how simple concepts for the programming of present waveforms have failed to be universally translated into clinical practice and ICD design.

References

1. Dillon SM (1992) Synchronized repolarization after defibrillation shocks. Circulation 85(5):1865-1878
2. Hodgkin AL (1938) The subthreshold potentials in a crustacean nerve fiber. Proc Royal Soc
3. Swerdlow CD et al (1996) Charge-Burping Theory Correctly Predicts Optimal Ratios of Biphasic Duration for Biphasic Defibrillation Waveforms. Circulation 94(9):2278-2284
4. Kroll MW (1994) A Model of the Single Capacitor Biphasic Defibrillation Waveform. PACE 17(11 Pt 1):1782-1792
5. Fast VG (2000) Nonlinear changes of transmembrane potential caused by defibrillation shocks in strands of cultured myocytes. Am J Phys 278:H688-H697

6. Mowrey KA (2002) Kinetics of defibrillation shock induced response: design implications for the optimal defibrillation waveform. Europace 4:27-39
7. Kroll MW Tchou PJ (2000) Testing of Implantable Defibrillator Functions at Implantation. In: Ellenbogen, Kay, and Wilkoff. Clinical Cardiac Pacing and Defibrillation WB Saunders New York 2000
8. Hamzei A et al (1999) Three capacitor multistep waveform lowers DFT. PACE NASPE Abstract Issue

Lessons from the Lower Energy Safety Study (LESS): Is One Ventricular Fibrillation Induction Adequate for ICD Implant?

S. L. Higgins

Introduction

As part of the routine implantable cardioverter defibrillator (ICD) insertion, termination of induced ventricular fibrillation is performed [1]. The primary function of such defibrillation threshold testing (DFT) is to determine an adequate safety margin for defibrillation. This is determined by serial DFT evaluations showing efficacy at energies at least 7-10 joules below the maximum available from the implanted device. Others use a two-fold safety margin as their implant criteria. If an adequate DFT safety margin is not achieved, measures are taken to optimize it including repositioning of the lead, reversing polarity or phase of the defibrillation pulse, adding a higher output generator or an additional lead [1-3].

ICD Physician Manuals provide a variety of guidelines for implant testing with all currently recommending more than one test of induced ventricular fibrillation (VF). For example, the Guidant Physician Manuals (St. Paul, MN, U.S.A.) recommend a step-down DFT beginning at 21 joules (J). If the DFT is 14 J or less, the physician can proceed with the implant. However, if the DFT exceeds 14 J, reconfirmation is recommended, once for 17 J and twice for 21 J or higher. A fundamental question arises as to whether a single DFT evaluation can be adequate to predict clinical success. Using data from the Lower Energy Safety Study (LESS), we will attempt to answer that question.

Background on LESS

The Lower Energy Safety Study (LESS) was performed at 32 investigational centers between April 1997 and December 1999. A total of 720 patients were enrolled with 636 completing all detailed DFT testing protocols. Patients were

Regional Cardiac Arrhythmia Center, Scripps Memorial Hospital, La Jolla, California, USA followed for a mean of two years, collecting conversion data for induced and spontaneous arrhythmias. Details of the LESS trial protocol and results are available elsewhere [4, 5]. The conclusion of the LESS trial was that a 5 J safety margin was acceptable if rigorous implant testing was performed. This rigorous testing was defined as a DFT ++ to signify step-down DFT evaluation to failure and then repeated two additional times with success. Figure 1 shows the testing required by the LESS protocol.

The LESS trial included rigorous step-down DFT evaluations, including double and triple repeat tests. Nevertheless, the results can be extrapolated to determine the potential results if less rigorous testing was applied. When this is performed, it is assumed that an additional 10 J (a total of over 15 J) of safety margin would be necessary to provide an adequate safety margin with just a single successful DFT shock. However, this extrapolation is a population based determination and may not result in an available energy level for testing.

As shown in Figure 1, the testing protocol in LESS began at 14 J. Therefore, we sought to answer the questions:

How well did success on the first shock at 14 J correlate to subsequent demonstration of a current "gold standard": 3 successes at 21 J or less?

How well did 2 successes without a failure at 17 J or less (which is already an accepted implant criteria) correlate to demonstration of 3 successes at 21 J or less?

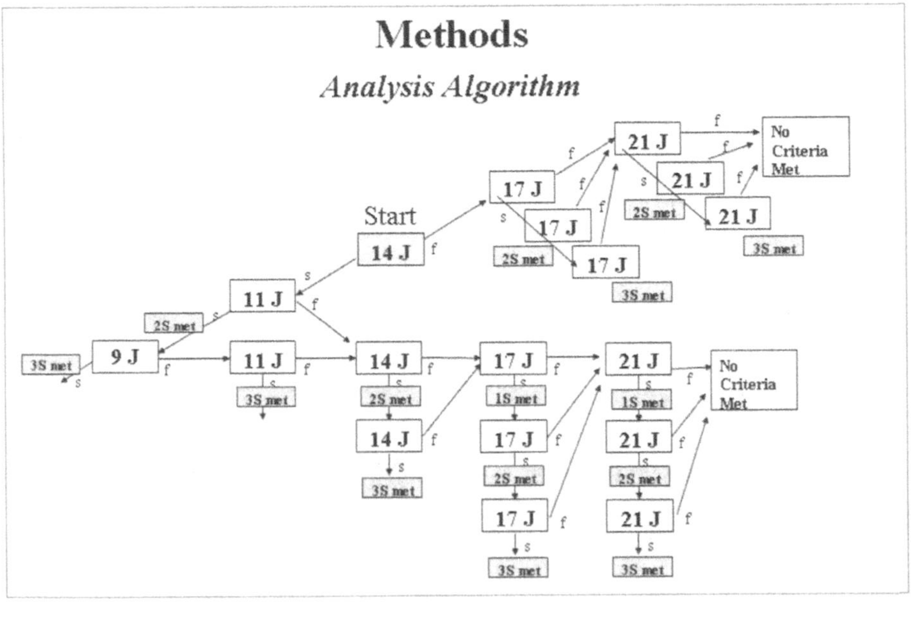

Fig. 1. A detailed analysis of the protocol required in the Lower Energy Safety Study. S refers to shock, 2S 2 shocks, 3S, 3 shocks; *s* (lower case) successful conversion of VF; *f*, failed conversion and *J*, joules. See text for details

Methods

The data from the LESS trial were evaluated retrospectively. Patients enrolled had a U.S. FDA approved indication for ICD implantation. All patients received a dual-coil defibrillation lead (ENDOTAK) and an active can pectoral pulse generator. Single right ventricular or dual chamber devices were implanted with none of the patients receiving a left ventricular lead. Generators were Guidant VENTAK Mini or AV devices (St. Paul, MN, USA).

Only patients who completed the entire testing protocol were included (see Fig. 1). The DFT was determined by induction of VF with the implanted ICD system, either with T-wave synchronous shock or 30 ms pacing algorithms. Only data from the induced VF episodes at implant were analyzed for this study. Testing began at 14 J and if the first shock was successful, then the energy was decreased on subsequent trials to 11, 9, 7, 5, and 2 J until a failure occurred. The DFT was defined as the lowest energy required to terminate VF once. After the DFT was obtained, the testing was repeated at this same energy to determine the DFT+ (defined as the lowest energy required to terminate VF on two consecutive tests without a failure) and the DFT++ (three consecutive tests).

For example, consider a patient who had successes at 14, 11, 9 and 7 J. A repeat at 7 J failed but two subsequent successes at 9 J were successful. This patient would be reported as having a DFT of 7 J and a DFT+ and DFT++ of 9J.

Continuous variables were expressed as mean ± standard deviation (SD). The differences between randomized groups were determined with Fisher's exact test with $p<0.05$ considered as statistically significant. Standard statistical definitions were utilized for comparisons such as positive predictive accuracy.

Results

As shown in Figure 2, the LESS trial enrolled a typical ICD implantation population. Further details are available in the primary publication [4]. Of the 720 patients enrolled in the LESS trial, 675 had testing that began at 14 J with some test data reported. Full testing as prescribed by the protocol was completed by 607 patients. Thus, data from 68 patients was excluded because it was incomplete (i.e., testing did not continue all the way to either a DFT++ or a failure at 21 J).

The original LESS trial evaluated the efficacy of implant DFT++ testing to predict successful conversion of spontaneously occurring tachyarrhythmias. A safety margin of 4-6 J was found to be adequate in predicting a greater than 99 % efficacy. For this investigation, we chose to use patients who had a 10 J safety margin with DFT++ testing as the "gold standard" or 21 J for the standard 31 J maximum output device. The findings with a single 14 J DFT evaluation are presented in matrix format in Figure 3. The test group refers to the patients

Age	66 ±12	**LV Ejection Fraction**	35±14 %
% Male	78%	**NYHA Class**	
ICD Indication		I	31%
VF	29%	II	44%
VT	49%	III	22%
NSVT (MADIT)	22%	IV	3%
Primary Tachyarrhythmia		**Primary Cardiac Disease**	
MVT	62%	Ischemic (CAD or CM)	74%
PVT/VF	22%	Non-Ischemic CM	14%
NSVT	12%	None	5%
other	3%	Other	6%
Secondary Arrhythmias		**Cardiac Surgical History**	
AF	19%	CABG	37%
Sinus bradycardia	9%	Other	19%
Heart Block	8%	none	43%
NSVT	11%		
		Anti-Arrhythmic Usage	29%

Fig. 2. Demographics of the LESS study population

"Test"
1S @ 14 Joules

	Pass 3S@ ≤21	**Fail 3S@ ≤21**
Pass 1S@14	**547**	**5**
Fail 1S@14	**43**	**12**

"Control"
2S @ ≤ 17 Joules

	Pass 3S@ ≤21	**Fail 3S@ ≤21**
Pass 2S@ ≤17	**584**	**5**
Fail 2S@ ≤17	**6**	**12**

Fig. 3. A matrix format showing efficacy of various DFT evaluations in comparison to the standard success rate with three sequential successes (DFT++) at 21 J or less. "Test" refers to the results with a single 14 J successful test. "Control" refers to the same comparison when patients had two successes at 17 J or less. *S*, successful conversion

who had a single DFT evaluation at 14 J. They are compared to the population who had a DFT++ determined at 21 J, as discussed. Similarly, the control patients who had a successful DFT+ determination at 17 J or less are compared to this same population. The positive predictive accuracy for the control evaluation was 99.2 % and for the test population, 99.1 % (p= NS).

Discussion

Since the advent of the ICD, implant defibrillation threshold testing has been utilized to predict clinical success of arrhythmia conversion. The term "safety margin" has been utilized to describe the difference between the implant DFT success level and the maximum energy available from the ICD. Prior to the LESS trial, the value of DFT testing was extrapolated from case report compilations [6-8]. Nevertheless, these retrospective reviews suggested that safety margins of 10 J determined at implant testing was reliable in predicting clinical efficacy. LESS was the first prospective evaluation of implant testing in predicting clinical efficacy. Although the DFT protocol was rigorous, a safety margin of 6 J or less was adequate when DFT++ was determined. However, the impractical aspects of performing multiple DFT evaluations during implant surgery have resulted in limited acceptance of the LESS protocol for routine implantations. Therefore, we reanalyzed the LESS results with a focus on the potential for a more practical implant testing protocol.

To understand better the results reviewed, it is necessary to understand the concept of predictive accuracy. This is reviewed in Figure 4. Positive predictive accuracy quantifies the reliability of one successful DFT evaluation at 14 J in predicting 3 successful shocks at 21 J (DFT++). When formulating a simplified implant testing scheme, positive predictive accuracy represents the most important statistic since a single successful test at 14 J must insure a safe implant if no further testing is performed. The positive predictive accuracy of 1 success at 14 J is the same as that for two successes at 17 J and statistically not different from three successes at 21 J. Thus, the added value of performing the first test at the lower value of 14 J makes this test essentially equivalent to the more rigorous protocol requiring three successes at the higher energy of 21 J.

Of the patients tested, 90 % succeeded on the first test at 14 J. Of those who failed, 75 % went on to succeed with two successes at 17 J or 21 J. Thus, with

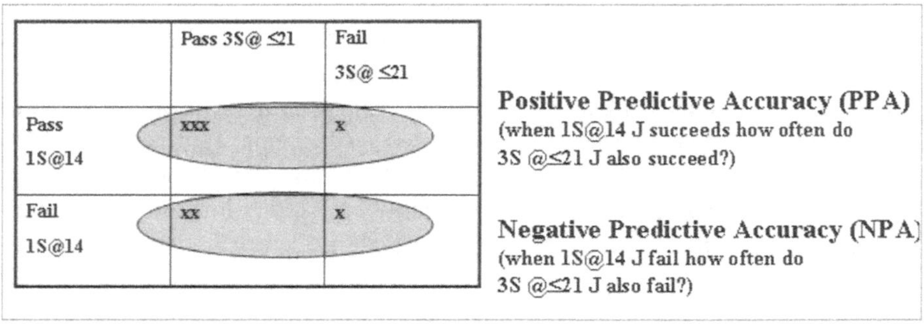

Fig. 4. A diagrammatic explanation of predictive accuracy and its application to matrix formats, such as shown in Figure 3

experienced implanters, 90 % of patients can be successfully implanted with one VF induction (at 14 J) and 97.5 % could be successfully implanted with two VF inductions, if the second shock after the failed 14 J was programmed to 21 J.

It is tempting to conclude that 97.5 % of patients would have an adequate safety margin without any implant DFT evaluation whatsoever. Of course, there are several limitations preventing this conclusion. It has been estimated that DFT evaluation has a mortality risk of less than 0.1 %. Thus, even if only 2.5 % or less of implants could benefit from operative DFT evaluation, routine use is still warranted. Statistical analysis of the positive predictive accuracy of no DFT testing versus the LESS standard of DFT+ < 21 J could not demonstrate equivalence ($p = 0.032$).

In addition, it is important to recognize that the LESS data comes from implanters at centers with extensive implant experience. This experience regarding lead positioning and other implant techniques is likely to correlate to a lower DFT. Before implantation without defibrillation testing can be recommended, further study is warranted.

This retrospective analysis of the LESS data does suggest that other standards can also be applied. Specifically, LESS suggests that two successes at 21 J should be adequate to ensure the new gold standard of three successes at 26 J. For implanters uncomfortable with performing a single DFT determination, this data regarding two successes at 21 J or less should be reassuring.

Conclusions

The Lower Energy Safety Study provides a wealth of data regarding implant defibrillation threshold testing and its relationship to clinically appropriate ICD device usage. However, the application of the recommended DFT++ testing to clinical practice is often impractical. In this study, the data was reanalyzed in regard to the potential success of less rigorous implant DFT evaluations.

We found that a single successful DFT conversion at 14 J is an acceptable screening method for implantation of a 31 J ICD. If the first shock at 14 J fails, two additional consecutive successes at 21 J or less should be demonstrated unless alternative measures are taken (lead repositioning, addition of subcutaneous array, etc.) [1, 3]. Using the suggested test scheme, approximately 90 % of patients could be implanted with a single VF induction and greater than 97 % of patients could be implanted with only 2 VF inductions. We recommend the use of the simplified implant protocol shown in Figure 5.

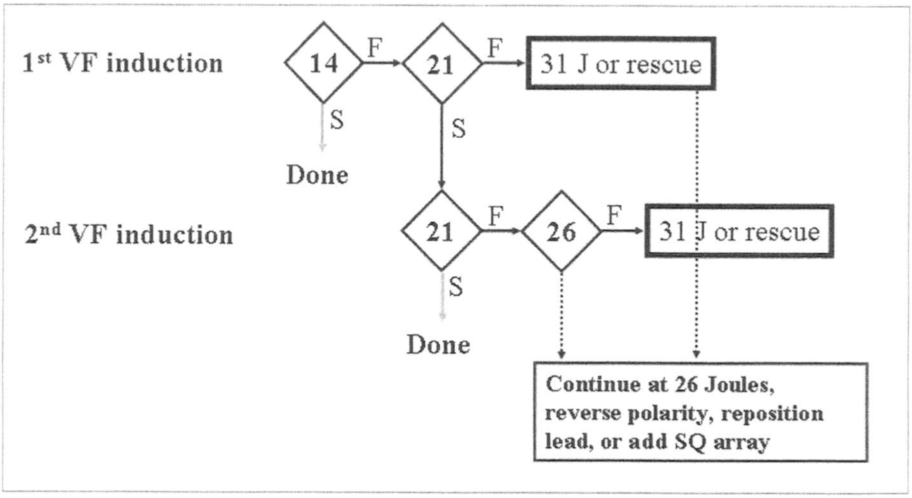

Fig. 5. Suggested new defibrillation threshold testing scheme. *F*, failure; *S*, successful conversion; *J*, joules; *SQ*, subcutaneous

References

1. Higgins SL (1997) The Implantable Cardioverter Defibrillator. A Videotape and Manual, Blackwell/Futura Publishing Co., Inc, Armonk, NY pp 46-49
2. Lang DJ, Heil JE, Hahn SJ et al (1995) Implantable cardioverter defibrillator lead technology: improved performance and lower defibrillation thresholds. PACE 18:548-559
3. Higgins SL, Alexander D, Kuypers C et al (1995) The subcutaneous array: A new lead adjunct for the transvenous ICD to lower defibrillation thresholds. PACE 18:1540-1548
4. Gold M, Higgins S, Klein R et al (2001) The effect of programmed energy safety margins on defibrillator efficacy: primary endpoint analysis from the low energy safety study (LESS). Circulation 104:11-772
5. Gilliam FR, Gold M, Higgins S et al (2001) Induced VF conversion testing predicts successful conversion of spontaneous VF: Results from the low energy safety study (LESS). PACE 24:611
6. Epstein A, Ellenbogen K, Kirk K et al (1992) Clinical characteristics and outcomes of patients with high defibrillation thresholds: a multicenter study. Circulation 86:1206-1216
7. Pinski S, Vanerio G, Castle L et al (1991) Patients with a high defibrillation threshold: clinical characteristics, management, and outcome. Am Heart J 122:89-95
8. Marchlinski F, Flores B, Miller J et al (1988) Relation of the intraoperative defibrillation threshold to successful postoperative defibrillation with an automatic implantable cardioverter defibrillator. Am J Cardiol 62:393-398

Inappropriate Defibrillator Therapies: Do Dual-chamber Devices Really Provide a Remedy?

T. Kurita[1], K. Satomi[1], A. Taguchi[1], W. Shimizu[1], K. Suyama[1], N. Aihara[1], S. Kamakura[1], K. Niwaya[2], J. Kobayashi[2]

Background

Inappropriate shock therapy from an implantable cardioverter defibrillator (ICD) is very painful for patients and may lead to a poor quality of life (QOL) and/or proarrhythmic effects. Excessively aggressive and specific programming of the ICD detection parameters with the aim of avoiding inappropriate therapy may result in a loss of its sensitivity (and in the worst case even to fatal underdetection of VF). Both sensitivity and specificity of the ICD's diagnostic functions are expected to be improved by atrial sensing, which provides a more complex algorithm for arrhythmia detection based on both ventricular and atrial activity [1–3]. On the other hand, the addition of an atrial lead may produce several adverse effects, such as extension of the operating time, higher risk of lead dislodgement, cardiac tamponade, and occlusion of the subclavian vein.

Purpose

The purpose of this study was to test the function of dual-chamber ICDs with reference to their accuracy in the detection of spontaneous tachyarrhythmias and to consider the proper indications and programming for single- and dual-chamber ICDs.

Patients

In Japan, the clinical use of precordial single-chamber ICDs was approved in February 1997 and the use of dual-chamber devices, in June 2000. From

[1]Division of Cardiology and [2]Division of Cardiovascular Surgery, National Cardiovascular Center, Osaka, Japan

February 1997 to January 2003, ICDs were implanted transvenously in 252 patients with VT/VF in our hospital. Dual-chamber devices were implanted in 71 of the 127 (55.9%) patients treated after their use was approved. The patients were divided into two groups: the single-chamber ICD group (S-ICD group; 181 patients, mean age 52 years, male/female ratio 146/35) and the dual-chamber ICD group (D-ICD group; 71 patients, mean age 59 years, male/female ratio 54/17). In the S-ICD group, Medtronic ICDs (models 7221CX, 7223CX, 7227CX, 7229) were implanted in 148 patients, and Guidant ICDs (MINI-IV 1796) in 33 patients. In the D-ICD group, Medtronic devices (models 7271, 7273) were implanted in all patients.

The indication for the dual-chamber ICDs were as follows; (1) bradycardia in 14/71 (20%), (2) supraventricular tachycardia in 13/71 (18%), (3) AV node conduction disturbances detected by an EP study in 12/71 (17%), (4) need for medication with β-blockers to treat heart failure in 12/71 (17%), (5) slower VT (heart rate < 150/min) in 3/71 (4%), and (6) other in 17/71 (24%).

Methods

We compared the incidence of inappropriate ICD therapy and complications (lead dislodgement, persistent pericardial effusion or cardiac tamponade, or wound infection) between the S-ICD and D-ICD groups. The inappropriate ICD therapy was defined as antitachycardia pacing and/or shock delivery during supraventricular tachycardia (SVT). All spontaneous episodes were classified as either appropriate or inappropriate therapy according to the decision of more than two physicians based on the stored electrograms recorded during the ICD therapy. We also evaluated the incidence of and reasons for generator exchanges of single- for dual-chamber ICDs.

Programming

The maximum cycle length for the VT detection interval was programmed to be 30–40 ms longer than that of the clinical VT, and the maximum VF detection cycle length was programmed at 280–300 ms in all ICDs. In the S-ICD group, the differential diagnostic functions for SVT, such as the sudden onset criteria or rate stability criteria, were principally programmed on. In the D-ICD group, all three SVT criteria (Medtronic PR-logic) for sinus tachycardia, AF/flutter, or other 1:1 SVTs were programmed on. The zone for the SVT criteria was programmed within the zone of the VT detection intervals.

Statistical Analysis

Student's t-test was used to compare the parameters between the two groups. A value of $p<0.05$ was defined as statistically significant.

Results

Inappropriate Therapy (Table 1)

The incidence of inappropriate ICD therapy did not significantly differ between the two groups [28/181 patients (15%) in the S-ICD group vs 9/71 (13%) in the D-ICD group; NS]. The causes of the inappropriate ICD therapy in the S-ICD and D-ICD groups were: (1) atrial fibrillation (AF) in 13/28 vs 3/9, NS; (2) sinus tachycardia in 4/28 vs 4/9, p=0.078; (3) oversensing of T-waves or electromyograms in 4/28 vs 1/9, NS; and (4) therapy delivery after spontaneous termination of VT/VF in 7/28 vs 1/9, NS, respectively for the two groups. Except for the inappropriate ICD therapy during sinus tachycardia, there was no significant difference between the two groups in the causes of inappropriate therapy.

Table 1. Inappropriate therapy after implantation of implantable cardioverter defibrillators (ICD)

	Single-chamber ICD	Dual-chamber ICD
Inappropriate ICD therapy in	28 (15%)	9 (13%)
AF	13	3
Sinus tachycardia	4	4
Oversensing	4	1
Therapy after spontaneous termination	7	1

Attempts to avoid the inappropriate therapy after the first event in the S-ICD group involved β–blocker administration in 4/28, reprogramming of the detection parameters in 15/28, and replacement of the ICD with a dual-chamber version in 4. Even after these attempts, 6/28 (21%) patients without an upgrade of the generator experienced recurrence of the inappropriate therapy.

In the D-ICD group, the additional attempts to avoid inappropriate therapy after the first inappropriate event were β-blocker therapy in 3/9 and reprogramming of the detection parameters in 4/9 patients. These attempts completely prevented the inappropriate ICD therapy in all patients thereafter.

Operating Time and Complications (Table 2)

The operating time was significantly shorter in the S-ICD group than in the D-ICD group (83 ± 30 min vs 104 ± 30 min, $p < 0.01$). The complications observed in the S-ICD and D-ICD groups were (1) lead dislodgement in 4/181 (2%) vs 2/71 (3%), NS; (2) persistent pericardial effusion or cardiac tamponade in 2/181 (1%) vs 4/71 (6%), $P = 0.057$; and (3) wound infection in 5/181 (3%) vs

0/71 (0%), NS, respectively, for the two groups. Except for the persistent pericardial effusion, there was no significant difference in the incidence of the complications between the two groups. No perioperative deaths were observed in either group.

Table 2. Operation time and complications associated with the ICD

	Single chamber ICD	Dual chamber ICD
Operation time (min)	83±30*	104±3
Complication		
Lead dislodgement	4 (1%)**	2 (3%)
Pericardial effusion	2 (1%)	4 (6%)
Wound infection	5 (3%)	0
Pneumothorax	1 (0.6%)	0
Skin necrosis	1 (0.6%)	1 (1%)
Total	14 (8%)	6 (8%)

*$p<0.01$, **$p=0.057$ vs dual-chamber ICD

Generator Replacement from a Single- to a Dual-chamber Device

In 8 cases in the S-ICD group, a generator replacement with insertion of a dual-chamber device was required, because of newly developed bradycardia in 4 and inappropriate ICD therapy in 4. In all these 8 patients, the subclavian vein was patent at the ICD implantation site and it was possible to insert an additional atrial lead through the same vessel.

Discussion

Inappropriate Therapy

As in other studies, it was not possible to demonstrate any clearly superior sensitivity of dual-chamber over single-chamber ICDs in the present study [1–3]. When only single-chamber ICDs were available (prior to June 2000 in Japan), a great deal of attention was devoted to avoiding inappropriate ICD therapy by producing a safety margin between the minimum cycle length of the SVT and the lower VT/VF detection interval during drug therapy, for example by giving β-blockers, digitalis, or calcium antagonists. Since introduction of dual-chamber ICDs there may have been a tendency to be less careful about avoiding this adverse effect and leave it to the dual-chamber device. It must be noted that even dual-chamber ICDs depend basically on the rate criteria for making a differential diagnosis between VT/VF and SVT. Particularly in the D-ICD group, missed diagnosis of sinus tachycardia was frequently observed, because prolongation of a relatively long PR interval caused P-wave sensing within the retrograde P-zone of the PR-logic algorithm (a PR interval > 50% of the RR interval) [3]. The newer Medtronic devices, which have the capability for programming more detailed SVT criteria, are expected to reduce the frequency of adverse events.

A much lower recurrence rate of inappropriate ICD therapy in the D-ICD group indicated that the dual-chamber ICDs had better flexibility and adaptability and were thus much better suited for making improvements to the programming after the first adverse event. Once enough has been learned about the characteristics of the dual-chamber ICD algorithm, it is possible to prevent inappropriate therapy even without the occurrence of an actual event.

Complications Associated with the Implantable Cardioverter Defibrillators

Although the implantation of a dual-chamber ICD takes approximately 20 min longer than the operation to implant a single-chamber ICD, the incidence of wound infection was no different between the two groups. The longer operation time for the dual-chamber ICD implantations was mainly taken up with maneuvering the atrial lead during the insertion. Persistent pericardial effusions or cardiac tamponades were relatively frequent in the D-ICD group. To obtain large atrial activity to eliminate the far-field R-wave sensing, several attempts were necessary to find an accurate atrial lead placement, and occasionally this resulted in the selection of the right atrial free wall as the appropriate site. This relatively difficult technique for atrial lead manipulation might be implicated in the higher incidence of atrial wall injuries and persistent pericardial effusions. Programmability of the blanking period for atrial sensing may be useful in cases with large far-field R-wave sensing.

References

1. Deisenhofer I, Kolb C, Ndrepepa G et al (2001) Do current dual chamber cardioverter defibrillators have advantages over conventional single chamber cardioverter defibrillators in reducing inappropriate therapies? A randomized, prospective study. J Cardiovasc Electrophysiol 12:134–142
2. Wilkoff BL, Kuhlkamp V, Volosin K et al (2001) Critical analysis of dual-chamber implantable cardioverter-defibrillator arrhythmia detection: results and technical considerations. Circulation 103:381–386
3. Kuhlkamp V, Wilkoff BL, Brown AB et al (2002) Experience with a dual chamber implantable defibrillator. Pacing Clin Electrophysiol 25:1041–1048

Should Antiarrhythmic Drugs Be Administered After First Appropriate ICD Shock, and If So, Which Ones?

G. Abali, K. Aytemir, A. Oto

Implantable cardioverter defibrillator (ICD) devices have been used for many years to prevent sudden cardiac death. Rapidly evolving ICD technology has widened the indications and clinical applications of these devices. Despite the technological advances, however, patients with ICDs are still at risk of sudden arrhythmic cardiac death. Furthermore, ventricular arrhythmias that require shock therapy, and inappropriate shocks triggered by supraventricular arrhythmias, adversely affect the quality of life of patients with implanted ICDs. However, many patients with ICDs have been discharged with no antiarrhythmic drug prescription. The addition of adjuvant antiarrhythmic drug treatment to ICD therapy is frequently required after the first shock therapy, to improve the quality of life of these patients.

Antiarrhythmic drugs have several potential interactions with ICD devices: beneficial, deleterious, and neutral (see Table 1). Also, patients with ICDs have structural heart diseases which necessitate using drugs other than antiarrhythmic ones. After the first appropriate shock therapy, recognizing important ICD and antiarrhythmic drug interactions and the patient's structural heart disease remains critical in the management of these patients.

Many patients with ICDs have a low ejection fraction due to ischemic, idiopathic, or other causes. They therefore need β-blocker therapy to prolong survival and prevent recurrent ischemic events, independent of any potential antiarrhythmic benefit. In patients with dilated cardiomyopathy, especially ischemic, β-blockers are the best choice of antiarrhythmic drugs after the first ICD shock. β-blockers have neutral effects on the defibrillation threshold. β-blockade has various advantages in patients with ICD. In a nonrandomized trial, β-blocker therapy reduced the incidence of ICD shocks and delayed the time to first ICD discharge, but had no effect on survival [1].

Amiodarone is a benzofuran derivative and is used for the treatment of patients with life-threatening ventricular arrhythmias when other drugs are

Department of Cardiology, Hacettepe University, Ankara, Turkey

Table 1. Drug–device interactions in ICD patients

Harmful interactions	Beneficial interactions
Increase in defibrillation threshold Slowing VT below the detection rate	Limiting the number of VT/VF episodes Slowing VT
Interference with VT detection by altering VT characteristics	Reducing inappropriate therapy due to supraventricular arrhythmia
Promoting resistance of VT to pacing termination	Decreasing defibrillation threshold
Promoting incessant slow VT	Treating symptomatic arrhythmia other than VT/VF
Sinus bradycardia or heart block requiring pacing	
QT prolongation	
1:1 conducted slow atrial flutter	

VT, Ventricular tachycardia; *VF*, ventricular fibrillation

ineffective or are not tolerated. A number of prospective, randomized, controlled trials have demonstrated improved survival with amiodarone therapy compared with placebo [2, 3]. It is the most frequently used antiarrhythmic drug in patients with left ventricular dysfunction. Among ICD recipients, 205–25% receive amiodarone at some time during follow-up in most large recent series [4]. The most common indications include treatment of atrial fibrillation and limitation of the frequency of episodes of symptomatic ventricular tachycardia or ventricular fibrillation.

Amiodarone can slow the ventricular tachycardia rate. This causes repeated attempts at antitachycardia pacing before delivery of an uncomfortable shock. After the drug is stopped the ventricular tachycardia rate will be increased, often necessitating reprogramming of the ICD. But the half-life of amiodarone is long, and the effect will be apparent for a further 1 or 2 months.

Another problem is the defibrillation threshold. In animal studies amiodarone may increase the defibrillation threshold [5]. This would cause failure of defibrillation in patients with ICDs. However, in a later study Kühlkamp et al. [6] showed that chronic amiodarone therapy does not constitute a particular risk of an inadequate defibrillation threshold in implantation of a defibrillator with biphasic shock. On the other hand, the stimulation threshold is raised in chronic therapy with amiodarone. Amiodarone is more effective than class I drugs in decreasing the number of ICD shocks [7]. Class I drugs also cause more symptomatic side effects.

Kettering et al. [8] designed a study to compare the efficacy of metoprolol and sotalol in preventing recurrences of sustained ventricular tachyarrhythmias and in reducing mortality in patients with an ICD. A total of 100 ICD-implanted patients were included in the study. Most of the patients were suffering from coronary heart disease and dilated cardiomyopathies. The mean left ventricular ejection fraction was 0.38 (SD±0.14). After withdrawal of prior antiarrhythmic medication, an electrophysiological study was performed in all patients and the indication for the implantation of an ICD was confirmed. Then patients were randomized to metoprolol or sotalol. The mean follow-up was 728 days. Thirty-three patients in the metoprolol group and the 30 patients in the sotalol group had at least one ventricular tachycardia/fibrillation episode during follow-up. None of these episodes was classified as torsades de pointes in the sotalol group. Nineteen patients in the metoprolol group and the 16 patients in the sotalol group were treated by shock therapy. Total mortality did not differ significantly between the two treatment groups. This study demonstrates that there is no significant difference between metoprolol and sotalol with regard to prevention of ventricular tachycardia/fibrillation recurrences and to total mortality in patients with an ICD. In disagreement with this study, Seidl et al. [9] showed that metoprolol was superior to sotalol with regard to the recurrence rate of ventricular tachyarrhythmias; no difference was found between the two groups in terms of total mortality.

Sotalol has β-blocker effects in addition to class III antiarrhythmic properties. Therefore it may be the drug of choice in patients with coronary heart disease and dilated cardiomyopathy who have an ICD. It has also been shown to reduce the defibrillation threshold [10]. Pacifico et al. [11] randomized 302 patients with ICD to receive either placebo or sotalol. The group receiving sotalol had a 48% risk reduction for delivery of shock. Sotalol can be used in patients with high defibrillation energy requirements. On the other hand, although sotalol has β-blocking properties, it does not prevent arrhythmic death in post-myocardial-infarction patients. Moreover, since it also has a negative inotropic effect, patients with dilated cardiomyopathy with ICD must be closely monitored during sotalol therapy. Sotalol can slow ventricular tachycardia, but the effect is modest and it is not likely that the tachycardia cycle length will be slowed below the programmed tachycardia zone.

Class Ic drugs such as flecainide and propafenone are relatively contraindicated for most patients with ventricular tachycardia or fibrillation and left ventricular dysfunction because of their negative inotropic and proarrhythmic effects.

Congenital long QT syndrome and hypertrophic cardiomyopathy are other reasons for ICD implantation. In these patient groups β-blockers are the first choice of antiarrhythmic drugs after the first shock therapy; amiodarone may be used as a second choice.

A special condition, Brugada syndrome, is another indication for ICD implantation. In this syndrome a genetic abnormality of the sodium channel has been identified that results in idiopathic ventricular fibrillation without any underlying cause. There is no known antiarrhythmic drug to prevent ventricular fibrillation in this syndrome. Only ICD therapy reduces the mortality.

Reduction in the defibrillation threshold, in the ventricular tachycardia rate to allow for antitachycardia pacing, and in the number of ICD discharges, and improvement in patients' quality of life are potential reasons for prescribing antiarrhythmic drugs for patients with ICDs. Table 2 summarizes the important interactions of antiarrhythmic drugs and ICDs.

Table 2. Antiarrhythmic drugs and ICD interactions

Drug	VT/VF prevention	Effects on DFT	VT modification	Advantages	Disadvantages
β+Blockers	Probably effective	None or decrease	May slow VT	Indication in coronary heart disease and congestive heart failure	Negative inotropy, bradycardia
Sotalol	Proven efficacy	May decrease	Moderately slows VT	Also has β+blocker activity	Negative inotropy, bradycardia
Amiodarone	Most probably effective	May increase	May slow VT, possibly below detection	Safe and tolerated in congestive heart failure	Bradycardia

DFT, Defibrillation threshold

Conclusions

ICDs have become an important therapeutic modality for patients with life-threatening ventricular arrhythmias. Despite the effectiveness and therapeutic sophistication of the ICD for terminating ventricular arrhythmias, antiarrhythmic drug therapy has been used in approximately half of ICD patients. However, antiarrhythmic drug therapy should only be instituted with an understanding of its potential harmful and beneficial effects on ICD therapy and the patient's underlying heart disease. There are not enough data to prove that antiarrhythmic drug treatment should be started after the first appropriate ICD shock.

References

1. Levine JH, Mellits D, Baumgartner RA et al (1991) Predictors of first discharge and subsequent survival in patients with automatic implantable cardioverter defibrillators. Circulation 84:558–566
2. Ceremuzynski L (1993) Secondary prevention after myocardial infarction with class III antiarrhythmic drugs. Am J Cardiol 72:82F
3. Julian DG, Camm AJ, Frangin G et al (1997) Randomised trial of effect of amiodarone on mortality in patients with left ventricular dysfunction after recurrent myocardial infarction: EMIAT. Lancet 349:667
4. Dorian P (1998) Interactions between implantable devices and pharmacological agents. Card Electrophysiol Rev 2:151–153
5. Epstein AE, Ellenbogen KA, Kirk KA et al (1992) Clinical characteristics and outcome of patients with high defibrillation thresholds. A multicenter study. Circulation 86:1206–1216
6. Kühlkamp V, Mewis C, Suchalla R et al (1999) Effects of amiodarone and sotalol on defibrillation threshold in comparison to patients without antiarrhythmic drug treatment. Int J Cardiol 69:271–279
7. Dolak GL for the CASCADE investigators (1994) Clinical predictors of ICD shocks. Am J Cardiol 73:237–241
8. Kettering K, Mewis C, Dörnberger V et al (2002) Efficacy of metoprolol and sotalol in the prevention of recurrences of sustained ventricular tachyarrhythmias in patients with an implantable cardioverter defibrillator. J Pacing Electrophysiol 25:1571–1576
9. Seidl K, Hauer B, Schwick N et al (1998) Comparision of metoprolol and sotalol in preventing ventricular tachyarrhythmias after implntation of ICD. Am J Cardiol 82:744–748
10. Dorian P, Newman D, Sheahan R et al (1996) D-sotalol decreases defibrillation energy requirements in humans. A novel indication for drug therapy. J Cardiovasc Electrophysiol 7:952–961
11. Pacifico A, Hohnloser SH, Williams JH et al (1999) Prevention of implantable defibrillator shock by treatment with sotalol. N Engl J Med 340:1855–1862

Quality of Life in Patients with ICD: Is It Improved or Worsened?

B. LÜDERITZ

Definition of Quality of Life

'Quality of life' has different meanings and entails different components, depending on the perspective of the investigator and the intention of any analysis. Although there is no exact definition of quality of life, there is an emerging consensus that quality-of-life assessment can be based on physical condition, psychological wellbeing, social activity, and everyday activity. These categories can then be further subdivided into a number of aspects such as mobility, self-care, family contact, intimacy, or negativity in terms of depression or anxiety. The approach to quality of life, therefore, must be multidimensional and involve a variety of investigatory tools (Table 1). The usefulness of many trials dealing with quality of life is limited by their unidimensional approach focusing only on restricted issues, e.g., functional status, excluding mental or psychological aspects or psychological features, leaving aside functional capacity. Future investigations of quality of life, moreover, will have to address a variety of health-associated sectors, including costs, working capacity, and social care, in addition to physical and mental integrity, since invasive therapies cause manifold interactions between the individual and the environment and vice versa. Quality-of-life research should, therefore, use an analytic model and comprehensively include predictors and response variables in a given time-frame in which the impact of therapy on quality of life is elicited [1].

The Implantable Cardioverter Defibrillator

The implantable cardioverter defibrillator (ICD) has demonstrably reduced the mortality of sudden cardiac death in patients with malignant ventricular tachyarrhythmias since its introduction into clinical practice. It has become the therapy of choice for patients with aborted sudden cardiac death or hemody-

Department of Medicine – Cardiology, University of Bonn, Bonn, Germany

Table 1. Assessment of quality of life: Medical Outcomes Study Short Form 36 (range 0–100, higher scores showing better functional status and wellbeing)

_	Role, physical
_	Vitality
_	Physical functioning
_	Social functioning
_	Mental health
_	Role, emotional
_	Bodily pain
_	General health

namically unstable ventricular tachyarrhythmias and various underlying heart diseases. Transvenous placement of the device became possible some time ago, followed by antitachycardia pacing and device miniaturization; the safety of the therapy in terms of reliability of hardware and software has meanwhile been demonstrated, and quality of life in patients with ICDs has gained increasingly in importance over the years. In the early period of ICD use, painless termination of ventricular tachycardia and the avoidance of inappropriate shocks were the main clinical points of interest, but today patient acceptance, coping behavior, and psychological integrity are increasingly focused on [2]. Quality-of-life assessment is of great importance in patients with ICDs, because it has been demonstrated that, although ICD therapy improves survival in patients who are at risk of sudden cardiac death, there are also several inherent problems, e.g., inappropriate shocks, fear of shock therapy, and the consciousness of the lifesaving character of the ICD [3–8]. The aim of ICD therapy is only fully achieved if patients regain the maximum possible flexibility, return to their normal range of activity, and are reintegrated into family and professional life. A large battery of measuring instruments is now in use to evaluate the quality of life in ICD patients, with the intention of obtaining targets and guiding approaches to support for this very selective patient population and providing interventional psychological tools [1].

Design of Quality of Life Measurement Scales

Measurement of quality of life should involve all aspects, subjective and objective, that can be affected by a therapy in each member of a patient population in either a positive or a negative way. This can be achieved only by the use of standardized instruments that have been validated. The primary issue for selection of a specific instrument is its expected performance in a required situation. The choice is guided by the instrument's psychometric properties, including validity, reliability, responsiveness, appropriateness to the question under scrutiny, use, and practical utility. The common measurement of quality of life is based on complex constructions including items, domains, scales, and instruments. An item is a single question, and a scale contains the available categories or other mechanisms for expressing the response to the question. For instance, a specific question might be answered by filling out an open-ended blank at the discretion of the patient, or several options, or a visual analogue line, where the patient places a quasidimensional mark. All three scales cited here are considered global, since no specific criteria are offered to the patient to demarcate the choice of categories or other expressions. A domain identifies a specific point of interest, such as functional capacity or digestion. This can include a response to single or multiple items.

The instrument itself is a collection of items that is used to gather the required information. An instrument can contain a global question or multiple items that can be categorized into different domains. For the measurement of quality of life, one or more instruments may be used. For a single instrument, the output result can be formed in two ways: either as a profile, preserving the components and citing them individually, or by aggregating the results to a single composite score. Some instruments offer both methods of presentation. The use of instruments and investigatory techniques is influenced by a number of factors: setting of the evaluation, type of questionnaire used (short form, clinic-based survey, mail-back survey), and others. There are two main types of instruments: *generic instruments* used for surveys in genereal populations to assess a variety of domains, and *disease-specific instruments* focusing on domains that are most relevant to a certain disease or condition under study. Disease-specific instruments are used for clinical trials to assess the influence of specific therapeutic interventions. An advantage of them is that they are restricted only to relevant dimensions for the specific disease, but are at a disadvantage in terms of comparability with other disease groups. It is possible to integrate both generic and disease-specific instruments by using a battery of scales and modular instruments, maintaining a core module to address both different disease groups and the therapy under investigation. Finally, studies have demonstrated that judgements on quality of life are highly subject and observer dependent. Therefore, a systematic approach to measuring quality of life is needed to allow for an improvement in health care professionals' evaluation of quality of life in all fields of medical therapy [1].

Quality of Life in Patients with Implantable Cardioverter Defibrillators

Patient acceptance of ICD therapy is influenced by a number of contributing factors, including the patient's preimplant medical history, socialization, environment, and technical aspects, such as number of shocks, battery location, device size/body size, and inappropriate shocks [2]. This means that a patient who easily adapts to the fact of an ICD implant itself may have a very low acceptance of the device during follow-up, depending on whether inappropriate or appropriate therapies are administered. A patient may also suffer from the fact that he is no longer allowed to drive or to work in his profession (e.g., as a mechanical engineer). Many patients do not experience shocks but live in constant fear of shocks. Therefore, quality-of-life measurements must address not only the obvious issues such as device-related, objective data, but also more subjective issues, including all the various perceptions of the individual patient.

In our own patient population, we investigated 57 (out of 763) patients with ICDs (Tables 2, 3) in a prospective pilot study, using a variety of quality-of-life issues [6, 8]. Eight different questionnaires were used to obtain information on general sociodemographic data and ICD implantation and therapy acceptance, personality (Freiburg Personality Inventory), and quality of life (MOS-SF 36 Inventory). In addition, the patients answered questionnaires on fear (State Trait Anxiety Inventory), complaints (Complaint List), depression (Beck Depression Inventory), and coping behavior.

The Coping Behavior Inventory evaluates the patient's reaction to the fact that he/she has a heart disease and to the changes in behavior during follow-up. In our patient population, 24 of 57 patients answered that they were used to the device after 2 months; the remaining 34 patients needed a longer period to adapt to the system (Fig. 1). The most frequent reply (20 patients) to the question of what their greatest fear was fear of ICD discharge, followed by fear of physical discomfort caused by the device, and finally restricted quality of life in professional, sports, and social activities. When asked whether they would recommend the device to other patients, the vast majority (56 of 57) answered in the affirmative (Fig. 2).

Shock incidence was found to be a very important factor that has a negative impact on quality of life, worsening the severity of depression, symptoms, and level of anxiety. In our own study population, experiencing more than five shocks caused a significantly higher level of anxiety in patients, independent of age or sex. These findings are consistent with the data of Dougherty and Hegel, who also found a significantly higher level of anxiety and depression in patients with $\leq$5 discharges than in patients without any appropriate or inappropriate discharge [7, 9, 10].

Table 2. Reasons for implantation of ICDs in patients treated at the University Hospital in Bonn ($N = 763$; 593 men, 170 women, age 63 ± 12 years; in all 1,140 devices were implanted, 372 being replacements)

Disease	*n*
Coronary artery disease	477
Idiopathic dilated cardiomyopathy	131
Hypertrophic (non)obstructive cardiomyopathy	14
Myocarditis	13
Arrhythmogenic right ventricular dysplasia	15
Idiopathic ventricular fibrillation	66
Long QT syndrome	4
Other	43

Table 3. ICD devices used (including replacements) in the 763 patients (May 2003)

Device	*n*	Device	*n*	Device	*n*	Device	*n*
AICD	60	7217 B	36	InSync ICD	24	Photon DR	16
PRX	45	7219 B, C, D, E	82	GEM III VR	31	Photon VR	12
Ventak P2	25	7220/1	23	GEM III DR	31	Atlas	7
Ventak Mini	53	7218	65	GEM III AT	33	Profile	24
Vental AV	31	7223	64	Marquis	23	Defender	50
PRIZM VR	27	Jewel AF	65	(Reveal)	28	Metrix	9
PRIZM DR	35	GEM DR	8	Cadence	3	Guardian ATP	11
Contak /Renewal	17	GEM SR	66	Cadet	3	Sentinel	4
Res-Q/ Micron	32			Contour	6		
Vitality	3	GEM II VR	41	Angstrøm	20	Phylax	1
		GEM DR	6	Belos	1	Alto DR	14

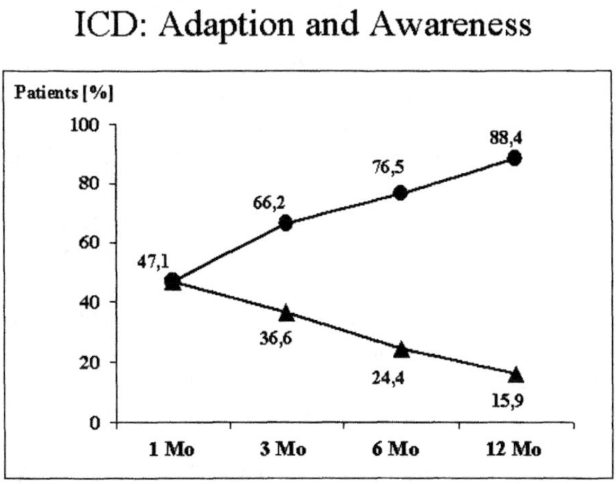

Fig. 1. Patient adaption to the implantable cardioverter defibrillator (ICD) and awareness of the device. There is a significant increase in adaption over the first 12 months after implant; awareness decreases continuously over time

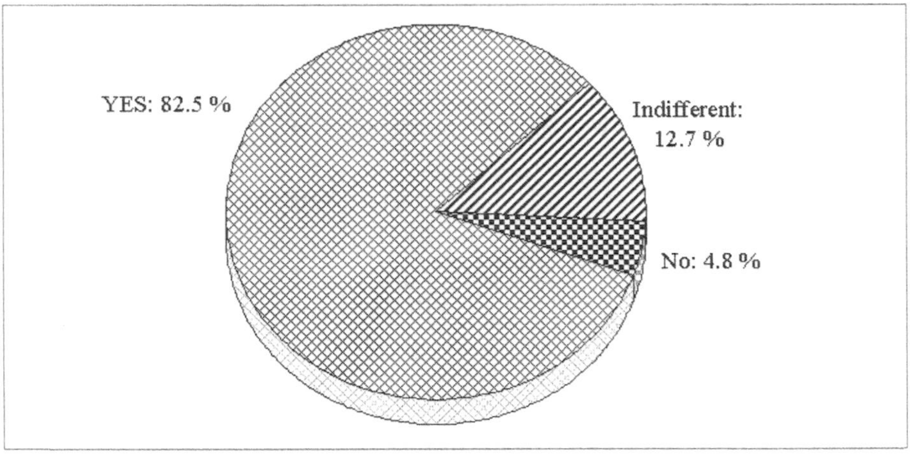

Fig. 2. Quality of life in ICD recipients. Replies to the question, "Was it worth having an ICD device implanted?"

References

1. Wolpert C, Jung W, Herwig S, Lüderitz B (2000) Quality of life in patients with implantable cardioverter-defibrillators. In: Aliot E, Clementy J, Prystowsky EN (eds) Fighting sudden cardiac death: a worldwide challenge. Futura, Armonk, pp 661–669
2. Sears SF, Conti JB (2002) Quality of life and logical functioning of ICD patients. Heart 87:488–493
3. Sears SF, Todaro JF, Lewis TS et al (1999) Examining the psychosocial impact of implantable cardioverter defibrillators: a literature review. Clin Cardiol 22:481–489
4. Vlay SC, Olson LC, Fricchione GL et al (1989) Anxiety and anger in patients with ventricular tachyarrhythmias: response after automatic internal cardioverter defibrillator implantation. Pacing Clin Electrophysiol 12:366–373
5. Lüderitz B, Jung W, Deister A, Manz M (1996) Quality of life in multiprogrammable implantable cardioverter-defibrillator recipients. In: Saksena S, Lüderitz B (eds) Interventional electrophysiology: a textbook. Futura, Armonk, pp 305–313
6. Kalbfleisch KR, Lehmann MH, Steinmann RT et al (1989) Reemployment following implantation of the automatic cardioverter defibrillator. Am J Cardiol 64:199–202
7. Dougherty CM (1995) Psychological reactions and family adjustment in shock versus no shock groups after implantation of internal cardioverter defibrillator. Heart Lung 24:281–291
8. Lüderitz B, Jung W, Deister A et al (1994) Patient acceptance of implantable cardioverter defibrillator devices: changing attitudes. Am Heart J 127:1179–1184
9. Hegel MT, Griegel LE, Black C et al (1997) Anxiety and depression in patients receiving implanted cardioverter-defibrillators: a longitudinal investigation. Intl J Psychiatry Med 27:57–69
10. Lüderitz B (2003) Quality of life in patients with ICD. In: Tse HF, Lee KLF, Lau CP (eds) Clinical cardiac pacing and electrophysiology. Monduzzi–MEDIMOND, Bologna, Italy, pp 157-163

OUT-OF-HOSPITALS CARDIAC ARREST AND PUBLIC ACCESS DEFIBRILLATION

Public Use of AEDs in Europe: Where Are We Now and Where Are We Going?

D. Chamberlain[1,2], L. Bossaert[3], S. Davies[4], M. Colquhoun[1,2]

The Potential for Automated External Defibrillators

Automated external defibrillators (AEDs) were introduced into clinical use in the early 1980s [1, 2], but acceptance was slow and it is only recently that their potential for community resuscitation has become widely appreciated. In Europe–as elsewhere–we remain a long way from the optimal use of an important technology. Sufficient experience has been gained, however, to show both the value of AEDs and their limitations, and to indicate where priorities for deployment might lie as their availability increases. The evidence confirming that we should encourage their widespread use is compelling. Whilst there may be a potential role for in-hospital use, the greatest contribution that AEDs can make towards improving survival from cardiac arrest lies outside hospital–for use in public places by persons who are not healthcare professionals.

Where Are We Now in Europe?

In many countries of Europe, the law has hindered the widespread use of AEDs. In many areas defibrillation is considered a medical responsibility. In some it can be delegated to nurses, whereas in others even this has not been deemed appropriate. The restriction has impacted adversely on important potential developments in resuscitation, but is slowly being addressed. In some countries the task has been easier than in others. At present (June 2003) the situation in various European countries for the use of *AEDs in public places* is as follows:

[1]Prehospital Emergency Research Unit, University of Wales College of Medicine and Lansdowne Hospital, Cardiff, UK; [2]Wales Heart Research Institute, Cardiff, UK; [3]Department of Intensive Care, University Hospital Antwerp, Edegem, Belgium; [4]Defibrillators in Public Places Initiative, Department of Health, London, UK

- No legal restriction: Norway, Republic of Ireland, Romania, United Kingdom.
- Law permits use: Austria, Iceland (soon), Italy, Sweden.
- Law does not cover unrestricted use: Belgium, Croatia, Denmark, Finland, Germany, Greece, Holland, Hungary, Poland, Portugal, Russia, Slovak Republic, Slovakia, Slovenia, Spain, Turkey.

However, the situation is complex and more favourable than is apparent from the above list. Some of the countries that still do not permit public use of AEDs by all-encompassing legislation do allow individuals to defibrillate (either with any defibrillators or with AEDs only), provided they have been trained appropriately or are acting under Good Samaritan provisions. These include Denmark, Finland, Germany, Greece, Hungary, Holland, Russia, Spain (in 4 of 17 provinces), Sweden (but only under medical control), and Switzerland. In all, some form of organized public-access defibrillation exists in at least 13 countries, with isolated initiatives in a few more. At least 11 countries have AEDs available in the homes of some high-risk patients.

The notion that defibrillation must remain in the hands of physicians does not explain all the reluctance to take advantage of automated defibrillation. General practitioners will witness patients with cardiac arrest more commonly than others outside the hospital environment. For these healthcare professionals at least, the case for possession of AEDs seems unassailable. Yet this is rare–if practised at all–in 10 European countries and is universal in none.

The slow development of community AED deployment in Europe is reflected in the paucity of papers on lay use–in contrast to the output from the United States, where enthusiasm has generally been greater. Notable, however, is a study from the Piacenza region of Italy [3], where AEDs were placed in high-risk locations, in lay-staffed ambulances, and in police cars. Unusually, 1,285 lay volunteers were trained in the use of AEDs without traditional education in cardiopulmonary resuscitation. During the first 22 months of the study, 354 cardiac arrests occurred, and the overall survival rate in the resuscitation attempts implemented by the trained volunteers was 3 times the success rate achieved by the traditional Emergency Medical System. The difference was due to the shorter response times. An important study of police defibrillation was undertaken in Amsterdam [4], but the results were generally disappointing because communication between the ambulance control centre and the police took longer than expected. Nevertheless, valuable lessons were learned, and future experience is likely to reflect improvements in procedures. The cost of a community programme was addressed in a 3-year prospective study in an urban emergency medical system in Helsinki [5]. Public sites with a previous incidence of at least one cardiac arrest per year were equipped with AEDs. 20 arrests were observed during the study, but the new system could be used in only seven of them. Although defibrillation was accomplished more rapidly in the AED group, none was discharged alive. The costs of training, administration, and supervision accounted for 85% of the budget. The authors cautioned that careful consideration should be given to costs before any major schemes are implemented.

The use of AEDs in most European countries has been cautious even in respect of emergency medical technicians. Experience has generally been favourable, however [6–10]. In France progress has been particularly cautious, but recent reports have drawn attention to the possible advantages of extending AED use to an informed and motivated public [11, 12]. Possible benefits have also been highlighted in Belgium [13].

The United Kingdom is fortunate in having had no legislation governing AED use, so that it has not been influenced by legal constraint. This is one explanation of why deployment outside hospitals and the conventional emergency service has progressed further than in other European countries. Other reasons include the influence of the Resuscitation Council (UK), which is the oldest organization of its type in Europe, the availability of funding from the British Heart Foundation (a major UK charity), and the central coordination of the Ambulance Service, which liaises closely with medical organizations with an interest in prehospital care.

True public use of AEDs in England (specifically) can be considered under two headings, those where the defibrillators are positioned in places of high risk with the intention that they be used 'on site', and those where they are kept for a more distant response that is nevertheless expected to be faster than can be provided by the conventional ambulance service. Many of the on-site units have been provided by the Department of Health to be used in public places [14], which have been identified by the ambulance services as being places where sudden cardiac death commonly occurs: most of these are airports and railway stations. Other units have been provided by charities and private organizations for use in sports facilities, rehabilitation areas, and industrial sites. These 'community' AEDs, which are intended for distant (rather than on-site) rescue, usually supplement responses by conventional ambulances and are usually under ambulance service control. Although they are integrated into the regular emergency system, they are nevertheless operated by volunteers and form part of a community, or public, system. The crucial difference is that for on-site units the AED is likely to be only a minute or two's walk away from the point of collapse and will be carried. The community units are likely to be transported by other means.

The two types of AED deployment–on site and community–entail very different costs and benefits, although the ratio between cost and benefit may not be very different. The term 'on site' has not been defined, but the expectation in England is for availability of a unit within 2 minutes' walking time from any collapse in the designated area. This implies that many units will be required within most airports and larger railway stations: for example, London's Gatwick airport has 45 units. The short response times ensure that a high rate of successful outcomes can be achieved–and this can justify the high capital cost. The community placements are intended to cover a very much wider area, so that capital cost is low but response times are relatively long, so that outcomes are correspondingly less favourable.

In England (figures from Resuscitation Council database, December 2002) the number of on-site AEDs was approximately 1,700. Over a period of 2 years (during which time the number of AEDs was building up progressively) 134 uses were recorded, 74% of which were for shockable rhythms, with most delays from collapse to 'pads-on' estimated to be in the range of 3–5 minutes. Twenty percent of the individuals who received shocks were discharged alive from hospital. The number of known community AEDs in the same period was 493. These were used for 222 resuscitation attempts, 35% of which were for shockable rhythms, with most delays in the 8- to 14-minute range. Only 3% of the individuals who received shocks were discharged alive. The AEDs had been deployed for varying periods, and no comparison based on accurate data for 'defibrillator-months' is available. But based on the data without correction for variations in deployment time, over a period of up to 2 years one successful discharge was obtained for every 63 on-site AEDs, and one successful discharge for every 82 community AEDs. One unit can, however, be expected to last up to 7 years, and the figures thus far were achieved in an average deployment time of little over 1 year. The cost–benefit ratio depends more on training strategies and infrastructure costs than capital outlay [5], however, and no appropriate analyses have yet been performed in England. The experience that has been gained and the improvements in success rate that recent scientific developments portend may ensure that these appear favourable when such analyses are undertaken.

Where Are We Going in Europe?

The use of AEDs in Europe is set to increase–but from a relatively low present position, so that there is much to be achieved. All the available evidence attests that AEDs can save lives that would otherwise be lost. They are inherently safe, and we know of no serious sequelae even when operators or bystanders have inadvertently received shocks from touching patients whilst shocks are being delivered or from other accidents. Analyses of downloads from large databases of attempted resuscitations have also shown satisfactory sensitivity to waveforms of ventricular fibrillation and 'shockable' ventricular tachycardia together with excellent specificity–which is perhaps more important in equipment designed for use by modestly trained individuals. Figures from Heartstart Scotland [15], with two analyses from 893 patients–involving 8,895 rhythm strips–showed that sensitivity is likely to be in the range of 90.3–94.4%, with specificity 99% or more. In Goteborg [16], analysis from 383 cases with 2,719 rhythm strips showed that specificity was 99.6%. Most failures to advise shocks could be ascribed either to fine waveforms or to human errors. A smaller Swedish study found a sensitivity of 93% and a specificity of 100% [17]. Whilst different models of AEDs have diverse algorithms, the science of pattern recognition is well understood and all new devices are tested against databanks of rhythms. Reliability has not been a major problem.

AEDs are also very simple to operate. One of the authors (D.A.C.) has not been challenged in his assertion that 'they are easier to use than a television set' (not a video recorder!). Although a recommendation is sometimes made for a 4-hour course of instruction for lay persons, this can only be justified if most of the time is taken to teach or refresh the skills in basic life support that are so much more complex [13]. One study showed that hospital staff trained only in basic life support were able to deliver sequential shocks in simulated arrests without any instruction in the use of the equipment [18], whilst another found that more than 40% of lay people were able to deliver shocks before any teaching on the technique [19]. Untrained American sixth-grade schoolchildren (10–11 years old) were able to use a device almost as quickly as trained professionals [20].

AEDs are not a panacea for countering the burden of premature cardiac death in the community. They can only be part of a system of prevention and care. The narrow time window for successful defibrillation will always limit their value, but this is so particularly because almost 80% of all cardiac arrests occur at home and relatively few in public places [21]. In this regard it is worth noting, however, that it is intrinsically more likely that the proportion dying at home is greater among those who are infirm than for those who are fit and active. This is confirmed by unpublished data from the UK Heart Attack Study (a major epidemiological survey of heart attacks in three UK cities over 3 years), which shows variation by age (Norris, personal communication). Among those aged under 55, 65% died at home–compared with 70% of those aged 56–64 and 79% of those aged 65–74. Any appreciable reduction in the incidence of sudden premature death at home requires multiple strategies in addition to better preventative measures: continuing education on rapid alert for possible cardiac pain, better arrangements for community AED programmes, the use of implantable defibrillators for the 10% known to be most vulnerable [21], a greater use of AEDs in homes [22], and also novel devices to counter collapse, which might be wearable [23] or used only if an emergency occurred.

No single plan can be made for optimal deployment of AEDs for all of Europe, but suggestions can be made for consideration in individual countries or regions. Assuming no legal restrictions remain in place, the use of AEDs in the public domain should be developed with clear objectives in mind and appropriate consideration for the cost–benefit ratio, which may be influenced by local factors. There is a clear advantage in having national or regional coordination and close liaison with–and control by–the local emergency service for community 'despatched' AED deployment. On-site AEDs should be expected in appropriate places for any of several reasons: to fulfil a duty of care (with prisons and factories as good examples); because cardiac arrests occur relatively frequently (as in airports and at busy railway stations); or because help is otherwise unobtainable (in commercial aircraft). The selection of suitable situations for community use and on-site units should be based on local epidemiological data.

Even with all these provisions, the contribution to countering premature sudden death will be relatively small in community terms. But as part of a broader strategy it should not be neglected. Moreover, better results can be expected in the future, with the likelihood that CPR before defibrillation [24] (and possibly after it) will improve immediate results. Simple algorithm adjustments in relation to delaying postshock analysis may give an associated benefit [25]. Further progress is likely as manufacturers appreciate the importance of very brief delays between the end of a compression sequence and the delivery of a shock: technical advances can make this possible. Real improvements in advanced life support for the management of patients after cardiac arrest are also in sight. Authorities have a responsibility to remove any legal barriers that preclude their widespread use by lay persons, and for physicians to press them to do so. An ideal scenario for 'where Europe should be going' with the public use of AEDs is becoming clear. It is for all of those in the field to ensure we do not lose the way.

Acknowledgements. Douglas Chamberlain's post is funded on an expenses-only basis by the Laerdal Foundation.

References

1. Jaggarao NS, Heber M, Grainger R, Vincent R, Chamberlain DA, Aronson AL (1982) Use of an automated external defibrillator-pacemaker by ambulance staff. Lancet II:73–75
2. Cummins RO, Eisenberg MS, Bergner L, Hallstrom A, Hearne T, Murray JA (1984) Automatic external defibrillation: evaluations of its role in the home and in emergency medical services. Ann Emerg Med 13:798–801
3. Capucci A, Aschieri D, Piepoli MF, Bardy GH, Iconomu E, Arvedi M (2002) Tripling survival from sudden cardiac arrest via early defibrillation without traditional education in cardiopulmonary resuscitation. Circulation 106:1065–1070
4. Koster RW (2002) Automatic external defibrillator: key link in the chain of survival. J Cardiovasc Electrophysiol 13:S92–S925
5. Kuisma M, Castrén M, Nurminen K (2003) Public access defibrillation in Helsinki-costs and potential benefits from a community-based pilot study. Resuscitation 56:149–152
6. Martens P, Calle P, Mullie A (1993) Do we know enough to introduce semi-automatic defibrillation by ambulancemen in Belgium? Eur J Med 2:430–434
7. Arntz HR, Oeff M, Willich SN, Storch WH, Schroder R (1993) Establishment and results of an EMT-D program in a two-tiered physician-escorted rescue system. The experience in Berlin, Germany. Resuscitation 26:39–46
8. Mols P, Clevenbergh P, Henry B, Decroly M, Langen C, Beaucarne E, Bruyninx J, Robert P, Labruyere JP, Flamand JP (1994) Semi-automatic external defibrillation. Eur J Emerg Med 1:210-213
9. Calle PA, Verbeke A, Vanhaute O, Van Acker P, Martens P, Buylaert W (1997) The effect of semi-automatic external defibrillation by emergency medical technicians on survival after out-of-hospital cardiac arrest: an observational study in urban and rural areas in Belgium. Acta Clin Belg 52:72–83
10. Herlitz J, Bang A, Holmberg M, Axelsson A, Graves JR, Lindqvist J, Holmberg S (1998) Rhythm changes during resuscitation from ventricular firbillation in relation to

delayed defibrillation, number of shocks delivered and survival. Resuscitation 34:17-22

11. Petit P (1999) Mort subite d'origine cardiaque : la chaîne de survie en France. Bull Acad Natl Méd 183:1581–1594
12. Kacet S, Zghal N, Kouakam C, Benameur N, Goldstein P (2002) Utílisatíon des défibrillateurs semi-automatique en-dehors de l'hôpital. Arch Mal Coeur Vaiss 95:945–949
13. Martens P, Calle P, Vanhaute O (1998) Theoretical calculation of maximum attainable benefit of public access defibrillation in Belgium. Belgian Cardio Pulmonary Cerebral Resuscitation Study Group. Resuscitation 36:161–163
14. Davies CS, Colquhoun M, Graham S, Evans T, Chamberlain D (2002) Defibrillators in public places: the introduction of a national scheme for public access defibrillation in England. Resuscitation 52:13–21
15. Sedgwick ML, Watson J, Dalziel K, Carrington DJ, Cobbe SM (1992) Efficacy of out of hospital defibrillation by ambulance technicians using automated external defibrillators. The Heartstart Scotland Project. Resuscitation 24:73–87
16. Herlitz J, Bang A, Axelsson A, Graves JR, Lindqvist J (1998) Experience with the use of automated external defibrillators in out of hospital cardiac arrest. Resuscitation 37:3–7
17. Jakobsson JG, Rehnqvist N, Nyquist O (1987) Experience with an automatic external defibrillator. Acta Anaesthesiol Scand 31:597–600
18. Domanovits H, Meron G, Sterz F, Kofler J, Oschatz E, Holzer M, Mullner M, Laggner AN (1998) Successful automatic external defibrillator operation by people trained only in basic life support in a simulated cardiac arrest situation. Resuscitation 39:47–50
19. Woollard M, Whitfield R, Smith A, Colquhoun M, Newcombe RG, Vetter N, Chamberlain D (2003) The acquisition and retention of skills in the use of the automated external defibrillator and CPR by lay responders: a prospective study. Resuscitation (in press)
20. Gundry JW, Comess KA, DeRook FA, Jorgenson D, Bardy GH (1999) Comparison of naive sixth-grade children with trained professionals in the use of an automated external defibrillator. Circulation 100:1703–1707
21. De Vreede-Swagemakers JJM, Gorgels APM, Dubois-Arbouw WI, van Ree JW, Daemen MJAP, Houben LGE, Wellens HJJ (1997) Out-of-hospital cardiac arrest in the 1990s: a population-based study in the Maastricht area on incidence, characteristics and survival. J Am Coll Cardiol 30: 1500–1505
22. Eisenberg MS (2000) Is it time for over-the-counter defibrillators? JAMA 284:1435–1438
23. Wellens HJJ, Gorgels AP, de Munter H (2003) Cardiac arrest outside of a hospital. How can we improve results of resuscitation? Circulation 107:1948–1950
24. Wik L, Hansen TB, Fylling F, Steen T, Vaagenes P, Auestad BH, Steen PA (2003) Delaying defibrillation to give basic cardiopulmonary resuscitation to patients with out-of-hospital ventricular fibrillation: a randomized trial. JAMA 289:1389–1395
25. Blouin D, Topping C, Moore S, Stiell I, Afilalo M (2001) Out-of-hospital defibrillation with automated external defibrillators: postshock analysis should be delayed. Ann Emerg Med 38:256–261

Use of AEDs by Lay People in Patients with Out-of-Hospital Cardiac Arrest: How Does It Impact Survival?

A. Capucci, D. Aschieri

Sudden cardiac arrest (SCA) claims an estimated 50 000 lives per year in Italy, representing a major public health problem. More people die each day of potentially reversible ventricular fibrillation (VF) than of any other cause of death, reversible or not. We know that restoring normal heart rhythm by a defibrillation shock not only saves life but is often followed by many years of active living. Unfortunately, most cardiac arrest does not occur in supervised places, and in more typical community settings victims of SCA rarely survive. Only 2%–5% of victims of SCA can be resuscitated with the commonly used emergency system of ambulances. The problem could be resolved simply by making defibrillation available to lay persons [1].

Defibrillation

Although (semi)automatic external defibrillators (AEDs) have been available in the United States for a long time [2], they have only recently been introduced in Europe. AEDs have become a suitable device for use by policemen and laymen. Placing AEDs in public places and training lay people in their use has given new hope in fighting sudden death and resulted in improved survival in cardiac resuscitation [3–8].

Preliminary experiences have suggested that a two-tier system involving a "first responder" with an AED who can arrive within 4–5 min may improve survival in comparison with a single-tier system that aims to deliver a fully trained paramedic in 8 min [9]. Seattle has achieved an average response time of 7 min and a VF survival rate of 30% [10]. In Rochester, Minnesota, response time averages 6 min and 45% survive [11].

When resuscitation in the community relies predominantly upon the ambulance service, every effort to improve survival rates seems to be useless.

Cardiology Department, "Guglielmo da Saliceto" General Hospital, Piacenza, Italy

Recently the data from the United Kingdom experience in training the ambulance crews better were published. The chances of a patient surviving SCA to be discharged from hospital alive did not appear to be affected by the paramedics' length of experience. The growing number of trained paramedics do not seem to improve the survival rate (14% in 1987–1989; 11.4% in 1992–1993) in either Scotland [12] or England [13].

Laypersons are the most likely to arrive first at the scene of an arrest.

Public Access Defibrillation

Public access defibrillation is the concept of placing AEDs in public and/or private settings where large numbers of people congregate or where people generally considered at high risk for heart attacks live or are found. All emergency first responder's vehicles and ambulances should be equipped with an AED. The American Heart Association has a goal of helping business and other facilities to establish public access defibrillation programs in order to reduce the time to defibrillation.

Therefore, most AEDs are designed to be used by nonmedical personnel such as police, fire service personnel, flight attendants, security guards, and other lay rescuers who have been properly trained. To fight SCA successfully, the goal should be to train many people in early defibrillation, and to provide them with AED which they can apply while awaiting for the medical emergency services to arrive. Early defibrillation gives the heart an opportunity to resume beating effectively. Of course, an AED only treats a fibrillating heart. In cardiac arrest without VF the heart does not respond to electrical current, but needs medication and breathing support instead. Also, AEDs are less successful when the victim has been in cardiac arrest for longer than a few minutes.

International Experience of Public Access Defibrillation

During the last 20 years, the experiences of several emergency departments in North American communities have been published and have demonstrated an increased discharge survival rate after out-of-hospital SCA treated by early defibrillation by police and paramedics: Table 1 summarizes the beneficial effects of this intervention. The lowest survival rates occurred in single-response systems and the highest rates in double-response systems, although there was considerable variation within each type of system. Hypothetical survival curves suggest that the ability to resuscitate is a function of the time, type, and sequence of therapy. Survival appears to be highest in double-response systems because ED is started early: the institutional emergency medical system is supported and coordinates the activation of organizations formed by lay volunteers equipped with an AED, who can provide first rescue and early defibrillation within 4–5 min. The development of this two-tier sys-

Table 1. High discharge survival rate after out-of-hospital ventricular fibrillation with early defibrillation by police and paramedics [14, 15].

Year	Locations	Before (%)	After (%)	Survival increase (-fold)
1980	Seattle, Washington	7	26	3.7
1984	Rural communities	3	19	6.3
1984	Iowa	3	19	6.3
1986	Southeast Minnesota	4	17	4.3
1986	Northeast Minnesota	2	10	5.0
1989	Wisconsin	4	11	2.8
1998	Indianapolis	8	14	1.7
1996	Rochester	–	49	
1998	Pittsburgh	3	26	8.6
2001	Piacenza	16	43	3.6

tem of early defibrillation has allowed the city of Seattle to achieve an average response time of 7 min and a survival rate of 26% for those with witnessed VF [14], and in Rochester, Minnesota, an average response time of 6 min with a 45% survival rate for witnessed VF [15]. If Rochester and Seattle's high survival rates could be achieved in Italy, as many as 10 000 unnecessary deaths could be prevented each year.

The most successful experience in public access defibrillation is the experience of Chicago airport [16]. In 16 of 21 cases of cardiac arrest the victims were successfully resuscitated. In 8 cases they were treated by lay people who had never before used an AED. A public videotape running in the airport was enough to teach them the AED application procedure.

In Las Vegas casinos (Clark County, Las Vegas, Henderson, Laughlin, Lake Tahoe, Philadelphia, Tunica) AED were publicly placed and security officers were trained in their use. One hundred five patients suffered a cardiac arrest, of whom 53% survived to hospital discharge. In 86% of cases the time from collapse to shock was 3.5±2.9 min. The survival rate was 74% when the time from collapse to first shock was less than 3 min and 49% when it was greater than 3 min. The recent experience in Las Vegas casinos confirms the strong relationship between time to first shock and survival rate [17].

First European Project of Public Access Defibrillation: Progetto Vita

Progetto Vita (Project Life) is the first European pilot project of early defibrillation by first responders in the community. The project started on 6 June 1999 in the city of Piacenza (99 878 inhabitants), where 39 AEDs were distributed according to a planned protocol involving 1285 trained lay volunteers (policemen, financial guards, municipal guards, firemen, railway station personnel, first aid volunteers, post office personnel, hazardous chemicals personnel). In particular, 12 police cars patrolling the town have AEDs in their equipment and can be called by the emergency medical service in all cases of suspected sudden cardiac arrest. This is termed a "code blue" call. Figure 1 shows the distribution of the AEDs in the town of Piacenza. Coordination of the project is the responsibility of the emergency department of the local hospital (cardiology department and 118 service).

In the previous 3 years, before starting the Progetto Vita, a mean of 107 episodes per year of SCD were recorded. Overall survival in all episodes of SCA was computed as 4.9%, with a mean time of intervention of the emergency medical system of 8 min. During the first 15 months after the start of Progetto Vita on 6 June 1999, 203 blue codes for suspected SCA were dispatched. In 106 cases, (52%), the volunteers arrived on the scene before the ambulance (mean intervention time: 5±1 min vs 6±2 min, respectively, $p<0.05$). Of the 203 cases, 197 were considered SCAs, and 63 of these were treated by volunteers of the Progetto Vita. In 40 of these 197 cases, shockable rhythms were detected, 16 of which were treated by the Progetto Vita volunteers, and 7 of these 16 patients were successfully defibrillated. Of the 24 patients treated by emergency medical personnel, only 4 were successfully defibrillated. Overall survival was 5.6% (11/197): survival improved from 2.9% (4/134) with emergency

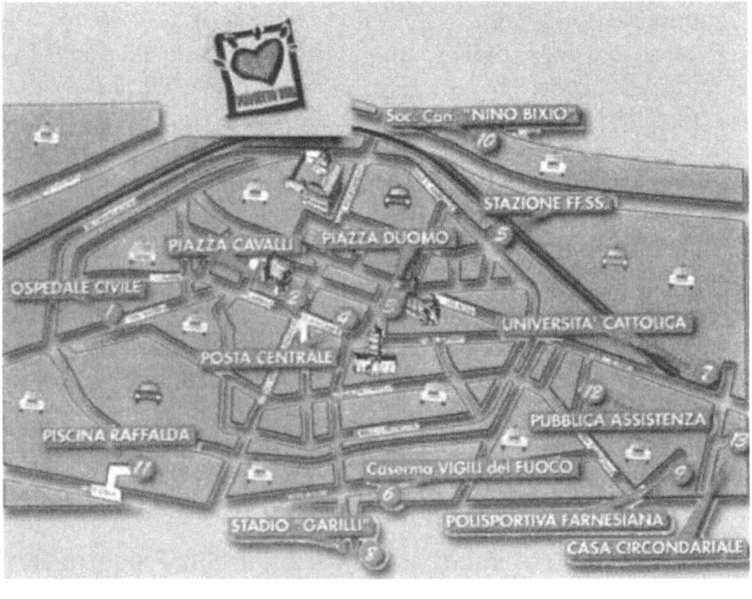

Fig. 1. Distribution of AEDs in the town of Piacenza

medical services intervention to 11.1% (7/63) when Progetto Vita was activated ($p<0.05$). The survival rate after "shockable" rhythm was 43.7% in the group treated by volunteers, vs 16.6 % in those treated by the emergency medical services ($p=0.05$).

Conclusions

Increasing rapid access to an AED to be used by lay people is likely to lead to higher survival from SCA. Mobile AEDs carried in police cars represent the better response to a SCA when the emergency system dispatcher includes police cars in a two-tier system of intervention. Ongoing studies are examining the benefit of having more widespread AEDs in the community.

References

1. Bayes de Luna A, Coumel P, Leclercq JF (1989) Ambulatory sudden cardiac death mechanisms of production of fatal arrhythmia on the basis of data from 157 cases. Am Heart J 117:151–159
2. Cummins RO, Eisemberg MS, Bergner L et al (1984) Automatic external defibrillation: evaluation of its role in the home and in emergency medical services. Ann Emerg Med 13:798–801
3. Weisfeldt ML, Keber RE, McGoldrick RP et al (1995) Public access defibrillation: a statement for healthcare professionals from the American Heart Association Task Force on the automatic external defibrillator. Circulation 92:2763–2772
4. Valenzuela TD, Roe DJ, Nichol G et al (2000) Outomes of rapid of rapid defibrillation by security officers after cardiac arrest in casinos. N Engl J Med 343:1206–1209
5. Page RL, Joglar JA, Kowal RC et al (2000) Use of automated external defibrillators by a US airline. N Engl J Med 343:1206–1209
6. Marenco JP, Wang PJ, Link MS et al (2001) Improving survival from sudden cardiac arrest: the role of the automated external defibrillator. JAMA 285:1193–1200
7. Myerburg RJ, Fenster J, Velez M et al (2002) Impact of community-wide police car deployment of automated external defibrillators on survival from out-of-hospital cardiac arrest. Circulation 106:1058–1064
8. Capucci A, Aschieri, Piepoli M et al (2002) Tripling survival from sudden cardiac arrest via early defibrillation, without traditional education in cardiopulmonary resuscitation. Circulation 106:1065–1070
9. Larsen MP, Eisemberg MS, Cummins RO, Hallstrom AP (1993) Predicting survival from out-of-hospital cardiac arrest: a graphic model. Ann Emerg Med 22:1652–1658
10. Eisenberg M, Horwood B, Cummins R et al (1990) Cardiac arrest and resuscitation: a tale of 29 cities. Ann Emerg Med 19:179–186
11. White RD, Asplin BR, Bugliosi TF, Hankins DG (1996) High discharge survival rate after out-of-hospital ventricular fibrillation with rapid defibrillation by police and paramedics. Ann Emerg Med 28:480–485
12. Guly UM, Mitchell RG, Cook R, Steedman DJ, Robertson CE (1995) Paramedics and technicians are equally successful at managing cardiac arrest outside hospital. BMJ *310:1091–1094*

13. Mackintosh AF, Crabb ME, Granger R, Williams JH, Chamberlin DA (1978) The Brighton resuscitation ambulances: review of 40 consecutive survivors of out-of-hospital cardiac arrest. BMJ 1:1115–1118
14. Eisenberg M, Horwood B, Cummins R et al (1990) Cardiac arrest and resuscitation: a tale of 29 cities. Ann Emerg Med 19:179–186
15. White RD, Asplin BR, Bugliosi TF et al (1996) High discharge survival rate after out-of-hospital ventricular fibrillation with rapid defibrillation by police and paramedics. Ann Emerg Med 28:480–485
16. Caffrey SL, Willoughby PJ, Pepe PE, Becker LB (2002) Public use of automated external defibrillators. N Engl J Med 347:1242–1247
17. Valenzuela TD, Roe DJ, Nichol G et al (2000) Outcomes of rapid defibrillation by security officers after cardiac arrest in casinos. N Engl J Med 343:1206–1209

In-Hospital Cardiac Arrest: Are We Well Enough Equipped and Prepared to Face It?

M. Santomauro[1], L. Ottaviano[1], A. Borrelli[1], C. Riganti[2], L. Quagliata[2], A. Costanzo[1], C. Liguori[1], D. Da Prato[1], M. Chiariello[1]

Sudden death is a real concern for nowadays medicine, especially as it can occur in people with no signs of disease at all. It can be the first symptom of an underlying problem. It may be defined as an unexpected event occurring with no warning signs, within less than an hour, in a person with a known but stable cardiac problem, or in a person with an unknown but pre-existing problem. Often a cardiac problem is the substrate for cardiac arrest (Table 1), but many other diseases can be the underlying cause of sudden death, which in 75% of cases is due to ventricular fibrillation or tachycardia, in 20% to bradyarrhythmia, and in 5% atrioventricular dissociation [1, 2]. In Italy it strikes more than 60 000 people per year, with a 10% overall mortality, 20% of which is made up of people with no previous signs of disease at all [1].

The chance of surviving a cardiac arrest depends strictly on the rapidity of intervention, and especially on correct execution of the four fundamental operations that represent the "chain of survival" [3]. First step is recognition of patient's unconsciousness and then the emergency system activation (naturally this step is referred to as "Out-of-hospital Emergency"), immediately followed by basic cardiopulmonary resuscitation, known as "Basic Life Support" (BLS) [4], which consists of sequences of chest compression and artificial ventilation. Defibrillation, the third step in the chain of survival, is the only treatment that can stop ventricular fibrillation or tachycardia, the main cause of death from cardiac arrest, while advanced cardiopulmonary resuscitation (CPR) or "Advanced Cardiac Life Support" (ACLS) is the last step. Since its discovery, external defibrillation has been the cornerstone of emergency cardiac care and the principal intervention in most successful resuscitations from full cardiac arrest.

A large body of out-of-hospital research [5–7] shows that rapidity of defibrillation is the most important determinant of survival in arrests due to shockable arrhythmias. Although most events occur outside hospitals, the problem is still a big concern inside the structure. In Italian hospitals, 85% of patients

Departments of [1]Cardiology and [2]Health Management, Federico II University, Naples, Italy

Table 1. Heart disease that may cause sudden cardiac death up to the age of 30 years and after the age of 30 years. The most frequent disease which causes sudden death below the age of 30 years is hypertrophic cardiomyopathy (50%), when the incidence of coronary artery disease is about 3%–20%. After the age of 30 years, the incidence of coronary artery disease is about 85%

Causes of sudden death < 30 years of age	%	Causes of sudden death > 30 years of age	%
Aortic stenosis	3–18	Coronary artery disease	85
Eisenmengeräs syndrome	15	Cardiomyopathy	10
Congenital cardiomyopathy	10	Valve disease	3
Hypertrophic cardiomyopathy	1–50	Electrical alternations	2
Right ventricular dysplasia	0–26		
Mitral prolapse	1–24		
Coronary artery disease	3–20		

admitted to general medicine departments suffer sudden death, whereas mortality is less than 10% for patients admitted to intensive care units. Survival rates of cardiac arrest patients outside critical care units remain about 15% at best, and survival is consistently lower on general units than in critical care areas [8, 9]. Explanations for this lack of progress usually involve comorbidity and unwitnessed arrests among patients on general units [9–14].

Defibrillation, in Italian hospitals, often occurs very late and with difficulty, either because of the lack of adequate means, i.e., defibrillators, or because of architectural and structural barriers which obstruct intervention. Sometimes the device is available only in specific departments of the hospital, and in some cases it is useless because it is not working or because staff are inexperienced in its use. Furthermore, in most cases intervention is carried out by a specialized team called out from other departments of the same hospital, usually after a long delay, which is even longer if no CPR has occurred in the meantime.

General unit nurses are in the most difficult position of anyone involved in the resuscitation effort. They are expected to respond immediately to unanticipated crises, unlike the members of the emergency team, who at least have a little time to collect their wits while in transit to the scene. More importantly, several factors preordain almost certain failure in the general unit nurse's primary designated task of initiating basic CPR and defibrillation. Performing basic CPR has been shown to be difficult for all levels of health care providers, even in nonstressful classroom simulations [15, 16]. Performance in an actual in-hospital cardiac arrest is harder and takes longer. In the emotionally stressful setting of an actual arrest, several preparatory steps must be taken: acquiring a respiratory barrier device, bringing a crash cart with cardiac board to the scene, and placing the cardiac board under the patient (a two-person task) [17,

18]. Starting ventilation, chest compressions, and defibrillation requires the coordinated actions of at least two people, because the use of pocket masks and most other barrier devices makes effective one-person CPR most difficult. Given these obstacles, effective CPR is rarely initiated before the emergency team arrives [19]. Expecting the general unit nurse to perform an excessively complex and difficult task in an emergency situation may cause a state of "learned helplessness" and increased dependence on the emergency team.

Early defibrillation programs can improve survival rates significantly by shortening the time from arrest to defibrillation. Improving the speed of in-hospital defibrillation may produce better results. If BLS-D is not given immediately and the ACLS team arrives in 7–10 min, the survival rate is about 20%. If BLSD is not given immediately and the ACLS team arrives after more than 10 min, the survival rate is very low (2%–8%) and survival is associated with irreversible brain damage. The gold standard is: with early activation of the ACLS team and immediate BLSD, the survival rate is about 80%–90% (Table 2).

The purpose of an in-hospital emergency service is to prevent sudden death due to cardiac arrest and, naturally, to avoid the complications of survived cardiac arrest, such as brain damage and kidney failure, within the limits of the whole hospital and among all its users (patients, visitors, students, staff). Complications and recovery from cardiac arrest are closely related to the time to intervention: it is well known that the chance of survival decreases by 10% with every minute that passes [20], and brain damage occurs after 4–5 min anoxia. In order to shorten intervention time and to avoid complications, the following are needed:

- Information and sensitization of staff,
- Hospital staff training in CPR and defibrillation techniques
- A hospital calling system for "hospital emergency"
- Selection and creation of an operative team
- Rational positioning of emergency trolleys within the hospital
- Standard procedures for all the staff
- Creation of a quality control system

Table 2. Percentage of survival with and without immediate basic life support and defibrillation (BLS-D). The survival rate is closely related to immediate performance of BLS-D

Action	Survival rate (%)
Early activation of ACLS team, no immediate BLSD (7–10 min)	20
Early activation of ACLS team, no immediate BLSD (>10 min)	2-8 + brain damage
Early activation of ACLS team, immediate BLSD	80–90

- A specific coordination center for in-hospital emergencies
- Retraining of the staff

The Naples Heart Project aims to achieve all nine of these requirements, through teaching materials, training courses, and the creation of a permanent in-hospital emergency team.

The Naples Heart Project [21, 22] began in July 2001, and since then it has already created about 835 BLS-D (CPR/basic life support and defibrillation) first responders among the hospital staff; 440 are physicians (fully trained or still in training), 310 nurses, and 85 administrative staff. Our first purpose is to train all general hospital nurses, physicians, and other working staff in BLS-D, a total of more than 3000 people. To achieve this, we have organized courses [23] based both on theory and practice, so that the participants can develop psychomotor ability and automated patterns, effective and focused enough to allow the rescuer to give the best aid he or she can. The teaching explains the rational basis of the chain of survival, providing basic cardiopulmonary resuscitation and defibrillation techniques courses, the practice part is intended to make the rescuer feel much more comfortable when aiding the victim.

The courses vary in material, length, and final test, depending on which group of participants they are intended for. We intend to keep the easiest and safest mode of intervention for nonmedical personnel, and to build in a little more specificity for physicians. All courses are held on one day. The course for administrative staff has a total duration of 6 h equally divided between theory and practice; they are trained to use a semiautomatic defibrillator, with no monitor for ECG, and with a voice system that guides the rescuer through all the steps of the chain of survival in sequence. These are, in fact, the only defibrillators they will be allowed to use, as stated by Monteleone's Law promulgated on 3 April 2001, which allows non-medical personnel [24] to use defibrillators but only semiautomatic devices. Courses for nurses (Fig. 1) last 8 h, they are given more information on the physiopathology and are trained in all the basic life support techniques and in use of the defibrillator. The courses for physicians are 10 h long, spending more time on physiopathology, epidemiology, and specific patterns of cardiac arrest. For all the groups we use biphasic wave defibrillators, as they use less energy than monophasic and have comparable effectiveness at a lower energy level. All the three groups have to take a final test, with basic questions and no ECG to interpret. Even though all participants so far have shown interest in the theory and practice, not all of them obtained a good grade at the final test; we had to re-enroll 40 in another session and have them re-tested, this time with positive results. Naturally, since nobody practices basic life support techniques or uses defibrillators daily (with a few exceptions), it is appropriate to repeat it at least once a year. For this reason we plan to keep it continuous and customary for all the personnel, including retraining after 1 year.

The Naples Heart Project training center also provides ACLS courses, in order to create an ACLS team to offer advanced cardiac life support any time anywhere in the hospital. ACLS courses are held over 2 days of 8 h, during

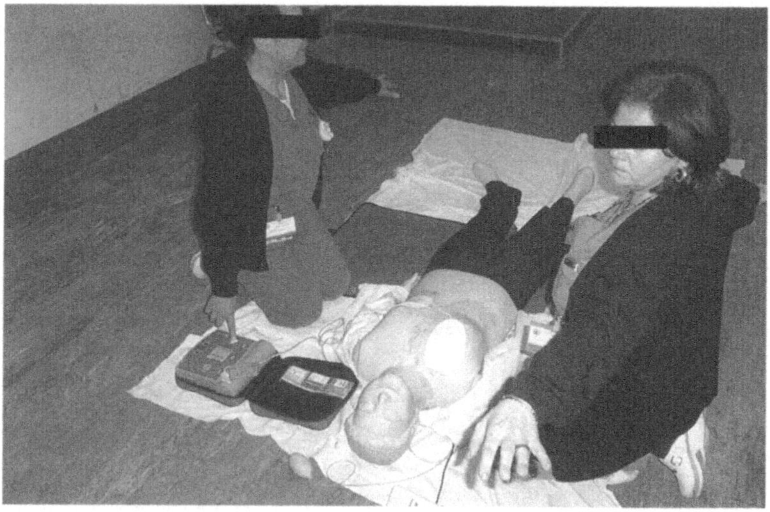

Fig. 1. Naples Heart Project BLS-D first responder course. Nurses' BLS-D training course

which physicians are trained in using manual defibrillators with external pacing capacity, drug administration for treatment of tachyarrhythmias and bradyarrhythmias, and airway intubation. To date we have organized several sessions with 25 participants per day; the number of participants has increased continuously from the month of July 2001 to May 2003 (Figs. 2, 3).

This Naples Heart Project was based on a feasibility study of in-hospital emergency services that aimed to evaluate and analyze structure planimetry, department and institutes position, internal practicability (features of buildings and preferred routes), staff numbers and distribution, the presence of a calling system for emergencies, and the instruments available. The aim is to find the best solution to make the chain of survival as fast and efficient as possible, in every place, at any time, and in all conditions in the hospital.

The Federico II University General Hospital has about 1200 beds divided among separate and independent institutes. Everyday several thousand people – patients, physicians, technical and administrative staff, visitors, students – live in this hospital. It is therefore necessary that anyone inside the general hospital must know all the hospital emergency programs. To make this possible we have created a leaflet about the hospital emergency service for patients and visitors, to be distributed in waiting rooms and at the main entrance, and with posters in every institute; and we have organized meetings and conferences for future BLSD providers such as physician, nurses, and administrative and technical staff. We are planning to set up a series of road signs (Fig. 4) throughout the hospital, with all the directions to the nearest defibrillation point.

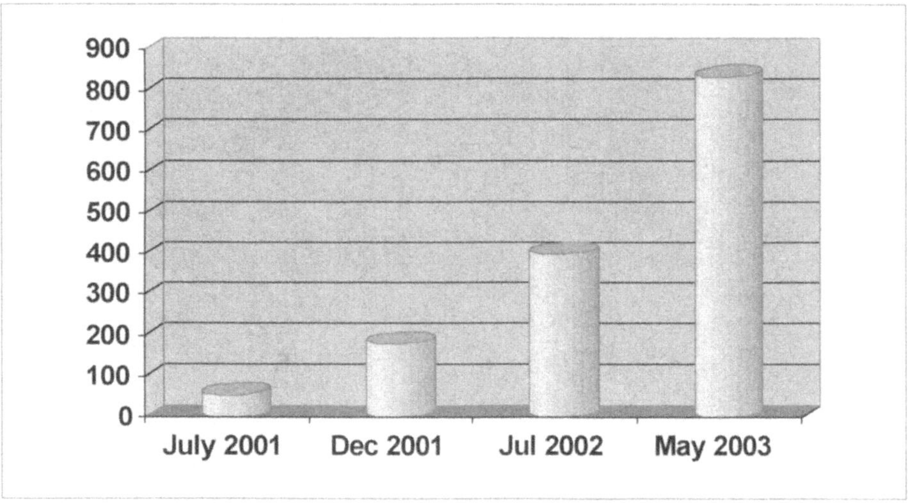

Fig. 2. Naples Heart Project's BLS-D first responders. The Naples Heart Project was begun in July 2001. Since then it has already created about 835 BLS-D first responders among the hospital staff; 440 were specialist physicians and physicians in training, 310 were nurses, and 85 were in the administrative staff

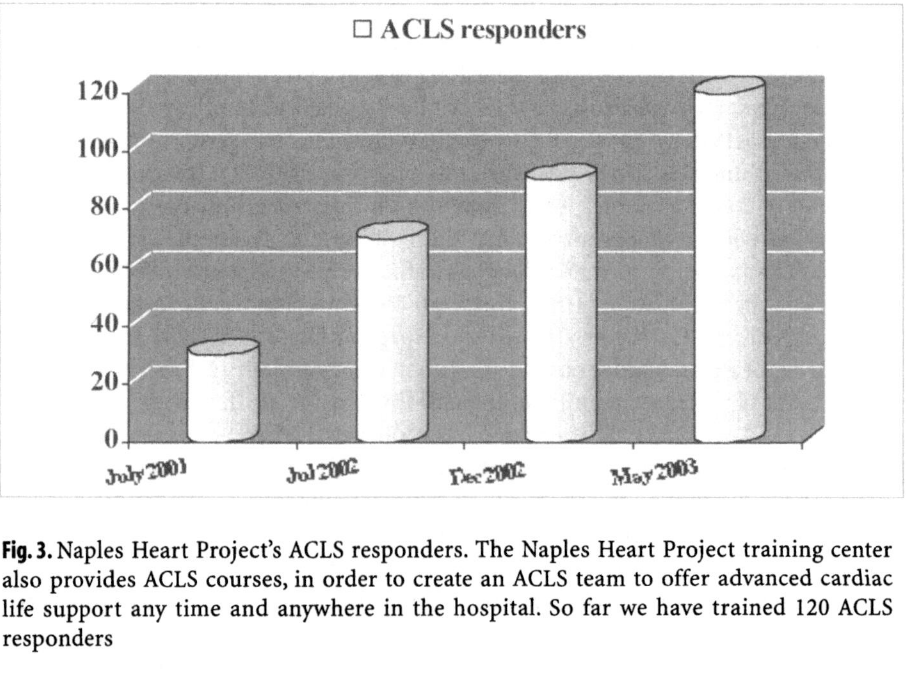

Fig. 3. Naples Heart Project's ACLS responders. The Naples Heart Project training center also provides ACLS courses, in order to create an ACLS team to offer advanced cardiac life support any time and anywhere in the hospital. So far we have trained 120 ACLS responders

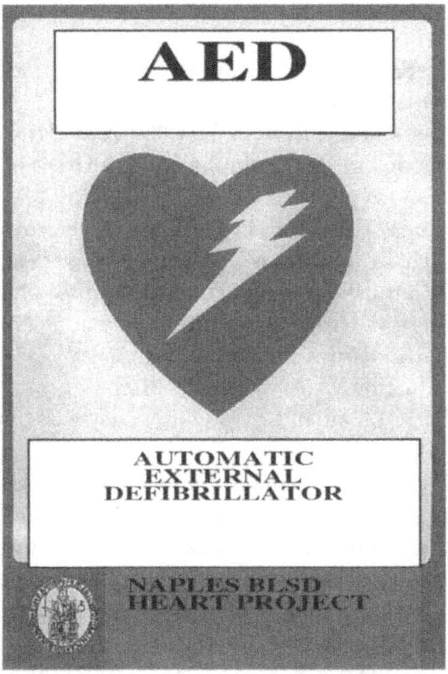

Fig. 4. Defibrillation point sign. The Naples Heart Project provides a series of road signs throughout the hospital with directions to the nearest defibrillation point

The project provides a rational distribution of semiautomatic defibrillators and materials, so as to have a defibrillator and a fully organized trolley for emergencies available on all floors, so that the delay due to access and transport of the material is greatly reduced; it has also been proposed to check the emergency trolley material and to maintain a checklist. In order to administer and coordinate the project, we will create the figure of an in-hospital emergency system leader whose role is to mediate contacts between the emergency team, training center, BLSD, and ACLS providers on one hand and the emergency coordination group (made up of a general manager, a medical manager, and a nursing manager) on the other hand.

In conclusion, an in-hospital emergency has to be understood not as a chaotic chain, but as an organized chain with standard protocols known by all the staff. It is necessary to organize training following a well-defined program with a fixed term, and the courses must give both theoretical and practical knowledge about emergencies. The Naples Heart Project, based on courses for BLS-D and ACLS responders and aimed at physicians, nurses, and other working staff at the general hospital, has this purpose. It is the first project in Italy of such a size and with such a purpose. It lays the basis for the development of a medical emergencies culture in both in-hospital and out-of-hospital scenarios.

References

1. Anonymous (1988) Vital statistics of the United States, 1988, vol 2, part A. National Center for Health Statistics, Hyattsville, Md
2. Bayes de Luna A, Coumel P, Leclercq JF (1989) Ambulatory sudden cardiac death: mechanism of production of fatal arrhythmia on the basis of data from 157 cases. Am Heart J 117:151–159
3. Cummins RO, Ornato JP, Thies WH, Pepe PE (1991) Improving survival from sudden cardiac arrest: the "chain of survival" concept. A statement for health professionals from the Advanced Cardiac Life Support Subcommittee and the Emergency Cardiac Care Commitee, American Heart Association. Circulation 83:1832–1847
4. Anonymous (1992) Guidelines for cardiopulmonary resuscitation and emergency cardiac care, I: introduction. JAMA 268:2172–2183
5. Myerburg RJ, Kessler KM, Zaman L et al (1982) Survivors of prehospital cardiac arrest. JAMA 247:1485–1490
6. Stoddard FG (1996) Public access defibrillation comes of age. Currents 7:1–3
7. Capucci A, Aschieri D, Piepoli MF, Bardy GH, Iconomu E, Arvedi M (2002) Tripling survival from sudden cardiac arrest via early defibrillation without traditional education in cardiopulmonary resuscitation. Circulation106:1065–1070
8. McGrath PB (1987) In-house cardiopulmonary resuscitation–after a quarter of a century. Ann Emerg Med 11:1365–1368
9. Dans PE, Nevin KL, Seidman CE, McArthur JC (1985) Inhospital CPR 25 years later: why has survival decreased? South Med J 78:1174–1178
10. Tunstall-Pedoe H, Bailey L, Chamberlain DA et al (1992) Survey of 3765 cardiopulmonary resuscitations in British hospitals (the BRESUS study: methods and overall results. BMJ 304:1347–1351
11. Lazzam C, McCans JL (1991) Predictors of survival of in-hospital cardiac arrest. Can J Cardiol 7:113–116
12. Bedell SA, Delbanco EF, Cook EF, Epstein FH (1983) Survival after cardiopulmonary resuscitation in the hospital. N EngI J Med 309:569–576
13. Hershey CO, Fisher L (1982) Why outcome of cardiopulmonary resuscitation in general wards is poor. Lancet 1:31–34
14. Grauer K, Cavallaro D (1993) ACLS–A comprehensive review. Mosby Lifeline, St Louis
15. Berden HJ, Hendrick JM, van Doornen JP et al (1993) A comparison of resuscitation skills of qualified nurses and ambulance nurses in The Netherlands. Heart Lung 22:509–515
16. Flesche C, Neruda B, Breuer S, Tarnow J (1994) Basic cardiopulmonary resuscitation skills: a comparison of ambulance staff and medical students in Germany (abstract). Resuscitation 28:S25
17. Kaye W, Mancini ME, Giuliano KK et al (1995) Strengthening the in-hospital chain of survival with rapid defibrillation by first responders using automated external defibrillators: training and retention issues. Ann Emerg Med 25:163–168
18. Grotta JC (1996) The importance of time. In: Proceedings of the National Symposium on rapid identification and treatment of acute stroke. The National Institute of Neurological Disorders and Stroke, Bethesda pp 5–9
19. Brown J, Latimer-Heeter M, Marinelli A et al (1995) The first 3 minutes: code preparation for the staff nurse. Orthop Nurs 14(3):35–40
20. Brenner BE, Kauffman J (1995) Response to cardiac arrests in a hospital setting: delays in ventilation (abstract). Circulation 92[Suppl 1]:761 (abs)

21. Santomauro M, Ottaviano L, Borrelli A et al (2002) Organization project for early semiautomatic in hospital defibrillation (heart project). Progress in Clinical Pacing, Rome, 3–6 December 2002, 46 (abs)
22. Santomauro M, Ottaviano L, Borrelli A et al (2003) Sudden cardiac death prevention through hospital early defibrillation: the Naples experience. Pacing Clin Electrophysiol 26:S186
23. American Heart Association in collaboration with the International Liaison Committee on Resuscitation (ILCOR) (2000) Guidelines 2000 for cardiopulmonary resuscitation and emergency cardiovascular care. An international consensus on science. Circulation 102[Suppl 1], pp 330-384
24. Kerber R, Becker L, Bourland J et al (1997) Automatic external defibrillators for public access defibrillation: recommendation for specyfing and reporting arrhythmia analysis, algorithm performance, incorporating new wave forms, and enhancing safety. Circulation 95:1677–1682

Mild Therapeutic Hypothermia for Treatment of Cardiac Arrest: Current Results and Future Perspectives

W. BEHRINGER, M. HOLZER, F. STERZ

Sudden cardiac arrest remains a major unresolved public health problem. It is still the leading cause of death, and few cardiopulmonary-cerebral resuscitation (CPCR) attempts on cardiac arrest victims result in neurologically intact long-term survivors [1, 2].

The pathogenesis of cerebral ischemia and post-ischemic encephalopathy are multifactorial and only partially understood [2–5]. Brain ischemia results in rapid loss of high-energy phosphate compounds [6] and generalized membrane depolarization with an increase in intracellular calcium and the release of large amounts of glutamate [4]. These mechanisms initiate multiple independent chemical cascades and fatal pathways during reperfusion, resulting in neuronal death due to necrosis and apoptosis [5]. Due to the multifactorial pathogenesis of post-arrest neuronal death, multifaceted treatment strategies or a combination of single-molecule targeted drugs is required to achieve survival without brain damage [7, 8].

Resuscitative Hypothermia

Hypothermia is "a state of body temperature which is below normal in a homeothermic organism" [9]. Accidental (uncontrolled) hypothermia is non-therapeutically altered body temperature in a homeothermic organism with its defense mechanisms like hypermetabolism, increased oxygen consumption, and shivering, associated with particular complications and requiring specific treatments. In contrast, therapeutic hypothermia, such as for cardiac surgery and neurosurgery, or resuscitation from cardiac arrest, necessitates controlled conditions to induce poikilothermia by insult or anesthesia and paralysis. In therapeutic hypothermia different degrees of cooling are defined: mild (36–33 °C), moderate (32– 28°C), deep (27–11°C), profound (10–6°C), and ultra-profound (5–0°C) hypothermia [2].

Department of Emergency Medicine, Vienna General Hospital, Austria

The benefit of protective/preservative cerebral hypothermia on outcome was shown as early as the 1950s [10–12]. Experimental and clinical trials were complicated by the injurious systemic effects of total body cooling, such as shivering, vasospasm, increased plasma viscosity, increased hematocrit, hypocoagulation, arrhythmias, ventricular fibrillation when temperatures dropped below 30 °C, and lowered resistance to infection during prolonged moderate hypothermia [9, 12–14]. The discovery in the late 1980s that even mild hypothermia is neuroprotective [8, 15, 16] led to renewed interest in this field. Resuscitative and preservative hypothermia for cardiac arrest was documented in a series of clinically reliable dog outcome studies with evaluation of brain histology at 3–4 days after the insult: moderate hypothermia gave some benefit for the brain, but had side effects for the heart [17]; mild hypothermia, which is safer and simpler than moderate hypothermia, improved function and brain histology after normothermic ventricular fibrillation cardiac arrest of 10–12 min without flow [18–22]; deep hypothermia via cardiopulmonary bypass after prolonged normothermic cardiac arrest did not improve function and worsened brain histology [20]; mild resuscitative hypothermia essentially normalized cerebral outcome after 11 min cardiac arrest no-flow when prolonged (12 h) and combined with measures promoting cerebral blood flow [22]; a 15-min delay in the initiation of brief (1–2 h) mild hypothermia after normothermic reperfusion did not improve functional outcome but did reduce histological damage [21]. Prolonged hypothermia, even if delayed, was effective in rats [23, 24].

While the benefit of intraischemic hypothermia on neuronal death is regarded as long-lasting [25], results regarding long-lasting effects of postischemic hypothermia have been more controversial. Brief (4 h) post-arrest mild hypothermia after normothermic incomplete forebrain ischemia in rats postponed neuronal damage but did not permanently salvage hippocampal neurons, while moderate intraischemic hypothermia gave lasting salvage of neurons at 2 months [26]. Minimal delay and long duration of mild hypothermia seem to be of critical importance. In gerbils, a 24-h duration of moderate hypothermia (32 °C), even when initiated 1 h after insult, was highly protective with respect to behavior and histologic damage at 30 days [27], whereas the neuroprotection was less when hypothermia was initiated 4 h after insult [28]; however, increasing the duration of hypothermia to 48 h resulted in long-lasting protection of neurons at 1 month, even when hypothermia was delayed by 6 h [29]. The long-lasting effect of delayed (6 h), prolonged (48 h) hypothermia (32–34 °C) on functional and histologic outcome at 1 month was confirmed in rats [30].

Clinical Trials with Hypothermia After Cardiac Arrest

The use of therapeutic hypothermia after cardiac arrest in patients was not introduced until the late 1990s, when Bernard et al. [31] showed that induced moderate hypothermia increased the number of patients with good outcome

(Glasgow Outcome Coma Scale category 1 or 2) compared with a historic control group (11 of 22, versus 3 of 22; $p < 0.05$), and reduced mortality (10 of 22 versus 17 of 22; $p < 0.05$). This was a nonrandomized study with a matched historical control group. Cooling was by surface cooling with ice packs over 12 h.

In the study of Yanagawa et al. [32], cardiac arrest survivors were cooled to a core temperature between 33 and 34 °C over 48 h, using water-filled cooling blankets in combination with alcohol. Three of 13 patients in the hypothermia group survived without disabilities as compared to 1 of 15 patients in the historical control group. A higher rate of pulmonary infection was observed in the hypothermia group, though pneumonia was not fatal in these patients.

In the pilot study of the European multicenter trial [33], 27 comatose patients who had been successfully resuscitated after ventricular fibrillation cardiac arrest were enrolled. Surface cooling was initiated within 62 ± 33 min after cardiac arrest with a water-filled blanket. The target temperature (33 ± 1 °C) was reached after 287 ± 145 min and was maintained for a further 24 h. Thereafter, patients were allowed to re-warm passively. The aim of this study was to investigate possible harmful side effects of mild therapeutic hypothermia and detected any complications related to treatment with mild hypothermia. As a secondary outcome parameter, neurological outcome was evaluated, using the cerebral performance category (CPC) score, subdivided into good outcome (CPC 1 or 2), poor outcome (CPC 3 or 4), or death at 6 months. Good neurological recovery was achieved in 14 (52%) patients, poor neurological recovery in 2 (7%) patients, and 11 (41%) patients died before discharge. This was a two-fold improvement in neurological outcome compared to historical controls.

Encouraged by the positive results of the feasibility studies described above, two prospective randomized clinical trials were conducted, and the results of these studies were published recently. In the Australian trial [34], 77 patients with return of spontaneous circulation after cardiac arrest of cardiac origin (ventricular fibrillation or pulseless ventricular tachycardia) were randomly assigned to treatment with hypothermia (33 °C core temperature over 12 h, cooled with ice packs) or normothermia. The primary outcome measure was survival to hospital discharge with sufficiently good neurological function to be discharged to home or to a rehabilitation facility. Good neurological outcome was achieved in 21 of 43 patients (49%) treated with hypothermia compared to 9 of 34 patients (26%) treated with normothermia ($p = 0.046$). After adjustment for baseline differences, the odds ratio for a good neurological outcome was 5.25 (95% confidence interval, 1.47–18.76; $p = 0.011$) for patients treated with hypothermia as compared to patients treated with normothermia. There was no difference in the frequency of adverse events, but hypothermia was associated with a lower cardiac index, higher systemic vascular resistance, and hyperglycemia.

In the European multicenter trial [35], 275 patients with restoration of spontaneous circulation after cardiac arrest of cardiac origin (ventricular fibrillation or pulseless ventricular tachycardia) were randomly assigned to therapeutic hypothermia (32–34 °C bladder temperature, cooled with cold air) over a period of 24 h, or to standard treatment with normothermia. All patients received standard intensive care according to a detailed protocol, including the use of sedation and muscle relaxation for 32 h. The primary end point was a favorable neurological outcome within 6 months after cardiac arrest, defined as CPC 1 or CPC 2; secondary end points were mortality at 6 months and the incidence of complications within 7 days. Favorable neurologic outcome was achieved in 75 of 136 patients (55%) in the hypothermia group as compared to 54 of 137 patients (39%) in the normothermia group (risk ratio, 1.40; 95% confidence interval, 1.08–1.81). Mortality at 6 months was 41% in the hypothermia group (56 of 137 patients died) as compared to 55% in the normothermia group (76 of 138 patients died; risk ratio, 0.74; 95% confidence interval, 0.58–0.95). No difference in the incidence of complications was observed between the two groups.

Future Perspectives

Cooling Methods

Delay in cooling can negate the beneficial effects of preservative and resuscitative hypothermia [21]. For this reason, a technique to induce hypothermia that is feasible in the prehospital setting has to be found. Surface cooling, as used in the two prospective randomized clinical trials described above [34, 35], proved to be very slow, needing up to 8 h to reach the target temperature. It needs to be determined whether faster cooling would have resulted in even better outcome.

Infusion of a large volume of ice-cold intravenous fluid in healthy humans changed core temperature by only 0.6°C (SD 0.1) [36], or by 2.5°C (SD 0.4) when a very large volume (40 ml/kg) was given [37]. Recently, 30 ml/kg of ice-cooled saline, given intravenously over 30 min, decreased core temperature by about 1.6°C in cardiac arrest survivors [38]. More invasive blood cooling techniques might be more powerful in inducing hypothermia, but can only be used by advanced emergency medical personnel, resulting in delay in starting. In dogs, veno-venous extracorporeal pump cooling proved to be quite efficient in rapidly inducing hypothermia [39], but this cooling technique requires a double-lumen venous catheter with portable miniaturized pump, heat exchanger, and cold source - device not yet available. Other novel endovascular cooling devices that use cold fluid pumped through a balloon at the tip of the catheter (inserted into the superior or inferior vena cava) are already in clinical use [40, 41]. This approach seems to be safe with the advantage of no fluid entering the circulation, though the cooling rate was only 1.0–1.9°C/h in cardiac arrest survivors (unpublished data).

Suspended Animation

About one half of out-of-hospital resuscitation attempts for sudden cardiac death fail to restore heartbeat, and these patients are given up in the field [1]. It is suspected that many of these deaths occur in patients with the potential for complete cardiac and cerebral recovery provided that prolonged cardiopulmonary bypass can be induced before loss of cerebral viability, to support the heart until it recovers from stunning, repair, or replacement [42, 43]. Cardiopulmonary bypass is not available in the field. Preservation of the organism is therefore needed until cardiopulmonary bypass can be initiated in the emergency department. In 1984, Bellamy et al. introduced the concept of "suspended animation for delayed resuscitation", starting with a focus on rapidly exsanguinating trauma patients. Suspended animation is "preservation of the organism during transport and surgical hemostasis, under prolonged controlled clinical death, followed by delayed resuscitation to survival without brain damage" [44].

Preservative hypothermia, induced and reversed with cardiopulmonary bypass before cardiac arrest, has been shown to preserve the organism for up to 15 min with mild hypothermia (34–36°C) [8], up to 20 min with moderate hypothermia (28–32°C) [10], up to 30 min with deep hypothermia (11–27°C) [45, 46], and up to 60 min with profound hypothermia (6–10°C) [47]. To preserve the brain rapidly with mild to moderate hypothermia until more prolonged preservation with profound hypothermic circulatory arrest could be induced and reversed by cardiopulmonary bypass [43, 47, 48], the use of an aortic cold saline flush, via a balloon catheter, was introduced [49–52]. In a clinically realistic exsanguination cardiac arrest dog outcome model, the induction of suspended animation by use of cold (4°C) aortic flush within the first 5 min of cardiac arrest was shown to preserve brain viability for a cardiac arrest time of 15 min [49], 20 min [50], 30 min [51], and 90 min, perhaps 120 min [52].

This approach of preserving the organism with rapidly induced mild to moderate cerebral hypothermia to buy time for transport to hospital also needs to be explored for normovolemic cardiac arrest patients who are temporarily resistant to conventional resuscitation attempts [42, 44]. The clinical scenario (modified after [42]) would be: (1) After cardiac arrest, a bystander will initiate basic life support and begin to induce cooling by exposure; (2) ambulance personnel arrive at the scene and start conventional advanced life support with hypothermic intravenous infusion with a vasoconstrictor and attempts at defibrillation; (3) if restoration of spontaneous circulation can not be achieved within 10 min, the emergency physician will further attempt cooling to achieve systemic temperatures as low as possible to preserve the brain and heart, leaving the patient in cardiac arrest for transport to the emergency department, where cardiopulmonary bypass will be initiated. This suspended animation hypothermic no-flow scenario during transport needs to be compared with hypothermic low-flow, i.e., continued external cardiac massage after cold aortic flush, and with normothermic low-flow, i.e. conventional external cardiac massage, in a large animal outcome study.

References

1. Eisenberg MS, Horwood BT, Cummins RO et al (1990) Cardiac arrest and resuscitation: a tale of 29 cities. Ann Emerg Med 19:179-186
2. Safar P, Behringer W (2003) Brain resuscitation after cardiac arrest. In: Layon AJ, Gabrielli A, Friedman W A (eds) Textbook of neurointensive care. Saunders, Philadelphia (in press)
3. Safar P (1997) Resuscitation of the ischemic brain. In: Albin MS (ed) Textbook of neuroanesthesia with neurosurgical and neuroscience perspectives. McGraw-Hill, New York, pp 557-593
4. Siesjo BK (1988) Mechanisms of ischemic brain damage. Crit Care Med 16:954-963
5. White BC, Sullivan JM, DeGracia DJ et al (2000) Brain ischemia and reperfusion: molecular mechanisms of neuronal injury. J Neurol Sci 179:1-33
6. Michenfelder JD, Theye RA (1970) The effects of anesthesia and hypothermia on canine cerebral ATP and lactate during anoxia produced by decapitation. Anesthesiology 33:430-439
7. Safar P (1986) Cerebral resuscitation after cardiac arrest: a review. Circulation 74:IV138-IV153
8. Safar P (1988) Resuscitation from clinical death: pathophysiologic limits and therapeutic potentials. Crit Care Med 16:923-941
9. Reuler JB (1978) Hypothermia: pathophysiology, clinical settings, and management. Ann Intern Med 89:519-527
10. Bigelow WG, Linsay WK, Greenwood WF (1950) Hypothermia: its possible role in cardiac surgery. Ann Surg 132:849-866
11. Rosomoff HL, Holaday A (1954) Cerebral blood flow and cerebral oxygen consumption during hypothermia. Am J Physiol 179:85-88
12. Dripps RD (1956) The physiology of induced hypothermia. National Academy of Science, Washington DC
13. Steen PA, Soule EH, Michenfelder JD (1979) Detrimental effect of prolonged hypothermia in cats and monkeys with and without regional cerebral ischemia. Stroke 10:522-529
14. Steen PA, Milde JH, Michenfelder JD (1980) The detrimental effects of prolonged hypothermia and rewarming in the dog. Anesthesiology 52:224-230
15. Busto R, Dietrich WD, Globus MY et al (1987) Small differences in intraischemic brain temperature critically determine the extent of ischemic neuronal injury. J Cereb Blood Flow Metab 7:729-738
16. Hossmann KA (1988) Resuscitation potentials after prolonged global cerebral ischemia in cats. Crit Care Med 16:964-971
17. Leonov Y, Sterz F, Safar P, Radovsky A (1990) Moderate hypothermia after cardiac arrest of 17 minutes in dogs. Effect on cerebral and cardiac outcome. Stroke 21:1600-1606
18. Leonov Y, Sterz F, Safar P et al (1990) Mild cerebral hypothermia during and after cardiac arrest improves neurologic outcome in dogs. J Cereb Blood Flow Metab 10:57-70

19. Sterz F, Safar P, Tisherman S et al (1991) Mild hypothermic cardiopulmonary resuscitation improves outcome after prolonged cardiac arrest in dogs. Crit Care Med 19:379-389
20. Weinrauch V, Safar P, Tisherman S et al (1992) Beneficial effect of mild hypothermia and detrimental effect of deep hypothermia after cardiac arrest in dogs. Stroke 23:1454-1462
21. Kuboyama K, Safar P, Radovsky A et al (1993) Delay in cooling negates the beneficial effect of mild resuscitative cerebral hypothermia after cardiac arrest in dogs: a prospective, randomized study. Crit Care Med 21:1348-1358
22. Safar P, Xiao F, Radovsky A et al (1996) Improved cerebral resuscitation from cardiac arrest in dogs with mild hypothermia plus blood flow promotion. Stroke 27:105-113
23. Coimbra C, Wieloch T (1994) Moderate hypothermia mitigates neuronal damage in the rat brain when initiated several hours following transient cerebral ischemia. Acta Neuropathol 87:325-31
24. Hickey RW, Ferimer H, Alexander HL et al (2000) Delayed, spontaneous hypothermia reduces neuronal damage after asphyxial cardiac arrest in rats. Crit Care Med 28:3511-3516
25. Green EJ, Dietrich WD, van Dijk F et al (1992) Protective effects of brain hypothermia on behavior and histopathology following global cerebral ischemia in rats. Brain Res 580:197-204
26. Dietrich WD, Busto R, Alonso O et al (1993) Intraischemic but not postischemic brain hypothermia protects chronically following global forebrain ischemia in rats. J Cereb Blood Flow Metab 13:541-549
27. Colbourne F, Corbett D (1994) Delayed and prolonged post-ischemic hypothermia is neuroprotective in the gerbil. Brain Res 654:265-72
28. Colbourne F, Corbett D (1995) Delayed postischemic hypothermia: a six month survival study using behavioral and histological assessments of neuroprotection. J Neurosci 15:7250-7260
29. Colbourne F, Auer RN, Sutherland GR (1998) Behavioral testing does not exacerbate ischemic CA1 damage in gerbils. Stroke 29:1967-1970
30. Colbourne F, Li H, Buchan AM (1999) Indefatigable CA1 sector neuroprotection with mild hypothermia induced 6 hours after severe forebrain ischemia in rats. J Cereb Blood Flow Metab 19:742-749
31. Bernard SA, Jones BM, Horne MK (1997) Clinical trial of induced hypothermia in comatose survivors of out-of-hospital cardiac arrest. Ann Emerg Med 30:146-153
32. Yanagawa Y, Ishihara S, Norio H et al (1998) Preliminary clinical outcome study of mild resuscitative hypothermia after out-of-hospital cardiopulmonary arrest. Resuscitation 39:61-66
33. Zeiner A, Holzer M, Sterz F et al (2000) Mild resuscitative hypothermia to improve neurological outcome after cardiac arrest. A clinical feasibility trial. Hypothermia After Cardiac Arrest (HACA) Study Group. Stroke 31:86-94
34. Bernard SA, Gray TW, Buist MD et al (2002) Treatment of comatose survivors of out-of-hospital cardiac arrest with induced hypothermia. N Engl J Med 346:557-563
35. Hypothermia After Cardiac ARrest Study Group (2002) Mild therapeutic hypothermia to improve the neurologic outcome after cardiac arrest. N Engl J Med 346:549-556
36. Baumgardner JE, Baranov D, Smith DS, Zager EL (1999) The effectiveness of rapidly infused intravenous fluids for inducing moderate hypothermia in neurosurgical patients. Anesth Analg 89:163-169
37. Rajek A, Greif R, Sessler DI et al (2000) Core cooling by central venous infusion of

ice-cold (4 degrees C and 20 degrees C) fluid: isolation of core and peripheral thermal compartments. Anesthesiology 93:629-637

38. Bernard S, Buist M, Monteiro O, Smith K (2003) Induced hypothermia using large volume, ice-cold intravenous fluid in comatose survivors of out-of-hospital cardiac arrest: a preliminary report. Resuscitation 56:9-13
39. Behringer W, Safar P, Wu X et al (2002) Veno-venous extracorporeal blood shunt cooling to induce mild hypothermia in dog experiments and review of cooling methods. Resuscitation 54:89-98
40. Keller E, Imhof HG, Gasser S et al (2003) Endovascular cooling with heat exchange catheters: a new method to induce and maintain hypothermia. Intensive Care Med 29:939-943
41. Dixon SR, Whitbourn RJ, Dae MW et al (2002) Induction of mild systemic hypothermia with endovascular cooling during primary percutaneous coronary intervention for acute myocardial infarction. J Am Coll Cardiol 40:1928-1934
42. Safar P, Tisherman SA, Behringer W et al (2000) Suspended animation for delayed resuscitation from prolonged cardiac arrest that is unresuscitable by standard cardiopulmonary-cerebral resuscitation. Crit Care Med 28:N214-N218
43. Safar P, Abramson NS, Angelos M et al (1990) Emergency cardiopulmonary bypass for resuscitation from prolonged cardiac arrest. Am J Emerg Med 8:55-67
44. Bellamy R, Safar P, Tisherman SA et al (1996) Suspended animation for delayed resuscitation. Crit Care Med 24:S24-S47
45. Hickey PR (1985) Deep hypothermic circulatory arrest: current status and future directions. Mt Sinai J Med 52:541-547
46. Livesay JJ, Cooley DA, Reul GJ et al (1983) Resection of aortic arch aneurysms: a comparison of hypothermic techniques in 60 patients. Ann Thorac Surg 36:19-28
47. Capone A, Safar P, Radovsky A et al (1996) Complete recovery after normothermic hemorrhagic shock and profound hypothermic circulatory arrest of 60 minutes in dogs. J Trauma 40:388-395
48. Tisherman SA, Safar P, Radovsky A et al (1991) Profound hypothermia (less than 10 degrees C) compared with deep hypothermia (15 degrees C) improves neurologic outcome in dogs after two hours' circulatory arrest induced to enable resuscitative surgery. J Trauma 31:1051-1061
49. Woods RJ, Prueckner S, Safar P et al (1999) Hypothermic aortic arch flush for preservation during exsanguination cardiac arrest of 15 minutes in dogs. J Trauma 47:1028-1036
50. Behringer W, Prueckner S, Safar P et al (2000) Rapid induction of mild cerebral hypothermia by cold aortic flush achieves normal recovery in a dog outcome model with 20-minute exsanguination cardiac arrest. Acad Emerg Med 7:1341-1348
51. Behringer W, Prueckner S, Kentner R et al (2000) Rapid hypothermic aortic flush can achieve survival without brain damage after 30 minutes cardiac arrest in dogs. Anesthesiology 93:1491-1499
52. Behringer W, Safar P, Wu X et al (2003) Survival without brain damage after clinical death of 60-120 mw in dogs using suspended animation by profound hypotermia. Crit Care Med 31:1523-1531

SYNCOPE: CURRENT EVALUATION AND MANAGEMENT

Distinguishing Syncope From Seizures: How Useful is the Clinical History?

R. S. Sheldon

Introduction

Transient loss of consciousness is a common clinical problem whose diagnosis frequently poses problems. About 20% of people faint at least once in their lives, probably 10% faint more than once [1], and it is the cause of 1-6% of emergency room visits [2]. The first diagnostic decision to be made is whether the patient has syncope or seizures. Although classic prodromal symptoms, such as convulsive activity, tongue-biting and physical trauma, are often used to diagnose a seizure disorder, this decision-making is based upon historical practice rather than quantitative evidence. The occurrence of convulsive syncope and of akinetic seizures has added to the difficulties of diagnosis. Finally, the pattern of diagnostic features may take several spells to emerge. The reliability of the diagnosis of the first loss of consciousness is surprisingly low [3], but this can be improved with preset diagnostic criteria [4].

Limitations of Current Diagnostic Approaches

Many clinicians are reluctant to trust the history of unconsciousness as a useful source of information. This has led to use of investigative tools that measure aspects of the central nervous system; ischemic, electrical, and structural aspects of the cardiovascular system; and various endocrinologic disorders [5, 6]. Most of these tests have limited diagnostic yield in unselected patients with a history of total loss of consciousness, most are expensive or invasive or both, and most continue to be used early in the diagnostic cascade. Are there other tests that might have a higher diagnostic yield?

Two relatively new diagnostic tools for syncope are tilt table tests and implantable loop recorders. Tilt tests have been enormously useful in the study

Cardiovascular Research Group, University of Calgary, Alberta, Canada

of neurally mediated syncope. They provide a diagnosis in most patients with syncope of uncertain origin, are useful tools in the study of its physiology and have provided diagnosed populations for natural history studies and clinical trials [2]. Implantable loop recorders record the ECG during syncope, and can therefore screen for arrhythmic causes of syncope and for neurally mediated syncope syndromes associated with transient bradycardias. They have established the diagnostic outcomes of patients at elevated risk for arrhythmic syncope, and have provided variable information about the heart rate of patients with probable neurally mediated syncope during their spells [7].

Tilt tests, although seemingly simple, are precariously balanced on a number of important variables [2]. Controlled studies have shown that the likelihood of positive studies in both syncope patients and control subjects depends on the angle and duration of headup tilt, whether a drug challenge is used, the type and dose of drug, the number of headup iterations during the tilt test, the volume status of the subject and the subject age. There is a variable correlation between the symptoms provoked by tilt testing and the subject's clinical symptoms, and widely variable and usually unvalidated hemodynamic criteria. Importantly, there is no gold standard population against which the test has been validated. This is important because different tilt test protocols appear to identify patient populations that do not overlap completely. Tilt test protocols, each with adequate specificities, are positive in populations that do not overlap. If they both have reasonable, albeit imperfect, accuracies, then which one is true? Can we diagnose patients with a test that appears to only diagnose a subset of truly positive patients? Finally, there appears to be an intractable trade-off between sensitivity and specificity. No single tilt test protocol now appears to function at a reliably high level.

The implantable loop recorder also has potential problems. It is a passive tool that relies on the patient having another syncopal spell. While this may be tolerable to many patients, it is not likely to be useful in patients with potentially fatal causes of syncope, and therefore its use may be practically restricted to patients with benign causes of syncope. Much of this may be vasovagal syncope, and in turn a large part may be associated with vasodepression rather than bradycardia [7, 8]. It is invasive and its utility depends upon its sensitivity and the consequences of a diagnosis. Therefore, the loop recorder is unlikely to find a niche in diagnosing patients with dangerous causes of syncope, and may simply detect sinus rhythm in many patients with vasovagal syncope.

Potential Usefulness of Diagnostic Histories

Many have felt that there is little to be learned from the symptoms associated with total loss of consciousness, since unconscious patients, by definition, do not remember their symptoms. However, quantitative histories and diagnostic scores are well known in other fields. They are known to improve diagnostic accuracy and there are known quantitative differences in the histories among patients with different causes of total loss of consciousness. Previous attempts at defining diagnostic criteria for unconsciousness syndromes of loss were limited by lack of quantitative data [9-11], lack of gold standard diagnostic groups [12, 13], lack of populations with both seizures and syncope [9, 11, 12, 14, 15], retrospective analyses [11, 13] and lack of translation of results into easily applied criteria [3, 4, 11, 12, 14, 15]. Recently several groups have turned to quantitative histories in attempt to resolve these problems.

Quantitative Histories

Both Calkins et al. and Alboni et al. reported that patients with different causes of syncope, such as ventricular tachycardia, complete heart block, and vasovagal syncope, have highly significant differences in the symptoms that accompany loss of consciousness [9, 10]. Although these differences in symptoms provide physicians with a sense of the differences among the groups, they do not provide them with simple tools that can be used in decision-making. These problems might be addressed with a quantitative analysis of the symptoms, expressed as a diagnostic point score. These point scores are likely to be quite useful. The reliability of the diagnosis of the first loss of consciousness is surprisingly low, but this can be improved with preset simple diagnostic criteria. This suggests that a structured questionnaire, if based on firm quantitative evidence, might be helpful in the assessment of the patient with total loss of consciousness.

The Syncope Symptom Study

We hypothesized that evidence-based diagnostic criteria could distinguish between syncope and seizures as causes of transient loss of consciousness. To test this, we performed the Syncope Symptom Study [16]. We administered a uniform questionnaire to 671 patients who were referred to three academic centers in Canada and Wales for assessment of transient total loss of consciousness. We first studied patients with securely defined diagnoses based upon conventionally accepted objective tests, then compared their responses to identify the historical features that most accurately correlated with their diagnoses. The causes of loss of consciousness were known satisfactorily in 539 patients and included complex partial epilepsy, primary generalized epilepsy, tilt-positive vasovagal syncope, ventricular tachycardia, and other diagnoses such as complete heart block and supraventricular tachycardias. The population was split randomly into 2 groups and the point score was developed using logistic regression analysis and receiver operator characteristic analysis in one subgroup. The point score was then validated in the second group.

The diagnostic features in favor of seizures included preceding emotional stress (1 point); déjà vu or jamais vu (1 point); head turning or unusual posturing or motor behavior during the spell (1 point each); or awakening confused (1 point) or with a cut tongue (2 points). Features in favor of syncope include a history of presyncope at other times (- 2 points), preceding diaphoresis (-2 points), or provocation by prolonged sitting or standing (- 2 points). The patient has seizures if the point score is ≥ 1, and syncope if the point score is < 1. Overall, the point score performed very well, diagnosing seizures with 94% sensitivity and 94% specificity. Interestingly, the addition of features such as the number of spells or the number of months the patients had had the symptoms did not improve the diagnostic accuracy of the score. Furthermore, the point score worked as well in patients with syncope of unknown cause as in patients with an established cause of syncope.

This study provided evidence for the partial validity of previous anecdotal approaches, and also illustrated the need for negative criteria. The classic seizure symptoms and signs of déjà vu, cut tongue, limb jerking and postictal confusion all contributed to the diagnosis of seizures. Symptoms of syncope such as prodromal diaphoresis, presyncope at other times, or provocation by prolonged sitting or standing often needed to be absent in order to diagnose of a seizure. We had anticipated that the relatively common occurrence of convulsive syncope might confound the analysis [17]. Indeed, 15% of our syncope patients had abnormal limb jerking noted by others. This was not a major problem. It may be because the classification scheme addresses it directly: to be diagnosed with epileptic seizures patients generally both have evidence of seizures, and lack of evidence of symptoms that are seen in patients with syncope.

The features that clinicians have used to diagnose seizures have included symptoms characteristic of specific syndromes. For example, diagnostic features of partial seizures include staring, lip smacking and repetitive facial jerks or grimacing, and prodromes of olfactory sensations, head turning or stiffening and a rising sensation in the abdomen. Signs of generalized seizures include tongue biting and tonic-clonic convulsions. Criteria for syncope similarly have been related to specific causes; examples include nausea, fatigue, and specific causal factors for vasovagal syncope. We anticipated that this might pose a problem in the derivation of the point score. To obviate this, we used a large patient population drawn from both neurology and cardiology clinics and inpatient services to establish criteria that would cover a range of syndromes.

These questions might help with diagnostic determinations. While we do not suggest that they supplant appropriate and targeted investigations in difficult cases, they may streamline initial patient assessment. This might be useful in a range of clinical and academic settings, and by preventing some unnecessary investigations they might reduce patient anxiety and morbidity as well as health costs [5, 6, 18, 19]. Similar analyses are underway to derive classification schemes for the various causes of syncope.

References

1. Chen LY, Shen WK, Mahoney DW et al (2002) Prevalence of self-reported syncope: An epidemiologic study from Olmsted County, MN. J Am Coll Cardiol 39:114A-115A (Abstract)
2. Benditt DG, Ferguson DW, Grubb BP et al (1996) Tilt table testing for assessing syncope. J Am Coll Cardiol 28:263-275
3. Hoefnagels WAJ, Padberg GW, Overweg J, Roos RAC (1992) Syncope or seizure? A matter of opinion. Clin Neurol Neurosurg 94:153-156
4. Van Donselaar CA, Geerts AT, Meulstee J et al (1989) Reliability of the diagnosis of a first seizure. Neurology 39:267-271
5. Linzer M, Yang EH, Estes III MA et al (1997) Diagnosing Syncope. Part I. Value of history, physical examination, and electrocardiography. Ann Int Med 126:989-996
6. Linzer M, Yang EH, Estes III MA et al (1997) Diagnosing Syncope. Part II. Unexplained syncope. Ann Int Med 127:76-87
7. Moya A, Brignole M, Menozzi C et al (2001) Mechanism of syncope in patients with isolated syncope and in patients with tilt-positive syncope. Circulation 104:1261-1267
8. Krahn AD, Klein GJ, Fitzpatrick A et al (2002) Predicting the outcome of patients with unexplained syncope undergoing prolonged monitoring. Pacing Clin Electrophysiol 25:37-41
9. Calkins H, Shyr Y, Frumin H et al (1995) The value of the clinical history in the differentiation of syncope due to ventricular tachycardia, atrioventricular block, and neurocardiogenic syncope. Am J Med 98:365-373
10. Alboni P, Brignole M, Menozzi C et al (2001) Diagnostic Value of History in Patients With Syncope With or Without Heart Disease. J Am Coll Cardiol 37:1921-1928
11. Wayne HH (1961) Syncope. Physiological considerations and an analysis of the clinical characteristics in 510 patients. Am J Med 30:418-438
12. Martin GJ, Adams SL, Martin HG et al (1984) Prospective evaluation of syncope. Ann Emerg Med 13:499-504
13. Day SC, Cook EF, Funkenstein H, Goldman L (1982) Evaluation and outcome of emergency room patients with transient loss of consciousness. Am J Med 73:15-23
14. Hopkins A, Garman A, Clarke C (1988) The first seizure in adult life. Value of clinical features, electroencephalography, and computerised tomographic scanning in prediction of seizure recurrence. Lancet 1:721-726
15. Commission on classification and terminology of the international league against epilepsy (1981) Proposal for revised clinical and electroencephalographic classification of epileptic seizures. Epilepsia 22:489-501
16. Sheldon R, Rose S, Ritchie D et al (2002) Historical Criteria That Distinguish Syncope From Seizures. J Am Coll Cardiol 40:142-148
17. Grubb BP, Gerard G, Roush K et al (1991) Differentiation of convulsive syncope and epilepsy with head-up tilt testing. Ann Int Med 115:871-876
18. Calkins H, Byrne M, El-Tassi R et al (1993) The economic burden of unrecognized vasodepressor syncope. Am J Med 95:473-479
19. Sutton R, Petersen M (1997) The economics of treating vasovagal syncope. PACE 20(II): 849-850

Diagnosis of Neurally Mediated Syncope: Might Use of the Implantable Loop Recorder Replace the Tilt-table Test?
A Positive View

A. Moya

The question addressed in this debate is whether implantable loop recording (ILR) could replace the tilt-table test (TTT) in the management of patients with syncope of unknown etiology.

First of all, let us define terms. In this debate we will refer to patients without structural heart disease and with normal ECG, because patients with syncope and structural heart disease, familial history of sudden death or abnormalities in baseline ECG, are at increased risk of having a cardiac origin of syncope [1], and in these patients the diagnostic strategy must be directed at assessing the degree of cardiac dysfunction and also at ruling out a possible arrhythmic cause of syncope, which in most cases will involve ECG monitoring and an electrophysiological study [2, 3].

Patients with syncope, absence of structural heart disease, and normal ECG have a very low probability of having a primary arrhythmia as a cause of syncope [4], and in these patients the most common etiology is a neuromediated mechanism. In addition, many such patients have a single syncopal episode or have clusters of episodes during limited periods of time, followed by long periods of remission, and only a minority of them have frequent and recurrent episodes that can affect their quality of life [5]. It has been shown that patients with syncope without evidence of structural heart disease have an excellent prognosis in terms of survival and cardiac events.

The etiology of the syncopal episodes can be found in the clinical history in some of these patients. Vasovagal syncope can be diagnosed if precipitating events such as fear, severe pain, emotional distress, instrumentation or prolonged standing are associated with a typical prodromal symptom. Situational syncope can be diagnosed if syncope occurs during or immediately after urination, defecation, coughing, or swallowing. Orthostatic syncope can be diagnosed when there is documented orthostatic hypotension associated with syncope or pre-syncope [6]. In some patients, especially in those older than 50,

Unitat d'Arítmies, Hospital General Universitari Vall d'Hebron, Barcelona, Spain

carotid sinus massage must be performed in order to recognize a carotid sinus syndrome that might be the cause of syncope [7]. When the diagnosis of syncope has been achieved by means of the clinical history or by carotid sinus massage, no further diagnostic tests are usually needed; however, in patients with recurrent and frequent syncopal episodes, and also in those who have experienced injuries related to syncope, some additional information about the behavior of heart rate and arterial blood pressure during syncopal episodes may be needed for its management.

In patients in whom the diagnosis has not been achieved after the initial evaluation, tilt-table testing (TTT) has been considered a useful tool. The objective of TTT is to trigger a vasovagal reaction, by means of orthostatic stress, in those patients who are prone to this type of reaction. There are several different protocols for TTT, varying in the degree of inclination, the duration of the test, the use of different provocative drugs, and the criteria applied to class a test as positive. Current guidelines recommend an inclination between 60° and 70°, with a baseline phase of at least 20 min and a maximum of 45 min [6]. If the baseline phase has been negative, the administration of nitroglycerine (400 μg s.l.) [8] or "low-dose" intravenous isoproterenol (1–3 μg/min is recommended to increase heart rate by 20–25% from baseline values) [9]. These protocols have been shown to have a good specificity, but the true sensitivity is unknown. Recently, data obtained from the ISSUE study have suggested that the sensitivity of TTT may be low [10]. This means that a positive response to TTT in a patient with syncope of unknown origin, absence of structural heart disease, and a normal ECG strongly suggests a vasovagal origin, but a negative response does not exclude this etiology. All this indicates that the contribution of TTT to the diagnosis of a vasovagal etiology of syncope in such patients is limited.

The positive responses to TTT have been classified as vasodepressor, cardioinhibitory, and mixed [11]. The impact of this classification on the follow-up and the management of these patients has not been demonstrated. Several authors have shown that the recurrence rate, the clinical follow-up, and the prognosis are the same irrespective of the type of response to TTT [12]. In addition, recent data obtained during the ISSUE study in eight patients with a positive TTT who had had an ILR implanted showed that there was no close correlation between the responses observed during TTT and during a spontaneous episode [10]. In this series there were two patients who had a severe cardioinhibitory response during TTT, and both patients showed a marked asystole during spontaneous syncope. In contrast, of the five patients who had a mixed response during TTT, three had an asystole during spontaneous syncope, one had sinus bradycardia, and the remaining patients had normal sinus rhythm. According to these data it can be concluded that the type of response to TTT during a positive response has a limited influence on the prognosis and management of patients with syncope.

All these data suggest that, in patients with syncope who have no structural heart disease and a normal ECG, the most frequent etiology is a neuromediated mechanism and that they are at a very low risk of major cardiac events, irrespective of the result of TTT. In this situation, if the patient has had a single syncope or infrequent syncopal episodes no specific treatment is needed, and the most reasonable approach is to reassure the patient about the benign nature of the disease and to give some advice on preventive measures. On the other hand, in those patients who have recurrent and frequent episodes, or who have sustained injury associated with syncope, some specific treatment must be considered. In these cases it is important to have the most accurate information about what happens during spontaneous episodes, and more specifically how the arterial blood pressure and heart rate behave, in order to select the most appropriate treatment. As shown before, the information obtained with TTT can be misleading as far as the exact origin and mechanism of syncope are concerned. Other tests, such as an electrophysiologic study, can be performed, but in the absence of structural heart disease and with a normal baseline ECG the diagnostic yield is extremely low. In these patients the implantation of an ILR gives a unique opportunity to record the ECG during any spontaneous syncopal episode, and this is probably the only way of ruling out a primary arrhythmia as a cause of syncope, which is extremely rare in patients without structural heart disease, or of recognizing some forms of vasovagal syncope with more or less severe cardioinhibitory responses. These findings can be helpful in selection of the proper treatment in these patients. In those cases in which no major changes in heart rate are observed during syncopal episodes, it can be difficult to differentiate a vasovagal mechanism from other clinical situations, such as psychogenic syncope [13], but in any case it makes it possible to rule out a severe rhythm disturbance, whether primary or secondary to a vasovagal origin.

Coming back to the question posed in the title, it can be considered that in patients with syncope, no structural heart disease, and normal ECG who have had only single or isolated episodes, clinical evaluation can be an adequate initial approach and TTT probably does not add any further information that would be useful for the prognosis or management. In contrast, those patients who have frequent or clinically severe episodes need specific treatment. In these cases, data obtained from TTT are not useful for use in therapeutic decision-making, for which data obtained from spontaneous syncopal episodes are usually needed; ILR could be helpful in these patients.

References

1. Martin TP, Hanusa BH, Kapoor WN (1997) Risk stratification of patients with syncope. Ann Emerg Med 29:459–466
2. Kaul U, Dev V, Narula J, Malhotra A, Talwar K, Bhatia M (1988) Evaluation of patients with bundle branch block and 'unexplained' syncope: a study based on comprehensive electrophysiologic testing and ajmaline stress. Pacing Clin Electrophysiol 11:289–297

3. Englund A, Bergfeldt L, Rehnqvist N, Astrom H, Rosenqvist M (1995) Diagnostic value of programmed ventricular stimulation in patients with bifascicular block: a prospective study of patients with and without syncope. J Am Coll Cardiol 26:1508–1515
4. Kapoor WN, Hanusa B (1996) Is syncope a risk factor for poor outcomes? Comparison of patients with and without syncope. Am J Med 100:646–655
5. Raviele A, Proclemer A, Gasparini G et al (1989) Long-term follow-up of patients with unexplained syncope and negative electrophysiologic study. Eur Heart J 10:127–132
6. Brignole M, Alboni P, Benditt D et al (2001) Guidelines on management (diagnosis and treatment) of syncope. Eur Heart J 22:1256–1306
7. Menozzi C, Brignole M, Lolli G et al (1993) Follow-up of asystolic episodes in patients with cardioinhibitory, neurally mediated syncope and VVI pacemaker. Am J Cardiol 72:1152–1155
8. Del Rosso A, Bartoletti A, Bartoli P et al (2000) Methodology of head-up tilt testing potentiated with sublingual nitroglycerin in unexplained syncope. Am J Cardiol 85:1007–1011
9. Morillo CA, Klein GJ, Zandri S, Yee R (1995) Diagnostic accuracy of a low-dose isoproterenol head-up tilt protocol. Am Heart J 129:901–906
10. Moya A, Brignole M, Menozzi C et al (2001) Mechanism of syncope in patients with isolated syncope and in patients with tilt-positive syncope. Circulation 104:1261–1267
11. Brignole M, Menozzi C, Del Rosso A et al (2000) New classification of haemodynamics of vasovagal syncope: beyond the VASIS classification. Analysis of the pre-syncopal phase of the tilt test without and with nitroglycerin challenge. Europace 2:66–76
12. Baron-Esquivias G, Pedrote A, Cayuela A, Valle JI, Fernandez JM, Arana E et al (2002) Long-term outcome of patients with asystole induced by head-up tilt test. Eur Heart J 23:483–489
13. Brignole M, Menozzi C, Moya A et al (2002) Nonarrhythmic syncope documented by an implantable loop recorder (an ISSUE substudy). Am J Cardiol 90:654–657

Unexplained Syncope: Can We Predict the Outcome of Prolonged Monitoring with the Implantable Loop Recorder?

A. D. Krahn, G. J. Klein, R. Yee, A. C. Skanes

Introduction

Syncope is a complex clinical symptom with multiple etiologies that are often difficult to discern. The major obstacles to diagnosis are the unpredictable and infrequent nature of events and the high spontaneous remission rate [1, 2]. Clinicians rely on clinical assessment and abnormal laboratory results to make a diagnosis by inference in many cases. Advances in long term cardiac monitoring techniques with the implantable loop recorders have added a powerful tool in the field for arrhythmia detection [3-9]. Optimal deployment of this technology is aimed to enhance diagnostic yield while directing scarce resources at patients with a high likelihood of device utilization [5, 10-12].

The Implantable Loop Recorder

The implantable loop recorder (ILR) is ideally suited to patients with infrequent recurrent syncope because it permits prolonged monitoring without external electrodes. The only commercially available implantable loop recorder at this time is manufactured by Medtronic (Reveal© - Minneapolis, MN). The ILR has a pair of sensing electrodes 3.7 cm apart on the shell, measures 6.1x1.9x0.8 cm, weighs 17 grams, and has a battery life of 14 months. It is inserted subcutaneously in the left chest using standard sterile technique and local anesthetic. It has been implanted in the right parasternal, subcostal and axillary regions with an adequate, albeit lower, amplitude signal. The recorded bipolar ECG signal is stored in a circular buffer capable of retaining 21 minutes of uncompressed or 42 minutes of compressed signal in 1 or 3 divided parts. Because the compressed signal quality is negligibly different from the

Division of Cardiology, University of Western Ontario, London, Ontario, Canada uncompressed signal, it is used most often to maximize the memory capacity of the device. The memory buffer is frozen using a hand-held activator provided to the patient. The episodes are downloaded after interrogation with a standard Medtronic 9790 pacemaker programmer. The current version of the device (Reveal Plus©) has programmable automatic detection of high and low heart rate episodes and pauses. The resultant memory configuration allows for division of multiple one-minute automatic rhythm strips in addition to 1-3 manual recordings. This permits automated backup of manual activations to detect prespecified extreme heart rates or pauses (typically < 30 bpm, > 160 bpm and pauses > 3 seconds). This also permits detection of asymptomatic heart rate changes that may influence clinical judgment as to the likely cause for syncope in the absence of symptomatic recurrence.

The implant procedure is similar to the creation of a smaller and more superficial pacemaker pocket. Cardiologists and cardiac surgeons have performed the implant in an operating room or in the electrophysiology or cardiac catheterization laboratory setting. An adequate signal can be obtained anywhere in the left thorax, without the need for cutaneous mapping [13]. Mapping does optimize the sensed signal, and is recommended in patients where automatic detection is desirable to prevent oversensing of T waves and double counting leading to automatic detection of high rate episodes. Right parasternal sites have been used to optimize p wave amplitude. The patient along with a spouse, family member or friend is instructed in the use of the activator at the time of implant. Use of prophylactic antibiotics is usually recommended to prevent pocket infection, similar to that for implantation of permanent pacemakers.

Initial Experience

The ILR was initially implanted in patients with recurrent unexplained syncope after extensive non-invasive and invasive testing was negative, including tilt and electrophysiologic testing [4, 6]. The device was very successful in establishing a symptom rhythm correlation (85%) in this difficult patient population that we previously had little to offer other than empiric therapy or reassurance. These results have been confirmed in a recent study assessing the selective use of electrophysiologic testing in combination with tilt testing in 184 patients with unexplained syncope [14, 15]. In the subgroup of 15 patients with negative tilt and electrophysiologic testing, the ILR provided a symptom rhythm correlation in 47%. These studies suggest that the ILR has a clear role as a test of last resort, but also call into question the utility of conventional testing in certain patient populations.

Subsequent studies have applied the ILR to less problematic patients populations with less extensive preimplant testing, lowering the postimplant likelihood of recurrence of syncope after implant to 30-70% [3, 7, 9]. Several studies have demonstrated the feasibility of the ILR in establishing a symptom rhythm correlation during long term monitoring [3, 6, 7, 16-18]. The largest of these studies combined data from 206 patients from 3 centers [3]. The majority of patients studied had undergone previous non-invasive testing and selective invasive testing, including tilt testing and electrophysiologic studies. Symptoms recurred during follow-up in 69% of patients days after device implant (Fig. 1). An arrhythmia was detected in 22% of patients. Sinus rhythm excluding, a primary arrhythmia was seen in 42% of patients and symptoms resolved without recurrence during prolonged monitoring in 31%. Bradycardia was detected more frequently than tachycardia (17% vs 6%), usually leading to pacemaker implantation. Failed activation of the device after spontaneous symptoms occurred in 4% of patients. In these patients, a symptom rhythm correlation was not obtained during the monitoring period.

The authors performed a multivariate analysis to predict recurrence of syncope and detection of bradyarrhythmia in an attempt to characterize patients that went on to pacemaker implant [3]. Logistic regression analysis of baseline variables found that age was the only independent variable that predicted need for pacing, associated with a 3% increase in risk per advancing year of age (odds ratio 1.027, p=0.026). Despite this finding, no age group could be identified in whom the likelihood of requiring pacing exceeded 30%. Logistic regression also found that patients with structural heart disease were less likely to experience recurrent symptoms during monitoring (49% vs. 78%, p=0.001), and that advancing age was associated with earlier recurrence of symptoms (p=0.01). No age group had an incidence of bradycardia requiring pacing greater than 30%, suggesting a limited role for empiric pacing in the unexplained syncope population.

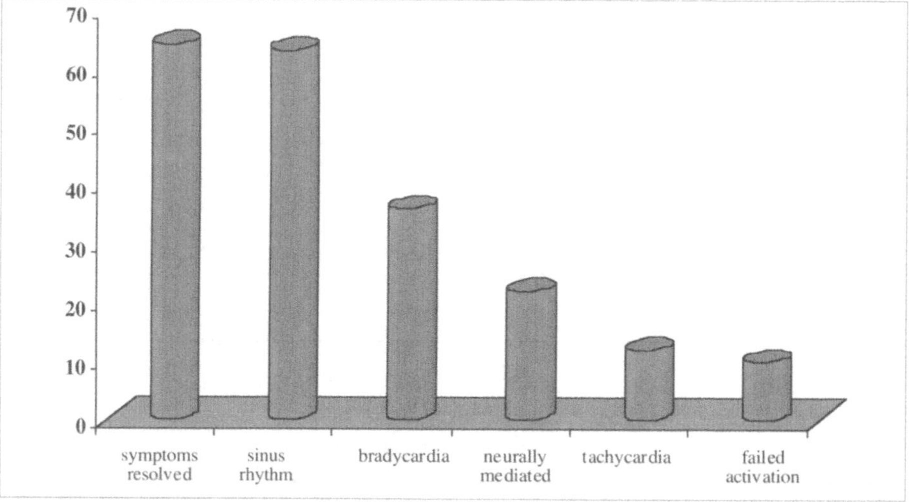

Fig. 1. Outcome in 206 patients undergoing prolonged monitoring with an implanted loop recorder for recurrent unexplained syncope. Symptoms recurred in 142 patients (69%), with a symptom-rhythm correlation determined in 132 (64%). Adapted from [3]

Predicting the Outcome of Prolonged Monitoring

A recent study examined a cohort of loop recorder patients baseline characteristics to develop a risk score to predict device utility [19]. This study identified three risk factors for syncope during the monitoring period: age less than 65 years, > 3 pre-implant syncopal episodes and absence of heart disease. The risk factor score (0-3) was associated with a progressive increased likelihood of device use (33%, 55%, 69% and 85% - Figure 2). Although the patients with the highest risk score were most likely to obtain a symptom rhythm correlation with the ILR, this utility is most likely to exclude an arrhythmia since these patients are likely to have neurocardiogenic syncope. Nonetheless, the pertinent negative is clinically very useful. The most difficult patients remain those with infrequent symptoms that may find it difficult to activate the device. Failed activation occurs in 4% of patients, and is weakly associated with age and uncertainty with technology [3]. The recent iteration of the device has automatic detection features that may allow detection of otherwise uncaptured events that are asymptomatic or associated with failed activation, further enhancing the diagnostic utility of the device.

Syncope resolves during long term monitoring in almost one third of patients despite frequent episodes prior to implantation of the loop recorder. This suggests that in these individuals the cause of syncope is self-limited, or reflects a transient physiologic abnormality. All reports using the ILR have suggested a low incidence of life-threatening arrhythmia or significant morbidity with a prolonged monitoring strategy. This verifies the generally good prognosis of recurrent unexplained syncope in the absence of severe left ven-

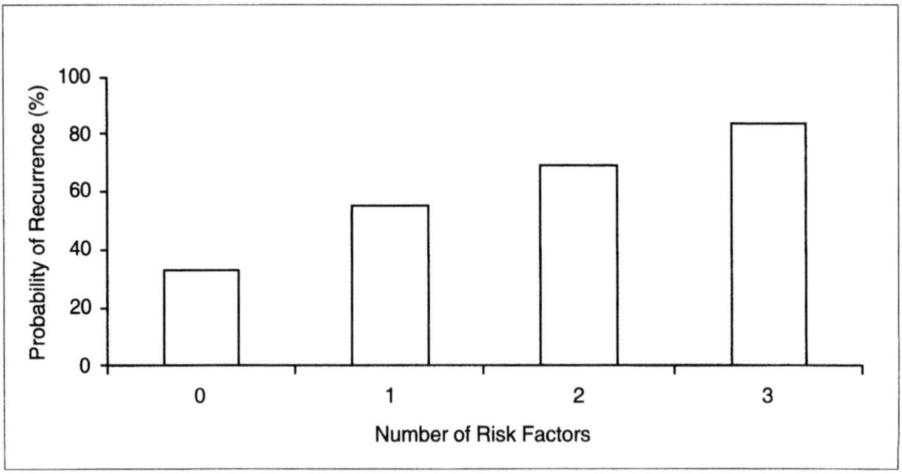

Fig. 2. Probability of recurrent symptoms during prolonged monitoring based on a simple risk factor score. Risk factors included age less than 65 years, absence of structural heart disease and more than 3 lifetime syncopal episodes. The likelihood of syncope during the ILR implant was 33% with no risk factors, 55% with one, 69% with two, and 84% with three

tricular dysfunction or when EP testing is negative, and the safety of a monitoring strategy. This finding was particularly striking in the negative electrophysiologic testing arm of the International Study on Syncope of Uncertain Etiology (ISSUE) study [20] (see below).

Recent Trials

The utility of prolonged monitoring in other populations has been shown in several recent studies using the ILR. In a study of atypical epilepsy, Zaidi et al studied 74 patients with ongoing seizures, despite anticonvulsant therapy, or unexplained recurrent seizures [21, 22]. They performed cardiac assessment including tilt testing and carotid sinus massage in all patients, and implantation of the ILR in 10 patients. Tilt testing was positive in 27% of patients, and carotid sinus massage was positive in 10%. Two of the 10 patients that subsequently underwent ILR monitoring demonstrated marked bradycardia preceding seizure activity; one due to heart block and the second due to sinus pauses. This study suggested that seizures that are atypical in presentation or response to therapy may have a cardiovascular cause in as many as 42% of patients, and that long term cardiac monitoring plays a role in select patients with atypical seizures.

In three recent studies from the ISSUE investigators, ILRs were implanted in 3 different groups of syncope patients to assess the spontaneous rhythm during spontaneous syncope after conventional testing [20, 23, 24]. The first study performed tilt tests in 111 patients with unexplained syncope suspected to be vasovagal, and implanted loop recorders after the tilt test regardless of result. Syncope recurred in 34% of patients in both the tilt positive and tilt negative group, with marked bradycardia or asystole the most common recorded arrhythmia during follow-up (46% and 62% respectively). The heart rate response during tilt testing did not predict spontaneous heart rate during episodes, with a much higher incidence of asystole noted than expected based on tilt response where a marked cardioinhibitory response is was uncommon. This study suggests that tilt testing is poorly predictive of rhythm findings during spontaneous syncope, and that bradycardia is more common in this population than previously recognized.

The second part of the ISSUE study performed long term monitoring in 52 patients with syncope and bundle branch block with negative electrophysiologic testing [24]. Syncope recurred in 22 of the 52 patients with conduction system disease. Long term monitoring demonstrated marked bradycardia mainly attributed to complete AV block in 17 patients, while it excluded AV block in 2. Three patients did not properly activate the device after symptoms. This study confirmed the previous view that negative electrophysiologic testing does not exclude intermittent complete AV block, and that prolonged monitoring or consideration of permanent pacing is reasonable in this population.

The third part of the ISSUE study examined the spontaneous rhythm in 35 patients with syncope and overt heart disease that had negative electrophysiologic testing [20]. The underlying heart disease was predominantly ischemic heart disease or hypertrophic cardiomyopathy with moderate left ventricular dysfunction. Although previous studies have suggested that patients with negative electrophysiologic testing have a better prognosis, there remains concern regarding the risk of ventricular tachycardia in this group. Importantly, only 2 of the 35 patients had severe left ventricular dysfunction (ejection fraction < 30%) that would have made them candidates for primary prevention of sudden death in keeping with the MADIT 2 Trial [25]. Symptoms recurred in 19 of the 35 patients (54%), with bradycardia in 4, supraventricular tachyarrhythmias in 5 and ventricular tachycardia in only 1 patient. There were no sudden deaths during 16±11 months of follow-up. This supports a monitoring strategy in patients with left ventricular dysfunction related to ischemic heart disease when EP testing is negative.

Finally, a single center prospective randomized trial compared early use of the ILR for prolonged monitoring to conventional testing in patients undergoing a cardiac workup for unexplained syncope [16]. Sixty patients (age 66±14 years, 33 male) with unexplained syncope were randomized to "conventional" testing with an external loop recorder, tilt and electrophysiologic testing or immediate prolonged monitoring with an implantable loop recorder with one year of monitoring. Patients were excluded if they had a left ventricular ejection fraction less than 35%. Patients were offered crossover to the alternate strategy if they remained undiagnosed after their assigned strategy. A diagnosis was obtained in 14 of 27 patients randomized to prolonged monitoring, compared to 6 of 30 undergoing conventional testing (52% vs. 20%, $p=0.012$). Crossover was associated with a diagnosis in 1 of 6 patients undergoing conventional testing, compared to 8 of 13 patients who completed monitoring (17% vs. 62%, $p=0.069$). Overall, prolonged monitoring was more likely to result in a diagnosis than conventional testing (55% vs. 19%, $p=0.0014$). Bradycardia was detected in 14 patients undergoing monitoring, compared to 3 patients with conventional testing (40% vs. 8%, $p=0.005$). These data illustrate the limitations of conventional diagnostic techniques for detection of arrhythmia, particularly bradycardia. Although there is clear selection bias in enrollment of patients referred to an electrophysiologist for workup, this study suggests that conventional testing has modest utility in patients with preserved left ventricular function.

When to Choose Prolonged Monitoring

The literature clearly supports the use of the implantable loop recorder in patients with recurrent unexplained syncope that have failed a non-invasive workup and continue to have syncope. This represents a select group that has been referred for further testing, where ongoing symptoms are likely and a symptom rhythm correlation is a feasible goal. Widespread early use of the ILR is likely to reduce the diagnostic yield as the prevalence of arrhythmias falls, supported by data from the RAST trial [14-16]. The optimal patient for prolonged monitoring has frequent recurrent symptoms suspicious for arrhythmia. After clinical assessment including determination of left ventricular function, a decision must be made if the clinical presentation is potentially life threatening. Primary and secondary prevention trials using implantable defibrillators support this practice. All reports using the ILR have suggested a low incidence of life-threatening arrhythmia or significant morbidity with a prolonged monitoring strategy. Conversely, there may be a low risk population where an ILR is not warranted. This would include patients without heart disease and a relatively low burden of syncope, in whom testing has a low yield and the diagnosis is almost certainly benign [15]. Cost considerations need to be accounted for in the decision to implant a monitor. The cost of the ILR is close to that of a basic single chamber pacemaker. Cost modeling and recent cost analysis suggests that the device is cost effective after non-invasive testing has been performed when a diagnosis is strongly sought after, comparing favorably to a conventional workup [5, 12].

Conclusions

Loop recorders have significantly improved our ability to the objective of obtaining rhythm symptom correlation physiologic data during spontaneous symptoms in patients with unexplained syncope. The implantable loop recorder is a especially useful tool for investigating patients with recurrent unexplained syncope when non-invasive tests are negative. The clinician should consider early use of the ILR when an arrhythmia is suspected, focusing on patients with a heavy syncope burden that are likely to experience recurrence.

Acknowledgements. Supported by Grant NA3397 from the Heart and Stroke Foundation of Ontario. Dr. Krahn is a Research Scholar of the Heart and Stroke Foundation of Canada.

References

1. Sra JS, Anderson AJ, Sheikh SH et al (1991) Unexplained syncope evaluated by electrophysiologic studies and head-up tilt testing. Ann Intern Med 114:1013-1019
2. Morady F, Shen E, Schwartz A et al (1983) Long-term follow-up of patients with recurrent unexplained syncope evaluated by electrophysiologic testing. J Am Coll Cardiol 2:1053-1059
3. Krahn AD, Klein GJ, Fitzpatrick A et al (2002) Predicting the outcome of patients with unexplained syncope undergoing prolonged monitoring. Pacing Clin Electrophysiol 25:37-41
4. Krahn AD, Klein GJ, Norris C, Yee R (1995) The etiology of syncope in patients with negative tilt table and electrophysiological testing. Circulation 92:1819-1824
5. Krahn AD, Klein GJ, Yee R, Manda V (1999) The high cost of syncope: cost implications of a new insertable loop recorder in the investigation of recurrent syncope. Am Heart J 137:870-877

6. Krahn AD, Klein GJ, Yee R, Norris C (1998) Final results from a pilot study with an implantable loop recorder to determine the etiology of syncope in patients with negative noninvasive and invasive testing. Am J Cardiol 82:117-119
7. Krahn AD, Klein GJ, Yee R (1999) Use of an extended monitoring strategy in patients with problematic syncope. Reveal Investigators. Circulation 99:406-410
8. Waktare JE, Malik M (1997) Holter, loop recorder, and event counter capabilities of implanted devices. Pacing Clin Electrophysiol 20:2658-2669
9. Nierop PR, van Mechelen R, van Elsacker A et al (2000) Heart rhythm during syncope and presyncope: results of implantable loop recorders. Pacing Clin Electrophysiol 23:1532-1538
10. Calkins H, Byrne M, el-Atassi R et al (1993) The economic burden of unrecognized vasodepressor syncope. Am J Med 95:473-479
11. Nyman JA, Krahn AD, Bland PC et al (1999) The costs of recurrent syncope of unknown origin in elderly patients. Pacing Clin Electrophysiol 22:1386-1394
12. Simpson CS, Krahn AD, Klein GJ et al (1999) A cost effective approach to the investigation of syncope: relative merit of different diagnostic strategies. Can J Cardiol 15:579-584
13. Krahn AD, Klein GJ, Yee R, Norris C (1997) Maturation of the sensed electrogram amplitude over time in a new subcutaneous implantable loop recorder. Pacing Clin Electrophysiol 20:1686-1690
14. Garcia-Civera R, Ruiz-Granell R, Morell-Cabedo S et al (2003) Selective use of diagnostic tests inpatients with syncope of unknown cause. J Am Coll Cardiol 41:787-790
15. Benditt DG, Brignole M (2003) Syncope: is a diagnosis a diagnosis? J Am Coll Cardiol 41:791-794
16. Krahn AD, Klein GJ, Yee R, Skanes AC (2001) Randomized Assessment of Syncope Trial : Conventional Diagnostic Testing Versus a Prolonged Monitoring Strategy. Circulation 104:46-51
17. Kenny RA, Krahn AD (1999) Implantable loop recorder: evaluation of unexplained syncope. Heart 81:431-433
18. Alboni P, Brignole M, Menozzi C et al (2001) Diagnostic value of history in patients with syncope with or without heart disease. J Am Coll Cardiol 37:1921-1928
19. Assar MD, Krahn AD, Kelein GJ et al (2002) Risk and timing of recurrent syncope in patients undergoing prolonged monitoring with an implantable loop recorder: Who really uses it and when? Circulation 106:436
20. Menozzi C, Brignole M, Garcia-Civera R et al (2002) Mechanism of syncope in patients with heart disease and negative electrophysiologic test. Circulation 105:2741-2745
21. Zaidi A, Clough P, Cooper P (2000) Misdiagnosis of epilepsy: many seizure-like attacks have a cardiovascular cause. J Am Coll Cardiol 36:181-184
22. Zaidi A, Clough P, Mawer G, Fitzpatrick A (1999) Accurate diagnosis of convulsive syncope: role of an implantable subcutaneous ECG monitor. Seizure 8:184-186
23. Moya A, Brignole M, Menozzi C et al (2001) Mechanism of Syncope in Patients With Isolated Syncope and in Patients With Tilt-Positive Syncope. Circulation 104:1261-1267
24. Brignole M, Menozzi C, Moya A et al (2001) Mechanism of Syncope in Patients With Bundle Branch Block and Negative Electrophysiological Test. Circulation 104:2045-2050
25. Moss AJ, Zareba W, Hall WJ et al (2002) Prophylactic implantation of a defibrillator in patients with myocardial infarction and reduced ejection fraction. N Engl J Med 346:877-883

Patients with Structural Heart Disease, Syncope of Unknown Origin and Suspected Ventricular Tachycardia: ICD Implantation or "Wait and See" Strategy?

C. Menozzi[1], N. Bottoni[1], M. Brignole[2]

Introduction

From a practical point of view it is useful to consider two different major determinants of outcome, namely the inducibility or not of ventricular tachyarrhythmias by means of premature ventricular stimulation and the presence or absence of a markedly depressed cardiac function. These two situations are variously combined.

Diagnostic Yield of Electrophysiological Study

Ventricular tachycardia may present in the form of syncope with or without palpitations or other accompanying symptoms. The major concerns about programmed electrical stimulation as part of an electrophysiological study for inducing clinically significant ventricular arrhythmia are its varying sensitivity (and specificity) in different clinical settings [1] and the lack of a standard protocol [2].

Inducibility

Generally speaking, programmed electrical stimulation is thought to be a sensitive tool in patients with chronic ischaemic heart disease (previous myocardial infarction) who are also susceptible to spontaneous monomorphic ventricular tachycardia. Conversely, the induction of a monomorphic ventricular tachycardia is thought to be a specific event that should guide therapy. For example, in the ESVEM trial [3], syncope associated with induced ventricular

[1]Department of Interventional Cardiology, Ospedale S. Maria Nuova, 4210 Reggio Emilia;
[2]Department of Cardiology and Arrhythmologic Centre, Ospedali Riuniti, Lavagna, Italy

tachyarrhythmias on electrophysiological testing indicated a high risk of death, similar to that of patients with documented spontaneous ventricular tachyarrhythmias. The specificity of induction of ventricular tachycardia has been questioned in patients with syncope and bifascicular block [4]. On the other hand, polymorphic ventricular tachycardia and ventricular fibrillation have previously been considered nonspecific findings, a concept that probably needs modification depending on the clinical setting. An example is seen in patients with Brugada syndrome, in whom the induction of polymorphic ventricular arrhythmias seems to be the most consistent finding [5, 6]. Another patient category, in which programmed electrical stimulation with induction of ventricular fibrillation is of unknown value, is made up of survivors of cardiac arrest with significant coronary artery disease who are undergoing coronary by-pass surgery [7, 8].

Noninducibility

The predictive value of noninducibility depends on the aetiology of the underlying heart disease, e.g., whether it is ischaemic or nonischaemic.

Link et al. [9] evaluated long-term follow-up in 68 consecutive patients with syncope who presented with coronary artery disease and had a negative invasive electrophysiological evaluation. After a mean follow-up of 30±18 months, there had been 2 sudden deaths, 1 episode of ventricular fibrillation and 1 of ventricular tachycardia in patients treated with an implantable cardioverter-defibrillator. All 4 arrhythmias occurred in patients with left-ventricular fractions of 25% or lower. Seventeen patients had recurrent presyncope or syncope. The authors conclude that in patients with coronary artery disease and syncope, noninducibility on electrophysiological study predicts a lower risk of sudden death and ventricular arrhythmias.

Conversely, programmed ventricular stimulation has a low predictive value in patients with nonischaemic dilated cardiomyopathy [10], and one study [11] on patients with unexplained syncope treated with implantable cardioverter-defibrillators (ICDs) showed a high incidence of tachyarrhythmic episodes during the follow-up despite an initially negative electrophysiological study. Brilakis [12], in a selected group of 17 patients out of a total of 54 affected by idiopathic dilated cardiomyopathy who received an ICD, observed an incidence of appropriate shocks at 1 year of 47% and 40% respectively, in patients with inducible and with noninducible sustained monomorphic ventricular tachycardia. In conclusion, programmed ventricular stimulation was not useful in risk stratification of patients with idiopathic dilated cardiomyopathy and syncope.

One study [13] evaluated the predictive value of a negative electrophysiological study in 35 patients with overt heart disease at risk of ventricular arrhythmias. These patients had previous myocardial infarction or cardiomyopathy with moderately low values for ejection fraction (mean 47±17) or nonsustained ventricular tachycardia, and underwent implantation of a loop recorder (ILR). During the follow-up, syncopal recurrences were never due to tachyarrhythmias, which were documented in only 1 patient and caused presyncope. Interestingly, the induction of polymorphic ventricular tachycardia or fibrillation during an electrophysiological study (which was regarded as a negative result) was of no value for predicting syncopal events or, in particular, ventricular tachyarrhythmias. Thus, in the absence of a severe pump dysfunction, negativity of the electrophysiological study predicts a low risk of ventricular tachyarrhythmias.

Cardiac Function

Markedly Depressed Cardiac Function

The advent of ICDs with improved documentation of arrhythmic events offers a safe and sensitive tool for follow-up in different high-risk populations. Seven studies [11, 14–19] have evaluated the utility of ICDs in highly selected patients with syncope. Link et al. [14] reported on 50 patients who had an appropriate device discharge rate of 22% after 1 year and 50% at 3 years of follow-up due to ventricular tachycardia/fibrillation. Among the 33 patients in the study conducted by Militianu et al. [15], an appropriate discharge of the device occurred in 36% over a period of 17 months. In these two studies the populations were comparable, including patients with ischaemic and with non-ischaemic cardiomyopathy, and the induction of ventricular fibrillation was also considered a positive result. Three studies concerned patients affected by coronary artery disease [16–18]. In the study by Mittal et al. [16], in which 67 consecutive patients with coronary artery disease, mostly with a prior myocardial infarction and a depressed ejection fraction (mean 37±13%), were evaluated, sustained monomorphic ventricular tachycardia was inducible in 43% of cases. During a follow-up of more than 1 year, 41% of inducible patients received an appropriate device discharge, and only 1 had a syncope relapse, which was not related to the ventricular arrhythmia. However, the total mortality was significantly higher in patients with inducible tachycardia than in those with non-inducible tachycardia, the actuarial 2-year survival rates being 84% and 45%, respectively. Andrews et al. [17] performed a retrospective case-control study in which 22 patients with unexplained syncope and inducible ventricular tachycardia were compared with a matched group of 32 patients with documented syncopal ventricular tachycardia. Almost all the patients had coronary artery disease with severe systolic dysfunction (mean ejection fraction 30%). After 1 year, a similar incidence of ICD discharges occurred in each of the two groups (57% vs 50%), suggesting that electrophysiological testing can identify patients with severe coronary artery disease at risk of life-threatening arrhythmias. In 178 patients with unexplained syncope, most of whom had inducible ventricular tachycardia/fibrillation and coronary artery disease and who were treated with ICDs, Pires et al. [18] observed a high recurrence of ventricular tachyarrhythmias (55% at 2 years) and a close correlation (85%) between recurrent syncope and ventricular arrhythmia and low mortality, which was comparable to the results in similar patients with documented sustained ventricular tachycardia/fibrillation. Two studies concerned patients affected by nonischaemic dilated cardiopathy [11, 19]. Knight et al. [11] performed a similar small retrospective case-control study in patients with nonischaemic dilated cardiopathy with severe systolic dysfunction (mean ejection fraction of 26%). Fourteen consecutive patients with unexplained syncope and a negative electrophysiological study were compared with a matched group of 19 patients with a documented cardiac arrest caused by ventricular tachyarrhythmia. After 2 years, approximately the same incidence of ICD discharges was observed in the two groups (50% vs 42%) and the relapses of syncope or presyncope were due primarily to ventricular fibrillation. The patients with more severe cardiomyopathy (ejection fraction of 20%) were more likely to receive an appropriate shock. Thus, in patients with very severe nonischaemic cardiomyopathy, risk stratification on a clinical basis seems superior to that based on the results of an electrophysiological study. Improved survival with ICD in respect of conventional therapy was observed in the study of Fonarow [19] in patients with nonischaemic advanced heart failure referred for heart transplantation (mean ejection fraction of 21%). Actuarial survival at 2 years was 85% in the 25 patients managed with an ICD and 67% in the 122 patients managed without. No patient with an ICD succumbed to sudden death, and an appropriate shock discharge occurred in 40% of these.

Finally, in a selected population of patients with advanced heart failure and a mean ejection fraction of 20%, the patients with syncope had a higher risk of sudden death (45% at 1 year) than those without (12% at 1 year); admittedly, the risk of sudden death was similar whether patients had supposed cardiac syncope or syncope from other causes [10].

Mildly Depressed Cardiac Function

When cardiac investigations are unable to support the initial suspect of cardiac syncope, the outcome seems to be favourable even if the diagnosis of the cause of syncope remains unexplained [9, 20–22].

In 68 patients with less severe coronary artery disease with a mean ejection fraction of 42±16, Link et al. [9] observed a low recurrence rate of syncope and all four episodes of arrhythmias or death occurred in patients with ejection fraction <25%.

In the aforementioned study conducted by Menozzi et al. [13] in patients with mildly depressed cardiac function and considered at risk of ventricular arrhythmias, the loop recorder showed that the syncopal recurrences during follow-up were never due to tachyarrhythmias, which were documented in only 1 patient and caused pre-syncope. Another study in which the ILR was used [23] included patients with structural heart disease as long as the ejection fraction was over 35%, and its results were not dissimilar.

Conclusions

Even in patients with overt heart disease, syncope is not necessarily an ominous finding and the outcome depends largely on the clinical features of the patients. It seems that only the inducibility of sustained ventricular tachycardia or a very depressed systolic function can predict a syncope attributable to ventricular arrhythmia and, conversely, their absence may predict a more favourable outcome. Table 1 shows the current recommendations embodied in the European Society of Cardiology Guidelines on Syncope, which reflect the above concepts [24]. Several data from the literature confirm that patients who

Table 1. Situations in which ICD therapy is likely to be useful (according to European Society of Cardiology Guidelines on Syncope [24])

Documented	Undocumented
Syncopal ventricular tachycardia or fibrillation without correctable causes (e.g., drug-induced) (class I, level A)	Syncope likely to be due to ventricular tachycardia or fibrillation
	Previous myocardial infarction and inducible sustained monomorphic ventricular tachycardia with severe haemodynamic compromise, in the absence of another competing diagnosis as a cause of syncope (class I, level B)
	Unexplained syncope in patients with depressed left ventricular systolic function in the absence of another competing diagnosis as a cause of syncope (class II, level B)
	Established long QT syndrome, Brugada syndrome, arrhythmogenic right-ventricular dysplasia, or hypertrophic obstructive cardiomyopathy, with a family history of sudden death, in the absence of another competing diagnosis for the cause of syncope (class II)
	Brugada syndrome or arrhythmogenic right ventricular dysplasia and inducible ventricular tachyarrhythmias with severe haemodynamic compromise in the absence of another competing diagnosis for the cause of syncope (class II)

undergo implantation of an automatic defibrillator according to these rules have a high incidence of spontaneous ventricular arrhythmias requiring device therapy and suppression of syncopal recurrences. In the other cases, which means the vast majority of patients with unexplained syncope and structural heart disease, a "wait-and-see" strategy seems advisable. In this context, implantation of a loop recorder is promising, providing guidance on a possible future therapy; this strategy of delayed therapy appears sufficiently safe and to involve a low risk [13].

References

1. Bigger JT Jr, Reiffel JA, Livelli FD, Wang PJ (1986) Sensitivity, specificity, and reproducibility of programmed ventricular stimulation. Circulation 73 [Suppl II]:73–78
2. Wellens HJJ, Brugada P, Stevenson WG (1986) Programmed electrical stimulation of the heart in patients with life-threatening ventricular arrhythmias: what is the significance of induced arrhythmias and what is the correct stimulation protocol? Circulation 72:1–7
3. Olshansky B, Hahn EA, Hartz VL, Prater SP, Mason JW (1999) Clinical significance of syncope in the electrophysiologic study versus electrocardiographic monitoring (ESVEM) trial. Am Heart J 137:878–886
4. Englund A, Bergfeldt L, Rehnqvist N, Åström H, Rosenqvist M (1995) Diagnostic value of programmed ventricular stimulation in patients with bifascicular block: a prospective study of patients with and without syncope. J Am Coll Cardiol 26:1508–1515
5. Alings M, Wilde A (1999) "Brugada" syndrome. Clinical data and suggested pathophysiological mechanism. Circulation 99:666–673
6. Brugada J, Brugada P, Brugada R (1999) The syndrome of right bundle branch block ST segment elevation in V1 to V3 and sudden death—the Brugada syndrome. Europace 1:156–166
7. Kelly P, Ruskin JN, Vlahakes GJ, Buckley MJ Jr, Freeman CS, Garan H (1990) Surgical coronary revascularization in survivors of prehospital cardiac arrest: its effect on inducible ventricular arrhythmias and long-term survival. J Am Coll Cardiol 15:267–273
8. Bergfeldt L (1999) CABG and ICD for all patients with hemodynamically significant ventricular arrhythmia and significant coronary artery disease? Do we know enough to decide—or to design a randomized trial? Pacing Clin Electrophysiol 22:1129–1131
9. Link M, Kim KM, Homoud M et al (1999) Long-term outcome of patients with syncope associated with coronary artery disease and nondiagnostic electrophysiologic evaluation. Am J Cardiol 83:1334–1337
10. Middlekauff H, Stevenson W, Stevenson L, Saxon L (1993) Syncope in advanced heart failure: high risk of sudden death regardless of origin of syncope. J Am Coll Cardiol 21:110–116
11. Knight B, Goyal R, Pelosi F et al (1999) Outcome of patients with nonischemic dilated cardiomyopathy and unexplained syncope treated with an implantable defibrillator. J Am Coll Cardiol 33:1964–1970
12. Brilakis E, Shen W, Hammill S et al (2001) Role of programmed ventricular stimulation and implantable cardioverter defibrillators in patients with idiopathic dilated cardiomyopathy and syncope. Pacing Clin Electrophysiol 24:1623–1630

13. Menozzi C, Brignole M, Garcia-Civera R et al (2002) Mechanism of syncope in patients with heart disease and negative electrophysiologic test. Circulation 105:2741–2745
14. Link MS, Costeas XF, Griffith JL et al (1997) High incidence of appropriate implantable cardioverter–defibrillator therapy in patients with syncope of unknown etiology and inducible ventricular tachycardia. J Am Coll Cardiol 29:370–375
15. Militianu A, Salacata A, Seibert K et al (1997) Implantable cardioverter defibrillator utilization among device recipients presenting exclusively with syncope or near-syncope. J Cardiovasc Electrophysiol 8:1087–1097
16. Mittal S, Iwai S, Stein K, Markowitz S, Slotwiner D, Lerman B (1999) Long-term outcome of patients with unexplained syncope treated with an electrophysiologic-guided approach in the implantable cardioverter-defibrillator era. J Am Coll Cardiol 34:1082–1089
17. Andrews N, Fogel R, Pelargonio G, Evans J, Prystowsky E (1999) Implantable defibrillator event rates in patients with unexplained syncope and inducible sustained ventricular tachyarrhythmias. J Am Coll Cardiol 34:2023–2030
18. Pires L, May L, Ravi S, Parry T, Lal V, Nino C (2000) Comparison of event rates and survival in patients with unexplained syncope without documented ventricular tachyarrhythmias versus patients with documented sustained ventricular tachyarrhythmias both treated with implantable cardioverter-defibrillator. Am J Cardiol 85:725–728
19. Fonarow G, Feliciano Z, Boyle N et al (2000) Improved survival in patients with nonischemic advanced heart failure and syncope treated with an implantable cardioverter-defibrillator. Am J Cardiol 85:981–985
20. Doherty J, Pembrook-Rogers D, Grogan W et al (1985) Electrophysiologic evaluation and follow-up characteristics of patients with recurrent unexplained syncope and presyncope. Am J Cardiol 55:703–708
21. Proclemer A, Gianfagna P, Fontanelli P et al (1987) Value of electrophysiologic testing in long term follow-up of patients with syncope of unknown cause. G Ital Cardiol 17:402–407
22. Kushner J, Hou W, Kadish A et al (2001) Natural history of patients with unexplained syncope and a nondiagnostic electrophysiologic study. J Am Coll Cardiol 14:391–396
23. Krahn A, Klein G, Yee R et al (2001) Randomized assessment of syncope trial. Conventional diagnostic testing versus a prolonged monitoring strategy. Circulation 104:46–51
24. Brignole M, Alboni P, Benditt D et al, for the Task Force on Syncope of the European Society of Cardiology (2001) Guidelines on management (diagnosis and treatment) of syncope. Eur Heart J 22:1256–1306

Vasovagal Syncope, Orthostatic Hypotension and Postural Orthostatic Tachycardia Syndrome: Is There a Connection?

A. Gonzalez-Hermosillo, M.F. Marquez, A. Kostine, K. Jauregui-Renaud, M. Cardenas

Introduction

Orthostatic intolerance is the development of symptoms during standing, which are relieved when the subject adopts a recumbent posture. Approximately 500,000 Americans are affected by this syndrome. Patients with orthostatic intolerance often complain of exercise intolerance, lightheadedness, dizziness, palpitations, disabling fatigue, blurred vision, headache, anxiety, depression, cold sweating, nausea, chest discomfort, and dyspnea. Sometimes these symptoms are prodromal for an impending syncopal event. Often, however, loss of consciousness occurs without warning. Presyncope or syncope is merely an extreme expression of this spectrum of symptoms.

Syncope (derived from the Greek words, 'syn' meaning "with" and the verb koptein meaning "to cut," or more appropriately in this case "to interrupt") is a symptom defined as a sudden temporary loss of consciousness and postural tone caused by cerebral hypoperfusion, with spontaneous recovery.

Over the last decade tilt-table testing has become widely accepted as a useful tool for diagnosing this disorder, while at the same time providing a controlled environment for observations and measurements. During the explosion of research that followed the introduction of the tilt table, it was noted that these episodic disturbances in autonomic nervous system tone could result in varying degrees of systemic hypotension. While these falls in pressure might not be sufficient to produce loss of consciousness, they could cause cerebral hypoperfusion sufficiently pronounced to be symptomatic.

Syncope is an important, common, medical problem elicited by conditions ranging from benign and self-limiting causes to chronic, recurrent, and potentially fatal causes. Neurally mediated syncope is the most common type of syncope. It has been estimated that up to 35% of syncopal events are vasovagal in nature.

Department of Cardiac Electrophysiology, Instituto Nacional de Cardiologia "Ignacio Chavez", Mexico City, Mexico

The clinical spectrum of dysfunction in orthostatic cardiovascular homeostasis includes conditions that are usually benign, such as a vasovagal syncope, postural tachycardia syndrome, dysautonomia, chronic fatigue syndrome, fibromyalgia, and severe forms of primary chronic autonomic failure with multisystemic involvement and severe orthostatic hypotension, such as pure autonomic failure and multiple system atrophy [1]. There is significant overlap in the symptoms, provoking speculation about a possible common autonomic substrate linking these disorders.

This paper is a review of the existing concepts concerning this disorder. Special emphasis is given to the relationship between vasovagal syncope (VVS) and postural orthostatic tachycardia syndrome (POTS), representing acute and chronic orthostatic intolerance, respectively.

Vasovagal Syncope

Vasovagal syncope occurs most frequently in young people and is characterized by premonitory signs and symptoms (lightheadedness, weakness, yawning, pallor, palpitations, headache, diaphoresis, visual blurring, impaired hearing, hyperventilation, and nausea). If the patient sits or lies down promptly syncope may be aborted. Observers who witness a syncopal episode will often report that the patient appeared pale or ashen in color, with cold skin and profuse sweating, dilated pupils, and occasionally urinary or fecal incontinence. Sometimes convulsions occur, indicating that the cerebral anoxic threshold has been reached. Although patients are not usually confused, during the postsyncopal period they may complain of nervousness, headache, fatigue, coldness, or dizziness. Some patients (particularly older ones) will give no history of any prodrome, and the episodes are then very abrupt and may lead to severe injury through the trauma associated with falling. Often, even frequent episodes that begin in adolescence will spontaneously abate by the time the patient reaches his or her mid-twenties. VVS can be precipitated by the sight of blood, loss of blood, sudden stressful or painful experiences, surgical manipulation, or trauma. What seems to distinguish this disorder from POTS is that between episodes these patients are quite normal and report few symptoms. There are others in whom the vagally mediated fall in blood pressure and heart rate will be sufficient to produce symptoms of cerebral hypoperfusion but will not lead to full loss of consciousness. The individuals will often present with complaints of mild orthostatic intolerance. The vasovagal response observed during tilt-table testing is characterized by an abrupt fall in systemic pressure, usually followed by a fall in heart rate.

The response of the cerebrovasculature to VVS has been investigated using transcranial Doppler (TCD) sonography of the middle cerebral artery. A number of studies have demonstrated that during tilt-induced VVS, cerebral arteriolar constriction and reduced cerebral blood flow velocity both occur before any cardiovascular changes and at the onset of hypotension and bradycardia

[2]. Recently, several investigators have reported cases of tilt-induced syncope resulting directly from cerebral vasoconstriction in the absence of systemic hypotension. This pattern is called "cerebral syncope" [3]. In patients with VVS, the detection of cerebral vasoconstriction by TDC before syncope allows the interruption of the test to avoid the risk of asystole [1]. There is little doubt that cerebral autoregulation fails to preserve cerebral blood flow during presyncope [4], but the conclusion that this is due to cerebral vasoconstriction, paradoxical or not, is controversial and does not reflect the complexity of events that take place before VVS. In our laboratory, we have confirmed that diastolic cerebral blood flow velocity is selectively decreased before the time of presyncope during head-up tilt in patients with VVS, in the absence of hypotension or bradycardia and without any significant change of the systolic cerebral blood flow velocity. In our practice, we stop the test at the onset of presyncope and return the patient to the supine position for ethical reasons. Therefore, we agree with Sung et al. [5] that in some patients abnormal baroreceptor responses triggered during orthostatic stress might result in a derangement of cerebral blood flow autoregulation, which might have an important role in the pathophysiology of VVS. The cerebral circulation is autoregulated in a complex way. It is possible that hyperventilation might lower the arterial carbon dioxide level and cause cerebral arteriolar constriction and syncope. It is also possible that hypocapnia contributes to the impairment of cerebral autoregulation during presyncope not through simple cerebral vasoconstriction, but by elevating cerebrovascular critical closing pressure and selectively impairing diastolic cerebral blood flow, thereby counteracting the effects of active cerebral vasodilatation [6].

A person's performance of vital and complex cerebral functions depends on an adequate cerebrovascular perfusion pressure, which under normal conditions is preserved by cardiovascular reflexes such as the baroreceptor reflex. Orthostatic stress, physical exercise, and other stimuli, such as emotion, pain and reflex mechanisms (micturition, defecation, deglutition, etc.) are among many activities that challenge cerebral perfusion and require the involvement of neurocardiogenic reflexes. After standing, between 500 and 800 mL of blood is trapped in the distensible veins below the level of the heart, plasma moves to the interstitial fluid, and venous return, cardiac output, and blood pressure decrease. These changes are detected by baroreceptors located in the arterial and cardiopulmonary regions. Information from the baroreceptors is then relayed to the central nervous system, where neuronal cell groups regulate reflex cardiovascular activity through changes in sympathetic and parasympathetic outflow. These changes are directed at restoring blood pressure and preserving cerebral perfusion during the challenge. The pathophysiology of neurally mediated syncope is still incompletely understood today. Our current knowledge is summarized below.

The precipitating events of syncope trigger a complex hemodynamic response. Several theories have been proposed to explain these hemodynamic events. The ventricular theory suggests that when baroreceptors detect a fall in blood pressure initiated by excessive venous pooling associated with upright posture or when a "hypersensitive" autonomic system over-responds to various stimuli, a reflex increase in the efferent sympathetic traffic with positive chronotropic and inotropic effects causes activation of mechanoreceptors that would normally fire only during stretch. This sudden surge in neural traffic to the brain stem mimics the condition seen in hypertension, thus provoking an apparently "paradoxical" sympathetic withdrawal with resultant parasympathetic predominance (Bezold–Jarish reflex), resulting in hypotension and bradycardia just before the syncope [1, 7]. VVS in humans, however, is probably triggered by mechanisms beyond those described by the Bezold–Jarish reflex. In animal models and in heart transplant patients, neurally mediated hypotension and bradycardia have been observed despite cardiac denervation [8]. Although it has been proposed that receptors in other cardiovascular regions may be excited by hypovolemia and trigger VVS, no experimental confirmation is available.

Another important premise of the ventricular theory is the presence of increased sympathetic tone. This idea is not supported by studies in VVS, which have shown that muscle sympathetic nerve activity (MSNA) does not increase before syncope. Mosqueda-Garcia et al. [9], found an attenuated sympathetic response to orthostatic stress characterized by a significantly blunted increase in MSNA, followed by a progressive decrease and total disappearance before syncope. It can be argued that recordings of MSNA may not reflect the noradrenergic changes evoked in other relevant regions (e.g., heart). During tilt, VVS patients exhibit variable responses in cardiac sympathetic function.

Recently, studies of heart rate variability (HRV) have provided noninvasive techniques with which sympathetic and parasympathetic activity can be assessed [10]. While some investigators have found that cardiac sympathetic tone increases before syncope [11, 12], others have found the opposite [13], or even evidence for both increase and decrease [14], depending on the individual subject. Two different patterns may be recognized in the cardiac autonomic changes preceding an occasional vasovagal event. The first pattern is characterized by a progressive increase in cardiac sympathetic modulation that leads to the sudden onset of bradycardia. The second pattern displays a gradual inhibition of sympathetic and a concomitant enhancement of vagal modulation of the heart period [8]. Currently, it is not clear whether differences in methodology, the selection of patients, or both, account for these discrepancies.

Attempts to evaluate sympathetic function with plasma norepinephrine in patients with VVS have also produced contradictory results. A blunted noradrenergic response combined with exaggerated adrenomedullary activation has been observed in VVS patients [15]. Confounding factors such as time of sampling, potential changes in norepinephrine clearance, and alterations in spillover to the general circulation are likely to account for these contradictory results.

Mosqueda-Garcia et al. [9] and Béchir et al [16] investigated baroreflex sensitivity. Subjects with recurrent VVS and positive tilt-table tests had lower cardiac baroreceptor sensitivity than controls under supine resting conditions or controls under orthostatic stress.

Postural Tachycardia Syndrome

Postural tachycardia syndrome is a disabling chronic disorder that primarily affects young women. This disorder is characterized by tachycardia and symptoms of cerebral hypoperfusion and sympathetic activation. The main complains are lightheadedness, blurred vision, palpitations, nausea, and fatigue. The symptoms become more markedly manifest with upright posture and are relieved by sitting or lying down. They are aggravated by body warming, stress, a meal, and exertion. Syncope is uncommon. Some patients have episodic symptoms at rest, usually early in the morning, and many also complain of always being cold. The heart rate alterations typically take the form of a persistent sinus tachycardia that occurs mainly while the subject is standing upright, although marked sinus arrhythmia may coexist. During head-upright tilt, these patients will display an increase in heart rate of greater than 30 bpm within the first 10 min, or achieve a maximum heart rate of 120 bpm associated with only mildly reduced blood pressure values. Pulse pressure may be excessively reduced, and with continued standing there may be acral coldness and venous prominence, resulting in blueness and even swelling of the feet. Occasionally, bradycardia and hypotension will be provoked in these patients during tilt-table testing.

Recently, a decrease in cerebral blood flow velocity with head-up tilt has also been shown in patients with POTS, suggesting that sympathetically mediated vasoconstriction in combination with increased ventilation causing hypocapnia could increase cerebrovascular resistance and explain the symptoms of cerebral hypoperfusion on standing [17, 18]. These findings may have clinical implications in patients with impaired orthostatic tolerance. Patients might benefit from interventions that modulate the ventilatory response to upright posture. We have observed that controlled breathing has a protective effect in patients with orthostatic intolerance during tilt testing [19].

In our laboratory, patients with VVS and those with POTS had different patterns in cerebral blood flow velocity during tilt testing. Patients with POTS had an earlier decrease and larger oscillations in the peak and trough systolic cerebral blood flow velocity in response to head-up tilt, despite well-sustained arterial blood pressure [20]. These observations indicate that in this group of patients regulation of cerebrovascular tone may be impaired, and this might therefore be a target for therapeutic interventions [21].

Some patients with POTS develop symptoms, despite a hypertensive response to standing, when diastolic blood pressure may increase by up to 50 mmHg [1]. Mitral valve prolapse detected by auscultation or by echocardiographic criteria is common. There is a danger of misdiagnosing the condition as inappropriate sinus tachycardia. In these cases, radiofrequency modification of the sinus node can make symptoms worse. This disorder can affect patients over a wide age distribution, ranging from children to the elderly. Some patients report the onset of symptoms after a variety of stresses, such as surgery, trauma, pregnancy, or a viral infection, but the majority state that their symptoms began in childhood and have progressively worsened over time. There is a cyclic nature of some patients' symptoms. Many women experience marked exacerbation of their complaints just prior to their menstrual periods.

While the etiology of POTS is still unclear, it is most likely that it represents a heterogeneous group of disorders with similar clinical characteristics [22]. The largest group of patients appears to have a mild form of idiopathic peripheral autonomic neuropathy ("partial dysautonomia"), in which an inability to increase peripheral vascular resistance during upright posture results in an excessive compensatory postural tachycardia [12]. Excessive venous pooling in the legs resulting in a reduction in ventricular preload has been reported, which in turn leads to baroreceptor unloading during upright posture with a resultant increase in sympathetic outflow [23]. Recent data have suggested that a reduction in circulating blood volume may have an important role in this disorder [24]. Furlan et al. [25] have combined tilt testing, MSNA, and HRV to provide moment-by-moment characterization of the hemodynamics and sympathetic traffic in patients with POTS. They found faster heart rates and increased sympathetic traffic to the blood vessels in the muscles (MSNA) during supine rest. On upright tilt the blood pressure did not change. The changes in central venous pressure with upright tilt were similar to the changes in control subjects, but the tachycardic response was exaggerated and the increase in MSNA blunted in POTS patients compared with normal subjects. The potentiated chronotropic response was accompanied by an attenuated sympathetic (presumed vasoconstrictor) response, thus ruling out hypovolemia alone as explanation. Increases in norepinephrine and the indices of sympathovagal modulation of the sinoatrial node (ratio of low-frequency to high-frequency components) were more pronounced in POTS, suggesting that any blunting of autonomic function was selective for postganglionic sympathetic efferent traffic to the lower extremities.

A second group of patients with POTS may have a component of β-receptor supersensitivity [26]. Many of these patients have high serum norepinephrine concentrations of at least 600 pg/mL on standing, and they also demonstrate exaggerated responses to adrenergic agonists. It is not clear whether this supersensitivity is primary in nature or due to a secondary denervation supersensitivity. Jacob et al. [27] reported that these patients demonstrate decreased norepinephrine clearance while standing as well as resistance to the norepinephrine-releasing effect of tyramine. In one severely affected family recent genetic studies demonstrated a mutation resulting in a deficiency of the norepinephrine transporter that otherwise clears it from the synaptic cleft [28]. Impairment of synaptic norepinephrine clearance could potentially result in a state of excessive sympathetic activation in response to physiological stimuli [12].

How do orthostatic changes in POTS compare to those seen in patients with VVS? In patients with VVS, upright tilt results in an initial increase in heart rate and a blunted increase in MSNA [15], a response similar to that seen in patients with POTS. In contrast to POTS, however, blood pressure, heart rate, and MSNA subsequently decrease dramatically in VVS [29]. POTS and VVS elicit similar symptoms, even though the blood pressure response in each of these conditions may be strikingly different. It may be that standing elicits different degrees of reflex neural inhibition in POTS and in VVS [30]. In POTS, the potentiated tachycardia acting (perhaps) via ventricular receptors may induce a partial and selective reflex inhibition of MSNA. Blood pressure is maintained by the faster heart rate. In VVS, postural change may elicit a more potent neural inhibitory reflex that results in initial inhibition and eventual disappearance of MSNA, with hypotension and bradycardia [30]. We have observed that with an increased stimulus intensity (such as is seen with isoproterenol or nitrate), POTS patients manifest hypotension and bradycardia similar to those seen in VVS.

Although no face-to-face comparative studies of the sympathovagal balance induced by orthostatic stress in patients with POTS and VVS have been published, the role of a strong vagal control in VVS might explain the differences found between the two disorders. Suzuki et al. [31], using the wavelet transformation technique to determine autonomic modulations on a per-second basis, found that vasovagal control clearly increased immediately prior to vasovagal syncope. Thus, in VVS this strong vagal modulation is able to overcome the initial sympathetic overactivity that is common to both disorders.

Orthostatic Hypotension and Dysautonomic Syncope

Orthostatic hypotension has been defined as a fall of more than 20 mmHg in systolic blood pressure within 3 min of standing. A smaller drop in blood pressure associated with symptoms may also be important. Some patients may have a slow but steady decline in blood pressure over a longer period of time (10–15 min) associated with symptoms, the so-called dysautonomic response [32]. This response is usually observed in elderly patients, although we have seen the pattern in young people [33]. In contrast to the purely vasovagal group, syncope is just one of a number of complaints and the patients rarely feel well; they often demonstrate other signs of autonomic dysfunction, such as abnormal sweating and impaired thermoregulatory control. As time goes on, some patients may develop a relatively fixed heart rate that shows little response to either postural change or exercise. In addition, some patients will develop a syndrome of supine hypertension that alternates with upright hypotension. It is important to note that any drugs the patient is taking that could produce hypotension should be identified. The physician should determine whether any medications could be contributing to the problem.

It is far beyond the scope of this chapter to review every autonomic disorder. Interested readers are referred to an excellent text on the subject [34].

Conclusions

Disturbances in autonomic tone and function can result in a wide variety of conditions that can ultimately culminate in the loss of consciousness. It is conceivable that the natural history of these disorders comprises transitions from one hemodynamic profile to another, supporting a possible common autonomic substrate. It is also possible that abnormalities within the central nervous system may play a pivotal role in the pathogenesis of orthostatic intolerance. Further, and more detailed, investigations will be necessary to expand our understanding of this heterogeneous group of disorders and to establish better diagnostic and therapeutic modalities.

References

1. Hermosillo AG (2001) Orthostatic hypotension, 2001. Cardiol Rev 9:339–347
2. Grubb BP, Gerard G, Roush K et al (1991) Cerebral vasoconstriction during head upright tilt-induced vasovagal syncope: a paradoxic and unexpected response. Circulation 84:1157–1164
3. Fredman CS, Bierman KM, Patel V et al (1995) Transcranial Doppler ultrasonography during head upright tilt-table testing. Ann Intern Med 123:848–849
4. Carey BJ, Manktelow BN, Panerai RB et al (2001) Dynamic cerebral autoregulatory responses to head-up tilt in normal subjects and patients with recurrent vasovagal syncope. Circulation 104:898–902
5. Sung RYT, Yu CW, Yam MC et al (2000) Cerebral blood flow during vasovagal syncope induced by active standing or head up tilt. Arch Dis Child 82:154–158
6. Carey BJ, Eames PJ, Panerai RB et al (2001) Carbon dioxide, critical closing pressure and cerebral hemodynamics prior to vasovagal syncope in humans. Clin Sci 101:351–358
7. Grubb BP, Kosinski D (2002) Evaluation and management of syncope. In: Ganz LI (ed) Management of cardiac arrhythmias. Humana, Totowa, NJ, pp 183–207
8. Fitzpatrick AP, Banner N, Cheng A et al (1993) Vasovagal syncope may occur alter orthotopic heart transplantation. J Am Coll Cardiol 21:1138–1141
9. Mosqueda-Garcia R, Burlan R, Tank J et al (2000) The elusive pathophysiology of neurally mediated syncope. Circulation 102:2898–2906
10. Malik M (1996) Task force of the European Society of Cardiology and the North American Society of Pacing and Electrophysiology. Heart rate variability: standards of measurement, physiological interpretation and clinical use. Eur Heart J 17:354–381
11. Lipsitz LA, Mietus J, Moody GB et al (1990) Spectral characteristics of heart rate

variability before and during postural tilt: relations to aging and risk of syncope. Circulation 81:1803–1810
12. Alehan D, Ayabakan C, Özer S (2002) Heart rate variability and autonomic nervous system changes in children with vasovagal syncope. Pacing Clin Electrophysiol 25:1331–1338
13. Morillo CA, Klein GJ, Jones DL et al (1994) Time and frequency domain analysis of heart rate variability during orthostatic stress in patients with neurally mediated syncope. Am J Cardiol 74:1258–1262
14. Furlan R, Piazza S, Dell'Orto S et al (1998) Cardiac autonomic patterns preceding occasional vasovagal reactions in healthy humans. Circulation 98:1756–1761
15. Mosqueda-Garcia R, Furlan R, Fernandez-Violante R et al (1997) Sympathetic and baroreceptor reflex function in neurally mediated syncope evoked by tilt. J Clin Invest 99:2736–2744
16. Béchir M, Binggeli C, Corti R et al (2003) Dysfunctional baroreflex regulation of sympathetic nerve activity in patients with vasovagal syncope. Circulation 107:1620–1625
17. Novak V, Spies J, Novak P et al (1998) Hypocapnia and cerebral hypoperfusion in orthostatic intolerance. Stroke 2:1876–1881
18. Jordan J, Shannon JR, Diedrich A et al (2000) Interaction of carbon dioxide and sympathetic nervous system activity in the regulation of cerebral perfusion in humans. Hypertension 36:383–388
19. Jauregui-Renaud K, Marquez MF, Hermosillo AG et al (2003) Paced breathing can prevent vasovagal syncope during head-up tilt testing. Can J Cardiol 19:698-700
20. Hermosillo AG, Jáuregui-Renaud K, Kostine A et al (2002) Comparative study of cerebral blood flow between postural tachycardia and neurocardiogenic syncope during head-up tilt test. Europace 4:369–374
21. Jacob G, Atkinson D, Jordan J et al (1999) Effects of standing on cerebrovascular resistance in patients with idiopathic orthostatic intolerance. Am J Med 106:59–64
22. Grubb B, Kanjwal M, Kosinski DJ. (2001) The postural orthostatic tachycardia syndrome: current concepts in pathophysiology diagnosis and management (review). J Interv Card Electrophysiol 5:9–16
23. Streeten DHP, Anderson GH Jr, Richardson R et al (1988) Abnormal orthostatic changes in blood pressure and heart rate in subjects with intact sympathetic nervous function: evidence for excessive venous pooling. J Lab Clin Med 111:326–335
24. Streeten DHP (1999) Orthostatic intolerance: a historical introduction to pathophysiology mechanisms. Am J Med Sci 317:78–87
25. Burlan R, Jacob G, Snell M et al (1998) Chronic orthostatic intolerance: a disorder with discordant cardiac and vascular sympathetic control. Circulation 98:2154–2159
26. Schondorf R, Low P (1993) Idiopathic postural tachycardia syndromes. In: Low P (ed) Clinical autonomic disorders. Little Brown, Boston, pp 641–652
27. Jacob G, Shannon J, Costa F et al (1999) Abnormal norepinephrine clearance and adrenergic receptor sensitivity in idiopathic orthostatic intolerance. Circulation 98:2154–2159
28. Shannon JR, Flattem Nl, Jordan J et al (2000) Orthostatic intolerance and tachycardia associated with norepinephrine-transporter deficiency. N Engl J Med 342:541–549
29. Morillo CA, Eckberg DL, Ellenbogen KA et al (1997) Vagal and sympathetic mechanisms in patients with orthostatic vasovagal syncope. Circulation 96:2509–2513
30. Narkiewicz K, Somers V (1998) Chronic orthostatic intolerance: part of a spectrum of dysfunction in orthostatic cardiovascular homeostasis. Circulation 98:2105–2107
31. Suzuki M, Hori S, Nakamura I et al (2003) Role of vagal control in vasovagal syncope. Pacing Clin Electrophysiol 26:571–578

32. Grubb BP, Karas B (1999) Clinical disorders of the autonomic nervous system associated with orthostatic intolerance: an overview of classification, clinical evaluation, and management. Pacing Clin Electrophysiol 22:798–810
33. Beck L, Pons M, Piot C et al (1999) A "dysautonomic" head-up tilt test pattern in elderly patients with neurocardiogenic syncope. Pacing Clin Electrophysiol 22:104–1012
34. Robertson D, Low PA, Polinsky RJ (1996) Primer on the autonomic nervous system. Academic Press, San Diego

Water Drinking to Prevent Orthostatic Hypotension and Neurally Mediated Syncope: Mechanisms and Benefits

C.J. Mathias, T.M. Young

Introduction

Water drinking is now recognized as having pressor effects even in normal subjects. In young subjects there is no change in blood pressure after water drinking, but in older subjects there is a rise in systolic blood pressure [1]. An even greater rise–in some cases over 30 mmHg–occurs in patients with orthostatic hypotension due to chronic autonomic failure (Fig. 1) [2]. Water alone, therefore, has appreciable cardiovascular effects in both normal and diseased man. The mechanisms of the pressor response remain unclear. Recognition of these effects of water is of importance in studies of cardiovascular and autonomic function. This review relates to the physiology and pathophysiology of water drinking, its ability to reduce orthostatic hypotension in autonomic failure, and its potential benefit when intermittent autonomic dysfunction causes orthostatic intolerance or syncope.

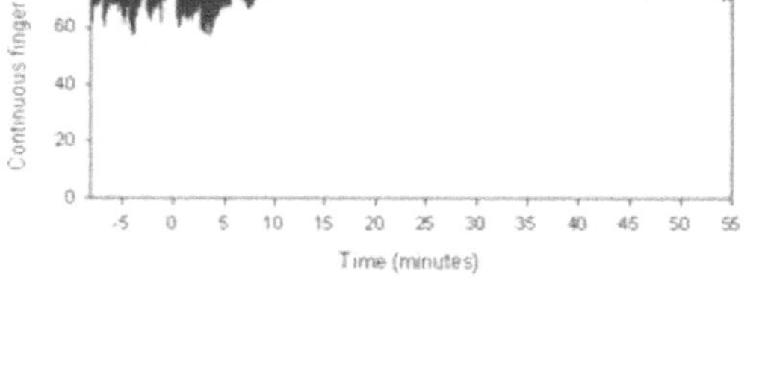

Fig. 1. Changes in blood pressure before and after 500 ml of distilled water ingested at time '0' in a subject with pure autonomic failure. Blood pressure is measured continuously using the Portapres II. From [2]

Neurovascular Medicine Unit, Imperial College London at St Mary's Hospital and Autonomic Unit, National Hospital for Neurology and Neurosurgery. London, and Institute of Neurology, University College London, London, UK

Physiological and Pathophysiological Responses to Water Drinking

In normal subjects aged between 25 and 40 years, water drinking does not change blood pressure [3, 4]. However, in older normal subjects (57 years) systolic blood pressure increases by 11 mmHg after 35 min [3]. In these studies, 480–500 ml water was ingested rapidly over a few minutes, with measurements made with the subjects in the seated position. The pressor response to water begins within 5 min of ingestion, reaches a peak at 30–35 min and wanes after 90 min. Plasma noradrenaline levels rise both in younger and older normal subjects. Muscle sympathetic nerve activity (MSNA) measured by microneurography in a peripheral nerve increases 20 min after ingestion, peaks at 30 min and returns to control levels at 50 min [4]. This was not reproduced in a later study [5].

The pressor effect of water drinking has been studied in two groups with primary autonomic failure, pure autonomic failure (PAF) and multiple system atrophy (MSA). In PAF, the autonomic nervous system only is involved, with a peripheral post-ganglionic sympathetic lesion; in MSA, there are associated neurological deficits (with parkinsonian and cerebellar signs), and the lesion is predominantly central and pre-ganglionic [6]. Systolic blood pressure rises by 37 mmHg in PAF and 33 mmHg in MSA after water [3]. This was confirmed in a study of 14 subjects with PAF with severe orthostatic hypotension, all of whom had substantial sympathetic denervation as based on a series of physiological and biochemical studies [2]. Even after ingestion of distilled water (as in the original studies Nashville tap water was used), blood pressure rises after a few minutes, peaks at 40 min and remains elevated for 35 min before returning to basal levels at 50 min. Systolic blood pressure increases by 18 mmHg (range 7–64 mmHg) and diastolic by 9 mmHg (range 5–37 mmHg). In a further study comparing responses in PAF and MSA [7], similar changes were noted but with different time courses in the two groups; blood pressure rises within 6 min in PAF, but takes 14 min in MSA.

Mechanisms of the Pressor Effect of Water Drinking

This still remains unclear. The various studies to determine why water drinking exerts a pressor effect are described below.

Regional Haemodynamics

In PAF, after water drinking there is no change in ejection fraction, stroke volume or cardiac output [2]. However, calculated total peripheral vascular resistance rises, favouring vasoconstriction as the haemodynamic mechanism responsible for the pressor response. The reasons for this could include reflex sympathetic activation through gastric distension. In normal subjects, graded gastric balloon distension raises MSNA and blood pressure [8]. However, when water is administered directly by mouth there is an initial and transient rise in blood pressure and heart rate but a decrease in MSNA [5], which does not rise above the baseline, unlike observations in an earlier study [4]. Furthermore, the same volume of water by stomach tube over 20 min causes no change in either MSNA or blood pressure in normal subjects [5]. When water at 9 °C or 24 °C is administered to patients with autonomic failure there is no difference in the pressor response [3].

Speed of Pressor Response

In PAF after water drinking, blood pressure and total peripheral vascular resistance rise relatively slowly, over minutes [2]; this rise occurs even later in MSA [7]. This is considerably slower than the pressor effects of reflexes, as observed in tetraplegics with high spinal cord lesions [9]. In such patients stimulation of viscera (urinary bladder and large bowel), or induction of skeletal muscle spasms, causes autonomic dysreflexia with a rapid rise in blood pressure within a few seconds. This is the result of spinal sympathetic reflex activity below the level of lesion and is not due to humoral effects [10]. Once the provoking stimulus is discontinued, blood pressure usually falls over a few minutes rather than rapidly because of impaired baroreflex activity and pressor supersensitivity [11].

The reasons for vasoconstriction, therefore, remain unclear. The long latency of the pressor response argues against neurally mediated reflexes and raises the possibility of the effects of vasoconstrictor substances released systemically or locally.

Vasoconstrictor Neurohumoral Substances

In normal subjects, plasma vasopressin and renin activity do not change after water drinking [3], making it less likely that they contribute to the pressor response. Plasma noradrenaline levels increase after water drinking in normal subjects [3, 4], but there is no correlation between the rise in plasma noradrenaline levels and the changes in blood pressure. Circulating plasma noradrenaline is more likely to reflect a rise in sympathetic nerve activity.

Water drinking may influence the levels of local vasoactive substances, with inhibition of vasodilators or increased levels of vasoconstrictors such as endothelin. This has not been studied.

Pharmacological Studies

In two MSA patients studied before and after ganglionic blockade with trimethaphan, plasma noradrenaline levels fell, indicating suppression of residual sympathetic nerve activity [3]. In neither was there a pressor response when water was administered after ganglionic blockade. This raised further the possibility of activation of sympathetic neural mechanisms. Further evidence in normal subjects was thought to favour this, as the pressor response to water was reported to be abolished by ganglionic blockade [3]. However, this evidence cannot be considered as it was performed only in younger subjects who did not have a pressor response to water.

The pharmacological effects of yohimbine, that acts on α_2 pre-synaptic receptors and stimulates the release of noradrenaline, are dependent on integrity of sympathetic nerve terminals. In patients with primary autonomic failure there is a correlation between the pressor response to yohimbine and to water drinking, suggesting that with less sympathetic denervation there is a greater pressor response [3]. This also implies the reverse: that with substantial sympathetic failure the pressor response to water drinking is less. However, in later studies in severely affected PAF [2] a marked pressor response to water ingestion also occurred.

Rehydration Affecting Intravascular and Extravascular Compartments

Fluid depletion is more likely to occur in patients with autonomic failure, for a variety of reasons. Sympathetic nerve activity influences renal tubular absorption of solutes, including sodium, and may account for urinary sodium and water loss in autonomic failure [12]. Furthermore, when supine these patients undergo a rise in blood pressure, sometimes to hypertensive levels. This increases renal perfusion and probably contributes to recumbency-induced polyuria [13, 14]). Overnight, when lying flat their body weight can fall by 1–1.5 kg, which worsens the degree of orthostatic hypotension and symptoms in the morning [15]. Correction of this fluid deficit is the basis of the nocturnal use of the vasopressin-2 agonist desmopressin which reduces overnight weight loss and is of benefit in reducing morning orthostatic hypotension and ensuing symptoms [15, 16].

Water drinking initially may raise plasma volume, but this is likely to be followed by redistribution from intravascular into extravascular spaces. The haematocrit has been used as a measure of plasma volume but a variety of factors can influence interpretation, especially in subjects with sympathetic denervation [12]. In normal subjects studied before, 30 and 60 min after water ingestion there is no change in the haematocrit [3]. However, the pressor effect of water occurs after 5 min and peaks at 30 min, making it likely that water redistribution had occurred when the first measurements were made after water drinking. In five persons with PAF, 500 ml of 5% dextrose also was infused but over a 60-min period; plasma volume increased by 5.3% and blood pressure by 18 mmHg, compared to 52 mmHg with oral water [3]. However, carbohydrate ingestion lowers blood pressure in autonomic failure [17], and the potential hypotensive effect of dextrose may have negated the pressor effect of this intravenous volume of water.

The reason for the different responses to water drinking in younger and older normal subjects is unclear. Older subjects are more likely to have renal tubule refractoriness to vasopressin, and thus may be relatively less fluid-replete than younger normal subjects. However, other factors, including less effective baroreceptors reflexes, or greater vascular responses to pressor stimuli, remain as possibilities.

Potential Benefits of Water Drinking in Autonomic Disorders

When the initial observations of the pressor effect of water were made, the possible benefits were postulated [18]. The effects of water on postural and post-prandial hypotension have since been studied in autonomic failure [7, 19]. After water drinking, standing blood pressure is raised by 31 mmHg systolic and 13 mmHg diastolic after 35 min. Post-prandial hypotension is reduced by drinking water immediately before a meal (from 43/20 to 22/12 mmHg after 90 min). In a further study comparing PAF and MSA, there were similar observations and water drinking reduced orthostatic hypotension; furthermore, there was a reduction in orthostatic symptoms in both groups [7]. Whether water drinking will benefit the many disorders that result in orthostatic hypotension [20] remains to be determined.

Water drinking also may benefit patients with intermittent autonomic dysfunction, as reported in children with vasodepressor syncope [21]. In normal adults, water drinking increases orthostatic tolerance (by 5 min) when tested using a combination of head-up tilt and lower body negative pressure [22]. Thus, water drinking may benefit subjects with vasovagal syncope, especially when provoked by standing still or in hot weather, when there is a greater likelihood of pooling or a reduction in fluid volume.

In the postural tachycardia syndrome, there is a substantial rise in standing heart rate (of over 30 bpm), usually without a fall in blood pressure. Studies in this group indicate that after water drinking the standing levels of blood pressure are not affected, but standing heart rate is lowered, by 15 bpm at 3 min and 12 bpm after 5 min [19]. The effects of water drinking on symptoms, however, were not reported.

Concluding Remarks

Drinking 500 ml of water does not raise blood pressure in young normal subjects but has a pressor effect in older subjects. There is an even greater response in patients with orthostatic hypotension due to primary chronic autonomic failure. The mechanisms of the pressor response remain unclear. Water drinking is effective in PAF and MSA in whom it reduces both orthostatic and post-prandial hypotension; furthermore it also reduces symptoms of orthostatic hypotension. Whether these benefits are offset by the expected later diuresis, especially in MSA, who often have urinary bladder disturbances, remains unclear.

There are many autonomic causes of syncope – vasovagal, carotid sinus hypersensitivity and situational. Vasovagal syncope is the most common form [23]. In such patients an increase in salt and fluid intake often reduces fainting and water may be of benefit. In the postural tachycardia syndrome, hypovolaemia may be a contributory factor. Water drinking does not raise the seated or standing blood pressure, but attenuates the postural rise in heart rate.

Thus, water ingestion may benefit both these groups with intermittent autonomic dysfunction. Whether this is likely to be more effective in the postural tachycardia syndrome, where symptoms often are directly related to standing , remains to be determined.

Acknowledgements. Dr Young is supported by the Autonomic Disorders Association Sarah Matheson Trust.

References

1. Jordan J, Shannon JR, Grogan E, Biaggioni I, Robertson D (1999) A potent pressor response elicited by drinking water. Lancet 353:723
2. Cariga P, Mathias CJ (2001) Human sympathetic denervation due to autonomic failure. Clin Sci 101:313–319
3. Jordan J, Shannon JR, Black BK et al (2000) The pressor response to water drinking in humans: a sympathetic reflex? Circulation 101:504–509
4. Scott EM, Greenwood JP, Gilbey SG, Stoker JB, Mary DA (2001) Water ingestion increases sympathetic vasoconstrictor discharge in normal human subjects. Clin Sci (Colch) 100:335–342
5. Endo Y, Yamauchi K, Tsutsui Y et al (2002) Changes in blood pressure and muscle sympathetic nerve activity during water drinking in humans. Jap J Physiol 52:421–427
6. Mathias CJ (2000) Disorders of the autonomic nervous system. In: WG Bradley, RB Daroff, GM Fenichel, CD Marsden (eds) Neurology in clinical practice, 3rd edn. Butterworth-Heinemann, Boston, USA, pp 2131–2165
7. Young TM, Mathias CJ (2003) Water ingestion and haemodynamic responses while seated and standing in subjects with chronic autonomic failure. Clin Autonom Res 13:122–123 (abs)
8. Rossi P, Andriesse GI, Oey PL et al (1998) Stomach distension increases efferent muscle sympathetic nerve activity and blood pressure in healthy humans. J Neurol Sci 161:148–155
9. Mathias CJ, Frankel H (2002) Autonomic disturbances in spinal cord lesions. In: Mathias CJ, Bannister R (eds) Autonomic failure: a textbook of clinical disorders of the autonomic nervous system, 4th edn. Oxford University Press, Oxford, pp 494–513
10. Mathias CJ, Christensen NJ, Corbett JL, Frankel HL, Spalding JMK (1976) Plasma catecholamines during paroxysmal neurogenic hypertension in quadriplegic man. Circ Res 39:204–208
11. Mathias CJ, Frankel HL, Christensen NJ, Spalding JMK (1976) Enhanced pressor response to noradrenaline in patients with cervical spinal cord transection. Brain 99:757–770
12. DiBona GF, Wilcox CS (2002) The kidney and the sympathetic nervous system. In: Mathias CJ, Bannister R (eds) autonomic failure: a textbook of clinical disorders of the autonomic nervous system, 4th edn. Oxford University Press, Oxford, pp 143–150
13. Schalekamp MADH, Man in't Veld AJ, Wenning GJ (1985) The second Sir George Pickering Memorial Lecture: What regulates whole body autoregulation? Clinical observations. J Hypertens 3:97–107

14. Kooner JS, da Costa DF, Edge W, Frankel HL, Bannister R, Peart WS, Mathias CJ (1987) Recumbency induces hypertension, diuresis and natriuresis in autonomic failure but diuresis alone in tetraplegia. J Hypertens 5[Suppl 5]:327-329
15. Mathias CJ, Fosbraey P da Costa DF, Thornley A, Bannister R (1986). The effect of desmopressin on nocturnal polyuria, overnight weight loss and morning postural hypotension in patients with autonomic failure. Br Med J 293:353–354
16. Mathias CJ, Young TM (2003) Plugging the leak-benefits of the vasopressin-2 agonist, desmopressin in autonomic failure. Clin Autonom Res 13:85–87
17. Mathias CJ, da Costa DF, McIntosh CM et al (1989) Differential blood pressure and hormonal effects following glucose and xylose ingestion in chronic autonomic failure. Clin Sci 77:85–92
18. Mathias CJ (2000) A 21st century water cure. Lancet 356:1046–1048
19. Shannon JR, Diedrich A, Biaggioni I et al (2002) Water drinking as a treatment for orthostatic syndromes. Am J Med 112:355–360
20. Mathias CJ (2002) To stand on one's own legs. Clin Med 2:237–245
21. Younoszai AK, Franklin WH, Chan DP, Cassidy SC, Allen HD (1998) Oral fluid therapy. A promising treatment for vasodepressor syncope. Arch Pediatr Adolesc Med 152:163–168
22. Schroeder C, Bush VE, Norcliffe LJ et al (2002) Water drinking acutely improves orthostatic tolerance in healthy subjects. Circulation 106:2806–2811
23. Mathias CJ, Deguchi K, Schatz I (2001) Observations on recurrent syncope and presyncope in 641 patients. Lancet 357:348–353

Physical Counterpressure Maneuvers to Prevent and Abort Vasovagal Syncope: A Novel Effective Treatment?

N. van Dijk, C.T.P. Krediet, I.G.J.M. de Bruin, J.J. van Lieshout, W. Wieling

Introduction

Vasovagal syncope is a common disorder characterized by reflex vasodilatation and bradycardia, resulting in a drop in systemic blood pressure and diminished cerebral perfusion. The episodes are usually provoked by patient-specific triggers, such as intense emotions or prolonged standing, and are self-limiting [1]. Up to half of the normal population experiences at least one episode of syncope during life. The vast majority of these episodes are of vasovagal origin [2, 3].

Although vasovagal syncope has a benign prognosis [4], quality of life may become seriously affected in patients with a high recurrence rate [5–7]. An intensive management strategy in patients with recurrent vasovagal syncope is therefore justified. However, current treatment options are limited [8]. To date, treatment of vasovagal syncope consists of explanation, reassurance, and recommendation of a high salt/fluid intake. Pacemaker therapy has been applied, but is controversial [8–10]. Although pharmacological interventions with drugs such as β-blockers and antidepressants (serotonin reuptake inhibitors) have been proposed, no long-term, multicenter, placebo-controlled studies have been able to show a benefit of the active drug over placebo [8]. The effectiveness of the specific α-adrenergic agonist midodrine on vasovagal syncope is promising [11], but needs further study. A major drawback of pharmacological treatment in vasovagal syncope is that patients become chronically dependent on medication for an intermittent disorder. This is costly and carries the risk of side effects.

Recently physical counterpressure maneuvers, i.e., crossing the legs and/or tensing the leg muscles, are proposed as a novel, safe, easy-to-apply and apparently cost-effective measure to combat or abort vasovagal syncope [12, 13]. In this review we will provide an overview of the therapeutic possibilities of physical counterpressure maneuvers in vasovagal syncope.

Academic Medical Centre, Department of Internal Medicine, Amsterdam, The Netherlands

History

Observations on the importance of intramuscular pressure and muscle tensing on orthostatic tolerance in patients prone to vasovagal syncope are buried in older case reports and case series. We will consider some of them in detail.

In the 1930s, Henderson et al. reported that *tonic* pressure in the skeletal muscles is essential for maintaining venous return of the blood to the heart [14]. A few years later Mayerson and Burch showed that patients with vasovagal syncope have a decreased skeletal muscle tone compared to normal subjects [15]. In 1947 Engel and Romano documented that *dynamic* muscle contractions could postpone or abort vasovagal fainting [16]. They suggested that this involved reinfusion of pooled blood to the thoracic region. The importance of reinfusion of venous blood was confirmed by experiments by Weissler et al. They demonstrated that inflating an antigravity suit, of the kind used by fighter pilots to prevent +*g*-induced loss of consciousness (G-LOC), could abort an impending vasovagal faint [17]. Inflation increased central venous pressure and cardiac output and the faint was aborted. Another procedure applied by pilots to prevent G-LOC is the anti-*g*-maneuver (tensing the leg and abdominal muscles) [18]. Newberry et al. described the beneficial effect of an anti-*g* maneuver to postpone a vasovagal reaction in a pilot, but this astute observation was overlooked [19]. The use of muscle tensing to prevent vasovagal fainting was rediscovered by psychologists in the 1980s. They demonstrated that in patients with vasovagal episodes due to injury/injection/blood phobia, applied body tension is effective to prevent syncope due to these anxiety-provoking stimuli [20]. The authors did not obtain actual blood pressure observations, however, and the findings were not picked up by clinicians taking care of patients with vasovagal syncope.

Inspired by observations that leg crossing and leg muscle tensing increase orthostatic tolerance in patients with autonomic failure [21, 22], Krediet et al. recently rediscovered the effectiveness of leg crossing and muscle tensing to postpone or abort vasovagal syncope [12]. Brignole et al. reported a similar effect of arm counterpressure maneuvers [13]. The latter based their maneuvers on the advice of the older generation of Italian general practitioners, to apply muscle tensing by hand gripping a wooden egg (used in the old days for darning socks) at the start of an impending faint [23].

Physiological Mechanisms

The magnitude of effect of the combination of leg muscle crossing and tensing on blood pressure during a vasovagal reaction is large (Fig. 1). Leg crossing and tensing induce a rise in systolic blood pressure during vasovagal syncope from an average pressure of 65 mmHg at the lowest point to 106 mmHg during the maneuver [12]. This rise is postulated to be caused by mechanical and

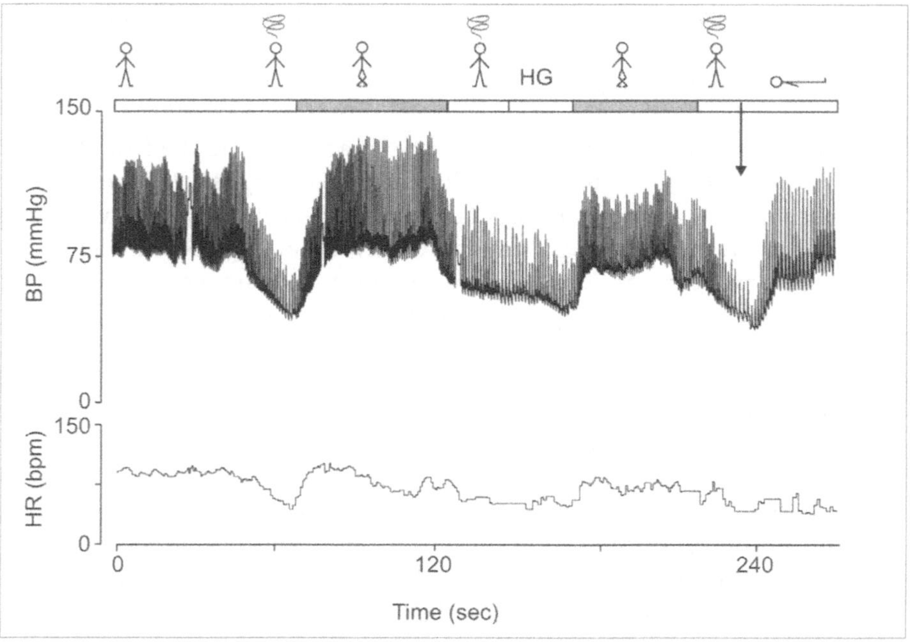

Fig. 1. Effects of leg crossing on blood pressure and heart rate during impending vasovagal syncope. Handgrip (HG) is not effective. *Arrow* indicates tilt-back

reflex effects [12]. The acute mechanical effect of reinfusion of pooled blood due to external skeletal muscle pressure causes a rapid increase in central venous pressure and cardiac output and consequently a rise in blood pressure and cerebral perfusion [24]. Furthermore, acute mechanical effects of kinking of large vessels in the legs could attribute to a rise in peripheral resistance [12].

Reflex effects of muscle tensing are likely to be involved in the rise of systemic blood pressure as well. Tensing of skeletal muscles is associated with activation of a central nervous drive (central command) resulting in withdrawal of vagal outflow to the heart and an instantaneous increase in heart rate [25, 26]. During maximal isometric muscle contractions, central command also induces a rise in sympathetic outflow to blood vessels and thus in peripheral resistance, with stabilization of blood pressure [26].

Tensing of skeletal muscles and the consequent stimulation of mechanical receptors in these muscles elicits a reflex increase in the muscle sympathetic nerve activity. Muscle chemoafferents are activated only after approx. 1 min of sustained muscle contractions. Activation of the muscle chemoreflex is therefore not likely to play an important role in the instantaneous blood pressure raising effect of physical counterpressure maneuvers [25]. Skeletal muscle contractions can also induce an instantaneous increase in heart rate by reducing vagal outflow to the heart (muscle–heart reflex) [27, 28]. The specific physiological effects underlying the ability to *abort* vasovagal syncope completely are currently under investigation.

Alternative physical counterpressure maneuvers applied to abort an impending faint are arm tensing and lower body tensing [13, 29]. Arm tensing consists of strong isometric contraction of the two arms, achieved by gripping one hand with the other and simultaneously abducting the arms [13]. The effects of arm tensing differ in our experience from simple hand gripping, which is ineffective in postponing vasovagal syncope (Fig. 1). We suggest that the effectiveness of arm tensing is based on the whole body tensing which is performed during these maneuvers. In present experiments we are focusing on the magnitude of the different physical counterpressure maneuvers on blood pressure during an impending faint.

When serious symptoms of an impending faint occur squatting or sitting down with the head bend between the knees can be applied [30]. The relative effectiveness of these different maneuvers needs further evaluation.

Patients report that the psychological effect of being able to control their symptoms has a major influence on their feelings of control and well-being [13]. This effect could be therapeutic in lowering the recurrence rate, since psychological uncertainty is conductive to vasodepressor syncope [31].

When and What to Apply?

Patients are usually well aware of the specific situations in which they are susceptible to syncope. In our current practice we instruct patients to apply leg crossing in these provocative situations as prophylaxis. A major advantage of leg crossing maneuvers is that they can be used inconspicuously in any social situation. Healthy people employ leg crossing unintentionally when standing still for a prolonged period of time ("cocktail party posture") [32]. Leg crossing can also be applied for the prevention of syncopal symptoms in a sitting position. Symptoms of an impending faint occurring during leg crossing can usually be diminished by applying tensing of the skeletal muscles of legs, abdomen, and buttocks.

When the combination of leg crossing and tensing does not relieve symptoms and a faint is imminent, we advise patients to squat immediately or sit or lie down as an emergency maneuver. Squatting is less embarrassing in public situations than lying down. Some patients apply a squatting-like maneuver by pretending to tie their shoe laces [32]. Patients should, however, be aware of the significant drop in blood pressure that occurs when arising after squatting, with reappearance of the symptoms. For this reason we instruct patients to rise with tensing of their muscles and to keep moving or to find a safe place to sit down immediately (Fig. 2).

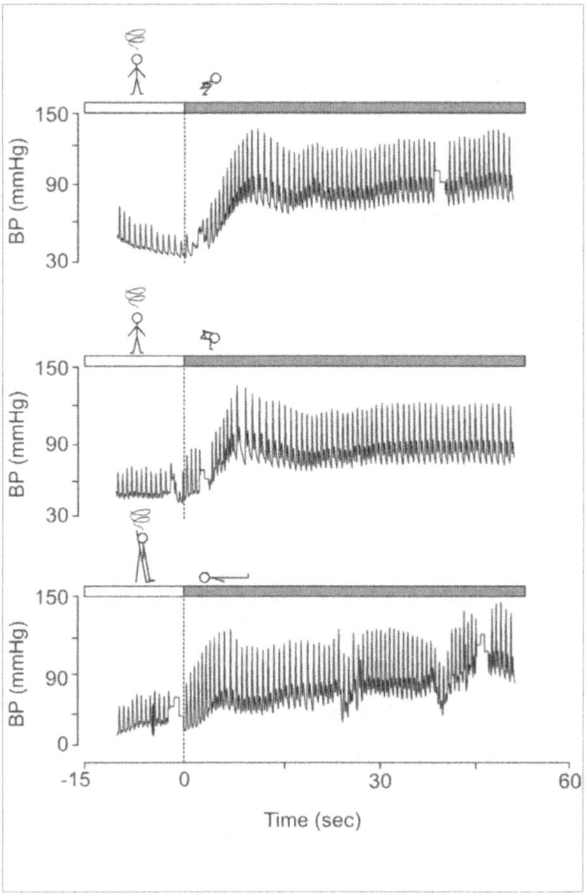

Fig. 2. Effects of squatting (*upper panel*), sitting with head bent between knees (*middle panel*), and lying down (*lower panel*) on blood pressure during impending vasovagal syncope

Training Patients in Counterpressure Maneuvers

Training enhances the effectiveness of leg crossing and muscle tensing [33]. Biofeedback on the performance of the maneuvers can be obtained using continuous Finapres® blood pressure recordings displayed on a computer screen [34]. During the session patients can observe directly the effects of the maneuvers on their blood pressure. The efficacy of the use of maneuvers like squatting is maximal without any training [33].

Training in physical counterpressure maneuvers can also be performed during tilt-table testing. When vasovagal syncope is induced for diagnostic purposes, patients apply (the previously instructed) maneuvers to postpone or even abort the episode. The laboratory surroundings give them maximal confidence in the efficacy of the maneuvers.

Conclusions

Physical counterpressure maneuvers such as leg-crossing with muscle tensing and arm tensing are effective measures to prevent or abort a vasovagal faint under laboratory conditions. Two small studies have shown effectiveness during daily life [12, 13]. A large, multicenter, randomized clinical trial is required to provide unambiguous evidence of the effectiveness of physical counterpressure maneuvers in the treatment of patients with recurrent vasovagal syncope.

References

1. Van Lieshout JJ, Wieling W, Karemaker JM, Eckberg DL (1991) Vasovagal syncope. Clin Sci 81:575–586
2. Wieling W, Ganzeboom KS, Krediet CT et al (2003) Initial diagnostic strategy in the case of transient losses of consciousness: the importance of the medical history. Ned Tijdschr Geneeskd 147:849–854
3. Ganzeboom KS, Colman N, Reitsma JB, Shen WK, Wieling W (2003) Prevalence and triggers of syncope in medical students. Am J Cardiol 91:1006–1008
4. Soteriades ES, Evans JC, Larson MG et al (2002) Incidence and prognosis of syncope. N Engl J Med 347:878–885
5. Linzer M, Pontinen M, Gold DT et al (1991) Impairment of physical and psychosocial function in recurrent syncope. J Clin Epidemiol 44:1037–1043
6. Rose MS, Koshman ML, Spreng S, Sheldon R (2000) The relationship between health-related quality of life and frequency of spells in patients with syncope. J Clin Epidemiol 53:1209–1216
7. Van Dijk N, Sprangers MA, Colman N, Wieling W, Linzer M (2003) Quality of life in syncopal patients. Proceedings of the 26th Annual Meeting of the Society of General Internal Medicine. J Gen Intern Med 18 Suppl 1:160
8. Brignole M, Alboni P, Benditt D et al (2001) Guidelines on the management (diagnosis and treatment) of syncope. Eur Heart J 22:1256–1306
9. Van Dijk N, Harms MP, Linzer M, Wieling W (2000) Treatment of vasovagal syncope: pacemaker or crossing legs. Clin Auton Res 10:347–349
10. Connolly SJ, Sheldon R, Thorpe KE et al (2003) Pacemaker therapy for prevention of syncope in patients with recurrent severe vasovagal syncope. Second vasovagal pacemaker study (VPS II): a randomized trial. JAMA 89:2224–2229
11. Kaufmann H, Saadia D, Voustianiouk A (2002) Midodrine in neurally mediated syncope: a double-blind, randomised crossover study. Ann Neurol 52:342–345
12. Krediet CT, Van Dijk N, Linzer M, Van Lieshout JJ, Wieling W (2002) Management of vasovagal syncope: controlling or aborting faints by legcrossing and muscle tensing. Circulation 106:1684–1689
13. Brignole M, Croci F, Menozzi C et al (2002) Isometric arm counter pressure maneuvers to abort impending vasovagal syncope. J Am Coll Cardiol 40:2053–2059
14. Henderson Y, Oughterson AW, Greenberg LA, Searle CP (1935) Muscle tonus, intramuscular pressure and the venopressor mechanism. Am J Physiol 114:261–268
15. Mayerson HS, Burch GE (1939) Relationships of tissue (subcutaneous and intramuscular) and venous pressures to syncope induced in man by gravity. Am J Physiol 126:258–269

16. Engel GL, Romano J (1947) Studies of syncope: IV. Biologic interpretation of vasodepressor syncope. Psychosom Med 9:288–294
17. Weissler AM, Warren JV, Estes EH Jr et al (1952) Vasodepressor syncope, factors influencing cardiac output. Circulation 15:875–882
18. Wood EH (1987) Development of methods for prevention of acceleration induced blackout and unconsciousness in World War II fighter pilots. Limitations: present and future. Physiologist 30(1 Suppl):S27–S30
19. Newberry PD, Hatch AW, MacDonald JM (1970) Cardio-respiratory events preceding syncope induced by a combination of lower body negative pressure and head-up tilt. Aerospace Med 41:373–378
20. Ost LG, Sterner U (1987) Applied tension. A specific behavioural method for the treatment of blood phobia. Behav Res Ther 25:25–29
21. Van Lieshout JJ, Ten Harkel AD, Wieling W (1992) Physical manoeuvres for combating orthostatic dizziness in autonomic failure. Lancet 11:897–898
22. Wieling W, Van Lieshout JJ, van Leeuwen AM (1993) Physical manoeuvres that reduce postural hypotension in autonomic failure. Clin Auton Res 3:57–65
23. Krediet CT, Van Dijk N, Linzer M, Van Lieshout JJ, Wieling W (2003) Management of vasovagal syncope: controlling or aborting faints by legcrossing and muscle tensing. Response Circulation 107:198e
24. Van Lieshout JJ, Pott F, Madsen PL, Goudoever J, Secher NH (2001) Muscle tensing during standing. Effects on cerebral tissue oxygenation and cerebral artery blood velocity. Stroke 32:1546–1551
25. Rowell LB, O'Leary DS (1990) Reflex control of the circulation during exercise: chemoreflexes and mechanoreflexes. J Appl Physiol 69:407–418
26. Thornton JM, Guz A, Murphy K et al (2001) Identification of higher brain centres that may encode the cardiorespiratory response to exercise in humans. J Physiol 533:823–836
27. Hollander AP, Bouman LN (1975) Cardiac acceleration in man elicited by a muscle-heart reflex. J Appl Physiol. 38:272–278
28. Gladwell VF, Coote JH (2002) Heart rate at the onset of muscle contraction and during passive muscle stretch in humans: a role for mechanoreceptors. J Physiol 540:1095–1102
29. Sabin N (2001) The use of applied tension and cognitive therapy to manage syncope (common faint) in an older adult. Aging Ment Health 5:92–94
30. Krediet CT, Wieling W (2003) Counter manoeuvers for vasovagal syncope. Europace 2003 (in press)
31. Engel GL (1978) Psychologic stress, vasodepressor (vasovagal) syncope, and sudden death. Ann Intern Med 89:403–412
32. Wieling W, Colman N, Krediet CT, Freeman R (2003) Nonpharmacological treatment of reflex syncope: a review. Clin Auton Res (in press)
33. Bouvette CM, McPhee BR, Opfer-Gehrking TL, Low PA (1996) Role of physical countermaneuvers in the management of orthostatic hypotension: efficacy and biofeedback augmentation. Mayo Clin Proc 71:847–853
34. Imholz BP, Wieling W, van Montfrans GA, Wesseling KH (1998) Fifteen years experience with finger arterial pressure monitoring: assessment of the technology. Cardiovasc Res 38:605–616

Isometric Arm Contraction at the Onset of Prodromal Symptoms: a New First-line Treatment for Vasovagal Syncope?

M. Brignole[1], F. Croci[1], C. Menozzi[2], A. Solano[1], P. Donateo[1], D. Oddone[1], E. Puggioni[1], G. Lolli[2]

Background

Vasovagal syncope is preceded by prodromal symptoms in about two-thirds of cases [1]. Prodromal symptoms are present in virtually all cases of tilt-induced vasovagal syncope, which occurs, on average, 1 minute after the onset of the prodromal symptoms [2]. During the prodromal phase, blood pressure falls markedly; this fall usually precedes the decrease in heart rate, which may be absent at least at the beginning of this phase [2, 3]. Hypotension is caused by vasodilatation in the skeletal muscles owing to the inhibition of sympathetic vasoconstrictive activity [2, 4–7]. Two recent clinical trials [8, 9] have shown that isometric maneuvers involving the legs or the arms can induce a significant increase in blood pressure during the phase of impending vasovagal syncope and allow the patient to avoid or at least delay the loss of consciousness in most cases. This effect seems to be mediated largely by sympathetic nerve discharge and vascular resistance increase during the maneuvers.

Leg Crossing and Muscle Tensing

Physical countermaneuvers were initially proposed for the management of orthostatic hypotension [10–13]. These mainly involve the muscles of the legs (leg-pumping and tensing, leg-crossing) or legs and abdomen (abdominal contraction, squatting).

The standard maneuver consists in leg-crossing combined with maximum tensing of the muscles in the legs, abdomen and buttock for the maximum tolerated time or until complete disappearance of symptoms is achieved (Fig. 1). The increase in orthostatic blood pressure is assumed to be due both to mechanical compression of the venous vascular bed in the legs and to a reflex

[1]Department of Cardiology, Arrhythmologic Centre, Ospedali del Tigullio, Lavagna; [2]Service of Interventional Cardiology, Department of Cardiology, Ospedale S Maria Nuova, Reggio Emilia, Italy

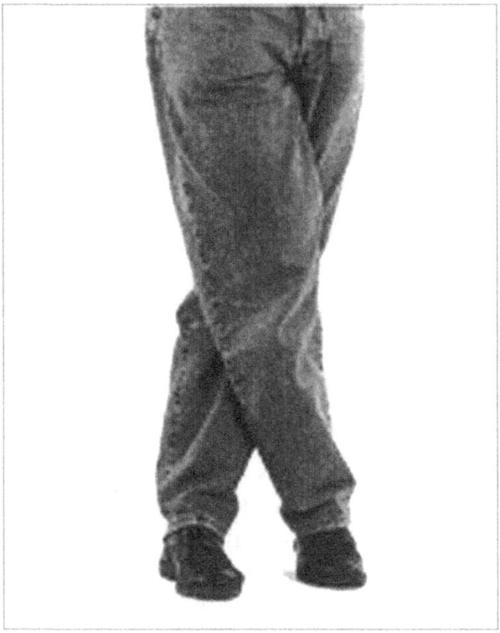

Fig. 1. Leg-crossing maneuver

increase in systemic vascular resistances resulting from the activation of mechanosensitive receptors in the muscles. In a very recent uncontrolled study [8], leg-crossing combined with muscle-tensing at the onset of prodromal symptoms, performed in 20/21 subjects, increased systolic blood pressure from 65±13 mmHg to 106±16 mmHg, postponed the faint by an average of 2.5 min. and in 5 subjects prevented vasovagal syncope; during the maneuvers symptoms disappeared in all patients.

Isometric Arm Counterpressure Maneuvers

Two isometric arm counterpressure maneuvers have been developed [9]. Handgrip consists in the maximal voluntary contraction of a rubber ball (approximately of 5–6 cm diameter) taken in the dominant hand for the maximum tolerated time or up to complete disappearance of symptoms (Fig. 2). Arm-tensing consists in the maximum tolerated isometric contraction of both arms, achieved by gripping one hand with the other and abducting (pushing away) the arms at the same time (Fig. 3).

Cardiovascular responses during handgrip have been previously studied in healthy and in hypertensive patients [8–10, 14–16], but not in fainting patients. Arm-tensing maneuvers have not been developed, earlier. Muscle sympathetic nerve discharge and vascular resistance increase during handgrip in healthy subjects [10, 16]. The increase in arterial pressure can be achieved by increased peripheral resistance alone in patients who lack the capacity to increase heart

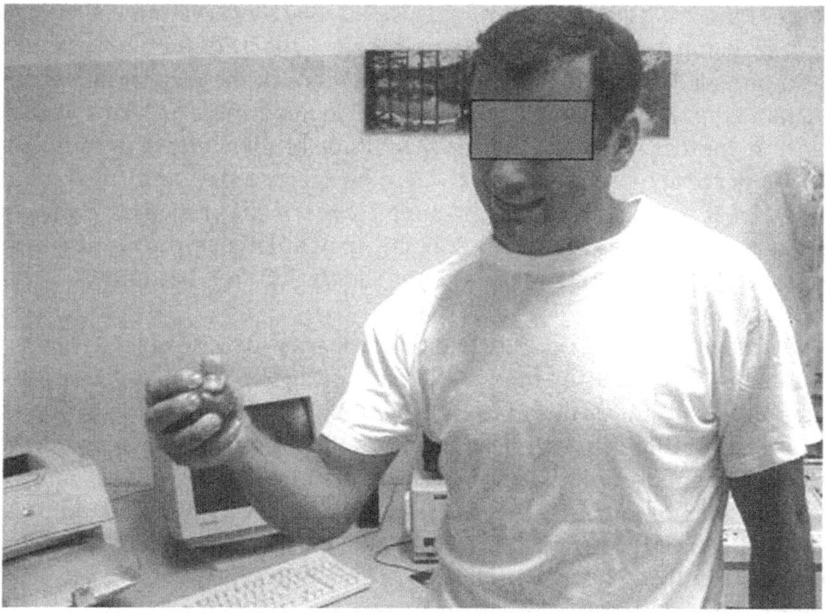

Fig. 2. Handgrip maneuver

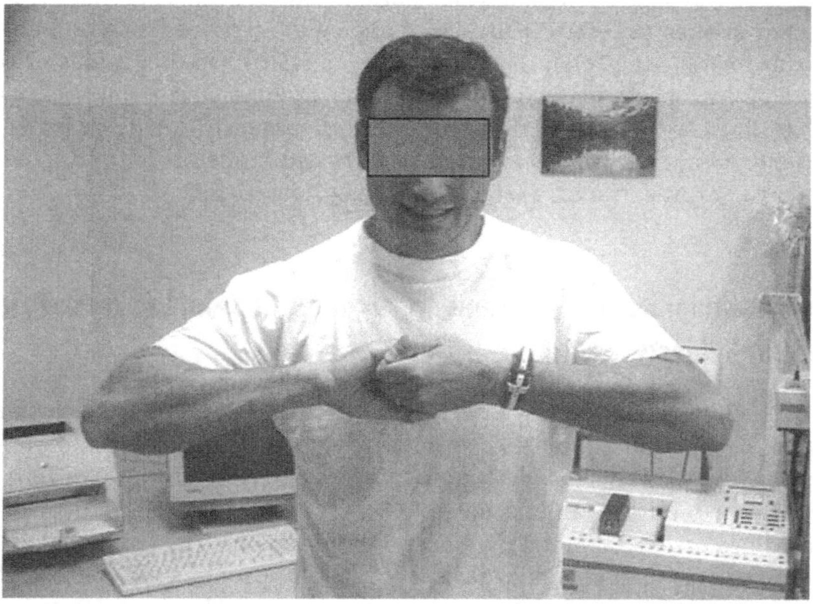

Fig. 3. Arm-tensing maneuver

rate or stroke volume because of surgical cardiac denervation following cardiac transplantation [17, 18] or pharmacological blockade with propranolol [8, 14]. In one study [18, 19] there was no difference in the magnitude of cardiovascular responses between handgrip performed with one and with both hands; in another study [19, 20] the magnitude of the increase in muscle sympathetic nerve activity was greater when the exercise was performed with two hands, but it was smaller than the simple sum of the responses evoked with each arm separately, suggesting that the sympathetic cardiovascular adjustments elicited by separate limbs are not simply additive, but rather exhibit an inhibitory interaction.

The effect of handgrip in attempted abortion of vasovagal syncope was evaluated in 23 patients by means of an acute single-blind, placebo-controlled, randomized, cross-over tilt-table efficacy study [9]. Handgrip was applied for 2 min, starting at the time of onset of symptoms of impending syncope. In the active arm, handgrip caused an increase in systolic blood pressure from 92±10 mmHg to 105±38 mmHg, whereas in the placebo arm, systolic blood pressure decreased from 91±11 mmHg to 73±21 mmHg (P=0.008). Heart rate behavior was similar in the two arms. In the active arm, 63% of patients became asymptomatic, versus 11% in the control arm (P=0.02); conversely only 5% of patients developed syncope, versus 47% of controls (P=0.01). A clinical follow-up feasibility study was also performed in 23 patients [9]. The patients were trained to self-administer arm tensing treatment or handgrip as soon as they experienced symptoms of impending syncope. During 12±4 months of follow-up (update January 2003), 16 patients experienced a total of 163 episodes of impending syncope (median 4 per patient, range 1–9). The 'treatment' was actually applied in 161/163 episodes of impending syncope (98%) and was successful in 160/161 (99%). Overall, 3 patients (13%) had 3 episodes of recurrence of syncope. No patients suffered injury or other adverse morbidity related to the relapses. A 4-scale semiquantitative questionnaire revealed that patient satisfaction was very good in 39% and moderately good in 61% of patients; no patients were partially satisfied or unsatisfied.

Cardiovascular Response to Handgrip, Arm-tensing and Leg-crossing in Healthy Subjects

In 32 healthy volunteers (mean age 44±12, 16 males), we evaluated the physiological response to 2 minutes of isometric contraction during standard handgrip, arm-muscle tensing and leg-crossing (as described above). The tests were performed on a tilt-table at 60°; ECG traces and noninvasive beat-to-beat recordings of arterial blood pressure were continuous. The sequential order of the maneuvers was randomized. Systolic blood pressure increased from 125±18 mmHg to 156±26 mmHg during handgrip, from 123±15 mmHg to 155±24 mmHg during arm-tensing and from 121±14 to 165±26 mmHg during leg crossing (P=0.02); diastolic blood pressure increased from 72±10 mmHg to

94±16 mmHg during hadgrip, from 73±11 mmHg to 97±17 mmHg during arm-tensing, and from 71±12 mmHg to 95±16 mmHg during leg-crossing (difference not significant); heart rate increased from 76±14 bpm to 84±16 bpm during handgrip, from 75±13 bpm to 86±15 bpm during arm-tensing and from 76±12 bpm to 92±18 bpm during leg crossing (P=0.04).

Thus, in healthy subjects systolic blood pressure, diastolic blood pressure, and heart rate increased to similar extents during handgrip and arm-tensing, whereas systolic blood pressure and heart rate increased more during leg crossing. Whether this greater increase has any clinical significance is unknown.

How Effective Are the Counterpressure Maneuvers?

While this approach seems to be very helpful in real life and patients are able to implement a counterpressure maneuver in the vast majority of attacks with a very high rate of success in relieving symptoms, we must nevertheless admit that most of these episodes would have resolved spontaneously without leading to syncope, even in the absence of the counterpressure treatment. Owing to the open design of the follow-up study, we are unable to establish the exact benefit of the treatment. The Physical Counterpressure Maneuver Trial (PC-Trial) is a multicenter, prospective, longitudinal randomized single blind clinical trial designed to address this question. The main hypothesis of the study is that, in patients with definite syncope and absence of significant structural heart disease, physical counterpressure maneuvers decrease the total syncope burden more than does the standard intensive conventional therapy consisting in explanation of the diagnosis, counseling advice, and increases of fluid and salt intake. Secondary end-points are: time to first syncopal recurrence; presyncope burden; and quality of life. The study will involve a minimum of 200 patients. Criteria for inclusion are: clinical diagnosis of classic neurally-mediated reflex syncope, based on the medical history or nonclassic diagnosis of neurally-mediated reflex syncope and a positive tilt-table test; three syncope episodes in the last 2 years or at least 1 syncopal spell in the last year and at least three episodes of presyncope in the last year; recognizable prodromal symptoms; and age 16–70 years. All patients will be checked by the attending physician at 1 and 12 months. Every 3 months follow-up checks will be made either during a regular visit or by telephone. The maximum follow-up period will be 18 months and the minimum, 6 months.

Practical Application

In the acute study [9], handgrip caused an abrupt rise in systemic blood pressure, which was already evident after 10 s. Consequently, symptoms of impending syncope disappeared in many patients and remained unchanged in others, and syncope was aborted. Conversely, in the control arm, blood pressure continued to fall slightly and about half of the patients developed syncope after a mean of 66 s. The benefits were maintained during the recovery phase, and only 20% of patients ultimately developed syncope (versus 58% in the control arm). This finding means that isometric arm contraction is able to abort syncope in most cases, even when the patient remains in the standing position. In real terms, this means that when symptoms of impending syncope occur the patient will have enough time to apply the counterpressure treatment before losing consciousness; in some cases the treatment will definitely abort the vasovagal reaction, while in others it will make it possible to delay syncope for the duration of the maneuver, thus allowing enough time to initiate other maneuvers to abort syncope (e.g. adopting a supine posture). This approach seems to be very helpful in real life. Indeed, during follow-up our patients were able to implement a counterpressure maneuver in 99% of cases and to relieve the symptoms in 99% of these. The treatment is therefore easy to perform, reliable, safe and well accepted by the patients, who expressed good levels of satisfaction. Admittedly, most of these episodes would have resolved spontaneously without leading to syncope even without the counterpressure treatment. Owing to the open design of the follow-up study, we are unable to establish the exact benefit of the treatment. A randomized trial should address this question. In any case, counter pressure maneuvers can be regarded as a first-line treatment in association with the other conventional measures usually recommended for vasovagal syncope (Appendix 1): namely, reassurance about the benign nature of the condition, training in the recognition of warning symptoms, avoidance of triggering events, adoption of maneuvers to abort the episode (e.g., supine posture), and avoidance of volume depletion and prolonged upright posture, etc. With regard to these latter treatment concepts, formal randomized studies are also lacking, but physiological evidence and clinical experience have been sufficient to warrant their inclusion in the available guidelines [20].

Leg-crossing seems to be slightly more effective in increasing blood pressure than the other two maneuvres. Whether this greater increase has any clinical significance is unknown. Conversely, arm exercises seem to be easier to perform in any situation than leg-crossing. Since arm-tensing does not require the use of any equipment, it seems more suitable, since it can be performed during daily life to abort spontaneous attacks. Anyway the three maneuvers should not be seen as rival treatments but rather as complementary therapies that can also be alternated by the patients during the vasovagal attack (Appendix 2).

Main Conclusion

Isometric arm contraction can abort impending vasovagal syncope by increasing systemic blood pressure. Chronic treatment based on self-administered arm counter pressure maneuvers is feasible, safe and well accepted by the patient. Arm counter pressure maneuvers can be proposed as a new first-line treatment for patients who are able to recognize prodromal symptoms before vasovagal syncope.

Appendix 1: Counseling Information (Optimal Standard Treatment) for Patients Prone to Vasovagal Syncope (or Fainting)

What Happens During Fainting?

With standing up from a supine position blood drops under the influence of gravity to the abdomen and legs. This means the heart cannot fill with as much blood as is necessary and the amount of blood the heart can pump around the body diminishes. Without countermeasures blood pressure will drop. Usually the body reacts with narrowing of the blood vessels in the abdomen and legs and by making the heart beat faster. Then more blood will stay in the upper part of the body and the blood pressure will rise again. These measures are taken by the involuntary nervous system; you cannot influence them actively. Some people display insufficient countermeasures in specific situations, which is why the fainting reaction occurs. Blood vessels then even become wider instead of narrower and a little later the heart rate slows down. The result of this faulty response is that the heart cannot pump enough blood to the brain; everything goes black before your eyes and/or you lose consciousness. By sitting or lying down you cause the heart to fill with blood and regain consciousness. Why this reaction happens more often to some people than to other is unknown.

When Does a Fainting Response Occur?

Most people know the circumstances in which they might faint. People who are susceptible to fainting reactions often display symptoms in the following situations:

- During emotional circumstances (seeing blood or being in pain)
- After a long period of standing (e.g. in a line or at a reception)
- In a warm atmosphere (in a sauna, warm weather, under a hot shower)
- Directly after exercise
- Directly after dinner or after too long without food
- During a period
- After too little rest
- During illness, nausea or fever.

Symptoms

The most important symptoms of people with fainting reactions are lightheadedness, seeing black spots and loss of consciousness. Before, during and after the episode people look pale, sweat profusely and are nauseous. After regaining consciousness the patient is often tired for a long time. Not all fainting reactions are accompanied by these typical responses.

Advice

Being susceptible to fainting reactions is not a serious disease, but can be very inconvenient and restrictive to yourself and people around you. The treatment of patients with fainting reactions consists of advice on what usually causes fainting reactions to diminish or even stop:

- It is important to understand completely what is going on with you. Do ask your physician for more explanation if you don't fully understand what fainting is or if you have any more questions.
- Try to find out in what circumstances you are susceptible to fainting and try to avoid them.
- If you recognise any symptoms of the fainting reaction sit down, or lie down if possible.
- Drink enough water and increase your salt intake.
- Avoid excessive use of alcohol.
- Make sure your body is in good shape, but do not exercise excessively.

Appendix 2: Instruction on Counterpressure Maneuvers

Purpose

Patients will be trained in different maneuvers. They will be advised to:

- Use leg-crossing as a preventive measure
- Use leg-crossing, handgrip and/or arm-tensing in case of symptoms of impending syncope. Patients will be instructed to maintain the maneuver they choose for as long as possible and eventually move on to a second/third maneuver if useful.

Session Protocol (Max. duration 1 hour):

- Explanation of purpose and session-program
- Renewed explanation of simple physiology and vasovagal reflexes
- Demonstration and explanation of the three maneuvers
- Instrumentation: Finapres attached to non dominant hand
- Practice of all three maneuvers using Finapres BP recordings as a biofeedback signal
- Offer of instruction sheet with photographs.

Maneuvers

Handgrip
Consists in maximal voluntary contraction of a rubber ball (approximately of 5-6 cm in diameter) held in the dominant hand for the maximum tolerated time or until complete disappearance of symptoms is achieved.

Arm-tensing

Consists in the maximum tolerated isometric contraction of the two arms, achieved by gripping one hand with the other and contemporarily abducting (pushing away) the arms for the maximum tolerated time or until complete disappearance of symptoms. It is not easy to perform this maneuver with the Finapres in place. It can be practiced without Finapres biofeedback or while gripping only three fingers of the instrumented hand.

Leg-crossing

Consists in leg-crossing combined with maximum tensing of muscles in the legs, abdomen, and buttock for the maximum tolerated time or until complete disappearance of symptoms is achieved.

References

1. Alboni P, Brignole M, Menozzi C et al (2001) The diagnostic value of history in patients with syncope with or without heart disease. J Am Coll Cardiol 37:1921-1928
2. Alboni P, Dinelli M, Gruppillo P et al (2002) Haemodynamic changes early in prodromal symptoms of vasovagal syncope. Europace 4:333-338
3. Brignole M, Menozzi C, Del Rosso A et al (2000) New classification of haemodynamics of vasovagal syncope: beyond the VASIS classification. Analysis of the pre-syncopal phase of the tilt test without and with nitroglycerin challenge. Europace 2:66-76
4. Mosqueda-Garcia R, Furlan R, Fernandez-Violante R et al (1997) Sympathetic and baroreceptor reflex function in neurally mediated syncope evoked by tilt. J Clin Invest 99:2736-2744
5. Morillo C, Eckberg D, Ellenbogen K et al (1997) Vagal and sympathetic mechanisms in patients with orthostatic vasovagal syncope. Circulation 96:2509-2513
6. Lipsitz LW, Mietus J, Moody GB, Goldberger AL (1990) Spectral characteristics of heart rate variability before and during postural tilt. Circulation 81:1803-1810
7. van Lieshout JJ, Wieling W, Karemaker JM, Eckberg DL (1991) The vasovagal response. Clin Sci 81:575-586
8. Krediet P, van Dijk N, Linzer M, Lieshout J, Wieling W (2002) Management of vasovagal syncope: controlling or aborting faints by leg crossing and muscle tensing. Circulation 106:1684-1689
9. Brignole M, Croci F, Menozzi C et al (2002) Isometric arm counter-pressure maneuvers to abort impending vasovagal syncope. J Am Coll Cardiol 40:2054–2060
10. Ten Harkel A, van Lieshout JJ, Wieling W (1994) Effects of leg muscle pumping and tensing on orthostatic arterial pressure: a study in normal subjects and patients with autonomic failure. Clin Sci 87:553-558
11. van Lieshout JJ, Ten Harkel A, Wieling W (1992) Physical manoeuvres for combating orthostatic dizziness in autonomic failure. Lancet 339:897-898
12. Bouvette CM, McPhee BR, Opfer-Gehrking TL, Low PA (1996) Role of physical countermaneuvers in the management of orthostatic hypotension: effcacy and biofeedback augmentation. Mayo Clin Proc 71:847-853
13. Wieling W, van Lieshout JJ, van Leuwen AM (1993) Physical manœuvres that reduce postural hypotension in autonomic failure. Clin Autonom Res 3:57-65
14. McAllister RG (1979) Effects of adrenergic receptor blockade on the response to iso-

metric handgrip: studies in normal and hypertensive subjects. J Cardiovasc Pharmacol 2:253-263

15. Verdecchia P, Brignole M, Delfino G, Queirolo C, De Marchi G, Bertulla A (1983) Systolic time intervals as possible predictors of pressure response to sustained beta-adrenergic blockade in arterial hypertension. Hypertension 5:140–146
16. Seals DR (1989) Sympathetic neural discharge and vascular resistance during exercise in humans. J Appl Physiol 66:2472–2478
17. Haskell WL, Savin WM, Schroeder JS et al (1981) Cardiovascular responses to handgrip isometric exercise in patients following cardiac transplantation. Circ Res 48:156-161
18. Grucza R, Kahn JF, Cybulski G, Niewiadomski W, Stupnicka E, Nazar K (1989) Cardiovascular and sympathoadrenal responses to static handgrip performed with one and two hands. Eur J Appl Physiol Occup Physiol 59:184-188
19. Seals DR (1989) Influence of muscle mass on sympathetic neural activation during isometric exercise. J Appl Physiol 67:1801-1806
20. Brignole M, Alboni P, Benditt D et al (2001) for the Task Force on Syncope, European Society of Cardiology. Guidelines on management (diagnosis and treatment) of syncope. Eur Heart J 22:1256

To Pace or not to Pace for Neurally Mediated Syncope: Do We Know the Answer? A Positive View

F. Giada, A. Raviele

Role of Pacing in Vasovagal Syncope

Single chamber VVI mode pacing proved to be ineffective in vasovagal syncope treatment [1], while several nonrandomized studies [2–4] showed a significant decrease in recurrence in patients who underwent dual chamber pacing. In the last few years, three randomized, noncontrolled studies have shown the efficacy of dual-chamber pacemaker implantation in reducing recurrence in patients with recurrent neuromediated syncope. The VPS study [5] demonstrated the effectiveness of rate-drop response pacemakers in patients affected by neurally mediated syncope who gave a positive response in the tilting test, presenting a varying cardoinhibitory component. The VASIS study [6], on the other hand, showed the effectiveness of a DDI-mode pacemaker with hysteresis in patients with neurally mediated syncope and positive tilting test with a marked cardoinhibitory component. Finally, the SYDIT trial [7] reported the superiority of pacemaker implantation over drug treatment with β-blockers.

Recently, the VPS II trial [8], a randomized, placebo-controlled study, was unable to demonstrate the superiority of active pacing over inactive pacing in patients with severe neurally mediated syncope.

Unsolved Questions About the Use of Pacemakers in Neurally Mediated Syncope

Possible Placebo Effect of the Pacemaker

Since the above-mentioned studies, except for VPS II, are uncontrolled (patients randomized to the control arm did not receive a pacemaker), the observed beneficial effects may be related to a placebo influence of the pace-

Cardiovascular Department, Umberto I Hospital, Mestre-Venice, Italy

maker. Thus, the decrease in syncope recurrence may be related to effective pacing activity as well as to a psychological sense of protection and safety provided by the implantation of the pacemaker.

Appropriate Patient Selection

A crucial point is the identification of those patients who stand to benefit particularly from pacemaker implantation. In this context, the role of the hemodynamic response during tilt-induced syncope needs to be clarified. The VASIS and SYDIT studies [6, 7], which enrolled patients with a marked cardoinhibitory component, showed a greater decrease in syncope recurrence during follow-up than did the VPS and VPS II trials [5, 8], which analyzed just few people with this characteristic among the enrolled patients.

The Vasovagal Syncope and Pacing Trial (Synpace)

The Synpace trial [9] was a multicenter, prospective, randomized, double-blind, placebo-controlled study started in April 2000 to resolve these issues. The main aim of the study was to compare the effect of active versus inactive pacing on syncope relapses in patients suffering from recurrent vasovagal syncope.

The primary end-point of the study was the first recurrence of syncope. Patients with severe vasovagal syncope and one syncopal recurrence after a positive tilt test were divided into two groups on the basis of their hemodynamic behavior during tilt-induced syncope: an asystolic group (development of asystole >3 s) and a mixed group (development of bradycardia < 60 beats per minute). Patients from both groups underwent implantation of a pacemaker and were randomized in a double-blind fashion to pacemaker *on* in DDD mode with rate-drop response or pacemaker *off* in OOO mode.

The interim analysis undertaken in September 2002 showed no significant treatment effect in favor of active pacing compared with inactive pacing. Thus, a decision was made to terminate enrollment and follow-up and to report study results as of October 2002. At that time, 29 patients (53 ± 6 years; 19 women) with recurrent vasovagal syncope (median 12 syncopes in the lifetime) had been enrolled. Asystolic response was present in 15 (52%) patients (mean asystole 13 ± 8 s). Of the 29 enrolled patients, 16 were randomized to pacemaker *on* (8 of the asystolic group and 8 of the mixed group), and 13 to pacemaker *off* (7 of the asystolic group and 6 of the mixed group). Every patient was followed up for a minimum of 4 months, with a median of 715 days (interquartile range 302–785 days). Follow-up data were available for all patients. Baseline clinical characteristics of patients with pacemaker *on* and patients with pacemaker *off* were similar.

In the intention-to-treat analysis there were no statistical differences between patients with pacemaker *on* and those with pacemaker *off* in the percentage who experienced syncope during follow-up in the total study population (50% vs 38%, p=ns), as well as in the mixed group (50% vs 50%, p=ns) and in the asystolic group separately (50% vs 29%, p=ns), nor in the probability of syncope-free survival as analyzed using Kaplan–Meier curves. The time to first syncope recurrence was slightly longer in patients with pacemaker *on* than in patients with pacemaker *off* in the total population (median 97 days vs 20 days, p=0.38), as well as in the asystolic group (median 97 days vs 11 days, p=0.06), while it was similar in patients with active pacing and those with inactive pacing in the mixed group (median 88 days vs 100 days, p=0.56). Considering all 29 patients together, the syncopal rate was significantly lower in the postimplantation period compared to the period before pacemaker implantation (0.06 ± 0.11 syncope/month vs 0.72 ± 0.68 syncope/month, p<0.001). However, no differences were found in the syncopal rate after pacemaker implantation between patients with pacemaker *on* and patients with pacemaker *off* in the total population (0.04 ± 0.06 vs 0.08 ± 0.15, p=ns), as well as in the mixed group (0.04 ± 0.06 vs 0.13 ± 0.20, p=ns) and in the asystolic group (0.05 ± 0.07 vs 0.04 ± 0.09). Finally, no statistical differences were observed between patients with pacemaker *on* and those with pacemaker *off* in the percentage who experienced presyncope during follow-up or in total number of presyncope episodes. Similar results were found in on-treatment analysis.

The only clinical variable able to predict syncope recurrence after pacemaker implantation was the number of syncopes in the lifetime. No deaths or severe syncope-related trauma occurred during the study.

The conclusions of the study were the following: active pacing is not superior to inactive pacing in preventing syncopal recurrence in patients with severe vasovagal syncope; the type of response shown during tilt testing has a limited value in predicting outcome.

Future Perspectives

One of the most important limitations of pacing in vasovagal syncope is timely detection of the onset of the neurally mediated reaction and triggering of pacing. Rate-drop response, like the other algorithms used in the studies mentioned above, is a sensing modality based on heart-rate reduction. It is possible that the use of different sensing modalities, such as those based on cardiac contractility [10] or respiratory changes [11], might yield better results in preventing syncopal relapse.

A crucial point in the use of permanent cardiac pacing in the treatment of vasovagal syncope is appropriate selection of the patients. It may be that the documentation of severe bradycardia/asystole during spontaneous syncope by means of an implanted loop recorder, rather than the observation of a cardioinhibitory response during tilt-induced syncope, can identify the patients who will benefit most from pacemaker implantation.

References

1. Benditt DG, Petersen M, Lurie KG et al (1995) Cardiac pacing for the prevention of recurrent vasovagal syncope. Ann Intern Med 122:204–209
2. Petersen MEV, Chamberlain-Webber R, Fitzpatrick AP et al (1994) Permanent pacing for cardioinhibitory malignant vasovagal syndrome. Br Heart J 71:274–281
3. Benditt DG, Sutton R, Gammage M, Fetter J, Markowitz T and the Rate-Drop Response Investigators (1997) Clinical experience with Thera DR rate drop response pacing algorithm in carotid sinus syndrome and vasovagal syncope. Pacing Clin Electrophysiol 20:832–839
4. Sheldon R, Koshman ML, Wilson W et al (1998) Effect of dual chamber pacing with automatic rate-drop sensing on recurrent neutrally mediated syncope. Am J Cardiol 81:158–162
5. Connolly SJ, Sheldon R, Roberts RS, Gent M (1999) The North American Vasovagal Pacemaker Study (VPS). A randomized trial of permanent cardiac pacing for the prevention of vasovagal syncope. J Am Coll Cardiol 33:16–20
6. Sutton R, Brignole M, Menozzi C et al on behalf of the Vasovagal Syncope International Study (VASIS) Investigators (2000) Dual-chamber pacing is efficacious in treatment of neurally-mediated tilt-positive cardioinhibitory syncope. Pacemaker versus no therapy: a multicentre randomized study. Circulation 102:294–299
7. Ammirati F, Colivicchi F, Santini M et al (2001) Permanent cardiac pacing versus medical treatment for the prevention of recurrent vasovagal syncope. Circulation 104:52–57
8. Connolly SJ, Sheldon R, Thorpe KE et al (2003) Pacemaker therapy for prevention of syncope in patients with recurrent severe vasovagal syncope (VPS II): a randomized trial. JAMA 289:2224–2229
9. Giada F, Raviele A, Menozzi C et al (2003) The Vasovagal Syncope and Pacing Trial (Synpace). A randomized, placebo-controlled study of permanent cardiac pacing for the treatment of recurrent vasovagal syncope. Pacing Clin Electrophysiol
10. Deharo JC, Peyre JP, Chalvidian T et al (2000) Continuous monitoring of an endocardial index of myocardial contractility during head-up tilt test. Am Heart J 139:1022–1030
11. Kurbaan AS, Erikson M, Petersen MEV et al (2000) Respiratory changes in vasovagal syncope. J Cardiovasc Electrophysiol 11:607–611

To Pace or Not to Pace for Neurally Mediated Syncope: Do We Know the Answer? A Negative View

O. OSEROFF

Introduction

The vasovagal or neurally mediated syncope (NMS) is a common disorder of the autonomic cardiovascular regulation, showing a substantial physical and social morbidity. This complex syndrome usually is caused by inappropriate reflex vasodilatation and bradycardia, of sporadic nature. However, a small percentage of patients present NMS as a chronic and recurrent disorder with an important impact on their quality of life. In such circumstances, as NMS becomes a risk for severe trauma, an adequate clinical assessment and careful selection of specific treatment is necessary.

Incidence

The reported incidence in a 10-year period for patients younger than 18 years is less than 15%, but for the population between 40 and 60 years old, the incidence rises to 20% and finally, for 70 years old individuals, the incidence is even higher. In 1997, half a million new patients had syncope in the United States, and 34% of them may have a recurrence in the short-term, being as almost half of them are unexplained and recurrent cases.

Etiology

Syncope is a symptom and not a disease itself, leading to a broad spectrum in terms of prognosis and risk, with regards to the pathophysiology that causes the syncope. Most of the published literature agree that NMS represents 24% of all causes of syncope, orthostatic syncope 11%, cardiac related are 18% (14% arrhythmic and 4% structural disease), non-cardiovascular origin is 12% and finally of unknown causes 34%.

Department of Cardiology, Hospital Castex, Buenos Aires, Argentina

Diagnosis

It is generally accepted that a positive response to the head-up tilt test (HUT) indicates that a neurally mediated mechanism may play a role in the genesis of the syncope. Recently, the increased use of HUT has shown a considerably high prevalence of relative bradycardia at the time of the syncope. This so-called "cardioinhibitory response", occasionally may be profound during the syncope induced by the HUT, and it is highly associated with more severe symptoms and predicts a poor response to the treatment [1]. The ISSUE study [2] compared the findings of a loop recorder implanted in 82 patients with isolated syncope and negative HUT, with 29 patients with a positive response. The medical history for both groups was similar for the recurrences (34%) and documented bradycardia (16% vs. 21% for negative and positive HUT respectively, p=ns).

It seems that spontaneous cardioinhibitory response is more frequent than is expected based on the HUT results, reflecting a low sensitivity and reproducibility of this diagnostic tool. Finally, the clinical characteristics and outcome also seems to be independent from the HUT response, but is still unclear if patients with severe bradycardia or asystole are a high risk subpopulation.

General Treatment

The sporadic and benign form of NMS does not require a specific therapeutic intervention. The educational need to change the lifestyle or to avoid situations that trigger the vagal reflex, as well as protecting actions at the moment of the faint, can be enough to prevent recurrences and complications.

On the other hand, empiric pharmacological therapy is considered the first option in prevention for recurrent NMS. Many drugs have been proposed as effective in the treatment of NMS and, in clinical practice, β-blockers currently are the most widely prescribed drug in preventing recurrences. Other used pharmacological agents are vasoconstrictors, volume expanders such as salt tablets or fludrocortisone, disopyramide, scopolamine, and recently serotonine uptake blockers. Moreover, long term compliance with drug therapy is far from satisfactory, either because of adverse effects or simply withdrawals.

The term "malignant NMS" characterizes patients with recurrent episodes with little or no prodrome, no recognizable triggers, marked bradycardia or asystole, and also older people whose abrupt faints are associated with important injuries. In certain circumstances, a small group of patients can be severely disabled, they may not be able to drive a car or perform a "potentially dangerous occupation". The individuals with this traumatic and recurrent form in whom physical injury or economic loss is a major concern, require careful clinical evaluation and a personal approach to treatment is mandatory.

Cardiac Pacing

The role of cardiac pacing for treatment of recurrent NMS remains controversial. Since patients with recurrent NMS are often resistant to medical treatment, permanent cardiac pacing has been proposed as an alternative long term therapy, and has become a valuable option when significant bradycardia is present. In fact, the usefulness of cardiac pacing, alone or in conjunction with drugs, for preventing symptoms, depends on the relative contribution of bradycardia to the hypotensive state. Equally critical is the ability of an implanted pacing system to recognize an imminent syncopal event and respond with an appropriately rate-drop response algorithm.

Clinical Trials

Several studies have evaluated the efficacy of pacemakers in the prevention of vasovagal episodes in the laboratory and clinical settings.

The first observational clinical experiments done with dual chamber pacing with rate-hysteresis (RH) or rate-drop response (RDR), showed an important reduction of symptoms between 80 and 92% during the follow-up period [3-4]. Pacemaker therapy was also able to reduce the positive HUT response performed after implantation [5].

The usefulness of DDI-RH versus DDD-RDR pacing [6] was compared on 20 patients with recurrent unexplained syncope, and a cardioinhibitory response to the HUT after one month of pharmacological treatment. After a mean follow-up of 17 months, the RDR group had lower syncopal recurrences, and most of them showed a negative HUT after the RDR pacemaker implant.

One of the first controlled randomized trials published was the VPS [7] that evaluated 54 patients with recurrent NMS and a positive HUT associated to a relative bradycardia. Timing of the first recurrence rises from 54 to 112 days ($p<0.0007$) with the use of RDR, and there was a relative risk reduction of 85.4% (70 vs. 22%, $p=0.00002$) in recurrence after the follow-up. In the VASIS trial [8], 42 patients were included and a benefit for patients with the RDR pacemaker was observed. Recurrence was 5% after a mean follow-up of 15 months compared with 61% after 5 months for patients with conventional drug therapy ($p=0.0006$). The Kaplan-Meier actuarial estimates of recurrence of syncope after 5 years were 6% in the RDR arm and 75% in the no pacemaker arm. The SYDIT study [9] compared medical treatment using beta-blockers with dual chamber RDR pacing, 93 patients were in follow-up for a mean of 1.4 years. The group assigned to RDR had a 4.3% recurrence after a mean of 390 days, and patients with beta-blockers showed a 25.5% recurrence after a mean of 135 days ($p=0.004$). Finally, the VPS-II [10] was the only double blind designed trial that compared DDD-RDR or sensing without pacing mode (ODO) in 100 patients. There was a 30% non significant relative risk reduction in the recurrence rate (42 vs. 33%) with the use of RDR.

Conclusions

Pacing for NMS should not be a first-line therapy, however, the main aspect for these individuals with this potentially disabling condition, is a need to reduce the frequency and severity of the attacks. In such a carefully selected population, correct tailoring of the pacemaker programming DDD-RDR can help the patient to recover his normal life activities.

Approximately 60% among this highly symptomatic, drug-refractory patients are expected to have another syncopal episode within one year, and require particular attention [11]. In such cases, pacing therapy with a RDR is probably a promising therapeutic option to reduce the incidence of potentially dangerous syncopal attacks. It has been demonstrated that RDR pacing markedly reduces the likelihood of recurrence and is more effective than pharmacological treatment with beta-blockers.

References

1. Lacroix D, Kouakam C, Klug D et al (1997) Asystolic cardiac arrest during Head-Up Tilt Test: incidence and therapeutic implications. PACE 20:2746-2754
2. Moya A, Brignole M, Menozzi C et al (2001) for the ISSUE Investigators. Mechanism of syncope in patients with isolated syncope and in patients with Tilt-positive syncope. Circulation 104:1261-1267
3. Petersen M, Chamberlain-Webber R, Fitzpatrick A et al (1994) Permanent pacing for cardioinhibitory malignant vasovagal syndrome. Br Heart J 71:274-281
4. Bendit D, Sutton R, Gammege M et al (1997) Clinical experience with Thera DR Rate-Drop Response pacing algorithm in carotid sinus syndrome and vasovagal syncope. PACE 20:832-839
5. Shah C, Thakur R, Xei B et al (1999) Dual chamber pacing for neurally mediated syncope with prominent cardioinhibitory component. PACE 22:999-1003
6. Ammirati F, Colivicchi F, Toscano S et al (1998) DDD pacing with rate drop response function versus DDI with rate hysteresis pacing for cardioinhibitory vasovagal Syncope. PACE 21:2178-2181
7. Connolly S, Sheldon R, Roberts R et al (1999) The North American Vasovagal Pacemaker Study (VPS). A randomised trial of permanent cardiac pacing for the prevention of vasovagal syncope. J Am Coll Cardiol 33:16-20
8. Sutton R, Brignole M, Menozzi C et al (2000) for the VASIS Investigators. Dual-Chamber pacing in the treatment of neurally mediated Tilt-Positive cardioinhibitory Syncope. Pacemaker versus no therapy: A multicenter randomised study. Circulation 102:294-299
9. Ammirati F, Colivicchi F, Santini M et al (2001) for the SYDIT Investigators. Permanent cardiac pacing versus medical treatment for the prevention of recurrent vasovagal syncope. A multicenter, randomized, controlled trial. Circulation 104:52-57
10. Connolly S, Sheldon R, Thorpe K et al (2003) Pacemaker therapy for prevention of syncope in patients with recurrent severe vasovagal syncope. JAMA 289:2224-2229
11. Sheldon R, Rose S, Flanagan P et al (1996) Multivariate predictors of syncope recurrence in drug-free patients following a positive tilt table test. Circulation 93:973-981

Patient-Activated Implantable Drug Pump for Treatment of Vasovagal Syncope: Is It Time for Clinical Use?

A. Raviele, F. Giada

Introduction

An implantable drug delivery system theoretically has a use in many arrhythmic situations, such as paroxysmal atrial fibrillation/atrial flutter, other supraventricular tachyarrhythmias, ventricular tachycardia, and vasovagal syncope. In this chapter the potential role of an implantable drug delivery system for treatment of vasovagal syncope is discussed.

The rationale for development of such a device is the following [1]. Vasovagal events, like many other autonomic nervous system disturbances, have a cyclic and unpredictable course with usually brief periods of symptom recrudescence (so-called clusters) alternating with sometimes very long periods of quiescence and asymptomatic status [2]. Thus, chronic therapy with drugs does not appear useful in the majority of cases and is often associated with significant or intolerable side effects as well as poor patient compliance, at least in young people [3]. Moreover, prevention of vasovagal reaction usually requires high drug plasma levels at the time of event occurrence that are difficult to reach with chronic oral administration [4]. As a matter of fact, drugs have only occasionally proved to be effective when evaluated in double-blind, randomized, placebo-controlled trials [5–9]. It is also noteworthy that electrical treatment with a pacemaker, even when effective, only rarely leads to complete elimination of symptoms [10–16], because of the hypotensive effects of the vasodepressor reflex that is present in practically all patients, generally precedes cardioinhibition, and is not amenable to correction or reversion by cardiac pacing [17–20].

For all these reasons, it seems logical and desirable to develop an implantable drug delivery system for treatment of vasovagal syncope. Such a device would allow the "on demand" delivery of a bolus of a vasoactive or cardioactive drug previously recognized to be able to abort vasovagal syncope,

Department of Cardiology, Umberto I Hospital, Mestre–Venice, Italy

possibly together with sequential pacing. However, there are a number of key issues to be addressed before implementation of such a device. They include the search for the most appropriate drug to be used for this purpose, the choice of a reliable marker of imminent vasovagal syncope, and the conception and building of the device. In order to afford these problems we planned an investigative study whose results are presented in this article.

Our research consisted of two parts [21, 22]. In the first part, we evaluated the efficacy and safety of phenylephrine (a fast-acting α-agonist agent with potent vasoconstrictor effect) as a potential drug to be used in a drug delivery system for treatment of vasovagal syncope; in the second part, we assessed the functioning during head-up tilt testing of an external prototype of a patient-activated drug delivery system that uses prodromal symptoms as a marker of imminent vasovagal syncope and phenylephrine as active drug.

Patient Population and Methods

A total of 27 patients were studied (26 women and 1 man, mean age 48 years), 17 of them during the first part of the study and 10 during the second part. The majority of these patients (78%) had no structural heart disease, whereas 6 patients (22%) had only mild hypertensive heart disease. All patients had frequently recurrent vasovagal syncopes (median number 20) with a median duration of symptoms of 10 years and with associated trauma in 50% of the cases. All were refractory to at least one drug chronically administered per os. Moreover, all patients had a reproducible positive response to at least two baseline head-up tilt tests performed according to the "Italian protocol" [22]: 20 min of upright tilt at 60° without medication plus 15 min after 400 μg of sublingual nitroglycerin spray. The type of response during baseline head-up tilt test was mixed in 13 cases (48%), vasodepressor in 10 cases (37%), and cardioinhibitory in 4 (15%).

Each patient underwent, after baseline evaluation, two other consecutive head-up tilt tests in the same day in a single patient-blind randomized fashion. In one a bolus of phenylephrine (1 mg in 1 ml of saline solution) was injected in the right atrium, through a catheter introduced via the right internal jugular vein, at the time the patient became symptomatic and blood pressure suddenly decreased by more than 50% compared to baseline values. In the other the same volume of placebo (1 ml of saline solution) was injected. During the first part of the study, carried out in 17 patients, drug and placebo were injected by the physician, using a syringe. In the second part of the study, carried out in 10 patients, phenylephrine and placebo were delivered by the patients themselves using an external modified version of a commercially available pharmacological pump (Algomed, Medtronic, Minneapolis, USA), at the time they experienced syncopal prodrome.

The Algomed system is a drug delivery system currently used for the delivery of pain-relieving drugs directly into the spinal area in patients with cancer or other painful diseases. The system consists of a drug reservoir connected to the control pad and the vascular catheter. For the present laboratory study, the catheter of the device was rendered suitable for the delivery of drug or placebo into the right cardiac chamber. The control pad consists of a reservoir fill port, a pumping chamber, and an activation valve. The patients must press the last two components to deliver a bolus of drug. During the test we disconnected the reservoir from the control pad and applied the control pad over the skin in the left subclavian region.

Results

All patients experienced a vasovagal reaction during both tilt tests, with phenylephrine and placebo injection. During the physician test, performed in 17 patients, phenylephrine administration led to an immediate raise of blood pressure in 15 cases, prevented syncope in 9 subjects, and restored consciousness in 6 subjects a few seconds after the injection, even though patients continued to be tilted up at the same angle. The efficacy of phenylephrine was 88%. In only 2 patients (12%) with severe cardioinhibitory response was the phenylephrine treatment unsuccessful. The drug was always well tolerated. In contrast, placebo did not prevent or abort syncope in any patient (efficacy=0%) and subjects had in all cases to be returned to the supine position for consciousness to be restored. The difference in efficacy between phenylephrine and placebo was highly significant ($p<0.001$). During the patient test, all 10 patients were able to perform appropriate activation of the drug delivery system at the time they experienced syncopal prodrome. The delivery of phenylephrine by means of the modified Algomed system was successful in avoiding or reversing tilt-induced syncope in every subject (efficacy=100%). The administration of placebo was not effective in any patient. Putting together the results of the physician test and the patient test, phenylephrine was successful in 25 cases (93%) and placebo in no case (0%)–a highly significant difference.

During the first part of the study, the mean values of systolic blood pressure, diastolic blood pressure, and heart rate at different times during the two head-up tilt tests performed with phenylephrine and placebo injection (with the patient in the supine position before tilt, just after start of tilt, at the onset of symptoms, and at the time of phenylephrine and placebo injection) were not significantly different. This suggests a similar extent of the vasovagal reaction during both tests. It is important to point out that the mean systolic blood pressure at the time of phenylephrine and placebo injection was quite low (about 60 mmHg) and that, at the same time, relative bradycardia was present compared to the time at which symptoms started (mean: 81–88 bpm vs 97 bpm). It is also noteworthy that the heart rate continued to decrease after phenylephrine injection (mean: from 81 to 68 bpm) as an expression of the activation of the baroreceptor reflex caused by the drug. Despite this, all patients but two fully recovered consciousness. The maximum values reached by systolic and diastolic blood pressure after phenylephrine injection were 176 and 100 mm Hg (mean), respectively. During the second part of the study, similar behavior of the mean values of systolic blood pressure, diastolic blood pressure and heart rate was observed.

In the physician test, the mean time between the onset of symptoms and the injection of phenylephrine or placebo did not differ significantly (69 s vs 59 s). After the injection of phenylephrine the drug effect started very soon (within 13±7 s) and all patients who recovered consciousness did it within a mean time of 32±17 s. The maximum effect of phenylephrine was observed after 90±35 s. The return to baseline values occurred in about 5 min. After the injection of placebo, the mean time for development of syncope was 32±23 s and tilt was stopped and patients returned to the supine position within 50±22 s. In the patient test, similar behavior was observed.

Conclusions

The results of this laboratory investigation led us to conclude that:

1. Phenylephrine is effective and safe in aborting tilt-induced syncope and may thus be proposed as an active drug in an implantable drug delivery system.
2. The prodromal symptoms are a reliable marker of imminent vasovagal syncope and may therefore be used as a "sensor" in a patient-activated drug delivery system.
3. The modified Algomed pump is an efficient prototype of a patient-activated drug delivery system for treatment of vasovagal syncope.

Obviously, further clinical studies are needed to confirm these laboratory results before implementing such a therapy in clinical practice.

References

1. Raviele A, Brignole M, Menozzi C et al (1997) Development of an implantable drug delivery system for the treatment of vasovagal syncope: a dream or a real prospect? In Raviele A (ed) Cardiac arrhythmias. Springer, Milan, pp 422–427
2. Sheldon R, Rose S, Flanagan P et al (1996) Risk factors for syncope recurrence after a positive tilt table test in patients with syncope. Circulation 93:973–981
3. Raviele A, Themistoclakis S, Gasparini G (1996) Drug treatment of vasovagal syncope. In: Blanc JJ, Benditt D, Sutton R (eds) Neurally mediated syncope: pathophysiology, investigations and treatment. Futura, Armonk, NY, pp 113–117
4. Kelly PA, Mann DE, Adler SW et al (1994) Low dose disopyramide often fails to prevent neurogenic syncope during head-up tilt testing. Pacing Clin Electrophysiol 11:1202–1206
5. Brignole M, Menozzi C, Gianfranchi L et al (1992) A controlled trial of acute and long-term medical therapy in tilt-induced neurally mediated syncope. Am J Cardiol 70:339–342

6. Morillo CA, Leicht JW, Yee R et al (1993) A placebo-controlled trial of intravenous and oral disopyramide for prevention of neurally mediated syncope induced by head-up tilt. J Am Coll Cardiol 22:1843–1848
7. Raviele A, Brignole M, Sutton R et al (1999) Effect of etilefrine in preventing syncopal recurrence in patients with vasovagal syncope. A double-blind, randomized, placebo-controlled trial. Circulation 99:1452–1457
8. Madrid AH, Ortega J, Rebollo J et al (2001) Lack of efficacy of atenolol for the prevention of neurally mediated syncope in a highly symptomatic population: a prospective, double-blind, randomized and placebo-controlled study. J Am Coll Cardiol 37:554–559
9. Flevari P, Livanis EG, Theodorakis G et al (2002) Vasovagal syncope: a prospective, randomized, crossover evaluation of the effect of propranolol, nadolol and placebo on syncope recurrence and patient's well-being. J Am Coll Cardiol 40:499–504
10. Petersen MEV, Chamberlain-Webber R, Fitzpatrick AP et al (1994) Permanent pacing for cardioinhibitory malignant vasovagal syndrome. Br Heart J 71:274–281
11. Benditt DG, Petersen M, Lurie KG et al (1995) Cardiac pacing for the prevention of recurrent vasovagal syncope. Ann Intern Med 122:204–209
12. Connolly SJ, Sheldon R, Roberts RS et al (1999) The North American Vasovagal Pacemaker Study (VPS): a randomized trial of permanent cardiac pacing for the prevention of vasovagal syncope. J Am Coll Cardiol 33:6–20
13. Sutton R, Brignole M, Menozzi C et al (2000) Dual-chamber pacing in the treatment of neurally mediated tilt-positive cardioinhibitory syncope. Pacemaker versus no therapy: a multicentre, randomized study. Circulation 102:294–299
14. Ammirati F, Colivicchi F, Santini M et al (2001) Permanent cardiac pacing versus medical treatment for the prevention of recurrent vasovagal syncope. Circulation 104:52–57
15. Connolly SJ, Sheldon R, Thorpe KE et al (2003) Pacemaker therapy for prevention of syncope in patients with recurrent severe vasovagal syncope (VPS II): a randomized trial. JAMA 289:2224–2229
16. Raviele A, Giada F, Menozzi C et al (2003) A randomized, double-blind, placebo-controlled study of permanent cardiac pacing for the treatment of recurrent tilt-induced vasovagal syncope. The Vasovagal Syncope and Pacing Trial (Synpace). Submitted for publication
17. Raviele A, Alboni P (1994) Syncope: an update on pathophysiology, diagnosis and therapy. G Ital Cardiol 24:1227–1260
18. Abboud FM (1986) Pathophysiology of hypotension and syncope. In: Hurst JW, Logue RB, Rackley CE et al (eds) The heart. Mc Graw-Hill, New York, pp 370–382
19. Sobel BE, Roberts R (1988) Hypotension and syncope. In: Braunwald E (ed) Heart disease. A textbook of cardiovascular medicine. Saunders, Philadelphia, pp 884–895
20. Benditt DG, Lurie KG, Adler SW (1995) Pathophysiology of neurally mediated syncope: peripheral and central mechanisms. In: Raviele A (ed) Cardiac arrhythmias. Springer, Berlin New York Milan, pp 102–109
21. Giada F, Raviele A, Gasparini G et al (2001) Efficacy of a patient-activated drug delivery system using phenylephrine as active drug in aborting tilt-induced syncope. Pacing Clin Electrophysiol 24:5 (abstract)
22. Raviele A, Giada F, Brignole M et al (2000) Comparison of diagnostic accuracy of sublingual nitroglycerin test and low-dose isoproterenol test in patients with unexplained syncope. Am J Cardiol 85:1194–1198

SICK SINUS SYNDROME:
CLINICAL ASPECTS AND PACING ISSUES

Genetics of Sinus Node Disease

E. Schulze-Bahr[1,2], D. Etzrodt[2], H. Wedekind[1,2], G. Breithardt[1,2], D. Isbrandt[3]

Introduction

Sinus node dysfunction (SND) is a major cause necessitating pacemaker implantation and accounts for approximately half of all patients requiring a pacemaker [1]. The term "sinus node dysfunction" is currently applied to a number of sinus nodal and atrial abnormalities that include persistent or intermittent sinus bradycardia, sinus node arrest or exit block, combined sinoatrial and atrioventricular conduction delay, and episodes of atrial tachyarrhythmias, sometimes together with periods of slow atrial and ventricular rates ("bradycardia-tachycardia syndrome"). Several of these ECG patterns can be often recorded in the same patient. The disease commonly occurs in adults with acquired heart disease, during antiarrhythmic therapy, or after surgically corrected congenital heart disease. In a significant portion of patients, however, SND appears in the absence of identifiable cardiac abnormalities or other associated conditions ("idiopathic" SND) [2]. A familial occurrence of idiopathic SND has been reported in some instances [3–5] and is also known for familial atrial fibrillation [2, 4, 5, 10].

These findings together with observations from twins suggest an important role for genetic factors in heart rate control [11]. As early as 1980, a publication by Havlik and coworkers, who investigated a large series of sets of male twins (n=355), reported findings suggesting that heart rate was under genetic control, by 54% of variation among individuals explained by heredity [12]. Later reports confirmed these findings and indicated a significant contribution of genetic effects on heart rate with a negligible contribution from common environmental effects [13–16]. In another large cohort of siblings of the Framingham study, heritability of heart rate and heart rate variability was assessed to estimate the contribution of genetic factors to their variance. After adjustment for covariation, it was estimated that even in the general popula-

[1]Department of Cardiology and Angiology, Hospital of the University of Münster, Münster; [2]Institute for Arteriosclerosis Research at the University of Münster, Molecular Cardiology, Münster; [3]Institute for Neural Signal Transmission, ZMNH, University of Hamburg, Germany

tion genetic factors may account for 13% –23% of the variation among heart rate and heart rate variability measurements [17]. Since signaling through the β_1-adrenergic receptor is one important determinant of heart rate regulation by the autonomous nervous system, Ranade and coworkers tested whether polymorphisms in the ADBR1 gene encoding this receptor are associated with resting heart rate. They reported that the 49G allele of the S49G polymorphism was significantly associated (p=0.0004) with resting heart rate, independently of other variables [18]. The data supported an additive model in which individuals heterozygous for the Ser49Gly polymorphism had mean heart rates intermediate to those of either type of homozygote, with Ser homozygotes having the highest mean heart rate and Gly homozygotes having the lowest, and thereby provided the first support for a link between common genetic variation and heart rate [18].

Pathophysiology of Sinus Node Activity

The sinoatrial node (SAN), located in the right atrial (RA) roof, is the physiological pacemaker in the human heart and is predominantly responsible for autonomous heart beat generation. The SAN has action potentials with a relatively positive maximum diastolic potential (≈–50 mV), a small phase-0 upstroke velocity (<2 V/s), and prominent phase-4 depolarization maintaining SAN pacemaker dominance. Since the SAN is composed of heterogeneous cells, action potential durations differ in the various regions of the SAN, being longest in the central zone to preserve SAN predominance. Pacemaking activity depends on a phase of spontaneous slow membrane depolarization that occurs between cardiac action potentials (phase 4, i.e., during diastole). Several time-dependent ionic currents apparently contribute to the course and slope of diastolic membrane depolarizations (Fig. 1). During phase 4, the "pacemaker current" I_f, an inward cationic (nonselective) current, and the L-type Ca^{2+} current (I_{CaL}), T-type Ca^{2+} current (I_{CaT}), and delayed rectifier K^+ current (I_K) are key currents that influence pacemaking activity. The maximum diastolic potential is potentially regulated by the background K^+ current I_{K1} and the transient outward current I_{to} [19], at least in the SAN of the guinea pig's heart. I_{CaL} underlies the action potential upstroke in the central SAN, whereas the Na^+ current I_{Na} has been proposed to contribute to subsidiary pacemaker activity in peripheral regions of SAN [20].

Heart rate control is achieved through control of SAN pacemaking by the autonomic nervous system: cholinergic or β-adrenergic stimulation either slows or accelerates the spontaneous SAN activity through regulation of the I_f and I_{CaL} currents [21]. β-Adrenergic stimulation positively shifts the voltage dependence of I_f activation, thereby accelerating diastolic depolarization [22–24]. Similarly, adrenergically induced increases in I_{CaL} conductance also enhance SAN phase-4 terminal depolarization [25, 26]. Conversely, a decrease

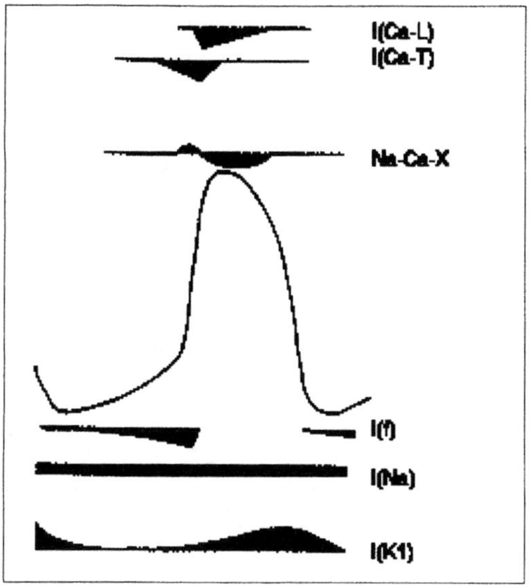

Fig. 1. SAN action potential and contributing ionic currents

in cellular cAMP levels (e.g., during muscarinic stimulation) leads to a decrease in I_f channel activity and thereby slows the heart rate. In addition, acetylcholine also activates the acetylcholine-sensitive K^+ current (I_{KACh}) and reduces I_{CaL} [25]. The particular activity of the hyperpolarization-activated nonselective cationic current I_f is cAMP-regulated, which involves direct interaction of cAMP with the cyclic nucleotide-binding domain (cNBD) of I_f channels and elicits a positive shift in the voltage dependence of I_f channel activation accompanied by an increase in current amplitude [22–24]. Abundance of the cNBD, either during introduced mutagenesis [27–30] or due to a naturally occurring mutation [31], indicates that the C-terminus of HCN channels makes an important contribution to the regulation of voltage- and cAMP-dependent channel gating and is associated with reduced I_f-mediated currents after cAMP stimulation.

Inherited Sinus Node Dysfunction

In 1960, Bacos and coworkers presented a family in which nine members of three generations exhibited an autosomal dominantly inherited form of nodal rhythm with bradycardia that tended to manifest paroxysms of atrial fibrillation in the fourth decade of life. Surawicz et al. published a follow-up of this family in 1988 [32, 33]. As previously predicted, affected individuals in subsequent generations had a slow heart rate with regular rhythm from birth, and developed intermittent atrial fibrillation with established atrial fibrillation requiring chronic treatment later. Some members of the third and fourth generations suffered from more symptomatic bradycardia at a younger age than their parents, which in some cases led to pacemaker implantation. Sudden death, presumably of cardiac origin, had occurred in one member of the third generation. Additional families were reported by Spellberg in 1971 [3], and Caralis and Varghese in 1976 [34]. Familial disorder of the sinoatrial node was also described by Nordenberg et al. in 1976 [35] and by Mackintosh and Chamberlain in 1979 [5, 36]. More often the sinus node abnormality is associated with conduction disturbances at the AV junction or in the distal conduction system. Lehmann and Klein in 1978 estimated that 2%–6% of cases that go by the jargonish term "sick sinus syndrome" (SSS) are inherited [4, 37]. In the family reported by Lehmann and Klein [4], mental retardation was associated. In another (rare) family case, brachydactyly was codominantly inherited. Ruiz de la Fuente and Prieto in 1980 described a new form of the heart–hand syndrome in three generations of a Spanish family with several instances of male-to-male transmission [38]. The hand abnormality was brachydactyly of subtype C, while the cardiac defect was intraventricular conduction defect in three individuals and sick sinus syndrome in one. Taken together, in some instances families are known with a congenital form of SND that is predominantly inherited in an autosomal dominant manner.

It is likely that slow and/or fast hyperpolarization-activated pacemaker (I_f) currents represent key determinants of spontaneous diastolic depolarization in the SAN. The fast component of I_f is most likely HCN2 and the slow, channel-dependent component HCN4 [39]. *HCN* genes have been suggested as candidates underlying disorders of heartbeat generation [40], since they are the molecular components of I_f ("pacemaker") channels [41]. Two of the four known genes encoding HCN channel subunits [39,42–44], *HCN2* and *HCN4*, are predominantly expressed in the heart [45]. We previously investigated the *HCN2* gene as a candidate for SND. However, we did not find *HCN2* gene mutations in a study population with "idiopathic" SND. In one of the index patients, however, who was characterized by sinus bradycardia at rest and chronotropic incompetence, a heterozygous 1-bp deletion mutation was detected that gave rise to a C-terminally truncated HCN4 protein (HCN4–573X) lacking the C-terminal cNBD domain [31]. The identified mutation eliminates the functionally important cNBD in the derived HCN4 subunit sequence due to a truncation of the C-terminus. Our in vitro expression data strongly support the notion that the patient suffered from SND due to the expression of mutant HCN4 channels, which are insensitive to intracellular cAMP and have altered activation and deactivation properties. Chronotropic incompetence is likely to occur when I_f channels cannot respond to increases in intracellular cAMP concentrations during β-adrenergic stimulation. The sinus bradycardia observed under resting conditions, on the other hand, might be explained by the altered deactivation kinetics of HCN4–573X channels; due to the extremely slow activation kinetics of HCN4 channels, cumulative current activation during repetitive heartbeat cycles, as demonstrated for KCNQ1 channels, might occur. Faster closure (deactivation) of I_f channels during sinus nodal action potentials may therefore decrease channel availability in the subsequent cycle, thereby slowing heart rate [31].

For familial atrial standstill, too, a genetic basis is now known. This is a rare arrhythmia that occasionally appears to be genetically determined. Criteria for the diagnosis of atrial standstill include absence of P waves on electrocardiogram, lack of response to atrial stimulation of the atria, and absence of an a wave in the jugular venous pulse and in the right atrial pressure pulse. Candidate gene screening revealed a novel mutation in the cardiac sodium channel gene *SCN5A* (D1275N) in a small family with autosomal dominant atrial standstill [46]. In addition, two closely linked polymorphisms were detected within regulatory regions of the gene for the atrial-specific gap junction protein connexin40 (Cx40) at nucleotides –44 (G→A) and +71 (A→G). Eight relatives were homozygous for both polymorphisms, which occurred in only approximately 7% of control subjects, and three of these relatives were affected by atrial standstill. The three living patients with atrial standstill exclusively coinherited both the rare Cx40 genotype and the SCN5A-D1275N mutation. It has been suggested that this rare Cx40 genotype is associated with a reduction in reporter gene assay when compared with the more common Cx40 genotype, and thus both the concurrence of a cardiac sodium channel mutation and rare polymorphisms in the atrial-specific Cx40 gene were responsible for the phenotype [46].

Patients with long QT syndrome of subtype 3 (linked to the cardiac sodium channel *SCN5A*), a heterogeneous disorder causing syncope and sudden death from ventricular arrhythmias, may also have intermittent signs of SND; in a large family reported by Grant et al. [47], some patients were characterized by an overlapping phenotype of Brugada syndrome, long QT-3 syndrome, and conduction system disease. In particular, one patient had atrioventricular block and sinus arrests, most likely as a consequence of conduction disease at the atrial level. Among the 25 affected patients (21 adults and 4 children) included in the study of the large French kindred, the average rate-corrected QT interval was 490 ms (for adults) and 465 ms (for children) compared with 380 ms and 403 ms in unaffected individuals. Sinus node bradycardia or junctional escape rhythm was diagnosed in all patients with LQT4. Episodes of atrial fibrillation were diagnosed in 12 adult patients but were absent during childhood. Positive linkage was obtained for markers located on chromosome 4q25–27. Very recently, it became clear that the gene linked with this peculiar phenotype is caused by an anchoring protein (*AnkyB*) gene mutation (E1425G). Since the initial description, Mohler et al. [48] reported that eight additional individuals had been born, of whom four carried the LQT4 haplotype. Sinus node abnormalities were diagnosed in utero in all affected members of the recent generation [48]. The mutation in ankyrin-B resulted in disruption in the cellular organization of the sodium pump, the sodium/calcium exchanger, and inositol-1,4,5-triphosphate receptors (all ankyrin-B-binding proteins), which reduced the targeting of these proteins to the transverse tubules as well as reducing the overall protein level. Ankyrin-B mutation also led to altered calcium ion signaling in adult cardiomyocytes that resulted in extrasystoles and provided a rationale for the arrhythmia. In this way, a novel mechanism for cardiac arrhythmia (with a broad phenotypic spectrum) due to abnormal coordination of multiple functionally related ion channels and transporters was reported for the first time [48].

Inherited Sinus Node Dysfunction in the Setting of Other Diseases

In addition to isolated forms of SND, a variety of cardiac and extracardiac disorders are known to be inherited and associated with SND. Especially for cardiomyopathies, the occurrence of arrhythmia may be the first sign of cardiac disease.

Familial hypertrophic cardiomyopathy (HOCM) with Wolff–Parkinson–White syndrome can be caused by mutation in the γ2 regulatory subunit of AMP-activated protein kinase (PRKAG2) [49, 50], potentially a glycogen storage disease [51], as well as the cardiac troponin I gene (TNNI3). Blair et al. [49] described mutations in PRKAG2, encoding the γ2 subunit of AMP-activated protein kinase (AMPK), in two families with severe HCM and Wolff–Parkinson–White syndrome in some affected individuals [49]. The mutations, one missense and one inframe single codon insertion, occur in highly conserved regions. Because AMPK provides a central sensing mechanism that protects cells from exhaustion of ATP supplies, the authors proposed that energy compromise may provide a unifying pathogenic mechanism in all forms of HCM. Reports that dominant mutations in PRKAG2, an enzyme that modulates glucose uptake and glycolysis, can cause HCM challenged the hypothesis that it is a disease only of the sarcomere. In addition to cardiac hypertrophy, individuals with PRKAG2 mutations frequently manifest electrophysiological abnormalities, particularly Wolff–Parkinson–White syndrome [50], atrial fibrillation, and progressive development of sinoatrial and/or atrioventricular conduction block. Although atrial fibrillation is common in HCM patients and becomes increasingly prevalent with disease duration, neither accessory pathway nor conduction system diseases are typical features of HCM. Thus, this disorder is a metabolic storage disease, in which hypertrophy, ventricular preexcitation, and conduction system defects coexist [51, 52].

Dilated cardiomyopathy (DCM) is a common disorder characterized by cardiac dilation and reduced systolic function that may uncommonly be associated with sinus node dysfunction in a familial manner [53]. Olson and Keating performed a general linkage approach to localize the disease gene in a large family with this phenotype. Linkage to chromosome 3p22–p25 was identified with a highly significant lod score of 6.09. So far, the gene for DCM associated with rhythm and conduction abnormalities is unknown in an approximately 30-cM candidate region. Although in arrhythmogenic right ventricular cardiomyopathy, a genetically determined cardiomyopathy involving primarily the right ventricle [54], a case with abnormalities of the sinus node, right atrium, and atrioventricular node was reported that, after careful investigation of biopsies taken from the right atrium, suggested that pathological changes may also extend into the atrium and atrioventricular node, thereby causing supraventricular rhythm disturbances [55].

Cardiac amyloidosis is part of a disease complex that results from deposition of unique twisted B-pleated sheet fibrils formed from various proteins by several different pathogenic mechanisms. Familial amyloidosis, inherited as an autosomal dominant trait, results from the production of a variant prealbumin protein termed transthyretin. More than 50 different point mutations have been described so far in the transthyretin (TTR) gene, and disease occurs in one of three clinical presentations: progressive neuropathy, cardiomyopathy, or nephropathy. Involvement of the heart is a common finding and is the most frequent cause of death in amyloidosis, predominantly in men; it is rare before the age of 30 years. Involvement of the cardiovascular system in amyloidosis can be most commonly found in the form of a restrictive cardiomyopathy, congestive heart failure due to systolic dysfunction, orthostatic hypotension, and/or abnormalities of cardiac impulse formation and conduction, e.g., atrial standstill due to atrial amyloid infiltration. Allensworth et al. [56] described three sibs below the age of 40 years with bradycardia, cardiac enlargement, and congestive heart failure. The electrocardiogram showed absent P waves with normal QRS configuration and duration. Stimulation of the atrium with a cardiac catheter or a pacemaker did not induce atrial depolarization.

Autosomal dominant Emery–Dreifuss muscular dystrophy (EDMD) and other forms of neuromuscular disorders may have electrophysiological abnormalities of the atria and atrioventricular node, and of infranodal conduction [57]. Patients with EDMD have a relatively high susceptibility to induced atrial flutter or fibrillation during electrophysiological studies, together with less frequent evidence of abnormal sinus node function and abnormal atrioventricular nodal or infranodal conduction. Atrial standstill is the unusual, potentially unique arrhythmia that sometimes occurs in EDMD patients. As an isolated disorder, partial or permanent atrial standstill has been reported in adults, rarely in children, and occasionally in families [58–60]. Classic Emery–Dreifuss muscular dystrophy is chromosome X-linked, and the genetic defect resides in the gene encoding emerin, a type II integral nuclear membrane protein that extends into the nucleoplasm from a transmembrane domain spanning the inner nuclear membrane [61]. By genetic linkage analysis, it became clear that even EDMD is genetically heterogeneous. Bonne et al. [62] identified the second locus for autosomal dominant EDMD on chromosome 1q11–q23 in a large French family by demonstrating mutations in the lamin A/C gene (LMNA) gene [62]. The LMNA protein is a component of the nuclear lamina, a fibrous layer on the nucleoplasmic side of the inner nuclear membrane thought to provide a framework for the nuclear envelope.

Conclusions

SND in absence of other cardiac disease ("idiopathic SND") is in part genetically determined and, especially in patients for whom this is the case, the family history may reveal other affected family members. The exact number of patients with idiopathic disease harboring gene mutations is unknown to date, since only a fraction of causative genes are known. In a variety of cardiomyopathies and neuromuscular disorders with a genetic background, SND may also occur in a familial manner and the arrhythmia may sometimes proceed to other clinical manifestations.

References

1. Lamas GA, Lee K, Sweeney M et al (2000) The mode selection trial (MOST) in sinus node dysfunction: design, rationale, and baseline characteristics of the first 1000 patients. Am Heart J 140:541–551
2. Sarachek NS, Leonard JL (1972) Familial heart block and sinus bradycardia. Classification and natural history. Am J Cardiol 29:451–458
3. Spellberg RD (1971) Familial sinus node disease. Chest 60:246–251
4. Lehmann H, Klein UE (1978) Familial sinus node dysfunction with autosomal dominant inheritance. Br Heart J 40:1314–1316
5. Mackintosh AF, Chamberlain DA (1979) Sinus node disease affecting both parents and both children. Eur J Cardiol 10:117–122
6. Beyer F, Paul T, Luhmer I, Bertram H, Kallfelz HC (1993) [Familial idiopathic atrial fibrillation with bradyarrhythmia. In German]. Z Kardiol 82:674–677
7. Brugada R, Tapscott T, Czernuszewicz GZ et al (1997) Identification of a genetic locus for familial atrial fibrillation. N Engl J Med 336:905–911
8. Chen YH, Xu SJ, Bendahhou S et al (2003) KCNQ1 gain-of-function mutation in familial atrial fibrillation. Science 299:251–254
9. Ellinor PT, Shin JT, Moore RK, Yoerger DM, MacRae CA (2003) Locus for atrial fibrillation maps to chromosome 6q14–16. Circulation 107:2880–2883
10. Bertram H, Paul T, Beyer F, Kallfelz HC (1996) Familial idiopathic atrial fibrillation with bradyarrhythmia. Eur J Pediatr 155:7–10
11. Van Hulle CA, Corley R, Zahn-Waxler C, Kagan J, Hewitt JK (2000) An exploration of the genetic and environmental etiology of heart rate in infancy and middle childhood. Twin Res 3:259–265
12. Havlik RJ, Garrison RJ, Fabsitz R, Feinleib M (1980) Variability of heart rate, P–R, QRS and Q–T durations in twins. J Electrocardiol 13:45–48
13. Hanson B, Tuna N, Bouchard T et al (1989) Genetic factors in the electrocardiogram and heart rate of twins reared apart and together. Am J Cardiol 63:606–609
14. Degaute JP, Van Cauter E, van de BP, Linkowski P (1994) Twenty-hour-hour blood pressure and heart rate profiles in humans. A twin study. Hypertension 23:244–253
15. Voss A, Busjahn A, Wessel N et al (1996) Familial and genetic influences on heart rate variability. J Electrocardiol 29(Suppl):154–160
16. Russell MW, Law I, Sholinsky P, Fabsitz RR (1998) Heritability of ECG measurements in adult male twins. J Electrocardiol 30(Suppl):64–68
17. Singh JP, Larson MG, O'Donnell CJ et al (1999) Heritability of heart rate variability: the Framingham Heart Study. Circulation 99:2251–2254

18. Ranade K, Jorgenson E, Sheu WH et al (2002) A polymorphism in the beta1 adrenergic receptor is associated with resting heart rate. Am J Hum Genet 70:935–942
19. Guo J, Mitsuiye T, Noma A (1997) The sustained inward current in sino-atrial node cells of guinea-pig heart. Pflugers Arch 433:390–396
20. Kodama I, Nikmaram MR, Boyett MR et al (1997) Regional differences in the role of the Ca2+ and Na+ currents in pacemaker activity in the sinoatrial node. Am J Physiol 272:H2793–H2806
21. Schram G, Pourrier M, Melnyk P, Nattel S (2002) Differential distribution of cardiac ion channel expression as a basis for regional specialization in electrical function. Circ Res 90:939–950
22. Brown HF, DiFrancesco D, Noble SJ (1979) How does adrenaline accelerate the heart? Nature 280:235–236
23 DiFrancesco D, Tortora P (1991) Direct activation of cardiac pacemaker channels by intracellular cyclic AMP. Nature 351:145–147
24. DiFrancesco D, Tromba C (1988) Inhibition of the hyperpolarization-activated current (if) induced by acetylcholine in rabbit sino-atrial node myocytes. J Physiol (Lond) 405:477–491
25. Irisawa H (1987) Membrane currents in cardiac pacemaker tissue. Experientia 43:1131–1135
26. DiFrancesco D (1993) Pacemaker mechanisms in cardiac tissue. Annu Rev Physiol 55:455–472
27. Wang J, Chen S, Siegelbaum SA (2001) Regulation of hyperpolarization-activated HCN channel gating and cAMP modulation due to interactions of COOH terminus and core transmembrane regions. J Gen Physiol 118:237–250
28. Wang J, Chen S, Nolan MF, Siegelbaum SA (2002) Activity-dependent regulation of HCN pacemaker channels by cyclic AMP: signaling through dynamic allosteric coupling. Neuron 36:451–461
29. Wainger BJ, DeGennaro M, Santoro B, Siegelbaum SA, Tibbs GR (2001) Molecular mechanism of cAMP modulation of HCN pacemaker channels. Nature 411:805–810
30. Viscomi C, Altomare C, Bucchi A et al (2001) C terminus-mediated control of voltage and cAMP gating of hyperpolarization-activated cyclic nucleotide-gated channels. J Biol Chem 276:29930–29934
31. Schulze-Bahr E, Neu A, Friederich P et al (2003) Pacemaker channel dysfunction in a patient with sinus node disease. J Clin Invest 111:1537–1545
32. Surawicz B, Hariman RJ (1988) Follow-up of the family with congenital absence of sinus rhythm. Am J Cardiol 61:467–469
33. Bharati S, Surawicz B, Vidaillet HJ Jr, Lev M (1992) Familial congenital sinus rhythm anomalies: clinical and pathological correlations. Pacing Clin Electrophysiol 15:1720–1729
34. Caralis DG, Varghese PJ (1976) Familial sinoatrial node dysfunction. Increased vagal tone a possible aetiology. Br Heart J 38:951–956
35. Nordenberg A, Varghese PJ, Nugent EW (1976) Spectrum of sinus node dysfunction in two siblings. Am Heart J 91:507–512
36. Mackintosh AF (1981) Sinoatrial disease in young people. Br Heart J 45:62–66
37. Lehmann H, Klein UE (1977) [Familial sinoatrial and atrioventricular arrhythmia causing an emergency case (author's trans)]. Med Klin 72:1379–1385
38. Ruiz dlF, Prieto F (1980) Heart-hand syndrome. III. A new syndrome in three generations. Hum Genet 55:43–47
39. Seifert R, Scholten A, Gauss R et al (1999) Molecular characterization of a slowly gating human hyperpolarization-activated channel predominantly expressed in thalamus, heart, and testis. Proc Natl Acad Sci USA 96:9391–9396

40. Ludwig A, Zong X, Hofmann F, Biel M (1999) Structure and function of cardiac pacemaker channels. Cell Physiol Biochem 9:179–186
41. Kaupp UB, Seifert R (2001) Molecular diversity of pacemaker ion channels. Annu Rev Physiol 63:235–257
42. Santoro B, Liu DT, Yao H et al (1998) Identification of a gene encoding a hyperpolarization-activated pacemaker channel of brain. Cell 93:717–729
43. Ludwig A, Zong X, Stieber J et al (1999) Two pacemaker channels from human heart with profoundly different activation kinetics. EMBO J 18:2323–2329
44. Vaccari T, Moroni A, Rocchi M et al (1999) The human gene coding for HCN2, a pacemaker channel of the heart. Biochim Biophys Acta 1446:419–425
45. Shi W, Wymore R, Yu H et al (1999) Distribution and prevalence of hyperpolarization-activated cation channel (HCN) mRNA expression in cardiac tissues. Circ Res 85:e1–e6
46. Groenewegen WA, Firouzi M, Bezzina CR et al (2003) A cardiac sodium channel mutation cosegregates with a rare connexin40 genotype in familial atrial standstill. Circ Res 92:14–22
47. Grant AO, Carboni MP, Neplioueva V et al (2002) Long QT syndrome, Brugada syndrome, and conduction system disease are linked to a single sodium channel mutation. J Clin Invest 110:1201–1209
48. Mohler PJ, Schott JJ, Gramolini AO et al (2003) Ankyrin-B mutation causes type 4 long-QT cardiac arrhythmia and sudden cardiac death. Nature 421:634–639
49. Blair E, Redwood C, Ashrafian H et al (2001) Mutations in the gamma(2) subunit of AMP-activated protein kinase cause familial hypertrophic cardiomyopathy: evidence for the central role of energy compromise in disease pathogenesis. Hum Mol Genet 10:1215–1220
50. Gollob MH, Green MS, Tang AS, Roberts R (2002) PRKAG2 cardiac syndrome: familial ventricular preexcitation, conduction system disease, and cardiac hypertrophy. Curr Opin Cardiol 17:229–234
51. Arad M, Benson DW, Perez-Atayde AR et al (2002) Constitutively active AMP kinase mutations cause glycogen storage disease mimicking hypertrophic cardiomyopathy. J Clin Invest 109:357–362
52. Gollob MH (2003) Glycogen storage disease as a unifying mechanism of disease in the PRKAG2 cardiac syndrome. Biochem Soc Trans 31:228–231
53. Olson TM, Keating MT (1996) Mapping a cardiomyopathy locus to chromosome 3p22–p25. J Clin Invest 97:528–532
54. Paul M, Schulze-Bahr E, Breithardt G, Wichter T (2003) Genetics of arrhythmogenic right ventricular cardiomyopathy–status quo and future perspectives. Z Kardiol 92:128–136
55. Nogami A, Adachi S, Nitta J et al (1990) Arrhythmogenic right ventricular dysplasia with sick sinus syndrome and atrioventricular conduction disturbance. Jpn Heart J 31:417–423
56. Allensworth DC, Rice GJ, Lowe GW (1969) Persistent atrial standstill in a family with myocardial disease. Am J Med 47:775–784
57. Hopkins LC, Jackson JA, Elsas LJ (1981) Emery-Dreifuss humeroperoneal muscular dystrophy: an X-linked myopathy with unusual contractures and bradycardia. Ann Neurol 10:230–237
58. Woolliscroft J, Tuna N (1982) Permanent atrial standstill: the clinical spectrum. Am J Cardiol 49:2037–2041
59. Ward DE, Ho SY, Shinebourne EA (1984) Familial atrial standstill and inexcitability in childhood. Am J Cardiol 53:965–967

60. Shah MK, Subramanyan R, Tharakan J, Venkitachalam CG, Balakrishnan KG (1992) Familial total atrial standstill. Am Heart J 123:1379–1382
61. Bione S, Maestrini E, Rivella S et al (1994) Identification of a novel X-linked gene responsible for Emery–Dreifuss muscular dystrophy. Nat Genet 8:323–327
62. Bonne G, Di Barletta MR, Varnous S et al (1999) Mutations in the gene encoding lamin A/C cause autosomal dominant Emery–Dreifuss muscular dystrophy. Nat Genet 21:285–288

Sleep Apnea: New Insights

M.G. Bongiorni[1], G. Giannola[1], E. Gronchi[1], E. Soldati[1], G. Arena[1], E. Hoffmann[2], M. Mariani[1]

Sleep apnea is the most common disorder of breathing during sleep. It is defined as repeated episodes of obstructive apnea and hypopnea during sleep, together with daytime sleepiness or altered cardiopulmonary function [1]. There are three syndromes of upper airway closure during sleep: obstructive sleep apnea (OSA), obstructive sleep hypopnea, and upper airway resistance. These three syndromes share two features: excessive daytime sleepiness and arousal associated with increased ventilatory effort in response to upper airway closure. The specific sites of narrowing or closure and upper airway dysfunction are influenced by the underlying neuromuscular tone, upper airway muscle synchrony, and the stage of sleep. Sleep apnea may be classified as two major forms: obstructive sleep apnea and central sleep apnea (CSA). Heart failure (HF) affects about 5 million people in the USA [2], and the largest epidemiologic studies in patients with HF found rates of prevalence of OSA of 37% and 11% respectively [3, 4]. Thus, OSA and CSA have a heavy impact on the health of these patients and on public health resources.

The pathophysiology of OSA [5] is shown in Figs. 1 and 2. During OSA, the effort against the occluded pharynx leads to a reduction of intrathoracic pressure. This reduction has three consequences: increases in left ventricular (LV) transmural pressure, in myocardial oxygen demand, and in venous return. The increased venous return leads to right ventricular (RV) distention, leftward shift of the interventricular septum, reduction of LV filling preload, and a consequent reduction in stroke volume. In addition, the increased LV transmural pressure results in a reduction of stroke volume through an increase of the LV afterload.

Apnea also stimulates the pulmonary stretch receptors, with a consequent increase in sympathetic nervous system activity that leads to an increase in heart rate, decrease in heart rate variability, vasoconstriction, and an increase in peripheral resistance and blood pressure with loss of vagal tone. The apnea

[1]Cardiothoracic Department, Cisanello Hospital, University of Pisa; [2]Division of Cardiology, Policlinic Hospital, University of Palermo, Italy

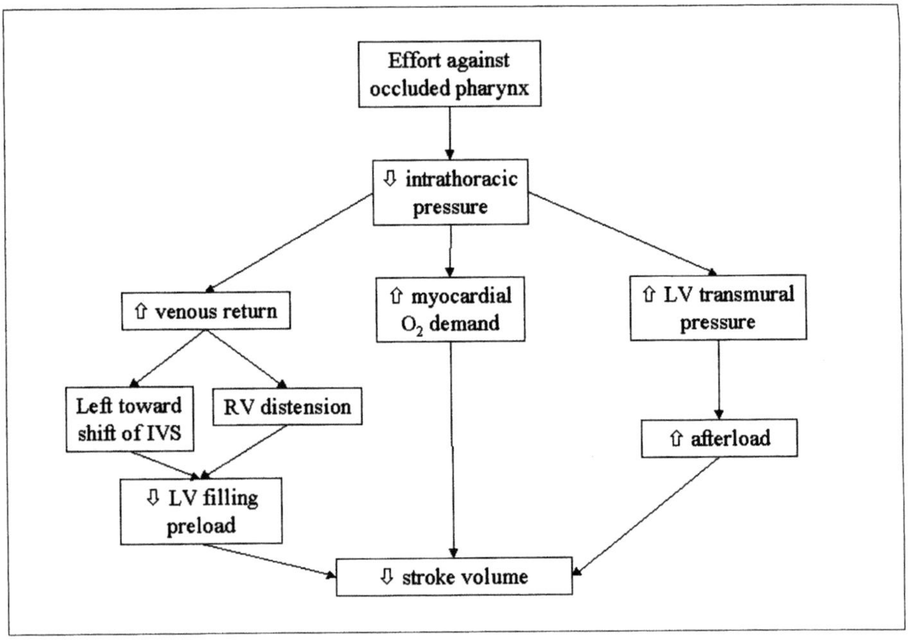

Fig. 1. Pathophysiology of OSA. *LV*, left ventricle; *RV*, right ventricle; *IVS*, interventricular septum

also causes hypoxia and hypercapnia and further augments sympathetic nervous system activity by stimulating peripheral and central chemoreceptors. All these features lead to myocardial ischemia, myocyte necrosis and apoptosis, arrhythmias, hypertrophy, failure, and increased mortality rates.

There is increasing evidence that inflammatory mediators such as C-reactive protein [6], oxidative stress [7], and vascular endothelial dysfunction [8] play important roles. In a great number of HF patients, OSA may play a role in the pathogenesis and progression of HF.

CSA is associated with Cheyne–Stokes respiration, a kind of periodic breathing in which central apneas and hypopneas alternate with periods of hyperventilation. Unlike OSA, CSA probably arises as a *consequence* of HF and should alert clinicians to the need to increase HF therapy.

The pathophysiology of CSA in HF [9] is outlined in Fig. 3. In HF patients, the pulmonary congestion stimulates pulmonary vagal irritant receptors, causing chronic hyperventilation and hypocapnia below the threshold level and apnea. Apnea, hypoxia, CO_2 retention, and arousal provoke periodic elevations in sympathetic activity (Fig. 2).

The main clinical significance of CSA in HF is the association with increased mortality [10], but there is no evidence that CSA may adversely influence HF or that it is a feature of poor cardiac function. From the pathophysiology it is easy to understand the greater risk of progression of myocardial failure, arrhythmias, and premature mortality. In a recent study it was

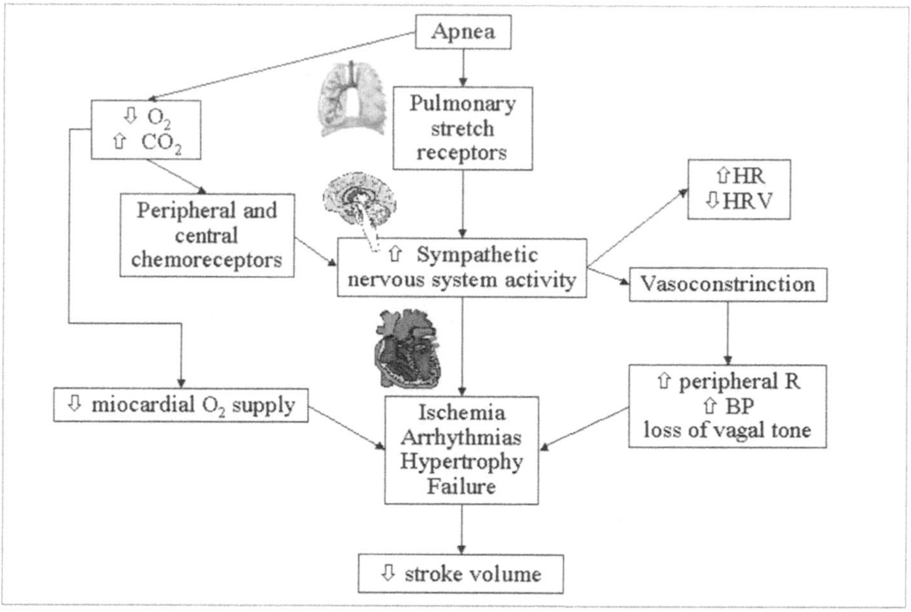

Fig. 2. Pathophysiology of OSA. *HR*, heart rate; *HRV*, heart rate variability; *R*, resistance; *BP*, blood pressure

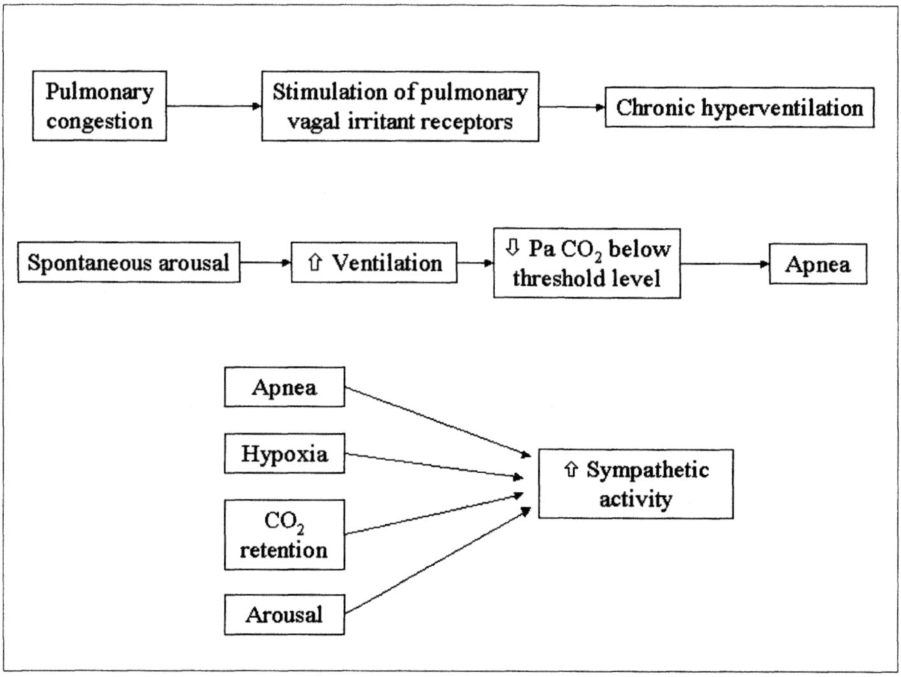

Fig. 3. Pathophysiology of CSA in HF

demonstrated that the ventilatory response to exercise is significantly augmented in HF patients with CSA compared with those without [11].

The treatments and the indications for treatment in the management of OSA in patients with HF remain to be established. General issues include weight reduction and abstinence from alcohol and sedatives, which predispose to pharyngeal collapse during sleep. Several studies support the use of continuous positive airway pressure (CPAP) via a nasal mask [12, 13]. CPAP alleviates OSA, improves sleep quality, reduces daytime sleepiness, augments neurocognitive function, lowers nocturnal and daytime blood pressure [14], reduces nocturnal and daytime sympathetic nervous system activity, increases heart rate variability, increases arterial baroreflex sensitivity, prevents recurrent hypoxia, reduces oxidative stress, increases endothelial-derived nitric oxide, and improves endothelially mediated vasodilation. Data to date support the use of CPAP only for patients with symptomatic OSA [15–17]. Mandibular advancement devices and surgical procedures (uvulopalatopharingoplasty and uvulopalatoplasty) are less effective [18–20].

A recent preliminary study [21] demonstrated that there is a high association between *Helicobacter pylori* infection and obstructive sleep apnea. This information may be important for future treatment strategies of the disease.

At present there is no consensus about how to treat CSA or indeed whether to treat it. What is certainly important is to treat the HF aggressively with diuretics, angiotensin-converting enzyme inhibitors, and ß-blockers. The next step is nocturnal supplemental oxygen and then the use of CPAP. This increases stroke volume and decreases LV afterload, preload, and cardiac sympathetic activity. In a recent study [22], Garrigue et al. evaluated the effect of using cardiac pacing to increase heart rate during sleep in 15 patients with CSA or OSA who had a cardiac pacemaker for symptomatic sinus bradycardia. All patients underwent three polysomnographic evaluations on consecutive nights (baseline and randomly spontaneous rhythm or dual chamber pacing mode with atrial overdrive) to analyze total duration and number of episodes of OSA and CSA. The overdrive pacing significantly reduced the number of episodes of OSA and CSA by more than 50%, reduced the number of arousals, and increased arterial oxyhemoglobin saturation without altering total sleep time. All these features returned to baseline when the pacemaker was turned off. Apnea is associated with hypoxemia, hypercapnia, bradycardia, and hypotension associated with increased vagal tone and variations in heart rate. The authors speculated that atrial pacing at high rate may counteract the enhanced vagal tone and may prevent the apnea, but were unable to suggest how. Their opinion was that cardiac pacing could be considered as an alternative to treatment with CPAP or oral theophylline.

Further larger studies will be required to determine the long-term benefit, how to select the right patients—in particular among those with no indications for pacemaker implantation—and what mechanisms are involved. Identification of the specific neural pathways involved may advance efforts to develop much-needed pharmacologic therapies for sleep apnea. These findings suggest that other therapies than mechanical maintaining of airway patency may be possible, and prevention of vagal tone may be a new proposal.

References

1. Strollo P, Rogers R (1996) Obstructive sleep apnea. N Engl J Med 334:99–104
2. Hunt H, Baker D, Chin M et al (2001) ACC/AHA guidelines for the evaluation and management of chronic heart failure in the adult: executive summary: a report of the American College of Cardiology/American Heart Association Task force on practice guidelines. Circulation 104:2996–3007
3. Sinn D, Fitzgerald F, Parker J et al (1999) Risk factor for central and obstructive sleep apnea I 450 men and women with congestive heart failure. Am J Respir Crit Care Med 160:1101–1106
4. Javaheri S, Parker T, Liming J et al (1998) Sleep apnea in 81 ambulatory male patients with stable heart failure: typrs and their prevalences, consequences, and presentations. Circulation 97:2154–2159
5. Bradley T, Floras J (2003) Sleep apnea and heart failure. Part I: obstructive sleep apnea. Circulation 107:1671–1678
6. Shamsuzzaman A, Winnicki M, Lanfranchi P et al (2002) Elevated C-reactive protein in patients with obstructive sleep apnea. Circulation 105:2462–2464
7. Dyugovskaya L, Lavie P, Lavie L (2002) Increased adhesion molecule expression and production of reactive oxygen species in leukocites of sleep apnea patients. Am J Respir Crit Care Med 165:934–939
8. Carlson J, Rangemark C, Hedner J (1996) Attenuated endothelium-dependent vascular relaxation in patients with sleep apnoea. J Hypertens 14:577–584
9. Bradley T, Floras J (2003) Sleep apnea and heart failure. Part II: central sleep apnea. Circulation 107:1822–1826
10. Lanfranchi P, Braghiroli A, Bosmini E et al (1999) Prognostic value of nocturnal Cheyne-Stokes respiration in chronic heart failure. Circulation 99:1435–1440
11. Arzt M, Harth M, Luchner A et al (2003) Enhanced ventilatory response to exercise in patients with chronic heart failure and central sleep apnea. Circulation 107:1998–2003
12. Massie C, Hart R (2003) Clinical outcomes related to interface type in patients with obstructive sleep apnea/hypopnea syndrome who are using continuous positive airway pressure. Chest 123:1112–1118
13. Mar J, Rueda J, Duran-Cantolla J et al (2003) The cost-effectiveness of nCPAP treatment in patients with moderate-to-severe obstructive sleep apnoea. Eur Respir J 21:515–522
14. Pepperell J, Ramadassingh-Dow S, Crosthwate N et al (2002) Ambulatory blood pressure after therapeutic and subtherapeutic nasal continuous positive airway pressure for obstructive sleep apnoea: a randomised parallel trial. Lancet 359:204–210
15. Flemons W (2002) Obstructive sleep apnea. N Engl J Med 347:498–504
16. McMahon J, Foresman B, Chisholm R (2003) The influence of CPAP on the neurobehavioral performance of patients with obstructive sleep apnea hypopnea syndrome: a systematic review. WMJ 102:36–43
17. Kaneko Y, Floras J, Usui K et al (2003) Cardiovascular effects of continous positive airway pressure in patients with heart failure and obstructive sleep apnea. N Engl J Med 348:1233–1241

18. Gotsopoulos H, Chen C, Quian J et al (2002) Oral appliance therapy improves symptoms in obstrucive sleep apnea. Am J Respir Crit Care Med 166:743–748
19. Engleman H, Mc Donald J, Graham D et al (2002) Continous positive airway pressure and mandibular repositioning splint. Am J Respir Crit Care Med 166:855–859
20. Meyer T, Woodson T (2003) Surgical management of snoring and obstructive sleep apnea. WMJ 102:28–31
21. Unal M, Ozturk L, Ozturk C et al (2003) The seroprevalence of *Helicobacter pylori* infection in patients with obstructive sleep apnoea: a preliminary study. Clin Otolaryngol 28:100–102
22. Garrigue S, Bordier P, Jais P et al (2002) Benefit of atrial pacing in sleep apnea syndrome. N Engl J Med 346:404–412

Remodeling of Sinus Node Function Produced by Supraventricular Tachyarrhythmias: What Are the Clinical Implications?

P.E. Vardas, H.E. Mavrakis

Introduction

The association of atrial fibrillation (AF) with sinus node dysfunction has been known for many years [1–4]. These abnormal atrial electrophysiological features may result from the same organic substrate [1–4]. A considerable body of experimental and human studies in the past 5 years have shown shortening of atrial refractoriness and repolarization and abnormal adaptation to rate as well as conduction slowing as a result of rapid atrial rates of certain duration. These changes are referred as atrial electrical remodeling [5–11]. Short-term rapid atrial rates induce these alterations in atrial electrophysiology via functional changes in ion channels and transporters. However, longer periods of atrial tachycardia result in changes in specific ionic current densities (I_{Ca}, I_{Na}) due to modified expression of the genes that determine the function of the responsible ionic channels [12–16].

Sinus Node Electrical Remodeling

Sinus node function has been implicated in the initiation, perpetuation, and recurrence of AF [17–19]. A reasonable question that arises is whether AF per se can affect the sinus node in the same way as it does the atrial myocardium. An experimental study conducted by Kirchoff and Allessie [20] showed that, although induced nonsustained AF can penetrate the sinus perinodal area and may interact with sinus pacemaker cells, it causes only minor overdrive suppression of automaticity. In contrast, Elvan et al. [21], in a dog study, found that pacing-induced persistent AF induces sinus node dysfunction in parallel with atrial electrical remodeling and that these disorders reverse gradually.

Human data are limited, although some studies have shown sinus node dysfunction to follow cardioversion in patients with AF [22, 23]. In a study including

Department of Cardiology, Heraklion University Hospital, Heraklion, Crete, Greece

12 patients with persistent lone AF, Kumagai et al. [22] assessed the sinus node function on the day after electrical conversion to sinus rhythm. They found that the mean corrected sinus node recovery time (CSNRT) of their patients was significantly longer than that of controls, and in nine of them (75%) it was abnormal (>525 ms). Tse et al. [23] also studied 11 patients with persistent AF 10 min after electrical conversion to sinus rhythm, and found similarly that these patients had significantly longer CSNRT than normal subjects or patients with paroxysmal AF. In that study abnormal CSNRT was found in 55% of patients with persistent AF.

In a recent study carried out in our department we investigated the temporal changes in sinus node function in post-cardioversion persistent AF patients and their possible relation with the recurrence rates of AF [24]. In 37 persistent AF patients internally cardioverted to sinus rhythm, CSNRT was assessed 5-20 min and 24 h after conversion at two pacing cycle lengths (PCL) of 600 ms and 500 ms. Fifteen patients (40.5%) relapsed during a 1-month follow-up. CSNRT values 5–20 min after conversion at PCL 600 ms (371±182 ms) and 500 ms (445±338 ms) were significantly higher than those of control subjects (278±157 ms, p=0.050, 279±130 ms, p=0.037 respectively). Significant temporal changes in CSNRT were also observed during the first 24 h following conversion (PCL 600 ms: 308±120 ms, p=0.034; PCL 500 ms: 340±208 ms, p=0.017). Similar data were obtained after autonomic blockade. Patients with abnormal CSNRT 5–20 min after cardioversion had higher recurrence rates (50%) than did those with normal function (37%), but this difference was not statistically significant.

Recently, Hadian et al. demonstrated in a human study that rapid atrial pacing, even for 10–15 min, significantly prolongs sinoatrial conduction time and CSNRT [25].

Mechanism of Sinus Node Depression

The mechanism of sinus node depression after conversion of atrial tachyarrhythmias in humans is not fully understood. Prolongation of SNRT after overdrive stimulation is probably due to a complex interaction between recovery of automaticity in nodal cells and sinoatrial conduction. Furthermore, it is well known that autonomic tone significantly affects sinus node automaticity. Recent data from our department [26] indicate increased vagal modulation in the initial post-cardioversion period, which may be responsible for the sinus node suppression that has been observed after electrical conversion of chronic AF. On the other hand, long-standing AF could cause prolonged overdrive suppression of the sinus node. Existing data are conflicting. Some studies [20, 27] suggest that the sinoatrial border exhibits entrance block at high atrial rates and thus the sinus node may be protected from overdrive suppression during AF. Indeed, in their study Kirchoff and Allessie [20] showed that during AF there is frequent local conduction block at the sinoatrial border. On the other hand, Elvan et al. [21] found significantly impaired sinus node function after 2–6 weeks of induced AF in dogs, which was more pronounced after autonomic blockade. These findings were interpreted as a feature of the AF-induced atrial electrical remodeling. In addition, a recent human study [28] including 10 patients with persistent atrial flutter and a mean CL of 257 ms showed significant reduction of CSNRT 3 weeks after termination of arrhythmia. However, AF results in significantly shorter FF intervals that may be blocked in the sinoatrial border, and thus the findings from the previous study cannot apply to patients with persistent AF. Furthermore, in our department, we examined the corrected return cycle length (CRC) curves after cardioversion of persistent AF. Although the first return cycle was prolonged, the pattern of these curves was not significantly affected. Abnormal CRC patterns suggest secondary suppression of the sinus node and have been observed in patients with sick sinus syndrome and abnormal intrinsic automaticity [29, 30].

Sinus Node Function, Abnormal Automaticity, and Recurrence of AF

The association of sick sinus syndrome with AF is well known [1–4]. Some authors suggest that bradycardia may enhance dispersion of excitability recovery and thus facilitate re-entrant arrhythmias [31]. Others have suggested that sinus dysfunction might predispose to ectopic atrial firings, producing conduction block and re-entry [32, 33]. In contrast, Nadeau et al. [18] observed that cholinergic AF was more readily initiated and sustained when an intact sinus node was present, while Kirchoff and Allessie [20] demonstrated a high incidence of dissociated activation of the normal sinus node fibers during AF that may result in sinoatrial echo beats contributing to AF perpetuation.

In our department we examined the possible role of suppressed sinus function in the recurrence of AF in postcardioversion patients [24]. We did not find any difference in sinus function between relapsed and nonrelapsed patients. However, the only factor among the clinical and electrophysiological parameters examined in this study that was found to have a role in recurrence was density of ectopic atrial beats (SVCd) in the postcardioversion period. Patients who relapsed had a significantly (p=0.001) higher number of atrial ectopic beats per hour (187±132) compared to those that did not (36±39), but there was no significant correlation of this parameter with CSNRT [24].

We also found that this parameter contains prognostic information, and that chronic AF patients who have more than 82 SVCd/h in the postcardioversion period are prone to relapse. It has been suggested that sinus node dysfunction can promote atrial ectopic activity [32, 33]. In contrast to those observations, in our study SVCd was not found to be related with sinus node function. Furthermore, no synergistic role of CSNRT with SVCd was identified. Thus, our findings do not support a role of the sinus node, either directly or indirectly, in the recurrence of AF. On the other hand, they are compatible with other studies claiming that enhanced automaticity per se, atrial stretch, and autonomic fluctuations are responsible for the high frequency of atrial ectopic beats [34, 35], as well as with those studies that point out the recently described role of ectopic foci in the pulmonary veins and other atrial sites in the initiation, perpetuation, and recurrence of AF in humans [36, 37]. Our data are also in accordance with the very recent observations of Waktare et al. [38], who found a higher density of ectopic atrial beats preceding initiation of AF paroxysms.

Clinical Implications

Involvement of the sinus node pacemaker in the electrical remodeling process has important pathophysiological and clinical implications. For example, if sinus dysfunction is a result of atrial electrical remodeling, it may be a reversible feature, and no further treatment for this abnormality would be necessary when it is observed in postcardioversion AF patients.

In our department [24] we assessed the temporal changes in sinus node function after cardioversion of persistent AF and found that it reaches control levels on the second day after cardioversion. We also observed that in four of our patients who had abnormal sinus node function CSNRT returned to normal levels on the 2nd day after cardioversion. In their experimental study, Elvan et al. [21] found that recovery of sinus node function after prolonged periods of AF exhibits a slower time course.

Since some of our patients did not have any significant improvement of sinus node function during the 24 h that followed cardioversion of chronic AF, we can speculate that in humans, too, recovery of suppressed sinus node function may be seen later in the postcardioversion period.

Recently, in a human study by Sparks et al., CSNRT decreased 35% at 600 ms and 44% at 450 ms, 3 weeks after catheter ablation of persistent atrial flutter [28]. In a similar study by Daoud et al., CSNRT decreased 25% 3 months after catheter ablation of persistent atrial flutter [39]. Recovery of sinus node function has also been demonstrated in patients with chronic AF in whom sinus rhythm is restored after the surgical maze procedure [40-41].

So we could hypothesize that, at least in some patients with chronic AF and flutter, the abnormal sinus node function observed in the postcardioversion period is a reversible feature that can be explained, at least in part, as a result of AF-induced electrical remodeling, since it resolves with time and is independent of autonomic function and other clinical or electrophysiological parameters. Thus, we believe that this possibility must be kept in mind when considering antibradycardia treatment in these patients after successful cardioversion or ablation.

Furthermore, when evaluating patients with suspected sick sinus syndrome, we must also consider that transient atrial tachyarrhythmias may also alter sinus node function [25].

References

1. Davies MJ, Pommerance A (1972) Pathology of atrial fibrillation in man. Br Heart J 34:520–525

2. Gomes J, Kang P, Matheson P, Gough W, El Sherif N (1981) Coexistence of sick sinus rhythm and atrial flutter–fibrillation. Circulation 63:80–86
3. Thery C, Gosselin B, Lekieffre J, Warebourg H (1977) Pathology of the sinoatrial node: correlations with electrocardiographic findings in 111 patients. Am Heart J 93:735–740
4. Bigger JT, Reiffel JA (1979) Sick sinus syndrome. Annu Rev Med 30:91–118
5. Wijffels MCEF, Kirchoff CJ, Dorland R, Allessie MA (1995) Atrial fibrillation begets atrial fibrillation. A study in awake chronically instrumented goats. Circulation 92:1954–1968
6. Goette A, Honeycutt C, Langberg JJ (1996) Electrical remodeling in atrial fibrillation. Time course and mechanisms. Circulation 94:2968–2974
7. Daoud EG, Bogun F, Goyal R et al (1996) Effect of AF on atrial refractoriness in humans. Circulation 94:1600–1606
8. Franz MR, Karasik PL, Li C, Moubarak J, Chavez M (1997) Electrical remodeling of the human atrium: similar effects in patients with chronic atrial fibrillation and atrial flutter. J Am Coll Cardiol 30:1785–1792
9. Pandozi C, Bianconi L, Villani M et al (1998) Electrophysiological characteristics of the human atria after cardioversion of persistent atrial fibrillation. Circulation 98:2860–2865
10. Yu W, Lee SH, Tai CT et al (1999) Reversal of atrial electrical remodeling following cardioversion of long–standing atrial fibrillation in man. Cardiovasc Res 42:470–476
11. Manios E, Kanoupakis E, Chlouverakis G et al (2000) Changes in atrial electrical properties following cardioversion of chronic atrial fibrillation: relation with recurrence. Cardiovasc Res 47:244–253
12. Gaspo R, Bosch RF, Bou-Abboud E, Nattel S (1997) Tachycardia induced changes in Na+ current in a chronic dog model of atrial fibrillation. Circ Res 8:1045–1052
13. Gaspo R, Bosch RF, Talajic M, Nattel S (1997) Functional mechanisms underlying tachycardia-induced sustained atrial fibrillation in a chronic dog model. Circulation 96:4027–4035
14. Daoud EG, Knight BP, Weiss R et al (1997) Effect of verapamil and procainamide on atrial fibrillation-induced electrical remodeling in humans. Circulation 96:1542–1550
15. Tieleman RG, De Langen C, Van Gelder IC et al (1997) Verapamil reduces tachycardia-induced electrical remodeling of the atria. Circulation 95:1945–1953
16. Fareh S, Villemaire C, Nattel S (1998) Importance of refractoriness heterogeneity in the enhanced vulnerability to atrial fibrillation induction caused by tachycardia-induced atrial electrical remodeling. Circulation 98:2202–2209
17. Page PL (1992) Sinus node during atrial fibrillation. To beat or not to beat. Circulation 86:334–336
18. Nadeau RA, Roberge FA, Billette J (1970) The role of the sinus node in the mechanism of cholinergic atrial fibrillation. Circ Res 27:129–138
19. Spach MS, Dolber PC, Heidlage JF (1989) Interaction of inhomogeneities of repolarization with anisotropic propagationin dog atria: a mechanism for both preventing and initiating reentry. Circ Res 65:1612–1631
20. Kirchoff CJ, Allessie MA (1992) Sinus node automaticity during atrial fibrillation in isolated rabbit hearts. Circulation 86:263–271
21. Elvan A, Wylie K, Zipes DP (1996) Pacing-induced chronic atrial fibrillation impairs sinus node function in dogs. Electrophysiological remodeling. Circulation 94:2953–2960
22. Kumagai K, Akimitsu S, Kawahira K et al (1991) Electrophysiological properties in chronic lone atrial fibrillation. Circulation 84:1662–1668

23. Tse HF, Lau CP, Ayers GM (1999) Heterogeneous changes in electrophysiological properties in the paroxysmal and chronically fibrillating human atrium. J Cardiovasc Electrophysiol 10:125–135
24. Manios E, Kanoupakis E, Mavrakis H et al (2001) Sinus pacemaker function after cardioversion of chronic atrial fibrillation: is sinus node remodeling related with recurrence? J Cardiovasc Electrophysiol 12: 800–806
25. Hadian D, Zipes D, Olgin J, Miller J (2002) Short-term rapid atrial pacing produces electrical remodeling of sinus node function in humans. J Cardiovasc Electrophysiol 13:584–586
26. Kanoupakis E, Manios E, Mavrakis H et al (2000) Relation of autonomic modulation to recurrence of atrial fibrillation following cardioversion. Am J Cardiol 86:954–958
27. Kerr CR, Strauss HC (1981) The nature of atriosinus conduction during rapid atrial pacing in the rabbit heart. Circulation 63:1149–1158
28. Sparks PB, Jayaprakash S, Vohra JK, Kalman JB (2000) Electrical remodeling of the atria associated with paroxysmal and chronic atrial flutter. Circulation 102:1807–1813
29. Jordan JL, Mandel WJ (1987) Disorders of sinus function. In: Mandel WJ (ed) Cardiac arrhythmias, their mechanisms, diagnosis and management. Lippincott, Philadelphia, pp 143–185
30. Desai JM, Scheinman M, Strauss HC, Massie B, O'Young J (1981) Electrophysiologic effects of autonomic combined blockade in patients with sinus node disease. Circulation 63:953–960
31. Han J, Millet D, Shizzoniti B, Moe GK (1966) Temporal dispersion of excitability in atrium and ventricle as a function of heart rate. Am Heart J 71: 481–487
32. Spach MS, Dolber PC, Heidlage JF (1989) Interaction of inhomogeneities of repolarization with anisotropic propagation in dog atria: a mechanism for both preventing and initiating reentry. Circ Res 65:1612–1631
33. Spach MS, Dolber PC, Anderson PAW (1989) Multiple regional differences in cellular properties that regulate repolarization and contraction in the right atrium of adult and newborn dogs. Circ Res 65:1594–1611
34. Solti F, Vecsey T, Kekesi V, Juhasz-Nagy A (1989) The effect of atrial dilatation on the genesis of atrial arrhythmias. Cardiovasc Res 23:882–886
35. Coumel P (1994) Paroxysmal atrial fibrillation: a disorder of autonomic tone? Eur Heart J 15:A9–A16
36. Haissaguerre M, Jais P, Shah DC et al (1998) Spontaneous initiation of atrial fibrillation by ectopic beats originating in the pulmonary veins. N Engl J Med 339:659–666
37. Chen SA, Hsieh MS, Tai CT et al (1999) Initiation of atrial fibrillation by ectopic beats originating from the pulmonary veins: electrophysiological characteristics, pharmacological responses and effects of radiofrequency ablation. Circulation 100:1879–1886
38. Waktare JE, Hnatkova K, Sopher M et al (2001) The role of atrial ectopics in initiating paroxysms of atrial fibrillation. Eur Heart J 22: 333–339
39. Daoud EG, Weiss R, Augostini RS et al (2002) Remodeling of sinus node function after catheter ablation of right atrial flutter. J Cardiovasc Electrophysiol 13:20–24
40. Tamai J, Kosakai Y, Yoshioka T et al (1995) Delayed improvement in exercise capacity with restoration of sinoatrial node response in patients after combined treatment with surgical repair for organic heart disease and the Maze procedure for atrial fibrillation. Circulation 91:2392–2399
41. Pasic M, Musci M, Siniawski H et al (1998) Transient sinus node dysfunction after the Cox-maze III procedure in patients with organic heart disease and chronic fixed atrial fibrillation. J Am Coll Cardiol 32:1040–1047

Drug-Induced Bradycardia: When Is a Pacemaker Warranted?

I.E. OVSYSHCHER, N. GULKO

Pacing and drug therapy may interact in cardiac patients in several ways, and one of them is when drug therapy induces bradycardia necessitating antibradycardia pacing. In this paper, several aspects of drug-induced bradycardia (DIB) will be discussed: definition, epidemiology, physiology, pathogenesis, drugs leading to bradycardia, clinical settings when DIB can require pacing, and management of DIB.

Definitions

There is no definition of bradycardia as a pathological cardiac rhythm. In this paper, we will use the definition: *bradycardia exists in adults when the heart rate is less than 60 bpm.*

Patients with DIB may be in sinus rhythm, any atrial rhythm, including slow atrial fibrillation (AF), nodal rhythm, or idioventricular rhythm.

Three kinds of bradycardia may be clinically observed:

1. Asymptomatic, benign
2. Asymptomatic, potentially malignant
3. Symptomatic

Asymptomatic bradycardia is potentially malignant when accompanied by:

1. Premature ventricular beats (PVBs) with short-long interval
2. Nonsustained ventricular tachycardia (VT)
3. QT prolongation [all three of these can deteriorate to VT/torsades de pointes (TDP)]
4. Low cardiac output (CO) and/or low left ventricular (LV) ejection fraction (EF), which can lead to progression or new heart failure (HF)

Symptomatic bradycardia is a rate that may create symptoms in a patient; another type of symptomatic bradycardia is asymptomatic patient bradycar-

Electrophysiology Research Laboratory, Faculty of Health Sciences, Ben Gurion University of the Negev, Beersheva, Israel

dia, which in turn creates symptoms in a physician, which can make him anxious and might impair his judgment.

Symptomatic bradycardia may be defined as a documented bradyarrhythmic event per se or bradyarrhythmia accompanied by a tachyarrhythmic event (TDP) that may be *directly responsible* for development of such clinical manifestations as:

1. Syncope
2. Near-syncope
3. Confusional state
4. HF, new or worsening (all these first four symptoms may be defined as severe symptoms)
5. Transient dizziness
6. Fatigue
7. Exercise intolerance (symptoms 5–7 may be defined as mild)
   All these symptoms may occur at rest and/or with exertion.
   Types of DIB after drug discontinuation may:
1. Disappear—this is transient bradycardia.
2. Continue—this is persistent bradycardia.
3. Not be expected to resolve.
4. Be expected to resolve.

In the recent guideline for pacing indications [1], all these terms are frequently used. In guideline was noted: "These terms are not specifically defined because the time element varies in different clinical conditions. The treating physician must use appropriate clinical judgment and available data in deciding when a condition is persistent or when it can be expected to be transient" [1].

Epidemiology

There are several sporadic reports, mostly regarding antiarrhythmic drugs (AAD) (Table 1.) In a recently published report [3] based on a study of 8770 postmyocardial infarction patients with recent-onset AF using a nested case-control design, 477 cases of bradyarrhythmia requiring a permanent pacemaker were matched (1:4) to 1908 controls. Multivariable logistic regression was used to estimate the odds ratio (OR) of pacemaker insertion associated with amiodarone use, controlling for baseline risk factors and exposure to sotalol, class I antiarrhythmic agents, β-blockers, calcium channel blockers, and digoxin. Amiodarone use was associated with an increased risk of pacemaker insertion (OR: 2.14, 95% CI). This effect was modified by gender, with a greater risk in women. Digoxin was the only other medication associated with an increased risk of pacemaker insertion (OR: 1.78, 95% CI). In 1005 patients with new-onset AF, amiodarone treatment significantly increased (more than three times) the rate of implantation of pacemakers [4].

In another recent report in 78 patients with a DDDRP system implanted for symptomatic bradycardia and paroxysmal or persistent AF, the bradycardia

Table 1. Incidence of significant drug-induced bradycardia (DIB): antiarryhthmic drugs administered for different indications. (Data collected from 31 studies, adapted from [2])

Drug	No. of patients	Incidence of DIB (%)
Disopyramide	96	5
Flecainide	227	0–14
Flecainide	52	14[a]
Propafenone	6018	1–4
Metoprolol	200	7
Sotalol	1946	1–17
Amiodarone	10 972	1–17
Amiodarone + digitalis	37	32
Amiodarone + carvedilol	109	6
Amiodarone + β-blocker	31	3
Quinidine + verapamil	102	7

[a]Pacemaker implanted; combination with amiodarone in 33 patients.

had been drug-induced in 33% of patients [2]. Development of DIB necessitating pacemaker implantation was found in 8% (2%–14%) of patients on a variety of AADs used for different indications and represents the most common proarrhythmic effect of antiarrhythmic therapy [2, 4, 5].

Physiology and Pathogenesis

Bradycardia may be symptomatic with heart rate 60 bpm and a patient may feel well with severe bradycardia of 30 bpm. The appearance of symptoms due to bradycardia depends on many factors, chiefly:

1. Coronary flow
2. Stroke volume (SV)
3. Cerebral perfusion

Coronary Flow

The physiologic determinants of coronary flow are diastolic perfusion pressure, heart rate, ventricular wall tension, dP/dt_{max}, and left ventricular end-diastolic pressure (LVEDP). With bradycardia the duration of diastole becomes longer such that the mean perfusion pressure progressively declines; on the other hand, myocardial oxygen consumption is directly related to heart rate, and slow rates are generally beneficial for the heart.

Stroke Volume

If the heart rate increases via sympathetic drive, the SV also increases, and as result the CO increases. If the heart rate is increased by the pacing, the SV does not change or even decreases, and as result the CO decreases [6].

Cerebral Perfusion

Cerebral perfusion mainly depends on CO. A key to understanding symptoms due to bradycardia is that for each patient there is a pathophysiologic turning point when bradycardia becomes dysfunctional regarding the trade-off between reduced coronary perfusion pressure and respectively coronary flow and diminished myocardial oxygen consumption, CO and cerebral perfusion.

Bradycardia usually exists due to chronotropic incompetence. Therefore, during exercise the heart rate may remain fixed or increase only insignificantly. There are such compensatory factors as increasing LVEDP, contractility (increased sympathetic activity), and SV, but at the expense of additional energy and an increase of mean VO_2 and as result, the coronary flow reduces.

Drugs Leading to Bradycardia

β-blockers, Ca antagonists, digitalis, antiarrhythmic drugs, tedisamil, cocaine and tegretol (carbamazepine) are all drugs that may lead to bradycardia. Clinical situations which could demand continuation of such drug(s), leading to bradycardia requiring pacing therapy, include:

Angina Pectoris

In patients managed by treatment with β-blockers and/or Ca antagonists, pacing may permit aggressive and more effective pharmacological therapy.

Rapid Atrial Tachyarrhythmia (RAT)

Induction of bradycardia by drugs is generally used for rate or rhythm control (Ca antagonists, digitalis, β-blockers, AADs such as amiodarone or sotalol). Several clinical situations may be observed:

1. Successful RAT suppression by drug(s) at the expense of bradycardia.
2. Unsuccessful RAT suppression by drug(s) with bradycardia; pacing may then permit higher doses of drugs when not previously tolerated due to bradycardia; higher drug doses may then suppress the arrhytmia.

Congestive HF

In patients treated by β-blockers and digitalis, pacing may permit effective pharmacological therapy.

Hypertrophic Obstructive Cardiomyopathy

Using Ca antagonists and/or β-blockers in combination with pacing may allow effective pharmacological therapy.

Hyperkalemia

Hyperkalemia with or without antiarrhythmic agents may lead to severe bradycardia.

Management of Drug-Induced Bradycardia

There are no guidelines for the management of DIB, neither are there any controlled studies regarding pacing in patients with DIB. Therefore, recommendations for using pacing in patients with DIB can only be based on expert opinions. The following guidelines may be suggested:

1. *Drug discontinuation and observation.* Patients with mild symptoms alleviated by rest should be managed by drug discontinuation and observation (if the drug cannot be discontinued, see below). Level of evidence: C.
2. *Drug discontinuation and supportive medical treatment.* Patients with a potentially malignant bradycardia and/or accompanied by mild symptoms that cannot be alleviated by rest and be expected to resolve within 24 hours should be managed by drug discontinuation (if drug cannot be discontinued, see below) and supportive medical treatment (atropine, isoproterenol, and/or specific antidote). Level of evidence: C.
3. *Drug discontinuation and temporary pacing.* Patients with DIB that may potentially be malignant and/or is accompanied by severe symptoms that cannot be alleviated by rest and supportive treatment should be managed by drug discontinuation (if drug cannot be discontinued, see below) and temporary pacing. Level of evidence: C.
4. *Drug continuation.*
   a) Patients in whom symptoms are resolving (e.g., transient symptomatic bradycardia) following drug titration and the drug continues to be effective could continue the treatment with a lower dose of the drug without pacing. Level of evidence: C.
   b) Patients with potentially malignant DIB or DIB accompanied by severe symptoms that cannot be alleviated by rest and supportive treatment, and when the drug should be continued, should be managed by temporary pacing and a gradual reduction of the dose of the drug, i.e., dose titration.
5. *Drug discontinuation/continuation and permanent pacing.* Patients with potentially malignant DIB and/or accompanied by any symptoms that cannot be alleviated by dose decreasing of the drug, discontinuation of the drug or drug cannot be discontinued, implantation of a permanent pace-

maker should be considered (persistent symptomatic bradycardia due to underlying conduction disease, provoked by drug [2]). Level of evidence: C.

References

1. Gregoratos G, Abrams J, Epstein AE et al (2002) ACC/AHA/NASPE 2002 guideline update for implantation of cardiac pacemakers and antiarrhythmia devices: summary article. Circulation 106:2145–61
2. Israel CW, Ehrlich JR, Barold SS et al (2002) Treatment of tachyarrhythmias with pacing and antiarrhythmic drugs. In: Israel CW, Barold SS (eds) Advances in the treatment of atrial tachyarrhythmias: pacing, cardioversion, and defibrillation. Futura, Armonk, NY, pp 305–323
3. Essebag V, Hadjis T, Platt RW et al (2003) Amiodarone and the risk of bradyarrhythmia requiring permanent pacemaker in elderly patients with atrial fibrillation and prior myocardial infarction. J Am Coll Cardiol 15:249–254
4. Reynolds MR, Hadjis T, Schwartzman DS et al (2003) Age and amiodarone use are important determinants of the need for permanent pacing among new onset AF patients (abstract). Pacing Clin Electrophysiol 26:1016, A350
5. Friedman PL, Stevenson WG (1998) Proarrhythmia. Am J Cardiol 82:50N–58N
6. Ovsyshcher I, Zimlichman R, Bondy C et al (1993) Measurement of cardiac output by impedance cardiography in pacemaker patients at rest: effects of various AV delay. J Am Coll Cardiol 21:761–767

Permanent Pacing Treatment: Conventional DDDR, Antitachycardia Pacing or Atrial Defibrillator?

M. Santini, R. Ricci, C. Pignalberi, M. Russo, B. Magris, L. Santini

Introduction

Atrial fibrillation is the most common arrhythmia in clinical practice and its incidence is increasing due to the aging of the population. It is associated with major clinical complications, such as heart failure, acute myocardial infarction, and stroke, and with impaired quality of life [1, 2]. Antiarrhythmic drugs have been widely used for cardioversion and maintenance of sinus rhythm, but they showed limited and usually temporary efficacy [3]. In consequence, several nonpharmacological therapies including physiological pacing, pacing prevention algorithms, antitachy pacing therapies, and low-energy internal cardioversion have been introduced to treat drug-refractory arrhythmias [4–6], and have been implemented in multifunction implantable devices.

Physiological Pacing

Antiarrhythmic benefits of atrial and dual-chamber pacing versus single-chamber ventricular pacing in reducing atrial fibrillation recurrences and in preventing progression to permanent atrial fibrillation have been clearly demonstrated in large prospective trials enrolling either patients with sinus node disease or unselected patients who are candidates for pacemaker implantation [7–9]. It has been also suggested that rate-responsive availability may maximize the effect of physiological pacing [10] by increasing the atrial pacing percentage and by preventing arrhythmias triggered by chronotropic incompetence. Furthermore, antibradycardia pacing may enhance the efficacy of antiarrhythmic drugs, by preventing drug-induced bradycardia and by allowing optimal drug dosage titration.

Department of Cardiology, San Filippo Neri Hospital, Rome, Italy

Pacing Prevention Algorithms

In the last years, several pacing prevention algorithms have been developed in order to increase the antiarrhythmic benefits of atrial pacing. Prevention algorithms include: (1) atrial overdrive algorithms designed to maintain a consistent atrial activation sequence by adjusting the atrial escape interval in order to remain just ahead of the intrinsic rate (atrial preference pacing); (2) pacing sequences following a premature atrial contraction aimed at avoiding short-long intervals (atrial rate stabilization); and (3) post-mode-switch overdrive pacing designed to prevent early recurrence of atrial tachyarrhythmias after termination of a previous episode. Early clinical studies, in which mainly patients with sinus node disease were enrolled, suggested a favorable effect of these new algorithms in atrial fibrillation prevention and in arrhythmia burden reduction, combined with good tolerance [11–13].

Multisite Atrial Pacing

Slow conduction in the right atrium and retrograde activation of the left atrium cause inhomogeneous dispersion of electrical activity with intra- and interatrial asynchrony [14]. The slow conduction has been recognized as be a determinant in the occurrence of paroxysmal atrial fibrillation [15, 16]. In these patients, multisite or single-site nonconventional permanent atrial pacing have been suggested in order to improve the activation sequence, to reduce the asynchrony in atrial activation, to pre-excite some areas potentially involved in re-entry circuits, and, finally, to reduce the dispersion of refractory periods. Biatrial synchronous pacing [17] and dual-site right atrial pacing [18], despite encouraging results in preliminary studies, did not in randomized trials demonstrate a definite superiority over conventional atrial pacing in preventing atrial fibrillation [19, 20]. Interatrial septal pacing at the Koch triangle level, which represents an area of anisotropic conduction, may prevent atrial fibrillation by lengthening of the coupling interval of premature atrial beats and by modifying the electrophysiological properties of the substrate. Effectiveness of this new technique, as compared with right atrial appendage pacing, has been demonstrated in small population controlled studies [21]. Finally, single-site pacing of the high interatrial septum at the Bachmann bundle level has been shown to be more effective than conventional atrial pacing in preventing progression to permanent atrial fibrillation [22].

Antitachycardia Pacing

It has been demonstrated that rapid atrial pacing delivered for treating atrial tachycardia or atrial flutter may be effective in restoring sinus rhythm in as many as 60%–90% of patients [23, 24]. Maximal effectiveness can be usually obtained by delivering antitachycardia pacing at a rate that is slightly greater than the atrial arrhythmia rate [25, 26]. Delivering some extrastimuli following a rapid pacing train may be more efficacious than overdrive atrial pacing at the same pacing cycle length in terminating atrial flutter [4]. High-frequency pacing may change atrial tachycardia in transient atrial fibrillation with later restoring of sinus rhythm. Effectiveness and safety of atrial antitachycardia pacing have been demonstrated in several clinical studies [27–29]. Atrial tachyarrhythmia detection was very good, with a positive predictive value of atrial detection ranging from 91% to 99%. The adjusted efficacy of atrial burst and ramp in treating regular atrial tachycardia ranged between 50% and 70%, while a 50-Hz burst was effective in treating less organized atrial tachyarrhythmias in 15%–25% of cases. It is worthwhile to stress that the atrial arrhythmia detected at very early onset was very commonly a well-organized atrial tachycardia, which is more suitable for antitachycardia pacing treatment. In fact, in all series it has been consistently observed that pacing therapy efficacy consistently increased as the atrial arrhythmia cycle lengthened. Furthermore, increasing the delay from arrhythmia detection to therapy delivery was associated with a significant reduction in efficacy. That was probably due to the fact that the majority of atrial tachyarrhythmias accelerated in a few minutes after onset. Finally, the safety of antitachycardia pacing therapy was excellent in all series, since no ventricular arrhythmia induction was observed in any case after antitachy pacing delivery.

Atrial Defibrillator

The efficacy and tolerance of endocavitary low energy cardioversion [30] led to the introduction of implantable multifunction devices capable of delivering atrial shock with the aim of interrupting atrial fibrillation early and preventing atrial remodeling, which is judged to be the main mechanism involved in persistence and recurrence of arrhythmia [31]. Despite documented good results in regard to therapy efficacy [32] and reduction of arrhythmia recurrence during follow-up [33], a stand-alone atrial defibrillator is no longer available for clinical implantation. The dual defibrillator combines the features of conventional dual-chamber defibrillators with the capability of preventing, detecting, and treating supraventricular tachyarrhythmias. Arrhythmia prevention is based on physiological pacing, rate responsive pacing, pacing prevention algorithms and multisite atrial pacing, when applicable. Arrhythmia therapies include atrial antitachy pacing and cardioversion. The efficacy of the dual defibrillator in treating spontaneous atrial tachyarrhythmias has been demonstrated in patients with [27, 34–36] or without [29] spontaneous major ventricular tachyarrhythmias. In particular, its atrial shock efficacy was very high when appropriately programmed. In fact, the ratio between the actually delivered shock energy and the atrial defibrillation threshold at implant and the delay between atrial fibrillation onset and shock delivery are the main determinants of success. Early delivery of at least twice the atrial defibrillation threshold represents the optimal programming. In regard to patient compliance, it should be stressed that shock tolerance is weakly related to the energy delivered and strongly dependent on the number of atrial shocks and their efficacy in restoring sinus rhythm. Highly symptomatic patients may tolerate the discomfort of shock if it is capable of stopping severe arrhythmia-related symptoms early.

Comments

The role of physiological pacing in atrial fibrillation prevention in patients with either sinus node disease or atrioventricular block has been definitely demonstrated in several major prospective randomized trials. Atrial fibrillation is a common event during the follow-up of paced patients, especially in those with devices implanted because of sinus node disease. On the other hand, sophisticated overdrive algorithms aimed at keeping rhythm control, suppressing premature atrial complexes, preventing short–long cycles, and preventing early recurrences of atrial arrhythmias have been demonstrated to be effective in reducing atrial fibrillation burden. Furthermore, antitachycardia pacing therapies and device-delivered atrial shock are documented effective tools and may represent a cost-effective approach by reducing the need for external cardioversion and hospitalizations. Prompt detection and interruption of atrial fibrillation episodes may reduce the electrophysiological remodeling process, thus increasing the sinus rhythm periods and preventing atrial fibrillation recurrences. The challenge for the next few years is to identify the best strategy for a selected group of patients. A multifunction implantable device equipped with all prevention and treatment features may be the optimal choice, especially for patients who need pacemaker implantation for symptomatic bradycardia. The higher cost of the device could be balanced by prevention of arrhythmia-related hospitalizations and reduced health care resource consumption. At any rate, controlled studies in this field, including comparison with radiofrequency ablation strategies and detailed cost-benefit analysis, are greatly needed.

References

1. Wolf PA, Abbott RD, Kannel WB (1991) Atrial fibrillation as an independent risk factor for stroke: The Framingham study. Stroke 22:983–988
2. Hamer ME, Blumenthal JA, McCarthy EA, Phillips BG, Pritchett ELC (1994) Quality of life assessment in patients with paroxysmal atrial fibrillation or paroxysmal supraventricular tachycardia. Am J Cardiol 74:826–829
3. Suttorp MJ, Kingma JH, Koomen EM et al (1993) Recurrence of paroxysmal atrial fibrillation or flutter after successful cardioversion in patients with normal left ven-

tricle function. Am J Cardiol 71:710–713

4. Hii JTY, Mitchell B, Duff HJ, Wyse DG, Gillis AM (1992) Comparison of atrial overdrive pacing with and without extrastimuli for termination of atrial flutter. Am J Cardiol 70:463–467
5. Baeriswyl G, Zimmerman M, Adamec R (1994) Efficacy of rapid atrial pacing for conversion of atrial flutter in medically treated patients. Clin Cardiol 17:246–250
6. Santini M, Pandozi C, Altamura G et al (1999) Single shock endocavitary low energy intracardiac cardioversion of chronic atrial fibrillation. J Interv Card Electrophysiol 3:45–51
7. Andersen HR, Nielsen JC, Thomsen PEB et al (1997) Long-term follow up of patients from a randomised trial of atrial versus ventricular pacing for sick-sinus syndrome. Lancet 350:1210–1216
8. Skanes AC, Krahn AD, Yee R et al, for the CTOPP Investigators (2001) Progression to chronic atrial fibrillation after pacing: The Canadian Trial of Physiologic Pacing. J Am Coll Cardiol 38:167–172
9. Lamas GA, Lee KL, Sweeney MO et al, for the Mode Selection Trial in sinus node dysfunction (2002) Ventricular pacing or dual chamber pacing for sinus node dysfunction. N Engl J Med 346:1854–1862
10. Sutton R (1999) Is rate response superior to single rate pacing in atrial arrhythmia control? Europace 1:211–212
11. Ricci R, Santini M, Puglisi A et al (2001) Impact of consistent atrial pacing algorithm on premature atrial complex number and paroxysmal atrial fibrillation recurrences in brady-tachy syndrome: a randomized prospective cross over study. J Interv Card Electrophysiol 5:33–44
12. Boriani G, Biffi M, Padeletti L et al (2001) Effects of consistent atrial pacing and atrial rate stabilization, two pacing algorithms to suppress recurrent paroxysmal atrial fibrillation in brady-tachy syndrome. Eur Heart J 3(Suppl. P):P7–P15
13. Camm J (2002) AF therapy study: preventive pacing for paroxysmal atrial fibrillation (abstract). Pacing Clin Electrophysiol 25:554
14. Simpson R, Foster JR, Gettes LS (1982) Atrial excitability and conduction in patients with interatrial conduction defects. Am J Cardiol 50:1331–1337
15. Cohen J, Scherf D (1965) Complete interatrial and intra-atrial block (atrial dissociation). Am Heart J 70:24–34
16. Castillo-Fenoy A, Vernant P (1971) Troubles de la conduction intra-auriculaire par bloc du faisceau de Bachmann. Arch Mal Coeur Vaiss 64:1490–1503
17. D'Allonnes GR, Pavin D, Leclercq C et al (2000) Long-term effects of biatrial synchronous pacing to prevent drug-refractory atrial tachyarrhythmia: a nine-year experience. J Cardiovasc Electrophysiol. 11:1081–1091
18. Saksena S, Prakash A, Hill M et al (1996) Prevention of recurrent atrial fibrillation with chronic dual-site right atrial pacing. J Am Coll Cardiol 28:687–694
19. Mabo P, Paul V, Jung W et al (1999) Biatrial synchronous pacing for atrial arrhythmia prevention: the SYNBIAPACE Study (abstract). Eur Heart J 20(Abs Suppl):4
20. Saksena S, Prakash A, Ziegler P et al, DAPPAF Investigators (2002) Improved suppression of recurrent atrial fibrillation with dual-site right atrial pacing and antiarrhythmic drug therapy. J Am Coll Cardiol 40:1140–1150
21. Padeletti L, Pieragnoli P, Ciapetti C et al (2001) Randomised crossover comparison of right atrial appendage pacing versus interatrial septum pacing for prevention of paroxysmal atrial fibrillation in patients with sinus bradycardia. Am Heart J 142:1047–1055
22. Bailin SJ, Adler S, Giudici M (2001) Prevention of chronic atrial fibrillation by pacing

in the region of Bachmann's bundle: results of a multicenter randomized trial. J Cardiovasc Electrophysiol 12:912–917
23. Macdonald P, Hackworthy R, Keogh A et al (1991) Atrial overdrive pacing for reversion of atrial flutter after heart transplantation. J Heart Lung Transplant 10:731–737
24. Peters RW, Shorofsky SR, Pelini M, Olsovsky M, Gold MR (1999) Overdrive atrial pacing for reversion of atrial flutter: comparison of postoperative with nonpostoperative patients. Am Heart J 137:100–103
25. Gloor HO, Fromer M, Kappenberger L (1986) Endocardial conversion of atrial flutter. Success rate of various stimulation protocols. Clin Prog Electrophysiol Pacing 4:67–75
26. Baeriswyl G, Zimmerman M, Adamec R (1994) Efficacy of rapid atrial pacing for conversion of atrial flutter in medically treated patients. Clin Cardiol 17:246–250
27. Adler SW, Wolpert C, Warman EN et al, for the Worldwide Jewel AF Investigators (2001) Efficacy of pacing therapies for treating atrial tachyarrhythmias in patients with ventricular arrhythmias receiving a dual-chamber implantable cardioverter defibrillator. Circulation 104:887–892
28. Ricci R, Pignalberi C, Disertori M et al (2001) Antitachycardia pacing therapy to treat spontaneous atrial tachyarrhythmias: the 7250 Dual Defibrillator Italian Registry. Eur Heart J 3(Suppl P):P25–P32
29. Gold MR, Sulke N, Schwartzman DS, Mehra R, Euler DE, for the Worldwide Jewel AF-Only Investigators (2001) Clinical experience with a dual chamber implantable cardioverter defibrillator to treat atrial tachyarrhythmias. J Cardiovasc Electrophysiol 12:1247–1253
30. Steinhaus DM, Cardinal DS, Mongeon L et al (2002) Internal defibrillation: pain perception of low energy shocks. Pacing Clin Electrophysiol 25:1090–1093
31. Wijffels M, Kirchhoff C, Dorland R, Allessie MA (1995) Atrial fibrillation begets atrial fibrillation. A study in awake chronically instrumented goats. Circulation 92:1954–1968
32. Wellens HJJ, Lau CP, Luderitz B et al (1998) Atrioverter: an implantable device for the treatment of atrial fibrillation. Circulation 98:1651–1656
33. Tse HF, Lau CP, Yu CM et al (1999) Effect of the implantable atrial defibrillator on the natural history of atrial fibrillation. J Cardiovasc Electrophysiol 10:1200–1209
34. Friedman PA, Dijkman B, Warman EN et al, for the Worldwide Jewel AF Investigators (2001) Atrial therapies reduce atrial arrhythmia burden in defibrillator patients. Circulation. 104:1023–1028
35. Schoels W, Swerdlow CD, Jung W et al, for the Worldwide Jewel AF Investigators (2001) Worldwide clinical experience with a new dual chamber implantable cardioverter defibrillator system. J Cardiovasc Electrophysiol 12:521–528
36. Ricci R, Pignalberi C, Disertori M et al (2002) Efficacy of a dual chamber defibrillator with atrial antitachycardia functions in treating spontaneous atrial tachyarrhythmias in patients with life-threatening ventricular tachyarrhythmias. Eur Heart J 23:1471–1479

HEMODYNAMICS AND CARDIAC PACING

Hemodynamic Assessment with Implantable Pacemakers
How Feasible and Reliable Is It?

R. CHIRIFE

Introduction

Hemodynamic assessment comprises the study of the two major functions of the heart: cardiac output (flow) and pressure, with a close interaction between the two governed by the peripheral resistance. Therefore, measurements related to pressure, volumes and flow are regarded as hemodynamic markers. Diagnostic sensors, such as high-fidelity catheter-tip manometers, provide accurate assessment of single-parameter cardiac function, but the intricate interaction between cardiac contractility, preload, vascular resistance and heart rate makes it very difficult for a single measurement to provide an accurate picture of heart function [1]. For example, isolated measurements of ventricular dP/dt will be of limited value for diagnosis, since this variable is strongly modulated by preload and afterload. This problem is further compounded when the sensor is to be permanently implanted within the heart in pacemakers or ICDs. With these devices it is generally thought preferable not to incorporate additional hardware attached to the pacing/defibrillator leads, and especially within the left heart chambers, because of the risk of clot embolization. With these concepts in mind, the idea of using intracardiac impedance sensors for hemodynamic assessment becomes very appealing, since no additional hardware is required on the pacing lead.

Sensors

At present, there are only two types of hemodynamic sensors available for implantable devices: pressure and impedance (volume) sensors. Although another type of device has been proposed (the intracardiac accelerometer, which detects heart sounds), the type of signal it detects means it cannot be considered a hemodynamic marker. The pressure transducer, which requires a

Hospital Fernández, Buenos Aires, Argentina

piezo-electric crystal in the lead, has not yet been found suitable for clinical application, but research is ongoing. Therefore, this presentation will deal primarily with intracardiac impedance sensors as hemodynamic markers.

Intracardiac Impedance

Impedance (or resistance) is the opposite of conductivity

In order to measure the impedance of blood to obtain an estimate of volume, at least one pair of electrodes is needed within the cardiac chambers [2, 3]. For example, standard pacemaker leads can be used to determine the impedance between two or more electrodes [4, 5]. The type of circuit used for this purpose is shown in Fig. 1. Since the intracardiac impedance changes are dynamic and of relatively small amplitude, the system used for impedance recording should have enough amplitude and time resolution. Although blood and tissues conduct electricity, they have different degrees of resistance (the blood has less resistance than the tissues), thus allowing the detection of volume changes. Larger volumes of blood will offer less resistance than smaller volumes, although the relationship is not linear (Fig. 2). In the example illustrated in Fig. 2 impedance was measured between the ring and the tip of a conventional pacing lead placed within an explanted dog's heart filled with anticoagulated blood. As the volume was changed by injecting or withdrawing blood, the resistance was measured and compared with that of the blood contained in the right ventricle.

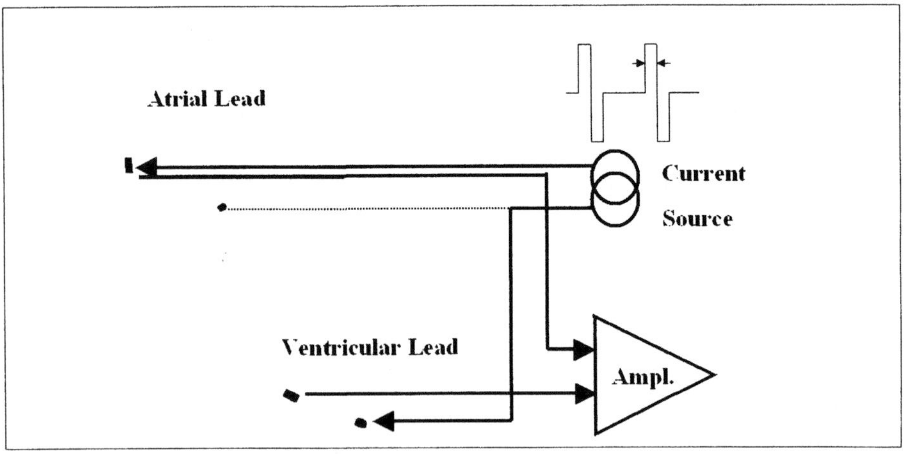

Fig. 1. Schematic of the connections needed for multipolar intracardiac impedance detection. In this example a transvalvular configuration is shown: the low-amplitude, constant-current source is driven to the atrial ring and ventricular tip electrodes and the resulting voltage detected between the atrial ring and ventricular ring. This configuration was shown to have the least wall motion artifact and the best correlation with intracardiac volumes

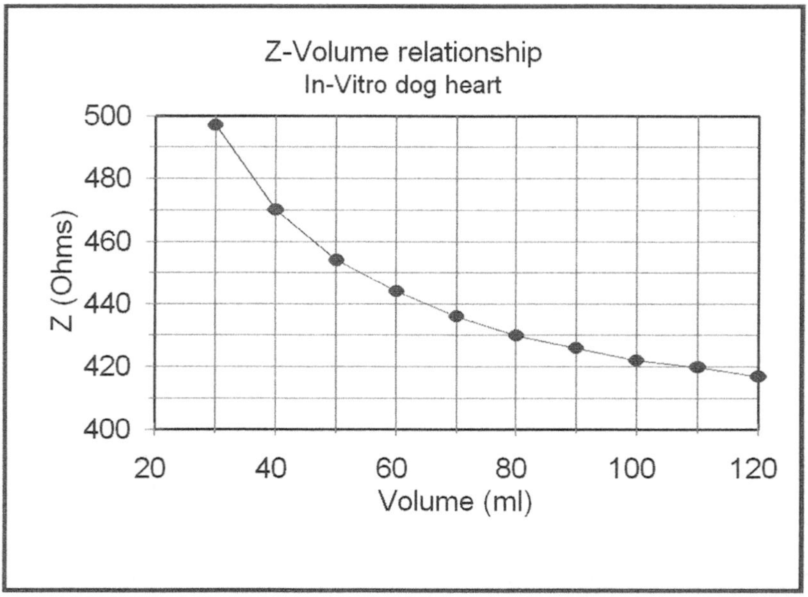

Fig. 2. Relationship between intraventricular volume and impedance (expressed in ohms). An explanted dog's heart was gradually filled with known amounts of blood, while the impedance between the ring and the tip of a pacing lead placed at the apex was measured. A nonlinear relationship was found

Different Types of Impedance Measurement

Earlier systems were based on the so-called AC-coupled method, which meant that only the changes of impedance were recorded, that is to say the peak-to-peak value of the change, with a tripolar electrode configuration (tip and two ring electrodes within the right ventricular cavity). This method allowed the estimation of relative stroke volume changes, rate of rise in ejection, and timing of events, such as measurement of the pre-ejection period [6]. CPI's Precept pacemaker (St. Paul, Minn., USA) embodied such a system for measurement of the pre-ejection period as a marker of cardiac contractility. A unipolar configuration (meaning the pacemaker can act as the ground electrode) may also reveal volume variations, but this configuration is far more sensitive to local wall motion, which can distort the volume waveform [7]. This approach is used in Biotronik's (Berlin, Germany) Inos CLS+ systems, in which analysis of the wall motion is used; other impedance configurations may be possible with this system [7]. The transvalvular impedance (TVI) configuration employs any combination of two to four electrodes from a combination of bipolar atrial and ventricular leads, an approach being developed by Medico (Rubano, Italy) [8]. A combination of more than two poles offers better rendering of volume changes and improved signal-to-noise ratio. By employing atrial and ventricular electrodes the system produces a waveform (Fig. 3).

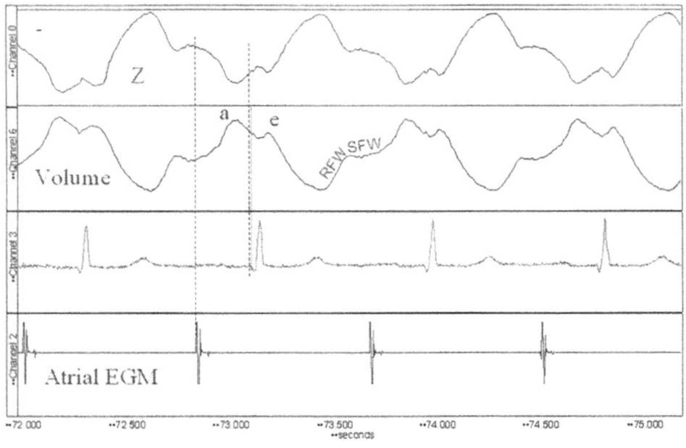

Fig. 3. Transvalvular impedance waveform is seen at the top. The reversal of the waveform in channel 2 has the typical volume waveform. After the atrial contraction (signaled by the atrial electrogram) there is an increase in volume (atrial kick), immediately followed by a rapid volume decrease corresponding to ventricular ejection. After ejection the rapid filling (RFW) and slow filling (SFW) waves are seen, ending with the atrial contraction of the next cycle

Limitations

Just as in the case of any other physiological measurement, spurious signals may contaminate the impedance waveform. Any distortion of the waveform is generally categorized as noise, which can be of various types:

a) Electronic noise related to the pacemaker circuitry is of random nature and high frequency and is generally removed by low-pass filtering or signal averaging.
b) Extracardiac noise is caused by changes in parallel resistance of the tissues surrounding the heart, such as lungs and diaphragm, and by motion of the heart related to postural changes. This type of noise can be significantly reduced by special algorithms.
c) Intracardiac noise is caused by atrial and/or ventricular wall motion and is noticeable after atrial contraction and after ventricular mechanical activation and early ventricular filling.

At present, noise reduction is achieved by different procedures: since for the calculation of cardiac preload and contractility only two parameters need to be extracted from the impedance and only single measurements, at the end of diastole (during isovolumic contraction) and at end-systole (during isovolumic relaxation), are required. These measurements are taken during time-specific windows where neither heart volume nor wall motion is changing, so that the effect of intracardiac noise is minimal. Averaging techniques, digital filters, and special algorithms to compensate for respiration and postural changes are now being used to improve the quality of the signal.

Hemodynamic Measurements

Since the detection of intracardiac impedance, whether intraventricular or transvalvular, may allow an estimation of relative volume change in the cardiac chambers, the question that arises is how to extract valuable hemodynamic information from it. As mentioned above, the peak-to-peak impedance change is a reflection of stroke volume change, but as is well known, this parameter is only one part of the picture of cardiac performance. The key parameters of cardiac function are *preload*, *afterload*, and *contractility*, and since the right ventricle is not exposed to the afterload offered by the peripheral resistance, and appraisal of preload and contractility is feasible from volume estimates, work has been done on assessing the feasibility of extracting these parameters from the intracardiac impedance waveform [4, 5]. The best *preload* marker is known to be the ventricular end-diastolic volume (EDV). This parameter requires no special calculation and in clinical practice beat-to-beat assessment of it by 2D echocardiography is possible. Radionuclide ventriculography is also adequate for EDV assessment, but no beat-to-beat measurement is possible. *Contractility* assessment is far more complex. There is no single measure of contractility that is not influenced by preload and/or afterload. In clinical practice, ejection fraction (EF) is probably the most frequently used parameter of contractile function. Since stroke volume (SV) is modulated both by contractility and by preload (Starling mechanism), obtaining the quotient between SV/EDV reduces the effect of preload, though not entirely abolishing it. In the right ventricle, where ejection faces a much lower and less variable load (pulmonary vascular resistance) than in the left ventricle, the calculation of contractility changes (not absolute values) may be less dependent on afterload.

Impedance Hemodynamics

In order to assess EDV with an impedance system, both the static and the dynamic resistances have to be measured. This is accomplished by DC coupling of the impedance measurement. The total value for intracardiac impedance at end-diastole will then be a marker of EDV, while the total impedance at end-systole will be a marker of end-systolic volume (ESV). With these two measurements it is then possible to calculate SV and EF. The total intracardiac impedance is composed of a static and a dynamic component. For a lead resistance of 500 Ω the static component is around 400 Ω. Fluctuations of impedance that take place above this "threshold" are due primarily to intracardiac volume changes and secondarily to changes related to extracardiac structures, such as wall motion and thoracic impedance changes caused by respiration. All of the impedance changes that are unrelated to intracardiac volume changes are considered noise. Ever since it was first incorporated into pacemakers in 1992, the impedance method has been subject to constant improvement and refinement aimed at reducing the level of noise and improving the detection of true hemodynamic markers of cardiac performance.

Measurement of Preload

End-diastolic volume of the right ventricle is considered to be one of the best markers of cardiac preload. The total value of end-diastolic impedance was tested in animal and human experiments with preload challenges, such as inferior vena cava occlusion in the dog or incremental pacing and isoproterenol to reduce diastolic filling in humans. Figure 4 shows how the impedance-derived estimation of end-diastolic volume follows a physiologically predictable response when intracardiac volume decreases as the balloon in the inferior vena cava is inflated. At the end of the occlusion, and upon release of the balloon, the expected overshoot is noted not only on the volume tracing but also on the arterial pressure record. Incremental pacing in humans causes a similar, albeit more attenuated, response (Fig. 5). Since preload changes in the absence of an inotropic stimulus are expected to provoke a reduction in stroke volume, this challenge allows the construction of typical Starling curves (Fig. 6).

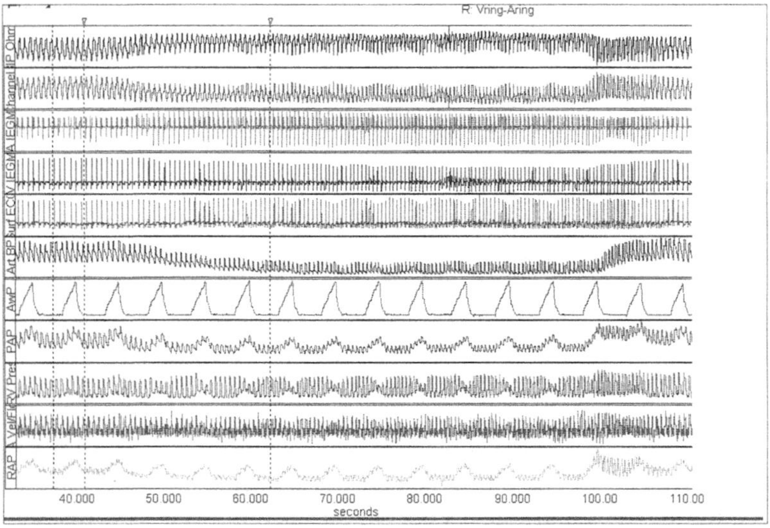

Fig. 4. Dog experiment. Continuous low-speed recording. An inflatable balloon was placed in the inferior vena cava to cause a sudden reduction in venous return to the right heart. Impedance (channel 1) was measured between the atrial and ventricular rings. At the point where the balloon was inflated, the expected reduction of end-diastolic volume is noted (channel 2). When the balloon was deflated an overshoot is noted on the volume waveform, indicating that impedance-derived volumes closely follow the expected physiological behavior. Channel 3 records the atrial EGM, channel 4, the ventricular EGM, and channel 5, the surface ECG; channel 6 records the arterial blood pressure, channel 7, the pulmonary wedge pressure (modulated by the respirator), and the last four channels, P.A. pressure, R.V. pressure, P.A. flow (electromagnetic flowmeter), and right atrial pressure

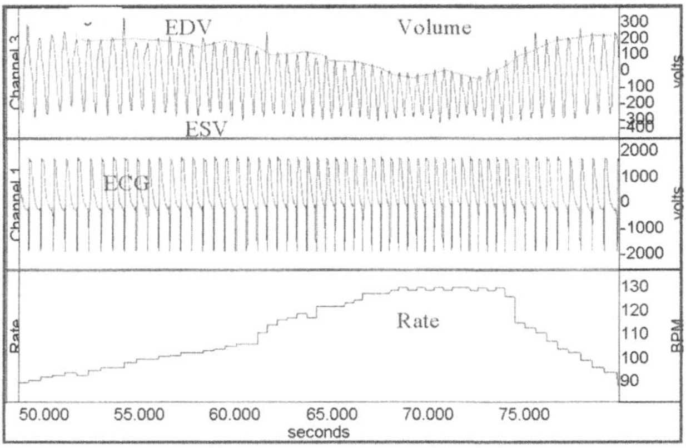

Fig. 5. Intraventricular impedance recorded from a patient during VVI pacing. The rate was increased from 90 to 130 ppm. End-diastolic volume decreases as the rate increases due to reduction of filling time. Accordingly, stroke volume also becomes smaller. End-systolic volume remains unchanged

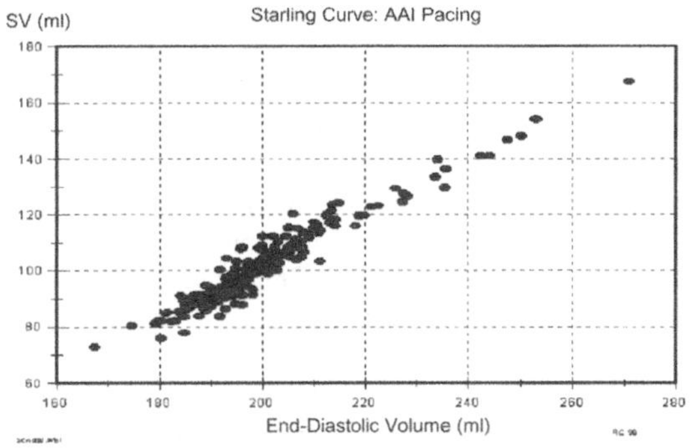

Fig. 6. Starling curve (relationship between SV and EDV)

Measurement of Contractility

Once the difficulties in obtaining an accurate assessment of contractility independent of preload and afterload were recognized, the model of preload correction of RV stroke volume was used. The SV/EDV ratio is aimed at removing the preload effect from SV (Starling), thus giving a widely used measure of contractility, the ejection fraction. Since the right ventricle (where impedance/volume measurements are taken) is a volume pump with very compliant afterload (the pulmonary vasculature), the effects of systemic afterload changes (in the arterial tree) are not apparent. Impedance-derived EF has been tested in animals and humans by comparison of the change in EF and the change in intrinsic heart rate under inotropic pharmacological stimulation.

Possible Applications of Hemodynamic Sensors

1. Physiological rate adaptation in patients with chronotropic incompetence.
2. Hemodynamic monitoring for the follow-up of patients with heart failure.
3. Discrimination of arrhythmia and its use as a marker of hemodynamic deterioration during tachyarrhythmias (in ICDs).
4. Hemodynamic upper rate limit control, to reduce the incidence of false-positive responses observed with motion sensors.
5. Hemodynamic monitoring in patients with neuro-cardiogenic syncope requiring a pacemaker.

In conclusion, hemodynamic assessment is feasible using intracardiac impedance. It offers reliable markers of preload and contractility by using standard pacing electrodes and no need for additional hardware on the leads.

References

1. Schlant RC, Sonnenblick EH (1994) Normal physiology of the cardiovascular system. In: Schlant RC, Alexander RW (eds) The heart, 8th edn. McGraw Hill, New York, pp. 113–151
2. Irnich W (1994) Impedance, conductance, resistance: definitions and measurement principles. In: Winter UJ, Klocke RK, Kubicek WG, Niederlag W (eds). Thieme, Stuttgart, pp 4–10
3. Baan J, de Jong TT, Kerkhof PLM, Moene RJ, van Dijk AD, van der Velde ET, Koops J (1981) Continuous stroke volume and cardiac output from intra-ventricular dimensions obtained with impedance catheter. Cardiovasc Res 15:328–334
4. Chirife R (1991) Acquisition of hemodynamic data and sensor signals for rate control from standard pacing electrodes. Pacing Clin Electrophysiol 14:1563–1565
5. Chirife R, Ortega DF, Salazar AI (1993) Feasibility of measuring relative right ventricular volumes and ejection fraction with implantable rhythm control devices. Pacing Clin Electrophysiol 16:1673–1683
6. Chirife R (1998) Physiological principles of a new method for rate responsive pacing using the pre-ejection interval. Pacing Clin Electrophysiol 11:1545–1554
7. Czygan G, Chirife R, Lippert M, Tentori MC, Mazzetti H (2002) Relative ventricular volume measurements by intracardiac impedance. Biomed Tech (Berl) 47 [Suppl 1] Pt 1:130–131
8. Di Gregorio F, Morra A, Finesso M, Bongiorni MG (1996) Transvalvular impedance (TVI) recording under electrical and pharmacological cardiac stimulation. Pacing Clin Electrophysiol 19:1689–1693

Hemodynamic Sensors: Their Impact in Clinical Practice

E. Occhetta[1], A. Magnani[1], M. Bortnik[1], G. Francalacci[1], F. Di Gregorio[2], C. Vassanelli[1]

Introduction

The need to adjust pacing rate to changing metabolic conditions has led to the development of different sensing systems that integrate the detection of atrial and ventricular electrical signals in permanent pacemakers [1]. All sensors currently available in the clinical setting assess the patient's metabolic demand indirectly. This is the case for activity sensors, which generally detect the intensity of body motion by an accelerometer, as well as for physiological sensors, which are sensitive to cardiac or respiratory parameters physiologically correlated to the cardiac rate. The activity sensors usually show good sensitivity and prompt rate-response, but may lack specificity, since they cannot distinguish between active and passive motion. Respiratory sensors are more specific, but they show a slow response, resulting in little sensitivity towards the rapid, small changes in a patient's activity which normally occur in daily life [2]. Cardiac sensors have to represent the best compromise between sensitivity and specificity, since the different aspects of cardiac function are regulated at the same time by the same controller, the autonomic nervous system (ANS). In patients with chronotropic incompetence, a pacemaker would restore normal rate control on the basis of relative changes in the inotropic, dromotropic, or bathmotropic regulation of the heart [3].

Cardiac Sensors

At present, cardiac sensors include Q-T or hemodynamic sensors. The Q-T sensor relies on the principle that the Q-T interval shortens as a function of the adrenergic input to the ventricular myocardium. Therefore, Q-T monitoring could give an insight into the overall sympathetic tone and allows corre-

[1]Division of Cardiology, School of Medicine, Università degli Studi del Piemonte Orientale, Novara, and [2]Medico Clinical Research, Rubano, Padua, Italy

sponding rate adaptation. The issue is complicated, however, since the Q-T interval is not dependent on adrenergic input alone, but is strongly influenced by the heart rate itself. Since the Q-T duration adapts automatically to the cycle length (shortening as the cardiac rate increases), this rate-responsive system is possibly affected by positive feedback and requires dedicated self-compensation algorithms [4].

Hemodynamic sensors detect changes in the hemodynamic performance of the heart, which partially depends on the ANS-induced inotropic regulation of myocardial fibers. Under physiological conditions, inotropic and chronotropic properties are controlled in order to synergistically modulate the cardiac output according to the metabolic demand. Once the required hemodynamic compensation has been achieved, the system is down-regulated [5]. Thanks to this intrinsic negative feedback, in the case of chronotropic incompetence, assessment of cardiac contractility would allow timely rate adaptation with reduced risk of overpacing [6].

Specific hemodynamic sensors have been designed to measure different expressions of the cardiac contraction strength. An implantable system sensitive to the maximum *dP/dt* in the right ventricle (RV) proved effective in a clinical trial [7], but was abandoned thereafter due to the long-term inconsistency of the sensor (a piezoelectric pressure transducer included in the pacing lead). Hemodynamic sensors that detect the mechanical action of the heart and blood flow have been proposed [8]. In clinical practice, peak endocardial acceleration (PEA) [9] and the rate of change of unipolar ventricular impedance [10] have been shown to correlate with the maximum RV *dP/dt* and are applied in currently used rate-responsive systems.

Peak Endocardial Acceleration

PEA is recorded by an accelerometer mounted in the tip of the pacing lead, which is sensitive to RV wall vibrations generated by the mechanical activity of the heart. The original PEA signal (PEA I) is detected during the isometric phase of systole and corresponds therefore to the first cardiac sound. The greater the contraction strength, the higher the amplitude of peak PEA I [9]. The pacing rate is regulated according to the PEA signal, being increased whenever the contraction strength increases and reduced if the contraction strength decreases (BEST-LIVING, Sorin, Italy). This algorithm allows rate-responsive pacing during physical exercise, mental stress, and activities of daily life [11, 12]. Interestingly, even if the sensor is located in the RV, the PEA I amplitude is determined by the contraction strength in the left ventricle (LV), where the systolic myocardial vibrations are generated [13].

Recently, another application of the intracardiac accelerometer has been reported. In addition to PEA I, the sensor can detect a further signal, which is designated as PEA II. PEA II is recorded during the isometric phase of diastole and corresponds to the second cardiac sound. Experimental studies indicate that the PEA II amplitude reflects the rate of rise of the pressure gradient across the aortic valve at the time of valve closure, which depends on both the rate of ventricular pressure reduction (negative LV dP/dt) and the afterload. For this reason, PEA II might provide information on LV diastolic function as well as on the trend of diastolic arterial pressure [14].

Ventricular Impedance

The main disadvantage of PEA recording comes from the need for a dedicated lead mounting the intracardiac accelerometer, which strongly limits the number of patients who could benefit from this sensor system. Electrical impedance measurement has been proposed as a valuable alternative: impedance can be assessed with standard pacing leads and is known to vary during the cardiac cycle as a result of changes in ventricular volume and myocardial structure. The rate of change of unipolar impedance (measured between the tip electrode in RV and the pacemaker can) during ventricular systole and the area under the signal are used as markers of cardiac contractility [15] to drive a rate-responsive pacemaker familiy (INOS, Biotronik, Germany). Clinical tests have demonstrated the reliability of this sensor during physical activity, as well as under conditions of mental stress [16, 17].

Since electrical impedance is inversely dependent on conducting volume, RV impedance was also applied to derive information on RV volume changes from diastole to systole, i.e., to assess the stroke volume (SV) [18]. However, SV and the other hemodynamic parameters related to the cardiac contraction strength (dP/dt_{max}, PEA I, ventricular impedance rate of change) are all strongly influenced by preload and afterload. As a consequence, they may reflect nonspecific, ANS-independent factors in addition to ventricular contractility. It is well known that the preload can change abruptly in daily life as a result of posture changes and skeletal muscle activity, thus affecting the force developed by the ventricle in systole and the SV, according to the Frank–Starling law. This reduces the reliability of all hemodynamic sensors during rest–activity transitions: in some instances, the compensatory inotropic reaction must overcome an opposite preload influence before the rate-response is triggered. This drawback could be eliminated only by assessing the instantaneous relationship between SV and preload, which is the most appropriate expression of contractility level in the heart [19].

Transvalvular Impedance

Cardiac impedance could be applied to detect changes in end-diastolic ventricular volume (EDV) as well as volume changes from diastolic to end-systolic conditions, provided that the absolute impedance is recorded instead of just peak-to-peak variation. This is possible if high-quality, stable, and noise-free impedance signals are derived. This goal has been achieved thanks to a new recording method whereby impedance is detected between the right atrium and the right ventricle, called transvalvular impedance (TVI).

TVI is a regular periodic waveform with a minimum value during atrial systole and a maximum at the end of the Q-T period [20, 21]. The minimum TVI, which is recorded close to the maximum ventricular filling, is sensitive to all conditions known to modify the preload. The maximum TVI, which is recorded when the ventricular systole is completed, corresponds to the minimal ventricular volume (end-systolic volume, ESV) and is sensitive to changes in cardiac contractility. The relative variations in EDV, ESV, SV, and ejection fraction (EF) define a cardiac inotropic index fully independent of preload effects, which is a direct expression of the ANS regulation of the heart [22, 23]. Even if TVI data are referred to the RV, the essential hemodynamic information holds for the systemic circulation as well, since under steady conditions the SV is the same in the pulmonary artery and the aorta. When the inotropic index was used to drive a rate-responsive stimulator (SOPHÓS EXT, Medico, Italy), the TVI-indicated pacing rate proved a precise replication of the individual sinus rate in patients with physiological chronotropic competence [24].

Clinical Impact of Hemodynamic Sensors

Rate-responsive pacing is just one of the many potential applications of hemodynamic sensors in implantable pacemakers. Clinical trials support the possible use of these tools to recognize the prodromes of neurally mediated syncope, and to trigger protective pacing [25, 26]. TVI has been proposed for beat-to-beat detection of mechanical ventricular activity and capture confirmation [20]. Hemodynamic sensors might assess contraction strength or SV in order to optimize the atrioventricular delay [27, 28]. In cardiac resynchronization therapy, they could provide indications about the most appropriate left ventricular pacing site, or the best interventricular delay to apply [29, 30]. Furthermore, hemodynamic sensors might play a role in the long-term monitoring of heart failure, helping the physician in the individual care of each patient. This last task would be quite appealing, especially if the diagnostic system gave information on the trend of the main hemodynamic variables such as the preload, the afterload, the SV, and the EF.
The new sensor based on TVI looks promising to play this important function in future hemodynamic pacemakers.

References

1. Lau CP (1993) Rate adaptive cardiac pacing: single and dual chamber. Futura, Mount Kisco, NY
2. Rossi P (1987) Rate responsive pacing: biosensor reliability and physiological sensitivity. Pacing Clin Electrophysiol 10:454–466
3. Occhetta E, Bortnik M, Francalacci G et al (2001) How reliable and effective are hemodynamic sensors to correct chronotropic incompetence? In: Raviele A (ed) Cardiac arrhythmias 2001. Springer, Milan, pp 586–594

4. Baig MW, Wilson J, Boute W et al (1989) Improved pattern of rate responsiveness with dynamic slope setting for the QT sensing pacemaker. Pacing Clin Electrophysiol 12:311–320
5. Pichelmaier AM, Braile D, Ebner E et al (1992) Autonomic nervous system controlled closed loop cardiac pacing. Pacing Clin Electrophysiol 15:1787–1791
6. Occhetta E, Francalacci G, Perucca A et al (1996) Improving exercise tolerance efficiently: how much sensor driven pacing is required? In: Santini M (ed) Progress in clinical pacing. Rome, pp 197–203
7. Bennett T, Sharma A, Sutton R et al (1992) Development of a rate adaptive pacemaker based on the maximum rate-of-rise of right ventricular pressure (RV dP/dtmax). Pacing Clin Electrophysiol 15:219–234
8. Daum DR, Jones BR, Lang DJ (2000) Hemodynamic sensors. Am J Cardiol 86(Suppl):95K–100K
9. Rickards AF, Bombardini T, Plicchi G et al (1996) An implantable intracardiac accelerometer for monitoring myocardial contractility. Pacing Clin Electrophysiol 19:2066–2071
10. Osswald S, Cron T, Gradel C et al (2000) Closed-loop stimulation using intracardiac impedance as a sensor principle: correlation of right ventricular dP/dtmax and intracardiac impedance during dobutamine stress test. Pacing Clin Electrophysiol 23:1502–1508
11. Langenfeld H, Krein A, Kirstein M et al (1998) Peak endocardial acceleration based clinical testing of the "BEST" DDDR pacemaker. Pacing Clin Electrophysiol 21:2187–2191
12. Clementy J, Kobeissi A, Garrigue S et al (2000) Validation by serial standardized testing of a new rate-responsive pacemaker sensor based on variations in myocardial contractility. Europace 3:124–131
13. Padeletti L, Perna AM, Michelucci A et al (1998) Contractility and peak endocardial acceleration (PEA) during experimental coronary occlusion. Arch Coeur Vaisseaux Cardiostim 98:17–3 (abstract)
14. Plicchi G, Marcelli E, Parlapiano M et al (2002) PEA I and PEA II based implantable haemodynamic monitor: preclinical studies in sheep. Europace 4:49–54
15. Schaldach M, Hutten H (1992) Intracardiac impedance to determine sympathetic activity in rate responsive pacing. Pacing Clin Electrophysiol 15:1778–1786
16. Witte J, Pichelmaier AM, Ebner E et al (1996) ANS controlled rate adaptive pacing. A clinical evaluation. Eur J Card Pacing Electrophysiol 6:53–59
17. Griesbach L, Gestrich B, Wojciechowski D et al (2003) Clinical performance of automatic closed-loop stimulation systems. Pacing Clin Electrophysiol 26(Pt.I):1432-1437
18. Chirife R, Ortega DF, Salazar A (1993) Feasibility of measuring relative right ventricular volumes and ejection fraction with implantable rhythm control devices. Pacing Clin Electrophysiol 16:1673–1683
19. Chirife R, Tentori MC, Mazzetti H et al (2001) Hemodynamic sensors: are they all the same? In: Raviele A (ed) Cardiac arrhythmias. Springer, Milan, pp 566–575
20. Di Gregorio F, Morra A, Finesso M et al (1996) Transvalvular impedance (TVI) recording under electrical and pharmacological cardiac stimulation. Pacing Clin Electrophysiol 19(Pt II):1689–1693
21. Gasparini M, Curnis A, Mantica M et al (2001) Hemodynamic sensors: what clinical value do they have in heart failure? In: Raviele A (ed) Cardiac arrhythmias. Springer, Milan, pp 576–585
22. Bongiorni MG, Soldati E, Arena G et al (2001) Hemodynamic sensors: what clinical value do they have in chronotropic incompetence? In: Raviele A (ed) Cardiac arrhythmias 2001. Springer, Milan, pp 595–601

23. Di Gregorio F, Curnis A, Pettini A et al (2002) Trans-valvular impedance (TVI) in the hemodynamic regulation of cardiac pacing. In: Mitro P, Pella D, Rybár R, Valocik G (eds) Cardiovascular diseases 2002. Monduzzi, Bologna, pp 53–57
24. Gasparini G, Curnis A, Mascioli G et al (2003) Clinical test of a pacing device driven by trans-valvular impedance. Pacing Clin Electrophysiol 26 (2–Pt II): S204 (abstract)
25. Deharo JC, Peyre JP, Ritter PH et al (1998) Treatment of malignant primary vasodepressive neurocardiogenic syncope with a rate responsive pacemaker driven by heart contractility. Pacing Clin Electrophysiol 21:2688–2690
26. Occhetta E, Bortnik M, Vassanelli C et al (2003) The DDDR closed loop stimulation for the prevention of vasovagal syncope: results from the INVASY prospective feasibility registry. Europace 5:153–162
27. Padeletti L, Porciani MC, Ritter P et al (2000) Atrioventricular interval optimization in the right atrial appendage and interatrial septum pacing: a comparison between echo and peak endocardial acceleration measurements. Pacing Clin Electrophysiol 23(11–Pt I):1618–1622
28. Ravazzi AP, Diotallevi P, Provera MF et al (2001) AV delay optimization using ventricular intracardiac impedance. Europace 2 [Suppl C]:C26 (abstract)
29. Bordachar P, Garrigue S, Reuter S et al (2000) Hemodynamic assessment of right, left, and biventricular pacing by peak endocardial acceleration and echocardiography in patients with end-stage heart failure. Pacing Clin Electrophysiol 23(11–Pt II):1726–1730
30. Bocchiardo M, Caponi D, Di Donna P et al (2003) Optimization of resynchronization therapy by intracardiac ventricular impedance. In: Gulizia M (ed) New advances in heart failure and atrial fibrillation. Springer, Milan, pp 411–415

Haemodynamic Pacing: When Is It Selectively Indicated?

J. Clémenty, S. Reuter, P. Bordachar, S. Garrigue, P. Jaïs, M. Haïssaguerre

Introduction

The determinant factors of cardiac output are systolic ejection volume and heart rate. Since the first pacemaker (PM) implantation in 1958, all the indications for PM implantation have been haemodynamic ones: heart rate stabilisation, exercise rate responsiveness, restoration of AV synchronisation (Table 1).

The incidence of congestive heart failure (CHF) has been rising for some years, to the extent that it is set to become the "epidemic of the next millennium". Dysregulation of the cardiac pump induced by myocardial fibrosis is associated with an impairment of the electrical cardiac influx propagation and has opened the way for nonbradycardia haemodynamic pacing aimed at improving the quality of life and prognosis of patients with CHF by mean of cardiac resynchronisation therapy (CRT).

Table 1. Electrical impairments with haemodynamic consequences and pacing modalities for haemodynamic improvement

CHF: Electrical disturbances	Haemodynamic pacing
	Rate responsive vs fixed rate
Cellular (channels, ions, proteins, etc.)	AAI (R) or DDD (R) vs VVI (R)
Inappropriate bradycardia or tachycardia	DDD + short AV delay vs tailored AV delay
Conduction delay	RVOT vs RV apex vs RV multisite pacing
- Intra-atrial	LV pacing
- AV	Biventricular pacing
- Intraventricular	Four-chamber pacing
	Nonexcitatory pacing

Hôpital Cardiologique, Université de Bordeaux, Pessac, France

CTOPP (and Others) vs MIRACLE (and Others)

Surprisingly, the recent pacing literature is characterised by conflicting results obtained with two different haemodynamic pacing approaches: AV delay preservation and CRT [1].

Numerous studies performed over a long period have established the deleterious effects of AV synchronisation loss, retrograde VA conduction inducing a decrease in cardiac output, AV valvular regurgitation, left atrial dilatation and neuro-hormonal disturbances.

Nonetheless, three large recent controlled trials including large cohorts of patients (PASE, CTOPP, UK-PACE) have not demonstrated any benefit of DDDR mode versus VVIR mode in all patients. Only younger patients or device-dependent patients or patients with PMs for sinus node disease are improved by dual-chamber devices [2].

The economic consequences of these studies (300 Euro per patient per day) might be expected to be contained by the short follow-up of the patients, the absence of impaired cardiac function in study patients, the additive cost of associated drugs (inotropic and antiarrhythmic drugs) and the necessity of upgrading VVI devices to DDD devices early in the follow-up for about 25% of the patients.

In contrast, all the controlled trials have established a significantly favourable effect of CRT, with an increase in cardiac output, systolic blood pressure, left ventricular ejection fraction, exercise tolerance and quality of life index [3]. CRT provides optimisation of AV contraction, right and left ventricular coordination, prolongation of left-ventricular filling time, improvement of septal motility, and reduction of the severity of mitral regurgitation. These results (Table 2) have been observed with short follow-up times (10–22 months).

Table 2. CRT: Results of controlled trials

Study	N	Changes in in NYHA class	Improvement in 6-min walking test (%)	Changes in VO_2 (%)	Changes in LVEF (%)
French pilot	125	−1.0	-	+42	+28
INSYNCH	103	−1.1	+20		-
PATH CHF	29	−1.2	+25	+24	-
MUSTIC	82	−0.8	+19	+10	+14
MIRACLE	453	−0.8	+17	+8	+21
Italian INSYCH	190	−1.0	+31	-	+24

LVEV, left-ventricular ejection fraction; *NYHA*, New York Heart Association; *VO_2*, oxygen uptake

It may be that the favourable results obtained in these trials, in which fewer than 1,000 patients were enrolled and were followed up for 1 or 2 years, do not reflect the effect in the thousands of patients each treated for several years outside clinical studies. In addition, the proportion of nonresponder patients must be estimated at about 20%, indicating technical limitations and the necessity for appropriate patient selection.

Patient Selection for CRT

Clinical Markers

In controlled studies the presence of a cardiomyopathy is a target factor, and no difference was observed in the efficacy of CRT efficiency between idiopathic and ischaemic cardiomyopathies.

CHF must be present. No study has established a potential preventive efficiency of CRT with respect to CHF. In controlled trials, only patients in NYHA classes III or IV are eligible, but small studies have found a beneficial effect of CRT in patients in NYHA class II. The mechanisms of action are not known, and AV pacing is probably useful to optimise CHF therapy (e.g. β-blockers and bradycardia).

The 6-minute walking test is not mandatory to check whether CRT is indicated. This test is closely correlated to the NYHA classification but provides an objective quantitative evaluation of the benefit of CRT [4].

The presence of mitral regurgitation is an important point for beneficial effects of CRT. Reuter et al. [5], in a retrospective study, have demonstrated that most patients who do not respond to CRT have nonsignificant mitral regurgitation. Mitral regurgitation is a marker of the alterations in left-ventricular shape in CHF: the most important is left-ventricular sphericity, and mitral regurgitation is the most severe. Remodelling induced by CRT is associated with a reduction in left ventricular sphericity [6].

The left-ventricular ejection fraction should be less than 35%.

Electrical Markers

Patients enrolled in controlled trials have a spontaneous QRS complex duration higher than 120 ms or a right-ventricle paced QRS complex duration of longer than 200 ms [7].

In the PATH-CHF II study, patients with a QRS duration longer than 150 ms show very fast improvement of their CHF (< 3 months), but after 6 months of follow-up, all the patients have improved, regardless of the QRS duration.

Some short studies have found an improvement for patients without QRS enlargement.

The left bundle branch block pattern is an important marker for CRT efficiency, but Garrigue et al. [8] have established a favourable effect of CRT in patients with the right bundle branch block pattern and an injection fraction <25%. Any improvement in a patient with the administration of CRT is unrelated to QRS narrowing by pacing; left-ventricular pacing has been shown to be equal in efficiency to biventricular pacing despite the preservation of a large, paced QRS complex.

Electrical markers are useful in patient selection, but are not absolutely mandatory [9].

Gold Standard for Patient Selection: Echocardiography

Echocardiography techniques provide the most reliable evaluation of the mechanical dispersion associated with CHF.

Echo-Doppler provides evaluation of the respective contributions of E- and A-waves to left-ventricular filling [10] and measurements of the pre-ejection time for the right and the left ventricles: the differences express the inter-ventricular conduction delay (n=< 40 ms).

Doppler tissue imaging (DTI) techniques provide an assessment of the difference in contraction time between the left ventricle different segments [11]. In a recent study, Yu et al. determined the index of synchronicity for 12 different segments of the left ventricle. CRT is efficient only in patients with a high value of this index (>32) before PM implantation [11].

In a previous study, Garrigue et al. demonstrated the absence of correlation between ECG abnormalities (bundle branch block, QRS duration) and the echocardiographic data on left-ventricular dys-synchronisation (Table 3). These results explain a possible improvement of cardiac function by CRT in

Table 3. Distribution of the ECG characteristics according to the different types of electromechanical ventricular asynchrony in the study population

ECG characteristic	Inter-V asynchrony alone	Intra-LV asynchrony alone	Inter-V and intra-LV asynchrony	Total asynchrony
Complete LBBB, (%)	07	55*	29	91
Complete RBBB, (%)	0	56*	27	82
Incomplete LBBB, (%)	02	44	10	56
Left anterior hemibloc, (%)	0	40	10	50
QRS width >120 ms, (ms)	06	56*	28	90
QRS width >140 ms, (ms)	08	51*	38	97
QRS width <120 ms, (ms)	02	46	10	58

*P<0.05, by a multivariate analysis of variance between the four types of asynchrony

patients with normal duration of the QRS complex and the absence of any correlation between CRT efficiency and narrowing of the QRS complex by CRT.

Conclusions

CRT is indicated only in patients with severe CHF despite optimal drug therapy. Patient selection should be based first of all on functional NYHA class and an objective evaluation of left-ventricular dysfunction by ejection fraction measurement. Because CRT is devoted to the correction of mechanical left-ventricular and interventricular dys-synchronisation, the next step in patient selection should be based on echocardiography techniques: Doppler evaluation of left-ventricular diastolic filling, electromechanical delay measurements and DTI assessment of segmental left-ventricular parietal asynergy [12]. After PM implantation, echocardiographic techniques allow precise programming of AV delay and VV delay [13].

Other studies will be necessary before CRT techniques can be extended to other classes of patients.

References

1. Parsonnet V (2000) Pace maker indication revisionism. Pacing Clin Electrophysiol 23:1197–1199
2. Lamas GA, Li KL, Sweeney MO (2002) Ventricular pacing or dual chamber pacing for sinus mode dysfunction. N Engl J Med 346:1854–1862
3. Abraham WT, Fisher WG, Smith AL et al (2002) Cardiac resynchronisation in chronic heart failure. N Engl J Med 346:1845–853
4. Demers C, Mackelvie RS, Negassa A et al (2001) Reliability validity and responsiveness of the six minutes walk test in patients with heart failure. Am Heart J 142:698–703
5. Reuter S, Garrigue S, Barold SS et al (2002) Comparison of characteristics in responder versus non responder with biventricular pacing for drug resistant congestive heart failure. Am J Cardiol 89 346–350
6. Kono T, Sabbah HN, Rosman H et al (1992) Left ventricular shape is the primary determinant of functional mitral regurgitation in heart failure. J Am Coll Cardiol 20:1594–1598
7. Cazeau S, Leclercq C, Lavergne T et al (2001) Effects of multisites biventricular pacing in patients with heart failure and intraventricular conduction delay. N Engl J Med 344:873–881
8. Garrigue S, Reuter S, Labeque JN et al (2001) Usefulness of biventricular pacing in patients with congestive heart failure and right bundle branch block. Am J Cardiol 88:1436–1441
9. Charles RG (2002) Cardiac resynchronisation therapy: when and for whom? Eur Heart J Suppl 4 [Suppl D]:D117–D121

10. Kindermann M, Frohlig G, Doerr T et al (1997) Optimizing the AV delay in DDD pace maker patients with high degree of AV block: mitral valve doppler versus impedance cardiography. Pacing Clin Electrophysiol 20:2453–2462
11. Ansalone G, Giannantoni P, Ricci R et al (2001) Doppler myocardial imaging in patients with heart failure receiving biventricular pacing treatments. Am Heart J 142:881–896
12. Yu CM, Fung WH, Lin H et al (2002) Predictors of left ventricular reserve remodeling after cardiac resynchronisation therapy for heart failure secondary to idiopathic dilated or ischemic cardiopathy. Am J Cardiol 1991:684–688
13. Gasparini M, Mantica M, Galimberti P et al (2002) Optimization of cardiac resynchronisation therapy: technical aspects. Eur Heart J Suppl 4 [Suppl 2]:D82–D87

Can Hemodynamic Sensors Ensure Physiological Rate Control?

G. Gasparini[1], A. Curnis[2], M. Gulizia[3], E. Occhetta[4], A. Corrado[1], G. Mascioli[2], L. Bontempi[2], G.M. Francese[3], A. Magnani[4], M. Bortnik[4], F. Di Gregorio[5], A. Barbetta[5], F. Monese[6], A. Raviele[1]

Introduction

Hemodynamic sensors are used mainly in clinical pacing to assess the inotropic state of the heart, with the aim of matching the pacing rate to the contractility level. If the patient's chronotropic competence is depressed, this approach should allow proper cardiac rate regulation based on the physiological correlation between inotropic and chronotropic function [1–4].

Hemodynamic sensors proposed in implantable pacemakers can detect different manifestations of the strength of cardiac contractions, such as the maximum ventricular dP/dt [5], the peak endocardial acceleration [6, 7], the pre-ejection interval [8, 9], the stroke volume (SV) [10, 11] and the systolic rate of change in ventricular impedance [12, 13]. It is well known that cardiac contraction strength depends on both the autonomic nervous system (ANS) regulation of myocardial contractility and the ventricular preload, according to the Starling law. Therefore, any expression of the contraction strength can be a timely and reliable reflection of the ANS input to the heart, only if a continuous preload assessment is provided in addition [14].

In recent years, a new hemodynamic sensing system based on transvalvular impedance (TVI) recording has been developed [15, 16]. TVI data can be converted into relative right-ventricular volumes [11], so that variations in preload (end-diastolic volume; EDV), end-systolic volume (ESV), SV and ejection fraction (EF) can be detected [17, 18]. The relationship between EDV and SV specifies the TVI-inotropic index (INX), which is a measure of cardiac contractility independent of ventricular preload and can be applied to derive the corresponding contractility-indicated pacing rate [19]. The present study has tested the rate-responsive (RR) behavior of an external DDD-R pacemaker driven by TVI during β-adrenergic pharmacological stimulation.

[1]O.U. of Cardiology, Umberto I Hospital, Mestre, Venice; [2]O.U. of Cardiology, Spedali Civili, Brescia; [3]O.U. of Cardiology, S. Luigi - S. Currò Hospital, Catania; [4]O.U. of Cardiology, Maggiore della Carità Hospital, Novara; Departments of [5]Clinical Research and [6]Research & Development, MEDICO SpA, Rubano, Padua, Italy

Materials and Methods

Twenty-five patients undergoing implantation of bipolar atrial and ventricular leads for permanent dual-chamber pacing were randomly selected for the study. Patients with ventricular or supraventricular tachyarrhythmias, coronary disease, dilated or hypertrophic cardiomyopathies, severe valve diseases, and any possible contraindication to the administration of a β agonist were excluded. After the conventional positioning procedure in the right heart and threshold measurements, atrial and ventricular leads were connected to an external cardiac stimulator (Sophós Ext, Medico, Italy), which provided DDD-R pacing based on TVI detection. The stimulator was connected to a PC (through an optically isolated serial cable) for real-time display of TVI waveform, pacemaker event markers, TVI-indicated rate, and actual cardiac rate. All the above data were also stored in the stimulator memory throughout the test and downloaded at the end of the session.

The TVI signal could be derived between the atrial ring electrode and either the ring or the tip ventricular electrode. After selection of the recording configuration, TVI was measured in 128 consecutive cardiac cycles in basal conditions (resting reference). The RR algorithm was then enabled, and β-adrenergic stimulation was induced by infusion of 2 μg/min isoproterenol (IPN). By monitoring SV as a function of EDV, the pacemaker automatically calculated the inotropic index (INX), which was converted to the TVI-indicated rate according to the equation:

$$\text{TVI rate} = \text{basic rate} + \text{resting rate} * \text{INX} * \text{rate gain}$$

where the rate gain is a programmable slope factor allowing individual tuning of the RR system.

In chronotropically competent patients, the basic rate was programmed at low values to prevent atrial pacing, thus allowing comparison of sinus rate and TVI trend rate during IPN administration. The sinus index (SNX) was defined as:

$$\text{SNX} = (\text{sinus rate} / \text{resting rate}) - 1$$

and the linear regression between INX and SNX at any time was calculated by standard data analysis tools.

Results

The majority of the patients studied (64%) were affected by conduction diseases without atrial disorders. During the tests, intrinsic AV conduction was present in 56% of the cases, while the remaining 44% underwent ventricular pacing. Atrial pacing was performed in 12% of patients only.

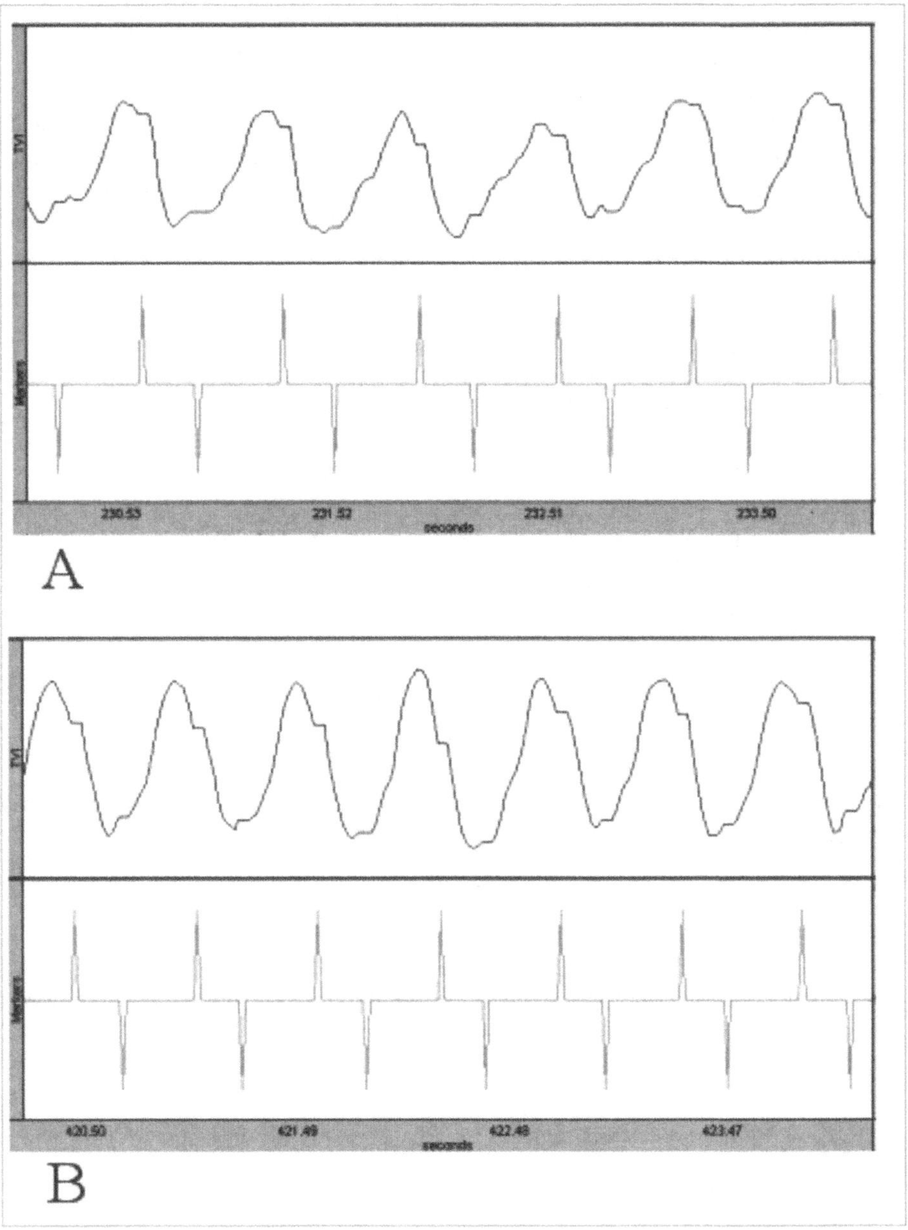

Fig. 1A, B. Transvalvular impedance (TVI; *upper tracings*) recorded between atrial and ventricular ring electrodes by the Sophós Ext stimulator, scaled in arbitrary units, and pacemaker event markers (*lower tracings*), indicating atrial sensing (*upward marker*) and ventricular sensing (*downward*) **A** in basal conditions and **B** during infusion of 2 µg/min isoproterenol. See text for detailed description

In the presence of chronotropic competence, β-adrenergic stimulation is expected to affect both sinus rate and ventricular contractility, with a similar time-course. Figure 1 shows an example of the TVI signal recorded by the Sophós Ext, in basal conditions (Fig. 1A) and during IPN infusion (Fig. 1B). The increase in intrinsic rate is accompanied by a substantial modification in TVI waveform, with higher end-systolic impedance, virtually unchanged end-diastolic impedance, and larger excursion from diastole to systole. This is interpreted by the RR system as an increase in SV, EF, and INX, and the pacing rate is modified accordingly.

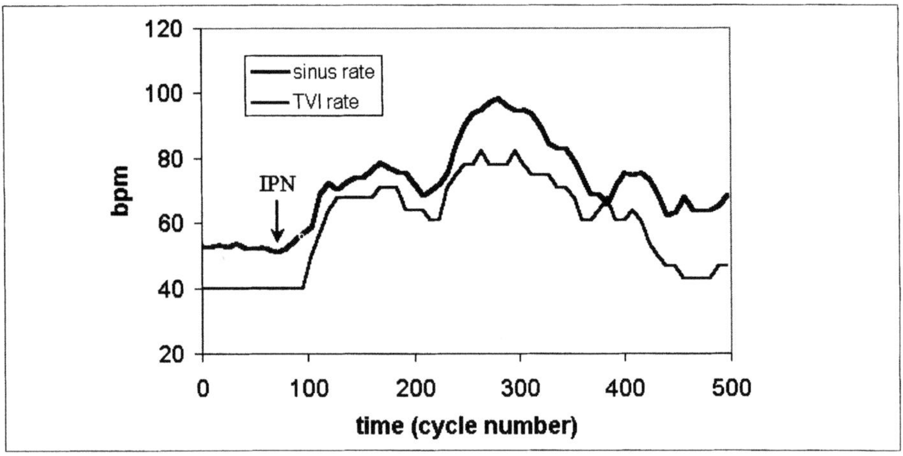

Fig. 2. Time-course of sinus rate (*thicker curve*) and TVI-indicated rate (*lighter curve*) during adrenergic challenge with isoproterenol (*IPN*)

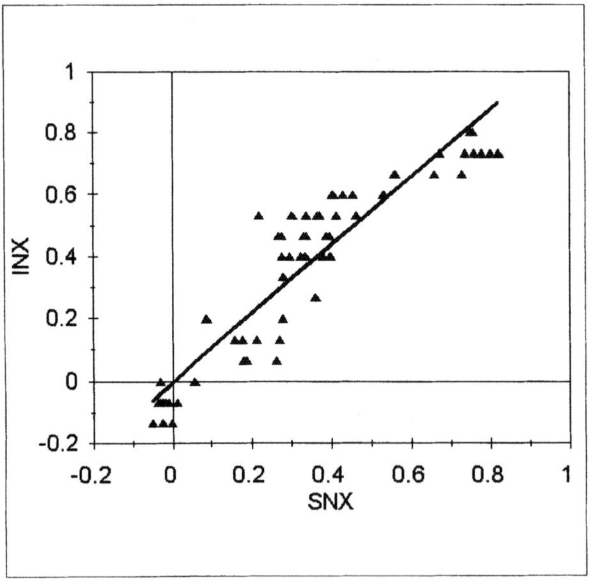

Fig. 3. Linear regression between sinus index (*SNX*) and inotropic index (*INX*) in the same patient as in Fig. 2. The regression line equation was: INX = 1.1*SNX - 0.007, where R^2 = 0.87

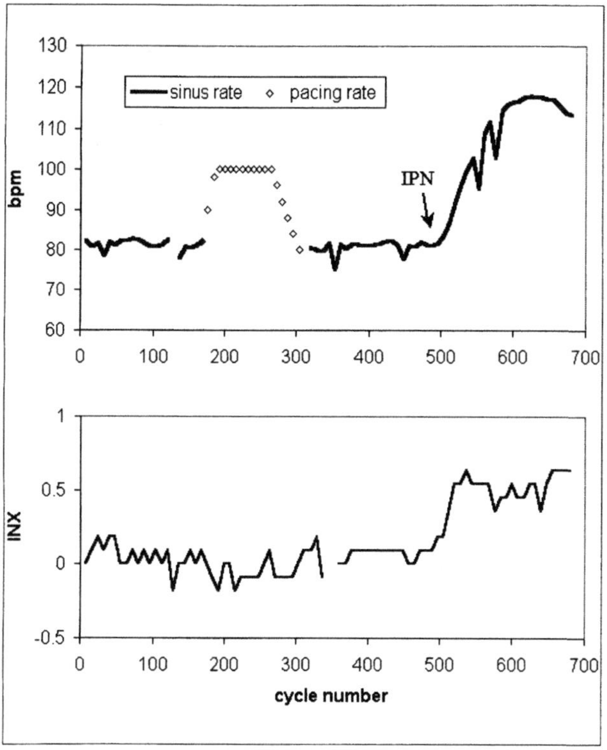

Fig. 4. *Upper panel*: time-course of sinus rate (*thick line*) and of pacing rate (*open symbols*) in a patient with chronotropic competence. The pacing rate was modified by basic rate reprogramming from 40 to 100 bpm, and then to 40 bpm again, after which the isoproterenol infusion (*IPN*) was started. *Lower panel*: time-course of the inotropic index (*INX*), which was unaffected by pacing rate changes and promptly increased during adrenergic stimulation

The trend of sinus rate and the TVI rate in a patient with normal sinus function is shown in Fig. 2. The increase in TVI rate closely mimicked the sinus rate increase, and a good correlation between INX and SNX was demonstrated ($r^2 = 0.87$; Fig. 3). In all patients who had a positive chronotropic response to IPN, the individual linear regression between INX and SNX had r^2 values in the range of 0.6–0.95. The slope coefficient ranged from 0.4 to 2.4, averaging 1.2 ± 0.7. The rate gain of the RR system was individually set in each patient to compensate for this variability, thus allowing one-to-one correspondence between TVI rate and sinus rate modifications.

The possible influence of the actual cardiac rate on INX and TVI rate was tested by basic rate reprogramming before IPN administration. An increase in cardiac rate induced by overdrive pacing, in the absence of a change in contractility, did not affect INX, which was only increased when β-adrenergic stimulation enhanced the ventricular inotropic tone (Fig. 4).

Discussion

The present study demonstrates that a good-quality TVI signal can be derived and processed by means of limited hardware and software resources that are fully compatible with the equipment and the allowed current drain of an implantable device. Thanks to the high stability and signal-to-noise ratio, TVI allows direct current (DC) recording, which means that no high-pass filtering is required. In such conditions, end-diastolic TVI is a preload marker, the peak-to-peak TVI excursion reflects the SV, and the relationship between the two specifies INX [17–19]. The stimulator Sophós Ext calculates INX in real time and reliably converts INX changes to pacing rate modifications. In patients with chronotropic competence, the TVI-indicated rate is consistent with the sinus rate trend during adrenergic challenge. On the other hand, in the absence of inotropic effects, INX is not sensitive to cardiac rate changes, indicating that the TVI-based RR system is free of positive feedback.

Our experience confirms that TVI is a promising new sensor, which can be integrated in a permanent pacemaker to gain information on cardiac hemodynamics and to drive an RR system ensuring physiological rate control.

References

1. Pichelmaier AM, Braile D, Ebner E et al (1992) Autonomic nervous system controlled closed loop cardiac pacing. Pacing Clin Electrophysiol 15:1787–1791
2. Clementy J, Kobeissi A, Garrigue S et al (2000) Validation by serial standardized testing of a new rate-responsive pacemaker sensor based on variations in myocardial contractility. Europace 3:124–131
3. Daum DR, Jones BR, Lang DJ (2000) Hemodynamic sensors. Am J Cardiol 86 [Suppl]:95K–100K
4. Occhetta E, Bortnik M, Francalacci G et al (2001) How reliable and effective are hemodynamic sensors to correct chronotropic incompetence? In: Raviele A (ed) Cardiac arrhythmias 2001. Springer-Verlag Italia, Milan, pp 586–594
5. Bennett T, Sharma A, Sutton R et al (1992) Development of a rate adaptive pacemaker based on the maximum rate-of-rise of right ventricular pressure (RV dP/dtmax). Pacing Clin Electrophysiol 15:219–234
6. Rickards AF, Bombardini T, Plicchi G et al (1996) An implantable intracardiac accelerometer for monitoring myocardial contractility. Pacing Clin Electrophysiol 19:2066–2071
7. Plicchi G, Marcelli E, Parlapiano M et al (2002) PEA I and PEA II based implantable haemodynamic monitor: pre clinical studies in sheep. Europace 4:49–54
8. Chirife R (1988) Physiological principles of a new method for rate responsive pacing using the pre-ejection interval. Pacing Clin Electrophysiol 11:1545-1554
9. Ruiter JH, Heemels JP, Kee D et al (1992) Adaptive rate pacing controlled by the right ventricular preejection interval: clinical experience with a physiological pacing system. Pacing Clin Electrophysiol 15:886–894
10. Wortel HJJ, Ruiter JH, De Boer HGA et al (1991) Impedance measurements in the human right ventricle using a new pacing system. Pacing Clin Electrophysiol 14:1336–1342
11. Chirife R, Ortega DF, Salazar A (1993) Feasibility of measuring relative right ventricular volumes and ejection fraction with implantable rhythm control devices. Pacing Clin Electrophysiol 16:1673–1683
12. Schaldach M, Hutten H (1992) Intracardiac impedance to determine sympathetic activity in rate responsive pacing. Pacing Clin Electrophysiol 15:1778–1786

13. Osswald S, Cron T, Gradel C et al (2000) Closed-loop stimulation using intracardiac impedance as a sensor principle: correlation of right ventricular dP/dt max and intracardiac impedance during dobutamine stress test. Pacing Clin Electrophysiol 23:1502–1508
14. Chirife R, Tentori MC, Mazzetti H et al (2001) Hemodynamic sensors: are they all the same? In: Raviele A (ed) Cardiac Arrhythmias. Springer-Verlag Italia, Milan, pp 566–575
15. Di Gregorio F, Morra A, Finesso M, Bongiorni MG (1996) Transvalvular impedance (TVI) recording under electrical and pharmacological cardiac stimulation. Pacing Clin Electrophysiol 19:1689–1693
16. Morra A, Panarotto D, Santini P, Di Gregorio F (1997) Transvalvular impedance (TVI) sensing: a new way toward the hemodynamic control of cardiac pacing. In: Vardas PE (ed) Europace '97. Monduzzi, Bologna, pp 529–533
17. Gasparini M, Curnis A, Mantica M et al (2001) Hemodynamic sensors: what clinical value do they have in heart failure? In: Raviele A (ed) Cardiac arrhythmias 2001. Springer-Verlag Italia, Milan, pp 576–585
18. Bongiorni MG, Soldati E, Arena G et al (2001) Hemodynamic sensors: what clinical value do they have in chronotropic incompetence? In: Raviele A (ed) Cardiac arrhythmias 2001. Springer-Verlag Italia, Milan, pp 595–601
19. Di Gregorio F, Curnis A, Pettini A et al (2002) Trans-valvular impedance (TVI) in the hemodynamic regulation of cardiac pacing. In: Mitro P, Pella D, Rybár R, Valočik G (eds) Cardiovascular diseases 2002. Monduzzi, Bologna, pp 53–57

Transvalvular Impedance: Does It Allow Automatic Capture Detection?

M.G. Bongiorni[1], E. Soldati[1], G. Arena[1], F. Di Gregorio[2], A. Barbetta[2], F. Monese[3], M. Mariani[1]

Introduction

Hemodynamic sensors of implantable pacemakers are designed to record the intensity of myocardial mechanical activity to allow estimation of the current state of the inotropic cardiac regulation [1]. This information is generally used to drive a rate-responsive system, relying on the physiological correlation between cardiac rate and contractility [2, 3]. However, the assessment of ventricular contraction based on hemodynamic evidence might also have important applications in the surveillance of pacing effectiveness [4]. Such a control system would enhance patient safety and allow a reduction in the stimulation energy, increasing the lifetime of the implanted device.

Hemodynamic validation of ventricular capture is an attractive prospect, which requires a sensitive and reliable hemodynamic sensor working on a beat-to-beat basis. Transvalvular impedance (TVI) is a good candidate for this task. TVI is the electric impedance as a function of time, recorded between an atrial and a ventricular electrode that can be either in contact with the myocardium or floating in the blood [5, 6]. Previous studies demonstrate that TVI is a low-noise, stable, periodic waveform, which is inversely related to the ventricular volume [7–9]. Indeed, TVI increases during the ventricular systole and decreases during passive and active ventricular filling, while it remains at the minimum diastolic level in the absence of ventricular ejection [5, 10, 11]. This feature has been applied in the design of an automatic capture recognition algorithm based on TVI, which was tested in the present study.

Materials and Methods

TVI was previously recorded by an external device connected to the pacing

[1]Cardiothoracic Department, Cisanello Hospital, University of Pisa; [2]Clinical Research Unit and [3]R&D Department, Medico Spa, Rubano (PD), Italy

leads during a pacemaker implantation procedure [5–11]. The TVI recorder generated high-frequency current and sampled the corresponding impedance signal, which was stored on hard disk with 1-KHz resolution for subsequent analysis and data processing. Since TVI proved to be a valuable tool allowing hemodynamic information to be obtained with standard pacing leads, an external DDD-R stimulator with the capability of real-time TVI recording and processing has recently been developed (Sophós Ext, Medico, Italy). TVI data are applied to regulate the pacer rate-responsive system and check for the presence of ventricular ejection at every beat. The automatic capture recognition algorithm compares the maximum TVI, recorded during the systolic time-window starting from a ventricular pacing spike, with a dynamic value referred to as the capture confirmation threshold (CCT). CCT is defined as a programmable percentage of the difference between average end-systolic and end-diastolic TVI in the preceding cycles (EsTVI, EdTVI), added to EdTVI. If end-systolic TVI in a given cycle ($EsTVI_i$) does not reach this level, ventricular pacing failure is assumed and the stimulator automatically increases the pulse energy to restore a correct response.

Although the Sophós Ext is an external device, it mimics the hardware and software characteristics of an implantable pacemaker, with a limited power supply. Therefore, the TVI sampling rate was reduced to 64 Hz in the intention of minimizing the current drain. We studied the TVI signal recorded with this restriction during pacemaker implantation in two patients, one with 1st-degree and one with 2nd-degree AV block, to find out the individual CCT that would ensure total sensitivity (100% recognition of pacing failures) matched with the best possible specificity (lowest prevalence of false alarms). TVI waveform and pacemaker event markers were displayed in real time on a PC screen and stored in the stimulator memory. In addition, the surface ECG was recorded throughout the test.

Results

In one patient, TVI was recorded between the atrial ring and the ventricular ring electrode by application of 45-μA-current pulses at 64 Hz. In spite of the reduced sampling frequency, the TVI signal recorded by Sophós Ext maintained a good signal-to-noise ratio suitable for beat-to-beat evaluation of ventricular activation. The overall average values of end-diastolic TVI and end-systolic TVI at rest were 367 and 396 Ω, respectively. The relative end-systolic TVI in each cardiac cycle ($relEsTVI_i$) was expressed by the ratio:

$$relEsTVI_i = (EsTVI_i - EdTVI) / (EsTVI - EdTVI)$$

The frequency distribution of $relEsTVI_i$ in a series of cardiac cycles (N=411) with regular ventricular capture during VDD pacing is shown in Fig. 1. A value of $relEsTVI_i$ between 0.85 and 1.2 was noticed in the vast majority of the cases (96% of cardiac cycles), while values lower than 0.65 were never observed. Therefore, CCT should have been set below 65% to obtain the maxi-

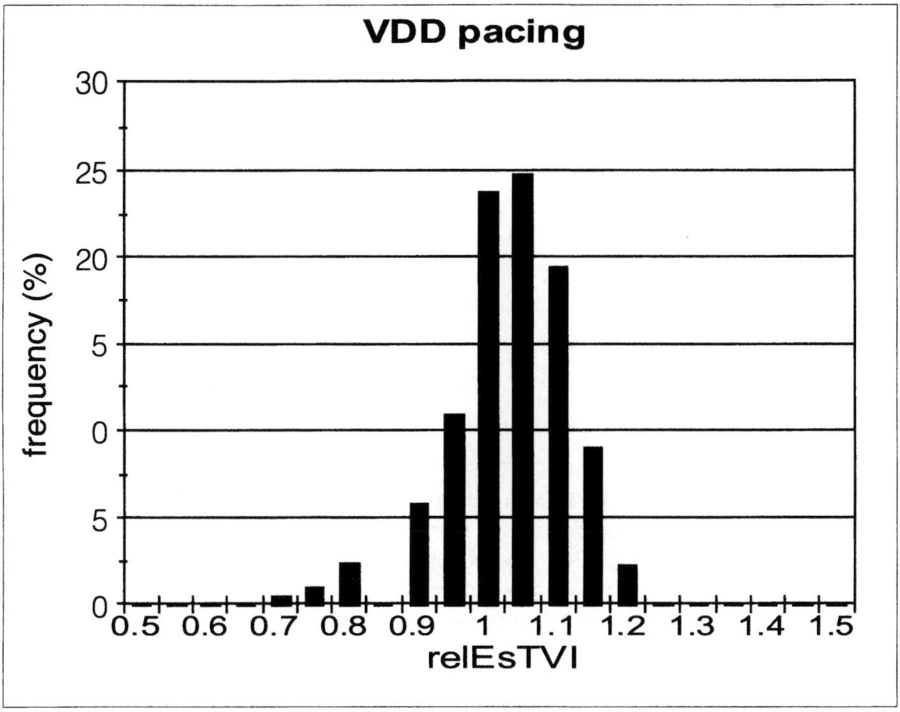

Fig. 1. Frequency distribution of relative end-systolic transvalvular impedance (*relEsTVI*) in the presence of regular ventricular capture (*N*=411). VDD pacing. See text for detailed explanation

mum specificity in capture recognition. Similar results were obtained in VVI pacing.

In the search for the minimum CCT that would allow proper detection of pacing failure, the ventricular threshold analysis was repeated ten times. The stimulator reduced the pacing energy stepwise until the spike was ineffective. If capture loss was recognized a special event marker was displayed, the procedure was broken, and the original pacing energy was automatically resumed. When CCT was programmed at a value between 50% and 62.5% all pacing failures were properly detected, both in VVI (Fig. 2) and in VDD pacing (Fig. 3), without false alarms. Conversely, if CCT was programmed at 37.5%, some failure episodes were missed.

In the second patient, TVI was recorded between the atrial ring and the ventricular tip electrode by the application of 30-μA-current pulses. End-diastolic and end-systolic TVI averaged 529 and 547 Ω, respectively, throughout the test. Total reliability in ventricular capture validation was obtained when CCT was set at 62.5%.

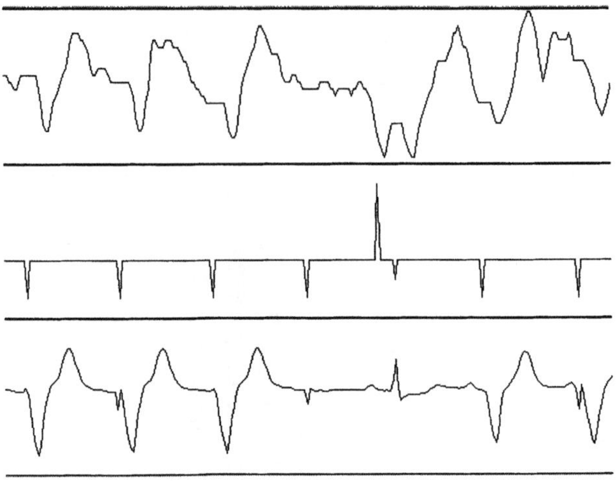

Fig. 2. Threshold analysis in VVI pacing at 100 bpm. *Tracings* from *top* to *bottom*: TVI, event markers, ECG III. *Deep downward markers*: ventricular pacing; *small downward marker*: ventricular sensing; *large upward marker*: ventricular pacing failure diagnosed by the device. Ventricular capture was obtained in the first three cycles, which showed regular TVI fluctuation. The fourth spike was ineffective: TVI did not reach the capture confirmation threshold throughout the post-spike systolic window, and the capture loss was properly recognized by the stimulator. After pacing inhibition due to a conducted QRS, the initial pulse energy was automatically resumed and regular ventricular capture was regained

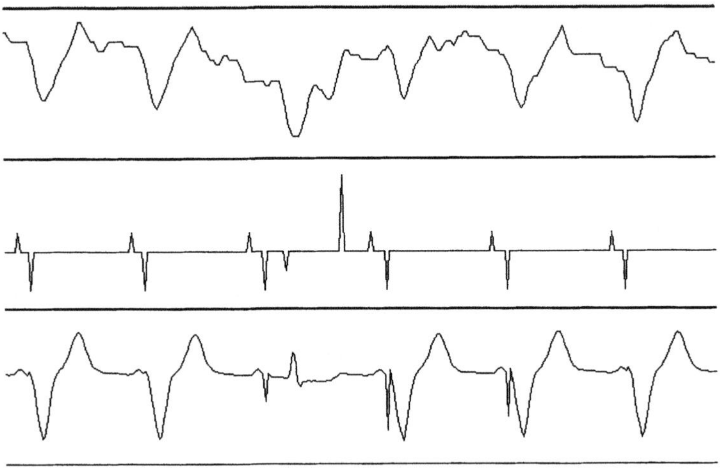

Fig. 3. Threshold analysis in VDD pacing. Sinus rate 82 bpm, AV delay 80 ms. *Tracings* from *top* to *bottom*: TVI, event markers, ECG III. *Small upward markers*: atrial sensing; *deep downward markers*: ventricular pacing; *small downward marker*: ventricular sensing; *large upward marker*: ventricular pacing failure diagnosed by the device. The third spike was ineffective and was followed by a delayed conducted QRS. The intrinsic ventricular activation was reflected by an increase in TVI, which reached the capture confirmation threshold after the post-spike systolic window and was therefore ignored by the system. The pacing failure alarm was activated, the pulse energy was automatically increased to the initial level, and regular ventricular capture was regained

Discussion

The automatic check of ventricular pacing effectiveness at every beat can improve the safety and reduce the energy cost of cardiac stimulation, allowing a reduction in battery size and/or an increase in pacemaker lifetime [12, 13]. The main strategy for capture recognition has been the early detection of the myocardial electric response after a pacing pulse. This is now possible, thanks to the progress in sensing amplifier technology, very fast pacemaker recharge processes, and the availability of pacing electrodes featuring low post-spike polarization [14, 15]. However, false alarms are often generated by undersensing of fusion beats [16, 17]. An alternative approach relying on hemodynamic sensors could prevent this inconvenience. Hemodynamic sensors can detect different parameters related to the pump function of the heart, such as ventricular pressure, endocardial acceleration, and cardiac impedance [18–21]. Therefore, stimulation effectiveness could be confirmed directly by any evidence of cardiac mechanical activation, provided that the sensor signal can be discriminated from the noise on a beat-to-beat basis. Furthermore, a hemodynamic control system could be applied not only to capture confirmation after pacing, but also to the validation of the pacemaker sensing function. An electrical signal resulting in pacing inhibition in the absence of hemodynamic effects should be regarded as an interference, possibly caused by cardiac far fields, myopotentials, or environmental electromagnetic phenomena [22]. In such conditions, the pacemaker might blank the ventricular sensing, switching over to an asynchronous or ventricle-triggered operating mode for a while.

Hemodynamic parameters reflecting processes typical of the isometric systole, such as maximum dP/dt and PEA I [18, 19, 23], can provide information on the ventricular contraction strength, but not on the actual systolic flow, which largely depends on the afterload and could even be absent if the pressure developed is too low to open the aortic valve. Ventricular ejection assessment seems more appropriate for pacing and sensing validation and can be obtained from cardiac impedance measurements by means of standard pacing leads [2, 20]. A previous study, based on intraventricular impedance recorded with a bipolar lead, demonstrated the high sensitivity of this approach in the recognition of capture loss. However, the specificity varied from 81% to 91% and multiparameter analysis was required for good discrimination [4]. Our study demonstrates that TVI allows quick recognition of ventricular ejection based essentially on evaluation of the absolute systolic impedance in each cardiac cycle. The algorithm can be run automatically and in real time, allowing 100% sensitivity and specificity if CCT is set in the range of 50–62.5%. Although additional tests are required to confirm this preliminary evidence, with special attention paid to the effects of posture, movement and breathing on the signal variability, TVI seems to be a valuable tool in the hemodynamic diagnosis of effective ventricular activity.

References

1. Daum DR, Jones BR, Lang DJ (2000) Hemodynamic sensors. Am J Cardiol 86 (Suppl):95K–100K
2. Chirife R, Tentori MC, Mazzetti H et al (2001) Hemodynamic sensors: are they all the same? In: Raviele A (ed) Cardiac arrhythmias 2001. Springer-Verlag Italia, Milan, pp 566–575
3. Occhetta E, Bortnik M, Francalacci G et al (2001) How reliable and effective are hemodynamic sensors to correct chronotropic incompetence? In: Raviele A (ed) Cardiac arrhythmias 2001. Springer-Verlag Italia, Milan, pp 586–594
4. Alt E, Kriegler C, Fotuhi P et al (1992) Feasibility of using intracardiac impedance measurements for capture detection. Pacing Clin Electrophysiol 15:1873–1879
5. Di Gregorio F, Morra A, Finesso M, Bongiorni MG (1996) Transvalvular impedance (TVI) recording under electrical and pharmacological cardiac stimulation. Pacing Clin Electrophysiol 19:1689–1693
6. Morra A, Panarotto D, Santini P, Di Gregorio F (1997) Transvalvular impedance (TVI) sensing: a new way toward the hemodynamic control of cardiac pacing. In: Vardas PE (ed) Europace '97. Monduzzi Editore, Bologna, pp 529-533
7. Gasparini M, Curnis A, Mantica M et al (2001) Hemodynamic sensors: what clinical value do they have in heart failure? In: Raviele A (ed) Cardiac arrhythmias 2001. Springer-Verlag Italia, Milan, pp 576–585
8. Bongiorni MG, Soldati E, Arena G et al (2001) Hemodynamic sensors: what clinical value do they have in chronotropic incompetence? In: Raviele A (ed) Cardiac arrhythmias 2001. Springer-Verlag Italia, Milan, pp 595–601
9. Di Gregorio F, Curnis A, Pettini A et al (2002) Trans-valvular impedance (TVI) in the hemodynamic regulation of cardiac pacing. In: Mitro P, Pella D, Rybár R, Valolik G (eds) Cardiovascular diseases 2002. Monduzzi Editore, Bologna, pp 53–57
10. Bongiorni MG, Soldati E, Arena G et al (1997) Transvalvular impedance as a marker of cardiac activity. In: Vardas PE (ed) Europace '97. Monduzzi Editore, Bologna, pp 525–528
11. Velimirovic DB, Calovic Z, Di Gregorio F et al (1998) Transvalvular impedance as a tool for atrial and ventricular capture detection. In: Santini M (ed) VIII International Symposium on Progress in Clinical Pacing—free papers. CEPI, Roma, pp 81–83
12. Boriani G, Biffi M, Branzi A et al (2000) Benefits in projected pacemaker longevity and in pacing related costs conferred by automatic threshold tracking. Pacing Clin Electrophysiol 23:1783–1787
13. Simeon L, Duru F, Fluri M et al (2000) The impact of automatic threshold tracking on pulse generator longevity in patients with different chronic stimulation threshold. Pacing Clin Electrophysiol 23:1788–1791
14. Clarke M, Liu B, Schüller H et al (1998) Automatic adjustment of pacemaker stimulation output correlated with continuously monitored capture thresholds: a multicenter study. Pacing Clin Electrophysiol 21:1567–1575
15. Lau C, Cameron DA, Nishimura SC et al (2000) A cardiac evoked response algorithm providing threshold tracking: a North American multicenter study. Pacing Clin Electrophysiol 23:953–959
16. Duru F, Bauersfeld U, Schüller H et al (2000) Threshold tracking pacing based on beat by beat evoked response detection: clinical benefits and potential problems. J Interv Card Electrophysiol 4:511–522
17. Candinas R, Liu B, Leal J et al (2002) Impact of fusion avoidance on performance of the automatic threshold tracking feature in dual chamber pacemakers: a multicenter

prospective randomized study. Pacing Clin Electrophysiol 25:1540–1545
18. Bennett T, Sharma A, Sutton R et al (1992) Development of a rate adaptive pacemaker based on the maximum rate-of-rise of right ventricular pressure (RV dP/dtmax). Pacing Clin Electrophysiol 15:219–234
19. Rickards AF, Bombardini T, Plicchi G et al (1996) An implantable intracardiac accelerometer for monitoring myocardial contractility. Pacing Clin Electrophysiol 19:2066–2071
20. Chirife R, Ortega DF, Salazar A (1993) Feasibility of measuring relative right ventricular volumes and ejection fraction with implantable rhythm control devices. Pacing Clin Electrophysiol 16:1673–1683
21. Osswald S, Cron T, Gradel C et al (2000) Closed-loop stimulation using intracardiac impedance as a sensor principle: correlation of right ventricular dP/dt max and intracardiac impedance during dobutamine stress test. Pacing Clin Electrophysiol 23:1502–1508
22. Pinski SL, Trohman RG (2002) Interference in implanted cardiac devices, part I. Pacing Clin Electrophysiol 25:1367–1381
23. Plicchi G, Marcelli E, Parlapiano M et al (2002) PEA I and PEA II based implantable haemodynamic monitor: pre clinical studies in sheep. Europace 4:49–54

What Are the Keys to Hemodynamic Improvement in Heart Failure Patients?

R. Ricci, G. Ansalone, C. Pignalberi, M. Russo, B. Magris, L. Santini , M. Santini

Introduction

Heart failure diagnosis has been growing world-wide during the last decade [1] because of population aging and because improved treatment for acute cardiac events prevents some early deaths, thus leading to chronic disease [2]. Cases of heart failure world-wide have been estimated to be as high as 22.5 million people (6.5 million of them in Europe and 4.8 million in the United States). The incidence of new cases has been calculated at 2 000 000 new patients per year (470 000 in Europe and 480 000 in the United States). Drug therapy may be effective in improving symptoms and survival [3–5], but the long-term prognosis of patients with heart failure is severely affected by the high incidence of progressive refractory heart dysfunction and sudden cardiac death [6]. Myocardial revascularization (through either percutaneous techniques or coronary artery bypass graft), valve disease surgery, and prevention and surgical treatment of congenital heart disease may play a major role in selected patients. Heart transplantation represents the gold standard for end-stage heart failure, but it cannot be made available to large populations. More recently, cardiac resynchronization therapy through atrio-biventricular pacing has been introduced with the aim of improving the electromechanical activation pattern of the heart [7, 8].

Cardiac Dyssynchrony

The keys to hemodynamic improvement in patients with advanced heart failure who are candidates for device therapy are the detection and treatment of cardiac dyssynchrony. Dyssynchrony may be localized either at the atrioventricular level (desynchronization between atria and ventricles), the interventricular level (desynchronization between the right and the left ventricle), or the intraventricular level (desynchronization among left ventricular walls). The last may involve

Department of Cardiology, San Filippo Neri Hospital, Rome, Italy either the longitudinal fibers, or the circumferential fibers, or the torsion and twisting fibers. Left bundle branch block with very wide QRS (≥150 ms) is usually the electrocardiographic pattern of ventricular dyssynchrony. Different degrees and types of cardiac dyssynchrony may coexist in individual patients. In heart failure patients the prevalence of ventricular dyssynchrony has been reported to be as high as 25%–30% [9, 10] and it has been associated with poorer survival [11]. Consequences of ventricular dyssynchrony include [12–14]:

- Delayed opening of the aortic valve as compared with the pulmonary valve (usually more than 40 ms)
- Delayed opening of the mitral valve as compared with the tricuspid valve
- Lengthening of pre-ejection time and isovolumetric relaxation time
- Reduction of left ventricular ejection time
- Shortening of diastolic filling time with E and A wave fusion
- Prolonged mitral regurgitation time with presystolic regurgitation
- Abnormal interventricular septal wall motion
- Reduced left ventricular dP/dt and reduced left ventricular ejection fraction
- Delayed activation of regional free wall segments which may follow the closing of the aortic valve, so that not only do they not contribute to the stroke volume, but they may also counteract ventricular filling

Recently, activation mapping of individual left ventricular segments has been extensively studied using various noninvasive techniques such as tissue Doppler imaging [15] or magnetic resonance imaging [16]. Since the 1970s, paradoxical motion of the interventricular septum has been proposed as the typical pattern in patients with left bundle branch block. As a matter of fact, various activation patterns have been observed in individual patients, and the lateral and/or the posterior wall of the left ventricle has been recognized as the most frequently delayed segment in this clinical setting [17]. According with the anatomical distribution of the left bundle branch fascicles, the greatest delay may be located in the inferior wall when the inferior fascicle is chiefly involved or in the lateral wall when the fibers of the superior fascicle are more damaged than those of the inferior one. The posterior wall may be regarded as a "border zone," whose activation pattern is dependent on the one fascicle or the other, owing to the variability and the complexity of the electromechanical activation in patients with left bundle branch block and heart failure. In some patients the delay in the activation of the posterior and lateral papillary muscle is directly involved in generating mitral regurgitation.

We evaluated regional activation of the left ventricle in a population of patients with nonischemic dilated cardiomyopathy [15]. Regional activation was classified according to four different qualitative patterns using tissue Doppler imaging. Pattern I was normal; pattern II, unsynchronized; pattern III, partially dyskinetic; and pattern IV, totally dyskinetic. At baseline, we observed a greater prevalence of normal and unsynchronized patterns in the interventricular septum and the anterior wall. Conversely, dyskinetic patterns were prevalent in the lateral and/or posterior walls. However, the site of most delayed activation may change in individual patients, so that in our opinion it should be investigated routinely before biventricular pacing implantation. In our series, we indeed demonstrated that discordance between the pacing site and the most delayed site could lead to a null effect or even deleterious effects on left ventricular performance. By contrast, concordance between these two sites allowed achievement of the greatest clinical and functional advantages [18].

Finally, in identifying the pathophysiology of patients with heart failure who may benefit from cardiac resynchronization therapy, the difference between the most dyskinetic area and the area with the greatest regional delay should be stressed. We cannot say whether it is more effective to pace the most delayed or the most dyskinetic region. For the time being, the former should be probably preferred, since it reflects the usual rationale of cardiac resynchronization therapy, while the latter should be avoided since it might not result in improvement, but rather in deterioration of the basal dyskinetic pattern. Furthermore, it should not be forgotten that in some patients the mechanical dysfunction per se may have greater influence than the electrical dysfunction on the severity of the electromechanical disease. In such a setting, correction of the electrical dyssynchrony may not lead to the expected results.

Conclusions

Cardiac dyssynchrony is an emerging cause of hemodynamic impairment in heart failure patients. It is associated with poor clinical outcome and may be responsible for progressive deterioration of cardiac function. Device therapy for cardiac dyssynchrony may allow optimal timing of atrial and ventricular contractions, simultaneous ejection from the right and left ventricles, and optimal resynchronization of the left ventricular walls. Preimplantation studies of cardiac dyssynchrony using a noninvasive technique such as tissue Doppler imaging may be very useful for optimal selection of candidates for cardiac resynchronization therapy, and may drive the choice of pacing site and individually tailored device programming. Clinical trials have demonstrated significant benefits of cardiac resynchronization therapy on heart functional class, exercise tolerance, quality of life, and hospitalizations in patients with advanced heart failure [19, 20]. In fact 25%–30% of them did not respond to device implantation. A deeper knowledge of the pathophysiology of heart failure together with individual study of dyssynchrony patterns may allow a reduction in the nonresponder rate and extension of the clinical benefits of cardiac resynchronization therapy.

References

1. Graves EJ (1991) Detailed diagnoses and procedures. National Hospital Discharge Survey, 1989. Vital and Health Statistics 1991. Series 13, no 107. National Center of Health Statistics, US Department of Health and Human Services. DHHS Publication No. (PHS)91-1768. US Government Printing Office, Washington, DC

2. Ho KKL, Pinsky JL, Kannel WB, Levy D (1993) The epidemiology of heart failure. The Framingham Study. J Am Coll Cardiol 22 (Suppl A):6A–13A
3. Hart SM (2000) Influence of beta blockers on mortality in chronic heart failure. Ann Pharmacother 34:1440–1451
4. Torp-Pedersen C, Kober L (1999) Effect of ACE inhibitor trandolapril on life expectancy of patients with reduced left ventricular function after acute myocardial infarction. TRACE Study Group. Trandolapril Cardiac Evaluation. Lancet 354:9–12
5. Baruch L, Anand I, Cohen IS et al (1999) Augmented short- and long-term hemodynamic and hormonal effects of an angiotensin receptor blocker added to angiotensin converting enzyme inhibitor therapy in patients with heart failure. Vasodilator Heart Failure Trial (V-HeFT) Study Group. Circulation 99:2658–2664
6. MERIT HF Study Group (1999) Effect of metoprolol CR/XL in chronic heart failure: metoprolol CR/XR randomized intervention trial in congestive heart failure (MERIT HF). Lancet 353:2001–2007
7. Cazeau S, Ritter P, Bakdach S et al (1994) Four chamber pacing in dilated cardiomyopathy. Pacing Clin Electrophysiol 17:1974–1979
8. Cazeau S, Ritter P, Lazarus A et al (1996) Multisite pacing for end-stage heart failure. Early experience. Pacing Clin Electrophysiol 19:1748–1757
9. Aaronson KD, Schwartz JS, Chen TM et al (1997) Development and prospective validation of a clinical index to predict survival in ambulatory patients referred for cardiac transplant evaluation. Circulation 95:2660–2667
10. Masoudi FA, Havranek EP, Smith G et al (2003) Gender, age, and heart failure with preserved left ventricular systolic function. J Am Coll Cardiol 41:217–223
11. Kearney MT, Zaman A, Eckberg DL et al (2003) Cardiac size, autonomic function, and 5-year follow-up of chronic heart failure patients with severe prolongation of ventricular activation. J Cardiac Fail 9:93–99
12. Grines C, Bashore T, Boudoulas H et al (1989) Functional abnormalities in isolated left bundle branch block: the effect of interventricular asynchrony. Circulation 79:845–853
13. Xiao H, Brecker S, Gibson D (1992) Effects of abnormal activation on the time course of left ventricular pressure pulse in dilated cardiomyopathy. Br Heart J 68:403–407
14. Xio Lee C, Gibson D (1991) Effects of left bundle branch block on diastolic function in dilated cardiomyopathy. Br Heart J 66:443–447
15. Ansalone G, Giannantoni P, Ricci R et al (2001) Doppler myocardial imaging in patients with heart failure receiving biventricular pacing treatment. Am Heart J 142:881–896
16. Prinzen FW, Wiman BT, Hunter WC, Faris OP, McVeigh ER (2000) Effects of single and biventricular pacing on the temporal and spatial dynamics of ventricular contraction (abstract). Circulation 102(II):161
17. Auricchio A, Klein H, Tockman B et al (1999) Transvenous biventricular pacing for heart failure: can the obstacles be overcome? Am J Cardiol 83:136D–142D
18. Ansalone G, Giannantoni P, Ricci R et al (2002) Doppler myocardial imaging to evaluate the effectiveness of pacing sites in patients receiving biventricular pacing. J Am Coll Cardiol 39:489–499
19. Cazeau S, Leclerq C, Lavergne T et al (2001) Effects of multisite biventricular pacing in patients with heart failure and intraventricular conduction delay. N Engl J Med 344:873–880
20. Abraham WT, Fisher WG, Smith AL et al, for the MIRACLE Study Group (2002) Cardiac resynchronization in chronic heart failure. N Engl J Med 346:1845–1853

Atrioventricular Delay in Heart Failure Patients: How to Manage It

H. O. Luttikhuis

Introduction

Since artificial heart stimulation started in the 1960s, with atrium and ventricle of the human heart being electrically connected in such a way as to give a haemodynamically optimal function, diastolic filling time has remained a challenge. In the 1970s, the physiologist Karloff advised that in congenital atrioventricular (AV) block in "normal hearts" an AV delay of 150 ms was needed according to physiological investigations. It is important to realize that during "right heart stimulation" we try to synchronize the left atrium and the left ventricle (LV).

The recent development of new techniques to stimulate the left ventricle (LV) on time relative to right ventricle (RV) activation has opened up new possibilities. The optimal contractile function of the LV has been thought to depend on programming of the optimal AV delay (OAVD). The OAVD itself depends on: (A) the inter- and intraatrial conduction time, (B) the AV nodal conduction time, (C) the inter- and intraventricular conduction times, (D) the heart rate or adrenergic status of the patient. The last reason (D) led to the integration of dynamic AV timing in DDD-R pacemakers; this means that the AV interval of the pacemaker decreases automatically with increasing heart rate. During cardiac resynchronisation therapy (CRT) for heart failure the interdependence of the V–V interval and OAVD is more complex and depends on A+B+C; it is perhaps better to say that the AV delay is different in every patient. Aurrichio et al. [1] therefore conclude: "[E]ven for the latter patients LV systolic function could be optimised by initialised selection of the AV delay."

Cardiac Thoracic Centre, The Isala Clinics, Zwolle, The Netherlands

Synchronising the Atria

In patients with P-waves lasting over 100 ms as a result of degenerative myocardial damage or medication (amiodarone), the intra- and interatrial conduction times are longer than normal (Fig. 1). In these circumstances, AV resynchronisation will require different AV timing for the right and left cardiac cycles (Fig. 2), which means four-chamber pacing with a "four-chamber" pacemaker.

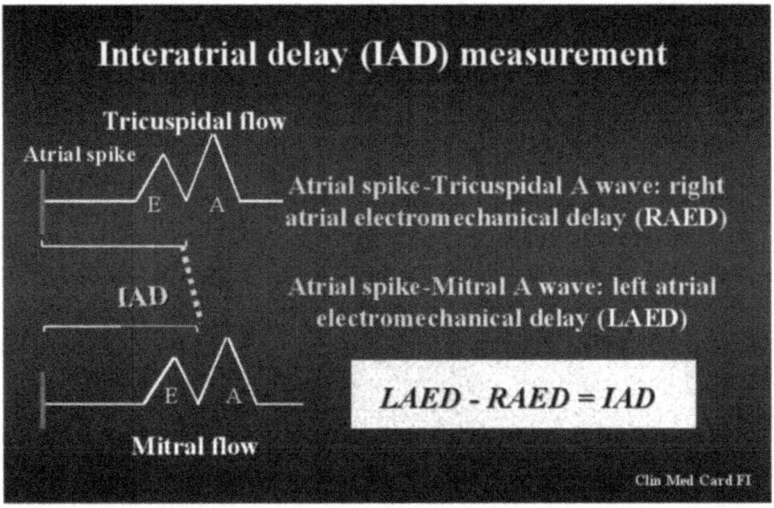

Fig. 1. Measurement of interatrial delay

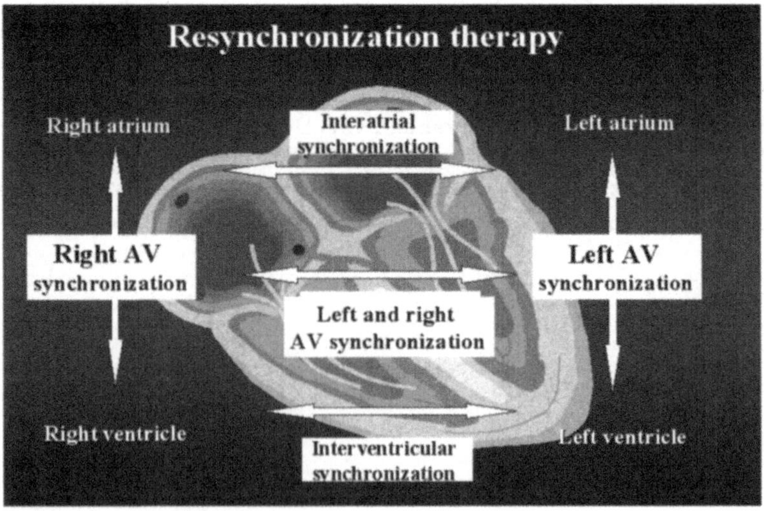

Fig. 2. Resynchronisation therapy

Padeletti et al. [2] have proved that low right atrial pacing (or low atrial septum or triangle of Koch) results in synchronisation of the interatrial delay with no decrease in the left and right diastolic filling times and thus without any decrease in cardiac output.

Intraventricular Conduction Time

In heart failure with intraventricular conduction delay (IVCD, see Fig. 3) there is an increase in isovolumetric contraction time (IVCT) and in isovolumetric relaxation time (IVRT) (Fig. 3), reducing the diastolic filling time (DFT) with consequent lowering of preload tension and cardiac output. Furthermore, this increase in IVCT and IVRT affects the timing of the AV delay. This means that the IVCD and IVRT have to be corrected before the OAVD can be programmed. The intraventricular conduction delay (IVCD) is defined as the prolonged contraction of the LV posterior wall after the opening of the mitral valve. The IVCD can be measured by tissue Doppler imaging of the posterior wall. In daily practice the IVCD is corrected by implanting a biventricular pacemaker (BV-pm) with the LV lead located at the posterolateral wall, unless the asynchrony is spotted at another site.

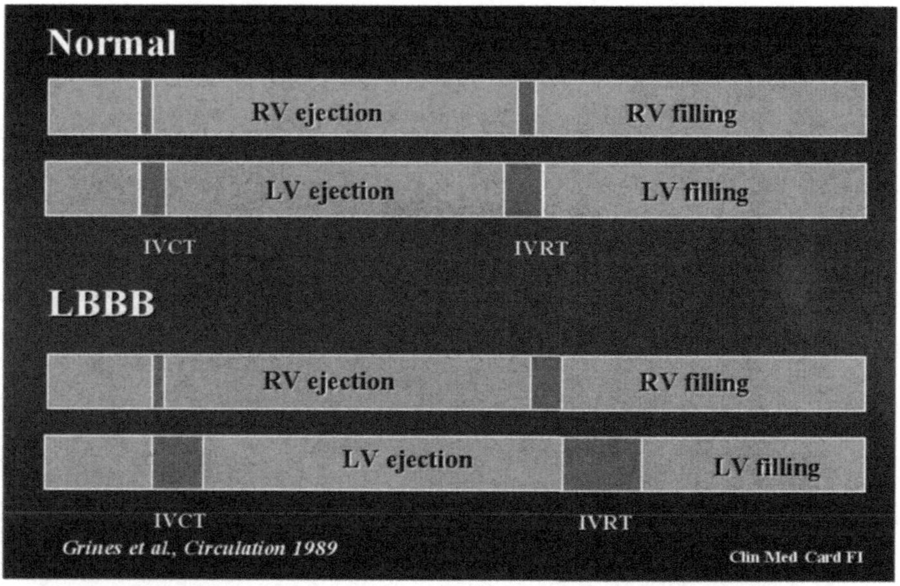

Fig. 3. Heart failure with intraventricular conduction delay (LBBB left bundle branch block)

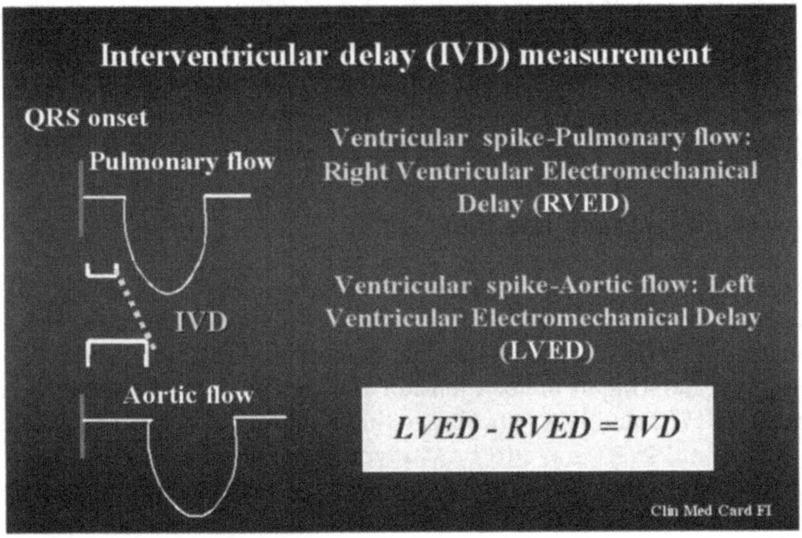

Fig. 4. Measurement of interventricular delay (IVD)

Interventricular Conduction Delay

The interventricular conduction delay (IVD) is defined as the time difference between the ventricular spike and the onset of LV ejection minus the onset of RV ejection (LVED–RVED=IVD) (Fig. 4). This results in a mechanical AV delay between the LV and the RV (Fig. 5).

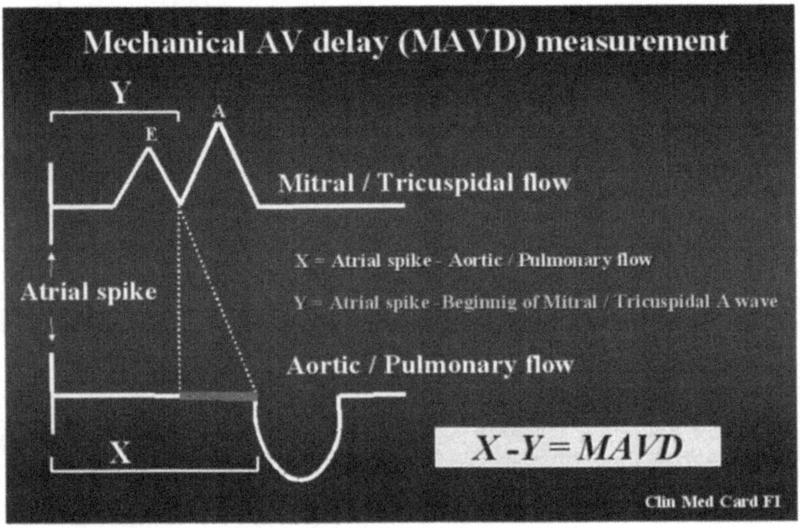

Fig. 5. Measurement of mechanical atrioventricular delay (MAVD)

Optimal Atrioventricular Delay

The optimal AV delay can be defined as the time that provides the longest diastolic filling period without abrupt interruption by the onset of the ventricular contraction (Ritter formula; see Fig. 6). The obvious inference that OAVD results in optimal cardiac output is true in only just under 60% of cases reported in the literature.

This means that "other" AV delays result in a higher cardiac output measured by echocardiography (velocity time integral).

The Sorin company has developed a special stimulation electrode (Best lead) with a sensor in the tip that can detect an electrical signal (peak endocardial acceleration, or PEA) during the isovolumetric contraction period; this signal represents myocardial contraction with a correlation coefficient of 0.86 relative to the inotropic state of the heart [2]. This haemodynamic sensor (PEA) makes it possible to quantify myocardial contractility and can be used for OAVD (Fig. 7) and for programming the V–V interval in CRT (Figs. 8, 9).

Thus, the definition of OAVD is confusing. Sawhney sees OAVD as the delay with the maximum VTI.

Data presented by van Gelder [3] at NASPE 2003 indicate that the maximum dP/dT occurs during fusion beats, which explains why LV pacing is reported in the literature as being as good as or even better than BV pacing. These findings ("fusion beats have the highest dP/dT") suggest that the AV conduction and the autonomous depolarisation of the septal part of the LV belong together and explain why well-timed LV depolarisarisation in LV pacing has a better result during VTI or dP/dT, or pulse pressure, or cardiac out-

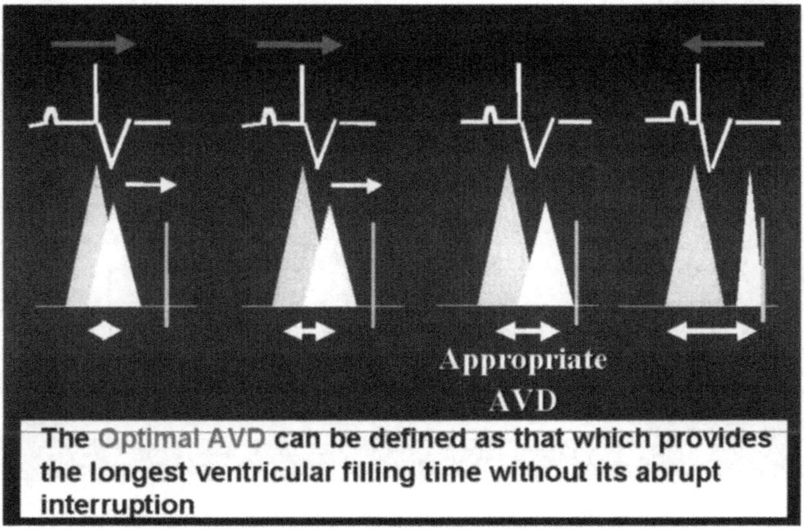

Fig. 6. Optimal AV delay (AVD) can be defined as the AVD that provides the longest ventricular filling time without abrupt interruption

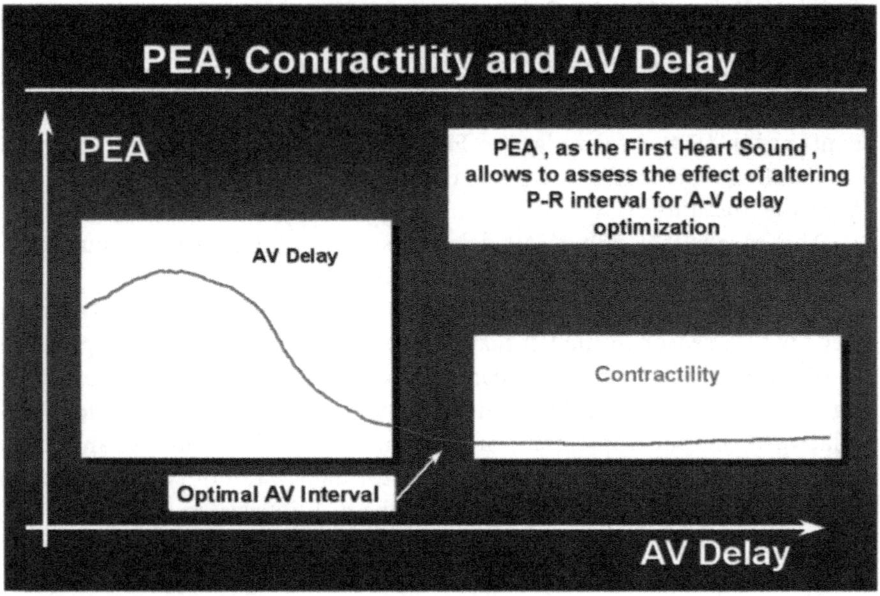

Fig. 7. Peak endocardial acceleration (PEA), contractility and AV delay

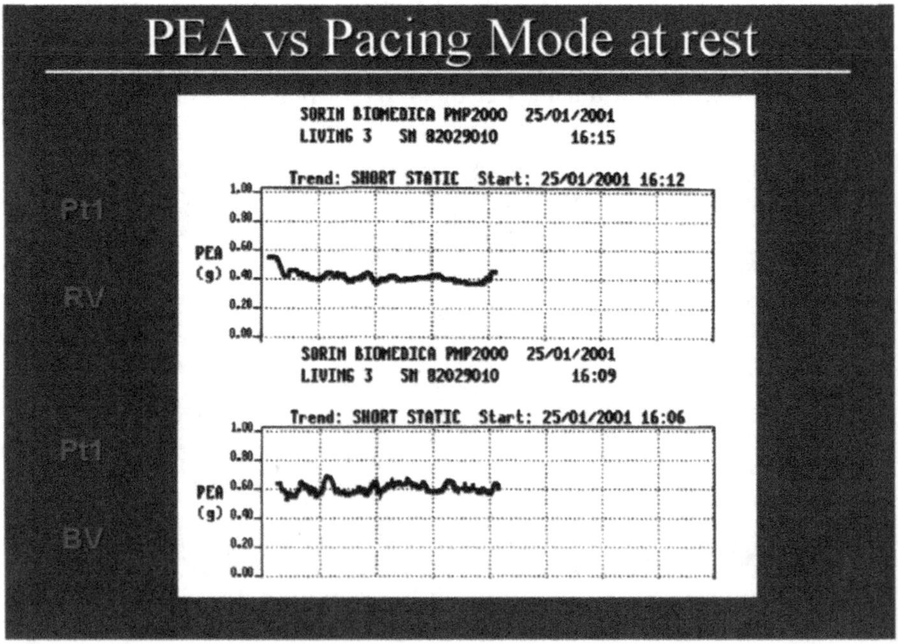

Fig. 8. PEA vs pacing mode at rest

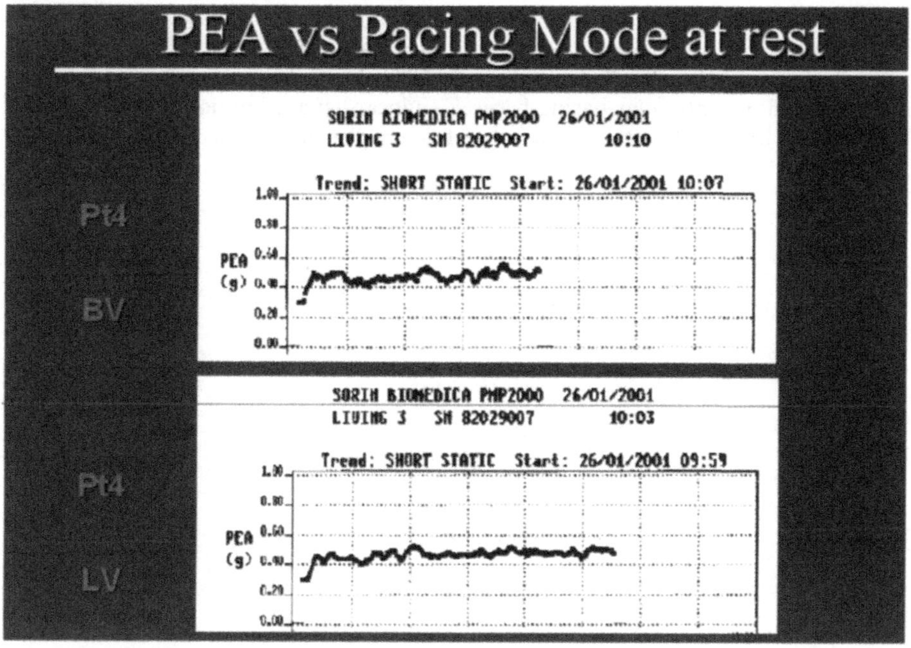

Fig. 9. PEA vs pacing mode at rest

put. This finding is restricted to patients with short or normal AVD (<220 ms). In patients with an abnormally long AVD accurate programming needed has to be found by echocardiography, because the LV septum is depolarised by the RV stimulation.

The PEA, which is closely correlated with the dP/dT of the LV, covers the OAVD (according to the Ritter formula in long AV delays) *and* the AV/septal depolarisation in normal AVDs, resulting in both situations in the haemodynamic OAVD. The programming of the CRT pacemaker (Best-Living) is therefore reliable and time saving both for the OAVD and for the finding of the V–V interval [4].

References

1. Auricchio A, Stellbrink C, Block M et al (1999) Effect of pacing chamber and atrioventricular delay on acute systolic function of paced patients with congestive heart failure. Circulation 99:2993
2. Padeletti L, Porciani M, Ritter P et al (2000) Atrioventricular interval optimization in the right atrial appendage and interatrial septum pacing: a comparison between echo and peak endocardial acceleration measurement. Pacing Clin Electrophysiol 23:1618-1622
3. van Gelder BM, Bracke FA, Meijer A (2003) The influence of intrinsic conduction on

left ventricular dP/at during biventricular pacing. Pacing Clin Electrophysiol 26:952 (abs)
4. Bordachar P, Garrique S, Reuter X et al (2000) Haemodynamic assessment of right, left and bi-ventricular pacing by peak endocardial acceleration and echocardiography in patients with end-stage heart failure. Pacing Clin Electrophysiol 23:1726-1730

Cardiac Resynchronisation and Haemodynamic Monitoring: the Living-CHF Study

J. Clémenty, for the BEST-CARE Study Group*

Introduction

Since multisite stimulation was first performed in heart failure (HF) [1], a few specific devices have been designed with capabilities for providing separated output control of pacing parameters for the right and left ventricular leads, as well as inter ventricular (VV) sequence programming. So far, there are no haemodynamic sensors to improve understanding of and follow up the effects of biventricular (BiV) stimulation and help in the programming of the resynchronisation parameters. In the meantime, Sorin Biomedica has developed the Living-BEST system, which is based on a sensor that is able to measure the amplitude of mechanical vibrations generated by the myocardium during the isovolumetric contraction of ventricles. The peak of endocardial acceleration (PEA) reflects events that produce vibrations that originate mainly in the left ventricle and are transmitted through the cardiac mass [2, 3]. It has been shown that PEA is correlated with contractility indexes, such as dP/dt_{max}, and is influenced by catecholamine levels. PEA variations are related to the capability of the myocardium to respond to adrenergic stresses. Human experiments [4, 5] have shown that PEA variation is greater during exercise with biventricular pacing than compared with to other modes, and it has been suggested that PEA might be used as a marker for selecting the position of ventricular pacing leads that provides the best haemodynamic effect. The version of the Living-BEST system designed specifically for biventricular pacing (Living CHF) has the capability of recording amplitudes and timings of PEA and providing real-time telemetry of the whole endocardial acceleration signal. Secondly, the device has the VV Interval programming feature, which can influence the efficacy of resynchronisation provided by biventricular stimulation. Recent studies [6-13] have been focused on improving understanding of the effects of cardiac resynchronisation therapy. Biventricular stimulation provides a more

Hôpital Cardiologique, Université de Bordeaux, Pessac, France homogeneous contraction of ventricles, which becomes faster and allows prolongation of the diastolic filling phase. Filling pressures are reduced with the frequent reduction in the mitral valve regurgitation. The most relevant parameter is the aortic pre-ejection interval [14], which has to become shorter to predict the beneficial effect of biventricular stimulation, and also the shortening in the contraction timing of the uncoordinated ventricular segments. In this context the use of a haemodynamic sensor is an interesting possibility as an analytic tool for the evaluation and optimisation of ventricular resynchronisation therapy.

Methods

The study protocol was approved by the local ethical committees. The patients included in the study had each had a severe cardiac heart failure (CHF) with dilated cardiomyopathy and the maximal tolerated drug therapy including β-blockers. Other inclusion criteria we are: QRS duration ≥ 150 ms, left-ventricular end-diastolic diameter (LVEDD) ≥ 60 mm, and left-ventricular ejection fraction (LVEF) ≤ 35%. A PR interval of 200 ms or more was been demanded for optimal AV delay optimisation by PEA measurements. The patients each had a DDDR pacemaker (Living CHF, Sorin Biomedica CRM, Saluggia, Italy) implanted. The programming configuration was DDDR, with the gravimetric sensor (GVM) activated for rate adaptation and the PEA sensor activated only for diagnostic information. Right atrial and ventricular leads were positioned with the standard configuration, while the left ventricular lead was introduced through the coronary sinus to reach a position where it would be effective in ventricular resynchronisation. This prospective observational study included three patient follow-ups: FU1 (during hospitalisation), FU2 (1 month after the implantation), and FU3 (3 months after the implantation). All patients underwent the following procedures: at FU1, AV delay optimisation by PEA, PEA, and echocardiographic parameters was measured at the following pacing configurations: RV, LV, BiV0 (VV interval = 0 ms), BiVC (VV interval = compensated, defined as the VV interval equal in value and opposite in sequence to the difference between left and right pre-ejection intervals as measured by echography). At FU2, PEA telemetry measurements were performed with the programmed configuration. At FU3, the procedure followed at FU1 for revision of PEA and echocardiographic measurements was applied again. The main echocardiographic parameters measured during follow-up were: LV pre-ejection interval (LPEI), RV pre-ejection interval (RPEI), aortic velocity-time integer (AoVTI), LV filling time (LFT) and the quantification of mitral valve regurgitation (MVR).

The aim of this study is to analyse the influence of timing parameter programming on haemodynamics, by means of PEA and echocardiographic data. It is important, moreover, to assess the possibility of using PEA data for the optimisation of AV delay and for analsis of the evolution of LV function.

Results

The study is in progress; we will present some preliminary observations made on the first patients who have received pacemakers (PMs); in 18 patients (mean age 72.9 ± 7.7 years) Living CHF systems have been implanted. All patients were in New York Heart Association (NYHA) functional class III. Twelve patients presented with a ischaemic LV dysfunction, while 6 patients showed an idiopathic LV dysfunction. All of them presented a long QRS duration (161.5 ± 17 ms), with a long PR interval (232.4 ± 34.6 ms). The mean LVEDD was 66.4 ± 6.0 mm and the LV ejection fraction (EF) was 26.54 ± 9.6 %. Figure 1 shows an example of the PEA curves during AV delay scanning automatic function at the different pacing configuration. As can be seen, the pattern changes significantly for the different pacing configurations, suggesting that varying the VV interval and/or sequence alters the overall cardiac mechanics. Recent studies have demonstrated that the optimal AV delay by PEA corresponds to the inflection point of the sigmoid curve fitting the PEA vs AV delay curve [15]. No statistically significant difference was found between the optimal AV delay defined in this way and that obtained by echocardiography (defined as the one that causes the longest diastolic filling time without interrupting the A-wave) in the preliminary series studied. Figure 2 shows the difference in the EA-IEGM signal between RV and LV pacing, which is

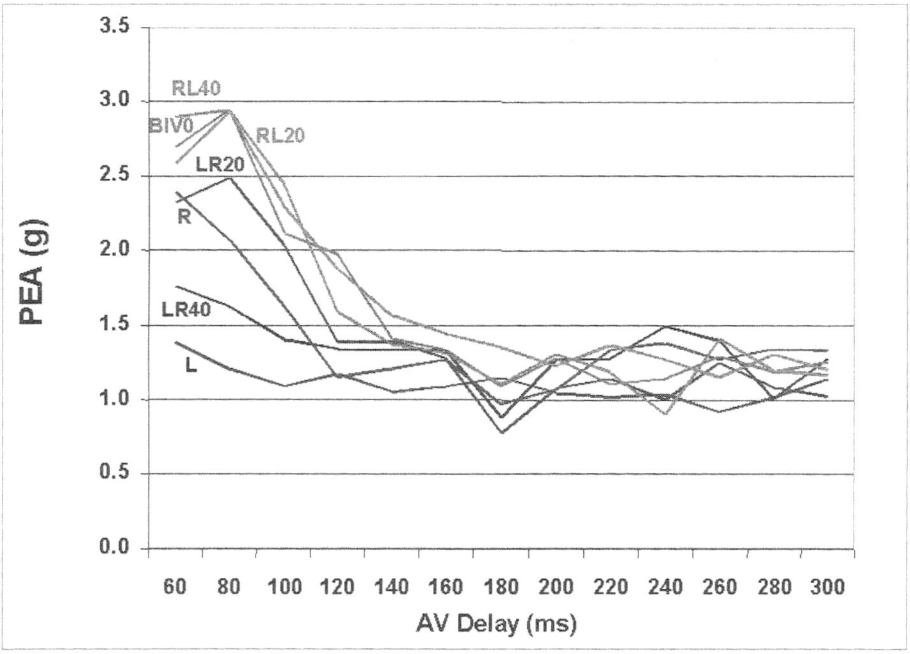

Fig. 1. PEA vs AV delay at different pacing configurations

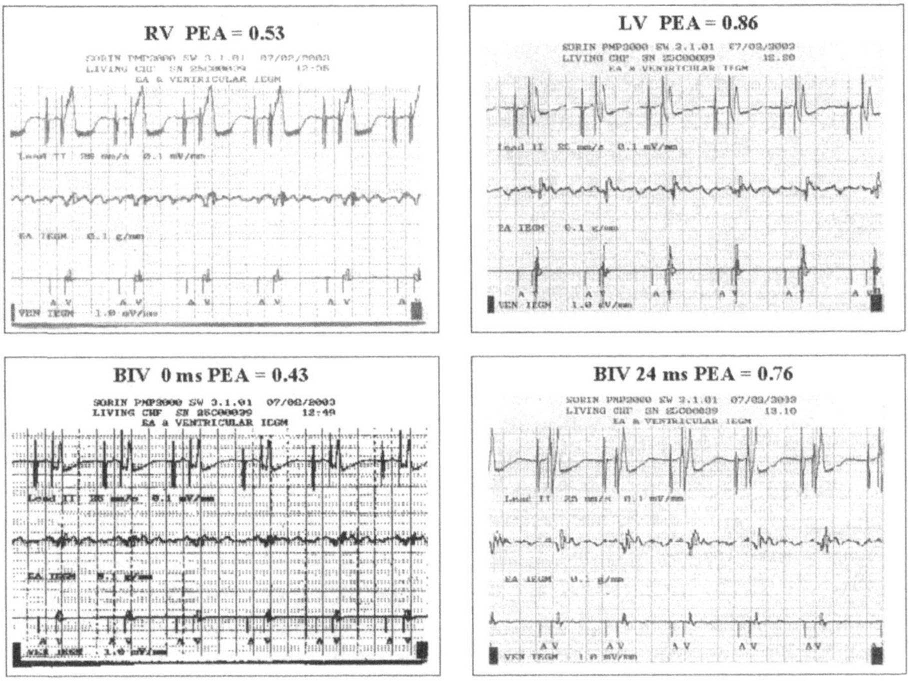

Fig. 2. EA signal with different pacing configurations

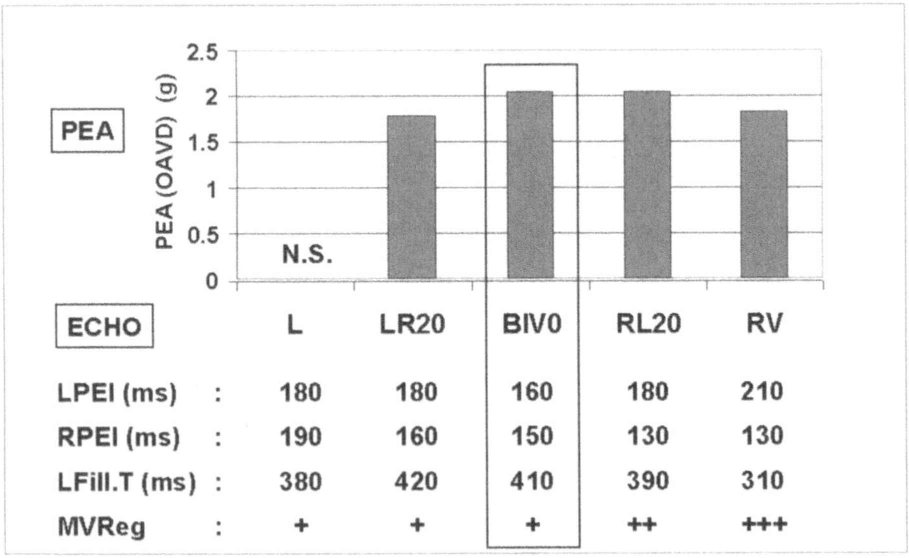

Fig. 3. PEA (OAVD) vs echocardiographic timings with different pacing configurations

of significant importance for the mechanical ventricular resynchronisation of the VV delay compensation in BiV pacing. Figure 3 summarises the relation between the PEA amplitude obtained at the OAVD and the best haemodynamic timing parameter configuration obtained by standard echocardiographic measurements (the shortest LPEI and RPEI intervals and the longest LV filling time, with the minimum mitral valve regurgitation). The clinical status of patients can be assessed from the maximum variation in PEA amplitude during a stress test. The correlation between Delta-PEA_{max} (g) and the maximum power developed by the patient is 0.83 (p=0.001).

Discussion

The aim of this study is to provide data to analyse each of the three ventricular pacing modes (RV, LV and BiV pacing) in patients with permanent pacing devices and the standard lead configuration. For this purpose, we selected patients in whom AV delay optimisation and VV interval programming were possible, so that we would be able to assess the influence of pacemaker timing on the haemodynamics. Because high-quality PEA recording can be consistently and safely obtained with the pacemaker that we used in this protocol, it was also important to determine whether or not PEA recordings taken in CHF failure patients might be of interest for myocardial contractility monitoring. Preliminary data show a good correlation between OAVD measured by PEA and echocardiography, even when the number of cases is too low for statistical significance. The capability of the system for obtaining the OAVD at different pacing configurations is of primary importance for assessing whether the combination of PEA amplitude and timing could be used for the determination of the best haemodynamic configuration.

Conclusions

This study confirms the feasibility and reliability of myocardial contractility monitoring with a permanent pacing device and opens up a new method for determination of the optimal pacing configuration for each heart failure patient. This study demonstrates the capability of the system for optimising AV delay and suggests that PEA real-time telemetry measurements could help in programming of the pacemaker timing parameters. Larger studies with longer-term follow-up are needed to confirm these preliminary results.

Appendix

BEST-CARE Study Group: S. Garrigue, Hôpital Haut-Lévêque, Bordeaux, France; P. Ritter, Clinique Bizet, Paris, France; J.C. Deharo, Hôpital Ste Marguerite, Marseille, France; L. Padeletti, Ospedale Careggi, Florence, Italy; P.P. Delnoy, Isala Klinieken, Zwolle, The Nederlands; J. Silvestre, Hospital La Paz, Madrid, Spain.

References

1. Cazeau S, Ritter P, Bakdach S et al (1994) Four-chamber pacing in dilated cardiomyopathy. Pacing Clin Electrophysiol 17:1974-1979
2. Rickards AF, Bombardini T, Corbucci G, Plicchi G (1996) An implantable intracardiac accelerometer for monitoring myocardial contractility. Pacing Clin Electrophysiol 19:2066-2071
3. Occhetta E, Perucca A, Corbucci G, Garberoglio B, Liverani L, Plicchi G (1995) Experience with a new myocardial acceleration sensor during dobutamine infusion and exercise test. Eur J CPE 5:204-209
4. Padeletti L, Porciani MC, Ritter P et al (2000) Atrioventricular interval optimization in the right atrial appendage and interatrial septum. Pacing Clin Electrophysiol 23:1618-1622
5. Reuter S, Garrigue S, Bordachar P et al (2002) Assessment of left ventricular pacing versus biventricular pacing in heart failure patients during exercise by using a hemodynamic sensor. Europace Cardiostim 3:A176
6. Bordachar P, Garrigue S, Reuter S et al (2000) Importance of QRS duration during multisite ventricular stimulation in heart failure: a hemodynamic noninvasive study using peak endocardial acceleration measurements. Pacing Clin Electrophysiol 23(II):636
7. Bordachar P, Garrigue S, Reuter S et al (2000) Hemodynamic assessment of right, left and biventricular pacing by peak endocardial acceleration and echocardiography in patients with end-stage heart failure. Pacing Clin Electrophysiol 23:1726-1730
8. Cazeau S, Ritter P, Lazarus A et al (1996) Multisite pacing for end-stage heart failure: Early experience. Pacing Clin Electrophysiol 19:1748-1757
9. Reuter S, Garrigue S, Bordchar P et al (2000) Intermediate–term results of biventricular pacing in heart failure: correlation between clinical and hemodynamic data. Pacing Clin Electrophysiol 23:1713-1717
10. Jaïs P, Takahashi A, Garrigue S et al (2000) Mid-term follow-up of endocardial biventricular pacing. Pacing Clin Electrophysiol 23:1744-1747
11. Lau C, Yu C, Chau E et al (2000) Reversal of left ventricular remodeling by synchronous biventricular pacing in heart failure. Pacing Clin Electrophysiol 23:1722-1725
12. Gras D, Mabo P, Tang T et al (1998) Multisite pacing as a supplemental treatment of congestive heart failure: preliminary results of the Medtronic Inc. InSync Study. Pacing Clin Electrophysiol 21:2249-2255
13. Leon A, Delurgio D, Fisher W et al (2001) Long term performance of a left ventricular lead to provide cardiac resynchronization. Pacing Clin Electrophysiol 24:643
14. Cazeau S, Leclercq C, Lavergne T et al (2001) Effects of multisite biventricular pacing in patients with heart failure and intraventricular conduction delay. N Engl J Med 344:873-880
15. Dupuis JM, Kobeissi A, Vitali L et al (2003) Programming optimal atrioventricular delay in dual chamber pacing using peak endocardial acceleration. Comparison with a standard echocardiographic procedure. Pacing Clin Electrophysiol 26(II):210-213

Heart Failure Therapy Driven by Implantable Sensors: What May We Expect?

G. Plicchi, E. Marcelli

Introduction

Despite significant improvements in medical therapy, the appropriate diagnosis and management of chronic heart failure (CHF) continues to offer many clinical challenges.

Although medical therapy with angiotensin-converting enzyme inhibitors and more recent β-blockers have shown beneficial effects on symptoms, hemodynamics, left ventricular systolic function, and survival, the relentless progression of underlying left ventricular dysfunction and periodic, severe symptomatic decompensation often requiring hospitalization remain essential features of the heart failure syndrome.

The recognition of decompensated heart failure is often delayed by the absence of clinical or radiographic signs consistent with elevated ventricular filling pressures and/or reduced cardiac output. Furthermore, treatment of patients with CHF may be inadequate because of the poor correlation between physical signs or symptoms and cardiac function [1]. Using hemodynamic implantable sensors to guide heart failure care is an attractive new approach for clinicians, but the research to discover effective ways to monitor the course of the disease and the response to treatment in patients with CHF is still ongoing. CHF therapy guided by information from an implantable hemodynamic sensor could be useful by providing early warning of an impeding severe exacerbation or, in the case of minor volume overload, confirming the patient's status and guiding the therapy; this could result in a substantial decrease in the need for health care utilization.

Continuous hemodynamic monitoring could also provide detailed information on CHF patients' status that might be helpful in their day-to-day management and would be superior to the one-off "spot measurements" typically

Biomedical Technology Unit, Department of Surgery and Transplantation, University of Bologna, Italy

used in CHF management and diagnosis, such as body weight and B-type natriuretic protein concentrations. Knowledge of left-sided cardiac filling pressure is important in the management of critically ill patients with cardiovascular diseases, and right heart catheterization with measurement of the pulmonary capillary wedge pressure (PCWP) provides a reliable estimation of the left-sided filling pressure in most clinical situations. However, pulmonary artery catheterization is an invasive procedure with known complications, and although it may be justified in acute settings, it does not have a role in the routine management of patients with stable CHF.

Recently, several new developments have taken place in pacing technology to treat selected patients with heart failure. These include biventricular pacing (cardiac resynchronization therapy, CRT) to correct abnormal patterns of left ventricular contraction and implantable cardioverter-defibrillators for treatment of malignant ventricular arrhythmias. Biventricular pacing in CHF patients aims to restore synchronous ventricular contraction. Delayed intraventricular depolarization causes dyssynchrony and an inefficient pattern of left ventricular contraction. Myocardial segments contracting at different times impair left ventricular function, cause a shorter diastole or overlapping systole/diastole, and aggravate functional mitral regurgitation. A number of studies have shown that biventricular or left ventricular pacing improves indexes of systolic function in patients with severe left ventricular systolic dysfunction, dilated cardiomyopathy (either ischemic or idiopathic), and a major left-sided intraventricular conduction disorder such as left bundle branch block. Ventricular resynchronization improves the sequence of electrical activation with resultant initiation of more coordinated, efficient left ventricular contraction coupled with reduced functional mitral regurgitation.

Of the numerous variables—pulse pressure (PP), LV$dP/dt_{max}$, myocardial oxygen consumption (MVO_2), PCWP—that have been used as indexes of the benefits of cardiac resynchronization [2–4], LV$dP/dt_{max}$, reflecting the contractile status of the heart, seems to be the most widely clinically accepted. Furthermore, Van Gelder et al. [5] recently used LV$dP/dt_{max}$ as parameter for the identification of the optimal atrioventricular (AV) delay in CRT. Although LV$dP/dt_{max}$ monitoring to optimize CRT in patients with CHF is intrinsically attractive and also helpful for the selection of responders to CRT therapy [6], the invasive nature of its measurement limits its field of application to acute settings or at the moment of the implantation of the device for CRT.

What is lacking in CRT is a means of continuously measuring the contractile status of the heart to monitor individual responses to CRT in patients with CHF with a view to optimal reprogramming of AVD and VV time in follow-up when heart remodeling occurs.

Heart Failure Therapy Driven by Implantable Sensors: State of the Heart

Pressure Sensor

Adamson et al. [7] recently reported results on the potential of an implantable hemodynamic monitoring device (Chronicle IHM, Medtronic) to provide continuous measurements of central hemodynamics in patients with CHF. The Chronicle Implantable Hemodynamic Monitor is a long-term implanted device designed to record ongoing right ventricular (RV) pressure, heart rate (HR), and other variables. The IHM consists of an implantable memory system, similar to the pulse generator of a pacemaker, that can be implanted subcutaneously in the prepectoral region, and of a pressure sensor in a modified pacemaker lead that is positioned in the right ventricle, preferably in the outflow tract. The pressure sensor uses the principle of variable capacitance to measure absolute pressure. The device continuously measures RV systolic and diastolic pressures (RVSP, RVDP), estimated pulmonary diastolic pressure (ePADP), maximum rate of change in pressure over time (*dP*/*dt*), HR, activity and temperature. The ePADP is derived from RV pressures at the time of the maximum *dP*/*dt*, the moment of the pulmonary opening.

The long-term effect of the IHM sensor has been recently investigated by Magalski et al. [8]: IHM devices were implanted in 32 patients with CHF (EF 29%±11%) and were tested with right heart catheterization at implantation and 3, 6, and 12 months later. The results showed no difference between IHM and catheter values at baseline or at 1 year, with high correlation coefficients. These findings are encouraging, but there may be some limitations concerning the application of measurements from the implantable device to specific patients [9]. Substantial variations likely to be of clinical importance were noted for individual determination of hemodynamic measures. Variations were more evident in the estimation of filling pressure, with differences of 10 mmHg between catheter and device measurements expected with some frequency; the errors involved both overestimation and underestimation. Conceivably, a favorable impact of therapeutic adjustments can be seen in groups of patients despite this degree of variation. The key issue may turn on safety. Treatments based on measurements with this degree of variation may result in symptomatic hypotension or adverse shifts in fluids balance in enough patients to cause concern despite an overall beneficial effect in a group of patients.

Intrathoracic Impedance Sensor

Recently Stadler et al. [10] reported results of the ongoing studies on the automated detection of decreases in intrathoracic impedance to predict CHF hospitalization. In this study, the intrathoracic impedance Z, measured between a right ventricular coil electrode and the can of an ICD, is being used to quantify fluid overload in patients with CHF. Thirty-three CHF patients with NYHA class III–IV function underwent implantation of a special pacemaker device and ICD lead. The results showed that, using a single threshold for all patients, the Z measurements allowed prediction of 12 out of 14 hospitalizations, with a median of 18.5 days warning before hospitalization. Due to the multifactor dependency of intrathoracic impedance, however, large clinical studies are needed to validate this approach.

Endocardial Acceleration Sensor

When the myocardium contracts isometrically, it generates vibrations that have audible components, which are responsible for the first heart sound. Both the audible and the nonaudible spectrum of these vibrations can be measured with an implantable endocardial accelerometer. The peak-to-peak value of these myocardial vibrations (peak endocardial acceleration, PEA), occurring in the isovolumic contraction phase, is an index of myocardial contractility, the directional changes of which mirror very closely changes in $LVdP/dt_{max}$ [11–16], the key parameter for evaluating the efficacy of resynchronization therapy.

For PEA assessment, a single-axis microaccelerometer sensor (BEST, Sorin Biomedica), encapsulated in rigid hermetic capsule and inserted inside the tip of a pacemaker lead, has been developed. The PEA has been recently used in the multicenter, randomized cross-over single-blind study WHERE (whole heart research) to evaluate the long-term progressive worsening of cardiac function in patients with chronic RV pacing. Preliminary results [17] showed a significantly larger left telediastolic diameter and lower PEA at the end of the paced ventricle condition compared to the spontaneous ventricle activation condition.

In a recent experimental study, we investigated the feasibility of PEA as a parameter by which to follow the progressive worsening of heart function during tachycardia-induced heart failure. Heart failure was induced in four sheep (mean body weight 67±5 kg) by means of rapid RV pacing (160 bpm) for 9±2 weeks. The PEA sensor was implanted at the apex of the right ventricle and connected to a biventricular pacer (Living CHF, Sorin), which allows telemetric transmission of the entire signal of the endocardial acceleration. At implantation time and at the end of the study, a pressure catheter (Millar) was inserted at the apex of the left ventricle to record LV systolic pressure (LVSP), LV end-diastolic pressure (LVEDP), and $LVdP/dt_{max}$. ECG and PEA in sinus rhythm and in RV rapid pacing were recorded during follow-up. Results showed that rapid RV pacing caused a worsening of cardiac function in all animals: $LVdP/dt_{max}$ (−69%±32), PEA (−56%±25), and LVEDP (+93%±23) (Fig. 1). These experimental results suggest that PEA is a reliable index by which to monitor and quantify the progressive worsening of cardiac function in heart

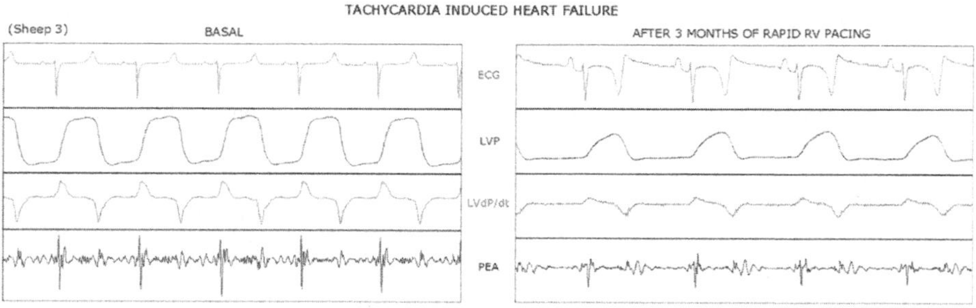

Fig. 1. ECG, LVP, LVdP/dt and PEA signals recorded at basal and after three months of rapid RV pacing

failure, and that it can be used at implantation and during follow-up for the optimization of CRT parameters: site, pacing configuration (biventricular or LV), VV timing, and AV interval.

The biventricular pacer (Living CHF, Sorin) with this unique capability to both give the therapy and assess its efficacy is now under clinical evaluation in Europe.

References

1. Sanders GP, Mendes LA, Colucci WS (2000) Noninvasive methods for detecting elevated left-sided cardiac filling pressure. J Card Fail 6:157–164
2. Kass DA, Chen CH, Curry C et al (1999) Improved left ventricular mechanism from acute VDD pacing in patients with dilated cardiomyopathy and ventricular contraction delay. Circulation 99:1567–1573
3. Auricchio A, Stellbrink C, Block M et al (1999) Effect of pacing chamber and atrioventricular delay on acute systolic function of paced patients with congestive heart failure. Circulation 99:2993–3001
4. Nelson GS, Berger RD, Fetics BJ et al (2000) Left ventricular or biventricular pacing improves cardiac function at diminished energy cost in patients with dilated cardiomyopathy and left bundle-branch block. Circulation 102:3053–3059
5. Van Gelder BM, Bracke FA, Meijer A (2003) The influence of intrinsic conduction on left ventricular dP/dt during biventricular pacing in cardiac resynchronization therapy. Pacing Clin Electrophysiol 26(4-Part II):952
6. Nelson GS, Curry CW, Wyman BT et al (2000) Predictors of systolic augmentation from left ventricular preexcitation in patients with dilated cardiomyopathy and intraventricular conduction delay. Circulation 101:2703–2709
7. Adamson PB, Magalski A, Braunschweig F et al (2003) Ongoing right ventricular hemodynamics in heart failure. J Am Coll Cardiol 41:565–571
8. Magalski A, Adamson P, Gadler F et al (2002) Continuous ambulatory right heart pressure measurements with an implantable hemodynamic monitor: a multicenter, 12-month follow-up study of patients with chronic heart failure. J Card Fail 8:63–70
9. Adams KF (2002) Guiding heart failure care by invasive hemodynamic measurements: possible or useful? J Card Fail 8:71–73

10. Stadler R, Wang L, Yu CM et al (2003) Automated detection of decreases in intrathoracic impedance to predict CHF hospitalization. Pacing Clin Electrophysiol 26 (4-Part II):932
11. Rickards AF, Bombardini T, Plicchi G (1996) An implantable intracardiac accelerometer for monitoring myocardial contractility. Pacing Clin Electrophysiol 19:2066–2071
12. Plicchi G, Marcelli E, Parlapiano M, Bombardini T (2002) PEAI and PEAII based implantable haemodynamic monitor: preclinical studies in sheep. Europace :49–54
13. Garrigue S, Bordachar P, Reuter S et al (2002) Comparison of permanent left ventricular and biventricular pacing in patients with heart failure and chronic atrial fibrillation: a prospective haemodynamic study. Heart 87:529–535
14. Dupuis JM, Kobeissi A, Vitali L et al (2003) Programming optimal atrioventricular delay in dual chamber pacing using peak endocardial acceleration: comparison with a standard echocardiographic procedure. Pacing Clin Electrophysiol 26 (1 part I):210–213
15. Padeletti L, Porciani MC, Ritter P et al (2000) Atrioventricular interval optimization in the right atrial appendage and interatrial septum pacing: a comparison between echo and peak endocardial acceleration measurements.Pacing Clin Electrophysiol 23(11 Pt 1):1618–22
16. Bombardini T, Gaggini G, Marcelli E et al (2000) Peak endocardial acceleration reflects heart contractility also in atrial fibrillation. Pacing Clin Electrophysiol 23:1381–1385
17. Padeletti L, Santini M, Ravazzi A et al (2003) Cardiac functionality evolution in patients with right ventricular pacing: the "WHERE" study. Pacing Clin Electrophysiol 26 (4-Part II):1100

CARDIAC RESYNCHRONIZATION THERAPY: MECHANISMS, TECHNICAL AND CLINICAL ASPECTS

Reverse Structural and Contractile Remodeling without Reverse Electrical Remodeling by Biventricular and Right Ventricular Apex Pacing in Dogs with Chronic AV Block

M. Peschar[1], M. A. Vos[2], F. W. Prinzen[1]

Introduction

Ventricular Pacing

During the last two decades an increasing body of evidence has built up that ventricular pacing causes abnormal, asynchronous electrical activation of the ventricles, and thereby also causes abnormal contraction patterns and reduced pump function [1]. During asynchronous contraction workload, myocardial blood flow and oxygen consumption are reduced in early-activated and increased in late-activated regions [1]. Long-term ventricular pacing induces ventricular dilatation and asymmetric hypertrophy, the latter due to local variation in myocyte size and proportional increase in collagen [2]. The latter study cited is an elegant demonstration that local myocardial load regulates local myocardial growth. However, the degree of hypertrophy appears to depend on the degree of initial hypertrophy. Left ventricular (LV) pacing in normal dog hearts induced circa 40% hypertrophy in the late-activated septum. In contrast, right ventricular (RV) pacing in hearts that were hypertrophying due to aortic banding showed no excessive hypertrophy in the late-activated LV free wall, but rather a reduction in hypertrophy of the early-activated septum [3]. Moreover, the asymmetry of hypertrophy appears to depend on the site of pacing: around 40% in case of LV pacing versus around 10% in the case of RV pacing.

Atrioventricular Block

The most classical application of ventricular pacing is to normalize heart rate in bradycardia, as induced by sick sinus node disease and atrioventricular (AV) block. Complete AV block causes a reduction in cardiac output and, as adapta-

[1]Departments of Physiology and [2]Cardiology, Cardiovascular Research Institute Maastricht, Maastricht, The Netherlands

tion to the decreased pump function, biventricular hypertrophy [4-9]. In addition, LV contractility is increased [4]. This increase is more pronounced at lower than at higher heart rates, resulting in a negative force-frequency relation (FFR). This alteration in contractile response is assumed to reflect changes in Ca^{2+} handling [5, 6]. However, these adaptations, which appear beneficial to maintain pump function, are accompanied by prolonged repolarization and increased risk of ventricular arrhythmias [7, 8].

Aim of the Study

The aim of the present study was to investigate the effect of normalization of load (pacing at physiological heart rate) and improvement of synchrony of activation (RV apex vs biventricular pacing) on reverse structural, contractile and electrical remodeling.

Methods

Experimental Protocol

The experiments were performed on 13 adult mongrel dogs of either sex and with a body weight of 30 ± 5 kg (mean ± SD). The dogs were randomly assigned to two groups: 8 weeks of complete AV block followed by either 8 weeks of RV apex pacing (RVa, n=7) or 8 weeks of simultaneous RVa and LV pacing (biventricular, BiV, n=6). Transvenous leads were positioned in the right atrium and RV apex alone (RVa group) or in combination with an epicardial lead positioned at the LV lateral free wall (BiV group). After 8 weeks of AV block the pacemaker was programmed to the VDD mode (atrial sensing and ventricular pacing with 100 ms AV delay) to restore physiological heart rate. Details of the induction of AV block and anesthetic regime have been published elsewhere [9].

Measurements

LV cavity volume and total and regional wall mass were determined using biweekly echocardiography [9]. The ratio of LV septum to free wall mass was used as an index of asymmetry of hypertrophy. QRS duration and QT time were measured in lead II of simultaneously recorded ECGs. Measurement of LV and RV action potential duration was performed using endocardially placed quadripolar electrodes to record monophasic action potentials (MAPs) at weeks 8 and 16 [8]. LV and RV action potential duration at 90% repolarization were measured [9]. QT time and action potential duration were corrected for heart rate according to the method of van de Water (QT_c and APD_c, respectively) [10]. At weeks 8 and 16 LV pressure was also measured, from which the maximum first positive (LV dP/dt_{max}) was calculated.

Results

Structural Remodeling

Within 8 weeks of AV block, the dogs developed around 25% LV hypertrophy (Fig. 1a). After onset of pacing, the decrease in LV mass was significant after 2 weeks of BiV pacing, but after 6 weeks of RVa pacing. After 8 weeks of pacing LV wall mass was comparable in both groups of paced hearts, being only 9 ± 14% (RVa) and 10 ± 9% (BiV) above the value before AV block. The LV septum to free wall ratio was significantly closer to 1 after BiV than after RVa pacing (Fig. 1b), indicating more uniform regression of hypertrophy during BiV pacing. After 8 weeks of AV block the LV cavity volume was increased by around 45%. Eight weeks of pacing at physiological heart rate decreased LV cavity volume by 28 ± 15% (RVa) and 13 ± 18% (BiV).

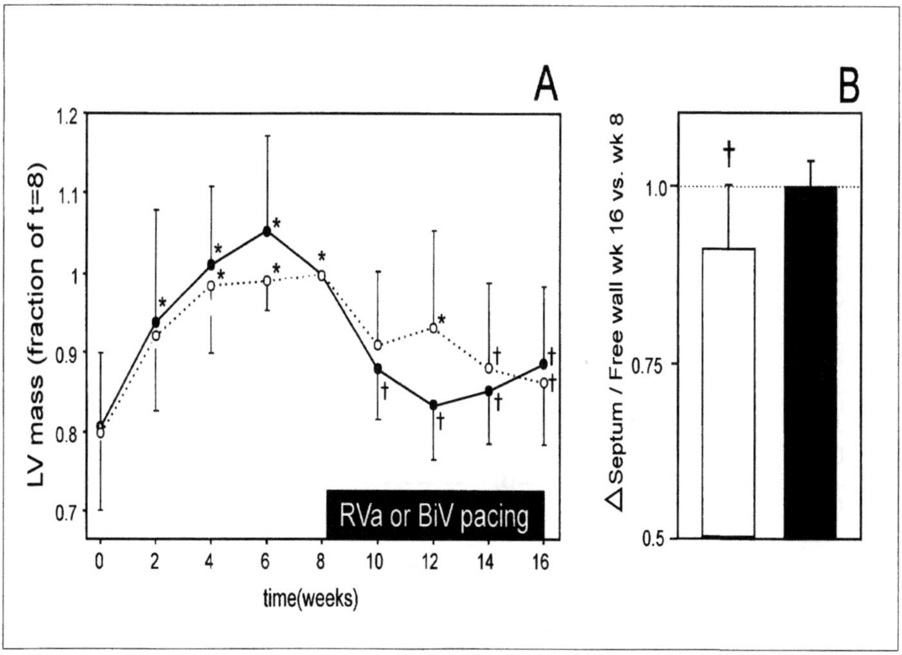

Fig. 1. A Time course of LV mass expressed as a fraction of their value at week 8, in the RVa (*open symbols*) and BiV groups (*closed symbols*). Changes in LV mass during 16 weeks of AV block (triangles) are from a previous study [9]. B Asymmetry index after 16 weeks expressed as a fraction of week 8 in the RVa (*white bar*) and BiV groups (*black bar*). * $p < 0.05$ vs SR (sinus rhythm at t=0) using ANOVA for repeated measurements; † $p < 0.05$ vs week 8 using group comparison

Contractile Remodeling

Reverse structural and contractile remodeling is illustrated in Fig. 2, where changes in LV$dP/dt_{max}$ were plotted against changes in LV end-diastolic volume, using the values at week 8 as a reference. For comparison, the values of these parameters at week 0 and 16 weeks of AV block, from a parallel study, were added to the figure. In both chronic pacing strategies, LV end-diastolic volume and LV$dP/dt_{max}$ decreased to near normal values, although end-diastolic volume tended to be larger in the BiV than in the RVa paced group. Reverse contractile remodeling was further evidenced by normalization of the slope and intercept of the FFR, as measured from LV$dP/dt_{max}$ over a wide range of paced heart rates. In both groups the FFR was negative at week 8 (RVa: -642±153, BiV: -662±444 mmHg) and was significantly less negative at week 16 (RVa: -339±112, BiV: -238±215 mmHg).

Electrical Remodeling

Acutely after onset of pacing, QRS duration was slightly, but not significantly, shorter in the BiV group than in the RVa group (96±16 ms vs 107±12 ms, respectively). No changes in QRS duration were observed in either group throughout the pacing period. Eight weeks of AV block prolonged QT_c time

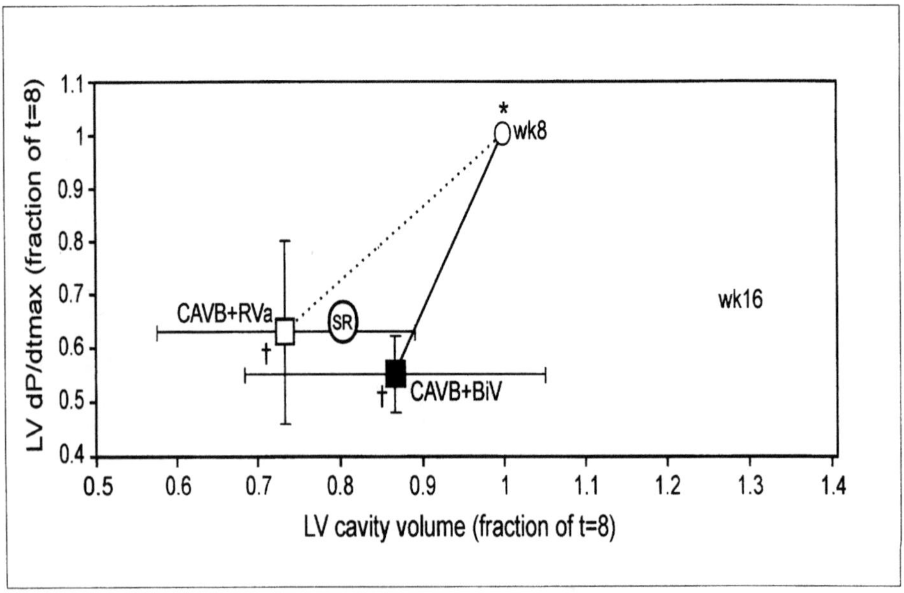

Fig. 2. Plot of LVdP/dtmax versus LV end-diastolic volume at weeks 8 and 16 in the RVa and BiV group. Values are expressed as a fraction of their value at week 8. Changes after 16 weeks of AV block (Δ) and during sinus rhythm (SR) are from a parallel study [9]. *$p < 0.05$ vs SR; †$p < 0.05$ vs week 8 using group comparison

(Fig. 3). Throughout the 8 weeks of pacing QT_C-time did not reverse to normal, despite regression of LV mass. The absence of reduction of repolarization time in both groups was confirmed by the MAP measurements, which showed comparable values of LV and RV APD_C at week 8 and 16 (Fig. 4).

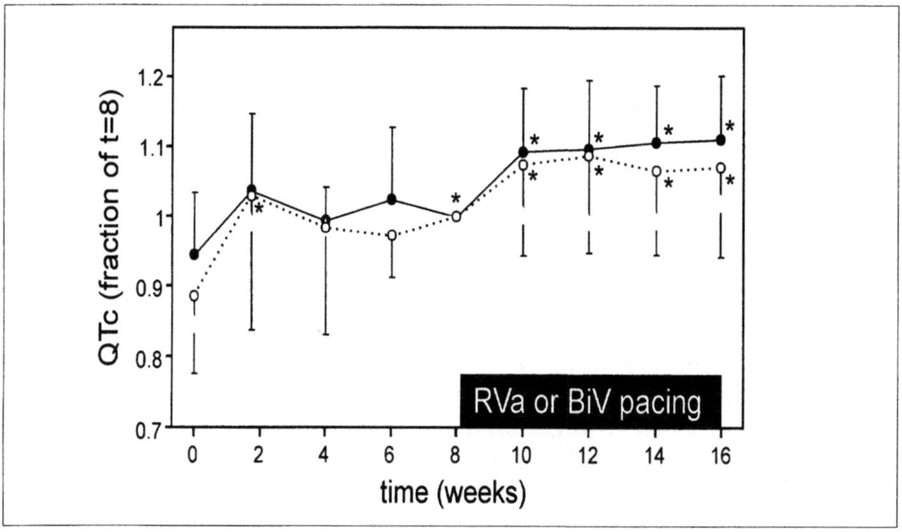

Fig. 3. Time-dependent changes of QT time corrected for heart rate [10] (QTc time) expressed as a fraction of its value at week 8. For symbols, see Fig. 1 legend. QTc data were obtained at idioventricular rhythm until week 8, thereafter during pacing. *$p <$ 0.05 vs SR using ANOVA for repeated measurements

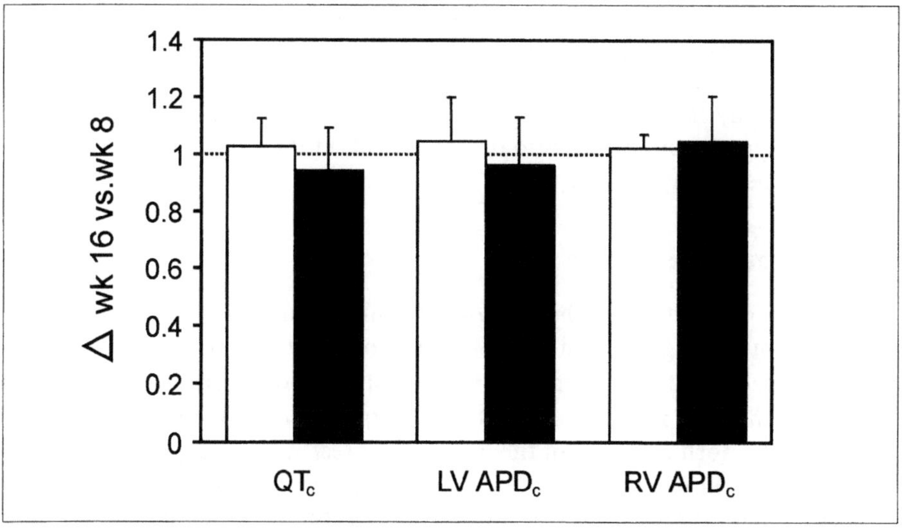

Fig. 4. QT_C time and LV and RV APD_C at week 16 as a fraction of their value at week 8 in the RVa (*white bars*) and BiV groups (*black bars*)

Discussion

In hearts that have become hypertrophied due to chronic bradycardia, normalization of the heart rate by ventricular pacing can cause reverse structural and reverse contractile remodeling, but not reverse electrical remodeling. Biventricular pacing leads to slightly but significantly quicker and more uniform regression of hypertrophy than RV apical pacing.

Reverse Structural Remodeling

Since the final degree of regression of hypertrophy in the present study was similar after BiV and after RVa pacing, the (a)synchrony of activation apparently does not play an important role. At first sight this seems remarkable, because asynchronous activation (LV pacing) in nonhypertrophic hearts leads to ventricular hypertrophy, especially in the late-activated areas [2]. Therefore, pacing bradycardiac hearts could have shown a mixture of reduction of LV mass due to increase of heart rate and an increase of LV mass due to asynchrony of activation. Apparently, in the situation of AV block, the normalization of heart rate is a stronger stimulus than the induction of asynchrony. Alternatively, the hypertrophic response to asynchronous activation could be less pronounced in hypertrophic hearts. This idea was supported by study where RVa pacing in pressure overload hypertrophy did not lead to (further) hypertrophy [3].

Although BiV pacing does not lead to QRS durations similar to those in sinus rhythm, activation of the LV is significantly more synchronous, as evidenced by MRI tagging [11]. The more synchronous LV activation in BiV pacing results in symmetrical regression of hypertrophy, as indicated by the LV septum to free wall ratio (Fig. 1b). The asymmetric regression of hypertrophy observed in RVa pacing is consistent with observations of asymmetric hypertrophy during single-site pacing in other studies [2, 3]. Therefore, asymmetry of hypertrophy is a characteristic effect of ventricular pacing, whereas the degree of hypertrophy appears to be dependent on the baseline situation (preexistent hypertrophy, bradycardia or not).

Reverse Contractile Remodeling

Restoration of heart rate in hearts with chronic AV block leads to reverse contractile remodeling, as evidenced by the normalization of the FFR after 8 weeks of pacing. It has been suggested that a decrease in SR Ca^{2+}-ATPase and/or an increase in Na^{+}/Ca^{2+} exchanger expression leads to a negative FFR [5, 6, 12]. The normalization of the FFR in the present study suggests a normalization of Ca^{2+} homeostasis and Na^{+}/Ca^{2+} exchanger current.

Only a few studies report on reverse contractile remodeling. Gerdes et al. showed that regression of hypertrophy after aortocaval shunt occlusion in rats was accompanied by a normalization of LV$dP/dt_{max}$ [13]. Reverse structural and reverse contractile remodeling do not necessarily run parallel, as demonstrated by Nakano et al., who showed that after valve replacement for mitral regurgitation, reverse contractile remodeling is not associated with regression of hypertrophy [14]. Longer action potential duration can lead to more Ca^{2+} influx, resulting in increased contractility. However, the reverse contractile remodeling despite unchanged action potential duration (see below) suggests that the latter does not contribute to contractility, at least not in this model.

Absence of Reverse Electrical Remodeling

The present study emphasizes that electrical remodeling may be less reversible than structural and contractile remodeling. In a previous study it was already shown that normalization of heart rate by RVa pacing does not lead to reverse electrical remodeling [9]. Here it is shown that, despite more synchronous electrical activation, BiV pacing, repolarization remains prolonged, as evidenced by prolonged QT_c time and LV and RV action potential duration. The lack of change of the repolarization parameters is independent of heart rate and activation sequence because the measurements during idioventricular rhythm, VDD pacing, and pacing at 100 beats/min show the same results.

In AV block the I_{to} current is reported to be unchanged [15]. Electrical remodeling in this model has been associated with an increased Na^+/Ca^{2+} exchanger current [16] and a decreased I_K current [15]. This decrease in I_K current is accompanied by downregulation of I_{Ks} protein [17] and mRNA [18]. Since reverse contractile remodeling implies normalization of the Na^+/Ca^{2+} exchanger current, irreversible changes in the K^+ channel are likely to be responsible for the absence of reverse electrical remodeling. This suggests that one gene is irreversibly changed, while other genes coding for structural and contractile proteins are reversibly altered.

The finding of poorly reversible electrical remodeling may also apply to other situations. For example, cardiac resynchronization therapy by BiV pacing often leads to reverse remodeling, expressed as reduction of LV cavity volume. However, reduction of life-threatening arrhythmias, which frequently occur in that particular patient category, has not yet been proven and, on the basis of the present data should not be assumed beforehand.

Conclusions

In canine hearts with bradycardia, normalization of heart rate by ventricular pacing leads to almost complete reverse structural and contractile remodeling. The degree of reverse remodeling is independent of the degree of synchrony of activation. However, electrical remodeling is not reversible, even when LV activation is more synchronous. Clinical studies should address this divergence in reverse remodeling to evaluate arrhythmogenic risk.

Acknowledgements. This study was financed by a grant from the Netherlands Heart Foundation (#95.043).

References

1. Prinzen FW, Peschar M (2002) Relation between the pacing induced sequence of activation and left ventricular pump function in animals. Pacing Clin Electrophysiol 25:484–498
2. van Oosterhout MF, Prinzen FW, Arts T et al (1998) Asynchronous electrical activation induces asymmetrical hypertrophy of the left ventricular wall. Circulation 98:588–595
3. van Oosterhout MF, Arts T, Muijtjens AM et al (2001) Remodeling by ventricular pacing in hypertrophying dog hearts. Cardiovasc Res 49:771–778
4. de Groot SH, Schoenmakers M, Molenschot MM et al (2000) Contractile adaptations preserving cardiac output predispose the hypertrophied canine heart to delayed afterdepolarization-dependent ventricular arrhythmias. Circulation 102:2145–2151
5. Hasenfuss G, Reinecke H, Studer R et al (1994) Relation between myocardial function and expression of sarcoplasmic reticulum Ca(2+)-ATPase in failing and nonfailing human myocardium. Circ Res 75:434–442
6. Houser SR, Piacentino V, Weisser J (2000) Abnormalities of calcium cycling in the hypertrophied and failing heart. J Mol Cell Cardiol 32:1595–1607
7. Swynghedauw B, Chevalier B, Charlemagne D et al (1997) Cardiac hypertrophy, arrhythmogenicity and the new myocardial phenotype. II. The cellular adaptational process. Cardiovasc Res 35:6–12
8. Vos MA, de Groot SH, Verduyn SC et al (1998) Enhanced susceptibility for acquired torsade de pointes arrhythmias in the dog with chronic, complete AV block is related to cardiac hypertrophy and electrical remodeling. Circulation 98:1125–1135
9. Peschar M, Vernooy K, Vanagt WYR et al (2003) Absence of reverse electrical remodeling during regression of volume overload hypertrophy in canine ventricles. Cardiovasc Res 58:510-517
10. van de Water A, Verheyen J, Xhonneux R et al (1989) An improved method to correct the QT interval of the electrocardiogram for changes in heart rate. J Pharmacol Methods 22:207–217
11. Wyman BT, Hunter WC, Prinzen FW et al (2002) Effects of single- and biventricular pacing on temporal and spatial dynamics of ventricular contraction. Am J Physiol Heart Circ Physiol 282:H372–379
12. Hasenfuss G, Schillinger W, Lehnart SE et al (1999) Relationship between Na+-Ca2+-exchanger protein levels and diastolic function of failing human myocardium. Circulation 99:641–648
13. Gerdes AM, Clark LC, Capasso JM (1995) Regression of cardiac hypertrophy after closing an aortocaval fistula in rats. Am J Physiol 268:H2345–2351
14. Nakano K, Swindle MM, Spinale F et al (1991) Depressed contractile function due to canine mitral regurgitation improves after correction of the volume overload. J Clin Invest 87:2077–2086
15. Volders PG, Sipido KR, Carmeliet E et al (1999) Repolarizing K+ currents ITO1 and IKs are larger in right than left canine ventricular midmyocardium. Circulation 99:206–210

16. Sipido KR, Volders PG, de Groot SH et al (2000) Enhanced Ca(2+) release and Na/Ca exchange activity in hypertrophied canine ventricular myocytes: potential link between contractile adaptation and arrhythmogenesis. Circulation 102:2137–2144
17. Volders PGA, Stengl M, Sipido KR et al (2002) Biophysical properties of downregulated IKs in canine ventricular hypertrophy. Biophys J 82:358a
18. Ramakers C, Dumaine R, Doevedans P et al (2000) Both KCNQ1 and KCNE1 expression is reduced in dogs with chronic AV–block. Eur Heart J 21(suppl S):239

How Are Perfusion and Adrenergic Innervation of the Left Ventricle Affected in Paced Patients?

E.N. SIMANTIRAKIS, P.E. VARDAS

Cardiac pacing, first introduced almost 45 years ago, is an established treatment for the prevention of symptomatic bradyarrhythmias. More recently, it has also proved valuable as an adjunct therapy in heart failure patients with ventricular conduction disturbances and, in some cases, in patients with hypertrophic cardiomyopathy. However, in patients with traditional indications cardiac pacing has been shown to be associated with "side effects", in particular when it results in atrioventricular and/or ventricular asynchrony [1]. On the other hand, in patients with dilated cardiomyopathy and bundle branch block, left ventricular (LV) or biventricular pacing improves LV systolic function [2] and quality of life [3, 4] and may decrease mortality [5] by resynchronizing ventricular contraction. Furthermore, in patients with ventricular hypertrophy and cavity obliteration during systole, right ventricular (RV) apical stimulation can increase cardiac systolic reserve [6], leading to clinical improvement [7, 8].

In order to examine the effects of artificial stimulation in greater depth and to explain the positive and/or negative implications for LV function, the impact of pacing on myocardial perfusion and adrenergic innervation has been investigated.

Myocardial Perfusion in Paced Patients

The RV apex is the most common site for ventricular stimulation, because of easy accessibility, lead stability and satisfactory sensing and pacing thresholds. However, the asynchronous electrical activation that this kind of stimulation causes impairs systolic and diastolic function and is associated with structural and histological changes in the ventricles. Recently, myocardial blood flow and perfusion have been studied during different kinds of pacing in animals and

Cardiology Department, Heraklion University Hospital, Heraklion, Crete, Greece

humans by means of positron emission tomography, ^{201}Tl scintigraphy and guidewire techniques. Most of these human studies found that a high percentage (46%–65%) of DDD paced patients showed perfusion defects in early activated regions close to the pacing site, while myocardial blood flow (MBF) and flow reserve changes were observed in the dominant coronary artery which mainly supplies these regions. Tse and Lau [9] found that RV apical pacing resulted in a high incidence of myocardial perfusion defects that increased with the duration of pacing. These myocardial perfusion abnormalities were associated with apical wall motion abnormalities and impaired global LV function. In a more recent study the same authors showed, in patients with complete heart block, that although at 6 months of pacing the incidence of myocardial perfusion defects and regional wall motion abnormalities, as well as the LV ejection fraction (LVEF), were similar during RV apical and RV outflow tract pacing, after 18 months the incidence of both perfusion defects (83% vs 33%) and regional wall motion abnormalities (75% vs 33%) was significantly higher, whereas LVEF (47±3% vs 56±1%) was significantly lower during RV apical than during RV outflow tract pacing [10]. We found similar results in our centre. In patients with complete heart block, paced for 32±19 months, 46.2% showed reversible perfusion defects on ^{201}Tl-dipyridamole myocardial scintigraphy [11]. However, 3 months of RV apical pacing were not enough to alter myocardial perfusion in patients with a narrow QRS complex paced for sick sinus syndrome [12], or those with ventricular conduction disturbances (right bundle branch block + left anterior fascicular block) paced because of trifascicular block [13]. A study by Skalidis et al. [14] found reduced coronary flow reserve in the defect-related artery, indicating impairment of microvascular flow in early activated regions. Similar results were reported by Nielsen et al. [15], who found that in patients with sick sinus syndrome chronic DDD pacing reduced inferior, septal and global mean MBF as well as LVEF. The latter reverted to baseline levels after the restoration of a normal ventricular activation sequence, despite the 22 months of permanent ventricular pacing that preceded the change. In a very recent study in our department, we reached similar conclusions, showing that left ventricular contractility, assessed by the conductance catheter method, and ventriculoarterial coupling improved after the restoration of a normal ventricular activation sequence in patients with long-term asynchrony because of RV apical stimulation [16]. Additionally, we found that after restoration of a normal ventricular activation sequence the blood flow in the dominant coronary artery increased, whereas the flow reserve in the artery decreased, suggesting that the changes in LV function were unrelated to changes in the coronary circulation. It is likely that both LV functional abnormalities and changes in coronary circulation are consequences of the altered ventricular activation sequence.

Results in animal studies are quite different from those in humans. Although acute ventricular pacing has been found to redistribute MBF within the LV wall [17, 18], in the long term regional differences in myocardial growth, due to the redistribution of workload by pacing, tend to equalize MBF distribution within the LV wall [19]. The authors suggested that these differences between animals and humans could be explained by the possible inability of the patients' myocardium to grow in proportion to the local differences in work. This could be related to pre-existing myocardial hypertrophy.

Although perfusion abnormalities induced by pacing need further elucidation regarding their clinical implications, they provide yet another reason for seeking more "physiologic" pacing sites. Especially for patients with concomitant coronary artery disease, who are not rare among candidates for cardiac pacing, perfusion abnormalities can worsen myocardial ischaemia and the clinical course of the disease.

In recent years myocardial perfusion and blood flow have been studied in patients paced for dilated and hypertrophic cardiomyopathy. In the former group of patients all the existing studies agree that although biventricular pacing improves septal oxidative metabolism, it does not significantly alter regional or global myocardial perfusion, which means that the haemodynamic and clinical improvement caused by biventricular pacing is not associated with any increase in oxygen demand [20–22]. In patients paced for hypertrophic obstructive cardiomyopathy, myocardial perfusion has been studied in an attempt to explain the mechanism of the anti-anginal effect of pacing. The results, however, are not consistent. Fananapazir et al. [23] found that 81% of 27 patients with hypertrophic obstructive cardiomyopathy had perfusion defects on exercise scintigraphy. After 8 weeks of DDD pacing, the abnormalities normalized or improved in 65%, but worsened in 17% of the patients. Another study by Posma et al. [24] found that the global perfusion reserve remained unchanged, whereas myocardial reserve became more homogeneously distributed. In this study perfusion reserve increased in three out of six patients but actually decreased in two during DDD pacing. Additionally, no relation was found between the individual effect of pacing on myocardial perfusion reserve and the clinical or haemodynamic responses to pacing.

Myocardial Adrenergic Innervation in Paced Patients

Cardiac myocytes and coronary circulation are innervated by both parasympathetic and sympathetic fibres. The dysfunction of the latter has been shown to play a pathogenetic role in a number of cardiac diseases, such as arrhythmias, cardiomyopathies and congestive heart failure. Recently, the development of radioactive tracers has facilitated the non-invasive assessment of the sympathetic innervation of the left ventricle, with single photon or positron emission tomography. [^{123}I]metaiodobenzylguanidine (^{123}I- MIBG), a guanethidine analogue that shares the same uptake, storage and release pathway as norepinephrine, has mainly been used in several studies examining myocardial adrenergic innervation in paced patients. Nakata et al. [25] were the first to show that ^{123}I-MIBG scintigraphic abnormalities occur in patients with implanted permanent pacemakers and that such abnormalities were more prominent under VVI than

DDD pacing mode, probably because of the worse haemodynamics that VVI mode entails. Later, Fukuoka et al. [26] found that long-term ventricular pacing, even in the presence of atrioventricular synchrony, accelerates cardiac sympathetic activity without affecting systemic sympathetic activity. In our department we studied left ventricular adrenergic innervation in several groups of paced patients. Apart from the global innervation, we also investigated the possibility of regional adrenergic disturbances by means of SPECT. Firstly we studied chronically paced patients (32±9 months), in DDD mode because of complete heart block. We found that the ^{123}I-MIBG uptake was significantly lower in paced patients than in normal subjects of similar age and sex [11]. Moreover, 89.7% of the patients presented regional abnormalities of ^{123}I-MIBG uptake, mainly in the early activated regions, indicative of increased sympathetic activity in these regions. These regional disturbances of the ^{123}I-MIBG uptake could not be attributed to coexisting perfusion disturbances, which were found in only 46.2% of patients. On the contrary, one might speculate that the lower workload in early activated regions leads in a compensatory way to increased sympathetic activity, which in its turn causes arterial constriction and decreases blood flow in some cases. Indeed, in this study we found that in regions with more severe ^{123}I-MIBG defects there was a higher probability of ^{201}Tl perfusion defects occurring. In a second study [12] we tried to overcome the limitation of the previous one, i.e. the unknown myocardial adrenergic activity before the pacemaker implantation. This study included patients with sick sinus syndrome and a narrow QRS complex, who underwent ^{201}Tl and ^{123}I-MIBG scintigraphic studies before and 3 months after the implantation of a pacemaker that was programmed so as to ensure complete ventricular capture. We found that, although myocardial perfusion did not change during this time period, there was a significant regional redistribution in ^{123}I-MIBG uptake. Such a redistribution was also found in patients with right bundle branch block and left anterior fascicular block after 3 months of DDD pacing [13]. Although the clinical significance of these findings needs further elucidation, they add another entry to the list of effects resulting from asynchronous ventricular activation. Furthermore, the global sympathetic acceleration and the regional adrenergic disturbances we described can contribute to the appearance of supraventricular and/or ventricular arrhythmias due to increased dispersion of refractoriness or to increased automaticity [27, 28].

Finally, in a recent, not yet published study we examined myocardial adrenergic innervation during RV apical and LV-based pacing in patients with chronic atrial fibrillation after atrioventricular junction ablation and with or without preserved LV function. We found that although disturbances of the adrenergic innervation of the left ventricle deteriorate during long-term RV apical pacing, they seem to reverse during pacing from the LV free wall or biventricular pacing, until they resemble those at baseline. These findings indicate that LV-based pacing ensures a more synchronous contraction and could have a positive impact on the up-regulation of β-adrenoreceptors in heart failure patients, by reducing the concentration of noradrenaline in myocardial tissue [29]. This, however, needs further investigation.

Conclusions

The altered ventricular activation sequence induced by pacing can have positive or negative implications, depending on the patient's disease and the kind of alteration. Although more studies are needed to elucidate the mechanisms and the clinical significance of changes in myocardial perfusion and adrenergic innervation, the findings to date have certainly increased our knowledge concerning the pathophysiology of the paced beat.

References

1. Rosenqvist M, Isaaz K, Botvinick EH et al (1991) Relative importance of activation sequence compared to atrioventricular synchrony in left ventricular function. Am J Cardiol 67:148–156
2. Kass DA, Chen CH, Curry C et al (1999) Improved left ventricular mechanics from acute VDD pacing in patients with dilated cardiomyopathy and ventricular conduction delay. Circulation 99:1567–1573
3. Linde C, Leclercq C, Rex S et al (2002) Long-term benefits of biventricular pacing in congestive heart failure: results from the MUltisite STimulation in cardiomyopathy (MUSTIC) study. J Am Coll Cardiol 40:111–118
4. Abraham WT, Fisher WG, Smith AL et al (2002) Cardiac resynchronization in chronic heart failure. N Engl J Med 346:1845–1853
5. Bradley DJ, Bradley EA, Baughman KL et al (2003) Cardiac resynchronization and death from progressive heart failure: a meta-analysis of randomized controlled trials. JAMA 289:730–740
6. Kass DA (2000) Mechanisms and efficacy of LV pre-excitation for patients with heart failure and supra-normal systolic function. Heart Fail Rev 5:357–365
7. Kappenberger LJ, Linde C, Jeanrenaud X et al (1999) Clinical progress after randomized on/off pacemaker treatment for hypertrophic obstructive cardiomyopathy. Pacing in Cardiomyopathy (PIC) Study Group. Europace 1:77–84
8. Maron BJ, Nishimura RA, McKenna WJ et al (1999) Assessment of permanent dual-chamber pacing as a treatment for drug-refractory symptomatic patients with obstructive hypertrophic cardiomyopathy. A randomized, double-blind, crossover study (M-PATHY). Circulation 99:2927–2933
9. Tse HF, Lau CP (1997) Long-term effect of right ventricular pacing on myocardial perfusion and function. J Am Coll Cardiol 29:744–749
10. Tse HF, Yu C, Wong KK et al (2002) Functional abnormalities in patients with permanent right ventricular pacing: the effect of sites of electrical stimulation. J Am Coll Cardiol 40:1451–1458
11. Simantirakis EN, Prassopoulos VK, Chrysostomakis SI et al (2001) Effects of asynchronous ventricular activation on myocardial adrenergic innervation in patients with permanent dual-chamber pacemakers; an I(123)-metaiodobenzylguanidine cardiac scintigraphic study. Eur Heart J 22:323–332

12. Marketou ME, Simantirakis EN, Prassopoulos VK et al (2002) Assessment of myocardial adrenergic innervation in patients with sick sinus syndrome: effect of asynchronous ventricular activation from ventricular apical stimulation. Heart 88:255–259
13. Simantirakis EN, Prassopoulos VK, Marketou ME et al (2003) Myocardial perfusion and adrenergic innervation in patients with RBBB and LAFB: the effect of altering the activation sequence with right ventricular apical pacing. Pacing Clin Electrophysiol 26:1202–1207
14. Skalidis EI, Kochiadakis GE, Koukouraki SI et al (2001) Myocardial perfusion in patients with permanent ventricular pacing and normal coronary arteries. J Am Coll Cardiol 37:124–129
15. Nielsen JC, Bottcher M, Nielsen TT, Pedersen AK, Andersen HR (2000) Regional myocardial blood flow in patients with sick sinus syndrome randomized to long-term single chamber atrial or dual chamber pacing–effect of pacing mode and rate. J Am Coll Cardiol 35:1453–1461
16. Simantirakis EN, Kochiadakis GE, Vardakis KE et al (2003) Left ventricular mechanics and myocardial blood flow following restoration of normal activation swquence in paced patients with long-term right ventricular apical stimulation. Chest (in press)
17. Prinzen FW, Augustijn CH, Arts T, Allessie MA, Reneman RS (1990) Redistribution of myocardial fiber strain and blood flow by asynchronous activation. Am J Physiol 259(2Pt2):H300–H308
18. Delhaas T, Arts T, Prinzen FW, Reneman RS (1994) Regional fibre stress-fibre strain area as an estimate of regional blood flow and oxygen demand in the canine heart. J Physiol 477(Pt 3):481–496
19. van Oosterhout MF, Arts T, Bassingthwaighte JB, Reneman RS, Prinzen FW (2002) Relation between local myocardial growth and blood flow during chronic ventricular pacing. Cardiovasc Res 53:831–840
20. Neri G, Zanco P, Zanon F, Buchberger R (2003) Effect of biventricular pacing on metabolism and perfusion in patients affected by dilated cardiomyopathy and left bundle branch block: evaluation by positron emission tomography. Europace 5:111–115
21. Nielsen JC, Bottcher M, Jensen HK et al (2003) Regional myocardial perfusion during chronic biventricular pacing and after acute change of the pacing mode in patients with congestive heart failure and bundle branch block treated with an atrioventricular sequential biventricular pacemaker. Eur J Heart Fail 5:179–186
22. Ukkonen H, Beanlands RS, Burwash IG et al (2003) Effect of cardiac resynchronization on myocardial efficiency and regional oxidative metabolism. Circulation 107:28–31
23. Fananapazir L, Dilsizian V, Bonow RO (1992) Dual chamber pacing relieves angina and improves myocardial perfusion abnormalities in patients with obstructive hypertrophic cardiomyopathy (abstract). Circulation 86(Supp I):I–273
24. Posma JL, Blanksma PK, Van Der Wall EE et al (1996) Effects of permanent dual chamber pacing on myocardial perfusion in symptomatic hypertrophic cardiomyopathy. Heart 76:358–362
25. Nakata A, Hirota S, Tsuji H, Takazakura E (1995) I–123 metaiodobenzylguanidine cardiac scintigraphy in patients with an implanted permanent pacemaker. Jpn Heart J 36:583–591
26. Fukuoka S, Nakagawa S, Fukunaga T, Yamada H (2000) Effect of long-term atrial-demand ventricular pacing on cardiac sympathetic activity. Nucl Med Commun 21:291–297

27. Dae MW, Lee RJ, Ursell PC, Chin MC, Stillson CA, Moise NS (1997) Heterogeneous sympathetic innervation in German shepherd dogs with inherited ventricular arrhythmia and sudden cardiac death. Circulation 96:1337–1342
28. Yoshioka K, Gao DW, Chin M (2000) Heterogeneous sympathetic innervation influences local myocardial repolarization in normally perfused rabbit hearts. Circulation 101:1060–1066
29. Bristow MR, Minobe W, Rasmussen R et al (1992) Beta-adrenergic neuroeffector abnormalities in the failing human heart are produced by local rather than systemic mechanisms. J Clin Invest 89:803–815

Cardiac Resynchronization Therapy: The Low Voltage Road or the High Voltage Road?

G. Boriani[1], M. Biffi[1], C. Martignani[1], C. Camanini[1], C. Valzania[1], I. Diemberger[1], D. Saporito[1], P. Bartolini[2], A. Branzi[1]

Background of Cardiac Resynchronization Therapy

Cardiac resynchronization therapy is an additional therapeutic option for heart failure patients that has became available in recent years and aroused great interest among both electrophysiologists and clinical cardiologists managing heart failure patients. The prevalence of conduction disturbances (QRS interval ≥120 ms) among patients with left ventricular dysfunction or overt heart failure has been found to range between 27% and 53% [1–3]. Upon analyzing subjects with varying degrees of functional impairment according to New York Heart Association (NYHA) functional class, wider mean QRS intervals were found in subjects with a higher degree of functional impairment [4]. In subjects with dilated cardiomyopathy the QRS interval was widened in electrograms recorded shortly before death as compared to recordings made a mean of 35 months before the terminal event [5]. In unselected patients, left bundle branch block was associated with increased risk of both total mortality and sudden death at 1 year [2]. In another study [6] a QRS duration >110 ms was associated with increased mortality independently of left ventricular ejection fraction. It is a matter for investigation to assess whether left bundle branch block with left QRS axis deviation is most closely related to left ventricular enlargement and left ventricular dysfunction or whether it carries additional prognostic implications [7]. In a recent paper [8], a widening of the QRS interval in patients with heart failure who were followed by a heart failure clinic was a definite and independent predictor of mortality. According to these data, analysis of the QRS interval may provide additional information as a basis for selecting candidates for nonpharmacological treatments.

[1]Istituto di Cardiologia, Università di Bologna, Azienda Ospedaliera S. Orsola-Malpighi, Bologna; [2]Laboratorio di Ingegneria Biomedica, Istituto Superiore di Sanità, Rome, Italy

Clinical Results with Cardiac Resynchronization Therapy

A series of studies with follow-ups ranging from 6 to 22 months have shown that cardiac resynchronization therapy can improve cardiac function, quality of life, and functional capacity (Table 1). The extent of improvement is in the range of 14%–28% for left ventricular ejection fraction, 17%–38% for exercise capacity in a 6-min walking test, and 8%–42% for peak oxygen consumption in a cardiopulmonary exercise test. This improvement has also been confirmed in the MIRACLE study, a double-blind randomized study with a 6-month follow up [9]. In the MIRACLE study patients randomized to undergo cardiac resynchronization therapy differed significantly from controls in terms of quality of life, since they more frequently reported an improvement (67% versus 39%) and less frequently a worsening (15% versus 27%).

In the MIRACLE study, cardiac resynchronization therapy was associated with a significant reduction both in hospitalizations and in the use of intravenous medications for worsening heart failure in comparison to controls. Overall the combined risk of a major clinical event (death or hospitalization for heart failure) was 40% lower in the resynchronization group than in the control group (p=0.03). A significant reduction in hospitalizations between the preimplantation and the postimplantation period was also reported [10].

A series of studies suggests that a process of reverse remodeling occurs in the months that follow the initiation of biventricular pacing. In the MIRACLE study [9], a double-blind randomized prospective study, patients who underwent cardiac resynchronization therapy had, compared to controls, a significant reduction in left ventricular diameters and an improvement in left ven-

Table 1. Cardiac resynchronization therapy in heart failure: results of a series of studies

Study	No. of patients	Follow-up (months)	Change in NYHA class at end of follow-up	6-min walking test (% change vs baseline)	VO_2 peak (% change vs baseline	LVEF (% change vs baseline)
French Pilot	125	22.0	–1.0	-	+42%	+28%
InSync	103	12.0	-1.1	+20%	-	-
Bad Oyenhauser	107	7.6	-1.0	+38%	+27%	-
InSync Italian Registry	190	10	-1.0	+31%	-	+24%
PATH-CHF	29	12.0	-1.2	+25%	+24%	-
MUSTIC	82	12.0	–0.8	+19%	+10%	+14%
MIRACLE	453	6.0	-0.8	+17%	+8%	+21%

LVEF, left ventricular ejection fraction; VO_2 peak, peak oxygen consumption

tricular ejection fraction that was also associated with a significant reduction in the area of mitral regurgitation. Reversal of left ventricular remodeling has been clearly demonstrated by Yu et al. [11], who serially studied the effects of biventricular stimulation during 3 months of pacing and 4 weeks of pacing withdrawal. The improvement in left ventricular ejection fraction, *dP/dt*, and myocardial performance index and the decrease in mitral regurgitation and ventricular volumes were pacing-dependent, since the withholding of pacing resulted in reversal of the observed improvement, with varying time courses.

Effects of Cardiac Resynchronization Therapy on Overall Survival and Role of Defibrillation Backup

A series of prospective randomized trials (ReLeVent, CARE-HF, and COMPANION) were designed to test the effects of cardiac resynchronization on mortality and to test the role of adding defibrillation capability to the implanted device [12]. The ReLeVent and CARE-HF studies are still ongoing, while the COMPANION study, a randomized controlled trial, was interrupted in November 2002, having proved the advantages (reduction of deaths and hospitalizations) of cardiac resynchronization therapy [12].

The primary end-point of COMPANION was a composite end-point including death or any hospitalization (including treatment with intravenous vasoactive drugs), and both cardiac resynchronization therapy and biventricular pacing with defibrillation backup were associated with a significant reduction (around 19%) in event rate compared to control at 12 months. One of the most interesting findings of COMPANION is related to the effect on survival: with regard to all-cause mortality, biventricular pacing with defibrillation backup was associated with a statistically significant 43% reduction at 12 months compared to controls while the 24% reduction obtained with biventricular pacing alone did not reach statistical significance [13].

Indeed, the question whether cardiac resynchronization therapy has to be associated with a defibrillation backup, and in which patients this is to be recommended, is a key question with clinical and economic implications.

As is known, cardioverter-defibrillators are a treatment of proven efficacy in appropriately selected patients, both in the setting of secondary prevention of sudden death after previous episodes of sustained ventricular tachyarrhythmias [14–17] and in the setting of primary prevention of sudden death in patients with coronary artery disease, previous myocardial infarction, and left ventricular dysfunction [18, 19]. In both settings, the patients with the most significant impairment in left ventricular dysfunction receive the greatest benefit in survival when treated with the defibrillator in comparison to conventional treatment ("the sickest patients benefit the most") [15, 16, 20]. All this evidence has to be translated into the setting of heart failure, where the proportion of deaths due to sudden death are proportionally higher in the lowest NYHA classes [21].

Today, devices able to deliver both biventricular pacing and the full spectrum of treatments for ventricular tachyarrhythmias (antitachycardia pacing, shock therapy) are available, but definite and specific indications for implanting these devices are lacking; usually, they are currently implanted when a class I indication for implanting a cardioverter-defibrillator is found in candidates for biventricular pacing. In these cases a reduction in the number of appropriate cardioverter-defibrillator interventions has been observed during biventricular pacing [22]. Since heart failure per se carries a risk of sudden death, a widening of indications is under investigation by prospective studies focused on the role of defibrillators in heart failure patients (SCD-HF) or, specifically, on the role of defibrillators with biventricular pacing capabilities [12, 23].

With regard to the indications for implanting a cardioverter-defibrillator for primary prevention of sudden death, there are important differences between ischemic heart disease and idiopathic dilated cardiomyopathy. For patients with coronary artery disease, the results of the MADIT II trial [19] related to postinfarction patients with left ventricular dysfunction (left ventricular ejection fraction ≤30%) with or without overt heart failure (NYHA functional class was I in 35%–39% and II in 34%–35% of enrolled patients) will obviously lead to increased use of devices with shock capabilities for patients in whom cardiac resynchronization therapy is indicated and who meet the inclusion criteria of this trial. For patients with idiopathic dilated cardiomyopathy and heart failure, the results of the CAT trial [13], a prospective controlled study performed in patients with dilated cardiomyopathy of recent onset with left ventricular dysfunction and in NYHA class II or III did not show any advantage of cardioverter-defibrillator therapy in terms of mortality, which was low both in patients who received such therapy and in controls. Another study, AMIOVIRT [24] compared amiodarone with the cardioverter-defibrillator in nonischemic cardiomyopathy and showed no differences in outcome.

For patients with idiopathic dilated cardiomyopathy, interesting data are provided by an observational study reported by Grimm et al. [25] in which patients with dilated cardiomyopathy, left ventricular ejection fraction equal to or below 30% and nonsustained ventricular tachycardia after cardioverter-defibrillator implantation had the same incidence of appropriate interventions as patients presenting with syncope or ventricular tachycardia/fibrillation. Although the study was not prospective, was uncontrolled, and used surrogate end-points, it may be useful for identification of a subgroup of patients with nonischemic cardiomyopathy who may potentially benefit from cardioverter-defibrillators for primary prevention of sudden death. Moreover, one of the important findings of the COMPANION trial is that the benefits of cardiac resynchronization therapy associated with defibrillation capabilities were observed in both ischemic and nonischemic patients, thus providing strong support for a widening of the indications for defibrillation therapy associated with biventricular pacing [23].

More data on the role of cardioverter-defibrillators without associated biventricular pacing in heart failure patients will be provided by the SCD-HF trial [12], in which treatment with a cardioverter-defibrillator is prospectively compared with amiodarone and controls in patients with NYHA class II or III function and left ventricular ejection fraction equal to or below 35%. The results of this trial, which is specifically devoted to heart failure patients, will surely influence the indications for implanting a cardioverter-defibrillator in such patients and therefore also for coupling defibrillation capabilities to biventricular pacing.

Conclusions

The answer to the question "Cardiac resynchronization therapy: the low voltage road or the high voltage road?" will have to wait for the results of prospective trials, but in our view the most promising road is high voltage one. This implies that cardiac resynchronization therapy will have to be delivered by a device which includes a ventricular defibrillation backup in case of ventricular tachyarrhythmias. In our view, the absence of powerful and sensitive stratifiers for the risk of sudden death strongly supports ensuring the availability of ventricular defibrillation backup whenever it is judged that a device for treating heart failure has to be implanted. In this perspective, as suggested by Jay Cohn [26] many years ago, ventricular tachyarrhythmias, and therefore even sudden death, have to be considered a typical component of the clinical expressions of heart failure. However, the indications for the use of devices with ventricular defibrillation capabilities must take into account possible exceptions, such as cases of very severe heart failure, in the absence of other potential therapeutic possibilities in the future (e.g., age not allowing inclusion in a transplant program, contraindications to any cardiac surgery), where implantation of a pacemaker for cardiac resynchronization may be proposed in the framework of a compassionate therapy aimed mainly at improving the patient's quality of life.

References

1. Aaronson KD, Schwartz JS, Chen TM et al (1997) Development and prospective validation of a clinical index to predict survival in ambulatory patients referred for cardiac transplant evaluation. Circulation 95:2660–2667
2. Baldasseroni S, Opasich C, Gorini M et al (2002) Left bundle-branch block is associated with increased 1-year sudden and total mortality rate in 5517 outpatients with congestive heart failure: a report from the Italian network on congestive heart failure. Am Heart J 143:398–405
3. Shamim W, Francis DP, Yousufuddin M et al (1999) Intraventricular conduction delay: a prognostic marker in chronic heart failure. Int J Cardiol 70:171–178
4. Stellbrink C, Auricchio A, Diem B et al (1999) Potential benefit of biventricular pacing in patients with congestive heart failure and ventricular tachyarrhythmia. Am J Cardiol 83:143D–150D

5. Wilensky RL, Yudelman P, Cohen AI et al (1988) Serial electrocardiographic changes in idiopathic dilated cardiomyopathy confirmed at necropsy. Am J Cardiol 62:276–283
6. Silvet H, Amin J, Padmanabhan S, Pai RG (2001) Prognostic implications of increased QRS duration in patients with moderate and severe left ventricular systolic dysfunction. Am J Cardiol 88:182–185, A6
7. Das MK, Cheriparambil K, Bedi A et al (2001) Prolonged QRS duration (QRS ≥170 ms) and left axis deviation in the presence of left bundle branch block: a marker of poor left ventricular systolic function? Am Heart J 142:756–759
8. Grigioni F, Carinci V, Boriani G et al (2002) Accelerated QRS widening as an independent predictor of cardiac death or of the need for heart transplantation in patients with congestive heart failure. J Heart Lung Transplant 21:899–902
9. Abraham WT, Fisher WG, Smith AL et al (2002) Cardiac resynchronization in chronic heart failure. N Engl J Med 346:1845–1853
10. Braunschweig F, Linde C, Gadler F et al (2000) Reduction of hospital days by biventricular pacing. Eur J Heart Fail 2:399–406
11. Yu CM, Chau E, Sanderson JE, Fan K et al (2002) Tissue Doppler echocardiographic evidence of reverse remodeling and improved synchronicity by simultaneously delaying regional contraction after biventricular pacing therapy in heart failure. Circulation 105:438–445
12. Cleland JG, Thackray S, Goodge L et al (2002) Outcome studies with device therapy in patients with heart failure. J Cardiovasc Electrophysiol 13:S73–91
13. Bansch D, Antz M, Boczor S et al (2002) Primary prevention of sudden cardiac death in idiopathic dilated cardiomyopathy: the Cardiomyopathy Trial (CAT). Circulation 105:1453–1458
14. The Antiarrhythmics versus Implantable Defibrillators (AVID) Investigators (1997) A comparison of antiarrhythmic-drug therapy with implantable defibrillators in patients resuscitated from near-fatal ventricular arrhythmias. N Engl J Med 337:1576–1583
15. Connolly SJ, Gent M, Roberts RS et al (2000) Canadian implantable defibrillator study (CIDS): a randomized trial of the implantable cardioverter defibrillator against amiodarone. Circulation 101:1297–1302
16. Connolly SJ, Hallstrom AP, Cappato R et al (2000) Meta-analysis of the implantable cardioverter defibrillator secondary prevention trials. AVID, CASH and CIDS studies. Antiarrhythmics vs Implantable Defibrillator study. Cardiac Arrest Study Hamburg. Canadian Implantable Defibrillator Study. Eur Heart J 21:2071–2078
17. Ezekowitz JA, Armstrong PW, McAlister FA (2003) Implantable cardioverter defibrillators in primary and secondary prevention: a systematic review of randomized, controlled trials. Ann Intern Med 138:445–452
18. Moss AJ, Hall WJ, Cannom DS et al (1996) Improved survival with an implanted defibrillator in patients with coronary disease at high risk for ventricular arrhythmia. Multicenter Automatic Defibrillator Implantation Trial Investigators. N Engl J Med 335:1933–1940
19. Moss AJ, Zareba W, Hall WJ et al (2002) Prophylactic implantation of a defibrillator in patients with myocardial infarction and reduced ejection fraction. N Engl J Med 346:877–883
20. Domanski MJ, Sakseena S, Epstein AE et al (1999) Relative effectiveness of the implantable cardioverter-defibrillator and antiarrhythmic drugs in patients with varying degrees of left ventricular dysfunction who have survived malignant ventricular arrhythmias. AVID Investigators. Antiarrhythmics Versus Implantable

Defibrillators. J Am Coll Cardiol 34:1090–1095
21. Metoprolol CR/XL Randomised Intervention Trial in Congestive Heart Failure (MERIT-HF) (1999) Effect of metoprolol CR/XL in chronic heart failure. Lancet 353:2001–2007
22. Higgins SL, Yong P, Sheck D et al (2000) Biventricular pacing diminishes the need for implantable cardioverter defibrillator therapy. Ventak CHF Investigators. J Am Coll Cardiol 36:824–827
23. Bristow M (2003) Cardiac resynchronization therapy reduces hospitalizations, and cardiac resynchronization therapy and implantable defibrillator reduce mortality in chronic heart failure. Results of the COMPANION trial. Late breaking clinical trials. American College of Cardiology 52nd Annual Scientific Session
24. Strickberger SA (2000) Multicenter randomized trial comparing amiodarone to implantable defibrillator in patients with nonischemic cardiomyopathy and asymptomatic nonsustained ventricular tachycardia: AMIOVIRT Trial. Circulation 102:2784
25. Grimm W, Hoffmann JJ, Muller HH et al (2002) Implantable defibrillator event rates in patients with idiopathic dilated cardiomyopathy, nonsustained ventricular tachycardia on Holter and a left ventricular ejection fraction below 30%. J Am Coll Cardiol 39:780–787
26. Cohn JN (1990) Mechanisms in heart failure and the role of angiotensin-converting enzyme inhibition. Am J Cardiol 66:2D–6D

Cardiac Resynchronization Therapy: What Are the Benefits of Digital Pacemakers?

G. Fröhlig[1], P. Wohlgemuth[2], N.M. van Hemel[3], A. Vincent[2]

While many applications in daily life switched from analogue to digital techniques long ago, pacemakers are only just entering the field of digital signal processing (DSP). Possible reasons for the late implementation of DSP are the widespread satisfaction with the technology already available and the difficult balance between calculating plus storing capacity and the energy constraints of small batteries. DSP, however, offers basic advantages that may also improve the performance of pacemakers.

The technique minimizes the variability in performance by limiting the tolerances in circuit design.

It becomes still more flexible, because it does not need dedicated hardware for any new functionality, can be upgraded by software injection, and allows for easy programmability.

It is essential for advanced pattern recognition, which enables the device to discriminate between signals of different origins and to analyze complex arrhythmias.

Basic Characteristics

The new platform includes a very fast processor, an extensive RAM memory, a high-resolution analogue-to-digital (AD) converter, and a speed-up telemetry circuit to display the sampled data in real time. Most importantly, the sampling rate of 800 Hz enables the AD converter to reproduce the frequency content of cardiac signals up to 400 Hz without any distortion. This accounts for the high-frequency components of atrial signals, which can specifically be picked up from minitip electrodes [1]. The digital filter can be deliberately tailored and even made programmable according to specific needs (lead tip geometry, fixed versus floating electrodes, etc.). Instead of only being sensed, the signal

[1]Medizinische Universitätsklinik, Innere Medizin III, Homburg, Germany; [2]Vitatron B.V., Arnhem, The Netherlands; [3]St. Antonius Hospital, Nieuwegein, The Netherlands

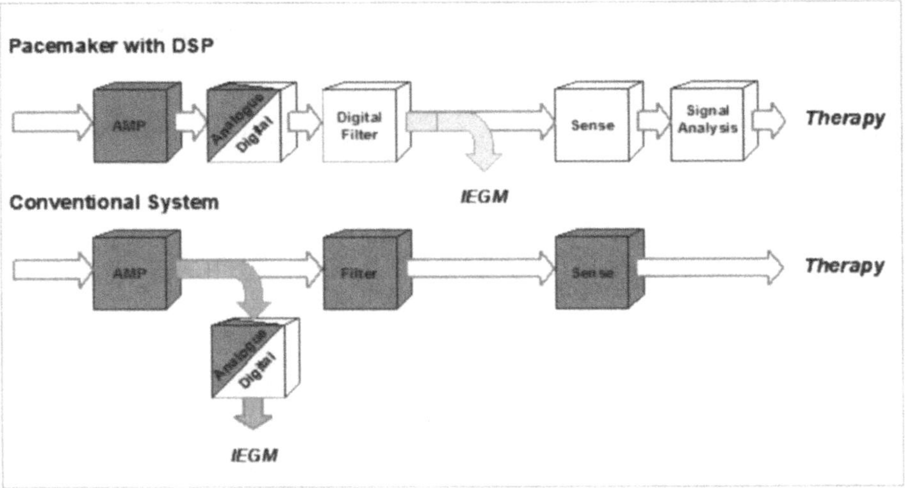

Fig. 1. Signal flow through the sensing circuitry of a DSP system and of a conventional system. IEGM telemetry in the DSP system displays signals after they have been digitized and filtered, just as they are "seen" by the detector circuitry; in the analogue system, telemetry is derived from the electronic path either before or after (not shown) filtering; since the signals have to be digitized before transmission, they will differ from the detector input. AMP, amplifier; Sense, detector circuitry

opens an analysis window, which is used to determine several EGM characteristics for operational discrimination and diagnostic storage. This includes the maximum amplitude beyond the triggering portion of intracardiac signals, which can be displayed in a histogram of beat-to-beat determination. Since the EGM telemetry branches off after digitizing and filtering, it displays the signals as "seen" by the sensing circuitry (Fig. 1) and allows for direct translation of "on-screen" EGM amplitudes into appropriate sensitivity settings.

Clinical Applications

Discrimination of Ventricular Far-field Signals in the Atrium

Depending on sensitivity settings and blanking times, far-field R-waves (FFRW) in the atrium have been found in up to 100% of patients [2, 3]. Despite some better rejection of these signals with short tip-to-ring spacing of bipolar leads, mode switches attributable to false tachycardia episodes and their storage in diagnostic counters can sometimes only be prevented by use of long blanking times. These, in turn, increase the risk of undersensing true atrial tachyarrhythmias.

Several techniques of intracardiac waveform analysis have been proposed, including morphology and adaptive filter-based algorithms to discriminate between antegrade and retrograde P-waves [4] and between P-waves and FFRW [5]. A digital signal processing implementation of correlation waveform analysis (CWA) has been reported [6], and such an algorithm has been successfully tested both offline and in real time [7]. Another promising technique is based on only two out of nine form parameters, which can be derived from DSP of atrial electrograms [8] (Fig. 2). The algorithm was tested offline using 100 recordings of intraoperative electrograms from 31 patients. EGMs were sampled with 8 bits and a sample rate of 800 Hz, filtered (15–180 Hz) and analyzed for slopes and amplitudes. The form parameters used were the most markedly negative values of the filtered signal and the slope signal. After an initial learning phase (first 30 s of each recording), the algorithm decided that the discrimination method was "applicable" in 33 and "not applicable" in 19 samples and that "no FFRW" was present in 48. If the method was applicable, the subsequent classification phase yielded 5 out of 1,352 false-negative FFRWs (sensitivity: 99.6%) and 0 out of 5,650 false-positive P-waves (specificity 100%). Lacking applicability was due to atrial fibrillation (11%), AV nodal rhythm (2%), atrial pacing only (1%), and an insufficient gap in the distribution histogram of the form parameters (5%).

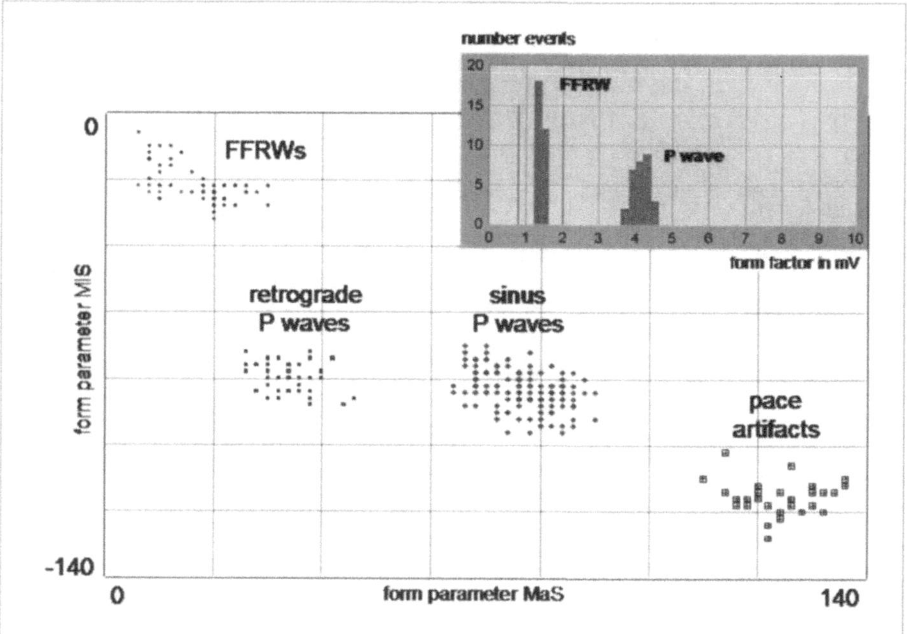

Fig. 2. Discrimination between atrial EGM components using two form parameters derived by DSP. The insert shows the histogram of a specific form factor distribution; a gap between P-wave and FFRW is mandatory for discrimination. *MaS*, maximum slope; *MiS*, minimum slope

Ischemia Detection in Ventricular EGMs

Using the inflation of a PTCA balloon during interventional procedures as a model of ischemia, correlation factors were calculated between three different EGM recordings (ventricular tip, ring and bipolar) and six limb leads (I-III, aVR-aVF). ST deviations from baseline were measured 80 ms after the J-point in the surface ECG and 110 ms after ventricular sensing in the intracardiac recording. Figure 3 shows the results of 4 of the 10 patients studied. It exemplifies the considerable variation in correlation factors depending on the intracardiac and surface lead configurations. While parameters that could be universally applicable are lacking, there is a highly significant correlation between the ST-segment variation in the limb leads and some of the intracardiac recordings in any case. The study is ongoing.

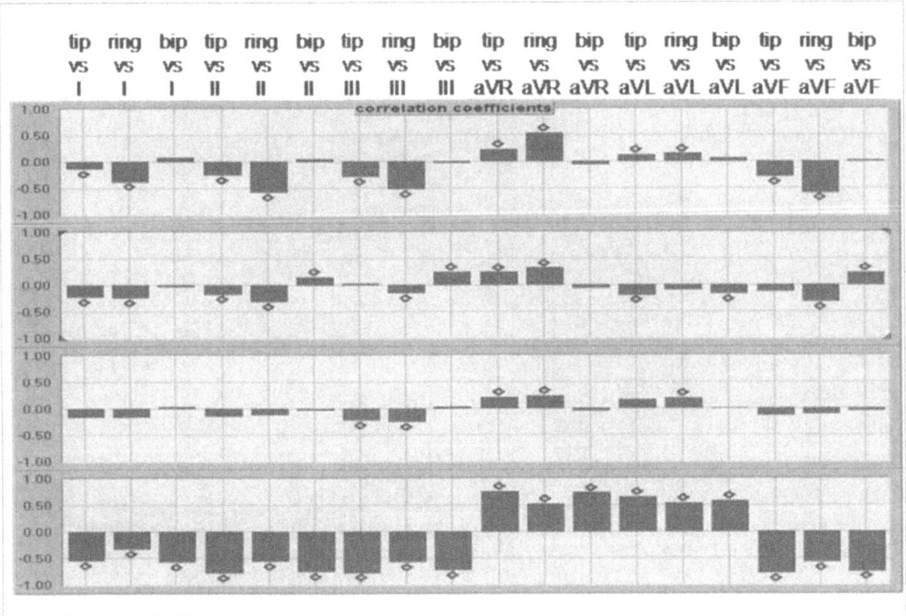

Fig. 3. Correlation coefficients between the ST deviation in three different intracardiac EGMs (tip, ring, bipolar) and six limb leads (see headline). ◊, significant. There is considerable variability in the results

Potential for Future Developments

The ability to discriminate between P-waves and FFRWs is essential for further developments.

Reliable recognition of remote signals or noise obviates the need for any blanking times reaching far beyond short pacing pulses, and it allows for permanent programming of high sensitivity levels (which obviates automatic sensitivity adjustments as well).

Using a specific set of form parameters, the algorithm may be used to identify retrograde P-waves and, by suspending atrial tracking, to prevent endless loop tachycardia.

The sensing configuration could be “combipolar” [9], which means it can record potential differences between one atrial and one ventricular electrode. While this arrangement minimizes myopotentials and EMI interference, the resulting EGM contains both P- and R-waves. Instead of utilizing simple timing criteria, the atrial and ventricular signals could be discriminated by DSP. The advantage of this solution is the opportunity to use unipolar leads and to benefit from their smaller dimensions and higher reliability than those of bipolar constructions.

Identifying rather than suppressing R waves in the atrium allows for measuring the AV interval from a single waveform and using it to control rate-adaptive algorithms [10].

Whether pacing termination algorithms or cardioversion are triggered in atrial arrhythmia will depend on a morphological differentiation between atrial flutter and fibrillation and on criteria of signal regularity. This type of EGM interpretation may be based both on pattern recognition and temporal signal evaluation.

In capture verification, waveform analysis may be better suited than simple threshold criteria to discrimination of the evoked response from polarization signals. This includes the capability for better definition and detection of the characteristics of fusion beats, which still pose a challenge to existing capture verification systems.

In summary, DSP is a logical step towards full analysis of complex intracardiac signals, which will improve the handling of hitherto unresolved problems in antibradycardia pacing.

References

1. Fröhlig G, Kindermann M, Seikat N, Wallbrück K, Böhm M, Schaldach M (2001) What pacemaker sense filters do discriminate best between P and far field R signals from atrial leads with different design? Pacing Clin Electrophysiol 24:663

2. Brouwer J, Nagelkerke D, den Heijer P, Ruiter JH, Mulder H, Begemann MJ, Lie KI (1997) Analysis of atrial sensed far-field ventricular signals: a reassessment. Pacing Clin Electrophysiol 20:916-922
3. Fröhlig G, Helwani Z, Kusch O, Berg M, Schieffer H (1999) Bipolar ventricular far-field signals in the atrium. Pacing Clin Electrophysiol 22:1604-1613
4. Throne RD, Jenkins JM, Winston SA, Finelli CJ, Di Carlo LA (1989) Discrimination of retrograde from anterograde atrial activation using intracardiac electrogram waveform analysis. Pacing Clin Electrophysiol 12:1622-1630
5. Sun W, Combs W, Panken E, Fotuhi P, Stangl K, Baumann G, Theres H (1999) Automatic and efficient R wave discrimination in the right atrium using a two-state hidden Markov model. J Cardiovasc Electrophysiol 10:343-350
6. Chiang CM, Jenkins JM, DiCarlo LA (1994) Digital signal processing chip implementation for detection and analysis of intracardiac electrograms. Pacing Clin Electrophysiol 17:1373-1379
7. Theres H, Sun W, Combs W, Panken E, Mead H, Baumann G, Stangl K (2000) P wave and far-field R wave detection in pacemaker patient atrial electrograms. Pacing Clin Electrophysiol 23:434-440
8. Van Hemel NM, Wohlgemuth P, Munnike D, Westendorp H, Engbers JG, Lawo T, Nebaznivy J, Taborsky M, Witte J (2003) Far field R wave discrimination by means of form analysis of atrial events. Pacing Clin Electrophysiol 26:930
9. Linde C, Markewitz A, Strandberg H, Larsson B, Binner L, Schuller H (2001) Combipolar sensing in dual chamber pacing: is there still a need for bipolar leads in the atrium? Pacing Clin Electrophysiol 24:1664-1671
10. Hexamer MP, Meine M, Kloppe A, Werner J (2002) Rate-responsive pacing based on the atrio-ventricular conduction time. IEEE Trans Biomed Eng 49:185-195

Cardiac Resynchronization Therapy: What Device Data Do We Need for Optimal Patient Treatment?

S. Sermasi[1], G. Corbucci[2], M. Marconi[1], M. Mezzetti[1], G. Piovaccari[1]

Introduction

The long experience of rate-responsive (RR) pacing and the technological advances in implantable devices form the basis for significant improvement of diagnostics for the treatment of atrial fibrillation (AF) or heart failure (HF) or both. In the past, the development of sensors for RR pacing gave the chance to investigate not only the effectiveness of physiological and mechanical sensors, but also long-term reliability and stability. Many sensors failed to demonstrate their long-term reliability and stability after implantation. For example, pressure sensors implanted in the right ventricle (RV) were totally surrounded by fibrosis after some months, making their membrane unreliable in detecting the true pressure. Similar problems were reported for oxygen saturation and pH sensors. Recently, pressure sensors for the RV have been proposed again for continuous monitoring of the hemodynamics of patients with HF: probably improvements in their technology have increased their long-term reliability. The strong competition for RR pacing in clinical practice has left in the market only the stable and reliable ones.

Today, a variety of mechanical sensors for motion detection and some physiological sensors such as for measuring QT interval, peak endocardial acceleration (PEA), and transthoracic/endocardial impedance (I) are available. The technological improvements in microelectronics are increasing the memory capacity of each device more and more, together with an acceptable current drain to guarantee an adequate length of life for the stimulators. These advances have a direct and immediate impact on the diagnostic functions mainly related to cardiac arrhythmias, since the sensors are basically the implanted leads.

The development of the diagnostic features for HF implies deep clinical research to understand what information can be achieved from the available

[1]Dipartimento delle Malattie Cardiovascolari, UO di Cardiologia, Ospedale Infermi, AUSL Rimini; [2]Vitatron Italia, Bologna, Italy

sensors. Again, the memory capacity of the implanted devices is crucial to store all the information coming from the sensors and to understand their clinical relevance.

Diagnostic Functions for AF

AF is the most common sustained rhythm disorder observed in clinical practice. Paroxysmal AF, without any associated heart disease, is a condition seldom related to an increased risk of embolic complications, reversible congestive heart failure, and can produce significant impairment of the quality of life. It is not a disease to treat by one single method, and the possible initiation mechanisms are difficult to identify by conventional diagnostics.

Certain conditions are required for AF to occur: a trigger to start the arrhythmia, spatial inhomogeneity in the refractory period, a region of unidirectional conduction block, a short wavelength to allow re-entry through the region of functional block, and sufficient atrial tissue mass to sustain a critical number of wavelets.

It is difficult to assess the efficacy of treatment, since AF may not be associated with evident symptoms and the majority of AF episodes are silent. The diagnostics of an implantable device can and should focus on the onset mechanisms and on the status and progression of AF. Especially when the patients are treated with drugs or pacing, it is very important to evaluate automatically the time to first onset of AF, as sinus rate begets sinus rate and AF begets AF. At the same time, it is necessary to store automatically parameters such as the number of transitions from sinus rate to AF (probably the most determining factor for symptoms), the duration of each episode (a determining factor for the risk of thromboembolic events), the total AF burden (which gives information on the stage of the disease), the incidence of premature atrial contractions in the last minutes before the onset of the AF episodes (to evaluate the relation between ectopic activity and AF episodes), and atrial and ventricular rate trends before the onset to evaluate the mechanism and the trigger of every episode. All this information is needed to evaluate the best strategy for AF prevention [1].

Heart Rate Variability

Heart rate variability (HRV) is a prognostic parameter for risk stratification for sudden cardiac death in post-myocardial-infarction patients. A decreased HRV has also been observed in patients with HF and chronotropic incompetence [2]. The significant decrease of HRV in HF patients with chronotropic incompetence suggests that chronotropic incompetence may relate to an abnormal autonomic influence on the heart of these patients. Monitoring of this parameter is feasible through an implanted device, which can continuously measure the spontaneous atrial cycles and store the data progression to a decreased HRV, making possible a therapeutic intervention.

A variety of methods for HRV measurement have been proposed, but some of them are too complex to be implemented in an implantable device. Spectral analysis of consecutive beats represents an interesting tool for HRV evaluation to be implemented in a standard computer, but it is too complex to be proposed for real-time analysis in an implanted device. A more appropriate a method could be based on the beat-to-beat variability of heart cycles, easily measurable by any device designed to store data or set appropriate therapies.

Physical Activity of the Patient

The reliability of mechanical sensors as accelerometers for motion detection has been proven in the past by many studies on RR pacing. The new indications for pacing in HF patients do not necessarily increase the use of the RR function since the large majority of these patients have a relatively high heart rate (HR). Thus they do not need activation of the RR function, except in the case of chronic AF and AV block or of an associated therapy with β-blockers inducing bradycardia. Therefore, these patients can benefit from daily physical exercise to improve their clinical status, and the amount of their daily activity can be measured automatically. Recently the so-called "activity log index" has been proposed to monitor the physical activity of HF patients implanted with a biventricular stimulator. The first results show that the same accelerometer normally used for the RR function gives a reliable indication of the patient's activity [3].

QT Interval

The long-term experience of evoked QT interval detection by implanted pacemakers makes continuous collection of data related to these physiological parameters easy and reliable. The QT interval reflects the process of ventricular de- and repolarization. It has been observed that prolongation and spatial inhomogeneity of the QT interval are linked to an increased susceptibility to ventricular tachyarrhythmias. Factors influencing QT interval are sex, HR, electrolyte status, autonomic tone, exercise, antiarrhythmic drugs, and ischemia. In addition, the QT interval changes in a circadian pattern.

A variety of applications of diagnostic and therapeutic functions could be proposed based on automatic and continuous QT interval assessment. It has been reported that ventricular arrhythmias are preceded by significant QT and QTc prolongation in patients with structural heart diseases. This phenomenon may facilitate the development of ventricular tachyarrhythmias [4]. Ventricular arrhythmias occurring in the setting of acquired long QT syndrome are often preceded by a pause followed by a markedly prolonged QT interval. An early beat (premature ventricular contraction) arising from the prolonged T-wave can initiate torsades de pointes. Many patients with permanent pacemakers, especially those with paroxysmal AF, often require antiarrhythmic drug therapy that could increase the risk of the long–short sequence leading to an arrhythmia. Although the electrophysiological mechanisms responsible for this pattern are a matter of debate, it is well documented that temporary pacing can prevent pauses and thus also the arrhythmias. The further information coming from the QT interval could additionally improve the timing of delivery of the pacing therapy by increasing the success of preventing pacing [5].

Biventricular pacing for patients with HF can prolong the QT interval and increase the transmural dispersion of repolarization. Biventricular pacing in patients with intrinsically heterogeneous ventricular myocardium can lead to the development of arrhythmias in a subset of them [6]. Of course, continuous automatic monitoring of this parameter could represent a substantial improvement of the patient's safety.

RV Pressure Sensor

Measurement of RV pressure has been proposed to chronically monitor the hemodynamic status of patients with HF. A previous approach was based on the use of a pressure sensor placed in the pulmonary artery, but the potential catheter instability at the distal end in the pulmonary artery makes such a system problematic. Ventricular arrhythmias induced by the catheter passing through the RV, and displacement of the tip forward into the pulmonary artery wedge position or backward into the RV, could represent an serious complication [7].

It is known that pulmonary artery end-diastolic and pulmonary artery wedge pressures are comparable in value to left ventricular end-diastolic pressure, and so they are important variables of the left ventricular preload in the majority of physiological and pathophysiological states. A specific algorithm for estimating the pulmonary artery end-diastolic pressure from a sensor in the RV has been developed [8]. The results from data obtained by monitoring RV pressure using a permanently implanted device in 28 adults with HF of varying degrees of severity have been reported: the suggestion is that an implantable device for long-term monitoring of HF progression is feasible [9, 10]. This technology will have a strong impact on the potentialities of biventricular stimulation devices.

PEA and Heart Sounds

PEA is measured by means of a microaccelerometer inserted into the tip of a RV pacing lead. The accelerometer is intrinsically insensitive to endocardial fibrosis since it detects inertial forces and not pressures. It has been proven that it represents the amplitude of the first heart sound (S1), a parameter that correlates to the left ventricular (LV) performance, even if it is allocated in the RV. In addition, it varies in correlation with the positive peak of LV *dP/dt*. Measurement of PEA is proposed to monitor LV contractility and to optimize the AV interval. These two features make it a specific parameter for patients with HF, both for monitoring and for optimizing electrical therapy. The same accelerometer can probably also detect the second heart sound (S2), which correlates to the negative peak LV *dP/dt* and to the aortic diastolic pressure [11].

Estimation of the pulmonary artery pressure by the spectral analysis of S2 was also proposed some years ago [12]. In addition, prognostic significance of a clearly audible fourth heart sound (S4) detected a month after an acute myocardial infarction has been hypothesized and an S4/S1 index has been proposed [13].

The possibility of chronically detecting and storing data from these signals could greatly improve the scientific knowledge and relevance of diagnostic information and the efficacy of therapies delivered.

Comment

For many patients affected by AF and/or HF, quality of life is very important, sometimes as important as improved survival. Again, HF is the most used diagnosis-related group (DRG) discharge diagnosis, AF the most frequently used arrhythmic DRG discharge diagnosis, and the incidence of AF increases with both age and worsening of functional HF class. The morbidity associated with AF and HF is principally related to hospitalization. This is the source of most of the costs for patient care. The advent of nonpharmacological or hybrid therapy with implantable devices seems to allow more sophisticated monitoring of patients. Additional improvements are still required, and future large-scale clinical trials must demonstrate that this technology can improve patients' quality of life and prevent hospitalizations compared with conventional monitoring [14].

References

1. Yang A, Hochhausler M, Schrickel J et al (2003) Advanced pacemaker diagnostics features in the characterization of atrial fibrillation: impact on preventive pacing algorithms. Pacing Clin Electrophysiol 26 (Part II):310–313
2. Fei L, Keeling PJ, Sadoul N et al (1996) Decreased heart rate variability in patients with congestive heart failure and chronotropic incompetence. Pacing Clin Electrophysiol 19 (Part I):477–483
3. Kadhiresan VA, Pastore J, Auricchio A et al (2002) A novel method – the activity log index – for monitoring physical activity of patients with heart failure. Am J Cardiol 89:1435–1437
4. Diem BH, Stellbtink C, Michel M et al (2002) Temporary disturbances of the QT

interval precede the onset of ventricular tachyarrhythmias in patients with structural heart diseases. Pacing Clin Electrophysiol 25:1413–1418
5. Pinski SL, Eguia LE, Trohman RG (2002) What is the minimal pacing rate that prevents torsades de pointes? Insights from patients with permanent pacemakers. Pacing Clin Electrophysiol 25:1612–1615
6. Medina-Ravell VA, Linkipalli RS, Yan GX et al (2003) Effect of epicardial or biventricular pacing to prolong QT interval and increase transmural dispersion of repolarization. Circulation 107:740–746
7. Anderson KM, Moore AA (1986) Sensors in pacing. Pacing Clin Electrophysiol 9:954–960
8. Reynolds DW, Bartelt N, Taepke R et al (1995) Measurement of pulmonary artery diastolic pressure from the right ventricle. J Am Coll Cardiol 25:1176–1182
9. Adamson PB, Magalski A, Braunshweig F et al (2003) Ongoing right ventricle hemodynamics in heart failure. J Am Coll Cardiol 41:565–571
10. Shabetai R (2003) Monitoring heart failure hemodynamics with an implanted device: its potential to improve outcome. J Am Coll Cardiol 41:572–573
11. Plicchi G, Marcelli E, Parlapiano M et al (2002) PEA I and PEA II based implantable haemodynamic monitor: preclinical studies in sheep. Europace 4:49–54
12. Chen D, Pibarot P, Honos G et al (1996) Estimation of pulmonary artery pressure by spectral analysis of the second heart sound. Am J Cardiol 78:785–789
13. Ishikawa M, Sakata K, Maki A et al (1997) Prognostic significance of a clearly audible fourth heart sound detected a month after an acute myocardial infarction. Am J Cardiol 80:619–621
14. Nohria A, Lewis E, Stevenson LW (2002) Medical management of advanced heart failure. JAMA 287:628–640

How to Identify Patients Most Likely to Respond to Cardiac Resynchronization Therapy

M. M. Gulizia, G. M. Francese

Introduction

Congestive heart failure (CHF) is one of the major healthy problems in Europe and the United States. It represents the major cause for hospital admission in the adult population with a prevalence from 0.4% up to 2% (22.5 million people world wide and 6.5 million in Europe; 747,000 in Italy). The incidence is 2 million patients per year world wide and 470,000 per year in Europe (66,000 in Italy) [1].

In addition to the clinical symptoms such as left ventricular dysfunction, reduced exercise tolerance, and impaired quality of life, these patients often have a markedly shortened life expectancy, with a further worsening in those with heart conduction defects [2–5]. From 1979 to 1996, mortality due to heart failure increased by 120%. The main causes of death are "sudden cardiac death" in 40% of cases, "pump failure" in 50%, and 10% with other causes.

In these last few years some well-designed pharmacological clinical trials with angiotensin converting enzyme (ACE) inhibitors or angiotensin II antagonists [6–9] and some β-blockers, such as carvedilol [10–13], metoprolol, [14, 15], or bucindolol [16], have shown reduction in the mortality and improvement of the clinical status in CHF patients. However, there was no improvement in the electrical conduction abnormalities often present in these patients.

Because some authors showed the uselessness of dual-chamber right-sided pacing [17–20], many others investigated the best pacing mode for CHF patients [23], finally demonstrating, only at the end of the 1990s, the role played by biventricular pacing compared with conventional pacing (right ventricular apex or right ventricular outflow tract) in increasing hemodynamic and functional status in CHF patients with left ventricular bundle branch block [24].

On the basis of this evidence, many other authors explored the role of

Cardiologia, Ospedale "S. Luigi–S. Currò", Catania, Italy

biventricular pacing as an adjunctive therapy to treat symptoms in patients with advanced CHF (NYHA class III–IV), dilated cardiomyopathy [left ventricular ejection fraction (LVEF) <35%, left ventricular end-diastolic diameter (LVEDD) ≥60 mm], and ventricular conduction disturbances (QRS >150 ms).

Although the first studies enrolled very small cohorts of patients, the results of the latest studies demonstrated the enhancing effect of cardiac resynchronization therapy (CRT) on heart hemodynamic performance, working ability, and quality of life in a larger number of patients with CHF and uncoordinated contraction [25–34].

The Pacing Therapies for Congestive Heart Failure Study (PATH-CHF) [35] and the Multisite Stimulation in Cardiomyopathies Study (MUSTIC) [36] were the two international studies that first, together with the preliminary data from the Italian InSync Registry (InSIR) [37], demonstrated that while the majority of patients "feel better" with CRT (and the benefit has an on-off effect), approximately 20%–30% will experience no clinical improvement with multisite pacing.

In the current cost-conscious health care environment, cost/effectiveness and cost/utility analysis of a new therapeutic strategy is increasingly used in order to implement a new option only when it really works. To date we have no certain way of telling who will benefit most from this therapy, and hence many investigators are looking for any features that predict the clinical response in the patient who is the optimal candidate for CRT.

Table 1 shows the patient selection of the major studies on CRT. All the studies reported in Table 1 demonstrated a statistical ($p<0.001$) improvement in mean NYHA class (almost one class of the classification) in the biventricular (BiV) paced population, as well an increase ($p<0.001$) in the mean distance walked in 6 min (with the exception of Contak ICD and InSync ICD trials). All these studies also showed an improvement in the quality of life of the patients by a reduction of more than 30% of the Minnesota Living with Heart Failure test score.

Furthermore, almost all studies observed (1) an increased peak oxygen consumption (VO_2) from baseline by a minimum of 8% to a maximum of 23%, (2) a statistically significant reduction in the length of hospital stay and in the overall number of hospitalizations, and (3) a reduction in the rate of hospitalizations per patient in the BiV-paced period [30–34, 38, 39].

However, although these published studies and many abstracts have shown that atriobiventricular pacing increases exercise capacity and quality of life in CHF patients with intraventricular conduction delay without a specific indication for conventional pacing, no definite indication has been given of any clinical routine practice predictors able to identify patients who will respond to CRT.

In order to assess the potential acute benefit of multisite cardiac pacing with optimized atrioventricular synchrony and simultaneous BiV pacing in patients with drug-refractory CHF, Leclercq et al. [40] performed an acute hemodynamic study in 18 patients with severe CHF (NYHA class III and IV)

Table 1. Proposed patient selection of the major studies on cardiac resynchronization therapy

Study (n random.) EF ≤ 35% for all	NYHA	QRS	Sinus	ICD	Status
MUSTIC AF (43)	III	>200*	AF	No	Published
PACMAN (328)	III	≥150	Normal	No	Enrolled?
MUSTIC SR (58)	III	>150	Normal	No	Published
VecToR (420)	II,IV	≥140	Normal	No	Enrolling
MIRACLE (453)	III,IV	≥130	Normal	No	Published
MIRACLE ICD (369)	III,IV	≥130	Normal	Yes	Presented
MIRACLE ICD II (186)	II	≥ 130	Normal	Yes	Complete
CARE HF (800)**	III,IV	≥120	Normal	No	Enrolling
COMPANION (>1600)	III, IV	≥120	Normal	No	Early term.
CONTAK CD (227)	III,IV	≥120	Normal	Yes	Reported
PATH-CHF (41)	III,IV	≥ 120	Normal	No	Published
PATH-CHF II (89)	III,IV	≥120	Normal	No	Presented

QRS, QRS duration at standard electrocardiogram; *Sinus*, patients in sinus rhythm (normal) or atrial fibrillation (AF); *ICD*, biventricular-ICD device implantation
* RV paced QRS; ** echo-based criteria for <150 ms

and major intraventricular conduction block (QRS duration 170±37 ms). They measured the pulmonary artery pressure, the pulmonary capillary wedge pressure (PCWP), and the cardiac index (CI) in different pacing configurations: atrial pacing (AAI) mode, used as reference, single-site right ventricular DDD pacing, and BiV pacing with the right ventricular lead placed either at the apex or at the outflow tract. The results of the study showed a significant increase in CI with BiV pacing compared with AAI or right ventricular DDD pacing (2.7 vs. 2 and 2.4 l/min per m^2, $p<0.001$). The PCWP also decreased significantly during BiV pacing compared with AAI (22 vs. 27 mmHg, $p<0.001$).

Although neither QRS duration, PR interval, or left axis deviation proved to be predictors for distinguishing between responders and non-responders to DDD BiV pacing, the authors identified a clinical predictive parameter in the LVEF ($p<0.036$) and an acute predictive parameter when they recorded an increase in cardiac output and decrease in PCWP by more than 10% during DDD BiV pacing compared with baseline (AAI mode).

In another acute study, Kass et al. [41] demonstrated the positive correlation between the baseline QRS duration and the percentage DdP/dtmax during left ventricle and BiV pacing. However, because of some discrepancies in the response to BiV pacing in some patients with wide QRS, the authors postulated that finding the optimal pacing site could play a major role in CRT.

The same results were found by Auricchio et al. [42], who underlined the importance of baseline QRS duration >150 ms, which was able to identify most of the acute responders to BiV pacing.

To determine whether some factors could predict the long-term clinical effectiveness of CRT, Alonso et al. [43] studied 26 patients with drug-refractory heart failure and wide QRS implanted with a BiV pacemaker. NYHA class, exercise tolerance, and LVEF were recorded at baseline and after pacemaker implantation. Patients were divided into two groups: group I, responders; group II, non-responders. QRS duration and axis at baseline and during biventricular pacing, interventricular conduction time, and left and right ventricular lead positions were compared between the two groups.

Only QRS duration during BiV pacing differed between the two groups, with a significantly shorter duration in group I than in group II (154±17 vs. 177±26 ms, p=0.016).

In a study on the sensitivity and specificity of QRS duration in predicting the acute benefit in CHF patients (PATH-CHF I and II) treated with CRT, Kadhiresan et al. [44] demonstrated that at smaller QRS duration thresholds the specificity tends to be lower, while accuracy was highest (80%) at a QRS duration of 155 ms, with positive and negative predictive values of 77% and 92%, respectively.

Performing a cardiac catheterization in 22 CHF patients with a dual-sensor micromanometer to measure LV and aortic pressure during sinus rhythm and LV free wall pacing, Nelson et al. [45] demonstrated that, although mechanical dyssynchrony is a key predictor for pacing efficacy in CHF patients with conduction delay, combining information about QRS and basal dP/dtmax provides an excellent tool for identifying maximal responders.

Other authors [46], speculating that pacing two sites with the longest conduction delay will result in the largest improvement in cardiac function in CHF, demonstrated that applying CRT in these sites does not necessarily produce better hemodynamic improvement in CHF patients.

Some authors [47] have hypothesized that the percentage increase in QRS duration at short atrioventricular delays during BiV pacing can distinguish responder from non-responder sites. Others [48] have demonstrated, in a group of 18 CHF patients in atrial fibrillation treated with BiV pacing compared with a group of 56 in sinus rhythm, that CRT improved both patient groups, suggesting that inter- and intraventricular resynchronization had a more-important effect than atrioventricular delay optimization.

In partial contrast with these results, in the analysis of 54 of 316 patients enrolled in the InSIR [49] who completed the 6-month Minnesota Quality of Life questionnaire or died of progressive heart failure during the 1st year after implantation, LVEDD was the only significant predictor of clinical outcome. The authors postulated that this could be due to the poor contractility reserve of a very dilated left ventricle, as shown by the LVEF percentage increasing only in the responder group.

Because of the limitations of surface ECG, in recent years different authors have proposed echocardiographic parameters able to indicate the presence of ventricular dyssynchrony [53–55]. In patients with a QRS duration of 120–150 ms it is possible to evaluate the presence of ventricular dyssynchrony by the presence of the following echo parameters: (1) a prolonged aortic pre-ejection delay (>140 ms), (2) an increased mechanical interventricular delay (>40 ms), and (3) a left ventricular segmental postsystolic contraction (LVPSC).

The first echo parameter is derived from the measurement between the onset of QRS complex and the beginning of the aortic flow on pulsed wave Doppler imaging. The second echo parameter is evaluated during pulsed wave Doppler imaging by the time difference between the onset of the pulmonary and the aortic flow. Finally, LVPSC is defined as the maximal local wall inward movement occurring after the start of the transmitral Doppler flow signal. This latter parameter can be usually assessed by either M-mode and/or tissue Doppler imaging (TDI), taking care to distinguish a passive movement from active local contraction.

The prolongation of the delay of these first two parameters determines a decrease in duration of left ventricular contraction and a decrease in regional ejection fraction, respectively. Hence, as described by other authors [54], a simple rule can be represented by the longer the aortic pre-ejection delay, and the shorter the left ventricular filling duration, the more advanced the ventricular dyssynchrony.

TDI can help to quantify the regional and global left ventricular function and also volumes. Tissue tracking (TT) and strain rate (STR) are two new modalities that can be derived from digitally recorded TDI loops of one or more heart beats. TT permits the visualization of the longitudinal motion amplitude in each myocardial segment during systole, while STR analysis can be used to determine whether this motion represents an active contraction or is merely passive.

In conclusion, many investigators are seeking reliable predictors of which CHF patients will benefit most from CRT. So far, the only certainty is that either BiV or LV pacing alone can significantly improve LV function in the short term and quality of life and exercise tolerance in the short-to-mid term in a large cohort of patients with intra- or interventricular conduction delay.

The main features of these patients are represented by a dilated cardiomyopathy, of ischemic origin or not, with a left ventricular end-diastolic diameter >55 mm (adapted to body surface index), a LVEF <35%, in III or IV NYHA functional class, under optimal medical treatment (ACE inhibitors/ATII antagonists, β-blockers, and diuretics), with a QRS duration of 130–150 ms or echo criteria for ventricular dyssynchrony.

The results of ongoing trials will perhaps clarify some aspects, such as the best LV pacing sites, when it is important to perform an acute test before the definitive implantation, how to manage patients with incomplete conduction defects or those with right bundle branch block, when to treat patients with atrial fibrillation, if the preimplantation TDI screening could improve the selection of candidates likely to benefit from CRT (a hypothesis that is currently being tested in a sub-study of the CARE-HF study [55]), and which patients are candidates for an ICD backup. These are in addition to the enthusiastic results coming from the preliminary reports of the COMPANION study.

References

1. Brown A, Cleland JGF (1998) Influence of concomitant disease on pattern of hospitalisation in patients with heart failure discharged from Scottish hospitals in 1995. Eur Heart J 1063–1069
2. Cohn JN, Johnson G, Ziesche S et al (1991) A comparison of enalapril with hydralazine-isosorbide dinitrate in the treatment of chronic congestive heart failure. N Engl J Med 325:303–310
3. Captopril Multicenter Research Group (1983) A placebo-controlled trial of captopril in refractory chronic congestive heart failure. J Am Coll Cardiol 2:755–763
4. Stevenson WG, Stevenson LW, Middlekauff HR et al (1996) Improving survival for patients with atrial fibrillation and advanced heart failure. J Am Coll Cardiol 28:1458–1463
5. Aaronson KD, Schwartz S, Chen T-M et al (1997) Development and prospective validation of a clinical index to predict survival in ambulatory patients referred for cardiac transplant evaluation. Circulation 95:2660–2667
6. Opie LH (1995) Fundamental role of angiotensin-converting enzyme inhibitors in the management of congestive heart failure. Am J Cardiol 75:3F–6F
7. Packer AC, Gheorghiade M, Young J et al (1993) Withdrawal of digoxin from patients with chronic heart failure treated with angiotensin-converting-enzyme inhibitors. N Engl J Med 329:1–7
8. The Acute Infarction Ramipril Efficacy (AIRE) Study Investigators (1993) Effect of ramipril on mortality and morbidity of survivors of acute myocardial infarction with clinical evidence of heart failure. Lancet 342:821–828
9. Cohn JN, Tognoni G, for the Valsartan Heart Failure Trial Investigators (2001) A randomized trial of the angiotensin-receptor blocker valsartan in chronic heart failure. N Engl J Med 345:16667–16675
10. Packer M (1998) Do beta-blockers prolong survival in chronic heart failure? A review of the experimental and clinical evidence. Eur Heart J 19 [Suppl B]:B40–46
11. Packer M, Bristow MR, Cohn JN et al (1996) The effect of carvedilol on morbidity and mortality in patients with chronic heart failure. N Engl J Med 334:1349–1355
12. Packer M, Coats AJS, Fowler MB et al, for the Carvedilol Prospective Randomized Cumulative Survival Study Group (2001). Effect of carvedilol on survival in severe chronic heart failure. N Engl J Med 344:1651–1658
13. Dargie HJ (2001) Effect of carvedilol on outcome after myocardial infarction in patients with left-ventricular dysfunction: the CAPRICORN randomised trial. Lancet 357:1385–1390
14. The Resolvd Investigators (2000) Effects of Metoprolol CR in patients with ischemic and dilated cardiomyopathy. The Randomized Evaluation of Strategies for Left Ventricular Dysfunction Pilot Study. Circulation 101:378–384
15. Goldstein S, Fagerberg B, Hjalmarson A et al, for the MERIT-HF Study Group (2001) Metoprolol controlled release/extended release in patients with severe heart failure: analysis of the experience in the MERIT-HF study. J Am Coll Cardiol 38:932–938
16. The Beta-Blocker Evaluation of Survival Trial Investigators (2001) Trial of the beta-blocker bucindolol in patients with advanced chronic heart failure. N Engl J Med

344:1659–1667
17. Hochleitner M, Hortnagl H, Ng CK et al (1990) Usefulness of physiologic dual-chamber pacing in drug-resistant idiopathic dilated cardiomyopathy. Am J Cardiol 66:198–202
18. Auricchio A, Sommariva L, Salo P et al (1993) Improvement of cardiac function in patients with severe congestive heart failure and coronary artery disease by dual chamber pacing with shortened AV delay. Pacing Clin Electrophysiol 16:2034–2043
19. Hochleitner M, Hortnagl H et al (1992) Long term efficacy of physiologic dual chamber pacing in the treatment of end stage idiopathic dilated cardiomyopathy. Am J Cardiol 70:1320–1325
20. Kataoka H (1991) Hemodynamic effect of physiological dual chamber pacing in a patient with end-stage dilated cardiomyopathy: a case report. Pacing Clin Electrophysiol 14:1330–1335
21. Gold MR, Feliciano Z, Gottlieb SS et al (1995) Dual-chamber pacing with a short atrioventricular delay in congestive heart failure: a randomized study. J Am Coll Cardiol 26:967–973
22. Linde C, Gadler F, Edner M et al (1995) Results of atrioventricular synchronous pacing with optimized delay in patients with severe congestive heart failure. Am J Cardiol 75:919–923
23. Brecker SJ, Xiao HB et al (1992) Effects of dual chamber pacing with short AV delay in dilated cardiomyopathy. Lancet 70:1320–1325
24. Blanc JJ, Etienne Y et al (1997) Evaluation of different ventricular pacing sites in patients with severe heart failure: results of an acute hemodynamic study. Circulation 96:3273–3277
25. Cazeau S, Ritter P et al (1994) Four chamber pacing in dilated cardiomyopathy. Pacing Clin Electrophysiol 17:1974–1979
26. Auricchio A, Stellbrink C et al (1999) Pacing therapies for congestive heart failure. (PATH-CHF study). Rational, design and endpoints of a prospective, randomized, multicentric study. Am J Cardiol 83:130–135
27. Saxon L, Boehemer J, Hummel J (1999) Biventricular pacing in patients with CHF: two prospective randomized trials (Vigor CHF). Am J Cardiol 83:120–123D
28. Saxon L, Kerwin WF, De Marco T et al (1998) The magnitude of sympathoneural activation in advanced heart failure is altered with chronic biventricular pacing. Arch Mal Coeur Vaiss 91:153
29. Gras D, Mabo P, Tang T et al (1998) Multisite pacing as a supplemental treatment of CHF: preliminary results of the Medtronic InSync study (NASPE abstr). Pacing Clin Electrophysiol 21:2249–2255
30. Abraham WT (2001) Late breaking clinical trial session at ACC 2001. Am Coll Cardiol 38:604–605
31. ACC (2002) Late breaking trials. J Am Coll Cardiol 40:13–14
32. Bristow MR, Feldman AM, Saxon LA, for the COMPANION Steering Committee and COMPANION Clinical Investigators (2000) Heart failure management using implantable device for ventricular resynchronization: comparison of medical therapy pacing, and defibrillation in chronic heart failure (COMPANION) trial. J Card Fail 6:276–285
33. Fergusson JJ III (2001) Meeting highlights. Highlights of the XXIII Congress of the European Society of Cardiology. Circulation 104:E111–E116
34. Medtronic InSync ICD cardiac resynchronization system. www.fda.gov
35. Huth C, Friedl A, Klein H, Auricchio A (2001) Pacing therapies for congestive heart failure considering the results of the PATH-CHF study. Z Kardiol 90 [Suppl 1]:10–15

36. Cazean S, Leclercq C, Lavergne T et al (2001) Effects of multisite biventricular pacing in patients with heart failure and interventricular conduction delay. N Engl J Med 344:873–880
37. Padeletti L, Porciani MC, Santini M et al (2001) InSync Italian Registry: long term clinical results of cardiac resynchronization. Europace [Suppl 2]:B58:787
38. Gulizia M, Ricci R, Lunati M et al (2001) InSync Italian Registry: does biventricular pacing impact on patients hospitalizations? Europace [Suppl 2]:B59:816
39. Auricchio A, Stellbrink C, Sack S et al (2001) PATH-CHF study: reduced hospitalization days due to heart failure. Europace [Suppl 2]:B49:471
40. Leclercq C, Cazeau S, Le Breton H et al (1998) Acute hemodynamic effects of biventricular DDD pacing in patients with end-stage heart failure. J Am Coll Cardiol 32:1825–1831
41. Kass DA, Chen CH, Curry C et al (1999) Improved ventricular mechanics from acute VDD pacing in patients with dilated cardiomyopathy and ventricular conduction delay. Circulation 30:1567–1573
42. Auricchio A, Stellbrink C, Block M et al (1999) Effect of pacing chamber and atrioventricular delay on acute systolic function of paced patients with congestive heart failure: the Pacing Therapies for Congestive Heart Failure Study Group: the Guidant Congestive Heart Failure Research Group. Circulation 99:2993–3001
43. Alonso C, Leclercq C, Victor F et al (1999) Electrocardiographic predictive factors of long-term clinical improvement with multisite biventricular pacing in advanced heart failure. Am J Cardiol 84:1417–1421
44. Kadhiresan V, Vogt J, Auricchio A et al (2000) Sensitivity and specificity of QRS duration to predict acute benefit in heart failure patients with cardiac resynchronization. NASPE II:555
45. Nelson G, Curry CW, Wyman BT et al (2000) Predictors of systolic augmentation from left ventricular preexcitation in patients with dilated cardiomyopathy and intraventricular conduction delay. Circulation 101:2703–2709
46. Butter C, Auricchio A, Stellbrink C et al (2001) Longer LV-RV delay may not yield better BiVRT outcome in HF. Europace [Suppl 2]:B11:649
47. Yu Y, Auricchio A, Butter C et al (2001) Assess effectiveness of BiVRT using surface QRS duration. Europace [Suppl 2] B11:770
48. Achilli A, Bocchiardo M, Sassara M et al (2001) Biventricular stimulation: comparison of results of sinus rhythm and chronic atrial fibrillation patients. Europace [Suppl 2]:B11:612
49. Montenero AS, Santini M, Lunati M et al (2001) InSync Italian Registry: baseline predictive factors of the clinical outcome. Europace [Suppl 2]:B49:613
50. Breithardt OA, Stellbrink C, Franke A, Balta O, Diem BH, Bakker P, Sack S, Auricchio A, for the PATH-CHF Study Group, and Pochet T, Salo R, for the Guidant Congestive Heart Failure Research (2002) Acute effects of cardiac resynchronization therapy on left ventricular Doppler indices in patients with congestive heart failure. Am Heart J 143:34–44
51. Sogaard P, Kim WY, Jensen HK, Mortensen P, Pedersen AK, Kristensen BO, Egeblad H (2001) Impact of acute biventricular pacing on left ventricular performance and volumes in patients with severe heart failure: a tissue Doppler and three-dimensional echocardiographic study. Cardiology 95:173–182
52. Cazeau S, Gras D, Lazarus A, Ritter P, Mugica J (2000) Multisite stimulation for correction of cardiac asynchrony. Heart 84:579–581
53. Yu CM, Chau E, Sanderson JE, Fan K, Tang MO, Fung WH, Lin H, Kong SL, Lam YM, Hill MRS, Lau CP (2002) Tissue Doppler echocardiographic evidence of reverse

remodeling and improved synchronicity by simultaneously delaying regional contraction after biventricular pacing therapy in heart failure. Circulation105:438–445
54. Gras D, Cebron JP, Brunel P, Leurent B, Bonus Y (2003) Selection of patients for cardiac resynchronization therapy. In: Gulizia M (ed) New Advances in Heart Failure and Atrial Fibrillation. Proceedings of the Mediterranean Cardiology Meeting. Springer-Verlag Italia, Milan, pp 237–241
55. Cleland JGF, Daubert JC, Erdmann E, Freemantle N, Gras D, Kappenberger L, Klein W, Tavazzi L, on behalf of the CARE-HF study steering committee and investigators (2001) The CARE-HF study (Cardiac Resynchronisation in Heart Failure study): rationale, design and end-points. Eur J Heart Fail 3:481–489

Upgrading from Right Ventricular Apical Pacing to Biventricular Pacing

M. H. SCHOENFELD

Introduction

It has been estimated that approximately 5% of the population worldwide suffers from congestive heart failure, of whom up to 30% may also have ventricular dyssynchrony resulting from intraventricular conduction delay [1, 2]. Recent work has demonstrated that biventricular pacing may be undertaken to achieve cardiac resynchronization, with resulting improvement in acute hemodynamics [3, 4] and sustained amelioration of heart failure symptoms [5-7]. A recent meta-analysis also indicates that cardiac resynchronization reduces mortality from progressive heart failure in patients with symptomatic impairment in left ventricular function [8], and recently reported late-breaking trials from the COMPANION investigators, as yet unpublished, substantiate this impression [9]. What remains unclear is the prevalence of symptomatic heart failure in patients with ventricular dyssynchrony due to right ventricular apical pacing, and whether revision to biventricular pacing in these patients will afford symptomatic relief and/or improved survival. It is the purpose of this chapter to assess the role of cardiac resynchronization in patients with paced rhythm from the right ventricular apex.

Evidence of Cardiac Decompensation from Right Ventricular Apical Pacing

It has long been appreciated that right ventricular pacing may result in severe regional left ventricular wall motion abnormalities. Boucher and co-workers analyzed 35 patients comparing sinus rhythm with ventricular pacing, noting the development of abnormal motion in septal, apical, and inferior walls, as well as cardiac dyssynchrony – the latter consisted of early right ventricular and anterobasal and posterobasal left ventricular motion with subsequent con-

Yale University School of Medicine; Cardiac Electrophysiology and Pacer Laboratory, Hospital of Saint Raphael, New Haven, Connecticut, USA

traction of the apex. This resulted in a deterioration in cardiac performance without significant change in ejection fraction [10]. More recent studies confirm this impression, with impaired left ventricular systolic and diastolic function demonstrated echocardiographically in young patients subjected to long-term right ventricular apical pacing [11], as well as an actual reduction in ejection fraction observed in sick sinus syndrome patients transitioning from sinus rhythm to long-term right ventricular pacing [12]. Acute hemodynamic studies in patients with severe heart failure were undertaken in patients who were temporarily paced from a variety of sites: right ventricular apex, right ventricular outflow tract, left ventricle, and right ventricular apex plus left ventricle (biventricular) [13]. Both left ventricular pacing alone and biventricular pacing resulted in a similar and significant improvement in pulmonary capillary wedge pressure and systolic pressure determinations V-wave amplitude compared with non-paced sinus rhythm and right ventricular apical or outflow tract pacing. In addition to improvements in systolic pressure and central venous pressure, left ventricular-based pacing also promoted a decrease in sympathetic nerve activity compared with right ventricular apical pacing in patients with left ventricular dysfunction [14]. What remains unclear is whether it is the intraventricular conduction delay per se, or something intrinsic to right ventricular pacing that is responsible for these findings. Some work suggests that mechanical dyssynchrony arising from left bundle branch block is greater in comparison with right ventricular apical pacing because a larger territory of myocardium is prematurely activated with the former [15]. Conversely, preliminary work would indicate that biventricular pacing resulted in a greater improvement in left ventricular ejection fraction in patients with pacer-induced intraventricular conduction delay compared to those with intrinsic left bundle branch block [16].

The purest way to evaluate the outcome of patients with right ventricular pacing in large clinical trials is to compare them with patients with preserved intact conduction through the atrio-ventricular node. Unfortunately, only one such study provides this comparison [17, 18]. Ventricular demand pacing in this study was associated with a higher occurrence of severe congestive heart failure compared with atrial demand pacing, both short- and long-term. This was accompanied by a decrease in left ventricular fractional shortening and increased dilatation of the left atrium.

In patients with atrial fibrillation and a rapid ventricular response, maintaining intact conduction has been compared with atrio-ventricular nodal ablation coupled with right ventricular pacing. In one large meta-analysis, ejection fraction improved in the patients undergoing AV node ablation, indicating a favorable outcome due to rate control, despite the resulting pacer-dependence [19]. The potential impact of underlying heart disease must, however, be considered. Thus, Ozcan et al. reported that a history of congestive heart failure was an independent predictor of death in patients undergoing AV node ablation [20]. In one small study group, pacer-dependence resulting from AV node ablation was associated with a significant deterioration in left ventricular ejection fraction [21].

In other large clinical trials, the incidence of heart failure has been examined in patients programmed to right ventricular pacing versus dual chamber pacing, with mixed outcomes. The Canadian Trial of Physiologic Pacing (CTOPP) reported no differences in the rates of hospitalizations for heart failure, even though the patients with dual chamber pacing were included with atrial-paced patients in the "physiologically paced" group [22]. How many of the dual-chambered patients were committed to atrial synchronous ventricular paced rhythm is unclear. In contrast, in the "Mode Selection Trial in Sinus-Node Dysfunction" (MOST), signs and symptoms of heart failure as assessed by a heart-failure score were less severe, with dual-chamber pacing compared with ventricular pacing [23]; once again, however, it is unclear how many of the dual chamber pacing group were actually in atrial-synchronous ventricular paced rhythm. Perhaps most noteworthy are the results from the DAVID trial. Defibrillator patients programmed to dual-chamber pacing (which resulted in atrio-ventricular paced rhythm in a majority) and back-up single chamber ventricular pacing set to an intentionally low rate so as to minimize right ventricular pacing were composed [24]. A significantly higher incidence of hospitalization for heart failure was observed in the former group. In contrast to the CTOPP and MOST trials, the DAVID investigators specifically addressed a group of patients with already impaired left ventricular function.

Evidence in Favor of Upgrading from Right Ventricular Apical Pacing to Biventricular Pacing

Based on the above observations, a number of reports have addressed the potential benefit of upgrading from right ventricular pacing to biventricular pacing [25-27]. These have been limited to patients who are ventricular paced in the setting of chronic atrial fibrillation. Leon et al. assessed the effects of biventricular pacing on ventricular function and heart failure course in pacer-dependent patients with chronic atrial fibrillation and prior AV junction ablation [25]. Twenty such patients with ejection fraction less than 36% were upgraded to biventricular pacing and demonstrated statistically significant improvements in NYHA functional classification (by 29%), increases in LV ejection fraction (by 44%), reductions of LV diastolic diameter (by 6.5%) and decrease in end-systolic diameter (by 8.5%). This was accompanied by a reduction in hospitalization by 81%. A case report demonstrated a reversed remodeling of cardiomyopathy after upgrading from ventricular rate-adaptive pacing (VVIR) to VVIR biventricular pacing in a pacer-dependent individual with atrial fibrillation and prior His-bundle ablation therapy [26]. Leclercq et al evaluated patients with NYHA class III symptoms and co-existent atrial fibrillation with a slow ventricular response. All patients had transvenous biventricular pacer implants [27]. A single-blind, randomized crossover study compared 37 of these patients programmed to right ventricular versus biventricular paced rhythm. Programming to biventricular pacing resulted in significantly improved exercise tolerance as assessed by mean distance walked, significant increases in peak oxygen uptake, and reduction in hospitalization by 70%.

Alternatives to Upgrading to Biventricular Paced Rhythm

Programmability affords alternative methods by which to minimize right ventricular pacing. Thus, patients may be set to a low backup rate, allowing sinus mechanism to prevail, as was the case in the majority of patients programmed to VVI pacing in the DAVID trial [24]. Programming to a longer AV interval in dual chamber systems may also allow for the emergence of intact conduction to the ventricle, albeit at times with some atrioventricular delay. Indeed, some pacing systems allow for positive atrio-ventricular interval hysteresis, automatically promoting a long AV interval to allow for native conduction (effectively AAI pacing), and a shorter AV interval when there is AV block [28-30]. In patients with impaired atrioventricular conduction, the balance must be weighed as to whether shorter AV intervals accomplished through right ventricular pacing are hemodynamically superior to maintaining a normal (though delayed) atrioventricular activation sequence in an effort to avoid the cardiac desynchronization associated with right ventricular pacing.

Feasibility and Methodology of Biventricular Pacing Upgrade

Leon and co-workers evaluated 60 patients with NYHA Class III and IV heart failure who underwent revision from right ventricular to biventricular pacing. The overall procedural success rate was 90%, with an 8.3% complication rate; successful upgrades resulted in statistically significant improvements in quality of life scores, NYHA class, and ejection fraction [31]. Thus, upgrade to biventricular pacing is both safe and efficacious.

It is often useful to perform venography to verify persistent patency of the subclavian system ipsilateral to the previous pacer site. If patency is confirmed, then passage of yet another lead through this system, ie. a coronary sinus lead, is feasible in an effort to upgrade for biventricular pacing. If the ipsilateral venous system is not patent, then the contralateral position will be required to achieve access. Under the latter circumstances, the newly implanted lead can be tunneled back to the original pocket site. Alternatively, the original system may be abandoned altogether, allowing for placement of the coronary sinus lead, new right ventricular (or ICD) lead and/or new atrial lead from the contralateral chest site.

In patients with an existing right ventricular pacing system, the implanter is typically free from one of the usual concerns associated with positioning a new biventricular pacing system, namely trauma to the right bundle, in patients with pre-existent left bundle branch block (with resultant asystole). Once the access is established, the coronary sinus lead is implanted as would be the case in any de novo biventricular system [32]. This entails cannulation of the coronary sinus either directly with a sheath, or, alternatively, by engaging the ostium with an electrophysiology catheter, as confirmed by left atrial recordings, and then guiding the sheath over the catheter. Coronary sinus balloon-occlusion venography through this sheath then allows for radiographic visualization of the coronary venous tree and guides the subsequent placement of the coronary sinus pacing lead in the lateral cardiac vein. Dislodgement of the chronically implanted right ventricular lead during coronary sinus lead placement should not be an issue, though great care should be undertaken to avoid trauma to the existing leads when percutaneous subclavian access is initially established.

What remains unclear is whether other lead positions in the right ventricle may allow for cardiac resynchronization without requiring biventricular coronary sinus lead placement. Some studies have prospectively evaluated the potential benefit, for example, of right ventricular outflow tract pacing [33, 34]. Victor et al. [33] examined 16 patients with complete AV block (6 patients with ejection fraction less than 40%) with chronically implanted pacemakers connected to two ventricular leads, using the atrial and ventricular ports for outflow tract and right ventricular apex respectively. After four months of pacing from one site, crossover to pacing from the alternative site was made with reassessment of NYHA class, LV ejection fraction, exercise time and maximal oxygen uptake. No symptomatic improvement or hemodynamic benefit was observed when comparing right ventricular outflow tract (RVOT) pacing to RV apical pacing. These authors did not, however, assess the potential benefit of pacing from both sites simultaneously. Buckingham et al. [34] examined 11 patients acutely undergoing elective electrophysiologic studies, comparing echo-derived cardiac outputs in sinus rhythm, AOO pacing, DOO pacing from the RV apex, DOO pacing from the RV outflow tract, and DOO pacing from both right ventricular sites. During DOO pacing, there was a trend for pacing in the right ventricular outflow tract or in both (right ventricular apex and outflow tract) sites to improve cardiac output when compared with right ventricular apical pacing. Narrowing of QRS from simultaneous pacing from both apical and outflow ventricular sites was also observed. Logistically, placement of a second lead in the right ventricular outflow tract to promote cardiac resynchronization is certainly easier. This approach could be considered if future studies demonstrate an associated long-term symptomatic improvement in patients with baseline left ventricular dysfunction and heart failure.

An important consideration is whether upgrade from right ventricular pacing to biventricular pacing should include upgrade to an ICD as well, i.e. not merely employing a pacer generator. Evidence from MADIT-II would indeed indicate that, in patients with an ischemic cardiomyopathy and left ventricular dysfunction (ejection fraction $\leq$ 30%), prophylactic ICD implantation improves overall survival [35].

Two other issues remain unexplored. The first is whether all "first time" patients who require de novo ventricular pacing should have a biventricular system implanted from the outset (as opposed to a right ventricular system), so as to preempt any potential concerns associated with chronic right ventricular pacing, whether or not they have previously demonstrated heart failure. The second question is whether chronic biventricular pacing may be used to preempt heart failure in patients with existing right ventricular pacing systems, but without previous left ventricular dysfunction and/or symptoms of heart failure.

Conclusions

Biventricular pacing has been used effectively to achieve cardiac resynchronization and thereby ameliorate symptoms of heart failure in patients with left bundle branch block and depressed ejection fraction. Its application to symptomatic patients with cardiac desynchronization, resulting from right ventricular apical pacing, has been less widespread, though initial results are highly encouraging. Upgrade from right ventricular apical pacing to a biventricular system is both safe and feasible. Additional clinical investigation will be required to substantiate the impression that such upgrade will result in long-lasting benefit. Other trials must be directed at equally difficult questions, such as whether the time-honored technique of right ventricular pacing should be abandoned for biventricular systems in all patients requiring pacing therapy.

References

1. Havranek EP, Masoudi FA, Westfall KA et al (2002) Spectrum of heart failure in older patients: results from the national heart failure project. Am Heart J 143:412-417
2. Kalinchak DM, Schoenfeld MH (2003) Cardiac Resynchronization: A Brief Synopsis, Part I: Patient Selection and Results from Clinical Trials. J Interventional Cardiac Electrophysiology (*in press*)
3. Blanc JJ, Etienne Y, Gilard M et al (1997) Evaluation of different ventricular pacing sites in patients with severe heart failure: results of an acute hemodynamic study. Circulation 996:3273-3277
4. Leclercq C, Cazeau S, LeBreton H et al (1998) Acute hemodynamic effects of biventricular DDD pacing in patients with end-stage heart failure J Am Coll Cardiol 32:1825-1831
5. Cazeau S, LeclercqC, Lavergne T et al (2001) Effects of multisite biventricular pacing in patients with heart failure and intraventricular conduction delay. N Engl J Med 344:873-880
6. Linde C, Leclercq C, Rex S et al (2002) Long-term benefits of biventricular pacing in congestive heart failure: results from the Multi-site Stimulation in Cardiomyopathy (MUSTIC) study. J Am Coll Cardiol 40:111-118
7. Abraham WT, Fisher WG, Smith AL et al (2002) Cardiac resynchronization in heart failure. N Engl J Med 346:1845-1853
8. Bradley DJ, Bradley EA, Baughman KL et al (2003) Cardiac resynchronization and death from progressive heart failure: a meta-analysis of randomized clinical trials.

JAMA 289:754-756
9. Cleland JGF, Thackray S, Goodge L et al (2002) Outcome studies with device therapy in patients with heart failure. J Cardiovasc Electrophysiol 13 (suppl):S73-S91
10. Boucher CA, Pohost GM, Okada RD et al (1983) Effect of ventricular pacing on left ventricular function assessed by radionuclide angiography. Am Heart J 106:1105-1111
11. Tantengco MV, Thomas RL, Karpawich PP (2001) Left ventricular dysfunction after long-term right ventricular apical pacing in the young. J Am Coll Cardiol 37:2093-2100
12. Paxinos G, Katritsis D, Kakouros S et al (1998) Long-term effect of VVI pacing on atrial and ventricular function in patients with sick sinus syndrome. PACE 21:728-734
13. Blanc JJ, Etienne Y, Gilard M et al (1997) Evaluation of different ventricular pacing sites in patients with severe heart failure: results of an acute hemodynamic study. Circulation 96:3273-3277
14. Hamdan MH, Zagrodzky JD, Joglar JA et al (2000) Biventricular pacing decreases sympathetic activity compared with right ventricular pacing in patients with depressed ejection fraction. Circulation 102:1027-3210
15. Xiao HB, Brecker SJ, Gibson DG (1993) Differing effects of right ventricular pacing and left bundle branch block on left ventricular function. Br Heart J 69:166-173
16. Patel AG, Singh A (2003) Resynchronization therapy produces greater improvement in left ventricular function in patients with pacer induced compared to those with intrinsic left bundle branch block. J Am Coll Cardiol (abs):113A
17. Andersen HR, Nielsen JC, Thomsen PE et al (1997) Long-term follow-up of patients from a randomized trial of atrial versus ventricular pacing for sick-sinus syndrome. Lancet 350:1210-1216
18. Nielsen JC, Andersen HR, Thomsen PE et al (1998) Heart failure and echocardiographic changes during long-term follow-up of patients with sick sinus syndrome randomized to single-chamber atrial or ventricular pacing. Circulation 97:987-995
19. Wood MA, Brown-Mahoney C, Kay GN, Ellenbogen KA (2000) Clinical outcomes after ablation and pacing therapy for atrial fibrillation: a meta-analysis. Circulation 101:1138-1144
20. Ozcan C, Jahangir A, Friedman PA et al (2001) Long-term survival after ablation of the atrioventricular node and implantation of a permanent pacemaker in patients with atrial fibrillation. N Engl J Med 344:1043-1051
21. Szili-Torok T, Kimman GP, Theuns D et al (2002) Deterioration of left ventricular function following atrio-ventricular node ablation and right ventricular apical pacing with permament atrial fibrillation. Europace 4:61-65
22. Connolly SJ, Kerr CR, Gent M et al (2000) Effects of physiologic pacing versus ventricular pacing on the risk of stroke and death due to cardiovascular causes. N Engl J Med 342:1385-1391
23. Lamas GA, Lee KL, Sweeney MO (2002) Ventricular pacing or dual-chamber pacing for sinus-node dysfunction. N Engl J Med 346:1854-1862
24. The DAVID Trial Investigators (2002) Dual-chamber pacing or ventricular backup pacing in patients with an implantable defibrillator. The Dual Chamber and VVI Implantable Defibrillator. (DAVID) Trial JAMA 288:3115-3123
25. Leon AR, Greenberg JM, Kanuru N et al (2002) Cardiac resynchronization in patients with congestive heart failure and chronic atrial fibrillation: effect of upgrading to biventricular pacing after chronic right ventricular pacing. J Am Coll Cardiol 39:1258-1263
26. Erol-Yilmaz A, Tukkie R, Schrama TA et al (2002) Reversed remodeling of dilated left

sided cardiomyopathy after upgrading from VVIR to VVIR biventricular pacing. Europace 4:445-449
27. Leclercq C, Walker S, Linde C et al (2002) Comparative effects of permanent biventricular and right-univentricular pacing in heart failure patients with chronic atrial fibrillation. Eur Heart J 23:1780-1787
28. Mayumi H, Kohno H, Yasui et al (1996) Use of automatic mode change between DDD and AAI to facilitate native atrioventricular conduction in patients with sick sinus syndrome or transient atrioventricular block. PACE 19:1740
29. Linde C (1997) The clinical utility of positive and negative AV/PV hysteresis In: Santini M (ed) Progress in Clinical Pacing 1996 Armonk, NY. Futura Media Services pp 339-345
30. Leclerq C, Gras D, LeHelloco A et al (1995) Hemodynamic importance of preserving the normal sequence of ventricular activation in permanent cardiac pacing. Am Heart J 129:1133
31. Baker CM, Christopher TJ, Smith PF et al (2002) Addition of a left ventricular lead to conventional pacing systems in patients with congestive heart failure: feasibility, safety, and early results in 60 consecutive patients. PACE 25:1166-1171
32. Kalinchak DM, Schoenfeld MH (2003) Cardiac Resynchronization: A Brief Synopsis Part II: Implant and Follow-up Methodology. J Interventional Cardiac Electrophys (*in press*)
33. Victor F, Leclercq C, Mabo P et al (1999) Optimal right ventricular pacing site in chronically implanted patients: a prospective randomized crossover comparison of apical and outflow tract pacing. J Am Coll Cardiol 33:311-316
34. Buckingham TA, Candinas R, Schlapfer J et al (1997) Acute hemodynamic effects of atrioventricular pacing at differing sites in the right ventricle individually and simultaneously PACE 20:909-915
35. Moss AJ, Zareba W, Hall WJ et al (2002) Prophylactic implantation of a defibrillator in patients with myocardial infarction and reduced ejection fraction N Engl J Med 346:877-883

Cardiac Resynchronisation Therapy in Patients with Atrial Fibrillation: Are Results as Good as in Patients with Sinus Rhythm?

C. LINDE

Introduction

In the last five years, controlled crossover trials and parallel comparisons of cardiac resynchronisation therapy (CRT) to control treatment have convincingly demonstrated symptomatic improvement in patients with severe heart failure and intraventricular conduction disturbances [1-5]. Almost all of these studies were performed exclusively in patients with sinus rhythm. There is, however, evidence from acute hemodynamic and long term studies that atrial fibrillation patients also benefit from CRT.

In a catheterisation study, Blanc et al demonstrated a hemodynamic benefit by temporary left ventricular based pacing in 23 patients, six of whom were in atrial fibrillation [6]. These observations were confirmed in a similar acute study by Etienne comprising 10 atrial fibrillation and 17 sinus rhythm patients [7]. In this study, left ventricular pacing and biventricular pacing provided the same benefit concerning pulmonary capillary wedge pressure, systolic blood pressure and mitral incompetence, irrespective of whether patients were in sinus rhythm or atrial fibrillation. These observations underline that ventricular resynchronisation, rather than AV-synchrony, was the explanation for the acute hemodynamic benefit. It is, however, not self-evident that acute hemodynamic improvements imply a long-term benefit.

The first early non-randomised study on CRT included atrial fibrillation patients. In the French pilot study, a beneficial effect by biventricular pacing was observed in 14 atrial fibrillation patients followed for a mean of 15 months [8].

What is the proof of a clinical benefit by CRT in atrial fibrillation patients in controlled studies? MUSTIC was a controlled crossover study aiming at evaluating symptomatic improvement by biventricular pacing compared to control pacing [1-3]. It is, so far, the only controlled study to have included

Department of Cardiology, Karolinska Hospital, Stockholm, Sweden

patients with atrial fibrillation. Patients were included if they had severe NYHA class association III heart failure in stable condition for at least one month and if they were on optimal medical treatment including ACE inhibitors and diuretics. The left ventricular ejection fraction had to be below 35% and the left ventricular end diastolic diameter > 60 mm. All patients had to have persistent (> 3 months) atrial fibrillation requiring a permanent pacemaker due to slow ventricular rhythm, either spontaneously or induced by a His-ablation. The paced QRS duration had to be > 200 ms. The study design is shown in Figure 1 [2]. A 6 week (non-ablated patients) to a 12 week (ablated patients) observation period in right ventricular (RV) ventricular inhibited rate-adaptive (VVIR) pacing was performed to verify stability of the heart failure condition and to allow for reversal of any tachycardia induced cardiomyopathy. The study began with a single-blind crossover comparison of three months each of biventricular pacing and right ventricular VVIR pacing, both at a basic rate of 70 bpm. Following the end of the crossover phases, patients were programmed according to their preferred study period and followed every three months for another six months. Patient characteristics are presented in Table 1. After the crossover phase, four of the patients preferred to be programmed to right ventricular VVIR pacing, while the rest preferred biventricular pacing. Forty-one patients completed the crossover period and 33 patients the 12 months follow up. The clinical results concerning the six minute walked distance, peak oxygen uptake, quality of life measured by the Minnesota Living with Heart Failure questionnaire are presented in Figure 2. Although there was no significant increase in the six minute walk distance at the end of the active crossover phase compared to the evaluation made at the start of the crossover, there was a significant increase at the 12 months follow up in biventricular pacing by a mean of 55 meters or 17% (p=0.004). The Minnesota score decreased by a mean of 14 points or 32% (p=0.002), whereas the peak VO_2 increased insignificantly by a mean of 1.1 ml/kg/min or 9% (NS). The NYHA class improved by a mean of 0.8 (p=0.0001). Hospitalisations for heart failure were three times less

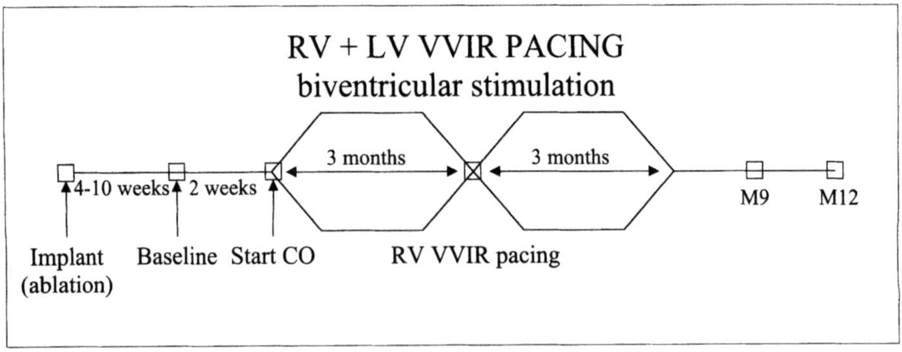

Fig. 1. The study design of the MUSTIC atrial fibrillation group. *CO*, cross over

Table 1. Baseline characteristics in the MUSTIC atrial fibrillation Group [2, 3]

Clinical Characteristics		Atrial fibrillation group n = 64
Mean age	(years)	65 + 9
Sex	(male/female)	52(81%) / 12(19%)
NYHA III		64 (100%)
Ischemic / non ischemic		17 (27%) / 47 (73%)
Drug treatment		
Ace inhibitor or AII blocker		64 (100%)
Diuretics		63 (98%)
Cardiac glycoside		36 (57%)
ß-blockers		14(22%)
Spironolactone		10(15%)
Amiodarone		14(22%)
Mean measurements		
LVEF	(%)	26 + 10
LVEDD	(mm)	68 + 7
MR area	(cm^2)	10.5 + 13.7
DFT	(ms)	349 + 95
ECG measurements		
Heart rate	(bpm)	74 + 5
QRS duration	(ms)	206 + 19
6-min walked distance	(m)	328 + 80
Peak VO_2	(ml/min/kg)	12.7 + 3.9

LVEF, left ventricular ejection fraction; *LVEDD*, left ventricular end-diastolic diameter; *MR*, mitral regurgitation; *DFT*, diastolic filling time

during biventricular pacing than during RV-VVIR pacing, and the left ventricular ejection fraction measured by radionuclides increased by a mean of 4 % (p=0.05). In a long-term follow up, Leclercq demonstrated that the benefits observed at one year were maintained in the 26 patients completing a 2 year follow up [9].

Over the duration of the study, the magnitudes of improvements in the sinus rhythm group were overall more impressive than for the atrial fibrillation group. There are a multitude of possible explanations to this finding. Among these are the high drop-out rate in the MUSTIC, attributed to events in the long-run in period (Fig. 1), and the heterogeneity of the atrial fibrillation group. Moreover, the potentially harmful effect of right ventricular pacing during the run-in could have contributed. Finally, to treat atrial fibrillation patients with biventricular pacing requires complete rate-control as not to allow for intrinsic rhythm obviating biventricular stimulation. In fact two patients in the MUSTIC were not paced due to insufficient rate control. Moreover, the paced QRS-duration during biventricular stimulation was in fact

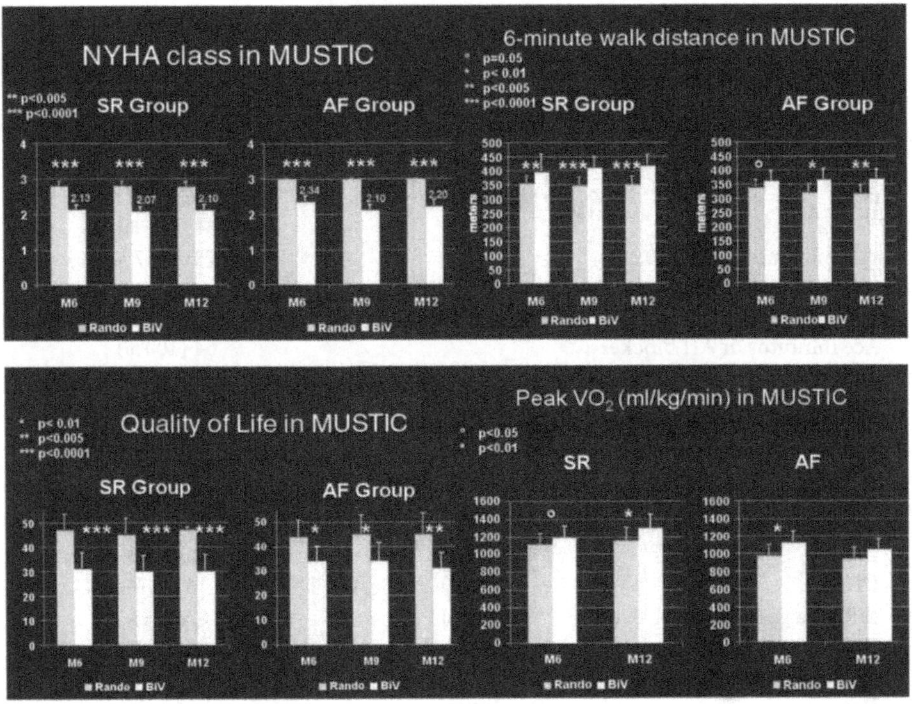

Fig. 2. Clinical results from the MUSTIC study concerning the six minute walk distance, peak VO_2, quality of life measured by the Minnesota Living with Heart Failure Questionnaire and the NYHA class in patients, after the active crossover phase in biventricular pacing (M6) and after 9 (M9) and 12 (M12) months in biventricular pacing compared to the same individuals at the time of randomisation. *Rando*, randomisation; *BIV*, biventricular pacing

longer in the atrial fibrillation group (170 ms) compared to the sinus rhythm group (156 ms). This could indicate that a lesser degree of ventricular synchronisation was obtained in the atrial fibrillation group.

Overall, the prevalence of atrial fibrillation in severe heart failure is 16 - 21%, as indicated by the CIBIS II [10] and MERIT HF [11] studies. Moreover, atrial fibrillation in heart failure becomes more prevalent with time, reflecting progressive remodelling of both the left ventricle and atrium. There is a strong consensus about the negative effect of atrial fibrillation on hemodynamics. However, its impact on prognosis remains controversial [12], although a clear survival disadvantage in combination with left bundle branch block was recently demonstrated by Baldasseroni et al. [13]. Therefore, atrial fibrillation patients are probably worse off both in terms of prognosis and hemodynamics.

The impact of CRT on survival remains to be proven. In the recently orally presented COMPANION trial, only the combination of CRT with an implantable cardioverter defibrillator (ICD) improved six month total mortality in NYHA class III heart failure patients [14]. The ongoing CARE-HF study will further elucidate whether CRT per se affects survival in these patients [15]. None of these studies, however, included patients with atrial fibrillation. The two year survival curves from the MUSTIC study do not indicate any worse survival rate in the atrial fibrillation compared to the sinus rhythm group, with a mean annual survival rate of 95.7 % at one year and 82.6 % at two years in the atrial fibrillation group and 87.9 % at one year and 77.6 % at two years in the sinus rhythm group [16].

Conclusions

Although the number of patients with atrial fibrillation participating in studies on CRT so far has been small, the evidence at large suggests that this treatment could be beneficial in these patients. This supports the initiation of a controlled long-term study on atrial fibrillation patients with heart failure and cardiac dyssynchrony. Such a study needs to compare the effects of CRT to optimal drug treatment both concerning heart failure and rate control.

Acknowledgements. Supported by the Swedish Heart and Lung Association.

References

1. Cazeau S, Leclercq C, Lavergne T et al for the Multisite stimulation in Cardiomyopthy (2001) Effects of multisite biventricular pacing in patients with heart failure and intraventricular conduction delay. N Engl J Med 12:873-880
2. Leclercq C, Walker S, Linde C et al (2001) Comparative effects of permanent biventricular and right univentricular pacing in heart failure patients with chronic atrial fibrillation. Eur Heart J 23:1780-1787
3. Linde C, Leclercq C, Rex S et al (2002) Long-term benefits of biventricular pacing in congestive heart failure. Results from the MUSTIC (Multisite STimulation in Cardiomyopathy) study. J Am Coll Cardiol 40:111-118
4. Auricchio A, Stellbrink C, Sack S et al (2002) Chronic effects of hemodynamically optimised cardiac resynchronisation therapy on patients with heart failure and ventricular conduction delay. J Am Coll Cardiol 39:2026-2033
5. Abraham WT, Fisher WG, Smith AL et al for the Miracle Investigators and Co-ordinators (2001) Multicentre InSync Randomised ClinicaL Evaluation (MIRACLE). Results of a randomised, double blind, controlled trial to assess cardiac resynchronisation therapy in heart failure patients. J Am Coll Cardiol 38:595-596
6. Blanc JJ, Etienne Y, Gilard M et al (1997) Evaluation of different ventricular pacing sites in patients with severe heart failure. Circulation 96:3273-3277
7. Etienne Y, Mansourati J, Gilard M (1999) Evaluation of left ventricular based pacing in patients with congestive heart failure and atrial fibrillation. Am J Cardiol 83:1138-1140
8. Leclercq C, Cazeau S, Ritter P, Alonso C, Gras D, Mabo P, Lazarus A, Daubert JC (2000) A pilot experience with permanent biventricular pacing to treat advanced heart failure. Am Heart J 140:862-870

9. Leclercq C, Linde C, Cazeau S et al (2002) Long term (2 years) clinical results of permanent biventricular pacing in patients with advanced heart failure and chronic atrial fibrillation: Results from the MUSTIC Trial. Pacing and Clin Electrophysiol 24:716
10. The CIBIS II Investigators and Committees (1999) The Cardiac Insufficiency Bisoprolol Study II (CIBIS II): a randomised trial. Lancet 353:9-13
11. MERIT-HF Study Group (1999) Effects of metoprolol CR/XL in chronic heart failure: Metoprolol CR/XL Randomised Intervention Trial in Congestive Heart Failure (MERIT.HF). Lancet 353:2001-2007
12. Middlekauff HR, Stevenson WG, Stevenson LW (1991) Prognostic significance of atrial fibrillation in advanced heart failure. Circulation 84:40-48
13. Baldasseroni S, de Biase L, Fresco C et al on behalf of the Italian Network on Congestive Heart Failure (IN-CHF) investigators (2002) Cumulative effect of complete left bundle branch block and chronical atrial fibrillation on 1-year mortality and hospitalisation in patients with congestive heart failure. Eur Heart J 23:1692-1698
14. Bristow MR for the Companion Steering Committee and Clinical Investigators (2000) Heart failure management using implantable devices for ventricular resynchronisation: Comparison of Medical Therapy, Pacing and Defibrillation in Chronic Heart Failure (COMPANION) Trial. J Cardiac Failure 6:276-285
15. Cleland JG, Daubert JC, Erdmann E et al (2001) The Care-HF study (Cardiac Resynchronisation in Heart Failure study): rationale, design and end-points. Eur J Heart Fail 3:481-489
16. Daubert C, Linde C, Cazeau S et al (2002) Mortality in patients included in the MUSTIC study: Long term (> 2 years) follow up. Pacing and Clin Electrophysiol 24:558A

Patients with Heart Failure and Right Bundle Branch Block or Nonspecific Intraventricular Conduction Disturbances
Can They Benefit from Cardiac Resynchronization Therapy?

S. Garrigue, P. Bordachar, S. Reuter, M. Hocini, P. Jaïs, M. Haïssaguerre, J. Clémenty

Introduction

Biventricular pacing (BVP) has recently been proposed for the treatment of patients with drug-resistant heart failure and long QRS duration [1–6]. The rationale for this suggestion is based on the high prevalence of inter- and intraventricular conduction delay among patients with heart failure [7-9] and on the resultant poor coordination of ventricular contraction and relaxation [9-11], which worsens the left-ventricular dysfunction. The purpose of BVP is to restore ventricular relaxation and contraction sequences as homogeneously as possible by providing right and left ventricular pacing simultaneously. Up to now, this specific pacing mode has been applied to heart failure patients with left bundle branch block (LBBB) to shorten the significant right-to-left interventricular delay with or without intraventricular asynchrony [12–14]. Recently, it was suggested that complete right bundle branch block (RBBB) should be considered as an independent predictor of mortality, and especially in heart failure patients, with the same weighting as LBBB [15]. Since not only marked right-to-left, but also left-to-right, interventricular delay observed on the surface electrocardiogram (ECG) worsens the burden of heart failure, there has been some speculation to the effect that BVP might also benefit patients with severe congestive heart failure and complete RBBB, on the basis that there may be a concomitant left-sided intraventricular conduction disorder that remains invisible on the surface ECG. Recently, several studies have suggested that the presence of a marked left intraventricular electromechanical delay is more likely than the QRS width to be the major criterion identifying patients who will respond to BVP [16-19].

In this chapter, we briefly review the different hypotheses that have been set up about multisite ventricular stimulation in patients affected by heart failure but without typical LBBB.

Hôpital Cardiologique du Haut-Levêque, Electrophysiology and Cardiac Pacing Department, University of Bordeaux, Pessac, France

Ventricular conduction disorders seen on the surface ECG as a prolonged QRS induce significant electromechanical abnormalities, and in particular significant intraventricular wall motion dyssynchrony [11, 16-22]. This means that, despite a longer duration of QRS, LVP may resynchronize the LV electrically, with the same hemodynamic effect as BVP. The lack of correlation between the LV activation time (recorded by optical mapping) and the QRS duration on the surface ECG (r=0.29; P=ns) in guinea pig experiments is likely to be similar in patients [23]. Prinzen et al. [22] also showed that it is the sequence of LV electrical activation rather than QRS shortening that determines whether or not BVP results in improved mechanical LV wall synchronization. This was confirmed by further studies showing that the ultimate benefit of BVP is mechanical (or electromechanical), an effect that does not necessarily correlate with alterations in ventricular activation [20–22].

Patients with Complete Right Bundle Branch Block

In our study, after 12 months of follow-up, 9 out of 12 patients with complete RBBB were clinically improved, with significantly higher performances in the maximal treadmill test after being resynchronized [16]. All these 9 patients had major intra-left-ventricular electromechanical disorders characterized by Doppler tissue imaging, but had nonetheless presented with complete RBBB rather LBBB. BVP markedly reduced the degree of intraventricular electromechanical asynchrony associated with a reduction of the interventricular delay. However, in the 3 patients who did not experience any improvement, BVP resulted only in shortening of the interventricular delay, with no effect on intra-left-ventricular electromechanical disorders. In fact, these nonimproved patients exhibited a much smaller degree of intra-left-ventricular asynchrony at baseline than the patients who did improve. This is consistent with data suggesting that advanced heart failure patients with major intraventricular delay (with or without interventricular delay) might be the optimal candidates for efficient BVP regardless of the presence of RBBB or LBBB. For the purpose of selection, Doppler tissue imaging technique allows noninvasive assessment of regional electromechanical coupling and might discriminate between patients with and without intra-left-ventricular asynchrony. Consequently, this technique might provide valuable information, since it offers the possibility of identifying good candidates for BVP.

As recently reported, instead of shortening the electromechanical delays present in all regions of the left ventricle, BVP may prolong some while shortening others, resulting in a time difference in the reduction of left ventricular wall activation [16–20]. Figure 1 shows in a patient that the electromechanical delay (EMD) of the left-ventricular free wall is 200 ms, while BVP results in its prolongation to 280 ms. Meanwhile, the EMD of the left-ventricular septal wall is 440 ms at baseline and shortens to 257 ms with BVP. Consequently, the prolongation of the free wall EMD associated with the shortening of the septal

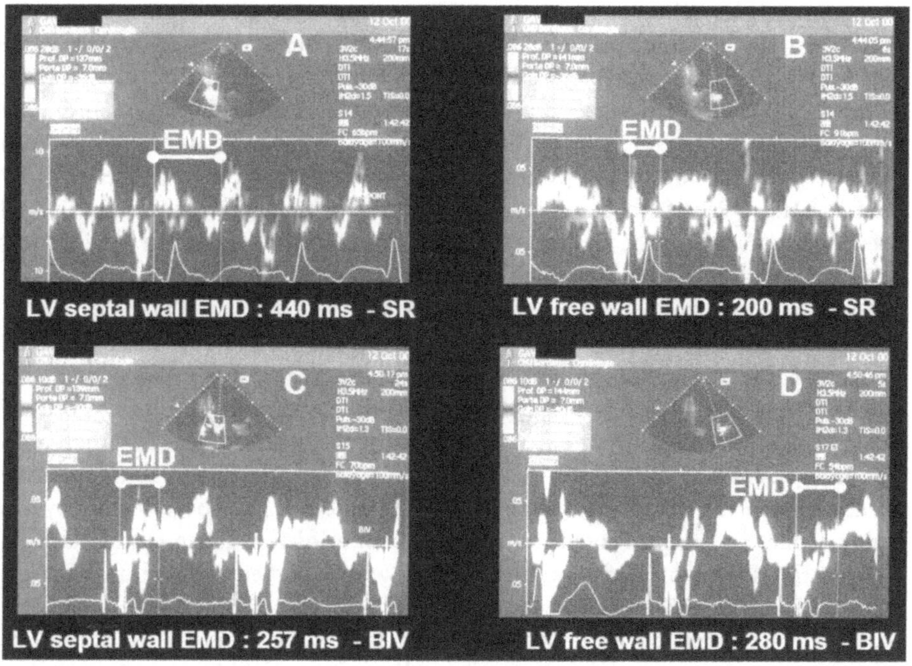

Fig. 1A–D. In this heart failure patient with complete right bundle branch block, the septal left ventricular electromechanical delay (EMD) decreased from A 440 ms with spontaneous rhythm (SR) to C 257 ms with biventricular pacing (BVP), while the free wall EMD increased from B 200 with SR to D 280 ms with BVP, resulting in better mechanical synchronization (183 ms vs 80 ms)

wall EMD results in a marked reduction of the time difference between the two, leading to more homogeneous left-ventricular activation. This may explain the decreased severity of mitral regurgitation in our population, which was accompanied by an increase in the aortic time–velocity integer without a consistent increase in the left-ventricular ejection fraction [16, 24].

Responder Patients According to Electromechanical Criteria and Not QRS Width

In initial studies of cardiac resynchronization therapy its efficacy was assessed on the basis of the acute hemodynamic response, as reflected, for example, in the first derivative of left-ventricular pressure or pulse pressure [6, 14]. However, the predictive value of acute hemodynamic improvement seen in chronic clinical or echocardiographic responses has not been established [25], and the invasive nature of the investigation limits the feasibility of serial assessment. In subsequent studies, responders were classified according to clinical improvements, such as NYHA class, quality-of-life score, or exercise tolerance [2–4, 12, 24]. Two studies conducted at the University of Rennes in France showed that clinical responders were associated with a much more significant shortening of QRS duration after BVP than were nonresponders [3, 26]. However, some of the patients concerned might have improved without substantial QRS width changes, since the standard deviation for QRS width reached ± 27 ms in the first study and ± 22 ms in the second. In other words, the QRS width might not be as sensitive as had been expected. In another study [24], clinical responders were associated with a smaller aortic time–velocity integral and more severe mitral regurgitation. In contrast, shortening of the QRS, which was observed in both groups, was not a predictor of clinical response [24]. Although clinical end-points are useful to assess the efficacy of BVP therapy, when used as predictors of successful therapy these end-points are limited by the subjective nature of patients' own evaluation (especially NYHA class and quality-of-life score), whereas placebo effects may also play a part in the perceived improvement. In addition, these studies did not assess the degree of systolic dyssynchrony, whose correction is in fact the primary benefit of BVP therapy [16, 17, 19].

Other studies [17, 18] have suggested that ECG criteria, including QRS duration and morphology, cannot predict resynchronization-induced LV reverse remodeling, and the reduction in end-diastolic volume has then been considered as a marker of efficient biventricular stimulation. Direct measurement of systolic dyssynchrony by echocardiography was shown to be the only independent predictor of reverse remodeling [18]. Responders not only had more severe systolic dyssynchrony at baseline, but had also improved significantly after 3 months of pacing. In contrast, systolic dyssynchrony worsened in nonresponders. A high baseline systolic dyssynchrony index was the only independent predictor of volumetric response: a value of 32.6 ms (+2 SDs from the mean in 88 normal controls) reliably differentiated responders from nonresponders [18] (Fig. 2). Therefore, these findings support the theory that systolic dyssynchrony is the main target of cardiac resynchronization therapy. Two recent long-term follow-up studies have suggested that it is the presence of left intraventricular, and not of left interventricular mechanical asynchrony that is an independent predictive factor of exacerbation of heart failure and even cardiac death [27, 28]. This observation underscores the fact that the role of major mechanical left-ventricular asynchrony predominates over that of QRS width. The presence of left-intraventricular asynchrony affects 56% of patients with a narrow QRS and more than 80% of patients with RBBB [28]. In addition, a recent study revealed that among patients with drug-resistant heart failure and a narrow QRS, cardiac resynchronization therapy could be beneficial in those who presented with a left-intraventricular mechanical asynchrony above 50 ms [29]. All these patients had a wider QRS with BVP than in their spontaneous rhythm, and yet the four left ventricular walls were better syn-

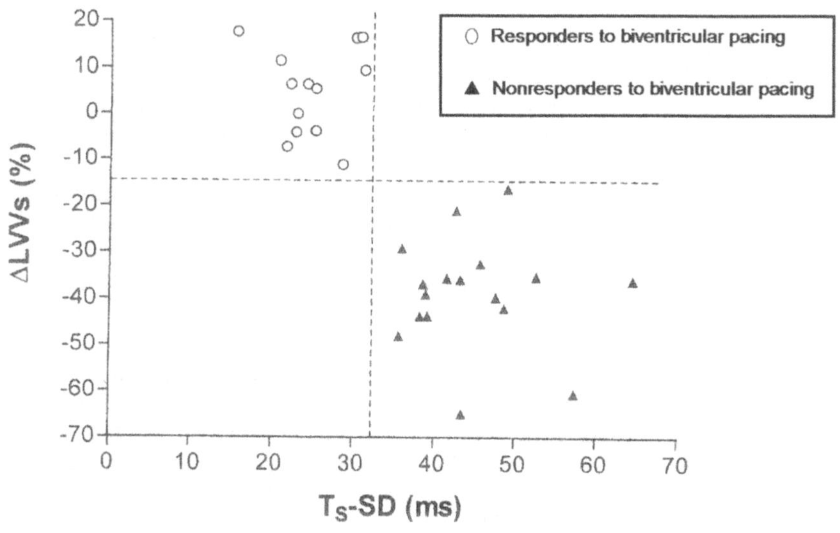

Fig. 2. Changes in left ventricular end-systolic volume (DLVVs) and severity of systolic dyssynchrony. The latter is represented by the standard deviation of the time to peak myocardial systolic contraction (T_S-SD). A difference of 2 standard deviations (32.6 ms, i.e., 95% of the studied population - N=30) was able to segregate responders to BVP completely from nonresponders

chronized. Consequently, heart failure patients who present with left-intraventricular mechanical asynchrony might be considered as responders to multisite ventricular pacing independently of the QRS width.

Consideration of left-ventricular pacing alone also illustrates the discrepancy between hemodynamic improvement and prolonged QRS [14, 30, 31]. Consequently, the left-ventricular pacing-induced large QRS width would represent the late activation of the right ventricle from the left ventricle.

Conclusions

Recent data suggest that echocardiography coupled with the tissue Doppler imaging technique is likely to be more selective and reliable than surface ECG for selecting responders to BVP. The presence of a left-intraventricular electromechanical asynchrony is the main parameter to be treated in heart failure patients; this new risk factor appears not to depend on QRS width and morphology, which means the indications for BVP can be extended to include patients with RBBB and even patients with a narrow QRS.

References

1. Cazeau S, Ritter P, Lazarus A et al (1996) Multisite pacing for end-stage heart failure: early experience. Pacing Clin Electrophysiol 19:1748-1757
2. Gras D, Mabo P, Tang T et al (1998) Multisite pacing as a supplemental treatment of congestive heart failure: preliminary results of the Medtronic InSync study. Pacing Clin Electrophysiol 21:2249-2255
3. Reuter S, Garrigue S, Bordachar P et al (2000) Intermediate-term results of biventricular pacing in heart failure: correlation between clinical and hemodynamic data. Pacing Clin Electrophysiol 23:1713-1717
4. Alonso C, Leclercq C, Victor F et al (1999) Electrocardiographic predictive factors of long-term clinical improvement with multisite biventricular pacing in advanced heart failure. Am J Cardiol 84:1417-1421
5. Bordachar P, Garrigue S, Reuter S et al (2000) Hemodynamic assessment of right, left and biventricular pacing by peak endocardial acceleration and echocardiography in patients with end-stage heart failure. Pacing Clin Electrophysiol 23:1726-1730
6. Auricchio A, Stellbrink C, Block M et al (1999) Effect of pacing chamber and atrioventricular delay on acute systolic function of paced patients with congestive heart failure. Circulation 99:2993-3001
7. Shamim W, Francis DP, Yousufuddin M (1999) Intraventricular conduction delay: a prognostic marker in chronic heart failure. Int J Cardiol 70:171-178
8. Wilensky RL, Yudelman P, Cohen AI et al (1988) Serial electrocardiographic changes in idiopathic dilated cardiomyopathy confirmed at necropsy. Am J Cardiol 62:276-283
9. Grines LC, Bashore TM, Boudoulas H, Olson S, Shafer P, Wooley CF (1989) Functional abnormalities in isolated left bundle branch block: the effect of interventricular asynchrony. Circulation 79:845-853
10. Xiao HB, Brecker SJ, Gibson DG (1992) Effects of abnormal activation on the time course of left ventricular pressure pulse in dilated cardiomyopathy. Br Heart J 68:403-407
11. Xiao HB, Lee CH, Gibson DG (1991) Effect of left bundle branch block on diastolic function in dilated cardiomyopathy. Br Heart J 66:443-447
12. Cazeau S, Leclercq C, Lavergne T et al (2001) Effects of multisite biventricular pacing in patients with heart failure and intraventricular conduction delay. N Engl J Med 344:873-880
13. Leclercq C, Cazeau S, Le Breton H et al (1998) Acute hemodynamic effects of biventricular DDD pacing in patients with end-stage heart failure. J Am Coll Cardiol 32:1825-1831
14. Kass DA, Chen CH, Curry C et al (1999) Improved left ventricular mechanics from acute VDD pacing in patients with dilated cardiomyopathy and ventricular conduction delay. Circulation 99:1567-1573
15. Hesse B, Diaz LA, Snader CE, Blackstone EH, Lauer MS (2001) Complete bundle branch block as an independent predictor of all-cause mortality: report of 7073 patients referred for nuclear exercise testing. Am J Med 110:318-319
16. Garrigue S, Reuter S, Labeque JN et al (2001) Usefulness of biventricular pacing in patients with congestive heart failure and right bundle branch block. Am J Cardiol 88:1436-1441
17. Yu CM, Chau E, Sanderson SE et al (2002) Tissue Doppler echocardiographic evidence of reverse remodeling and improved synchronicity by simultaneously delaying regional contraction after biventricular pacing therapy in heart failure. Circulation 105:438-445

18. Yu CM, Fung WH, Lin H et al (2003) Predictors of left ventricular reverse remodeling after cardiac resynchronization therapy for heart failure secondary to idiopathic dilated or ischemic cardiomyopathy. Am J Cardiol 91:684-688
19. Ansalone G, Giannantoni P, Ricci R et al (2002) Doppler myocardial imaging to evaluate the effectiveness of pacing sites in patients receiving biventricular pacing. J Am Coll Cardiol 39:489-499
20. Leclercq C, Kass DA (2002) Retiming the failing heart: principles and current clinical status of cardiac resynchronization. J Am Coll Cardiol 39:194-201
21. Wyman BT, Hunter WC, Prinzen FW, McVeigh EA (1999) Mapping propagation of mechanical activation in the paced heart with MRI tagging. Am J Physiol 276:H881-H891
22. Prinzen FW, Hunter WC, Wyman BT, Mc Veigh ER (1999) Mapping of regional myocardial strain and work during ventricular pacing: experimental study using magnetic resonance imaging tagging. J Am Coll Cardiol 33:1735-1742
23. Garrigue S, Reuter S, Efimov IR et al (2003) Optical mapping technique applied to biventricular pacing: potential mechanisms of ventricular arrhythmias occurrence. Pacing Clin Electrophysiol 26:197-205
24. Reuter S, Garrigue S, Barold SS et al (2002) Comparison of characteristics in responders versus non-responders with biventricular pacing for drug-resistant congestive heart failure. Am J Cardiol 89:346-350
25. Stellbrink C, Breithardt O, Franke A et al (2001) Impact of cardiac resynchronization therapy using hemodynamically optimized pacing on left ventricular remodeling in patients with congestive heart failure and ventricular conduction disturbances. J Am Coll Cardiol 38:1957-1965
26. Lecoq G, Leclercq C, Alonso C et al (2003) Value of baseline and paced ECG to predict the clinical response to cardiac resynchronization therapy in patients with severe heart failure (abstract). Pacing Clin Electrophysiol 26:1019
27. Fauchier L, Marie O, Casset-Senon D et al (2002) Interventricular and intraventricular dyssynchrony in idiopathic dilated cardiomyopathy: a prognostic study with Fourier phase analysis of radionuclide angioscintigraphy. J Am Coll Cardiol 4:2022-2030
28. Garrigue S, Lafitte S, Bader H et al (2002) Relationship between QRS characteristics and the presence of inter- and intraventricular dyssynchrony: direct implications in heart failure patient management by using the echocardiographic tissue Doppler imaging technique (abstract). Circulation 106:556
29. Turner MS, Bleasdale R, Mumford CE et al (2003) Coronary sinus pacing improves mechanical synchrony in heart failure patients with normal QRS duration <120 ms despite the absence of electrical dyssynchrony (abstract). Pacing Clin Electrophysiol 26:1119
30. Etienne Y, Mansourati J, Gilard M et al (1999) Evaluation of left ventricular based pacing in patients with congestive heart failure and atrial fibrillation. Am J Cardiol 83:1138-1140
31. Touiza A, Etienne Y, Gilard M et al (2001) Long-term left ventricular pacing: assessment and comparison with biventricular pacing in patients with severe congestive heart failure. J Am Coll Cardiol 38:1966-1970

Which Left Ventricular Stimulation Site Is Best for Cardiac Resynchronisation Therapy?

F. Nacci[1], F. Fino[1], E. Spennati[2], V.F. Napoli[3], S. Favale[1]

In the last few years, cardiac resynchronisation therapy has been proposed as a way of restoring a physiological interventricular and left intraventricular activation sequence in patients with severely symptomatic left ventricular (LV) systolic dysfunction and left bundle branch block (LBBB). In this population haemodynamic and clinical benefits have been confirmed.

In patients with LBBB, LV activation follows right ventricular (RV) activation. Therefore, opening and closing of the aortic valve and opening of the mitral valve are delayed, while the RV sequence of events remains unchanged. This leads to an inversion of the normal sequence of RV and LV systole and diastole, an abnormal movement of the interventricular septum and a shortened LV filling time [1–4]. As a result, LV end-systolic diameter is increased and LV ejection fraction and +dp/dt are reduced, as are cardiac output and mean arterial pressure [5, 6].

The haemodynamic effects of LBBB in subjects with LV systolic dysfunction are enhanced because myocardium lacks the usual compensatory ability to hypercontract [7].

Studies on endocardial mapping [8, 9] have shown that in subjects with ischaemic or nonischaemic LV systolic dysfunction with LBBB or during stimulation at the RV apex, the basal posterior or posteroinferior LV wall is the area of delayed activation, except in the subgroup of subjects with septal scarring. On the basis of these data the lateral and posterolateral walls are the preferred sites for LV stimulation in biventricular systems.

Many studies have investigated the efficacy of LV stimulation at the epicardial or endocardial surface of the lateral or posterolateral wall, alone or together with RV stimulation. All published studies show acute improvement in LV systolic function parameters.

In their study, Blanc et al. [10] enrolled subjects with both ischaemic and nonischaemic dilated cardiomyopathy assigned to NYHA class III or IV

[1]U.O. di Cardiochirurgia, Dipartimento di Emergenza e Trapianti d'Organo, Ospedale Consorziale Policlinico, Università di Bari; [2]Divisione di Cardiologia, Presidio Ospedaliero Civile, Ostuni; [3]Divisione di Cardiologia, IRCCS "S. Maugeri", Cassano Murge, Italy

despite the highest tolerated drug dosage (ACE inhibitors, diuretics and digoxin) who had presented with first-degree atrioventricular (AV) block and/or LBBB. LV stimulation was performed using an endocardial lead retrogradely positioned at the level of the LV lateral wall. Subjects underwent VDD stimulation (VVI in cases with atrial fibrillation) at the level of the RV outflow tract, at the LV lateral wall and, in the case of biventricular stimulation, at the level of the RV apex and LV lateral wall with AV delay at 100 ms. Twenty-three subjects were evaluated. Compared with baseline values, with LV stimulation there were a significant improvement in systemic systolic arterial pressure (+7%) and decreases in pulmonary capillary wedge pressure (–22%) and in mean V wave amplitude (–35%). These values were not significantly different from those obtained with biventricular stimulation.

Leclercq et al. [11] evaluated subjects with both ischaemic and nonischaemic dilated cardiomyopathy qualifying them for assignment to NYHA class III or IV despite treatment at the maximum tolerated dosage with ACE inhibitors and diuretics, and with LV ejection fraction <35%, LV end-diastolic diameter >60 mm, who were in sinus rhythm and had intraventricular conduction disturbances and QRS duration >120 ms. LV stimulation was at the ostium of the lateral or posterolateral cardiac vein. DDD stimulation was performed at the RV apex, at the RV outflow tract, at the LV lateral wall and, in the case of biventricular stimulation, both at the level of the RV apex and at the LV lateral or posterolateral wall, with the AV delay varying depending on the subject. Eighteen subjects were evaluated. Compared with baseline values, biventricular stimulation brought about a significant improvement in cardiac index (+35%) and decreases in pulmonary capillary wedge pressure (–18.5%) and in V-wave amplitude (–21%).

The subjects of the study conducted by Kass et al. [12] had ischaemic or nonischaemic dilated cardiomyopathy classified in NYHA class III or IV despite the highest tolerated drug dosage (ACE inhibitors, diuretics and digoxin) and were in sinus rhythm with an AV delay >150 ms. The LV stimulation site was at the middle of the lateral cardiac vein or the anterior cardiac vein. Subjects underwent VDD stimulation at the LV apex, at the upper or mid-right interventricular septum, at the LV free wall and, in the case of biventricular stimulation, at the RV apex or right interventricular septum and the LV free wall. Three or four AV delays were studied, differing by 25–30 ms from each other, the longest being 20–70 ms shorter than the intrinsic AV delay. Eighteen subjects were evaluated. Compared with baseline values, LV stimulation led to a significant improvement in +dp/dt (+23.7%), peak systolic pressure (+5.7%) and pulse pressure (+18%). Biventricular stimulation values were also significantly increased: +12.8%, +3.2% and +14.6%, respectively.

Like the other studies, the PATH-CHF I study [13] involved subjects with ischaemic or nonischaemic dilated cardiomyopathy, who were categorised in NYHA class III or IV despite optimised medical therapy and were in sinus rhythm with AV delay >150 ms and QRS duration >120 ms. LV stimulation was performed by way of an epicardial lead positioned on the surface of the apex or, rarely, of the LV mid-lateral wall by lateral thoracotomy. Subjects underwent VDD stimulation with five different AV delays equally distributed between 0 ms and the intrinsic AV delay minus 30 ms. Retrospective analysis [14] of intraoperative haemodynamic tests performed in the first 25 patients enrolled was the only attempt at identifying any association between LV stimulation site and percentage change in LV +dp/dt and aortic pulse pressure. In this evaluation the percentage increase in LV + dp/dt and aortic pulse pressure averaged over all AV delays obtained at the mid-lateral wall were greater than at any other LV stimulation site, while the results obtained at the mid-anterior wall were poorer than at any other LV region.

Many other clinical studies have investigated the efficacy of LV stimulation at the epicardial or endocardial surface of the lateral or posterolateral walls, in some cases also combining it with RV stimulation. They showed an improvement in symptoms, in quality of life, in functional capacity, in number of admissions to hospital and, more recently, in mortality in long-term follow-up [15–23]. No clinical study has been performed to assess the correlation between LV stimulation site and benefits at follow-up. The MUSTIC study [15] has provided some more data on the implantation procedure.

MUSTIC inclusion criteria were: ischaemic or nonischaemic LV systolic dysfunction, LVEF <35%, LV end-diastolic diameter >60 mm, NYHA class III or IV despite treatment at the maximum tolerated dosage with at least ACE inhibitors and diuretics, in sinus rhythm and with a QRS duration >150 ms. This was a crossover study of atriobiventricular stimulation with optimal AV delay vs inactive stimulation (VVI at 40 beats/min), each for a period of 3 months, in random order. Pacemakers were implanted transvenously. The lead for LV stimulation was placed in a tributary of the coronary sinus. The target LV stimulation site was the mid-lateral wall. Other stimulation sites on the lateral or posterolateral walls were also accepted. The great cardiac vein and the middle cardiac vein were used only when the first-named sites were inaccessible. Implantation of the lead for LV stimulation was attempted in 64 subjects, with a 92% success rate, and a lateral position was obtained in 80% of subjects, with a mean stimulation threshold of 1.4 V. During atrioventricular stimulation the primary end-point of 6-min walking distance showed a 23% improvement (399.2 vs 325.7 m) compared with the inactive stimulation phase. Moreover, the Minnesota score decreased by 32% (29.6 vs 43.2) and peak VO_2 increased by 8% (16.2 vs 15.0 ml/kg per min) with active pacing. During the first 3 months of the study three subjects with active atriobiventricular stimulation were admitted to hospital owing to worsening of their cardiac insufficiency, as against nine subjects with inactive stimulation. At the end of the study 85% of patients preferred atriobiventricular stimulation and 4%, inactive stimulation, while 10% had no preference.

These results were confirmed by data analysis in respect of patients definitively programmed to atriobiventricular stimulation with optimal AV delay at 12 months of follow-up [22]. At that time the 6-min walking distance had improved by 20% over that at the time of randomisation (418 vs 348 m), the

Minnesota score had decreased by 36% (30 vs 47), peak oxygen uptake was greater by 11% (16.6 vs 14.9 ml/kg per min, difference not statistically significant), and NYHA class was 0.7 lower (2.1 vs 2.8). The frequency of hospital admissions attributable to worsening heart failure during biventricular stimulation was one-seventh that during inactive stimulation, and the total mortality was 85% (there were no deaths related to stimulation). These data support the lateral wall as the option of first choice for the placement of leads for LV stimulation.

Surgical implantation of an electrocatheter for LV stimulation makes it possible to optimise the stimulation site; however, lateral thoracotomy is associated with significant operative mortality and postoperative morbidity and mortality and can only be used as a second-choice approach [24]. The transvenous procedure is associated with negligible morbidity and mortality. However, lead placement in the coronary sinus and cardiac tributary veins limits the choice of stimulation site. Target positions may not be reached owing to anatomical obstructions, coronary sinus dissections, lead instability, high stimulation thresholds, and diaphragmatic stimulation. The success rate of transvenous LV lead placement varies between 86% and 92% in different studies [15–18, 25–27].

Technological progress in LV pacing leads has facilitated access to the coronary sinus and the positioning at different levels of the various branches, thus enabling correlations between the LV stimulation site and the related clinical benefits.

References

1. Grines CL, Bashore TM, Boudoulas H (1989) Functional abnormalities in isolated left bundle branch block. Circulation 79:845–853
2. Hultgren HN, Craige E, Fujii J (1983) Left bundle branch block and mechanical events of the cardiac cycle. Am J Cardiol 52:755–762
3. Takeshita A, Basta LL, Kioschos JM (1974) Effect of intermittent left bundle branch block on left ventricular performance. Am J Med 56:251–255
4. Kingma I, Tyberg JV, Smith ER (1983) Effects of diastolic transseptal pressure gradient on ventricular septal position and motion. Circulation 68:1304–1314
5. Bramlet DA, Morris KG, Coleman RE et al (1983) Effect of rate-dependent left bundle branch block on global and regional left ventricular function. Circulation 67:1059–1065
6. Bourassa MG, Boiteau GM, Allenstein BJ (1962) Hemodynamic studies during intermittent left bundle branch block. Am J Cardiol 10:792–799
7. Herman MV, Heinle RA, Klein MD et al (1967) Localized disorders in myocardial contraction: asynergy and its role in congestive heart failure. N Engl J Med 277:222–232
8. Vassallo JA, Cassidy DM, Miller JM et al (1986) Left ventricular endocardial activation during right ventricular pacing. J Am Coll Cardiol 7:1228–1233
9. Hatala R, Savard P, Tremb̀oay G et al (1995) Three distinct patterns of ventricular activation in infarcted human hearts: an intraoperative cardiac mapping study during sinus rhythm. Circulation 91:1480–1494

10. Blanc JJ, Etienne Y, Gilard M et al (1997) Evaluation of different ventricular pacing sites in patients with severe heart failure. Circulation 96:3273–3277
11. Leclercq C, Cazeau S, Le Breton H et al (1998) Acute hemodynamic effects of biventricular DDD pacing in patients with end-stage heart failure. J Am Coll Cardiol 7:1825–1831
12. Kass DA, Chen C, Curry C et al (1999) Improved left ventricular mechanisms from acute VDD pacing in patients with dilated cardiomyopathy and ventricular conduction delay. Circulation 99:1567–1573
13. Auricchio A, Stellbrink C, Sack S et al (1999) The pacing therapies for congestive heart failure (PATH-CHF) study: rationale design, and endpoints of a prospective randomized multicenter study. Am J Cardiol 83:130D–135D
14. Auricchio A, Klein H, Tockman B et al (1999) Transvenous biventricular pacing for heart failure: can the obstacles be overcome? Am J Cardio 83:136D–142D
15. Cazeau S, Leclercq C, Lavergne T et al (2001) Effects of multisite biventricular pacing in patients with heart failure and intraventricular conduction delay. N Engl J Med 344:873–880
16. Abraham WT, Fisher WG, Smith AL et al (2002) Cardiac resynchronization therapy in chronic heart failure. N Engl J Med 346:1845–1853
17. (2002) Contak CD Guidant cardiac resynchronization therapy defibrillator system including the CONTAK CD pulse generator and the EASYTRAK left ventricular coronary venous lead. Summary of safety and effectiveness. www.fda.gov
18. (2001) Medtronic Insync ICD cardiac resynchronization system. www.fda.gov
19. Stellbrink C, Breithardt O, Franke A et al (2001) Impact of cardiac resynchronization therapy using hemodynamically optimized pacing on left ventricular remodeling in patients with congestive heart failure and ventricular conduction disturbances. J Am Coll Cardiol 38:1957–1965
20. Abraham W, Hayes D, Sackner-Bernstein J et al (2002) Cardiac resynchronization therapy reduces the risk of hospitalization for heart failure and the length of stay: results from the MIRACLE trial (abstract). Eur Heart J 23 [Suppl]:3
21. Auricchio A, Stellbrink C, Sack S et al (2002) Long-term clinical effect of hemodynamically optimized cardiac resynchronization therapy in patients with heart failure and ventricular conduction delay. J Am Coll Cardiol 39:2026–2033
22. Linde C, Leclercq C, Rex S et al (2002) Long-term benefits of biventricular pacing in congestive heart failure: results from the multisite stimulation in cardiomyopathy (MUSTIC) study. J Am Coll Cardiol 40:111–118
23. Bristow MR, Saxon LA, Boehmer J et al (2003) ACC Late-breaker preliminary results. Communication, March 2003.http://www.acc.org
24. Cazeau S, Ritter P, Lazarus A et al (1996) Multisite pacing for end-stage heart failure: early experience. Pacing Clin Electrophysiol 19:1748–1757
25. Ricci R, Ansalone G, Toscano S et al (2000) Cardiac resynchronization: materials, technique and results. The InSync Italian Registry. Eur Heart J 2 [Suppl J]:J6–15
26. Pappone C, Auricchio A, Schalij M et al (2001) Can transvenous left ventricular leads be used as standard treatment for heart failure patients? The European experience with the first 1000 over-the-wire lead implants (abstract). Pacing Clin Electrophysiol 24:619
27. Baker CM, Christopher TJ, Smith PF et al (2002) Addition of a left ventricular lead to conventional pacing systems in patients with congestive heart failure: feasibility, safety, and early results in 60 consecutive patients. Pacing Clin Electrophysiol 25:1166–1171

Permanent His Bundle Pacing: A Good Unconventional Mode of Right Ventricular Pacing?

E. Occhetta, M. Bortnik, G. Francalacci, A. Magnani, C. Piccinino, C. Vassanelli

Introduction

Atrial fibrillation (AF) is the most common arrhythmia, affecting more than 1% of the general population [1], and it is usually associated with several different cardiac and noncardiac conditions, including hypertension, ischemic heart disease, cardiomyopathy, and valvular heart disease. In some patients without structural heart disease it is called "lone atrial fibrillation." Atrial fibrillation can be classified as paroxysmal when it terminates spontaneously, persistent when it requires pharmacological or electric cardioversion to be terminated, and permanent when all attempts to terminate it fail.

In patients with AF, the restoration and maintenance of sinus rhythm is the primary therapeutic goal; for patients with recurrent AF, the two available pharmacological strategies are rhythm or rate control and anticoagulation. At present nonpharmacological strategies include:

1. Electrical procedures for arrhythmia prevention (single-site or multisite atrial pacing with specific, currently available algorithms)
2. Electrical procedures which terminate AF (low-energy intracardiac cardioversion)
3. Ablation procedures which modify atrial substrate or eliminate triggering sites (particularly in the pulmonary venous system)

Ablate and Pace Strategy

When the above-mentioned clinical approaches are ineffective and patients still complain of severe symptoms, ablation of the atrioventricular (AV) node and permanent pacing are effective in controlling the ventricular rate. This

Division of Cardiology, School of Medicine, Università degli Studi del Piemonte Orientale, Novara, Italy palliative treatment does not eliminate the electrophysiologic substrate of the disease or the need for anticoagulation, but it alleviates symptoms and improves the quality of life. Implantation of a pacemaker (PM) is generally required as the majority of patients who undergo radiofrequency catheter ablation of the AV junction are pacemaker-dependent [2].

The procedure is quite simple, with a high success rate (>95%) and a very low complication rate (<2%). In patients with permanent AF, a single-chamber VVIR PM is used for permanent pacing; patients with paroxysmal AF require a DDDR system with extended diagnostic and therapeutic functions with respect to AF.

Randomized trials have shown the beneficial effects of this procedure on quality of life in symptomatic patients with fast and irregular ventricular response during episodes of paroxysmal AF [3]. This therapeutic approach does not eliminate the risk of progression to chronic AF, which can be reduced by concomitant drug treatment [4] and currently available pacing techniques and algorithms aimed at prevention of AF or at the reduction of the AF burden [5].

In patients with chronic AF, the clinical benefits are less established: previous nonrandomized trials have shown an improvement in quality of life after regularization of the ventricular rate after "ablate and pace therapy." However, Brignole et al. [6] in a randomized trial reported only a slight, nonsignificant improvement in quality of life, while no differences were observed in objective hemodynamics and functional parameters of performance.

Hence, "ablate and pace" should not be considered as the first-choice therapy in patients with paroxysmal or chronic AF, but should be restricted to patients in whom all pharmacological and nonpharmacological therapies aimed to preserve sinus rhythm or to control the ventricular rate failed.

Physiological Ventricular Pacing

One of the most important perplexities about the ablate and pace therapy stems from the need from a PM implantation, which is usually performed through an endocardial lead positioned in the apex of right ventricle. Right ventricular pacing from the apex is known to result in asynchronous ventricular contraction, with particularly delayed left ventricular activation, interventricular motion abnormalities, negative inotropic effects, and structural changes in the left ventricle. Moreover, the occurrence of functional mitral regurgitation related to right ventricular apical pacing has been reported [7, 8].

With the introduction of active fixation leads, other stimulation sites such as the right ventricular outflow tract were tested to improve left ventricular performance. De Cock et al. [9] showed a significant increase in cardiac index when pacing was performed from the right ventricular outflow tract compared to the apex; Gold et al. [10] did not observe any significant improvement in hemodynamic parameters in patients with severe heart failure. More recently, bifocal right ventricular pacing seems to induce better hemodynamic results [11].

It has been supposed that biventricular pacing can improve the contraction synchrony of the left ventricle in cases of severe contractile dysfunction, by improving its global performance; the main issue of this procedure is left ventricular access. The two alternative options have clear drawbacks: the epicardial approach requires a surgical thoracotomy, and left ventricular pacing through the coronary sinus is sometimes difficult because of the great anatomic variability of the cardiac vein system. Clinical benefits of biventricular stimulation in patients with advanced heart failure are evident in the results of randomized trials: MUSTIC [12], PATH-CHF [13], and MIRACLE [14].

An ongoing prospective randomized trial (OPSITE) [15] has been designed to evaluate if left ventricular pacing (and biventricular pacing) is better than right ventricular pacing in patients with permanent atrial fibrillation treated with ablate and pace therapy.

The clinical benefits of biventricular pacing have been described only in patients with a wide QRS interval (≥150 ms); no data are available in patients with normal His-Purkinje activation and wide QRS due to forced right ventricular apical pacing. In this context, high right ventricular septal pacing could provide significant hemodynamic improvement.

Permanent Direct His Bundle Pacing

Deshmukh et al. [16] have shown the safety and efficacy of permanent direct His bundle pacing after AV junction ablation. The study group included 18 patients who had a history of chronic AF, dilated cardiomyopathy (left ventricular ejection fraction <40%), NYHA functional class III or IV, and narrow QRS complexes before ablation. Permanent His bundle pacing was feasible and long-term safe in 12/18 patients (65%); QRS was persistently narrow. At a mean follow-up of nearly 2 years, the authors found a significant improvement in both hemodynamic function and NYHA class, but it is not clear whether most of the benefit derived from rate control or from the endocardial stimulation site.

Padeletti et al. [17] also noted an improvement in contractility (detected by the peak endocardial acceleration, PEA) and hemodynamic performance during acute His bundle pacing, compared to conventional right ventricular pacing.

Shwaab [18] recently confirmed the feasibility of septal permanent stimulation, with a narrow QRS interval in 83/120 patients (69%), without any pacing and sensing problem and no lead dislodgment. He also documented a tendency toward a greater QRS reduction when the high septum was stimulated as compared to pacing of mid or apical parts of the right ventricular septum. In patients undergoing AV junction ablation, the safety of this procedure nevertheless still remains a major concern as the long-term lead stability has not been completely established; the need for standard right ventricular apical back-up pacing is still unclear.

Clinical Study

Aims and Patient Selection

We have planned a prospective randomized study [19] aimed at:

- Evaluating the feasibility and long-term safety of permanent His bundle pacing (high right ventricular septum) and the concomitant need for back-up apical stimulation in patients with chronic AF after AV node ablation
- Comparing the effects of permanent His bundle pacing to those of conventional right apical stimulation on quality of life and on hemodynamic function

Patients are considered for this study if they have:

- A clear indication for AV node ablation because of chronic AF and a rapid drug-resistant ventricular rate
- Underlying structural heart disease (ischemic disease, hypertrophy, dilated cardiomyopathy, etc.)
- Narrow QRS complexes (<120 ms) even during a high ventricular rate

Methods

Before the procedure all the patients enrolled undergo:

- Quality of life and functional class assessment via the Minnesota Living with Heart Failure questionnaire, 6-min walking test, and/or VO_2 exercise test
- 24-hour Holter monitoring
- Complete echocardiographic evaluation including systolic and diastolic left ventricular function and valvular assessment

AV node radiofrequency ablation is performed by a standard method, in order to achieve a stable AV block with an escape rhythm of >30 bpm and narrow QRS; after the procedure, the quadripolar His monitoring lead is left in place to guide the subsequent high septal permanent pacing.

A conventional bipolar lead is placed in the right ventricular apex and the correctness of its position assessed by routine parameters (pacing threshold, lead resistances, and R wave amplitude). Through the same approach, a second bipolar screw-in lead is advanced and positioned, using a steerable stylet (Locator, St. Jude Medical), in the high right ventricular septum, as proximal as possible to the mapping His quadripolar catheter.

Correctness of the screw-in lead position is evaluated by means of the same routine parameters as used for the apical pacing; absence of atrial fibrillation potential far fields must also be detected. Then septal and conventional leads are connected, respectively, to the "atrial" and "ventricular" DDDR PM plugs. The device is programmed in DDDR mode with a short AV delay. If His high septal pacing is effective, ventricular apical stimulation falls in the ventricular refractory period; if His stimulation fails, due to lead dislodgment and/or threshold increase, ventricular pacing is guaranteed by the conventional apical lead.

After 1 month, patients are randomly assigned to two periods of 6 months with the PM programmed in VVIR (conventional apical ventricular stimulation) and DDDR (septal ventricular stimulation) modes respectively. At the end of each period a complete re-assessment of quality of life, functional class, echocardiographic parameters, and 24-h Holter monitoring is performed.

Preliminary Results

Since September 2001, 15 patients have been enrolled; a high right ventricular septal position has been successfully achieved in 14 subjects; in 1 patient the failure was possibly related to the presence of mitral and aortic mechanical prosthetic valves [20]. We obtained a good stimulation threshold (0.6 ± 0.1 V) in all cases, without any complication and with acceptable fluoroscopic exposure times (16 ± 9 min; range 8–40 min). At the time of implantation, QRS was significantly shorter with His pacing (121 ± 14 ms) than with apical pacing (180 ± 19 ms).

During the follow-up period, one patient has dropped out of the study as he had an ICD implanted because of the occurrence of ventricular fibrillation 5 days after the procedure, unrelated to His-septal pacing. In one patient a minor lead dislodgment was observed with persistent good septal and apical ventricular pacing. No abnormal threshold increases have been observed.

Out of 13 patients so far enrolled in the trial, 7 completed the two study periods with cross-over randomization (6 months with apical stimulation and 6 months with His stimulation), 2 have completed the first, and 4 are still in the first period. The results of the 7 patients who have completed the study are shown in Table 1.

Table 1. Results of 7 patients with completed data of follow up

	Baseline	Apical pacing	Septal pacing
NYHA class	2.3 ± 0.4	2.0 ± 0.1	1.8 ± 0.3*
Symptoms score	27.8 ± 12.2	16.3 ± 8.3*	13.1 ± 9**
Distance covered in 6-min walk (m)	349 ± 30	339 ± 70	433 ± 84**
LVEF (%)	54.3 ± 6.9	49 ± 3.2	51 ± 5.3
Mitral regurgitation	1.6 ± 0.3	1.7 ± 0.4	1.5 ± 0.5
Tricuspid regurgitation	1.5 ± 0.4	1.5 ± 0.8	1.3 ± 0.4
PAP (mmHg)	8.3 ± 3.4	36.0 ± 10*	30.8 ± 5.3

*$p < 0.05$, septal or apical pacing versus baseline
**$p < 0.05$, septal pacing versus baseline and apical pacing

Conclusions

We expect that the final results of the present study will confirm whether AV node ablation and "physiological" pacing through appropriate right and left ventricular synchronization can improve not only quality of life but also hemodynamic function in patients with chronic atrial fibrillation and narrow QRS complexes.

References

1. Benjamin EJ et al (1994) Independent risk factors for atrial fibrillation in a population-based cohort. The Framingham Heart Study. JAMA 271:840-844
2. Curtis AB et al (2000) Prevalence and characteristics of escape rhythms after radiofrequency ablation of the atrioventricular junction: results from the registry for AV junction ablation and pacing in atrial fibrillation. Am Heart J 139:122-125
3. Brignole M et al (1997) Assessment of atrioventricular junction ablation and DDDR mode-switching pacemaker versus pharmacological treatment in patients with severely symptomatic paroxysmal atrial fibrillation. A randomized controlled study (PAF). Circulation 96:2617-2624
4. Brignole M et al (2002) An evaluation of the strategy of maintenance of sinus rhythm by antiarrhythmic drug therapy after ablation and pacing therapy in patients with paroxysmal atrial fibrillation (PAF 2). Eur Heart J 23:892-900
5. Gaita F et al (2000) PIPAF study: improvements during a multi-site atrial pacing experience. Europace Suppl 1(suppl D):D218 (abstract)
6. Brignole M et al (1998) Assessment of atrioventricular junction ablation and VVIR pacemaker versus pharmacological treatment in patients with heart failure and chronic atrial fibrillation. A randomized controlled study. Circulation 98:953-960
7. Sassone B et al (2001) Pacemaker-induced mitral regurgitation: prominent role of abnormal ventricular activation sequence versus altered atrioventricular synchrony. Ital Heart J 2:441-448
8. Disney PJS et al (2003) Biventricular pacing for severe mitral regurgitation following atrioventricular nodal ablation. Pacing Clin Electrophysiol 26[2-Pt I]:643-644
9. De Cock CC et al (1998) Hemodynamic benefits of right ventricular outflow tract pacing: comparison with right ventricular apex pacing. Pacing Clin Electrophysiol 21:536-541
10. Gold MR et al (1997) The acute hemodynamic effects of right ventricular septal pacing in patients with congestive heart failure secondary to ischemic or idiopathic dilated cardiomiopathy. Am J Cardiol 79:679-681
11. Zamparelli L, Cioffi L, Di Costanzo A et al (2003) Dual-site right ventricular pacing in heart failure patients. In: Gulizia M (ed) New advances in heart failure and atrial fibrillation. Springer, Milan, pp 401-404
12. Cazeau S et al, for the MUSTIC Study Investigators (2001) Effects of multisite biventricular pacing in patients with heart failure and intraventricular conduction delay. N Engl J Med 344:873-880
13. Auricchio A et al, for the PATH-CHF Study Investigators (2002) Long-term clinical effect of hemodynamically optimized cardiac resynchronization therapy in patients with heart failure and ventricular conduction delay. J Am Coll Cardiol 39:2026-2033
14. Sutton MJSJ et al, for the MIRACLE Study Investigators (2003) Effect of cardiac

resynchronization therapy on left ventricular size and function in chronic heart failure. Circulation 107:1985-1990

15. Brignole M, Gammage M (2001) An assessment of the optimal ventricular pacing site in patients undergoing "ablate and pace" therapy for permanent atrial fibrillation. Europace 3:153-156
16. Deshmukh P et al (2000) Permanent, direct His bundle pacing. A novel approach to cardiac pacing in patients with normal His-Purkinje activation. Circulation 101:869-877
17. Padeletti L et al (2000) Permanent His bundle pacing in man: a comparison with right ventricular apical pacing. Pacing Clin Electrophysiol 23:679 (abstract)
18. Shwaab B et al (2001) Septal lead implantation for the reduction of paced QRS duration using passive fixation leads. Pacing Clin Electrophysiol 24:28-33
19. Occhetta E et al (2002) "Ablate and pace" in chronic atrial fibrillation: intraventricular high septal VVIR pacing to perform a "physiological" ventricular synchronization. Gior Ital Aritmol Cardiostimol 5(suppl 1):256-260
20. Occhetta E et al (2003) Permanent hisian pacing after AV node RF ablation in chronic atrial fibrillation: preliminary results of a feasibility and efficacy study. Pacing Clin Electrophysiol 26 (4-part II):1121 (abstract).

Cardiac Resynchronization Therapy: Is Atrial Resynchronization Important with Biventricular Pacing?

F. Di Pede, G. Gasparini, M. Celestre, G. Zuin, B. De Piccoli, A. Raviele

Cardiac resynchronization therapy performed with biventricular pacing has been recognized as one of the most promising techniques in the treatment of patients with congestive heart failure [1–3]. Many papers demonstrate significant hemodynamic improvement in patients with severe left ventricular dysfunction and left bundle branch block treated with VDD biventricular pacing and shortened atrioventricular (AV) delays [1–4]. The concept is that biventricular pacing may be an effective pacing modality by synchronizing contraction of the right and left ventricles, leading to improvement of cardiac performance and reduction of mitral regurgitation. Some authors have emphasized the importance of optimization of the stimulation site during ventricular resynchronization therapy and concluded that a posterior/lateral/posterior-lateral left ventricle lead position in combination with a right ventricle apex lead position provides more consistent hemodynamic improvements [5]. Recently published trials have shown a substantial improvement in symptoms, cardiac function, and functional capacity and a less consistent effect on hospitalization, but no convincing evidence for a reduction in cardiac mortality [4]. However, cardiac resynchronization probably is not yet optimal, and many technical and physiopathological concepts are under debate. The subject of this paper is the importance of atrial resynchronization and, consequently, the importance of optimization of the AV delay on both the right and the left sides of the heart.

Importance of AV Delay

Nowadays it is widely recognized that the results of acute hemodynamic and echocardiographic studies suggest the need for optimization of the AV delay during ventricular resynchronization therapy. Auricchio et al. [3] have demon-

Department of Cardiology, Umberto I Hospital, Mestre–Venice, Italy

strated that the greatest acute hemodynamic improvement occurs only within definite AV delays. Ritter et al. [6] proposed a simple method based on Doppler echocardiography of transmitral flow to calculate the optimal AV delay in order to provide the longest left ventricular filling time. However, we do not have data confirming the need for AV delay optimization on a long-term basis. Recently published data show that biventricular pacing is also beneficial in patients with atrial fibrillation in whom mechanical atrial contraction is absent [7]. However, the clinical benefits in this population seem to be less than in patients in sinus rhythm, suggesting that biventricular pacing acts mainly through ventricular resynchronization and AV delay optimization probably has a minor role in improving cardiac performance.

Importance of Right Ventricular Performance

In clinical practice, the optimal AV delay is determined on the basis of left ventricular performance, and the optimization of right ventricular filling is not adequately addressed in the setting of ventricular resynchronization therapy. The importance of right ventricular function on exercise capacity and survival in heart failure patients is shown in the results of recently published studies [8–10]. It is well known that right ventricular function depends on pulmonary artery pressure, and as a general rule increased pulmonary artery pressure is coupled with reduced right ventricular systolic function and poor prognosis. Since pulmonary artery pressure depends on left ventricular function, right ventricular function seems mainly related to left ventricular function, which is a well known prognostic factor. However, the importance of right ventricular function as independent predictor of exercise capacity and survival in a population of advanced heart failure patients has been recognized [9]. These data emphasize the necessity of evaluating right heart hemodynamic variables to define the hemodynamic status of patients with heart failure and may be the background for studies aimed at improving right heart hemodynamics by optimizing right AV mechanical delay.

Interatrial Delay

Patients with congestive heart failure frequently have conduction delays at the atrial level in addition to the AV and intraventricular level. This may be the substrate for arrhythmias and may have hemodynamic consequences. Actually, in patients with prolonged interatrial and interventricular conduction time treated with DDD pacing, left and right AV mechanical delays may be substantially different, as recently shown [11]. Particularly in patients treated with biventricular stimulation, pacing at the right atrium appendage produced shorter left than right mechanical AV delay [11]. Therefore, optimizing right mechanical AV delay may cause nonoptimal left mechanical AV delay and vice versa. Other authors [12] have observed that atrial pacing from conventional atrial sites may determine significant prolongation of the interatrial conduction time, potentially leading to further changes in left and right AV delays in comparison with AV delays obtained during VDD pacing. For this reason, pacing at the right atrial appendage does not allow AV delay optimization in both the right and the left sides of the heart in patients with spontaneous or induced interatrial conduction delay.

Atrial Resynchronization

Multisite atrial pacing and septal atrial pacing have been attempted to synchronize atrial activation and contraction. Single-site right atrial septal pacing effectively shortens P wave duration [13]. In unselected patients right atrial septal pacing reverses the physiological right-to-left atrial contraction sequence to a left-to-right sequence [13]. Therefore, atrial septal pacing shortens interatrial delay by anticipating left atrial activation, but does not synchronize right and left atrial contraction. On the basis of echocardiographic measurements, it has been observed that combined interatrial septum pacing and biventricular pacing produces similar left and right mechanical AV delays by reducing both interatrial and interventricular delays [11]. These similar AV delays were due to a greater left mechanical AV delay in patients paced at the interatrial septum than in patients paced at the right atrial appendage. Therefore, biventricular pacing with biatrial resynchronization can lead to similar right and left AV mechanical delays and probably make feasible the optimization of AV delays of the right and left sides of the heart.

The SAVERT Study

We designed a study (SAVERT: value of *s*eptal *a*trial pacing in patients eligible for *v*entricular *r*esynchronization *t*herapy) to investigate the acute hemodynamic effect on cardiac performance of atrial resynchronization therapy (performed by stimulating at the low interatrial septum) combined with biventricular stimulation in patients who need ventricular resynchronization therapy for congestive heart failure. The hypothesis behind this study is that atrial stimulation at the interatrial septum provides an acute hemodynamic improvement in comparison with pacing at the classical site (right atrial appendage), particularly in patients characterized by interatrial conduction disturbances. The main objective of this study was to compare the acute effect on cardiac function of two different atrial pacing sites, right atrial appendage and low interatrial septum, during ventricular resynchronization therapy using DDD pacing. The results of this study will answer the question of whether atrial resynchronization may confer further acute hemodynamic benefit on patients undergoing ventricular resynchronization therapy.

The inclusion criteria for the study were: NYHA function class 2 or higher; left ventricular ejection fraction 35% or less, QRS duration 150 ms or more, dilated cardiomyopathy of any etiology, left bundle branch block pattern or IVCD and absence of second- or third-degree AV block.

All patients had clinical indication for biventricular pacing. The mean age was 70±7 years, 67% of patients were male, and ischemic heart disease was present in 60% of cases. The mean NYHA class was 2.5±0.5, the mean LVEF was 29±4%, the mean QRS duration was 184±16 ms. The hemodynamic study was performed during the implantation session. Two atrial leads were placed at the right atrial appendage and low interatrial septum. The ventricular leads were placed at the right ventricular apex and left ventricular free wall. The pacing protocol consisted of 50 beats in AAI mode with atrial pacing at the right atrial appendage followed by 50 beats in biventricular DDD mode with atrial pacing at the right atrial appendage (DDD-RAA) or at the low interatrial septum (DDD-LIS) at four different AV delays. The acute hemodynamic response was evaluated by LV+*dP*/*dt*, aortic pulse pressure (PP). The optimal AV delay was determined by both LV+*dP*/*dt* and PP. One patient could not be tested due to a limited dissection of the coronary sinus intima and another patient was excluded due to invalid data. Eleven patients had the LV lead in the lateral or posterolateral vein and two patients in the anterolateral vein. The optimal AV delays during DDD-RAA and DDD-LIS pacing were 202±61 ms and 159±45 ms, respectively ($p<0.01$, paired *t*-test). The average (±SE) %LV+*dP*/*dt* increases with DDD-RAA and DDD-LIS pacing with respect to the baseline in AAI mode at the optimal AV delay were 22.7±4.3% and 19.5±4.3%, respectively ($p<0.01$). The difference between %PP increase during DDD-RAA and during DDD-LIS (12.2±2.0 vs 11.5±1.9%) was not significant. These results show that both pacing configurations improve the contractile function, while the increase in LV+*dP*/*dt* with DDD-RAA was significantly larger than with DDD-LIS.

In conclusion, our data do not support the concept that atrial resynchronization obtained by low interatrial septum pacing leads to a further acute hemodynamic benefit in patients who are candidates for cardiac resynchronization therapy. However, our patients were not selected on the basis of the presence of large interatrial delay. Therefore, it is possible that in some patents with large interatrial delay, low interatrial septum pacing could be beneficial. The lack of additional benefits of atrial resynchronization with low interatrial septum pacing may be due to nonphysiological activation of the atria in response to septal or multisite atrial stimulation. In patients in sinus rhythm, impulses travel from the sinus node to the AV node and, consequently, contraction proceeds in a craniocaudal direction, while stimulation of other sites of the atria, such as the coronary sinus or low interatrial septum, may generate a different sequence of contraction leading to unpredictable hemodynamic effects. We cannot rule out that other sites in the atria could be more effective than the low interatrial septum.

Finally, these data demonstrate that the translation of the electrophysiologic or echocardiographic concept of atrial resynchronization to hemodynamics requires caution.

References

1. Blanc JJ, Etienne Y, Gilard M et al (1997) Evaluation of different ventricular pacing sites in patients with severe heart failure. Circulation 93:3273–3277
2. Leclercq C, Cazeau S, Le Breton H et al (1998) Acute emodynamic effects of biventricular DDD pacing in patients with end stage heart failure. J Am Coll Cardiol 32:1825–1831
3. Auricchio A, Stellbrink C, Block M et al (1999) Effect of pacing chamber and atrioventricular delay on acute systolic function of paced patients with congestive heart failure. Circulation 99:2993–3001
4. Cleland JGF, Ghosh J, Khan NK et al (2003) Multi-chamber pacing: a perfect solution for cardiac mechanical dyssynchrony? Eur Heart J 24:384–390
5. Auricchio A, Butter C, Stellbrink C et al (2000) Effect of left ventricular stimulation site on the systolic function of heart failure patients during ventricular resynchronization therapy. Pacing Clin Electrophysiol 23(4part II):589 (abstract 147)
6. Ritter P, Dib JC, Lelievre T et al (1994) Quick determination of the optimal AV delay at rest in patients paced in DDD mode for complete AV block. Eur JCPE 4:A163
7. Linde C, Leclerq C, Rex S et al (2002) Long-term benefits of biventricular pacing in congestive heart failure: results from the multisite stimulation in cardiomyopathy study. J Am Coll Cardiol 40:111–118
8. Di Salvo TG, Mathier M, Semigran MJ, Dec GW (1995) Preserved right ventricular ejection fraction predicts exercise capacity and survival in advanced heart failure. J Am Coll Cardiol 25:1143–1153
9. De Groote P, Millaire A, Foucher-Hossein C et al (1998) Right ventricular ejection fraction is an independent predictor of survival in patients with moderate heart failure. J Am Coll Cardiol 32:948–954
10. Ghio S, Gavazzi A, Campana C et al (2001) Independent and additive prognostic value of right ventricular systolic function and pulmonary artery pressure in patients with chronic heart failure. J Am Coll Cardiol 37:183–188
11. Porciani M C, Sabini A, Colella A et al (2002) Interatrial septum pacing avoids the adverse effect of interatrial delay in biventricular pacing: an echo Doppler study. Europace 4:317–434
12. Parravicini U, Mezzani A, Bielli M (2000) DDD pacing and interatrial conduction block: importance of optimal AV interval setting. Pacing Clin Electrophysiol 23:1448–1450
13. Kindermann M, Schwaab B, Berg M, Fröhling G (2000) The influence of right atrial septal pacing on the interatrial contraction sequence. Pacing Clin Electrophysiol 23:1752–1753

Impact of Cardiac Resynchronization Therapy on Mortality: What Do We Expect from Ongoing Trials?

M. Lunati, M. Paolucci, G. Magenta, G. Cattafi, R. Vecchi, M. Schirru, T. Di Camillo

Introduction

Cardiac resynchronization therapy (CRT), a device-based therapy applied in the context of continuing conventional medical treatment for patients with advanced heart failure (HF) and dyssynchronous left-ventricular (LV) contraction, improves cardiac function and quality of life, but its effects on mortality were uncertain until 2003.

There are two mechanisms of death in patients with HF:

1. Sudden death (SD) attributable to cardiac arrhythmias;
2. Medically refractory progressive HF.

Patients with HF in NYHA class 2 generally die suddenly, while patients whose HF falls in NYHA class 4 generally die from irreversible HF.

Prolongation of the QRS interval (in particular complete left bundle branch block; LBBB) is associated with a significant increase in mortality, and CRT can remove the negative prognostic effect of LV dyssynchrony that is manifested in the ECG in the pattern of LBBB.

The full results of the trials addressing the effects of CRT on mortality in patients with HF and LV dyssynchrony will give us and the regulatory authorities convincing clinical evidence that this new technology ought to change medical practice in HF.

What We Know

In a recent meta-analysis, Bradley et al. [1] tried to determine whether CRT reduces cardiac mortality from progressive HF. The four randomized clinical trials (RCT) considered were:

S.C. Elettrofisiologia, Dipartimento Cardio-Toraco-Vascolare "A. De Gasperis", A.O. Niguarda-Cà Granda, Milano, Italy

1. The Contak CD [2] trial, in which 490 patients were randomized;
2. The Insync ICD [3], in which 554 patients were randomized;
3. The Multicenter Insync Randomized Clinical Evaluation (MIRACLE) [4], in which 532 patients were randomized;
4. The Multisite Stimulation in Cardiomyopathies Trial (MUSTIC) [5], in which 58 patients were randomized.

The mean LV ejection fraction (EF) ranged from 21% to 23%, and the majority of patients had ischemic cardiomyopathy; the mean QRS duration ranged from 158 to 176 ms.

Baseline ACEi or ARBs ranged from 87% to 96%; β-blocker use ranged from 28% to 60%; and patients with conventional indication for ICDs were included in the Contak CD and Insync ICD trials. Each patient was randomized to a "CRT on" or a "CRT off" group. Follow-up during the randomized phases ranged from 3 to 6 months in duration.

When the data from all the RCTs were pooled, CRT was found to be associated with a statistically significant 51% reduction in mortality from progressive HF, the mortality rates being 1.7% for CRT patients vs 3.5% for controls (OR: 0.49; 95% C.I. 0.25–0.93).

Moreover, CRT was associated with a trend towards lower all-cause mortality (OR: 0.77; 95% C.I. 0.51–1.18). CRT had no clear impact on ventricular tachycardia (VT) and ventricular fibrillation (VF) (OR:0.92; 95% C.I. 0.67–1.27).

The conclusions of the meta-analysis were:

- CRT, acting through a significant reduction of the most common mechanism of death (irreversible HF) in HF patients, may have a substantial impact on mortality.
- CRT shows a trend towards reducing all-cause mortality, even if we do not know the exact additive role of β–blockers and ICD.

At the ACC meeting in Chicago, March 2003, Bristow et al. [6] presented the results of the COMPANION (Comparison of Medical Therapy, Pacing and Defibrillation in Chronic Heart Failure) trial, which was halted prematurely in November 2002 when the trial's DSMB projected that the study would reach its primary end-point ahead of schedule.

COMPANION is a parallel RCT in 1,600 patients with moderate/severe HF (NYHA 3-4, LV EF ≤ 35%), ischemic or nonischemic cardiomyopathy, and QRS duration > 120 ms, PR >150 ms.

Patients were randomized in a 1:2:2 fashion to an optimal medical treatment for HF (β-blockers + ACEi or ARBs + diuretics + spironolactone ± digoxin), optimal medical treatment + CRT, or optimal medical treatment + CRT with ICD.

The primary end-point of the trial, a composite of all-cause deaths and all-cause admissions to hospital, over 12 months was significantly reduced by 19% in both the CRT and the CRT/ICD arms.

CRT was associated with a nonsignificant trend towards reduction of 23.9% in all-cause mortality, and CRT with ICD was associated with a highly significant reduction of 43.4% in all-cause mortality, a secondary end-point of the study. Moreover, the investigators found no difference in outcomes between ischemic and nonischemic patients.

These very preliminary data of the COMPANION trial are of course very exciting (it is the first trial to demonstrate reduction in morbidity + mortality by CRT or CRT/ICD and also the first trial to demonstrate a reduction in all-cause mortality by CRT/ICD in a general HF population), albeit incomplete (the outcome of the dropout patients, the rate of crossover, and the numbers of deaths in the different treatment arms are still unknown, for example) or somewhat inconclusive. (Approximately 80% of all the events contributing to the primary end-point were related to all-cause admissions to hospital, a "soft" end-point that could be open to patient and investigator bias; nor is it yet clear how patients should be selected for an ICD, which is very costly in terms of money and morbidity, or whether other treatments might be just as effective).

Only a few days ago, another trial examining the efficacy and safety of devices combining CRT and ICD capabilities was published: the MIRACLE ICD trial [7, 8], in which 369 patients with LV EF <35%, QRS duration >130 ms, NYHA class III–IV, and high risk of life-threatening ventricular arrhythmias were randomized. In the study report, Young et al. [7] demonstrated that patients assigned to CRT+ICD experienced a greater improvement in quality-of-life score (–17.5 vs –11) and functional class (–1 vs 0) than did patients assigned to ICD only, but in contrast with previous studies there was no difference in distance walked in 6 min (55 m vs 53 m), in LV size and function, in overall HF status, or in rates of hospital admission (these findings underscore the importance of better performance in patient selection, better placement of the LV lead tip, and better programming of the device).

Importantly, the trial showed that CRT does not interfere with ICD function. Finally, while the trial was not specifically designed to address the question of whether CRT+ICD therapy decreases mortality, no statistical difference in survival between the treatments was observed.

What We Will Know in the Near Future?

The results in terms of the impact of CRT on mortality seem to be very promising, but as we have seen, there is still some uncertainty, which we hope will disappear when we know the results of the CARE HF trial [9] and of the SCDHeFT trial [10] even if CRT is not applied in the last-named study.

The primary outcomes of the CARE HF Study, in which 800 patients were enrolled, are death plus hospital admission due to major cardiovascular events, judged by a blinded committee. In 2004, the results of the trial will give robust evidence of any morbidity and/or mortality benefit of CRT. Moreover CARE HF is one of the largest studies in terms of patient numbers, and particularly of patients randomized to the control groups, of duration of follow-up, and of reduced investigator biases.

Finally, in the SCDHeFT (Sudden Cardiac Death HF Trial) enrollment has just been completed of 2,500 patients with dilated cardiomyopathy of any etiology (class II–III, EF ≤35%) randomized to placebo, amiodarone, or ICD, followed up for a minimum of 2.5 years. The primary aim of the study is to compare all-cause mortality.

References

1. Bradley DJ, Bradley EA, Baughman KL et al (2003) Cardiac resynchronization and death from progressive heart failure. A meta-analysis of randomized clinical trials. JAMA 289:730–740
2. US Food and Drug Administration (2002) Summary of safety and effectiveness: Guidant Contak CD CRT-D system (report). Available at http://www.fda.gov/cdrh/pdf/ p010012.html
3. US Food and Drug Administration (2002) Summary of safety and effectiveness: Medtronic Insync ICD Model 7272 (report). Available at http://www.fda.gov/ohrms/dockets/ac/02/briefing/3843b2.htm
4. Abraham WT, Fisher WG, Smith AL et al (2002) Cardiac resynchronization in chronic heart failure. N Engl J Med 346:1845–1853
5. Cazeau S, Leclerq C, Lavergne T et al (2001) Effects of multisite biventricular pacing in patients with heart failure and intraventricular conduction delay. N Engl J Med 344:873–880
6. Bristow MR, Saxon LA, Boehmer JP et al (2003) Cardiac resynchronization therapy reduces hospitalization and cardiac resynchronization therapy and an implantable defibrillator reduces mortality in chronic heart failure: results of the COMPANION trial. Paper presented at: American College of Cardiology 52nd Annual Scientific Session, 30 March to 2 April 2003, Chicago
7. Young JB, Abraham WT, Smith AL et al (2003) Combined cardiac resynchronization and implantable cardioversion defibrillation in advanced heart failure. The MIRACLE ICD Trial. JAMA 289:2685–2694
8. Bradley DJ (2003) Combining resynchronization and defibrillation therapies for heart failure. JAMA 289:2719–2721
9. Cleland JGF, Daubert JC, Erdmann E et al (2001) The CARE-HF study: rationale, design and end-points. Eur J Heart Failure 3:481–489
10. Klein H, Auricchio A, Reek S et al (1999) New primary prevention trials of sudden cardiac death in patients with left ventricular dysfunction: SCD-HEFT and MADIT II. Am J Cardiol 83:91D–97D

COMPANION Study: Rationale

D. S. Cannom

The heart failure pandemic afflicts 5 million people in the United States, accounts for 900,000 hospitalizations and causes or contributes to 300,000 deaths per years [1-3]. Pharmacologic therapy reduces heart failure progression, morbidity and mortality but still leaves many patients with symptoms and shortened survival. Thus any new modality such as cardiac resynchronization therapy (with or without backup defibrillation) has important implications for patient clinical status and, perhaps, survival.

The major completed controlled trials of cardiac resynchronization therapy (CRT) and CRT with an implantable cardioverter defibrillator (CRT-D) have similar inclusion criteria: New York Heart Association (NYHA) symptoms of class II to IV, left ventricle ejection factor (LVEF) < 35 %, prolonged QRS duration (> 120-150 msec), exclusion of patients having pacemaker indications and stability of medical therapy for heart failure prior to their enrollment [4]. These studies asked limited investigational questions since their purpose was to achieve FDA approval for device market release. Thus, the studies were designed to evaluate the safety and efficacy of CRT or CRT-D compared to no CRT/CRT-D for a period of 3-6 months. Morbidity and mortality were not a primary or secondary endpoint of any of these studies with the exception of the COMPANION and CARE-HF trials. The majority of the completed trials identified functional status, exercise capacity and quality of life as primary efficacy endpoints.

CRT appears to have a favorable effect on functional status and quality of life. It is associated with significant improvement in exercise capacity. Its effect on systolic function is improved, with little effect on diastolic function or LV mass. However, study durations have been short. Data on hospitalization was not consistent and only the MIRACLE trial demonstrated a reduction in hospitalization heart failure [5].

The need for a more comprehensive randomized clinical trial that addressed the critical issues of morbidity (i.e. hospitalization for congestive

Department of Cardiology, Good Samaritan Hospital, Los Angeles, California, USA heart failured (CHF)) and mortality was apparent. COMPANION was the largest and most ambitious resynchronization trial ever undertaken and the first to study the composite endpoint of death and hospitalization as its primary endpoint [6]. All COMPANION patients were on a maximal medical regimen so that any benefits of CRT could be attributed to the device.

The COMPANION study was a parallel, randomized, open-label, 3-arm study undertaken in 128 centers throughout the United States. Inclusion criteria consisted of the following:

- NYHA class III or IV heart failure
- normal sinus rhythm
- QRS duration of > 120 ms and PR interval > 150 ms
- left ventricular ejection fraction ≤ 35 %
- left ventricular end-diastolic dimension ≥ 60 mm

All patients required hospitalization for heart failure within 12 months prior to randomization. Again, all patients received Optimal Pharmacological Therapy (OPT) consisting of a beta-blocker for > 3 months (unless they were intolerant); a diuretic if needed; an angiotensin-converting enzyme inhibitor or an angiotensin receptor blocker; and spironolactone (for 1 month) with or without digoxin (Fig. 1).

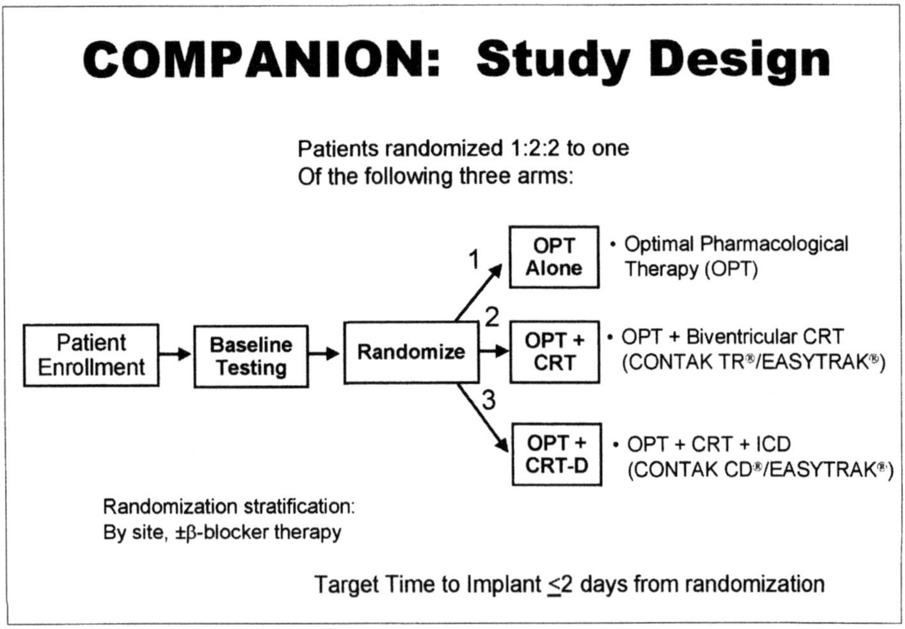

Fig. 1. COMPANION Randomization Scheme. Shown is the COMPANION study design. After baseline testing and surmising medical therapy, there was a 1:2:2 randomization to optimal pharmacological therapy (OPT), OPT plus a biventricular chronic resynchronization device, or OPT and a chronic resynchronization device with an ICD

The ratio for randomization was 1:2:2. For every one patient randomized to OPT alone (controls), two were randomized to OPT plus biventricular CRT and two to OPT plus CRT with ICD (CRT-D). Randomization was stratified based on study center and beta-blocker therapy. Target time to implant was ≤ 2 days from randomization [6].

The primary composite endpoint of COMPANION was all-cause death and all-cause hospitalization (except elective admissions for CRT to CRT-D, including treatment for decompensated heart failure with vasoactive drugs for a period of > 4 hours in an urgent-care setting). Secondary endpoints included all-cause mortality, hospitalization due to heart failure and maximal exercise. Tertiary endpoints included submaximal exercise and quality of life.

It was statistically forecast that an enrollment of 2200 patients would be required to see the 1000 events required for the study's predefined primary endpoint. However, enrollment was halted at 1634 patients in November 2002 after the study's Data and Safety Monitoring Board reported that the prespecified number of events had been achieved. Final and complete data collection and analysis of the COMPANION study are still ongoing, including a cost analysis. Enrollment had been extremely slow in the last months of the trial due to the availability of market released CRT devices. However, the very high event rate in the OPT arm allowed achievement of the endpoint (see below).

The data from the COMPANION trial has not been published; yet, the preliminary data as presented at the American College of Cardiology March 2003 is of extreme interest. It appears that CRT alone has a positive effect on rehospitalization while CRT-D has a substantial impact on mortality reduction (see above). Both ischemic and nonischemic populations benefit equally from the therapy. More sophisticated analysis–including effects on LV function and remodeling and the nature, if any, of the interaction between the ICD and CRT–await the publication of the the main study and the many substudies to follow.

References

1. Hunt SA, Baker DW, Chin MH et al (2001) ACC/AHA Guidelines for the evaluation and management of chronic heart failure in the adult: executive summary. Circulation 104:2996-3007
2. Cleland JGF, Khand A, Clark AL (2001) The heart failure epidemic: exactly how big is it? Eur J Heart Fail 22:623-626
3. Kannel WB, Belanger AJ (1991) Epidemiology of heart failure. Am Heart J 121:951-957
4. From Resynchronization Therapy for Heart Failure Expert Consensus Conference held at NASPE's 23rd Annual Scientific Session (2002) held in San Diego, California.
5. St John Sutton MG, Plappert TJ, Abraham WT et al (2002) Cardiac resynchronization therapy results in improvement in echocardiographic parameters in heart failure patients: evidence from MIRACLE and MIRACLE ICD trials. J Cardiac Fail (8(4):abstract 034

6. Bristow MR, Feldman AM, Saxon LA (2000) Heart failure management using implantable devices for ventricular resynchronization: comparison of medical therapy, pacing, and defibrillation in chronic heart failure (COMPANION) trial. J Card Fail 6:276-285

Pharmacological Therapy in COMPANION Study: Compliance and Dosage

A. Boccanelli, G. Cacciatore

Physiopathological Basis of Pharmacological Therapy for Congestive Heart Failure

A widely used definition of heart failure is 'failure of the heart to maintain systemic perfusion commensurate with the requirements of metabolizing tissues.' This definition and view of myocardial failure dominated the development of medical treatment strategies for the clinical syndrome of heart failure between the mid-1960s and the mid-1980s (the cardiorenal model), and the pharmacological approaches in this period were designed to bring about an acute increase in the performance of weakened heart muscle. Myocardial systolic dysfunction is best demonstrated as a downward and rightward shift in the Frank–Starling relation or a plot of preload or resting length versus myocardial performance. It was largely because positive inotropic agents can acutely shift the cardiac output/preload relation upward and to the left that the initial attempts to improve the natural history of chronic heart failure (CHF) took the form of these types of pharmacological therapy.

As physicians began to perform careful hemodynamic measurements, it became apparent that heart failure was associated with a reduced cardiac output and excessive peripheral vasoconstriction. This latter realization led to development of the cardiocirculatory or hemodynamic model, according to which heart failure arises largely as a result of altered pumping capacity of the heart and excessive peripheral vasoconstriction.

Between 1986 and 1993, multiple clinical trials were conducted with vasodilators, positive inotropic agents, or 'inodilators' as strategies for enhancing systolic performance, and all resulted in worsening of the natural history of CHF. Furthermore, the disappointing clinical outcome of these trials appears to have been due to long-term adverse effects on the heart, inasmuch

Cardiology Department, San Giovanni Hospital, Rome, Italy

as many or most aspects of the clinical syndrome of heart failure–such as exercise tolerance, symptoms, and hemodynamics–were initially improved by these agents. Although the precise nature of the adverse cardiac effects of these agents is not known, an acceleration of the processes leading to arrhythmic/ sudden death was observed in some studies. In addition, a common feature of agents that increase myocardial performance by pharmacological means is that they use components of β-adrenergic pathways to increase contractility or they indirectly activate neurohormonal/autocrine-paracrine compensatory mechanisms in response to vasodilatation. Thus, although the cardiorenal model provided the rational basis for the use of diuretics to control the volume status of patients with heart failure, and the cardiocirculatory model provided the rational basis for the use of inotropes and intravenous vasodilators to augment cardiac output, these medications all carried the potential to produce adverse effects on the biology of the heart, without prolonging the life of patients with moderate to severe heart failure.

On the basis of the above arguments, it has become apparent that heart failure can no longer be defined in simple hemodynamic terms. Indeed, what has become increasingly apparent is that at some point in the overall pathogenesis of heart failure, the disease will progress independently of the patient's hemodynamic status [1]. Heart failure may be viewed as a progressive disorder that is initiated after an index event either damages the heart muscle, with a resultant loss of functioning cardiac myocytes or, alternatively, disrupts the ability of the myocardium to generate force. Regardless of the nature of the initiating event, the feature that is common to each of these index events is that they all produce a decline in the pumping capacity of the heart. In most instances, patients will remain asymptomatic or minimally symptomatic following the initial decline in pumping capacity of the heart, or will develop symptoms only after the dysfunction has been present for some time. Thus, when viewed within this conceptual framework, left-ventricular (LV) dysfunction is necessary but not sufficient for the development of the syndrome of heart failure.

Many compensatory mechanisms are activated in the setting of cardiac injury, which are able to sustain and modulate LV function for periods ranging from days to months or even years: early activation of the sympathetic nervous system and salt- and water-retaining systems in order to preserve cardiac output, and activation of a family of vasodilatory molecules, including natriuretic peptides, prostaglandins (PGE_2 and $PGEI_2$), and nitric oxide.

At some point patients will become overtly symptomatic, with a resultant striking increase in morbidity and mortality. Why this transition to symptomatic heart failure occurs, exactly how it occurs, and whether it occurs in all patients with LV dysfunction remain unknown. What is known, however, is that the transition to symptomatic heart failure is accompanied by further activation of neurohormonal and cytokine systems, and also a series of adaptive changes within the myocardium, which are collectively referred to as LV remodeling. Although there are further modest declines in the overall pumping capacity of the heart during the transition to symptomatic heart failure, the weight of experimental and clinical evidence suggests that heart failure progression occurs independently of the hemodynamic status of the patient. Accordingly, it becomes difficult to ascribe the transition to symptomatic heart failure to worsening LV function alone.

Thus, heart failure should be viewed as a neurohormonal model [2], in which disease progresses as a result of the overexpression of biologically active molecules that are capable of exerting toxic effects on the heart and circulation. Thus far, a variety of proteins, including norepinephrine, angiotensin II, endothelin, aldosterone, and tumor necrosis factor (TNF) have been implicated as some of the potentially biologically active molecules whose biochemical properties are sufficient to contribute to disease progression in the failing heart. Many of the so-called classic neurohormones, such as norepinephrine and angiotensin II, are synthesized directly within the myocardium, and thus act in an autocrine and paracrine manner. Furthermore, molecules such as angiotensin II, endothelin, and TNF are peptide growth factors and/or cytokines produced by a variety of nucleated cell types within the heart, including cardiac myocytes, and thus do not necessarily have a neuroendocrine origin. Nonetheless, the important unifying concept that arises from the neurohormonal model is that the overexpression of biologically active molecules can contribute to disease progression independently of the hemodynamic status of the patient, by virtue of the direct toxic effects that these molecules exert on the heart and circulation. The evidence in support of this point of view is derived from two lines of investigation. First, many experimental models have shown that pathophysiologically relevant concentrations of neurohormones are sufficient to mimic some aspects of the heart failure phenotype. Secondly, data generated from clinical trials indicate that antagonizing neurohormones lead to clinical improvement in patients with heart failure. In particular, ACE inhibitors and β-blockers have shown their ability to prevent the progression of pump dysfunction that characterizes the natural history of heart failure. Unexpectedly and remarkably, β-blockade may substantially improve pump function in the long term. It is important to emphasize that the beneficial effects of these treatments are not pharmacological but rather are due to favorable effects on the biology of the failing heart [3]. Thus, one logical explanation for why heart failure progresses is that long-term activation of a variety of neurohormonal mechanisms produces direct end-organ damage within the heart and circulation. Accordingly, progressive activation of neurohormonal mechanisms may explain why heart failure can develop insidiously many years after an acute myocardial infarction, despite the absence of ongoing ischemia. The neurohormonal model also explains why the so-called heart failure phenotype appears to be remarkably consistent in patients with different etiologies of their heart failure, insofar as disease progression is ultimately driven by very similar portfolios of biologically active molecules, regardless of the immediate cause.

Drug Therapy for Heart Failure

Drugs available for the management of heart failure will be reviewed with reference to the clinical trials (Table 1).

Table 1. Drugs for heart failure: their effects on quality of life and survival

Drugs	Quality of life	Survival
Digitalis	↑	↔
Inotropes	↑	↓
Diuretics	↑	?
ACE inhibitors	↑	↑
Direct vasodilators	↑	↔
β–blockers	↔→↑	↑
Calcium-channel blockers	↔	↔
Amiodarone	↔	↔

Inotropic Agents

A series of trials have shown that digitalis can exert beneficial effects on functional capacity, symptoms, and LV function. The effect of digoxin on survival of patients with heart failure was the primary end-point of DIG Trial, in which 6800 patients with LV ejection fraction (EF) <45% who were already taking an ACE inhibitor and a diuretic were enrolled [4]. Follow-up at 3–5 years showed no net impact on all-cause or cardiovascular mortality, with a lower incidence of mortality from progressive heart failure (–12 %) offset by an increased risk of presumably arrhythmic death. There was a substantial favorable effect of digoxin on the combined end-point of death or hospital admissions for worsening heart failure (–28 %).

On these grounds, digitalis is now considered a useful drug in the treatment of heart failure, not only as an agent able to increase reduced myocardial contractility, but rather as a drug able to decrease sympathetic nervous system activity and catecholamine sensitivity.

Unlike all other inotropic drugs, digitalis is recommended and widely used in patients with persistent symptoms after optimized therapy with ACE inhibitors and diuretics.

Inotropic agents such as β–adrenergic agonists and phosphodiesterase inhibitors are reserved for patients with acutely decompensated heart failure, patients refractory to standard oral therapy, and patients on transplant waiting lists. In such conditions even drugs that have not shown favorable effects on mortality have improved morbidity and quality of life in the short term.

Diuretics

Diuretics are deemed essential in the treatment of heart failure, as they bring about a rapid improvement in both clinical and hemodynamic terms in most patients with CHF. Benefits induced by diuretics are due not only to the increased renal water and sodium excretion, but also to hemodynamic changes. Indeed several studies have shown that clinical improvement induced by diuretic therapy is associated with a favorable hemodynamic profile (venodilatation, reduced ventricular filling pressure, and improvement of cardiac performance).

Although their effects on long-term survival of patients with heart failure have never been studied or documented, most of the patients in trials of ACE inhibitors and β–blockers in which significantly reduced mortality was demonstrated were taking diuretic drugs. However, knowledge of both potential problems and potential benefits can lead to safer and more effective use of these agents.

Renin-Angiotensin System Inhibitors in Congestive Heart Failure

The most important advance in treatment of congestive heart failure during the last two decades has been the utilization of ACE inhibitors. After the publication of the results of the Consensus Study [5], the SOLVD Treatment [6] and the V-HeFTII Trials, ACE inhibitors became a standard of care for symptomatic patients with reduced EF. This recommendation was strengthened by a meta-analysis of 32 published and unpublished studies involving 7105 patients and 1320 fatal events. Overall there was a 23% reduction in deaths and a 35% decrease in deaths plus hospital admission for heart failure. The SOLVD Prevention Trial, conducted in parallel with the SOLVD Treatment Trial, focused on patients with an EF $\leq$ 35% and few symptoms or none at all. Although there was no significant reduction in mortality (risk reduction 8%), there was a highly significant 37% decrease in the risk of developing overt heart failure and a 44% reduction in the risk of hospitalization for heart failure. Indeed, the mortality curves from the treatment trial appear similar to those in the prevention trial, shifted 18 months to the right. Taken together, these studies support the impression that ACE inhibitors slow the progression both of LV dilatation and dysfunction and of worsening symptoms and prognosis.

For patients who are intolerant of ACE inhibitors, angiotensin receptor antagonists are an effective alternative. Like ACE inhibitors, these drugs reduce systemic vascular resistance and LV filling pressure and increase the cardiac index, while effects on exercise duration and symptoms are modest. The ELITE Study suggested a survival benefit of losartan over captopril, but ELITE II failed to demonstrate the superiority of angiotensin receptor blockade. For heart failure patients who remain symptomatic with ACE inhibitor therapy the addition of an angiotensin receptor antagonist theoretically has the potential for maximal blockade of activation of the renin–angiotensin system (RAS). The recently completed Val-Heft Trial examined >5000 patients with mild to moderate heart failure and showed that valsartan, when added to an ACE inhibitor, reduced the frequency of admission to hospital with heart failure by 28% but had no effect on mortality. A trend toward worse outcome was observed in patients taking a β–blocker in addition to an ACE inhibitor and an angiotensin receptor blocker. The CHARM Study is currently under way to evaluate the survival benefit of candesartan when added to an ACE inhibitor. An important arm of the study will address optimal RAS blockade in patients with diastolic heart failure.

Despite treatment with an ACE inhibitor or angiotensin receptor antagonists, patients with heart failure may demonstrate elevated aldosterone levels. Mechanisms of 'aldosterone escape' include alternative stimuli for aldosterone synthesis (e.g., adrenocorticotropic hormone and endothelin), potassium-dependent aldosterone secretion, and reduced aldosterone clearance. Recent evidence suggests that spirololactone, an aldosterone receptor blocker, is safe and effective in treating patients with heart failure. The RALES study, in which > 1600 patients with severe heart failure and low EF were randomized to receive spironolactone or placebo, was stopped early because of a 30% reduction of mortality in the spironolactone group [7]. In addition, spironolactone improved symptoms and reduced the number of admissions to hospital for heart failure.

Direct Vasodilators

The augmented preload and afterload in patients with heart failure led us to consider whether direct vasodilator drugs might be useful. Some of these are active on the arterial system (minoxidil, hydralazine, prazosin, calcium-channel blockers) and others on the venous system (nitrates), while still others have a mixed action (nitroprusside, flosequinan, ACE inhibitors).

Overall, the results obtained with direct vasodilators in the treatment of congestive heart failure have not been definitely convincing. The PROFILE Trial (Prospective Randomized Flosequinan Longevity Evaluation) was stopped prematurely because of an excess of mortality in the group of patients treated with flosequinan. The FIRST (Flolan International Randomized Survival Trial) showed a similarly unfavorable effect of epoprostenol on long-term survival.

In contrast, V-HeFTI (Vasodilator Heart Failure Trial I) showed that with the combination of hydralazine and isosorbide dinitrate (mean doses 270 and 136 mg/day, respectively) mortality was significantly lower (–34%) than with digitalis and diuretics or with conventional therapy plus prazosin. The results of this trial showed for the first time that a pharmacological treatment could have a positive influence on the survival of patients with CHF. The results obtained were initially attributed to hemodynamic changes induced by the combination of hydralazine and isosorbide dinitrate. Subsequently, however, it was realized that different mechanisms could explain the clinical efficacy of the combination of these two drugs: an antiremodeling effect of nitrates and a reduction of nitrate tolerance induced by hydralazine.

Important considerations about the efficacy of direct vasodilators compared with ACE inhibitors emerged from the results of V-HeFTII. In this trial the combination of hydralazine and isosorbide dinitrate did not have such a favorable effect on survival as did enalapril (total mortality −28%, sudden death −19%), but its effect on LV function and exercise capacity was better than that of enalapril.

Calcium-channel blockers, despite the favorable hemodynamic changes they can induce, were not able to improve the morbidity and mortality of patients with CHF, because of their negative inotropic effect and unfavorable neurohormonal activation. It was suggested that second- and third-generation calcium-channel blockers could be better tolerated and more effective because of their selectivity and lesser negative inotropic effect. In V-HeFTIII the use of felodipine was not associated with any clinical improvement; nor did any significant difference in mortality from placebo emerge on comparison. In the PRAISE trial (Prospective Randomized Amlodipine Survival Evaluation) amlodipine induced a positive trend in mortality (−16%) and had a particularly significant effect (−46%) in the subgroup of patients with idiopathic dilated cardiomyopathy. However, the PRAISE II trial was not able to confirm these results. Finally, MACH I (Mortality Assessment in Congestive Heart Failure) showed that the use of mibefradil, a selective T-calcium-channel blocker, was associated with an increase in mortality, so that the drug was withdrawn.

β-Blockers

After ACE inhibitors, β–blockers are the other class of drugs for which a favorable influence on the natural history of CHF has been ascertained. While they were initially regarded as contraindicated in CHF, during the two last decades it has been clearly demonstrated that they can improve functional class and LV structure and function.

While CIBIS I (Cardiac Insufficiency Bisoprolol Study I), the MDC Trial (Metoprolol in Dilated Cardiomyopathy), and the ANZ Trial (Australia/New Zealand Heart Failure Research Collaborative Study Group) did not demonstrate any clear effect of bisoprolol, metoprolol and carvedilol, respectively, on mortality, larger studies have shown a definite effect of β–blockers on mortality. Indeed, the US Carvedilol Heart Failure Trials Program demonstrated a large reduction in mortality (−6 5%, $p < 0.001$), a significantly lower frequency of hospitalization for cardiovascular reasons (−27%), and a significantly lower combined risk of death plus hospitalization for cardiovascular causes in the treatment group than in the placebo group [8]. In CIBIS II the risk reduction in overall mortality was 34%, the decrease in sudden death amounted to 44%, and the frequency of need for admission to hospital in heart failure was reduced by 36%. In MERIT-HF (Metoprolol CR/XL Randomized Intervention Trial in Congestive Heart Failure) similar results were obtained: reduced mortality (–35%), with reductions in both sudden death (–41%) and death from worsening heart failure (–49%). In a meta-analysis of 22 trials involving 10135 patients with CHF, the odds ratio for death 0.65 with β–blockers and the odds ratio for hospitalization for heart failure was 0.64. These ratios translate into 3.8 lives saved and 4 admissions to hospital avoided for every 100 patients treated for 1 year.

The large clinical trials touched on above were conducted mainly in patients with mild to moderate CHF, and only 5% of the patients included in the meta-analysis were in NYHA class IV. The effects of β–blocker therapy in severe CHF has recently been studied in the COPERNICUS (Carvedilol Prospective Randomized Cumulative Survival) Trial, in which 2289 patients with III–IV NYHA class CHF and with EF < 25% were enrolled [9]. The trial was stopped prematurely because of a significant 35% reduction in the risk of death and a 24% reduction in combined risk of death and hospitalization in the treatment group compared with placebo. Beneficial effects of carvedilol were also observed in a subgroup of high-risk patients, meaning those with LV EF ≤ 15% or at least three hospitalizations for heart failure in the previous year.

In the BEST trial (Beta Blocker Evaluation of Survival Trial), patients with NYHA classes III and IV were randomly assigned to placebo or bucindolol. Although the survival analysis showed a trend in favor of the β–blocker, it was not statistically significant. This result is surprising in the face of all the other trials, but it is not jarring as it first appears. First, the confidence interval around the primary end-point of death from any cause overlaps those of other trials. Secondly, an improvement in survival was observed in nonblack patients. Finally, results for many of the secondary end-points favored bucindolol, which induced a decrease in the mortality form cardiac causes, the combined end-point of death from any cause or from cardiac transplantation, and in hospital admissions for heart failure.

Therefore, on the grounds of the results of these two studies and of the favorable results obtained in the CAPRICORN (Carvedilol Post-Infarct Survival Control in LV Dysfunction) trial, in which patients with postischemic LV dysfunction were randomized to carvedilol or placebo, β–blockers have clearly shown their ability to decrease mortality in a wide spectrum of systolic heart failure, ranging from mild to severe heart failure. However, the introduction of β–blockers into the therapy requires strict selection criteria for the patients, who must be in a consolidated stable condition with no need for intensive care, in a euvolemic state (without cardiac disease-related rales, ascites or more than minimal edema despite optimal treatment with diuretics). Furthermore, administration of β–blockers requires careful surveillance of the patient during the titration phase, for which hospitalization may sometimes be required, and the dose must be gradually escalated according to a strategy consistent with our understanding of the support of the failing heart by the adrenergic nervous system. Finally, contraindications must be kept in mind (reactive airways disease, sinus node dysfunction, abnormalities in cardiac conduction system, etc.).

Antiarrhythmic Drugs

An unsolved problem in the management of patients with CHF is the treatment of ventricular arrhythmias and prevention of sudden death. The most favorable results have been obtained with β–blockers: in CIBIS II and MERIT-HF bisoprolol and metoprolol reduced the rate of sudden death (-44% and -41%, respectively). Therefore, the most appropriate therapy seems to be a wide use of β–blockers, combined with the use of amiodarone in patients with frequent and complex arrhythmias, in whom the implantation of an antiarrhyhmic implantable cardioverter defibrillator (AICD) is not indicated. These two drugs have a synergetic effect and are generally well tolerated when administered at low doses.

In contrast, the use of class I antiarrhythmic drugs is absolutely contraindicated owing to their negative inotropic effect and to their demonstrated negative effect on survival.

Pharmacological Treatment of Chronic Heart Failure in Clinical Practice

Guidelines for the pharmacological treatment of CHF [10] indicate that in patients with asymptomatic LV dysfunction (NYHA class I), the only therapy whose efficacy has been clearly ascertained is treatment with ACE inhibitors. Therefore, these drugs must be administered to all patients with this condition, as they have shown their ability to prevent or delay the development of overt heart failure.

In symptomatic patients (NYHA II–IV) the conventional therapy is a combination of ACE inhibitors and diuretics, with digitalis in addition in persistently symptomatic patients. The dose of the ACE inhibitor used must be progressively escalated up to the maximal tolerated dose. In contrast, the dose of diuretic can be adapted to the individual patient's clinical condition, varying with the signs of peripheral and pulmonary fluid retention.

In the light of the results of the mortality trials with β–blockers published since compilation of the most recent guidelines, these drugs have assumed a well-defined role in the treatment of patients with CHF. Indeed, β–blockers are indicated in all patients with symptomatic LV systolic dysfunction, apart from any patients with clear-cut contraindications. Therapy with β–blockers must be started early, in stable patients already receiving optimized therapy with ACE inhibitors, diuretics, and digitalis if necessary. Low initial doses must be increased slowly and progressively (start low and go slow), with careful clinical monitoring, up to the maximal tolerated dose. Angiotensin receptor antagonists have not proved superior to ACE inhibitors, and it is not yet certain whether their addition to ACE inhibitors and/or β-blockers offers any advantage. Therefore, at the moment, their utilization is limited to patients with contraindications to or intolerance of ACE inhibitors. Since publication of the RALES study, use of an aldosterone receptor antagonist such as spironolactone has been considered indicated in patients with severe CHF who are already receiving optimized treatment. Future studies will address the role of such antagonists in less advanced cases of CHF. In the past, the combination of hydralazine and isosorbide dinitrate was suggested as an alternative therapy for patients who were intolerant of ACE inhibitors. At present, angiotensin receptor antagonists have been introduced but this combination has not been officially recommended. However, nitrates can be used in patients who are refractory to optimized treatment and in patients with heart failure and angina. Although therapy with inotropic nondigitalis drugs is generally not recommended, the administration of these drugs has a well-defined role in patients refractory to conventional oral treatment and in patients with multiorgan failure who are on a transplant waiting list. In these circumstances the main goal of therapy is quality of life (reduction of symptoms) rather than quantity of life (prolonging survival).

Conclusions

Although large clinical trials have shown that medical therapy can prevent LV dysfunction from degenerating into overt heart failure and can slow the progression of the clinical disease to the most severe forms of refractory heart failure, we are now facing a marked increase both in the prevalence of heart failure and in its morbidity and mortality. It has been estimated that heart failure affects 4.6 million patients in the United States, with 550,000 new cases each year, and 22.5 million patients throughout the world. Almost 1 million patients with a primary diagnosis of heart failure are discharged from U.S. hospitals each year, making this condition the most common reason for hospitalization in the Medicare (≥65 years) population. The 5-year mortality is about 50%, and from 1979 to 1998 heart failure deaths increased by 135%. There are an estimated 3 million outpatient visits, and the annual total cost of this disease has reached $ 21 billion. Because of the aging of the population these numbers can be expected to rise.

The apparent paradox can be explained by the efficacy of modern treatment of heart disease in reducing acute deaths from acute myocardial infarction, arrhythmias and complications of arterial hypertension. Furthermore, as we all live longer, there is a growing population of older people who are more vulnerable to the development of heart failure because of the loss of myocytes caused by apoptosis.

Other issues can explain the discrepancy: for example the slow introduction of new drugs into clinical practice. Notwithstanding the definite recommendation that ACE inhibitors be used in all forms of LV dysfunction, these drugs are still not uniformly prescribed and are often used at too-low doses. The same is true for β–blockers. It is assumed that one-third of patients in whom they are indicated do not receive ACE inhibitors and that two-thirds do not receive β–blockers.

Furthermore, beyond the indications included in guidelines, the medicamentous treatment of the individual patient must be tailored according to the etiology of his or her heart disease and the pathophysiology of heart failure. Because of the fluctuating nature of the disease, in which overt heart failure alternates with relative improvement, close follow-up is needed so that the use of individual drugs can be adapted to the patient's needs in each phase of the conditions. The efficacy of the medical treatment also depends on correct information supplied to the patient and the family on the severity of the disease, the potential benefits and risks of the therapy, and the necessity for strict compliance with the drug therapy and the prescribed lifestyle. Patients followed up in multidisciplinary programs definitely do better: their stays in hospital are fewer and shorter and they have a better quality of life than do patients followed up as part of a conventional care program.

Over the next few years, progress in the pharmacological treatment of CHF can be expected to result from more vigorous attempts at prevention of coronary heart disease, which is its most common cause, wider utilization of the currently available therapies, development of new blockers of neurohumoral mediators and cytochines and, finally, from novel therapies such as myocyte and gene replacement.

References

1. Mann DL (1999) Mechanisms and models in heart failure. Circulation 100:999–1008
2. Packer M (1992) The neurohormonal hypothesis: a theory to explain the mechanism of disease progression in heart failure. J Am Coll Cardiol 20:248–254
3. Eichhorn EJ, Bristow MR (1996) Medical therapy can improve the biologic properties of chronically failing heart: a new era in the treatment of heart failure. Circulation 94:2285–2296
4. The Digitalis Investigation Group (1997) The effect of digoxin on mortality and morbidity in patients with heart failure. N Engl J Med 336:525–533
5. The CONSENSUS Trial Study Group (1987) Effects of enalapril on mortality in severe congestive heart failure. Results of the Cooperative North Scandinavian Enalapril Survival Study (Consensus). N Engl J Med 316:1429–1435
6. The SOLVD Investigators (1991) Effect of enalapril on survival in patients with reduced left ventricular ejection fractions and congestive heart failure. N Engl J Med 325:293–302

7. Pitt B, Zannad F, Remme WJ et al for the Randomized Aldactone Evaluation Study Investigators (1999) The effect of spironolactone on morbidity and mortality in patients with severe heart failure. N Engl J Med 341:709–717
8. Packer M, Bristow MR, Cohn JN et al for the US Carvedilol Heart Failure Study Group (1996) The effect of carvedilol on morbidity and mortality in patients with chronic heart failure. N Engl J Med 334:1349–1355
9. Packer M, Coats AJS, Fowler MB et al (2001) Effect of carvedilol in severe chronic heart failure. N Engl J Med 344:1651–1658
10. Remme WJ (1997) The treatment of heart failure. (The Task Force of the Working Group on Heart Failure of the European Society of Cardiology) Eur Heart J 18:736–753

The Lesson from the COMPANION Study: How Large Is the Patient Population That May Benefit?

E.G. Gronda, M. Mangiavacchi, D. Pini, L. Genovese, L. Tomaello, B. Andreuzzi, A. Municinò

Nearly 5 million persons living in the United States have heart failure, with 550 000 new cases diagnosed annually. Heart failure is the only cardiovascular disease in which the prevalence is increasing; projections suggest that prevalence will increase two- to three-fold by the year 2010 [1]. This increase is probably the result of aging of the population and the successful treatment of acute coronary syndromes.

In addition to its increasing prevalence, heart failure continues to be characterized by frequent morbidity and unacceptably high mortality despite substantial advances in drug therapy [2]. Heart failure generally leads to death by one of two mechanisms: sudden death, or death from progressive heart failure. The relative proportion of patients dying from these two mechanisms varies with severity of heart failure. Patients with mild heart failure most commonly die suddenly, while patients who survive to the advanced stages of heart failure predominantly die of progression of heart failure – a gradual loss of ventricular function that leads to inadequate systemic perfusion and death.

A common finding in advanced heart failure is abnormal electrical activation or electrical ventricular dyssynchrony in an electrocardiogram. Ventricular dyssynchrony is manifested as prolongation of the QRS interval, often in the pattern of left bundle branch block. Prolongation of QRS interval has been associated with decreased cardiac function and increased mortality, and occurs in about 25% patients in the real-world heart failure population [3].

In recent years cardiac pacemakers have been modified in an effort to correct ventricular dyssynchrony, a treatment referred to as cardiac resynchronization therapy (CRT). Unlike traditional right ventricular pacing, cardiac resynchronization uses a left ventricular lead that is usually positioned in a coronary vein. The left ventricular lead ensures stimulation of the left ventricle at the time of right ventricular depolarization. Cardiac resynchronization enhances cardiac function, decreases myocardial oxygen consumption,

U.O. di Cardiologia Clinica e di Terapia dell'Insufficienza Cardiaca, Istituto Clinico Humanitas, Rozzano, Milan, Italy increases functional capacity, and improves quality of life. The effect of cardiac resynchronization on mortality, however, is uncertain. Moreover, it is not well established whether this therapy is able to affect positively both sudden death and heart failure death in the different clinical settings. Recent data from the literature address the possibility that CRT can decrease progression of heart failure and the related mortality [4].

One of the most burning controversies in the heart failure arena remains whether or not CRT and implantable cardioverter-defibrillators (ICDs) can provide real benefit in addition to optimized medical treatment including β-blockers, as heart failure patient populations enrolled in clinical trials present different severities of heart failure at the time of randomization. A useful insight into the consistency of prognosis and benefits from tested therapy in heart failure populations can be provided by comparing patient population characteristics and annual mortality rates in the published trials on advanced heart failure population.

Reviewing data from the RALES trial [5], it is worth noting that in the treatment arm only 90 patients enrolled as in NYHA class III–IV also received β-blockers, and that in this group 1-year mortality was 14% in comparison to 20% among patients not receiving β-blockers. These data are consistent with the annual mortality rate in 313 NYHA class IV patients (14.4%) treated with β-blockers in MERIT-HF, CIBIS 1994, CIBIS II trials[6].

Due to the need to better define the severity of heart failure and the efficacy of therapies, new criteria by which to assess the prognosis of heart failure have been proposed that include the number of hospital admissions for heart failure in the year before the patient's enrolment in the study [7]. In the COPERNICUS trial (Carvedilol Prospective Randomized Cumulative Survival study), a subgroup of 308 patients with advanced heart failure have been enrolled after recent or repeated hospital admissions due to worsening symptoms of heart failure [8]. In this patient population with more advanced heart failure, 1-year mortality was 24% in the placebo arm superimposable on the control arm population of the RALES trial, and 16% in the treated arm, providing proof of a benefit of β-blocker therapy in this setting, but also confirming that hospitalization for heart failure itself entails a worse prognosis, with annual high mortality rate despite β-blocker administration.

It is noteworthy that in post-myocardial-infarction patients with or without heart failure who have a reduced left ventricular ejection fraction (LVEF), placement of an ICD was shown to significantly improve survival in MADIT II (the second Multicenter Automatic Defibrillator Implantation Trial) [9]. However, all patients in this study had an ischemic etiology of their heart failure, and the use of an ICD alone was associated with evidence of increased heart-failure-related hospitalization. Thus, the COMPANION (Comparison of Medical Therapy, Pacing, and Defibrillation in Chronic Heart failure) trial has been designed to test the hypothesis that CRT, either alone or combined with an ICD (CRT-D), would significantly reduce all-cause mortality and all-cause hospitalization in heart failure patients.

The study was designed to be large enough to have mortality as an endpoint [10]. Patients averaged close to 67 years of age, LVEF was in the range of 22%, 70% had left bundle branch block, and QRS averaged 158 ms. In approximately 55%–60% of patients, an ischemic etiology underlays the heart failure. There were no significant differences in baseline variables between the three study groups.

An important aspect of the COMPANION trial was that all events that occurred after randomization counted toward the final endpoint. Inclusion criteria were: NYHA class III–IV heart failure symptoms, a QRS duration of 120 ms or greater, sinus rhythm, a PR interval greater than 150 ms, a LVEF of 35% or less, and LVEDD equal to 60 mm or greater. Patients were required to be on treatment with a stable dose of β-blockers for at least 3 months and stable doses of ACE inhibitors and diuretics, with or without digoxin. Patients eligible for enrollment in the trial had to have been hospitalized for heart failure for at least 1 month and not more than 12 months prior to enrollment. Trial patients were randomized in a 2:2:1 manner to receive either a CRT pacemaker, CRT in conjunction with an ICD (CRT+), or optimal pharmacologic therapy (OPT).

In the control arm were 308 patients; 66% were on treatment with β-blockers and 55% receiving spironolactone. In this group 1-year mortality was 19%. This mortality rate seems consistent with mortality reported in equivalent β-blocker cohorts with unstable advanced heart failure and therefore represents a reliable control group.

COMPANION Trial Results

The primary endpoint of the trial for both the CRT and CRT+ patients groups was a composite of all-cause mortality and hospitalization. The Data and Safety Monitoring Board stopped enrollment on 18 November 2002, when more than 1000 endpoints in a total of 1520 patients had been reached with a median follow-up of 16 months. The mean age of the patients in the trial was 66 years, 67% were male, and approximately 85% of the patients were in NYHA functional class III. The mean LVEF was 22%, the mean QRS duration was 156–159 ms, and left bundle branch block was present in approximately 70% of patients.

As mentioned, the primary endpoint was a composite of all-cause death and hospitalization. Approximately 67% of the patients in the OPT group met this endpoint during follow-up. The investigators reported that in the CRT group there was an 18.6% reduction in the combined endpoint compared with OPT, which was significant (p=0.015). The results were also favorable in the CRT+ group, in which there was a 19.3% reduction in the combined endpoint vs OPT, which was also significant (p=0.005).

Death occurred in 19% of patients in the OPT group, and there was a significant (43%) reduction in mortality with CRT+ vs OPT (p=0.002). On the other hand, CRT alone was associated with a 24% reduction in mortality compared with OPT, but this reduction did not meet statistical significance (p=0.12). Of note, both patients with ischemic and those with nonischemic cardiomyoprithy appeared to benefit from CRT.

While previous trials of CRT such as InSync and MIRACLE (Multicenter InSync Randomized Clinical Evaluation) [11] have shown improvements in functional status and quality of life, COMPANION is the first trial to show that the therapy is associated with a reduction in mortality. Mortality alone was significantly reduced in the CRT+ arm. We do not yet have any information regarding the breakdown of sudden cardiac death versus heart failure deaths in the trial, but certainly ICD therapy in conjunction with CRT could be expected to have an impact on both. CRT therapy by itself did not significantly reduce mortality, but the trend was toward a reduction, and there was a significant impact on combined hospitalization and mortality. This trial as well as the previously mentioned meta-analysis of several resynchronization trials [4] showed that hospitalizations are reduced in patients receiving CRT. Although no formal cost-effectiveness analyses have been conducted yet, a marked reduction in hospitalization for heart failure at follow-up will have a positive impact on the cost-benefit ratio of the therapy.

With the number of clinical trials previously reported that show functional improvements in patients receiving CRT, and the new information on reduction in mortality and hospitalizations deriving from COMPANION and other trials, CRT has become firmly established as an effective treatment for patients who have significant symptoms from heart failure despite OPT.

It is noteworthy that the mean age of the enrolled population is consistent with the age of the general heart failure population, and that the number of women is higher than in previous heart failure trials. On the basis of these observations, we can estimate that patients in NYHA class III–IV with a recent history of heart failure progression requiring supplementary intravenous therapy can undergo ICD or ICD combined with CRT treatment in order to reduce adverse events, which seem to peak at 12–18 months after hospital admission or hospital-like treatment, having an incidence of 40%–60% per year [12] .

In Lombardy, the population numbers about 9 million people and the number of hospital admissions for heart failure based on a DRG 127 coding were 35 000 in 1997 [13], with per years increase of 8% comparing the numbers of hospitals amissions in the previous years, according with other european reports [14]. This data may provide evidence that in the general population about 4000 heart failure hospital admissions occur per million inhabitants every year. Considering that diastolic dysfunction has been reported as the second cause of heart failure hosital admissione [15], it can be estimated that about 60% of heart failure patients seen in medical wards suffer because of systolic dysfunction. In this population, the prevalence of left or right bundle branch block is about 30% while a left ventricular ejection fraction below 30% is present in half of them regardeless of the aetiology (ischemic versus non ischemic) [3]. In this setting COMPANION criteria for CRT and CRT + ICD implantation can be easily fulfilled.

References

1. Bonneaux L, Barendregt JJ, Meeter K et al (1994) Estimated clinical morbidity due to ischemic heart disease and congestive heart failure: the future rise of heart failure. Am J Public Health 84:20-28
2. Stewart S, MacIntire K, Hole DJ, Capewell S, McMurray JJV (2001) More malignant than cancer? Five-year survival following a first hospital admission for heart failure. Eur J Heart failure 3:315–322
3. Baldesseroni S, Opasich C, Gorini M et al (2002) Left bundle branch block is associated with increased 1 year sudden and total morality rate in 5517 outpatients with congestive heart failure: a report from the Italian Network on Congestive Heart failure. Am Heart J 143:398–405
4. Bradley DJ, Bradley EA, Baughman KL et al (2003) Cardiac resynchronization and death from progressive heart failure. A meta-analysis of randomized controlled trials. JAMA 289:730–740
5. Pitt B, Zannad F, Remme WJ et al (1999) The effect of spironolactone on morbidity and mortality in patients with severe heart failure. N Engl J Med 341:709–717
6. Whorlow SL, Krum H (2000) Meta-analysis of beta blocker therapy on mortality in patients with NYHA Class IV chronic congestive heart failure. Am J Cardiol 86:886–889
7. Packer M (2001) Proposal for a new clinical end point to evaluate the efficacy of drugs and devices in the treatment of chronic heart failure. J Card Fail 7:176–182
8. Packer M , Coats AJS, Fowler MB, Katus HA, Krum HB et al (2001) Effect of carvedilol on survival in severe chronic heart failure. N Engl J Med 344:1651–1658
9. Moss AJ, Zareba W, Hall JW (2002) Prophylactic implantation of a defibrillator in patients with myocardial infarction and reduced ejection fraction. N Engl J Med 348:877–883
10. Bristow MR, Feldman AM, Saxon LA, for the COMPANION Steering Committee and COMPANION Clinical Investigators (2000) Heart failure management using implantable devices for ventricular resynchronization: Comparison of Medical Therapy, Pacing, and Defibrillation in Chronic Heart failure (COMPANION) trial. J Card Fail 6:276–285
11. Abraham WT, Fisher WG, Smith AL et al (2002) Cardiac resynchronization in chronic heart failure. N Engl J Med 346:1845–1853
12. Metcalfe C, Thompson SG, Cowie MR, Sharples LD (2003) The use of hospital admission data as a measure of outcome in clinical studies of heart failure. Eur Heart J 24:105–112
13. Gronda E, Mangiavacchi M, Andreuzzi B et al (2002) A population-based study on overt heart failure in Lombardy (survey of hospitalization in 1996 and 1997. Ital Heart J 3(2):96–103
14. Bellotti P, Badano LP, Acquarone N et al, for the OSCUR Investigators (2001) Specialty related differences, in clinical profile management and outcome of patients hospitalized for heart failure: the OSCUR Study. Eur Heart J 22:596–604
15. Ahmed A, Roseman JM, Duxbury AS et al (2002) Correlates and outcomes of preserved left ventricular systolic function among older adults hospitalized with heart failure. Am Heart J 144:365-372

PACEMAKER/ICD COMPLICATIONS: DETECTION AND MANAGEMENT

How to Detect and Manage Pacemaker/ICD Failure and Infections

M.G. Bongiorni, G. Arena, E. Soldati, G. Giannola, E. Gronchi, G. Sgarito, M. Mariani

Background

Device therapy involving pacemakers for bradyarrhythmias and implantable cardioverter defibrillators (ICDs) for tachyarrhythmias has undergone a surprising evolution. System failure and infection, however, are still possible complications. In contrast to the relative frequency of lead failure, either as a result of implantation error or of deterioration of the lead materials, primary malfunction of the pulse generator is rare. The key to diagnosing device failure lies in meticulous assessment of the integrity of the leads and an understanding of the timing cycles of the specific device, which is facilitated by access to bidirectional telemetry. Infection is another complication of implanted devices; it is reported to occur in 0–19% of patients with pacemakers [1, 2] and in 2%–7% of patients with ICDs.

Management of complications ranges from abandonment of a failed lead and reimplantation of a new lead to removal of all inflammatory tissue, removal of all implanted devices, and reimplantation of new devices. In the early 1980s, before the development of successful low-morbidity techniques for extracting leads, every attempt was made to salvage the chronic pacemaker site or, at least, to leave the leads in place if the site had to be abandoned. Removal of long-term implanted leads was considered only when the complication was life-threatening. During the past 10 years, however, effective, low-morbidity techniques have evolved for transvenous extraction of leads [3], facilitating the management of complications relating to long-term implanted leads.

Diagnosis of Pacemaker/ICD Failure

The assessment of patients with a suspected pacemaker/ICD system problem must aim to gather as much information as possible. This includes the indica-

Cardiothoracic Department, Cisanello Hospital, University of Pisa, Italy

tions for device implantation, the operative record of the implantation procedure, and the model of all portions of the implanted system; in addition, the programmed parameters and data measured are absolutely crucial to correct evaluation of the device. Many devices have special programming features that may appear as malfunctions to clinicians not completely familiar with the particular system under scrutiny.

Even in the current high-technology environment of implanted devices, the history and physical examination continue to be important. The patient should be asked about symptoms relating to potential device malfunction. These include presyncope, syncope, palpitations, slow or fast pulse rates, pain or erythema around the implanted devices, fevers, chills, night sweats, and extracardiac stimulation. It is also important to obtain any history of trauma to the area where the device is located, exposure to intense electromagnetic signals or therapeutic radiation, use of electrocautery or defibrillation (internal or external), or any programming changes by other medical personnel. In otherwise asymptomatic ICD patients, repeated shocks may suggest false signal detection.

Physical maneuvers may be useful to unmask an intermittent symptom or malfunction during an examination. Positional changes (sitting or standing up) or having the patient perform in-place exercise or isometric maneuvers may accelerate the heart rate to allow observation of sensing (correct tracking and inhibition). Manipulation of the device and lead may disclose an intermittent lead fracture, loose connection, or insulation failure that was not evident while the patient was lying quietly on the examination table. Other helpful maneuvers include movement of the patient's ipsilateral arm (reaching overhead or reaching behind the back) and isometric exercise (pressing hands together in front of the chest or reaching around the chest to scratch the opposite side), and, in the case of an abdominal implant, having the patient do situps is helpful in identifying an intermittent problem. If the patient develops symptoms during the induced abnormal behavior, and these symptoms reproduce those that occurred spontaneously, there is a high likelihood that the cause of the symptoms has been identified.

An ECG tracing with the magnet applied to the pulse generator should also be performed. This provides information about the status of the battery and, if the device was otherwise inhibited, allows a quick assessment of capture and whether the output was being delivered to the appropriate chamber. If no output is seen during application of the magnet, several possibilities should be considered: the battery may be depleted, the device may be nonfunctional, or an open circuit (such as a lead fracture) may be present. In some models, the magnet response is programmable and can be turned on or off. If the magnet function is disabled, placement of a magnet over it does not result in an overt change in its demand behavior. Alternatively, the magnet may not have been positioned properly or an inappropriate magnet may have been used.

The programmed settings should be both retrieved and printed by telemetry. Printing is important because it documents the initial settings and serves as a reference in case the clinician wishes to restore the device to the same settings when the evaluation is complete. If measured telemetry is available, these data should be requested and printed. The same recommendation holds for models that have extensive histograms, trend data, or other diagnostic counters. After the mode and rate have been verified, an evaluation of the remaining programmed parameters is appropriate. The identified output, pulse width, sensitivity, and refractory periods should be reviewed for each channel and correlated with the ECG. The presence and status of any special programmable features should be checked. The latter includes rate-modulation behavior, ELT prevention and termination algorithms, hysteresis, search hysteresis, time-of-day-dependent or circadian sensor-based rate changes, rate-adaptive atrioventricular (AV) delay, differential paced and sensed AV delay, rate smoothing, and others. Other diagnostic information is now routinely available in all ICDs, including charge times, capacitor reformation times, and high-voltage lead impedance.

Lead impedance is one of the most important elements of the measured data. Proper interpretation of lead impedance, however, is dependent on the manufacturer and model of the lead used, the method of measurement, and the historical values of the individual lead's impedance. The other parameters of the lead's performance, including pulse voltage, pulse charge, pulse energy, and current, should also be correlated with the measured impedance. A marked discrepancy between observed and expected values may identify a telemetry error or measurement error within the pacemaker rather than a primary problem with the lead. It is prudent to repeat the measurements several times if a conflict is noted.

ICD leads serve dual functions; the construction of the ICD leads is therefore more complex than that of the pacemaker leads. Two types of sensing leads have been developed: (1) a true bipolar sensing lead, with an independent defibrillation coil on the same electrode; and (2) an integrated bipolar lead, in which the distal electrode and the most proximal coil to the distal electrode are used as the sensing electrode pair. The additional wire conductors requiring independent insulation mandate electrodes of greater diameter and complexity and, by inference, provide greater potential for complications. These electrodes are more prone to crush fracture or insulation material failures. To test the integrity of the right ventricular electrode, the operator needs to interrogate the sensing and pacing as well as the defibrillation conductors. Sensing and pacing function is tested by using the external programmer. Sensing in sinus rhythm and during ventricular tachycardia and ventricular fibrillation is analyzed to assess sensing integrity. Oversensing in sinus rhythm may occur as a result of a very small ventricular signal, large T waves, far-field sensing of P waves, interference due to a fractured conductor, or "noise" from a loose terminal pin set-screw. The integrity of the high-voltage electrodes can be verified on the basis of the analysis of impedance values and delivered energies during an ICD shock. It is also possible to administer a low-energy shock in sinus rhythm to obtain the high-voltage lead impedance. Such testing is discouraged in an outpatient setting because of the discomfort that even a low-energy shock is likely to cause to the patient. Less invasive means of testing the highvoltage lead integrity are now present in some ICDs.

If a system problem is suspected, posteroanterior and lateral chest radiographs should be obtained. It is usually best to request a slightly overpenetrated exposure to visualize the intracardiac segment of the pacing leads for position and integrity. Requesting a thoracic spine exposure technique provides optimal penetration for visualization of the pacing leads. It is recommended that, whenever possible, chest radiographs taken after the implantation be compared with the current radiographs. The film should be inspected for evidence of conductor disruption, insulation failure, as inferred from a deformity in the conductor coil because the insulation is radiolucent, proper lead placement in the generator connector block, electrode perforation, and dislodgment or malpositioning of a lead. Close attention should be paid to the infraclavicular area, where pressure from the clavicle and first rib may cause lead failure. In some cases, overlapping leads or leads overlying other structures may make it difficult to visualize a deformity of the conductor coil. If a problem is suspected, multiple views including oblique and uncommon views may be required.

On occasion, a fluoroscopic evaluation of the patient may be useful. This shows many of the mechanical or positional problems and defects listed earlier. It also provides a dynamic view of the lead system, facilitating identification of excessive electrode movement consistent with an unstable lead, or there may be insufficient slack so that respiratory movement causes traction on the lead and tension at the electrode–tissue interface. Either of these would provide an explanation for an intermittent capture or sensing problem.

Diagnosis of Pacemaker/ICD Infection

Infections involving implanted devices are challenging, not only because of the severity and duration of the inflammatory reaction, but also because of the sequelae. Local infection presents a spectrum that ranges from contaminated tissue to cellulitis with marked tissue loss. Acute infections after an initial implantation in normal tissue are rare and usually result from some breach of technique, contaminating the pocket with a virulent bacterium. For example, inadvertent contamination of the pocket or devices with *Staphylococcus aureus* will probably cause an acute infection. Most surgical sites are contaminated by mainly nonvirulent bacteria, such as *Staphylococcus epidermidis*, and do not become infected. The body's defenses can eradicate a small inoculum of these bacteria. However, a large inoculation or the presence of a culture medium such as devitalized tissue or hematoma can negate the body's defenses, and an infection will ensue. Most infections begin after an invasive reintervention procedure, usually after replacement of a new device (pulse generator or lead) back into the old pocket. Again, during a surgical procedure, tissue is normally exposed to some degree of contamination, such as skin bacteria, but some chronic pockets cannot tolerate even minimal levels of contamination without developing an infection. Sometimes the infection may be occult, causing no signs or symptoms. In these low-grade infections some sort of balance is usually reached between the bacteria and the body's defenses. Such chronic infections are usually caused by *Staphylococcus epidermidis*. On pocket exploration, exuberant fibrous tissue with or without an exudative effusion is found; granulation tissue may also be present. A chronic draining sinus may stabilize a chronic infection; if the infected material drains through the skin, the cavity is decompressed, the concentration of bacteria and their toxins is decreased, and the cellulitis resolves.

When the suppurative effusion decompresses into the blood, bacteremia causing septicemia and endocarditis may develop. The diagnosis of endocarditis related to pacemaker lead infection should be systematically considered in patients with fever, a history of local complications, or pulmonary pathology after device insertion. Generally, two different clinical presentations are described [4]: the acute form, with an early presentation with sepsis, often in conjunction with local signs of infection, and a chronic form beginning several months later. The presentation may be atypical and the presenting symptoms may occur late after the last intervention at the implantation site. Fever and chills are the most frequent symptoms; other symptoms may be asthenia, wasting, septic shock, and/or arthralgia. Pulmonary complications include septic embolism, pulmonary abscess, recurrent bronchitis (with fever, cough, and expectoration), and pleural effusion. One rare manifestation may be a history of spondylitis.

Blood results often show erythrocyte sedimentation rate and C-reactive protein (CRP) increase as well as leukocytosis due to an increase in polymorphonuclear cells. Blood cultures are often positive: as already mentioned, staphylococci are responsible for the vast majority of these infections, especially *S. epidermidis* in the chronic form and *S. aureus* in the acute form [5, 6]. Preoperative antibiotic therapy may account for negative blood cultures; moreover, the amorphous material (slime) that is universally found in staphylococcal colonies may also be responsible for these negative cultures, by isolating the lead and the germ from the culture material [7].

For diagnosis of endocarditis the imaging method currently used is echocardiography. In a review of published reports, Kugener et al. [8] reported the results of transthoracic echocardiography (TTE) obtained in 42 cases of permanent endocavitary lead infection. The sensitivity of the technique was poor, and it provided a positive diagnosis in only 15 of the cases reviewed (36%). This low sensitivity can be explained by the use of the TM mode in the earliest cases. However, more recent papers [4, 9] reported diagnosis of vegetations along implanted leads in only 23–30% of cases. With the two-dimensional mode, the main technical difficulties—apart from poor echogenicity in some patients—were the echoes induced by the leads, which interfere with the visualization of small structures. In addition, when vegetation was visualized, it was generally not possible to determine whether there was tricuspid valve endocarditis, lead infection, or both.

Transesophageal echocardiography (TEE) is at present the gold-standard diagnostic tool for pacemaker/ICD endocarditis: Cacoub et al. [10] demonstrated that TEE was diagnostic or suggestive in 23/24 patients (96%), compared with 22% for TTE ($p<0.0001$). Surgical findings were in accordance with TEE findings in 87% of patients of that series. Similar results have been reported by Klug et al. [4], who noted that TEE findings were concordant with surgical findings in 92% of patients. In the series reported by Victor et al. [9], the sensitivities of TTE and TEE were 30% and 96% respectively. The specificity and positive predictive value of TEE were both 100%. The negative predictive value of TEE was 94%.

A recent, very promising technological improvement in the field of diagnosis is intracardiac echography, performed using catheters provided with an echo transducer at the tip. Intracardiac echography can allow the relationships between leads and most anatomical structures to be determined better than with TEE [11].

Ventilation perfusion pulmonary scintigraphy may be used to reveal pulmonary septic embolism, which can be expected in about 20% of patients, particularly in those with long-standing sepsis. In cases of fever without any other diagnostic finding, the use of scintigraphy with radionuclide-labeled leukocytes may show high-intensity absorption in the mediastinum, suggestive of pacemaker endocarditis.

Management of Pacemaker/ICD Failure or Infection: Indications for Removal

The management of pacemaker/ICD complications involves several approaches, from simply reprogramming in the case of pseudomalfunction to removal of the entire hardware. The present paper will not systematically discuss all the approaches, but will focus on the indications and techniques for transvenous removal, which require particular facilities and training.

The indications for lead removal are generally described according to the Byrd classification [12]. The categories "mandatory," "necessary," and "discretionary" have served well during the developmental phase of lead extraction technology and physician skills.

Mandatory indications: leads must be removed. Mandatory conditions are those in which leaving the leads in place would be life-threatening or disabling, such as septicemia, endocarditis, lead migration (e.g., perforating, causing arrhythmia, causing emboli), device interference (e.g., abandoned implantable defibrillator lead), or obliteration of all usable veins.

Necessary indications: leads should be removed. Necessary conditions are those in which lead removal would correct a problem or prevent a life-threatening situation from developing, but the existing problem is not considered life-threatening. Examples are pocket infection, chronic draining sinus, erosion, vein thrombosis, lead migration (not presently causing life-threatening problem), potential device interference, and lead replacement (e.g., supernumerary, extract and implant thrombosed vein).

Discretionary indications: leads may be removed. Discretionary conditions are those in which it is preferable to remove the leads but in which it would rarely be considered a medical necessity, e.g., cases of pain, malignancy, lead replacement (e.g., lead abandoned for less than 3–4 years).

In 2000 a North American Society of Pacing and Electrophysiology (NASPE) Policy Conference was held which established indications, facilities, and training for chronically implanted lead transvenous removal [13].

Transvenous Techniques for Lead Removal

To date the most extensive experience has been with the use of *mechanical sheaths* and *powered sheaths.*

Mechanical sheath dissection was introduced into clinical practice by Byrd in the late 1980s [14]. The most widely used extraction system is supplied by Cook Vascular Inc. This system is provided with locking stylets and dilator sheaths; they are used as a first choice when the proximal end of the lead is exposed (superior approach). The technique in the case of the superior approach consists of a combination of traction by the locking stylet, mechanical dilation of adherences by the dilating sheaths, and countertraction at the tip of the lead by the outer telescopic sheaths. A transvenous workstation with a tip deflecting wire, Dormier basket, and loop retriever is the first choice of tool in the case of totally intravascular leads (inferior approach). The most recent results from the US Extraction Database were reported for 6420 leads in 4090 patients [15]; 93% of leads were completely extracted, 5% were partially extracted, and 2% were not removed. Major complications occurred in 1.6% of patients, including a 0.2% mortality rate.

The VascoExtor system by VascoMed consists of a locking stylet with a remote control anchoring mechanism at the tip. A rotating motor can be applied to the stylet in order to facilitate advancement or withdrawal of the stylet; the system can be used on a wide range of coil lumen dimensions. A dilator sheath and a transfemoral workstation provided with a snare-loop catheter for intravascular lead extraction are also available. In a multicenter European study [16], removal attempts were made for 150 leads. Complete removal was possible in 122 cases (81%), partial removal was possible in 18 cases (12%), and failure to remove the lead occurred in 10 cases (7%). There were no serious complications associated with the procedure. None of the patients died.

Powered sheath techniques were developed in the 1990s using a source of energy (excimer laser, radiofrequency) to make dissection of binding sites faster and easier. Laser energy is delivered at the edge of a special sheath; the circumferential zone of optic fibers at the end of the sheath delivers a 308-nm laser beam that is effective for about 1 mm. In an ideal situation, the sheath is passed over the lead, vaporizing each binding site until the sheath reaches a point about a few millimeters from the heart wall. The lead is then removed from the heart wall using countertraction.

A recent paper reported the US experience with laser sheaths [17]; 2561 pacing and defibrillator leads were treated in 1684 patients in 89 centers. Ninety percent of the leads were completely removed, 3% were partially removed, and the remaining leads failed to be removed. Major perioperative complications (tamponade, hemothorax, pulmonary embolism, lead migration, and death) were observed in 1.9% of patients, with in-hospital death in 13 (0.8%). Minor complications were seen in an additional 1.4% of patients. In the European multicenter experience [18], 179 leads in 149 patients were extracted in 11 centers. Complete extraction of 89.5% of the leads was achieved, 6% were partially extracted, and 4.5% of the extractions failed. Complications were few but included one ventricular perforation that did not need surgery; two other perforations were related to the reimplantation of leads and required surgery.

Radiofrequency energy powers the electrosurgical sheaths, which are used to ablate the encapsulating fibrous tissue in a manner similar to the laser sheath method. The electrosurgical sheath works as a bipolar electrosurgical cutting instrument, similar to the conventional devices used for hemostasis and cutting. The electrical arc sited at the tip of the sheath cuts the fibrous tissue. An outer sheath is used as a workstation and for counterpressure and countertraction. This technique is presently under clinical evaluation in the US; early reports showed effectiveness and safety similar to those with mechanical and laser extraction.

Although the results of the mechanical sheath and the powered sheath techniques are similar, the duration of procedures and, consequently, of radiation exposure are shorter using powered sheaths; on the other hand, the powered techniques are more expensive. In the near future the cost/benefit ratio of both types of techniques will require careful evaluation. Probably, most procedures could be performed by mechanical techniques, while powered sheath techniques could be reserved for selected difficult cases.

Technological advances in transvenous lead removal can be achieved by modifying the techniques and the approaches as well as improving the materials. In our personal experience [19, 20] and in many reports [21], it was observed that the success rate of removal was strongly affected by the presence of free-floating leads, calcified scar tissue, or the impossibility of advancing a stylet into the lead. In presence of these factors, an approach through the right internal jugular vein presents some advantages. Most free-floating leads can be exposed via the jugular approach and can thus be subjected to a standard procedure for exposed leads. In addition, the straight course of the lead from the jugular vein to the right atrium or ventricle allows dilation along the longitudinal axis of the lead, allowing easier dilation and countertraction. These conditions appeared to increase the effectiveness of mechanical dilation and to reduce the risk of complications. Following these observations we developed a jugular approach (removal of leads from the internal jugular vein) for free-floating and difficult exposed leads [22].

Finally, another recent technological improvement in the field of transvenous removal is the use of intracardiac echography (ICE), performed using catheters with an echo transducer at the tip. The use of ICE during transvenous removal procedures can allow the relationships between leads and most anatomical structures to be determined better than with fluoroscopy; it can be very useful either to detect the presence of vegetations and their outcome during dilation, or to monitor the possible occurrence of complications. However, because of the costs, the need for an additional venous puncture and a dedicated operator, ICE will probably be of most use in selected cases, such as: difficult leads, multiple leads, suspicion of vegetation, old leads, or free-floating leads [23].

Lead Extraction: Personal Experience

Since December 1989, we have managed 831 patients (609 men, mean age 66.6 years, range 6–93 years) with 1342 leads (mean pacing period 66.11 months, range 1–336 months). There were 1231 pacing leads (PL; 765 ventricular, 454 atrial, and 12 coronary sinus leads) and 111 defibrillating leads (DL; 95 ventricular, 5 atrial, and 11 superior vena cava leads). The indications for removal were class I in 33.9 % and class II in 66.1% of the leads (Fig. 1). We performed

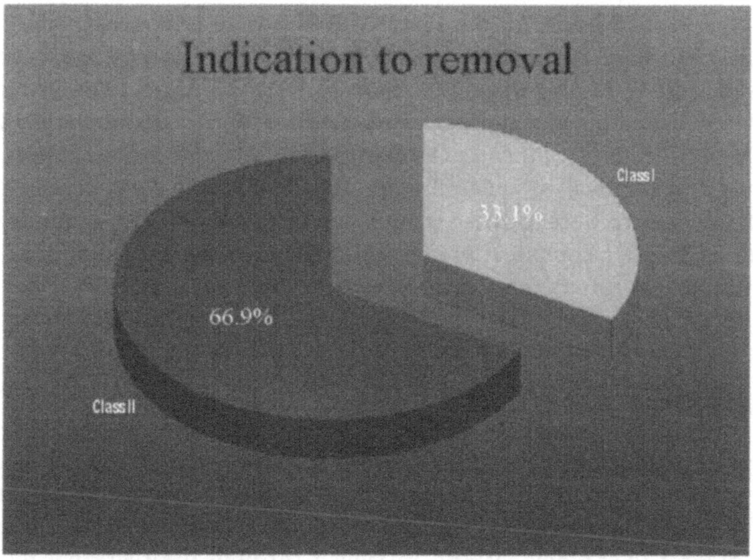

Fig. 1. Indications for lead removal according to NASPE class

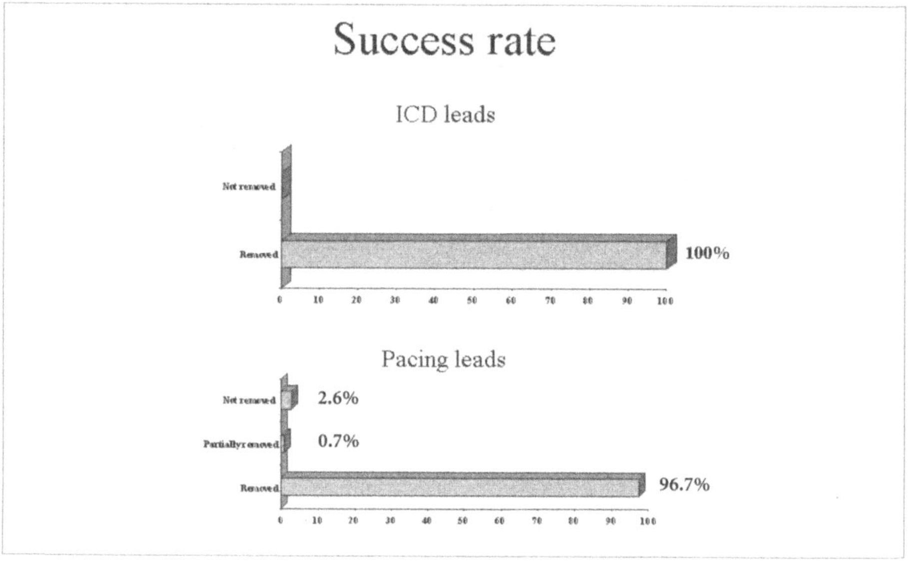

Fig. 2. Success rate for removal of ICD and pacing leads respectively

mechanical dilation using the Cook Vascular extraction kit and, if necessary, other intravascular tools (catchers and lassos, Osypka). As mentioned above, since 1996 we have developed a new approach using the internal jugular vein for use in the case of free-floating leads or when removal through the implant vein was not possible (difficult exposed leads). The transvenous mechanical removal technique was not applicable in 14 leads (1.04%). Removal was attempted in 1328 leads. All the 111 DL (100%) were removed. Of the remaining 1217 PL, 1177 (96.7%) were totally removed, 8 (0.7%) were partially removed, and 32 (2.6%) were not removed (Fig. 2). From 1996 onwards, the newly introduced jugular approach was used for 36 free-floating and 122 difficult exposed leads (i.e., those not removed via the conventional approaches), allowing the removal of 156/158 leads (98.7%). Major complications in the overall experience were: cardiac tamponade (6 cases, or 0.45%, with death in 1 case, or 0.12%). No complications directly related to the jugular approach were observed.

Conclusions

The management of pacemaker/ICD-related complications requires a spectrum of knowledge and techniques. Clues to the problem and its cause are found in the patient's history, physical examination, and the various diagnostic tests integral to the devices and retrieved through bidirectional telemetry. When a "software problem" is detected, reprogramming may be enough to solve it; when a "hardware problem" is present (malfunctioning or infection), the solution may range from replacement of devices or the repositioning or insertion of a new lead to the extraction of leads. Some of these procedures have the potential for tearing the heart and veins, precipitating a life-threatening complication. To minimize the incidence of these complications and to ensure a satisfactory resolution, training in these procedures, and the availability of surgical support should a problem arise, is essential.

References

1. Rettig G, Doenecke P, Sen S et al (1979) Complications with retained transvenous pacemaker electrodes. Am Heart J 98:587–594
2. Parry G, Goudevenos J, Jameson S et al (1991) Complications associated with retained pacemaker leads. Pacing Clin Electrophysiol 14:1251–1257
3. Byrd CL (2001) Advances in device lead extraction. Curr Cardiol Rep 3:324
4. Klug D, Lacroix D, Savoye C et al (1997) Systemic infection related to endocarditis on pacemaker leads: clinical presentation and management. Circulation 95:2098–2107
5. Choo MH, Holmes DR, Jr, Gersh BJ et al (1981) Permanent pacemaker infections: characterization and management. Am J Cardiol 48:559–564
6. Morgan G, Ginks W, Siddons H et al (1979) Septicemia in patients with an endocardial pacemaker. Am J Cardiol 44:221–224
7. Peters G, Saborowski F, Locci R et al (1984) Investigations on staphylococcal infection of transvenous endocardial pacemaker electrodes. Am Heart J 108:359–365
8. Kugener H, Rey JL, Tribouilloy C et al (1993) Infectious endocarditis on permanent endocavitary pacemakers: value of echocardiography and review of the literature (in French). Ann Cardiol Angeiol (Paris) 42:331–338
9. Victor F, De Place C, Camus C et al (1999) Pacemaker lead infection: echocardiographic features, management, and outcome. Heart 81:82–87
10. Cacoub P, Leprince P, Nataf P et al (1998) Pacemaker infective endocarditis. Am J Cardiol 82:480–484
11. Arena G, Bongiorni MG, Soldati E et al (2002) Usefulness of intracardiac echography for transvenous leads extraction. Pacing Clin Electrophysiol 25(4 Pt II):545
12. Byrd CL, Schwartz SJ, Hedin N (1992) Lead extraction. Indications and techniques. Cardiol Clin 10:735–748
13. Love CJ, Wilkoff BL, Byrd CL et al (2000) Recommendations for extraction of chronically implanted transvenous pacing and defibrillator leads: indications, facilities, training. North American Society of Pacing and Electrophysiology Lead Extraction Conference Faculty. Pacing Clin Electrophysiol 23(4 Pt 1):544–551
14. Byrd CL, Schwartz SJ, Hedin NB et al (1990) Intravascular lead extraction using locking stylets and sheaths. Pacing Clin Electrophysiol 13(12 Pt 2):1871–1875
15. Byrd C, Wilkoff BL (2002) Techniques and devices for extraction of pacemaker and implantable cardioverter-defibrillator leads. In: Ellenbogen KA, Kay GN, Wilkoff BN (ed) Clinical cardiac pacing and defibrillation. Saunders, Philadelphia
16. Alt E, Neuzner J, Binner L et al (1996) Three-year experience with a stylet for lead extraction: a multicenter study. Pacing Clin Electrophysiol 19:18–25
17. Byrd CL, Wilkoff BL, Love CJ et al (2002) Clinical study of the laser sheath for lead extraction: the total experience in the United States. Pacing Clin Electrophysiol 25:804–808

18. Kennergren C (1999) Excimer laser assisted extraction of permanent pacemaker and ICD leads: present experiences of a European multi-centre study. Eur J Cardiothorac Surg 15:856–860
19. Bongiorni MG, Soldati E, Arena G et al (1998) The transvenous removal of definitive electrocatheters for stimulation and defibrillation: the indications, methods and results (in Italian). Cardiologia 43:1105–1109
20. Bongiorni MG, Arena G, Soldati E et al (1999) Lead extraction: how easy and safe is it today? In: Raviele A (ed) Cardiac arrhythmias 1999. Springer, Milan
21. Bracke F, Meijer A, Van Gelder B (2002) Extraction of pacemaker and implantable cardioverter defibrillator leads: patient and lead characteristics in relation to the requirement of extraction tools. Pacing Clin Electrophysiol 25:1037–1040
22. Bongiorni MG, Soldati E, Arena G et al (2001) Percutanous extraction of infected pacemaker/ICD leads: which technological advances and results? In: Raviele A (ed) Cardiac arrhythmias 2001. Springer, Milan
23. Bongiorni MG, Arena G, Soldati E et al (2001) Pacemaker/ICD lead infection: what are the main intracardiac echocardiographic features? In: Raviele A (ed) Cardiac arrhythmias 2001. Springer, Milan

Pacemaker/ICD Lead Extraction Using the Excimer Laser Sheath: What Are the Advantages and What Are the Risks?

G. Gasparini, A. Rossillo, F. Giada, A. Corrado, A. Raviele

Introduction

Since 1965 transvenous lead implantation for cardiac pacing has been the routine treatment for bradyarrhythmias. At the end of 1980s, the implantable cardioverter defibrillator (ICD) was considered the first-line therapy for tachyarrhythmia management, and in recent years new ICD indications for the primary prevention of sudden death have been added. Moreover, biventricular pacing for the treatment of congestive heart failure has been recently introduced. Thus, the number of implantable devices with a growing number of leads is increasing day after day.

On the other hand, the need to remove leads for different problems is increasing, too. The original Byrd classification [1] of the indications for lead removal into three categories (mandatory, necessary, and discretionary) has now been replaced by a classification into three categories according to the authors' agreement about lead removal [2]. Early leads were bulky, and if infection, exit block, or any other malfunction occurred, simple traction on the lead with varying degrees of force was enough to separate it from vascular and endocardial adhesions. Because the lead bodies were large and strong and implant durations relatively short, rates of successful removal were high. Later, leads became smaller in diameter and more fragile and remained implanted for longer periods, so that traction became less effective while the risk of internal tears, bleeding, and breaking of the lead increased. For these reasons special instruments to extract long-term implanted pacing and defibrillator leads were developed.

The first specialized tools included a stylet that locked to the tip of the lead with a variety of steel and plastic mechanical dissecting sheaths (the Cook system). Applying counter-traction on the locking stylet, fibrosis and vascular adhesions are mechanically dissected by advancing the sheath along the lead

O.U. of Cardiology, Umberto I Hospital, Mestre–Venice, Italy

body. When the sheath reaches the tip of the lead it prevents ventricular or atrial wall avulsion. A success rate (leads completely removed) of 87% in 1299 patients, with fatal or near-fatal complications in 2.5% of patients (0.6% deaths), was reported with the Cook system [3]. Later, some improvements were made in distal grip of the stylet by Cook and VascoMed [4]. In a small series of 34 patients the VascoExtor system was able to completely remove leads in 32 patients (94%) and no complications were observed [5]. Recently, a new lead locking device (LLD) with a thin cylindrical metallic braid has been developed. After introduction of the stylet within the lead as far as the tip, the proximal end of the braid is released and expands radially to completely fill the lumen of the conductor coil along its entire length. This permits traction of the LLD and the lead as a unit. Kennergren and co-workers [6] reported a success rate (leads completely removed) of 95% in 57 patients, the LLD being used in conjunction with sheaths and other instruments of extraction by very experienced investigators; no major complications were observed.

The Excimer Laser Sheath

Endocardial lead implantation for cardiac pacing and, even more, for defibrillation stimulates a dense fibroelastic reaction at the electrode–myocardial interface. This fibroelastic tissue contains both fibrous connective tissue and elastic tissue, and extends up the lead producing a ring surrounding the lead along its entire length, especially in the venous course. In particular, ICD leads differ from standard bradycardia pacing leads because they are stiffer, larger, with exposed coil; moreover, it seems that shocks delivered by the coil determine a focal electrical injury around it. Both these aspects contribute to the fibroelastic tissue reaction [7]. Given the more intense inflammatory reaction and larger fibrous sheaths that encase ICD leads and attach to intracardiac structures, such as the tricuspid valve, more complicated extraction is to be expected.

Recently, in order to improve the success rate of lead extraction when the fibroelastic reaction is particularly strong and the risk of tearing of the cardiac and vessel walls is high, the excimer laser sheath has been introduced. The laser sheath consists of thin inner and outer polymer walls between which a single layer of optical fibres (82, each with a core diameter of 100 μm) has been spirally wrapped. At the distal tip of the sheath the fibres present a single circumferential ring of light sandwiched between the inner and outer walls. At the proximal end of the sheath the fibres pass through a connecting cable to the laser generator. There are three different sizes of sheath: 12, 14, and 16 French (outer diameter) [8]. The CVX-300 Excimer XeCl Laser System (Spectranetics, Colorado Springs, Colorado, USA) provides laser energy by a xenon chloride laser with a wavelength of 308 nm at repetition rate of 25–40 Hz and a fluence (output energy per unit area of fibre) at the distal tip set to values between 30 and 60 mJ/mm [2]. It is a cool cutting laser (50 °C) with a very limited absorption depth: at a tissue depth of approximately 0.06 mm, 64% of the energy is absorbed and at 0.18 mm 95% is absorbed. The energy is absorbed by lipids and proteins and not by water. Thanks to these characteristics the excimer laser is capable of disrupting, with a combination of photochemolysis and photothermal ablation, the fibrotic sheaths around leads immediately in contact with the device tip, producing particles no larger than 5 μm, while not damaging other leads or the blood vessels [9].

Efficacy and Complications: Literature Data

The first experiences of expert investigators with the use of the excimer laser sheath were reported in 1998. The laser system was considered efficacious for complete lead removal. Kennergren [10] used the excimer laser sheath to remove 50 leads in 45 patients and reported a success rate of 93% without major complications. In the same year Bracke et al. [11] published their experience with the laser sheath on 32 leads on which extraction failed with other different tools; 81% of them were successfully removed using the excimer laser sheath, but two major complications occurred: a small tear in the right atrial appendage with acute pericardial tamponade, and tearing of the left internal mammary artery, probably due to its aberrant position anteriorly to the subclavian vein, both surgically resolved. The importance of the learning curve has been noted by these authors, considering that five out of six failures occurred in the first half of their series. Afterwards, the results of the PLEXES trial were published by Wilkoff and co-workers [12]. This was the first randomized trial in which excimer laser sheath extraction was compared to non-laser lead extraction in 465 chronically implanted pacemaker leads (301 patients). The success rate was 94% in the laser group and 64% in the non-laser group (p=0.001). Moreover, 88% of the non-laser failures were resolved by the laser tools. There were five complications (3.2%) in the laser group, three of which required intervention (1 death, 0.6%), although none of them were considered to be directly related to the application of laser energy. Another important experience of a European multi-centre study with the excimer laser sheath was reported by Kennergren (on behalf of the PLESSE investigator group) [13] on 179 leads (17 ICD leads) in 149 patients. The overall success rate was 89.4%; there was only one ventricular perforation directly related to the extraction procedure and that did not require open chest surgery. The efficacy and complications using the three different laser sheath sizes were compared by Epstein et al. [14] on 1285 leads in 863 patients. No significant differences in success rate (89%, 86%, and 90% with the 12-, 14-, and 16-French sizes, respectively) or complications (3%, 4%, and 6%, with death in 2, 4, and 1 patients, respectively) were reported. Subsequently, other single-centre experiences in pacemaker and ICD lead extraction with the excimer laser sheath were reported, with success rates ranging from 84% to 100% and major complications ranging from 0% to 5.5% [15–18]. Finally, the total experience, from 1995 to 1999, in the United States with using the excimer laser sheath on 2561 pacing and defibrillator leads (1684 patients from 89 centres) was reported by Byrd and co-workers [19]: 90% success rate with major complications (haemopericardium with tamponade, haemothorax, pulmonary embolism, lead migration) in 1.9% of patients (including 0.8% in-hospital deaths), and minor complications in an additional 1.4% of patients.

Comments

The large number of devices implanted annually worldwide will inevitably increase the numbers of lead extractions. The fibrosis which is generally found subcutaneously at the venous entry and at the upper portion of the superior vena cava as well as at the electrode–myocardium interface increases over time. The longer the time from implantation, the potentially less efficacious is lead extraction by direct traction [20]. The excimer laser sheath is an important tool that can disrupt this fibroelastic tissue, freeing the lead which can then be easily removed. The high success rate in removing old leads, ICD leads, and, often, leads that have failed to be extracted with other removal tools, confirms its effectiveness. However, this technique may be burdened by potentially life-threatening complications and sometimes deaths, even though they too are not directly related to the laser energy application, but linked to the extraction procedure itself. Indeed, complications observed with excimer laser sheath extractions are no more frequent than those observed with other extraction tools [3]. In any case, authors suggest performing the extraction in an operating room with a surgical standby.

It is important to underline that complications are strictly linked to operator experience. Undoubtedly, the excimer laser sheath should preferably be used in centres where one operator generally has plenty of experience in lead extraction and is able to use any other instruments of extraction to complete the procedure. In fact, the use of other tools via the femoral, right subclavian, or jugular vein to remove lead fragments is necessary to further improve clinical outcome. Moreover, because the technique is relatively expensive [15], a stepwise protocol for extraction should be suggested, using traction first, in particular when the time from implantation is relatively short [20]. Finally, the excimer laser sheath might be used to create ipsilateral venous access in the case of an obstructed vein, to insert a new lead [21].

Conclusions

Extracting pacemaker and ICD leads has been simplified with the use of the excimer laser sheath. Its efficacy is over 90% in the majority of papers, while major complications are seen in about 2% of patients. However, the cost of the system and the intrinsic risks of the procedure suggest that the excimer laser sheath should be used in problematic extractions by expert operators in centres that are able to resolve life-threatening complications.

References

1. Byrd CL, Schwartz SJ, Hedin N (1992) Lead extraction: indications and techniques. Cardiol Clin 10:735–748
2. North American Society of Pacing and Electrophysiology Lead Extraction Conference Faculty (2000) Recommendations for extraction of chronically implanted transvenous pacing and defibrillator leads: indications, facilities, training. Pacing Clin Electrophysiol 23:544–551
3. Smith HH, Fearnot NE, Byrd CL et al (1994) Five-year experience with intravascular lead extraction. Pacing Clin Electrophysiol 17II:2016–2020
4. Tyers GFO (2000) Lead extraction methods (abstr). Europace 1(suppl):D45
5. Manolis AS, Maounis TN, Vassilikos V, Chiladakis J, Melita-Manolis H, Cokkinos DV (2001) Ancillary tools in pacemaker and defibrillator lead extraction using a novel lead removal system. Pacing Clin Electrophysiol 24:282–287
6. Kennergren C, Schaerf RHM, Duncan Sellers T et al (2000) Cardiac lead extraction with a novel locking stylet. J Interv Cardiac Electrophysiol 4:591–593
7. Epstein AE, Kay GN, Plumb VJ, Dailey SM, Anderson PG (1998) Gross and microscopic pathological changes associated with nonthoracotomy implantable defibrillator leads. Circulation 98:1517–1524
8. Reiser C, Taylor K (1997) Excimer laser catheter for pacing lead removal. Soc Photooptic Instrum Eng Proc 2970:80–84
9. Reiser C, Taylor K, Lippincott R (1998) Large laser sheaths for pacing and defibrillator lead removal. Lasers Surg Med 22:42–45
10. Kennergren C (1998) First European experience using excimer laser for the extraction of permanent pacemakerleads. Pacing Clin Electrophysiol 21:268–270
11. Bracke FA, Meijer A, van Gelder B (1998) Learning curve characteristics of pacing lead extraction with a laser sheath. Pacing Clin Electrophysiol 21:2309–2313
12. Wilkoff BL, Byrd CL, Love CJ et al (1999) Pacemaker lead extraction with the laser sheath: results of the Pacing Lead EXtraction with the Excimer Sheath (PLEXES) trial. J Am Coll Cardiol 33:1671–1676
13. Kennergren C, on behalf of the PLESSE (Pacing Lead Extraction Surveillance Study in Europe) investigators group (1999) Excimer laser assisted extraction of permanent pacemaker and ICD leads: present experiences of a European multi-centre study. Eur J Cardiothoracic Surg 15:856–860
14. Epstein LM, Byrd CL, Wilkoff BL et al (1999) Initial experience with larger laser sheaths for the removal of transvenous pacemaker and implantable defibrillator leads. Circulation 100:516–525
15. Levy T, Walker S, Paul V (1999) Initial experience in the extraction of chronically implanted pacemaker leads using excimer laser sheath. Heart 82:101–104
16. Parsonnet V, Roelke M, Trivedi A, Rizvi SA, Pervez A (2001) Laser extraction of entrapped leads. Pacing Clin Electrophysiol 24:329–332
17. Bracke FA, Meijer A, van Gelder B (2001) Endovascular extraction techniques. Part 3: results and indications in patients with an ICD. Neth Heart J 9:117–122
18. Gilligan DM, Dan D (2001) Excimer laser for pacemaker and defibrillator lead extraction: techniques and clinical results. Lasers Med Sci 16:113–121

19. Byrd CL, Wilkoff BL, Love CJ, Duncan Sellers T, Reiser C (2002) Clinical study of the laser sheath for lead extraction: the total experience in the United States. Pacing Clin Electrophysiol 25:804–808
20. Bracke FA, Meijer A, van Gelder B (2002) Extraction of pacemaker and implantable cardioverter defibrillator leads: patients and lead characteristics in relation to the requirement of extraction tools. Pacing Clin Electrophysiol 25:1037–1040
21. Bracke FALE, Meijer A, van Gelder LM (2002) Use of a laser sheath to obtain venous access in pacemaker lead-related obstruction without extraction of the lead. Europace 4:67–68

How to Detect and Treat Superior Vena Cava Obstruction Caused by Multiple Pacing/ICD Leads?

G. Chiarandà[1], A. Busà[2], G. Muscio[1], A. Lazzaro[3], L. Cavarra[1], T. Regolo[4]

Epidemiology

Superior vena cava (SVC) obstruction caused by permanent implantation of leads for pacemakers or defibrillators is not infrequent, having been observed in 35–45% of all cases, and in 20% of cases total occlusion is found 2 years after the intervention [1–3]. Such a high prevalence is observed only if patients are subjected to venography 1 year after implantation, because thrombosis is asymptomatic in the majority of cases owing to the development of collaterals.

The diagnosis of SVC obstruction is generally made during the revision of the implantation, when new leads have to be inserted [4]. In fact, SVC thrombosis is clinically apparent only in 0.2–5% of cases [5–7], when it manifests as SVC syndrome, or pulmonary embolism, or sudden death resulting from tricuspid occlusion. SVC syndrome is very rare, its incidence ranging from less than 0.01% (2 out of 1,000 implantations) to 0.40% [2, 6, 7–11]. In his review of the literature, Blackburn found only 25 cases among more than 1 million patients who had undergone implantation [12]. No data are available about the rate of SVC obstruction after explantation of pacing leads, since venography is not generally performed at follow-up and the development of collaterals hides clinical findings [13]. The prevalence of occlusion after the implantation of ICD has not been extensively studied. A recent paper found a stenosis of the major subclavian in 75%, and total obstruction in 7%, of subjects with one-chamber defibrillators who had no signs of venous obstruction [14].

Predisposing Mechanism and Physiopathology

The pathogenesis of lead-induced venous obstruction seems to involve several factors, which include (1) endothelial damage induced by the lead(s); (2) for-

[1]Divisione di Cardiologia con UTIC, Augusta (SR); [2]Divisione di Cardiologia, Vittoria (RG); [3]Divisione di Cardiologia con UTIC, Caltagirone (CT); [4]Istituto di Cardiologia, Ospedale Ferrarotto (CT), Italy

eign-body reaction with inflammation, fibrosis and thrombosis; (3) a postoperative state of hypercoagulability; and (4) extension and propagation of thrombi from ligated veins or fibrous stenosis [8, 15]. Fibrous stenosis generally develops just over the right atrium [11]; occlusion starts where the leads are in contact with the vessel wall or in spots where the lead loses its insulating surface [16]. The onset of venous obstruction seems to be associated with several predisposing factors, such as (1) infected leads [17]; (2) retained leads; (3) repeated pacemaker implantation [11]; (4) vessel wall trauma during implantation; (5) dual-chamber devices [2]; and (6) loss of insulation of leads. The effect of the number and size of leads is controversial, and while Goudevenos et al. report them as a risk factor [17], Bauset in a recent paper refutes this [11]. ICD leads, which are larger than pacing leads and also include shock coils, induce occlusion in a low percentage of cases almost comparable to that seen with pacing leads [8, 14]. According to Sticherling et al. [14], it is not clear why ICD leads with diameters up to 3.93 mm and/or the presence of two or more leads are not predictors of occlusion; the authors conclude that the maximum size does not seem to be a major risk factor in occlusion, in contrast to the use of three or more leads. No differences in the incidence of thrombosis were found between cephalic vein or subclavian vein approaches, or between various insulating materials used for leads [8], although some authors suggest that polyurethane is less thrombogenic than silicone [16, 18]. The onset of venous obstructions is thought to take place an average of 6 [9] to 15 [11] months after lead implantation, though it has also been observed immediately after [19]. Venous thrombosis without stenosis may occur early (< 1 year); late stenosis (> 1 year) can happen with or without thrombosis [9].

Symptoms

The clinical presentation is influenced by the magnitude and functionality of the collaterals developed. Usually, the onset is insidious and the patient remains asymptomatic; when a revision of the pacing device is needed the diagnosis becomes evident [20]. The time to symptom occurrence can also be several years after pacemaker implantation; symptoms can be minimal or completely absent.

In SVC syndrome, symptoms include bloating and acute edema of head, face, upper arms and chest, headache, dizziness, dyspnea, chest or upper arm pain and numbness, nonpulsatile distension of veins in the neck and shoulders, prominent collaterals in these regions, and facial discoloration and cyanosis, all of which are worsened by lying down or leaning forward [21].

Diagnosis

It is important to distinguish SVC syndromes due to lead-induced thrombosis from those that have other causes (e.g., malignancies, which count for about 90% of all cases). For this reason careful history-taking and a physical examination are needed. A chest radiogram can exclude the majority of malignancies (bronchogenic carcinoma in 80% of cases). CT, spiral CT, digital image subtraction phlebography and NMR are currently the diagnostic procedures of first choice, having high sensitivity and specificity, while venography is no longer the principal imaging technique but is very useful in the preparation for surgical correction [11]. Doppler echocardiography can detect absence of flow in the obstructed veins, i.e. in the SVC [22].

Therapy

Given the low prevalence of this pathology, in the face of the high number of pacemaker and ICD implantations, and the lack of randomized controlled trials, too little experience is available for a consensus on the best treatment to be possible. Hence, the approach to each case is conditioned mainly by the expertise in the various surgical and percutaneous techniques in the hospital the patient is referred to.

Anticoagulation

A conservative medical treatment was used in the past with some success in SVC syndrome, but at present, owing to the high incidence of recurrence, it is used mainly as an adjunctive treatment in SVC syndrome induced by lead implantation, especially when the thrombosis is located under a stenosis in the SVC or when leads cannot be explanted. In a recent study on ten patients with SVC syndrome treated with sodium heparin plus oral anticoagulants, this treatment was successful in only 3, all of whom had early thrombosis (< 1 year), probably without stenosis. Some good results have been obtained in patients with collaterals. Since the associated morbidity is low, anticoagulation could be a feasible first-line therapy; more aggressive approaches could still be chosen if severe symptoms persisted after anticoagulation. At this time, there is no consensus on the role of anticoagulation after stenting or vascular surgery [11].

Thrombolysis

This approach was suggested in 1974 [23]. The duration of symptoms before the onset of thrombolytic therapy is a strong predictor of success: this intervention is effective only when applied acutely, its success rate being 88% when it is performed sooner than 5 days after the onset of the thrombosis, but only 25% when it is performed more than 5 days after [24]. The best results are obtained within the first week. In each case, thrombolysis remains useful as a way of attenuating symptoms, disclosing the morphology of lesions and optimizing further percutaneous or surgical interventions [11]. The most common medications used are urokinase and rtPA delivered in situ by way of infusion catheters.

Percutaneous Endovascular Procedures

Angioplasty

Angioplasty [25] with or without stenting [26] was introduced in 1986. Stenting is performed in patients with residual fibrotic stenosis, generally after thrombolysis, since angioplasty alone would carry a high rate of early restenosis in these circumstances. It is contraindicated in patients recently treated for pacemaker infection and in patients with septicemia or positive hemocultures [13]. Total occlusion of the SVC is not a contraindication. Stents with a less tight metal scaffold carry a lower risk of thrombosis [27].

A strategy of thrombolysis and angioplasty with stenting has given an 85% technical success rate [28]. Complications of this strategy include bleeding attributable to thrombolysis and anticoagulation, stent migration, and occlusion. Angioplasty has also been performed after failed surgery.

There is currently no evidence to suggest that compression of the pacemaker leads by the stent can damage their functionality [11]; it is thought that since leads are encapsulated in the vessel wall by the tissue reaction there may be no direct contact between stent and leads [29].

Furthermore, there are concerns about the outcome of any lead explantation, which could be made difficult by the presence of the stent [11]. At present, no prospective randomized clinical trials relating to the role of stenting in lead-induced SVC syndrome are available, so that the indications for such techniques are still not well defined. There is no evidence that stenting has any advantage over angioplasty alone, except when angioplasty alone has failed. The critical point is long-term patency, since SVC syndrome is a benign condition and long-term survival is expected.

Surgery

Invasive surgery through a sternotomy remains the gold standard, but is now reserved for patients with debilitating symptoms and evidence of long-term obstruction. The aims of the surgical procedures are to get rid of SVC obstruction and stenosis and to explant endocardial leads and implant epicardial [11] or transfemoral [13] leads if needed. The type of procedure selected is determined by the degree and extension of the secondary fibrotic stenosis. Implants of autologous tissue from the pericardium are used for cavoplasty; as an alternative it is possible to perform a bypass from the jugular or the innominate vein to the right atrium, using an autologous spiral vein, or to construct a Dacron graft [11], especially in patients without residual indications for pacing, near-complete caval stenosis, and retrograde azygos flow. Such an intervention could be the procedure of first choice in patients of this kind [30].

References

1. Stoney W, Addestone R, Alford W et al (1996) The incidence of venous thrombosis following long-term transvenous pacing. Ann Thorac Surg 22:166–170
2. Mazzetti H, Daussaut A, Tentori C et al (1993) Superior vena cava occlusion and/or syndrome related to pacemaker leads. Am Heart J 125:831–837
3. Antonelli D, Turgeman Y, Kaveh Z, Artoul S (1989) Short-term thrombosis after transvenous permanent pacemaker insertion. Pacing Clin Electrophysiol 12:280–282
4. Spittel PC, Vliestra RE, Hayes DL et al (1990) Venous obstruction due to permanent transvenous pacemaker electrodes: treatment with percutaneous transluminal balloon venoplasty. Pacing Clin Electrophysiol 13:271–274
5. Phibbs B, Marriot H (1985) Complications of permanent transvenous pacing. N Engl J Med 22:1428–1432
6. Porath A, Avnun L, Hirsch M, Ovsysshcher I (1987) Right atrial thrombus and recurrent pulmonary emboli secondary to cardiac pacing; a case report and short review of literature. Angiology 38:267
7. Bogart DB, Collins RH, Montgomerie MA, Dombek SJ, Earnest JB, Fischer EH (1985) Shock late after implantation of a permanent transvenous cardiac pacemaker. Am J Cardiol 55:1241–1242
8. Spittell P, Hayes D (1992) Venous complications after insertion of a transvenous pacemaker. Mayo Clin Proc 67:258–265
9. Kar AK, Ghosh S, Majumdar A, Mondal M, Dutta I (2000) Venous obstruction after permanent pacing. Indian Heart J 52:431–433
10. Lin CT, Kuo CT, Lin KH, Hsu JS (1999) Superior vena cava syndrome as a complication of transvenous permanent pacemaker implantation. Jpn Heart J 40:477–480
11. Bauset R (2002) Pacemaker-induced superior vena cava syndrome: a case report and review of management strategy. Can J Cardiol 18:1229–1232
12. Blackburn T, Dunn M (1988) Pacemaker-induced superior vena cava syndrome: consideration of management. Am Heart J 116:893–896
13. Newall N, Stables R, Palmer N, Ramsdale D (2002) Treatment of superior vena caval obstruction following permanent pacemaker extraction. Pacing Clin Electrophysiol 25:1780–1783
14. Sticherling C, Chough SP, Baker RL et al (2001) Prevalence of central venous occlusion in patients with chronic defibrillator leads. Am Heart J 141:813–816
15. Goto Y, Abe T, Sekine S, Sakurada T (1998) Long-term thrombosis after transvenous permanent pacemaker implantation. Pacing Clin Electrophysiol 21:1192–1195
16. Stokes K, Chem B, Anderson J et al (1995) The encapsulation of polyurethane-insulated transvenous cardiac pacemaker leads. Cardiovasc Pathol 4:163–171
17. Goudevenos JA, Reid PG, Adams PC, Holden MP, Williams DO (1989) Pacemaker induced superior vena cava syndrome: report of four cases and review of the literature. Pacing Clin Electrophysiol 12:1890–1895
18. Palatianos GM, Dewanjee MK, Panoutsopoulos G et al (1994) Comparative thrombogenicity of pacemaker leads. Pacing Clin Electrophysiol 17:141–145
19. Furman S, Hayes DL, Holman DR (1993) A practice of cardiac pacing. Futura, New York
20. Pavia S, Wilkoff B (2001) The management of surgical complications of pacemaker and implantable cardioverter-defibrillators. Curr Opin Cardiol 16:66–71
21. Tan CW, Vijitbenjaronk P, Khuri B (2000) Superior vena cava syndrome due to permanent transvenous pacemaker electrodes: successful treatment with combined thrombolysis and angioplasty. A case report. Angiology 55:963–969

22. Fernandez Vazquez E, Ortega Antelo M, Merlos Navarro S, Martin-Vivaldi Martinez F, Jimenez Lozano G (2002) Superior vena cava syndrome secondary to intracavitary implantation of a pacemaker. Arch Bronconeumol 38:336–338
23. Williams D, Demos N (1974) Thrombosis of superior vena cava caused by pacemaker wire and managed with streptokinase. J Thorac Cardiovasc Surg 68:134–137
24. Gray BH, Olin JW, Graor RA, Young JR, Batholomew JR, Ruschhaupt WF (1991) Safety and efficacy of thrombolytic therapy for superior vena cava syndrome. Chest 99:54–59
25. Sherry CS, Diamond NG, Meyers TP, Martin RL (1986) Successful treatment of SVC syndrome by venous angioplasty. AJR Am J Roentgenol 147:834–935
26. Charnsangavej C, Carrasco CH, Wallace S, Wright KC, Ogawa K, Richli W, Gianturco C (1986) Stenosis of the vena cava: preliminary assessment of treatment with expandable metallic stents. Radiology 161:295–298
27. Oudkerk M, Kuijpers T, Schmitz P et al (1996) Self-expanding metal stents for palliative treatment of superior vena cava syndrome. Cardiovasc Intervent Radiol 19:146–151
28. Crowe MT, Davies CH, Gaines PA (1995) Percutaneous management of superior vena cava occlusions. Cardiovasc Intervent Radiol 18:367–372
29. Teo N, Sabharwal T, Rowland E, Curry P, Adam A (2002) Treatment of superior vena cava obstruction secondary to pacemaker wires with balloon venoplasty and insertion of metallic stents. Eur Heart J 23:1465–1470
30. al-Saman MM, Fares AM, Rabee HM (2000) Extra-anatomical long-saphenous conduit for decompression of superior vena cava syndrome. Eur J Vasc Surg 19:426–427

Lead-Related Thrombi in Patients with Pacemaker/ICD: What Is the Prevalence, Clinical Significance, and Recommended Management?

R.M. Polimeni[1], G. Meduri[1], A. Amato[1], D. Baccellieri[2]

The presence of thrombi on a permanent pacemaker lead is a rare complication of pacing. The reported cases relate to axillary subclavian vein thrombosis or the onset of thrombi at different sites on the permanent pacemaker lead [1–3]. Clinically, thromboembolic complications related to permanent cardiac pacing may affect the upper arm, axillary, subclavian or jugular veins, right atrium, and pulmonary circulation [4, 5].

There is a relative paucity of data on this subject, so the prevalence of these late complications of permanent pacing is unknown. Most of the information dates back to the 1970s; only a few cases were reported in 1990s [6–8].

A comprehensive study regarding the prevalence and significance of lead-related thrombi in patients with implantable cardioverter-defibrillators (ICDs) has been recently published by Chow et al. [9]. In a series of 185 consecutive patients who received ICDs, lead-related thrombi were detected in 25% of the patients by transesophageal echocardiography (TEE) at a mean of 4 months after ICD implantation. This is the first study to report the prevalence of ICD lead-related thrombi: an unexpected value if compared with the clinical behavior of these patients.

Chow et al. report different locations on the ICD leads where thrombi congregated: the right atrial–superior vena cava junction (25%), the right atrial body (36%), the tricuspid annulus (25%), the right ventricle, the ostium of the coronary sinus and superior vena cava. Thrombi were significantly ($p<0.01$) more often present in patients with polyurethane leads (35%) than in patients with silicone leads (20%). ICD lead-related thrombi were more common in patients not on anticoagulation treatment.

As far as the optimal diagnostic assessment of lead-related thrombi in patients with pacemakers and ICDs is concerned, TEE should be performed because of its better resolution and the detailed visualization of the superior vena cava and right atrium. This method avoids the limitations related to a

[1]U.O. di Cardiologia, UTIC, Ospedale S. Maria degli Ungheresi, Polistena (RC), and [2]U.O. di Chirurgia Vascolare, Policlinico Universitario G. Martino, Messina, Polistena (RC), Italy

poor acoustic window and reverberations produced by the pacemaker or ICD lead.

The incidence of lead-related thrombosis is probably underestimated in clinical practice: large studies are needed to define the its true prevalence, the clinical incidence of pathological manifestations, and the optimal therapy. In the case of an uninfected thrombus attached to a pacemaker or ICD lead, the optimal treatment depends on the clinical manifestation, size and shape of the thrombus, and the alternative approaches, which include thrombolysis and surgery [2, 3, 5, 10, 11]. Prophylactic anticoagulation could be necessary in ICD patients if the results reported by Chow et al. are confirmed by a large clinical trial, performance of which would be desirable in the near future. Increasing symptoms of dyspnea and right-sided heart failure should prompt a high index of suspicion of pulmonary embolism in patients with transvenous pacemaker or ICD leads: in these cases a complete diagnostic workup to detect possible lead-related thrombi becomes necessary.

References

1. Swinkels BM, Oudeophuis AJM, Zegers ES et al (2001) Recurrent pacemaker lead induced axillary subclavian vein thrombosis. Pacing Clin Electrophysiol 24:910–911
2. Zegers ES, Oudeophuis AJM, Meursing BTJ et al (2000) Successful treatment of subclavian vein thrombosis with thrombolysis after pacemaker implantation. Cardiologie 7:11–14
3. Hicken GJ, Ameli FM (1998) Management of subclavian axillary vein thrombosis: a review. Can J Surg 41:13–25
4. Spittel PC, Hayes DL (1992) Venous complications after insertion of a transvenous pacemaker. Mayo Clin Proc 67:258–265
5. Wierzbowska K, Krzeminska-Pakula M, Marszal-Marciniak M et al (2001) Symptomatic atrial pacemaker lead thrombosis: detection by echocardiography and successful surgical treatment. Pacing Clin Electrophysiol 24:391–393
6. Kinney EL, Allen RP, Weidner WA et al (1979) Recurrent pulmonary emboli secondary to right atrial thrombus around a permanent pacing catheter: a case report and review of the literature. Pacing Clin Electrophysiol 2:196–202
7. Nicolosi GL, Charmet PA, Zanutti D (1980) Large right atrial thrombosis: rare complication during permanent transvenous endocardial pacing. Br Heart J 43:199–201
8. Harcombe AA, Newell SA, Ludman PF et al (1998) Late complications following permanent pacemaker implantation or elective unit replacement. Heart 80:240–244
9. Chow BJW, Hassan AH, Chan KL, Tang AJL (2003) Prevalence and significance of lead related thrombi in patients with implantable cardioverter-defibrillators. Am J Cardiol 91:88–90
10. Cooper CJ, Dweik R, Gabbay S (1993) Treatment of pacemaker-associated right atrial thrombus with 2 hour rTPA infusion. Am Heart J 126:228–229
11. De Vries H, Inversen S, Zimmermann W et al (1991) Chronic thromboembolic cor pulmonale in pacemaker-associated right atrial thrombi. Pulmonary thromboendarterectomy with removal of electrodes as a life-saving measure. Dtsch Med Wochenschr 116:294–298

Effects of Electromagnetic Interference on Implanted Cardiac Devices

M. L. Blitzer, M. H. Schoenfeld

Introduction

Cardiac pacemakers and defibrillators are remarkable devices with the ability to provide marked symptom relief and life-saving therapy. An ever-expanding list of indications continues to enlarge the pool of patients who live with implantable devices. Intrinsic to the function of these devices is the ability to sense intra-cardiac signals. An unfortunate by-product is the potential for electromagnetic energy in the environment to interact with and disturb the normal functioning of these devices. This chapter will review the way electromagnetic interference (EMI) can affect cardiac devices and then discuss specific situations and optimal techniques to minimize the chance of untoward interaction.

Electromagnetic interference can occur with energy anywhere along the full electromagnetic spectrum, although interaction is most likely with radio or microwave frequencies. The three most feared sequelae are 1) inhibition of ventricular pacing output in pacemaker-dependent patients, 2) inappropriate triggering of implantable cardiac defibrillator (ICD) shock therapy and 3) damage to the system (device). The first, in theory, could result in lethal asystole. Fortunately, in practice, most reports of ventricular inhibition occur for only 1 or, at most, a few beats. This could be due to the brevity of the source of interference (e.g. electrocautery bursts in the operating room) or the brevity of the time the patient is in range of the source of interference (e.g. walking through an anti-theft detector at the entrance to a store).

The chance of EMI-induced pacing inhibition is further limited by noise reversion modes [1]. The specifics of these algorithms vary by manufacturer, but all are based on the concept that rapid frequencies are unlikely to originate in the heart; therefore, rapid signals reset "noise sampling" windows, eventually resulting in asynchronous pacing. Noise reversion algorithms are quite effective in pacemakers but are infrequently applied within cardiac defibrillators whose primary purpose is to successfully detect the rapid signals of ven-

Cardiac Electrophysiology and Pacer Laboratory, Hospital of Saint Raphael; Yale University School of Medicine, New Haven, Connecticut, USA

tricular tachycardia and ventricular fibrillation.

The frequency of inappropriate ICD shock therapy in response to EMI has been substantially reduced with recent generations of devices as "committed" treatment has been replaced by re-confirmation algorithms. With the earlier algorithms, the EMI needed only to last for sufficient time to trigger "detection" of ventricular tachycardia (VT), while with the newer algorithms, the EMI must persist, at least intermittently, during charging and pre-shock redetection in order to cause an inappropriate shock.

Other common but less dangerous forms of interaction include triggering of rapid pacing or inappropriate mode switching, asynchronous pacing or transient suppression of ventricular tachycardia (VT) sensing. While sensing of EMI on the ventricular channel can inhibit output, the same EMI on the atrial channel can result in rapid ventricular tracking. Fortunately, the rate of ventricular pacing is limited to the programmed upper rate limit of the device. Sensing of very rapid impulses on the atrial channel can result in mode switching with the resulting potential for "pacemaker syndrome" related to loss of atrio-ventricular (AV) synchrony.

Asynchronous pacing can occur in a pacemaker if it is exposed to a static magnetic field. It usually requires roughly a 10 Gauss strength magnetic field to close the reed switch. Fortunately, this is rarely of clinical import as decades of purposeful magnet application during trans-telephonic monitoring have demonstrated. The probability of an inadvertent pacing impulse falling on the T wave and triggering VT is miniscule.

That same magnetic field elicits an entirely different response when applied to a defibrillator. In this instance, reed switch closure has no effect on pacing function but instead transiently inhibits VT detection and treatment. Importantly, some defibrillators may be more permanently deactivated if the magnetic field remains constant for greater than thirty seconds. This may be noted in some device models by a change in R wave synchronous beeping tones to a continuous tone. There have been reports of "hidden" magnetic fields from Bingo wands [2] and stereo speakers inadvertently deactivating certain defibrillators. Recently, more manufacturers have been incorporating speakers into ICDs which sound when a magnet field of sufficient strength to close the reed switch are encountered to "warn" the patient and allow him to remove himself from his present environment.

Other EMI interactions with cardiac devices are rare but cannot be ignored. This includes the possibility of inducing current flow along the lead producing ventricular capture [3], or increased pacing thresholds from a "burn" at the electrode-myocardial interface. Permanent damage to the circuitry of the device from strong electric current remains possible but has been minimized with filtering circuitry such as Zener diodes which shunt current flow away from the internal circuitry. More commonly, a momentary "spike" may trigger an electric (Power-On) reset particularly with pacemakers where a device may revert to more "primitive" settings such as VVI or VOO. Most commonly, this will require specific programming commands to restore the prior settings.

While programmers communicate with cardiac devices via radio-frequency energy, it is exceedingly rare for EMI to directly result in device re-programming as most companies require a specific RF "handshake" between the two before re-programming is permitted.

Electrocautery

The use of intraoperative electrocautery remains one of the most common sources of EMI/cardiac device interaction. Virtually all of the above-mentioned interactions are possible. Obviously, the most concerning are those of EMI-induced ICD shocks and EMI-induced pacer inhibition. A careful pre-op assessment of pacer dependency, frequency of tachyarrhythmias and shocks and exact programmed parameters is critical. The use of cautery should be minimized with individual pulses limited to 1-2 seconds and with sufficient time between pulses to minimize possible hemodynamic effects of cautery-induced pacing inhibition [4]. Bipolar electrocautery has markedly reduced interaction with cardiac devices and is theoretically preferable but its decreased efficacy on hemostasis compared to unipolar electrocautery limits its enthusiastic use among surgeons. With unipolar cautery, it is important to place the grounding pad away from the device such that current flow from tip to pad is drawn away from, not towards, the device. ICDs, in general, should have their tachycardia functions turned "off" either with formal reprogramming of the device pre- post-surgery or with continuous magnet application. However, there is potential for permanent reprogramming of certain defibrillators with continuous magnet application. Additionally, there is the risk for unsecured magnets to be dislodged from their position adjacent to the device during surgery thereby obviating their function. The recently released Medtronic Smart Magnet® represents a small advance in this area since caregivers can be reassured as to the correct positioning of the magnet by a series of lights on top of the magnet which remain lit as long as the magnet remains in the correct position. Rapid access to external defibrillators must be assured in patients with peri-procedural ICD de-activation.

In general, patients with pacemakers who are not pacer-dependent do not require specific reprogramming. In contrast, in patients who are pacer-dependent, consideration should be given to reprogramming to an asynchronous mode or magnet application. Telemetry should be carefully watched for pacemaker inhibition. It is often useful to have a second means of monitoring the pulse as electrocautery can often create sufficient artifact on the ECG monitor to render it useless. Following the arterial line pressure tracing or the deflections on the pulse oximeter are often very helpful. Rather than creating a fixed set of intraoperative rules, the most important aspect of management is an awareness that potential interactions can occur, an understanding of how to avoid and correct potential problems and good communication between surgeon, anesthesiologist and staff.

MRI

Magnetic resonance imaging (MRI) presents a complicated array of fixed and variable magnetic fields and radiofrequency pulse sequences. This creates a wide range of potential interactions with cardiac devices. These include reed switch closure, pacing inhibition, inappropriate ICD discharges and rapid pacing. The latter can either be initiated either from the pulse generator or, independently, by the induction of current flow along the lead. Other potential interactions can result in a rise in pacing thresholds or the induction of torque on the generator itself. Recent devices have less ferro-magnetic material in the housing and, therefore, are subject to less rotational and translational forces [5]. Similarly, the metal alloy present within the leads has virtually no ferrous material and, therefore, has minimal potential for dislodgement. Prior to initial device placement, the implanter should always consider if an MRI is likely to be necessary in the near future and, if possible, schedule the imaging prior to implantation.

In general, the presence of a permanent pacemaker (PPM) or ICD should be considered an absolute contraindication to MRI. If an MRI is suggested in a patient with an implanted device, other imaging modalities should be explored. There is some limited data on the use of MRI in patients with pacemakers (and even less in those with ICDs). In very rare situations, use of an MRI may be considered but only with close coordination and discussion among electrophysiologist, radiologist and patient. Factors that may decrease the likelihood of complications include the use of less powerful MRI machines, imaging of extremities (i.e. device not within gantry), careful reprogramming of the device, selection of spin sequences, peri-procedural monitoring and restriction of scans to non pacemaker-dependent patients [6].

DC Cardioversion

Cardioversion produces the largest energy pulse of any source likely to be encountered. Devices have built-in protective mechanisms such as zener diodes designed to shunt energy away from the delicate device circuitry when sensed energy exceeds certain values. Nonetheless, in rare cases, particularly with older pacemakers, irreversible circuitry damage can occur. Other potential complications include triggering reset mode and inducing current flow down the lead resulting in elevated pacing thresholds (usually transient). Problems may be minimized by using the least required energy. Use of more efficient biphasic defibrillators may help in that regard. The pads should be placed at least 5 cm from the implanted device [7]. Antero-posterior pad positioning is ideal when trying to keep the shocking vector perpendicular to the vector between device and lead. Often, the ICD itself can be utilized to deliver the shock. Using an external defibrillator with back-up pacing capabilities is prudent in pacer-dependent patients particularly those who have older devices.

Radiotherapy

The primary issue with radiotherapy is potential damage from the ionizing radiation to silicone oxide insulators within the semiconductors [8]. This can result in random component failure and premature battery depletion. Most problems occur with thoracic radiation (i.e. breast or lung cancer) where the device would be within the radiation field. In these instances the device may need to be abandoned in favor of a new lead/device system elsewhere or lead extenders can be used to move the generator to the ipsilateral abdomen or contralateral pectoral region.

Even if the device is not directly within the radiation field, it should be shielded. Intensified device testing both during treatment as well as for several months afterward is important. There should be a low threshold to implant a new generator if any significant abnormality is noted. As always, particular care should be taken in pacemaker-dependent patients.

Transcutaneous Electric Nerve Stimulation

Transcutaneous electric nerve stimulation (TENS) is an increasingly common treatment for various musculoskeletal disorders. The induced electrical field has the potential for interacting with pacemakers and causing pacing inhibition, particularly when placed near to unipolar pacing systems [9]. Fortunately, clinically important interactions are rare. There have been numerous reports, however, of TENS resulting in inappropriate defibrillator shocks [10]. The initial session should therefore be performed with ICD personnel observing for any interaction and with the device programmed to "monitor-only" mode. The authors recently had a patient in whom formal observation of the TENS procedure showed no interaction with the device. However, the patient became frustrated with the lack of treatment results and turned the TENS unit, on his own, to maximal output. This immediately resulted in delivery of a shock.

Anti-Theft Surveillance Systems

Anti-theft detection systems are becoming ubiquitous in retail centers around the world. Several different technologies are used to detect metal alloy-containing tags on retail merchandise. The greatest number of interactions have been reported with the acousto-magnetic technology [3]. "Worst case" testing has been done in which patients linger within the fields closely apposed to the gates. In these situations, there are reports of sensing irregularities causing rapid pacing or pacing inhibition in pacemaker patients and inappropriate shocks in ICD patients. However, the frequency of clinically relevant symptoms in real life situations has been extraordinarily rare. Patients should be reassured that, as long as they walk through the store thresholds without either lingering or leaning directly against the gates, that there is minimal risk of harm [11].

Cellular Telephones

Use of cellular technology has exploded worldwide over the last decade with hundreds of millions of current users. Digital technology has usurped analog as the dominant worldwide system. Even within the spectra of digital telephony, several distinct systems are available which vary in band spectrum, power usage and modulation techniques. Power output of a given phone can vary markedly depending on its proximity to cellular towers. Regions with greater density of cell towers generally use less of the maximal output of the telephone than more sparsely populated regions, but other factors, such as the density of cell use in a given area at a given moment in time, also have important effects.

In one large study, the most common interactions with pacemakers was tracking interference sensed on the atrial channel followed by asynchronous pacing and ventricular inhibition. The only clinically significant effects were noted when the cell phone (while "on") was held directly over the device. There were no important interactions noted with the cell phone placed at the ipsilateral ear. Untoward effects were seen more commonly with dual chamber devices [12].

The presence of feed-through filters, which are present in virtually all modern day devices, markedly diminish the potential for EMI. All pacemaker patients should be cautioned to avoid placing a cell phone in a shirt or jacket pocket overlying the generator. Some recommend using the ear contralateral to the device for use, although this is likely not necessary except with high-powered fixed cellular devices, such as those in cars and boats.

Testing of cell phones in patients with ICDs has been less extensive than with pacemakers but a reasonably sized database is emerging. In general, interference has been extraordinarily rare and limited to situations with phones held within one inch of the ICD. Reed switch activation leading to VT underdetection and erroneous shock therapy are theoretically possible. Similar recommendations to pacemaker patients apply.

Airport Security Devices

Walk-through metal detectors have been extensively tested for potential interaction with implanted devices. In general, careful observation has not revealed any alteration in normal pacemaker/defibrillator behavior nor have patients reported symptoms [13]. On the other hand, metal detectors can easily pick-up the ferrous material in the device case. This is particularly relevant at the enhanced sensitivity settings that most airport detectors have been using in recent years.

If a hand held detector is used, greater potential for problems exists. There is a report of an inappropriate ICD shock being triggered as well as an incident of inadvertant reversion to a "monitor-only" mode secondary to prolonged contact between device and detector [1]. There is minimal chance for interactions if the patient requests that the airport worker limit the time the detector is near the implanted device. If patient or security expresses any concern over these parameters, a hand search is a safe and reasonable alternative.

Conclusions

Electromagnetic energy is ubiquitous in daily life. Careful design of implanted devices has successfully kept the potential for important interactions to a minimum. This has greatly enhanced the quality of life of device recipients. Many patients return to work full-time and travel widely. Nonetheless, EMI will only increase in the future as emerging technologies such as higher powered cellular telephones, new laptop computer communication protocols and even wireless credit-card readers become widely disseminated. Databases, which reach relevant parties with updated information on new device interactions, will be important to avoid problems. Continuing communication among device manufacturers, physicians, patients and regulatory bodies will be critical.

References

1. Pinski SL, Trohman RG (2002) Interference in implanted cardiac devices, Part I. PACE 25:1367-1381
2. Ferrick KJ, Johnston D, Kim SG et al (1991) Inadvertant AICD inactivation while playing bingo. Am Heart J 121:206-207
3. McIvor ME, Reddinger J, Floden E et al (1998) Study of pacemaker and implantable cardioverter defibrillator triggering by electronic article surveillance devices (SPICED TEAS). PACE 21:1847-1861
4. Madigan JD, Choudhri AF, Chen J et al (1999) Surgical management of the patient with an implanted cardiac device: Implications of electromagnetic interference. Annals of Surgery 5:639-647
5. Gimbel JR, Johnson D, Levine PA et al (1996) Safe performance of magnetic resonance imaging on five patients with permanent cardiac pacemakers. PACE 19:913-919
6. Sommer T, Vahlhaus C, Lauck G et al (2000) MR imaging and cardiac pacemakers: In vitro evaluation and in vivo studies in 51 patients at 0.5 T. Radiology 215:869-879
7. Goldschlager N, Epstein A, Friedman P et al (2001) Environmental and drug effects on patients with pacemakers and implantable cardioverter/defibrillators: A practical guide to patient treatment. Arch Intern Med 161:649-655
8. Pinski SL, Trohman RG (2002) Interference in implanted cardiac devices, Part II. PACE 25:1496-1509
9. Eriksson M, Schuller H, Sjolund B (1978) Hazards from transcutaneous nerve stimulation in patients with pacemakers. Lancet 1:1319

10. Philbin DM, Marieb MA, Aithal KH et al (1998) Inappropriate shocks delivered by an ICD as a result of sensed potentials from a transcutaneous electronic nerve stimulation unit. PACE 21:2010-2011
11. Mugica J, Henry L, Podeur H (2000) Study of interactions between permanent pacemakers and electronic antitheft surveillance systems. PACE 23:333-337
12. Hayes DL, Wang PJ, Reynolds DW et al (1997) Interference with cardiac pacemakers by cellular telephones. New Engl J Med 336:1473-1479
13. Cooperman Y, Zarfati D, Laniado S (1988) The effect of metal detector gates on implanted permanent pacemakers. PACE 11:1386-1387

Subject Index

Ablation 11, 159, 177, 271, 293
    balloon 173
    catheter 107, 195, 205, 215, 285, 357, 433, 451
    cryothermal 2, 189, 285
    linear 221
    of atrial fibrillation 149
    radiofrequency 215
Accessory pathway 89, 285
ACE inhibitors 93
Age 599
AICDs 469, 527
Alpha-antagonist agents 659
Amiodarone 301
Angiotensin receptor blockers 93
Antiarrhthmia theraphy 541
Anticoagulation 71, 231
    level 235
    protocol 205
Antitachycardia pacing 697
Antithrombotic therapy 127
Arrhythmia 177, 379, 427, 655, 767
    supraventricular 141
Atrial
    arrhythmias 301
    defibrillator 697
    fibrillation 11, 23, 29, 43, 51, 71, 79, 93, 99, 117, 107, 127, 137, 159, 173, 177, 189, 195, 205, 215, 221, 231, 235, 301, 697
        arrhythmogenesis 149
        classification 127
        non-valvular 11
        post-operative 43
    flutter 257, 271
        acute treatment 257
    resynchronization 851
    tachycardia 293
Autonomic failure 625
Autonomic nervous system 641

Bionic therapy 117
Biventricular pacing 753, 815
BLS-D 569
Body surface potential maps 387
Brugada Syndrome 335, 339
Brugada-Type ECG 331

Cardiac
    arrest 563
    arrhythmias 309
    dyssynchrony 741
    function 705
    ion channels 379
    mapping 357
    pacing 141, 651, 655, 679
    resynchronization 805
    resynchronization therapy 741, 823, 837, 861, 877
    surgery 43, 415
Cardiovascular drugs 99
Cardioversion 51, 71, 93, 235
    electrical 79
Clinical trials 469, 489
Coffee 309
Congenital heart disease 293
Congestive heart failure 117, 805
Contractility 705, 767
Conversion therapy 51
Coronary
    artery disease 405
    revascularization 405
Cost-effectiveness 489
CPAP 679
Cryotherapy 177

Death 857
Defibrillation 469, 519, 527, 555
early 563, 569
Diagnosis 589, 599
Diagnostic functions 799
Drug therapy with ICD 541
Dual-chamber pacing 137, 697

Early recurrences 79
Ejection fraction 397
Electrical cardioversion 79
Electroanatomic mapping 433
ECG 335
Electromagnetic interference 911
Electrophysiological testing 481
Electrophysiology 379
study 387, 463, 469, 481
Embolic events 205
Excimer laser sheath 897
External defibrillator 555, 563

First responder 555

Gene mutations 379
Genetics 667
Guidelines 127

Handgrip 641
Heart
failure 107, 741, 823, 837, 851, 857, 861, 877
rate 99
transplantation 427
Hemodynamics 705, 741,
High-density pulmonary vein mapping 149
Hypertension 23
Hypertrophic cardiomyopathy 371, 29
Hypertrophy 767
left ventricular 371

Ibutilide 257
Impedance 705
Implantable defibrillators 141, 405, 427, 463, 469, 481, 489, 519, 527, 541, 837, 877, 885
economics 497
failure 885
implant complications 893
infections 885
lead extraction 897
Incisional tachycardia 293
Inherited cardiomyopathy 339
Intracardiac echocardiography 451
Isometric exercise 641
Isthmus 271

Laser energy 173
Lead extraction 885, 897
new technologies 897
Left atrial appendage 71
Left ventricular
dysfunction 481
pacing 753
stimulation 837
Long term follow-up 823
Loop recorders 589, 599

Management algorithm 43
Mapping 271
Microwave ablation 215
Mutation 667
Myocardial infarction 397

Naples Heart Project 569
Nervous system autonomic 655
Neurally-mediated syncope 625, 651
Non-responders 741
Non-invasive markers 469
Non-sustained ventricular tachycardia 481
Normal hearts 11

Oral anticoagulants 231
Orthostatic hypotension 625
Overdrive 679

Pacemaker 705, 837, 885
failure 885
implant complications 897
infections 885
lead extraction 897
therapy 655, 799
Pacing 107, 767
prevention algorithms 697
preventive 137
right ventricular 815
transesophageal 257
Parasympathetic nervous system 117
Peak endocardial acceleration 753
Physical counterpressure maneuvers 633
Post-myocardial infarction 481
Postural tachycardia syndrome 625

Prevalence 331
Prognosis 29
Public access 555
Pulmonary vein 173, 177, 159, 189
isolation 159
stenosis 149

Quality of life 107

Rate control 117
versus rhythm control 127
Re-entry 271
Resynchronization therapy 857
Reverse remodeling 767

Seizures 589
Sensors 799
Sick sinus syndrome 137
Signal averaged ECG 387
Sinus node disease 667
Sleep apnea 679
Sport activity 11
Stroke prevention 231
Substrate modification 221
Sudden death 335, 339, 379, 397, 405, 463, 469, 497, 541, 563, 569, 861, 877
Surgery 221, 293
Syncope 589, 599, 641

Therapy responders 805
Thromboembolic risk 235
Thromboembolism 231
Thrombus formation 205
Tilt test 589, 659, 641
Transesophageal
echocardiography 71
pacing 257
Treatment 633
T-wave alternans 387

Valvular heart surgery 301
Vasovagal syncope 633, 655
therapy 659
Ventilation 679
Ventricular
arrhythmias 141, 387, 415
fibrillation 335, 415, 527, 541, 563
idiopathic 339
resynchronization 741, 823, 837, 851, 857, 861, 877
tachycardia 357, 397, 415, 433, 451, 489

Water 625
Waveforms 519

GPSR Compliance

The European Union's (EU) General Product Safety Regulation (GPSR) is a set of rules that requires consumer products to be safe and our obligations to ensure this.

If you have any concerns about our products, you can contact us on ProductSafety@springernature.com

In case Publisher is established outside the EU, the EU authorized representative is:

Springer Nature Customer Service Center GmbH
Europaplatz 3
69115 Heidelberg, Germany

Batch number: 10607186

Printed by Printforce, the Netherlands